Urologic Surgery

Consultant Editor

WILLIAM H. BOYCE, M.D.

Professor and Chairman, Section of Urology
Bowman Gray School of Medicine
Winston-Salem, North Carolina

105 Contributors

Third Edition

Urologic Surgery

Editor

JAMES F. GLENN, M.D.

Professor of Surgery (Urology) and Dean of the School
Emory University School of Medicine
Atlanta, Georgia

J. B. Lippincott Company

Philadelphia · Toronto

The authors and publisher have exerted every effort to ensure that drug selection and dosage set forth in this text are in accord with current recommendations and practice at the time of publication. However, in view of ongoing research, changes in government regulations, and the constant flow of information relating to drug therapy and drug reactions, the reader is urged to check the package insert for each drug for any change in indications and dosage and for added warnings and precautions. This is particularly important when the recommended agent is a new or infrequently employed drug.

Acquisitions Editor: Edward B. Hutton, Jr.
Sponsoring Editor: Sanford Robinson
Manuscript Editor: Rachel Bedard
Indexer: Gene Heller

Art Director: Maria Karkucinski
Designer: Patrick Turner
Production Assistant: George V. Gordon
Compositor: Monotype Composition Company
Printer/Binder: Halliday Lithograph

THIRD EDITION

3 5 6 4 2

Library of Congress Cataloging in Publication Data

Main entry under title:

Urologic surgery.

   Includes bibliographies and index.

   1. Genito-urinary organs—Surgery. I. Glenn, James F. (James Francis), 1928– II. Boyce, William H.
RD571.U75   1983   617'46   82-22954
ISBN 0-06-140923-5

List of Authors

EDITOR

JAMES F. GLENN, M.D.
Professor of Surgery (Urology) and Dean of the School
Emory University School of Medicine
Atlanta, Georgia

Chapter 1

CONSULTANT EDITOR

WILLIAM H. BOYCE, M.D.
Professor and Chairman, Section of Urology
Bowman Gray School of Medicine
Winston-Salem, North Carolina

Chapter 16

CONTRIBUTING AUTHORS

SAMUEL S. AMBROSE, M.D.
Professor of Surgery (Urology)
Emory University School of Medicine
Atlanta, Georgia

Chapter 51

E. EVERETT ANDERSON, M.D.
Professor of Urology
Duke University Medical Center
Durham, North Carolina

Chapter 15

JULIAN S. ANSELL, M.D.
Professor and Chairman, Department of Urology
University of Washington School of Medicine
Seattle, Washington

Chapter 65

THOMAS P. BALL, M.D.
Brigadier General, USAF (MC)
Consultant in Urology to Surgeon General
United States Air Force
Staff Urologist, Wilford Hall Medical Center
Associate Clinical Professor of Urology
University of Texas Health Science Center
San Antonio, Texas

Chapter 97

LYNN H. W. BANOWSKY, M.D.
Professor of Surgery/Urology
Chief, Section of Renal Transplantation
University of Texas Health Sciences Center
San Antonio, Texas

Chapter 35

ZORAN L. BARBARIC, M.D.
Professor of Radiology
UCLA Medical School, Center for Health Sciences
Los Angeles, California

Chapter 20

JOHN M. BARRY, M.D.   *Chapter 28*
Professor of Surgery and Chairman, Division of Urology
School of Medicine
Oregon Health Sciences University
Portland, Oregon

A. BARRY BELMAN, M.D., M.S.   *Chapter 98*
Professor of Urology and Child Health and Development
George Washington University School for Health Sciences
Chairman, Department of Pediatric Urology
Children's Hospital National Medical Center
Washington, D.C.

SAUL BOYARSKY, M.D.   *Chapter 42*
Professor of Genitourinary Surgery
Washington University School of Medicine
St. Louis, Missouri

WILLIAM H. BOYCE, M.D.   *Chapter 16*
Professor and Chairman, Section of Urology
Bowman Gray School of Medicine
Winston-Salem, North Carolina

WILLIAM BRANNAN, M.D.   *Chapter 56*
Chairman, Department of Urology
Ochsner Clinic
New Orleans, Louisiana

CHARLES B. BRENDLER, M.D.   *Chapter 59*
Assistant Professor of Urology, Brady Urological Institute
The Johns Hopkins Hospital
Chief of Urology, Baltimore City Hospitals
Baltimore, Maryland

HERBERT BRENDLER, M.D.   *Chapter 86*
Professor and Chairman, Department of Urology
Mount Sinai Medical Center
New York, New York

PAUL L. BUNCE, M.D.   *Chapter 105*
Professor of Surgery (Urology)
University of North Carolina School of Medicine
Chapel Hill, North Carolina

C. EUGENE CARLTON, M.D.   *Chapter 24*
Professor and Chairman, Department of Urology
Baylor College of Medicine
Houston, Texas

CULLEY C. CARSON III, M.D.   *Chapter 18*
Assistant Professor of Urology
Duke University Medical Center
Durham, North Carolina

GEOFFREY D. CHISHOLM, M.D., CH.M., F.R.C.S., F.R.C.S.E.   *Chapter 19*
Professor of Surgery, University of Edinburgh
Honorary Consultant Urological Surgeon
Western General Hospital
Edinburgh, United Kingdom

ABRAHAM T. K. COCKETT, M.D.   *Chapter 43*
Professor of Urological Surgery
Chairman, Division of Urology
University of Rochester Medical Center
Rochester, New York

ALVIN D. COUCH, M.D.   *Chapter 95*
Chief, Urological Surgery Section
Veterans Administration Medical Center
Asheville, North Carolina

DAVID A. CULP, M.D.   *Chapter 79*
Professor and Head of the Department of Urology
University of Iowa College of Medicine
Iowa City, Iowa

D. PATRICK CURRIE, M.D.   *Chapter 73*
Clinical Assistant Professor of Urologic Surgery
Bowman Gray School of Medicine
Chief, Section of Urologic Surgery
Forsyth Memorial Hospital and Medical Park Hospital
Winston-Salem, North Carolina

CHARLES J. DEVINE, JR., M.D.   *Chapter 76*
Professor and Chairman, Department of Urology
Eastern Virginia Medical School
Norfolk, Virginia

PATRICK C. DEVINE, M.D.   *Chapter 82*
Professor of Urology, Eastern Virginia Medical School
Norfolk, Virginia

JAMES H. DEWEERD, M.D.   *Chapter 21*
Emeritus Consultant, Department of Urology, Mayo Clinic
Anson L. Clark Professor of Urology Emeritus
Mayo Medical School
Rochester, Minnesota

JOHN P. DONOHUE, M.D.   *Chapter 37*
Professor and Chairman, Department of Urology
Indiana University Medical Center
Indianapolis, Indiana

DAVID M. DRYLIE, M.D.   *Chapter 96*
Professor of Surgery and Chief, Division of Urology
University of Florida College of Medicine
Gainesville, Florida

JOHN W. DUCKETT, M.D.   *Chapter 4*
Associate Professor of Urology
University of Pennsylvania School of Medicine
Director of Pediatric Urology, The Children's Hospital of Philadelphia
Philadelphia, Pennsylvania

HERBERT B. ECKSTEIN, M.D., M.CHIR., F.R.C.S.   *Chapter 48*
Consultant Surgeon, Hospital for Sick Children
London, England

RICHARD M. EHRLICH, M.D.   *Chapter 60*
Professor, Department of Surgery, Division of Urology
UCLA Medical Center
Los Angeles, California

WILLIAM R. FAIR, M.D.   *Chapter 88*
Professor and Chairman, Division of Urology
Washington University School of Medicine
Urologic Surgeon-in-Chief, Barnes and Associated Hospitals
St. Louis, Missouri

DONALD P. FINNERTY, M.D.   *Chapter 102*
Assistant Professor of Surgery (Urology)
Emory University School of Medicine
Atlanta, Georgia

ELWIN E. FRALEY, M.D.   *Chapter 81*
Professor and Chairman, Department of Urologic Surgery
University of Minnesota College of Health Sciences
Minneapolis, Minnesota

GERALDO DE CAMPOS FREIRE, JR., M.D.   *Chapter 52*
Assistant Professor of Urology
Faculty of Medicine of the University of Sao Paulo
Sao Paulo, Brazil

FLOYD A. FRIED, M.D.   *Chapter 54*
Professor of Surgery and Chief, Division of Urology
University of North Carolina School of Medicine
Chapel Hill, North Carolina

WILLIAM L. FURLOW, M.D.   *Chapter 83*
Professor of Urology, Mayo Medical School
Consultant, Department of Urology
Mayo Clinic and Mayo Foundation
Rochester, Minnesota

JOSÉ-MARÍA GIL-VERNET, M.D.   *Chapter 14*
Professor and Chairman of Urology
Facultad de Medicina
Universidad de Barcelona
Barcelona, Spain

RUBEN F. GITTES, M.D.   *Chapter 3*
Elliott Carr Cutler Professor of Urological Surgery
Harvard Medical School
Boston, Massachusetts

JAMES F. GLENN, M.D.   *Chapter 1*
Professor of Surgery (Urology) and Dean of the School
Emory University School of Medicine
Atlanta, Georgia

DAVID W. GODDARD, M.D.*   *Chapter 87*
Attending Urologist, Halifax General Hospital
Daytona Beach, Florida

EDMOND T. GONZALES, JR., M.D.   *Chapter 46*
Director of Pediatric Urology, Texas Children's Hospital
Professor of Urology
Baylor College of Medicine
Houston, Texas

SAM D. GRAHAM, JR., M.D.   *Chapter 6*
Assistant Professor of Urology
Emory University School of Medicine
Atlanta, Georgia

JOHN T. GRAYHACK, M.D.   *Chapter 5*
Herman Kretschmer Professor and Chairman of Urology
Northwestern University Medical School
Chicago, Illinois

S. LEE GUICE III, M.D.   *Chapter 23*
Pediatric Urologist, Ochsner Medical Institutions
New Orleans, Louisiana

EARL HALTIWANGER, M.D.   *Chapter 50*
Associate Professor of Surgery (Urology)
Emory University School of Medicine
Chief of Urology
Atlanta Veterans Administration Medical Center
Atlanta, Georgia

LLOYD H. HARRISON, M.D.   *Chapter 22*
Professor of Surgery (Urology)
Bowman Gray School of Medicine
Winston-Salem, North Carolina

RICHARD H. HARRISON III, M.D.   *Chapter 103*
Clinical Professor of Surgery (Urology)
Texas A&M University Health Center and Texas A&M University Medical School
Bryan, Texas

---

* Deceased

W. HARDY HENDREN, III, M.D.   *Chapter 53*
Chief of Pediatric Surgery, Massachusetts General Hospital
Professor of Surgery, Harvard Medical School
Boston, Massachusetts

HARRY W. HERR, M.D.   *Chapter 72*
Associate Attending Surgeon, Urologic Service
Memorial Sloan-Kettering Cancer Center
Associate Professor of Surgery
Cornell University Medical College
New York, New York

CLARENCE V. HODGES, M.D.   *Chapter 49*
Professor of Surgery/Urology
J. A. Burns School of Medicine, University of Hawaii
Honolulu, Hawaii

JACK HUGHES, M.D.   *Chapter 38*
Attending Urologist, Durham General Hospital
Clinical Associate Professor, Duke University Medical Center
Durham, North Carolina

JOSEPH J. KAUFMAN, M.D.   *Chapter 25*
Professor of Surgery/Urology
Chief, Division of Urology
UCLA School of Medicine
Los Angeles, California

PANAYOTIS P. KELALIS, M.D.   *Chapter 45*
Professor of Urology, Mayo Medical School
Chairman, Department of Urology
Mayo Clinic and Mayo Foundation
Rochester, Minnesota

DIETER KIRCHHEIM, M.D.   *Chapter 71*
Clinical Associate Professor of Urology
University of Washington Medical School
Seattle, Washington

STEPHEN A. KRAMER, M.D.   *Chapter 77*
Instructor in Urology, Mayo Medical School
Consultant, Department of Urology
Mayo Clinic and Mayo Foundation
Rochester, Minnesota

R. LAWRENCE KROOVAND, M.D.   *Chapter 99*
Associate Professor of Urology
Wayne State University School of Medicine
Associate Director of Pediatric Urology
Children's Hospital of Michigan
Detroit, Michigan

DAVID F. PAULSON, M.D.   *Chapter 58*
Professor and Chairman, Division of Urology, Department of Surgery
Duke University Medical Center
Durham, North Carolina

HARPER D. PEARSE, M.D.   *Chapter 9*
Associate Professor of Surgery/Urology
Head, Urologic Oncology
University of Oregon Health Sciences Center
Portland, Oregon

ALAN D. PERLMUTTER, M.D.   *Chapter 100*
Professor of Urology
Wayne State University School of Medicine
Chief, Department of Pediatric Urology
Children's Hospital of Michigan
Detroit, Michigan

PAUL C. PETERS, M.D.   *Chapter 92*
Professor and Chairman, Division of Urology
The University of Texas Southwestern Medical School
Dallas, Texas

MICHAEL G. PHILLIPS, B.H.S., PA-C   *Chapter 29*
Assistant Director
Alabama Regional Organ Bank
Department of Surgery, University of Alabama
Birmingham, Alabama

JAMES M. PIERCE, JR., M.D.   *Chapter 70*
Professor and Chairman, Department of Urology
Wayne State University School of Medicine
Detroit, Michigan

VICTOR A. POLITANO, M.D.   *Chapter 41*
Professor and Chairman, Department of Urology
University of Miami School of Medicine
Miami, Florida

ROBERT K. RHAMY, M.D.   *Chapter 2*
Professor of Urology
Vanderbilt University School of Medicine
Nashville, Tennessee

CHARLES J. ROBSON, M.D.   *Chapter 7*
Professor of Surgery (Urology) and Chairman of the Division of Urology
University of Toronto
Chief of Urology, Toronto General Hospital
Toronto, Canada

OSCAR SALVATIERRA, JR., M.D.   *Chapter 33*
Chief, Transplant Service
Professor of Surgery and Urology
University of California
San Francisco, California

PETER L. SCARDINO, M.D. *Chapter 67*
Professor of Surgery/Urology
Medical College of Georgia, Augusta
Director of Education for Urology, Memory Medical Center
Savannah, Georgia

CLAUDE C. SCHULMAN, M.D. *Chapter 47*
Chairman, Department of Urology, University Clinics of Brussels
Erasme Hospital, University of Brussels
Brussels, Belgium

JOSEPH W. SEGURA, M.D. *Chapter 90*
Associate Professor in Urology, Mayo Medical School
Consultant, Department of Urology, Mayo Clinic
Rochester, Minnesota

SHERIDAN W. SHIRLEY, M.D. *Chapter 62*
Clinical Professor of Surgery (Urology)
University of Alabama School of Medicine
Birmingham, Alabama

HILLIARD F. SIEGLER, M.D. *Chapter 34*
Professor of Surgery, Professor of Immunology
Duke University Medical Center
Durham, North Carolina

MATTHEW S. SMITH, M.D. *Chapter 55*
Department of Urology
Watson Clinic
Lakeland, Florida

BRUCE H. STEWART, M.D. *Chapter 104*
Chairman, Division of Surgery
Member, Department of Urology
Cleveland Clinic Foundation
Cleveland, Ohio

RALPH A. STRAFFON, M.D. *Chapter 85*
Chairman, Department of Urology
Cleveland Clinic Foundation
Cleveland, Ohio

RICHARD T. TURNER-WARWICK, D.M.(Oxon), M.CH., F.R.C.S., F.A.C.S. *Chapter 68*
Senior Urological Surgeon
The Middlesex Hospital, St. Peter's Hospital,
and The Royal National Orthopaedic Hospital
Senior Lecturer, The London University Institute of Urology
Director of Urological Studies, The Middlesex Hospital Medical School
London, England

DAVID C. UTZ, M.D. *Chapter 89*
Anson L. Clark Professor of Urology
Mayo Medical School
Consultant, Department of Urology
Mayo Clinic and Mayo Foundation
Rochester, Minnesota

KENNETH N. WALTON, M.D. *Chapter 17*
Professor and Chairman, Section of Urology
Emory University School of Medicine
Atlanta, Georgia

R. KEITH WATERHOUSE, M.D. *Chapter 61*
Professor and Chairman, Department of Urology
Downstate Medical Center, State University of New York
Brooklyn, New York

GEORGE D. WEBSTER, M.B., F.R.C.S. *Chapter 66*
Assistant Professor of Urology, Duke University Medical Center
Durham, North Carolina

JOHN L. WEINERTH, M.D. *Chapter 32*
Associate Professor of Urology and General Surgery
Duke University Medical Center
Durham, North Carolina

JOSEPH K. WHEATLEY, M.D. *Chapter 36*
Assistant Professor of Surgery (Urology)
Emory University School of Medicine
Atlanta, Georgia

JOHN E. A. WICKHAM, M.S., M.B., B.SC., F.R.C.S. *Chapter 12*
Director of the Academic Unit, Institute of Urology
University of London
Consultant Surgeon, St. Peter's Hospitals
Senior Consultant Urologist, St. Bartholomew's Hospital
London, England

CHESTER C. WINTER, M.D. *Chapter 78*
Professor of Urology
Ohio State University College of Medicine
Columbus, Ohio

JOHN R. WOODARD, M.D. *Chapter 8*
Professor of Surgery (Urology)
Emory University School of Medicine
Chief, Urology Section, Henrietta Egleston Hospital for Children
Atlanta, Georgia

BRADFORD W. YOUNG, M.D. *Chapter 64*
Chairman, Department of Urology Presbyterian Hospital of the Pacific Medical Center
San Francisco, California

JOHN D. YOUNG, JR., M.D *Chapter 39*
Professor and Head, Division of Urology University of Maryland School of Medicine
Baltimore, Maryland

Preface

The first edition of *Urologic Surgery* made its appearance in 1969, the second edition, in 1975. Now, in 1983, we present a revised and expanded third edition. On this occasion, it is incumbent upon us to acknowledge the advances that have taken place in urological surgery during the scant 14 years since the inception of this work.

Improvements have been wrought in every phase of urologic surgery and in all of the parasurgical areas. Advances in anesthesia, antibiosis, medical techniques, and diagnostic capability can be enumerated at length. As simple but explicit examples of such progress, we can point to the use of sodium nitroprusside for blood pressure control during surgery, aminoglycosides that have revolutionized antibacterial therapy, the use of beta-adrenergic blockade in pheochromocytoma, and the emergence of computed tomography scanning as a preferred diagnostic imaging technique. These represent but a few of the remarkable advances of the past few years.

In concert with these developments, urologic surgery has become more sophisticated. There is no doubt that we are accomplishing more effective radical surgery in the management of malignant diseases than ever before. Reconstructive techniques, including heroic urethroplasties and urinary undiversion, have been altered significantly during the past decade. Pediatric urology and the surgical correction of congenital defects have shown outstanding progress, and pediatric urology now stands as a well-defined subspecialty of our discipline. Physiological surgery, such as resolution of urinary incontinence or implantation of inflatable penile protheses, has entered the armamentarium of the urologic surgeon.

In the preface to the first edition, I expressed the hope that *Urologic Surgery*, by constituting the basis for further surgical innovation, might render itself obsolete. Indeed, that very thing has happened, and the fondest wish now for the third edition is that it, in turn, will be rendered obsolete by still further progress in our discipline.

JAMES F. GLENN, M.D.

From the Preface to Second Edition

Our objective has been to develop a volume which deals explicitly and specifically with urologic surgery, focusing upon technical details, surgical problems, pitfalls to be avoided, and management complications. The new and revised second edition has been expanded to seventy-one chapters, each written by an authority recognized as eminently proficient in that respective area. Some chapters of the first edition have been subdivided, elevating certain sections to chapter status in an effort to provide broader coverage. Recent innovations in surgical technique and some of the less common surgical problems have been included in this revision.

Most of the original authors of *Urologic Surgery* have joined in the effort of producing the second edition and have rendered enthusiastic support of this expansion and revision. In addition, we have been joined by outstanding urologic surgeons from Canada, Great Britain, Europe, South Africa, and South America, lending international authority and expertise to this volume.

There are and will continue to be differences of opinion in surgical matters, and these differences constitute areas of intellectual controversy, most often leading to advances in surgery. Rather than provide a bland and noncontroversial approach, our editorial policy has been to recognize the differences of opinion and encourage each author to present his own views, based upon experience and personal preference. In instances in which controversy is of significant degree, the variations in approach to urologic surgical problems will be evident in this text, hopefully stimulating the reader to examine his own opinions in these given areas.

The evolution of a textbook is rather like fathering a child: conception is a pleasant and enjoyable task, gestation requires several months of patience, labor may be somewhat exhausting, but delivery is attended by a great sense of satisfaction. It is only when the final product is taken home that the sleepless nights begin, and it is then that the critical parental eye is cast upon all the deficiencies that should have been so obvious from the beginning. The first edition of *Urologic Surgery* was neither malformed nor retarded, but it was clear that the opportunity existed for reorganization and improvement. It is the collaborative hope of all the contributors, the editors, and artists that the second edition represents a substantial advance.

JAMES F. GLENN, M.D.

*U*rologic Surgery has been designed to satisfy a definite need in the field of urology. While numerous texts deal with the spectrum of urologic diseases and their etiology, pathology, diagnosis, and general treatment, no text deals explicitly with surgical considerations. A number of atlases project the technical aspects of urologic surgery, but there have been no previous efforts to amplify the problems and the rationale of specific urologic procedures.

The philosophy which has guided the authors of this volume is one which is fundamental to the many outstanding urologic training programs in this country: Urologists are—first and foremost—surgeons, and excellence in urologic surgery can be achieved only through diligent and exhaustive application to both the fundamentals of surgery and the advancing technology of the urologic specialist. It is our purpose to present the spectrum of urologic surgery and to focus upon the technical aspects of our craft. Since no individual can be thoroughly familiar with every aspect of our growing specialty, recognized authorities in various phases of urologic surgery have joined their knowledge and skill to produce this volume. The authors have worked with medical illustrators of exceptional capability to provide new and comprehensive understanding of surgical anatomy and the specific challenges of urologic surgery. Our success in providing a detailed work of wide scope will be measured by the reader.

It is hoped that this volume will provide insight not only for the resident student of urologic surgery but also for the experienced practitioner of the surgical arts in urology. It is recognized that not all urologic surgeons will be called upon to perform all the procedures described, but familiarity and competence in assessing the efficacy and advisability of these operations must lie within the sphere of every urologist. Finally, it is the most sincere ambition of the authors that this book constitute a basis for further surgical innovation and advances. The greatest of satisfaction will be achieved when this volume is rendered obsolete by such progress.

JAMES F. GLENN, M.D.

Acknowledgments

The editor acknowledges with gratitude the collaboration and cooperation of the 104 additional authors who have joined in preparation of this third edition of *Urologic Surgery*. Further, special gratitude is extended to William H. Boyce, friend and confidant, advisor and critic, consultant editor and master surgeon, whose innovative ideas are expressed in many ways in this volume.

The superb quality of illustrative material in this third edition reflects the expertise of many medical artists to whom we are grateful, but special recognition must be given to Charles H. Boyter, Patsy A. Bryan, and others of our staff in Medical Illustration here at Emory University School of Medicine.

I remain deeply indebted to many colleagues, past and present: my many former residents who have participated in this edition, the faculty at Duke who continue to lend so much to this work, and my associates in urology here at Emory who have all contributed to this improved volume.

Finally, I must acknowledge the expertise and assistance of my own secretarial staff, the splendid editorial capabilities of our publishers, and the outstanding cooperation and support of the J. B. Lippincott Company, which has become the medical branch of our long-time publishers, Harper & Row.

Contents

Urologic Surgery

Nonfunctional Adrenal Tumors and Aldosteronism

James F. Glenn

1

The surgical cure of aldosteronism constitutes a major challenge. The firmly established indications for adrenal surgery are primary malignancies, endocrine control of metastatic malignant diseases, benign tumors, and functional cortical and medullary indications. Primary aldosteronism due to adenoma or focal hyperplasia, with or without associated metabolic disorders, may account for a very substantial percentage of cases of hypertensive disease.[32]

On the basis of autopsy findings of so-called benign nonfunctioning adrenal adenomas in hypertensive patients, estimates have been made which suggest that as many as 2 million patients in the United States alone may suffer hypertension due to aldosteronism. To date, only a small fraction of this number of patients has been identified, but diagnostic methods are improving.

The observations of Liddle and associates[29] suggest that there may be another as yet unrecognized steroid hormone that is sometimes responsible for hypertension.[3] Indeed, Gunnells and colleagues[23] have reported improvement in five of seven patients with hypertension, low renin–angiotensin levels, and no evidence of aldosteronism when these patients underwent bilateral adrenalectomy.

HISTORICAL NOTES

The history of adrenal surgery constitutes a fascinating chapter in the evolution of modern urologic practice. A relation between adrenal tumor, hirsutism, and obesity was first recognized by William Cooke in 1756. Subsequent to this, particularly during the nineteenth century, there were reports of genital and other somatic aberrations associated with adrenal tumors. However, even Hippocrates and John Hunter had recognized the clinical syndrome of hirsutism and secondary sex changes in women.

The first successful removal of an adrenal tumor was accomplished by Thornton in 1889, operating on a 36-year-old woman with hirsutism and virilizing changes. A huge tumor of approximately 20 lb was removed *en bloc* with the left kidney, but the fact that the tumor was of adrenal origin was not recognized until many years later when it was examined by other observers.

In 1914 the first planned operation for adrenal tumor, resulting in complete cure, was accomplished by Sargent, although this was not recorded until the paper of Gordon Holmes in 1925. The tumor was apparently a benign right adrenal adenoma some 17 cm in size, inducing Cushing's syndrome.[24]

Other isolated case reports followed. In 1924, Collett recorded surgical cure of adrenal adenoma causing adrenogenitalism in a 1½-year-old girl.[14] Charles H. Mayo may have been the first to remove a pheochromocytoma in 1927.[30] In 1945, Huggins reaffirmed earlier work by himself and by Scott, advocating total bilateral adrenalectomy in patients with disseminated prostatic cancer.[25] In 1955, Conn documented primary aldosteronism as a cause for hypertension,[15] and 10 years later Conn and Nesbit had successfully alleviated severe hypertension of primary aldosteronism (sometimes due to adenomas of only a few millimeters in diameter) in the absence of associated hypokalemic alkalosis observed in their earlier cases.[16]

Classification of Adrenal Disorders

Various classifications of the surgical diseases of the adrenal have been proposed, and none is entirely satisfactory.[6] Surgical diseases of the adrenal gland may be categorized according to benign or malignant potential, the presence or absence of abnormal hormonal activity, the endocrine manifestations of adrenal disease, or the anatomic tissue of origin of the adrenal tumor.[10]

A modification of the anatomic classification of adrenal abnormalities is recommended here as a basis for surgical consideration. Surgical diseases of the adrenal may be subdivided into those of cortical origin, those of medullary origin, and those of nonadrenal origin (Table 1-1).

Nonfunctioning tumors of the adrenal constitute

TABLE 1-1. Surgical Diseases of the Adrenal Gland

Diseases of the adrenal cortex
  Congenital adrenal hyperplasia
  Idiopathic bilateral adrenal hyperplasia
  Secondary adrenocortical hyperplasia
  Focal nodular hyperplasia
  Benign cortical adenoma
  Adrenocortical adenocarcinoma
  Aldosteronoma
  Feminizing tumors
Diseases of the adrenal medulla
  Benign pheochromocytoma
  Malignant pheochromocytoma
  Neuroblastoma, sympathogonioma
  Ganglioneuroma
  Neurofibroma
  Extra-adrenal paraganglioma
Heterologous adrenal disorders
  Neonatal adrenal hemorrhage
  Idiopathic, infectious, or hemorrhagic cysts
  Metastatic malignancy
  Fibroma, lipoma, myoma, myelolipoma
  Hemangioma, lymphangioma, hamartoma

---

an area of special interest, because the lack of any endocrine abnormality often delays diagnosis. Carcinoma of the adrenal, for example, is frequently diagnosed on the basis of metastatic disease, often to bone. This diagnosis prompts a search for the primary, nonfunctioning malignancy, which is discovered by various radiographic techniques. Similarly, nonfunctioning metastatic carcinoma *to* the adrenals is common; carcinoma of the lung is a notorious offender, and metastases in the adrenals often grow to enormous size before detection.[41]

Benign nonfunctioning cortical adenomas were once thought to be common. However, with the recognition of aldosteronism, most often due to adenoma of the adrenal cortex, it now must be acknowledged that most of the lesions previously considered to be benign nonfunctioning adenomas may well have been aldosteronomas. A few benign adenomatous lesions may still exist.[1]

Other benign nonfunctioning lesions include ganglioneuroma, the various forms of adrenal cysts, and the rare tumors listed in Table 1-1.

Indications for Surgery

The mere presence of anatomic or histologic abnormalities of the adrenal does not necessarily constitute an indication for surgery.[10] On the contrary, some of these diseases are best managed by medical means, particularly congenital adrenal hy-

perplasia, or the adrenogenital syndrome. It is conceivable that additional medical measures of control will evolve during the next decade, perhaps providing control of still other functional but benign disease processes, such as aldosteronism.[9]

Calcification of the adrenal gland does not necessarily constitute an indication for surgery, particularly in adults, but the incidence of calcification of neuroblastoma in infants and children puts the burden on the surgeon, who must differentiate between tumor and benign calcification. Whether to operate on benign adrenal cysts in an elderly patient without symptoms of functional adrenal disease, pain, weight loss, or other manifestations of organic illness is a speculative matter. In this situation the surgeon must make a judgment based on probabilities and calculated risks. However, most diseases of the adrenal that confront the urologic surgeon demand operative intervention.

Special consideration should be given to carcinoma of the adrenal. Functional adrenal malignancy produces florid Cushing's syndrome, but a large number—perhaps a majority—of patients with carcinoma of the adrenal have a nonfunctioning tumor, very often manifesting by metastatic disease. The issue is whether adrenalectomy is indicated in the presence of metastatic malignancies, and it is generally accepted that removal of a primary, particularly a large adrenal, lesion should be accomplished if technically feasible. Subsequent treatment of metastatic disease by chemotherapy, o,p'-DDD, or other appropriate therapy, may be facilitated by removal of the primary. It should be remembered that virtually any mass identified in the adrenal may represent primary nonfunctioning carcinoma, and all diagnostic and therapeutic measures should be taken in such instances; discovery of an adrenal mass on routine intravenous pyelography or other abdominal radiographic study should precipitate intensive diagnostic efforts.

Nonfunctioning adrenal tumors that constitute indications for surgery include the rare so-called nonfunctioning adenomas, because these may be malignant lesions. Many adrenal cysts also should be operated on, often merely because of the size of the lesion, which causes compression or displacement of surrounding viscera.[18,26] Metastatic tumors of the adrenal should rarely be operated on, but very often an adrenal mass is demonstrated and there is no known primary. In such instances, it is justifiable to remove the metastatic lesion of the adrenal in order to establish a histologic diagnosis in the search for the primary disease. Similarly, removal of adrenal fibromas and lipomas may be justified for diagnostic purposes alone.

Aldosterone tumors are perhaps the most fascinating of all the surgical diseases of the adrenal.[28] Classically, the syndrome associated with primary aldosteronism consists of hypertension, hypokalemia and alkalosis, hypernatremia, increased urinary potassium loss and diminished urinary sodium excretion, decreased glucose tolerance, carpopedal spasms, and mental disturbances that range from anxiety to frank psychoses. Recently, it has been documented that aldosteronism may exist in its early stages without alteration of potassium and sodium balance, although abnormal glucose tolerance tests may be observed.

Overt aldosteronism with hypertension and the classic metabolic alterations is most often due to a single adenoma of the adrenal; ectopic adrenal adenoma, lying beneath the capsule of the kidney, has been reported on only one occasion. Diffuse bilateral focal hyperplasia of the adrenals is seen in adults and quite often in the unusual cases of aldosteronism in children.

Childhood adrenal disorders, in addition to pheochromocytoma, neuroblastoma, congenital adrenal hyperplasia, and Cushing's disease, include various benign or malignant cysts, the most common being the benign nonfunctioning inclusion cyst.[35] Of particular importance is neonatal adrenal hemorrhage; at birth, the combined weight of the adrenals is 9 g, 0.25% of total body weight, compared with 12 g, 0.17% of adult weight.[8] The neonatal adrenals are quite vascular, and the trauma of even a normal delivery may predispose to hemorrhage, usually presenting a flank mass, later calcifying (Fig. 1-1). If neonatal adrenal hemorrhage is bilateral, acute adrenal insufficiency may ensue.[19,27]

Clinically, other diseases of the adrenal may not be readily appreciated. However, the presence of an adrenal mass demonstrated by the diagnostic methods discussed below may be sufficient indication in itself for surgical exploration.

Diagnostic Methods

Clinical acumen in evaluating the syndromes of adrenal disease may lead to accurate diagnosis. However, the use of radiographic and laboratory procedures results in the refinement of diagnosis and frequent localization of the tumor, enabling better surgical and medical management for the patient.

The diagnosis of primary aldosteronism by laboratory methods is becoming more refined and more generally available.[31] In the presence of advanced disease, demonstration of increased urinary potassium and decreased urinary sodium excretion, hypernatremia, hypokalemia, and alkalosis is diagnostic. A diminished glucose tolerance is evident in most of these patients, and certain forms of diabetes may be manifestations of aldosteronism.[22]

There are four forms of primary aldosteronism: (1) aldosteronoma, which accounts for 80% to 90% of aldosteronism; (2) idiopathic aldosteronism due

FIG. 1-1. Adrenal calcification may be due to neonatal adrenal hemorrhage as seen here in the left adrenal gland, or it may be the result of infection, infarction, or tumor.

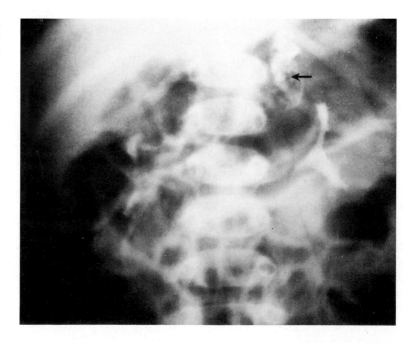

to adrenocortical hyperplasia type A; (3) hyperaldosteronism due to adrenocortical hyperplasia type B; and (4) hyperaldosteronism in children, which is remediable with glucocorticoid administration. Our focus is on the first form, which is due to discrete adenoma and is the only one that constitutes an indication for surgery.

The electrolyte and acid–base disorders of aldosteronism are easily explained by hyperexcretion of aldosterone, but the exact mechanism of hypertension in aldosteronism remains poorly understood. Signs and symptoms of aldosteronism are indistinguishable from those of essential hypertension, but the diagnosis is virtually established by laboratory findings of hypokalemia (serum potassium of less than 3.5 mEq/liter), alkalosis (serum bicarbonate value of more than 30 mEq/liter), and hyperkaluria (in excess of 30 mEq/24 hr). Hypervolemia due to water restriction may be seen, and there may be relative anemia due to this dilutional effect. Some patients exhibit polyuria and a fixed specific gravity of approximately 1.010. Elevated urinary aldosterone excretion (normal range 5 μg/24 hr to 19 μg/24 hr) is virtually diagnostic of aldosteronism. Measurement of plasma aldosterone levels is less reliable than 24-hr urinary excretion values, because plasma levels ordinarily vary on a diurnal basis and in response to upright or supine posture. Demonstration of low plasma renin activity provides corollary diagnostic confirmation. An additional diagnostic test is the administration of spironolactone, which acts by competing with aldosterone for the receptor sites in target tissues, correcting both the hypertension and the metabolic abnormalities in patients with aldosterone-producing adenomas; patients with idiopathic hyperaldosteronism do not respond.

Radiographic diagnostic methods are indispensable in the evaluation of suspected adrenal disease. A plain film may reveal calcification in the region of the adrenal, seen in conjunction with tumors, prior hemorrhage, or inflammatory reaction (Fig. 1-1). Intravenous urography may disclose kidney displacement or distortion of the collecting system due to impingement by adrenal tumor. Retrograde pyelography may be necessary to confirm such findings, particularly if malignant adrenal tumor has rendered the ipsilateral kidney nonfunctional.

More sophisticated urologic techniques include the use of planography or nephrotomography, with or without concomitant intravenous urographic contrast medium. Retroperitoneal gas insufflation contrast studies have long been advocated, and may be accomplished by presacral or perinephric insufflation of 95% carbon dioxide (Fig. 1-2). The use of air or gases other than carbon dioxide is unsatisfactory because of poor resorption and the hazards of embolism and subcutaneous or mediastinal emphysema. Tumors as small as 1 cm to 2 cm in diameter can be localized by a judicious

FIG. 1-2. Preoperative localization of adrenal tumors may be accomplished through urography or planography, although the most effective method may be retroperitoneal carbondioxide insufflation **(A),** here delineating a large right suprarenal mass. A typical benign adrenal adenoma with surrounding adrenal tissue **(B)** was removed through a unilateral posterior rib approach.

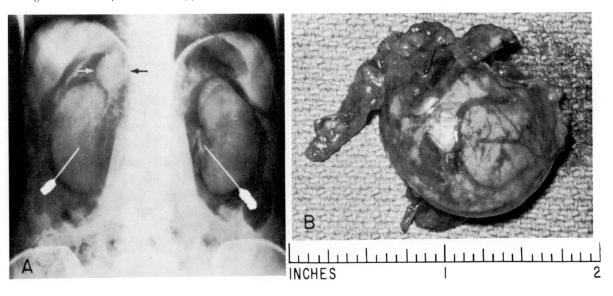

combination of intravenous pyelography and retroperitoneal perinephric carbon dioxide contrast studies.

Vascular diagnostic methods are often worthwhile. Abdominal and selective adrenal angiography may be performed (Fig. 1-3), seeking the tumor stain or blush that persists in the highly vascular adrenal tumors. The method of percutaneous retrograde femoral-aortic catheterization is preferred, because translumbar aortography requires introduction of the needle through an area potentially involved by the disease process.[17]

Retrograde catheterization of the vena cava may be accomplished under fluorographic control for the collection of blood samples at levels from the iliac vein up to the superior vena cava. These samples can be assayed for relative concentration of steroids or catechols, and preoperative localization of tumor may be effected, particularly in pheochromocytoma. With the catheter in position, cavography or renal venography can aid in tumor localization (Fig. 1-4).

Adrenal venography may be useful in diagnosing small tumors of the adrenal (1 cm or less).[12] Adrenal vein catheterization may be extremely useful in localizing aldosteronomas, and elevations of venous aldosterone values above the normal range of 1.4 nmol/dl to 33.6 nmol/dl essentially confirm the diagnosis and localize the tumor. In such instances, with the venous catheter *in situ* gentle retrograde injection of small amounts

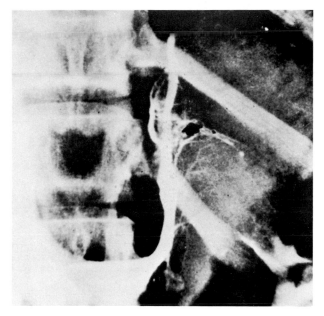

FIG. 1-4. In adrenal venography, selective catheterization of the main adrenal vein permits retrograde injection, here demonstrating a 1-cm aldosteronoma of the left adrenal gland.

contrast material may be judiciously administered. As seen in Figure 1-4, small aldosteronomas can be visualized by this technique.

Computed tomography (CT) is the most sophisticated and accurate method of diagnostic localization of adrenal tumors.[33] Although tumors of less than 1 cm in diameter are difficult to visualize, the technique offers many possibilities for potentiation, particularly if radioactive iodine-cholesterol agents that localize in the adrenal can be compounded for use in conjunction with CT scanning. Large tumors of the adrenal (Fig. 1-5) are readily visualized without contrast enhancement.[39]

CONTRAINDICATIONS TO SURGERY

Benign nonfunctioning lesions of the adrenal may very well be managed conservatively. It is imperative, however, that the surgical decision be based on certain knowledge that the tumor mass in question constitutes no threat by virtue of malignancy, size, potential for hemorrhage, or infection, or as a manifestation of extra-adrenal disease. Ideally, simple uncomplicated cysts of the adrenal could be watched and treated conservatively. However, most adrenal tumors that come to the attention of the surgeon have already progressed to a size that may demand surgical intervention.

The most inflexible contraindication to adrenal

FIG. 1-3. Adrenal angiography may be accomplished by flush aortograms, here demonstrating a large right adrenal pheochromocytoma, or by selective adrenal arterial catheterization.

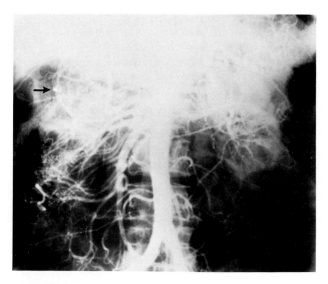

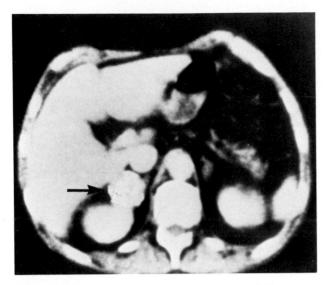

FIG. 1-5. In this CT scan, a large tumor of the right adrenal is evident anteromedial to the kidney and somewhat behind the vena cava.

surgery is, of course, inadequate evaluation and preparation of the patient. In general, crises that might prompt emergency adrenal exploration are few. Even the presence of severe hypertension due to pheochromocytoma does not constitute an emergency, because sustained and paroxysmal hypertension can be controlled by parenteral or intravenous phentolamine and β-blockers. Complete clinical, chemical, and anatomic diagnostic steps can and should be taken in virtually every instance of surgical disease of the adrenal, and adrenal surgery under other circumstances cannot be recommended.

Anatomy of the Adrenals

EMBRYOLOGIC CONSIDERATIONS

The adrenal gland, consisting of cortex and medulla, arises from both mesodermal elements (cortex) and ectodermal elements (medulla). Developmentally, the first traces of the adrenal cortex are evident in the 6-mm embryo at approximately the fourth week of life, with rapid growth to the eighth week, at which time the adrenal is as large as the fetal kidney. Ectodermal medullary tissues are evident in 16-mm embryos, with primitive sympathetic ganglion cells migrating to the medial aspect of the primitive cortical mass, where they are subsequently enfolded.[11]

Adrenal cortical tissue arises from dorsal cells

of the blastema cords at the medial borders of the mesonephric bodies; ventral cells of the same region give rise to testicular interstitial cells or ovarian theca cells. This common embryologic origin of adrenal and gonadal tissue accounts for the observation of adrenal rests in gonadal structures—rests that may undergo hyperplasia in the adrenogenital syndrome and that may prompt misdiagnosis of interstitial cell tumors.

Histologic differentiation of adrenal and gonadal tumors is often extremely difficult. Ectopic adrenal tissue, cortical and medullary, may be found virtually anywhere in the retroperitoneal space, the embryologic site of the mesonephric blastema, and the neural crest.

The ectodermal sympathetic ganglion cells that constitute the adrenal medulla arise from the same primordial neural crest that is the origin of the sympathetic chain. It is hence understandable that pheochromocytoma (tumor of the adrenal medulla) and paraganglioma (tumor of the sympathetic system) have identical histologic characteristics and clinical manifestations.

The adrenal of the 8-week embryo approximates the size of the kidney, and even at term the adrenal is extremely large, about one third the size of the kidney, and is a highly vascular and friable organ. Regression in adrenal size proceeds rapidly during the first month of life. The extremely large size and vascular, friable nature of the neonatal adrenal may account for the high incidence of adrenal hemorrhage in the newborn, probably due to trauma at delivery. Quite often, the mass occasioned by neonatal adrenal hemorrhage is misdiagnosed as Wilms' tumor or neuroblastoma.

SURGICAL ANATOMY

The adrenal glands are situated at the medial aspect of the upper poles of the kidneys (Fig. 1–6). The average adult adrenal measures approximately 4 cm by 3 cm by 1 cm and weighs 3 g to 6 g, with the average weight per pair of adult adrenals ranging as high as 15 g. The normal gland is yellowish and triangular, flattened or concave on its renal aspect, and sometimes semilunar as it approximates the large vessels. The atrophic gland is thin and pale, usually readily recognizable; the hyperplastic gland may be difficult to identify, grossly or histologically, except by its large size.[34]

Benign adrenal tumors and some malignant adrenal tumors are encapsulated, firmer than the usual friable normal gland, and generally have the golden yellow appearance that exaggerates the color characteristics of normal adrenal tissue. Such

FIG. 1-6. Anatomic relations of adrenal glands, as revealed by CT scanning

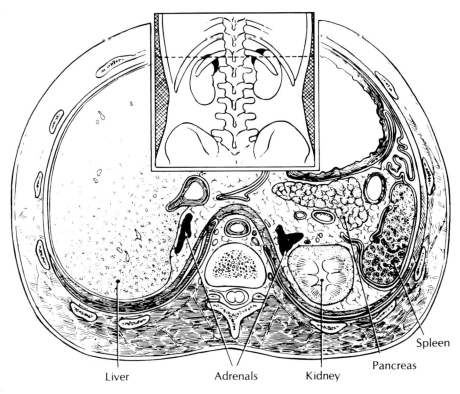

Liver   Adrenals   Kidney   Pancreas   Spleen

tumors may be located in any portion of the gland or may replace the entire adrenal. Malignant adrenal tumors may be infiltrative and invasive, involving all contiguous structures, including the kidney, great vessels, liver, diaphragm, posterior abdominal musculature, peritoneum and its contents, and the pancreas. The adrenals lie within the perinephric fascia of Gerota with the kidneys, and they are surrounded by loose connective tissue and fat. The connective tissue forms a pseudocapsule that facilitates surgical mobilization.

The blood supply of the adrenals is quite variable from side to side and from patient to patient, and it is relatively independent of renal circulation (Fig. 1-7). The major arterial supply of the adrenal, consisting of as many as 50 small branches, is derived from the aorta, the renal artery, and the inferior phrenic artery, with occasional supply on the left from the splenic artery.

Venous return is much more constant than arterial supply; the main right adrenal vein arises from the hilum of the gland medially and empties directly into the vena cava, and the left main adrenal vein joins the inferior phrenic to empty into the left renal vein. Appreciation of the multiplicity of arteries is essential to hemostasis during dissection of the gland, and knowledge of the usually constant venous drainage enables mobilization of the pediclelike vein for final clamping and ligation in removal of the gland.

Damage to contiguous structures must be avoided in surgical dissection (Fig. 1-8). The right adrenal gland lies close to the liver superiorly and anteriorly, the vena cava medially, and the kidney inferolaterally. Dense attachment of the vena cava causes great difficulty in mobilization, and careful identification of the vena cava is essential to prevent or control hemorrhage. On the left, the gland lies somewhat lower on the superior medial aspect of the kidney, closer to the renal pedicle; caution must be taken in exposing the inferior surface of the gland to prevent damage to the renal artery and vein. The posterior aspect of the stomach and the tail of the pancreas approximate the left adrenal surface and in the presence of malignancy may be involved by tumor.

HISTOLOGIC ANATOMY

The intrinsic appearance of the adrenal gland is that of a structure folded upon itself, the cortex enveloping the medulla. In dissection of hyperplastic adrenals, the outer cortical layers may separate from the medial medullary region because of excessive friability of hyperplastic glands.

Grossly, it is impossible to differentiate the zones

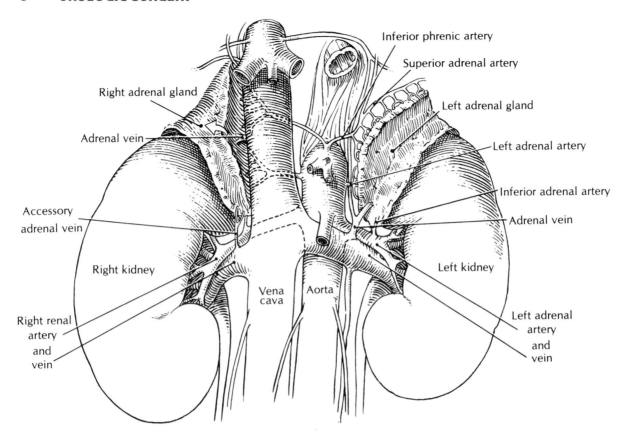

FIG. 1-7. The usual blood supply of the adrenal glands is pictured here (anterior view), but a highly variable pattern of vascular supply and drainage can be anticipated.

of the adrenal cortex at surgery. Histologic identification of the various zones is possible on section, and, from the outside inward, the three vaguely defined layers of zona glomerulosa, zona fasciculata, and zona reticularis are evident, with medullary tissue located centrally. A loose fibrous stroma surrounding the entire gland can be appreciated histologically, but it is sometimes defined grossly, aiding in mobilization of the adrenal.

Histochemical study of the adrenal has helped our understanding of the endocrine function of the gland, and enzymatic defects of the adrenal leading to malfunctional states can now be identified. The chromaffin reaction of the medulla seems to be proportional to catechol content, and diagnosis of pheochromocytoma is invalid without a positive chromaffin reaction. In the adult adrenal, total lipid content represents about 20% of weight, with cholesterol—the basic steroid building block—accounting for about 8% of weight. These values are much lower—4% and 1%, respectively—in neonates.

Hazards of Adrenal Surgery

ADRENAL INSUFFICIENCY

In this era of adequate corticosteroid replacement therapy, adrenal insufficiency should not occur with surgery. It is the practice of most surgeons undertaking adrenal exploration for virtually any reason to prepare the patient with supplementary cortisone acetate, usually in a dosage of 100 mg/day for 2 days before surgery, 100 mg immediately before surgery, and 100 mg intravenously during the immediate postoperative period. Steroid dosage from that point can be determined on the basis of the actual surgery accomplished.

In some cases of adrenal surgery, corticosteroid supplementation is not routine. Exploration for neuroblastoma usually does not require cortisone, and adrenocorticoid preparation of patients to be explored for pheochromocytoma is optional, because only 10% to 15% of pheochromocytomas or paragangliomas originate from multiple sites and so may require bilateral total adrenalectomy.

There are few immediate ill effects of adrenocorticoid supplementation, although susceptibility

FIG. 1-8. Relative surgical relations of adrenals, viewed through an anterior abdominal approach

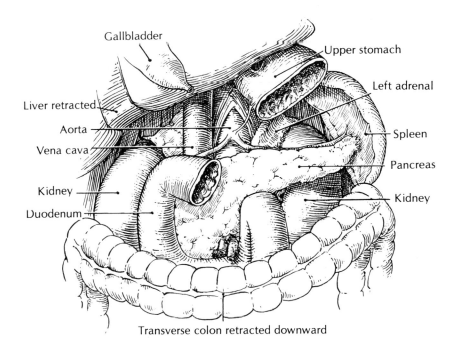

Gallbladder

Upper stomach

Left adrenal

Liver retracted

Aorta

Spleen

Vena cava

Pancreas

Kidney

Kidney

Duodenum

Transverse colon retracted downward

to micro-organisms may be increased. The use of cortisone derivatives in the preoperative, operative, and postoperative phases may also prompt the use of prophylactic broad-spectrum antibiotics.

SURGICAL HEMORRHAGE

The adrenal glands are extremely vascular, as noted in the discussion of blood supply, and the approach to the adrenals through Gerota's fascia and the perinephric adipose tissue necessitates dissection of a relatively vascular field. Thus constant and meticulous attention must be given to hemostasis. Many surgeons routinely use metal neurosurgical hemostatic clips, which afford good control. Under appropriate anesthesia, the electrocautery is extremely useful, particularly in managing venous and arteriolar bleeding in the perinephric fat of the obese patient.

Hemorrhagic tendencies may be accentuated in some patients with surgical disease of the adrenal. The newborn infant with neonatal adrenal hemorrhage offers an extremely vascular field for surgery, and hemorrhagic diatheses in the newborn must also be suspected. Preparation of such patients with supplementary menadione (vitamin K), fresh whole blood in transfusion, and the usual supportive measures is strongly indicated in such situations.

The most serious hemorrhagic problems in adrenal surgery result from damage to the great vessels encountered, particularly the vena cava, aorta, and vessels of the renal pedicle. Obviously, attention to details of dissection will avoid such injury. When such vascular injury occurs, the use of standard vascular instruments for control enables appropriate and effective repair. Atraumatic arterial silk is generally used.

BLOOD PRESSURE ALTERATIONS

Control of alterations in blood pressure during and after adrenal surgery often poses a challenge. Although hypotensive difficulties are rarely encountered in most surgical diseases of the adrenal, pheochromocytoma may present significant and serious pressor problems. Whole blood and plasma volume expanders should be used without hesitation when hypotension is encountered during or after the removal of pheochromocytoma or paraganglioma.

Problems resulting from the extensive and prolonged use of vasoconstrictors include possible oliguria, anuria, and vasospasm at the site of injection; cerebral ischemia; and potential peripheral vascular complications secondary to circulatory insufficiency.[7]

Hypertensive responses except during the manipulation of a pressor tumor are uncommon, and in such a situation the use of phentolamine is advisable. Cardiac arrhythmias may accompany acute hypertensive states. Halothane anesthetic agents have been recommended as useful in avoiding the cardiovascular complications. A major advance in anesthesia for patients undergoing adrenal surgery in the presence of hypertension, as seen with pheochromocytoma, has been the advent of sodium nitroprusside infusion, providing moderate hypotension, stability of blood pressure, and decreased tendency to bleeding.

PLEURAL OR PERITONEAL INJURY

Opening the pleural or peritoneal cavities during the course of adrenal exploration carries no peculiar risks. Although surgeons have attempted to avoid entry into these spaces, no particular hazards are incurred by such excursions if proper closures are effected. Incision of the peritoneum during flank, transthoracic, or posterior exploration of the adrenal may be desirable, affording access through the abdominal cavity for manual exploration of the contralateral adrenal area, the para-aortic area, and the true pelvis.

Entry into the pleural cavity necessitates no special therapeutic measures under modern anesthesia, which includes intubation with controlled respiration. Under such circumstances, airtight closure of the pleura and diaphragm may be effected with the lung in full controlled expansion. Generally, it is unnecessary to use chest tube drainage, although the use of a multi-eyed catheter for a period of 24 hr of water-seal suction may be desirable in some instances.

On many urologic services, it is routine practice to obtain a postoperative roentgenogram of the chest, frequently in the recovery room, to assess the possibilities of pleural entry and pneumothorax. If significant quantities of air or fluid are evident within the chest cavity, needle aspiration is usually sufficient, but occasionally secondary introduction of a chest catheter may be necessary. Atelectasis should be avoided because it increases the possibility of pneumonia, a serious complication, particularly in patients receiving supplementary corticosteroid therapy.

Surgical Approaches

FLANK APPROACH

Surgical approach to the adrenal glands through a standard flank incision is advocated by many authorities and accounts for most of the early successful adrenalectomies. It has the advantage of relative simplicity and great familiarity to urologic

surgeons, and permits ample visualization of the kidney and adrenal. Even in situations of bilateral adrenal involvement, Harrison and others may use the standard flank approach, effecting definitive surgery on one side, repositioning the patient in the contralateral flank position, and completing the operation with exposure and appropriate surgery of the opposite adrenal gland.[6] There are two basic disadvantages of the flank approach. First, only one of the adrenals can be visualized at any one time, and a decision for total removal, subtotal adrenalectomy, extirpation of the encapsulated tumor, or no surgical intervention must be made without knowledge of the condition of the contralateral adrenal. Second, the standard flank approach below the rib margins may give low access to the perinephric space, rendering total mobilization of the kidney necessary in order to provide visualization of the adrenal, and in some instances the adrenal may be quite high under the rib cage. These technical difficulties may be obviated by the modified flank incision, made over the 11th or 12th ribs with resection of the underlying rib to provide more cephalad exposure of the adrenal area.[5,40] Of course, when an extra-adrenal tumor such as pheochromocytoma or paraganglioma or a neuroblastoma is suspected, the flank approach may be definitely inferior to abdominal exploration.

Technique

With the patient under appropriate endotracheal anesthesia, the usual kidney position is effected with extreme lateral flexion (Fig. 1-9). The table is gradually broken to approximately 30 degrees, and further flexing may be effected as the operation proceeds. The kidney bar is generally not elevated until after the flank has been incised and the retroperitoneal space has been entered.

The usual incision is oblique, curving downward and anteriorly in parallel with the terminal ribs, and is 20 cm to 30 cm in length, depending on body build of the patient; the more obese patients require greater incisional exposure. The incision may be subcostal, or if rib resection has been elected, may overlie the 11th or 12th rib. Tenth rib resection is not recommended for the flank approach.

Care should be taken to identify the ilioinguinal and iliohypogastric nerves, retracting them from the field to prevent damage. If associated vessels are injured, ligation should be effected with fine black silk rather than electrocautery hemostasis, because the latter may induce attendant nerve injury. The external oblique and internal oblique muscles are divided in the direction of the incision

FIG. 1-9. The lateral or flank approach to the adrenal may be accomplished in several ways: **(A)** 11th- or 12th-rib resection; **(B)** classic subcostal approach; **(C)** modified hockeystick incision of Young; **(D)** 10th-rib resection with patient in usual flank position.

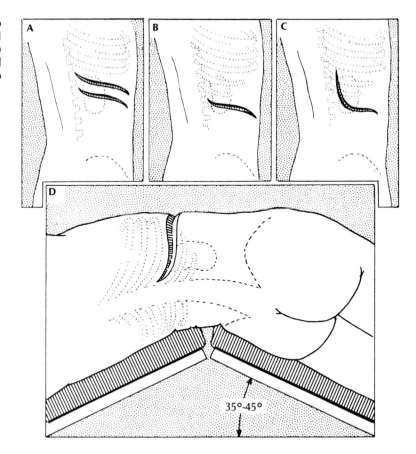

anteriorly, and the underlying transversalis musculature may be split in the direction of its fibers.

Resection of the terminal portion of the 11th or 12th rib requires periosteal incision and elevation using the usual periosteal elevators and the Doyen clamp. The periosteum in the rib bed is then exposed to a distance of about two thirds of the length of the rib, and the rib is resected at its posterior angle. The rib bed is incised anteriorly, exposing retroperitoneal fat, and more posterior division of the rib bed periosteum can be effected bluntly to retract the diaphragmatic reflection and underlying pleura superiorly by gentle manual deflection, preventing pleural entry.

In the subcostal approach, the lumbar fascia at the small triangle is first incised, with dissection and separation proceeding anteriorly. Once this has been done, Gerota's fascia is identified, opened, and retracted, enabling dissection of the perinephric fat. The kidney is exposed (Fig. 1-10), and downward traction is exerted with a broad Deaver retractor. A Mikulicz pad or a sponge is used to prevent injury to the kidney itself.

The Turner Warwick technique of supracostal incision may be used in the standard flank approach.[37] Incision is made in the relatively avascular area just above a rib, usually the 12th or the 11th, and division of the costovertebral ligaments enables direct exposure of the adrenals without rib resection or renal displacement. Witherington has reported a technical advance that further enhances the supracostal approach.[40]

When the kidney is drawn downward in the operative field, the adrenal is similarly displaced downward and into view. Dissection of the perinephric fat at the superior pole of the kidney should proceed sharply and under direct vision. The golden yellow color and consistency of the adrenal, poorly encapsulated, is dissimilar from normal perinephric fat, which is whiter and more glistening. Overt tumors may be readily palpable and visible when the adrenal is drawn down into view. Hyperplastic adrenals, on the other hand, may be more densely adherent to the surrounding fat.

As dissection proceeds, hemostasis is effected with silver clips or with fine silk ligature, preferably 4-0 or 3-0. As the adrenal is developed, the mul-

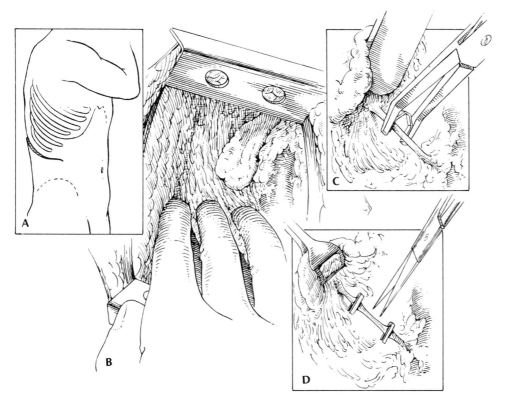

FIG. 1-10. In the subcostal approach to the adrenal, **(A)** the incision is made at the level most appropriate for exposure. **(B)** The kidney is retracted inferiorly and the adrenal is exposed. **(C)** Metal hemostatic clips may be used. **(D)** The vessels are divided between clips.

tiplicity of arteries supplying the gland must be controlled, preferably by hemostatic clips, but in some instances by using right-angle clamps, division, and ligature with fine silk. The adrenal gland may be fully exposed on its anterior, posterior, and lateral surfaces before a decision is reached regarding advisability of total extirpation. However, the adrenal should not be separated from its medial, superior, or inferior attachments until determination has been made about the ultimate course of surgery.

Once a surgical decision has been reached, complete dissection of the gland may be effected. On the left, the gland lies in close proximity to the aorta, which is readily identified and which enables a somewhat more vigorous dissection than does the vena cava on the right. The fibrous periadrenal connective tissue may be grasped with an Allis forceps or Babcock clamp, permitting lateral retraction, and medial mobilization is effected with a bronchial dissector. The larger arteries are clamped and ligated with silk; smaller vessels may be controlled with multiple hemostatic clips.

The final area of dissection is the hilum of the gland, from which the major adrenal vein issues, entering the vena cava on the right and the renal vein on the left. This vessel should be carefully exposed, doubly clamped, divided, and ligated with silk.

After removal of the gland, the adrenal fossa should be carefully observed for evidence of bleeding. A pack of sponges may be inserted for a few minutes to permit vessel retraction, and a Gelfoam sponge may be inserted into the fossa if necessary. The aorta on the left and the vena cava on the right must be inspected before closure to ensure that no injury has been incurred.

Finally, the superior pole of the kidney, which has been retracted during surgery, must be examined for possible lacerations. If capsular tears have been incurred, closure is accomplished with a running or interrupted suture of medium chromic catgut in preference to silk. Replacement of the perinephric fat around the superior pole of the kidney is desirable, and Gerota's fascia may be closed in the usual fashion or left open. Drains are not used.

The flank musculature, fascia, and the perios-

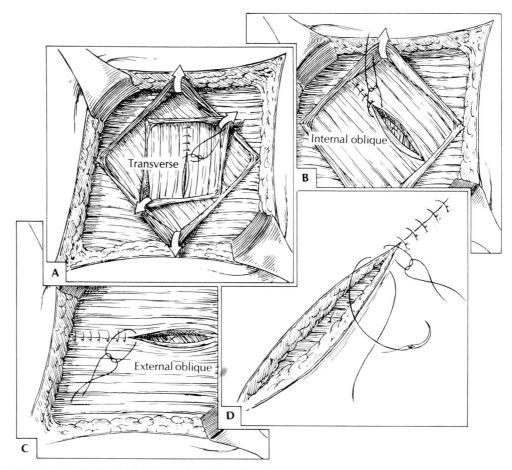

FIG. 1-11. In the flank approach to the adrenal, muscular layers and fascia can be closed with running sutures of catgut, although interrupted sutures of absorbable or nonabsorbable material can be used.

teum of the rib bed are closed with either interrupted sutures of medium silk or running or interrupted sutures of medium chromic catgut (Fig. 1-11). Subcutaneous tissues are closed with interrupted mattress sutures of fine plain catgut, and skin closure is effected according to the surgeon's preference, usually with interrupted sutures of fine black silk. Occlusive dressings are applied.

Postoperatively, it is desirable that the patient be kept on the back or on the operated side so that the perinephric space will be obliterated, further discouraging any hemorrhagic tendencies.

THORACOLUMBAR AND TRANSTHORACIC APPROACHES

The thoracolumbar approach to the adrenal gland, modified from that advocated by Chute, Soutter, and Kerr for renal surgery,[13] and the transthoracic transdiaphragmatic approach advocated by Gar-

lock and others are similar in characteristics and may be considered simultaneously.[36] Such approaches to the adrenal have the advantage of providing excellent exposure and an opportunity to palpate the thoracic sympathetic chain in cases of pheochromocytoma when a rare paraganglioma of the chest may be encountered. Ready access is also gained to the abdominal cavity, which can be opened widely for manual or visual exploration. The disadvantages are that the contralateral adrenal is not accessible through such a unilateral approach and the somewhat extensive exposure renders closure more tedious and time-consuming.

Technique

In the transthoracic transdiaphragmatic approach, the patient is placed in the extreme lateral position, the operating table is hyperextended, and the kidney bar is used (Fig. 1-12). When the thoracolumbar incision is used, the patient may be in a lateral or modified 45-degree lateral position, again

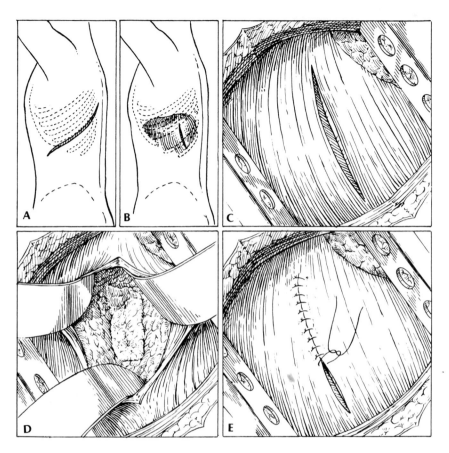

FIG. 1-12. A transthoracic, transdiaphragmatic approach to the adrenal is accomplished with the patient in the usual lateral position. **(A)** A 10th-rib incision is made. **(B** and **C)** The underlying diaphragm is incised in the direction of its fibers. **(D)** Excellent exposure of the left adrenal can be achieved, but exposure of the right adrenal is difficult because of interposition of the liver. **(E)** The diaphragm can be closed by a single- or double-layer running suture of chromic catgut or an interrupted suture of nonabsorbable material.

with the table hyperextended, giving access to the abdomen.

Incision is made over the 10th or 11th rib, beginning posteriorly and carrying forward to the tip of the rib, or curving downward through the abdominal muscles in the thoracolumbar approach. Hemostasis is effected with electrocautery or ligature. The musculature is divided in the direction of the incision, and the periosteum of the rib is incised and elevated. In the transthoracic approach, as much of the rib is resected as is conveniently possible, whereas with the thoracolumbar approach, the distal two thirds of the rib may be resected (Fig. 1-13). The rib bed is incised and the pleural cavity is entered.

The diaphragm is retracted and incised to enable entry into the retroperitoneal space or the abdominal cavity. Two incisions may be made in the diaphragm, one laterally between the lumbocostal arch and the tendinous portion of the left leaflet, providing access to the adrenal area, and a second anterior diaphragmatic incision parallel with muscular fibers, extending between the left leaflet and the attachment to the costal cartilages, enabling incision of the peritoneum and abdominal exploration. The diaphragm may be divided with a single incision, preferably extending from the lateral margin medially as far as is necessary to afford exposure.

In the thoracolumbar incision, the peritoneum and its contents are displaced anteriorly by gentle deep retraction, the lateral wound margins being held by self-retaining retractors of the usual and available variety. By either method of exposure, the perinephric fascia may be incised medially, enabling prompt access to the anteromedial aspect of the upper pole of the kidney and the adrenal area. Palpation generally discloses tumor immediately, and the thickened hyperplastic gland usually is easily discernible. Dissection of the perinephric fat and gentle exposure of the adrenal gland are effected in the manner just described, and hemostasis, isolation of the adrenal, and final ligation of the hilar vasculature are accomplished in routine fashion.

The thoracolumbar and transthoracic transdiaphragmatic incisions should not be closed until the peritoneum has been opened and the contralateral adrenal gland palpated. A peritoneal incision also provides an opportunity for manual inspection of

FIG. 1-13. In the thoracolumbar approach to the adrenal, **(A)** the incision is made over the 10th or 11th rib and extended inferiorly into the lumbar flank region, providing excellent deep exposure **(B)** of the kidney and the adrenal.

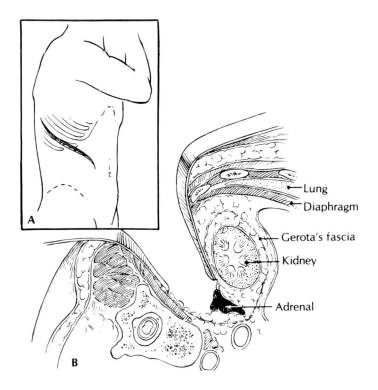

the pelvic organs, the para-aortic area, and the mesentery. Such investigation may obviate the need for a second exploration of the contralateral adrenal gland, shortening the operating time and rendering convalescence less tedious.

Closure of these exposures requires considerable attention to detail. The peritoneotomy is closed with a running suture of medium chromic catgut. The perinephric fat and fascia should be replaced and may be sutured if desired. The diaphragmatic incisions are closed in two layers, preferably with medium silk mattress sutures.

In general, it is desirable to use chest catheter suction drainage for 24 hr or more when the thoracic cavity has been exposed. The pleura should not be closed until a multi-eyed chest catheter has been positioned, either through the incision or through a stab wound in the intercostal space immediately above or below the level of the incision. The pleura is then closed with fine silk or chromic catgut, with the lung under positive-pressure expansion. Pleural closure is facilitated by incorporation of the periosteum in the suture. The overlying musculature, the subcutaneous tissue, and the skin are then closed in the usual fashion. Drains other than the advocated chest catheter are not used.

In thoracolumbar or transthoracic exposure on the right, the liver poses an anatomic barrier to effective abdominal exploration; accordingly, in exploratory procedures, an initial approach from the left is advocated.

POSTERIOR OR SIMULTANEOUS BILATERAL APPROACH

The posterior approach to the adrenal gland is probably the simplest and most expeditious method. The posterior procedure was popularized by Young more than 30 years ago; a number of modifications and improvements in this technique are now recommended.[20]

The advantages of posterior exposure of the adrenals include the relative lack of morbidity, the fact that both adrenals can be exposed simultaneously, and the ease and speed with which the procedure can be accomplished from a technical standpoint. The disadvantages of the method are the required prone jackknife position, which can embarrass respiration and provide some anesthetic difficulties; the relatively small operative field in which to work; and the inaccessibility of the abdominal cavity if further exploration is indicated or required. Because the operation is entirely retroperitoneal, no major body cavities need be entered, and the thorax and the abdomen remain intact.

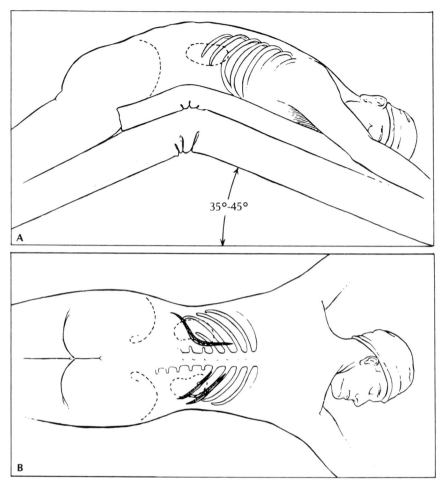

FIG. 1-14. The posterior approach to the adrenal provides the opportunity for unilateral or simultaneous bilateral exposure. **(A)** The patient is positioned prone on a flexed operating table. **(B)** The choice of surgical incisions depends on individual preference.

Technique

General endotracheal anesthesia is required. For the posterior approach the patient is then placed in the prone position with the kidney rest immediately under the inferior margin of the anterior rib cage, and the table is flexed to the modified jackknife position at about 35 degrees (Fig. 1-14). The kidney rest may be elevated subsequently if further flexion is desired or necessary, although elevation of the bar may make ventilation somewhat more difficult. The entire lower thoracic and lumbar back is prepared in a standard fashion, and drapes are applied to expose the lower rib cage bilaterally.[2]

Young advocated bilateral hockeystick incisions, beginning just below the costovertebral angle of the 12th rib some two and three finger-widths lateral to the spine on each side. The vertical component of the incision extends downward and then laterally, terminally paralleling the course of the 12th rib. Superficial musculature is incised,

and the paravertebral musculature may be retracted medially using the special Young retractor. The kidneys are exposed and retracted downward and laterally, drawing the adrenals into view.

Currently, it is more advantageous to use a straight oblique incision immediately over a rib, which is then resected to enable entry into the retroperitoneal space. Generally, either the 11th or 12th rib is resected, depending on the relative location of the adrenal as determined by prior pyelography or retroperitoneal gas contrast studies. Eleventh rib resection is preferred because it gives most direct access to the adrenal, but resection of the 12th rib may be quite satisfactory and is less likely to result in pleural damage (Fig. 1-15). The Turner Warwick supracostal incision may be used above the selected rib in any case, displacing the rib inferiorly by retraction.[37]

The electrocautery is used for coagulation of subcutaneous vessels. Skin towels are applied either with towel clips or running silk suture. Musculature is divided sharply in the line of the incision

FIG. 1-15. Used in all surgical approaches, rib resection involves incision and elevation of the periosteum from the underlying rib, with subsequent removal of as much rib as is technically possible, to provide medial access to the adrenal area.

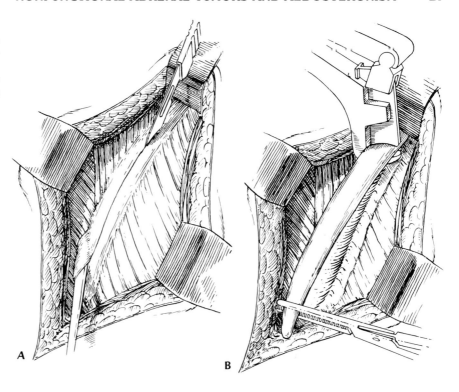

A   B

immediately over the underlying rib, and vessels are clamped and ligated with fine black silk. The periosteum of the selected rib is then incised and stripped from the rib in the usual manner.

As much as possible of the rib is resected, and the cartilaginous tip of the rib is grasped with a Kocher clamp to permit elevation for introduction of rib-cutting instruments. The medial paraspinal musculature may be retracted considerably to permit maximal exposure for resection of the rib.

Incision of the fibrous rib bed is made at the lateral terminus of the periosteum, permitting blunt dissection posteromedially, which allows superior displacement of the diaphragm and pleura and avoids entry into the thorax. If the thoracic cavity is entered, closure may be accomplished immediately or may be deferred until the conclusion of the procedure. Under forced ventilatory inspiration, obliterating the pleural space, the pleura itself is closed with running suture of atraumatic medium catgut. The diaphragm may be closed with multiple interrupted fine silk mattress sutures.

In entering the rib bed, care must be exercised to avoid injury to the infracostal vessels and nerves. Use of the cautery in the vicinity of these structures should be avoided because neuralgias may result. Musculature lateral to the tip of the resected rib may be divided bluntly or sharply to develop greater exposure.

Gerota's fascia is then incised, enabling visualization of the perinephric fat. Dissection of the area is accomplished bluntly and sharply until the posterior aspect of the upper pole of the kidney can be visualized. It is unnecessary to mobilize the entire kidney, but the upper pole may be completely freed of surrounding fat, enabling the placement of a deep curved retractor, covered by a knit sock, over the upper pole of the kidney for downward retraction.

In a unilateral approach, the Finochietto retractor with deep or shallow blades may be used to provide ample exposure. In the simultaneous bilateral approach, the blades of the Finochietto retractor may be reversed and the retractor may be used to compress the two lateral bundles of paravertebral musculature, effecting maximal medial exposure in each wound (Fig. 1-16).

With the kidneys drawn inferiorly by gentle retraction, the suprarenal fat is bluntly dissected until the golden yellow adrenal tissue is first identified. By palpation, the extent of the adrenal gland can be determined, facilitating further dissection and exposure. In general, tumors of 1 cm or more in greatest diameter are readily palpable at this point. The hyperplastic gland may be considerably enlarged, but its friable nature and the occasional adherence of periadrenal fat may make delineation of the gland difficult. Many aldosterone

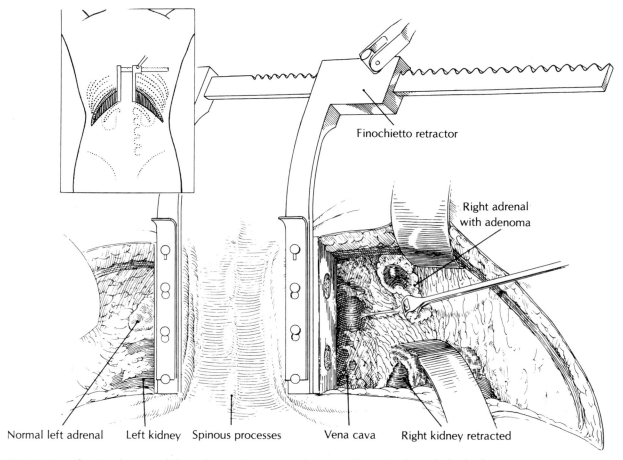

Finochietto retractor

Right adrenal
with adenoma

Normal left adrenal   Left kidney   Spinous processes   Vena cava   Right kidney retracted

FIG. 1-16. The simultaneous bilateral posterior approach, generally made through the bed of the 11th rib, is facilitated by use of a self-retaining retractor (*inset*), providing exposure for inspection of both adrenals before the surgical decision is made.

tumors are quite small, and hence palpation and even visualization may afford no localizing clues.

Standard practice involves complete posterior and lateral exposure of the glands initially with dissection of the superior aspect of the adrenals following. Hemostasis is maintained by the application of metal clips as the dissection proceeds. Multiple small arteries will be encountered; major venous drainage is almost always confined to the single large vein issuing from the hilum of the adrenal.

On the left, the adrenal is then dissected medially, the arterial supply being isolated and divided as dissection proceeds. After removing the periadrenal fat and retracting the kidney downward, the adrenal is readily visualized (Fig. 1-17). The final phase of left adrenal dissection comprises the identification, clamping, and division of the vein as it empties into the renal vein. Right-angle clamps may be preferred for this maneuver. Lig-

ation is done with medium black silk, and the gland can then be severed from its fibrous attachments and delivered.

On the right, the adrenal is isolated from the upper pole of the kidney and from the renal pedicle before the medial attachments to the vena cava are approached. With lateral traction exerted by a long Babcock clamp, dissection of the medial aspect of the gland may proceed from above downward or from below upward. When the adrenal vein is encountered, it is clamped, divided, and ligated in the usual fashion, permitting the ready delivery of the adrenal from the fossa.

The most frequently encountered difficulties in the posterior approach consist of injuries to the vena cava on the right or the renal vein on the left, or lacerations of either kidney. Vascular injuries are best controlled by right-angle vascular clamps of any variety, permitting running suture of the vesical wall with 4-0 atraumatic arterial silk.

FIG. 1-17. A left adrenal tumor is exposed through a posterior approach with the kidney retracted inferiorly.

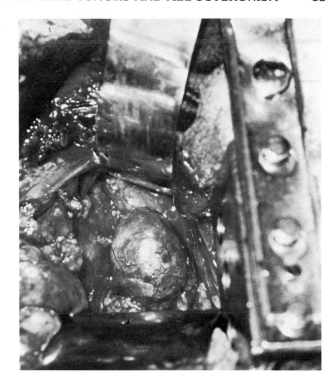

Lacerations of the kidneys, usually due to vigorous retraction, can be repaired by simple running through-and-through suture using atraumatic medium Vicryl with an interposed segment of perinephric fat, isolated for the purpose of cushioning the suture line. Mattress sutures may be preferred but generally are unnecessary.

The fossa must be carefully inspected to ensure that there is no bleeding. Minor bleeding may be controlled by the insertion of a small Oxycel or Gelfoam sponge. The kidneys are allowed to return to their normal positions, and the perinephric fat is drawn up and over the upper pole of each kidney, virtually obliterating the adrenal space. Gerota's fascia may be closed or not, depending on surgical preference. No drains are used.

The incision is closed in layers, using multiple interrupted sutures of medium black silk for all fascial and muscular layers, fine black silk or fine plain catgut for subcutaneous fat, and multiple interrupted fine silk sutures for the skin. A dry, sterile, occlusive dressing is used, and in the case of simultaneous bilateral exposure, an overriding abdominal binder may be affixed as the patient is taken from the operating table to a recovery bed.

In cases in which pleural injury has been incurred or is suspected, a postoperative chest film should be obtained in the recovery room to assess possible lung collapse.

TRANSABDOMINAL APPROACH

The most expeditious approach to adrenal surgery may be through the abdomen in some cases. Neuroblastoma, frequently infiltrating and extraadrenal, is encountered in infants and small children, and transabdominal exploration and extirpation provide the most convenient surgical method. The transabdominal approach is particularly effective in dealing with pheochromocytoma, which may be bilateral (in 10%–15% of the patients) or have origin in chromaffin tissue in the sympathetic chain extrinsic to the adrenal gland (in 15% or more of the patients).

The transabdominal approach is preferred in secondary or tertiary operations performed for reexploration of patients who have had previous surgery for adrenal carcinoma, pheochromocytoma, or other similar disease. Finally, the transabdominal approach is most efficacious in dealing with large tumors of 8 cm to 10 cm in diameter or greater.

The advantages of the transabdominal approach is that it provides access to both adrenal glands, the abdominal viscera, and the entire retroperitoneal space through a single incision. Positioning is simplified, in that the usual supine abdominal position is used. The disadvantages are that such exposure is surgically tedious and time consuming,

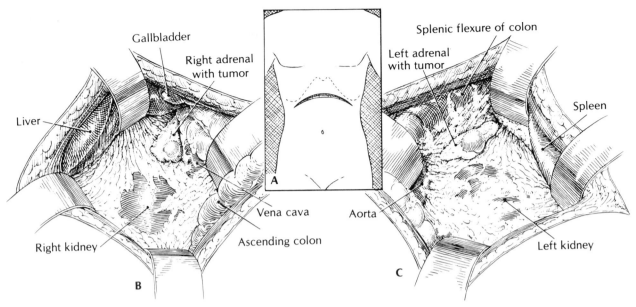

FIG. 1-18. Transabdominal approach to the adrenal. **(A)** A curving transverse subcostal incision provides excellent transabdominal exposure of adrenals. **(B)** On the right, the posterior peritoneum is incised lateral to hepatic flexure, the colon is retracted medially, the liver is retracted superiorly, and care is taken to displace the duodenum medially before incising the renal fascia. **(C)** On the left, similar exposure is effected by incision of the posterior peritoneum lateral to the descending colon and division of the splenocolic attachment with superior retraction of the spleen and medial retraction of the colon.

that mobilization of the adrenal glands themselves through an abdominal incision is technically difficult, and that postoperative morbidity is higher than with the extraperitoneal approaches owing to the concurrent ileus, which is generally more protracted in an anterior approach.

Obviously, the transabdominal approach is not necessary when the problem is one of discrete adrenal abnormality, such as bilateral hyperplasia or even aldosteronism; in these cases the extraperitoneal approaches offer greater simplicity and equivalent results with diminished morbidity.

Technique

The incision used for the transabdominal approach may be left to surgical preference. Many surgeons consider a vertical midline or paramedian rectus incision to be satisfactory, but we prefer a transverse upper abdominal incision, curving in parallel with the inferior costal margin (Fig. 1-18). In the latter approach, both recti are transected a few centimeters below the xiphoid process, and lateral musculature is similarly incised, providing ample exposure. In infants and children, a straight transverse upper abdominal incision, usually about one or two finger-widths above the umbilicus, is

preferred; the incision should be generous, extending lateral to the rectus muscles on each side.

If adrenal tumor has been localized by appropriate diagnostic studies prior to surgery, the surgeon may judiciously use only a unilateral subcostal incision (Fig. 1-19), deferring extension of the incision to the contralateral side until further exposure of the opposite adrenal proves necessary. If the unilateral transabdominal incision is used, the patient's ipsilateral arm should be elevated over and across the upper thorax, and the involved flank can be elevated with sandbags or by positioning of the table (Fig. 1-20).

The electrocautery may be used for hemostasis. Silk ligature is preferred for control of larger vessels, although absorbable ligature may be used. When the abdominal cavity is entered, thorough manual exploration is accomplished initially. Both adrenal areas should be palpated, and the surgeon should then direct his attention to the entire posterior retroperitoneal space.

Once manual examination has been effected in the transabdominal approach, the adrenals themselves may be exposed (see Fig. 1-18). The approach to the left adrenal gland is less complicated than that to the right adrenal, and consequently, unless

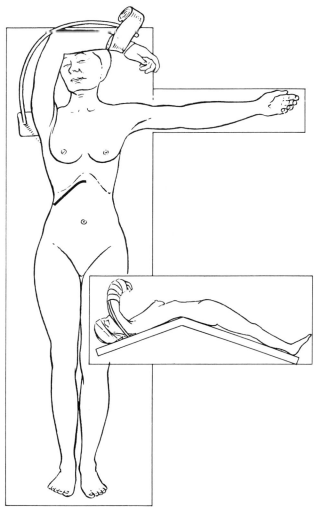

FIG. 1-19. The unilateral abdominal approach may be used for large unilateral adrenal tumors.

FIG. 1-20. (A) Lateral view of patient positioned for unilateral abdominal approach shows hyperextension with ipsilateral arm elevated. (B) View of patient from foot of table shows slight rotation of table.

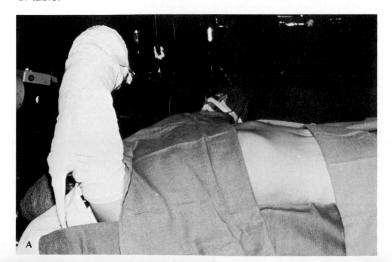

there is palpable evidence of a right adrenal abnormality, the left gland is exposed initially.

In infants and extremely thin persons, the small intestine may be retracted superiorly, permitting exposure of the posterior abdominal peritoneum at the level of the renal vessels, just below the celiac axis. A vertical incision with blunt dissection of the posterior peritoneum provides access to the retroperitoneal space, where Gerota's fascia may be opened, enabling mobilization of the kidney and the attendant adrenal gland. Routine adrenalectomy is generally a simple matter in such cases.

The body build of the average patient will require more extensive mobilization of the viscera to approach the left adrenal. The splenic flexure of the colon is retracted medially, and incision is made in the posterior peritoneum lateral to the colon in vertical fashion. It is almost always advisable to divide the splenocolic ligament to enable maximum mobilization of the colon.

Blunt and sharp dissection is effected, Gerota's fascia is opened, and the perinephric fat is dissected to expose the anterior surface of the kidney. Fat,

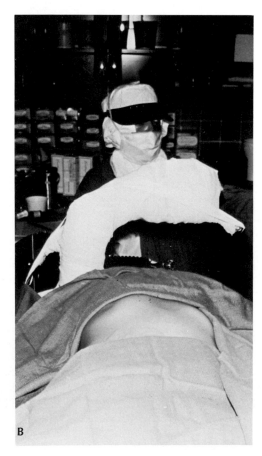

fascia, and anterior viscera are then retracted medially, enabling blunt and sharp dissection of the suprarenal fat until the adrenal gland is exposed. Here again, the specific problems encountered relate to potential injury to the kidney, its major vessels, or the abdominal aorta. In addition, the location of the spleen is such that the transabdominal approach may demand splenic retraction, and this may cause splenic laceration.

Occasionally, splenectomy is necessary to enable

FIG. 1-21. **(A)** An intravenous pyelogram demonstrates inferior displacement of the right kidney by a large suprarenal mass (a nonfunctional benign adrenal adenoma). **(B)** A selective adrenal arteriogram shows irregular calcification of the tumor and no significant neovascularization. **(C)** A radiograph of the removed tumor reveals calcification. **(D)** Areas of hemmorhage and calcification are seen in a cut section of the 12-cm adenoma.

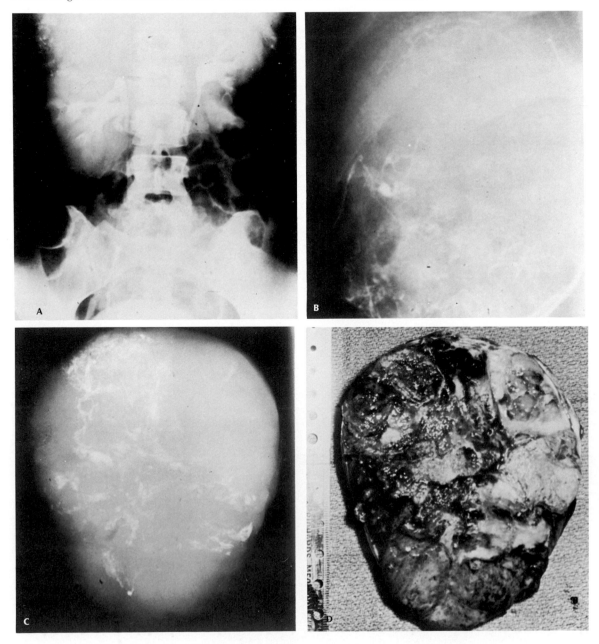

adequate visualization in the left upper quadrant, and judicious removal of the spleen in such instances is justified. In some cases, it may prove expeditious to approach the left adrenal through the lesser sac, displacing the stomach to the left.

Transabdominal exposure of the right adrenal is more tedious than exposure of the left, although the right gland lies somewhat lower than the left. On the right side, the size and configuration of the liver and the contiguity of the duodenum with the anterior renal surface constitute the major surgical hazards. The ascending colon at the level of the hepatic flexure is retracted medially, vertical incision is made in the posterior peritoneum lateral to the colon, and Gerota's fascia is entered, enabling dissection of the perinephric fat.

The liver is retracted superiorly, taking care to avoid injury to the inferior hepatic surface and gallbladder. With a Deaver or Harrington retractor placed from the left into the perinephric space, the anterior surface of the kidney can be exposed. The adrenal gland is found to lie just superior to the kidney, often somewhat posterior to the vena cava. The usual dissection and hemostasis are accomplished. The major attachment of the gland is to the vena cava, and great care must be exercised in medial dissection of the right adrenal.

The posterior peritoneal incisions, in the midline or on either side, are closed with running suture of medium atraumatic catgut, usually 3-0 chromic. Viscera displaced for purposes of adrenal exposure generally return to their normal position and with such posterior closure. The anterior peritoneum is similarly closed with running suture of absorbable material. All viscera that have been vigorously retracted must be carefully examined for injury, particularly spleen and liver. Such lacerations are generally repaired with medium chromic catgut over cushioning fat, which may be obtained from the perinephric space; Gelfoam or Oxycel may be used.

Closure of the abdominal incision, vertical or transverse is begun with running suture of absorbable synthetic suture for peritoneum and posterior fascia, followed by multiple interrupted silk sutures; through-and-through sutures are used for musculature, mattress sutures for fascia, and fine interrupted sutures for subcutaneous tissues. Skin may be closed with a choice of suture, usually fine black silk. Drains are not used, and occlusive dressings are applied.

When the transabdominal approach to adrenal surgery is used, many surgeons use nasogastric suction as a routine measure. Certainly, the increased difficulties with paralytic ileus justify such measures. Introduction of the nasogastric tube on the evening prior to surgery facilitates decompression of the bowel and consequent technical facility in mobilization of the intestine at the time of surgery. Nasogastric suction so used should be continued for 24 hr to 48 hr postoperatively to facilitate convalescence.

Preoperative and Postoperative Management

The specifics of preoperative and postoperative management of the patient undergoing adrenal surgery depend, quite naturally, on the pathology prompting surgical intervention. Adequate hydration, nutritional balance, and reconstitution of adequate blood volume and hemoglobin levels are prerequisites to any surgical intervention. Definitive preoperative localization of adrenal tumors is of obvious advantage to patient and surgeon alike.

Massive nonfunctioning adrenal tumors constitute a special challenge.[4,38] In such cases, a surgeon may not be able to assess contralateral adrenal function and may not even know whether a contralateral adrenal exists. Therefore, it is desirable to institute preoperative corticosteroid replacement therapy, something that can be initiated within 24 hr of the planned procedure. With the security of preoperative preparation, very large tumors can be approached with confidence (Fig. 1-21).

Primary aldosteronism presents a situation in which medical judgment is extremely important. Most aldosterone-secreting tumors are unilateral adenomas, but bilateral tumors and bilateral focal hyperplasia occur with such frequency that total bilateral adrenalectomy may be imperative in many cases. Furthermore, progressive numbers of instances of normokalemic aldosteronism due to extremely small adrenal tumors can be anticipated; the surgeon may be unable to identify the tumor grossly, and bilateral adrenalectomy may be required. In primary aldosteronism, it is good practice to effect preliminary corticosteroid supplementation and replacement therapy.

Total adrenalectomy of the involved gland remains the procedure of choice in aldosteronism due to primary adenoma. In many cases, the affected adrenal will not only exhibit the solitary adenoma but also display areas of focal hyperplasia (Fig. 1-22), which could become autonomous adenomas with time. Consequently, total removal of the affected gland, most often the left adrenal, is indicated. If the patient should exhibit future evidence of aldosteronism, only the remaining contralateral adrenal gland need be explored.

In total adrenalectomy, reimplantation of auto-

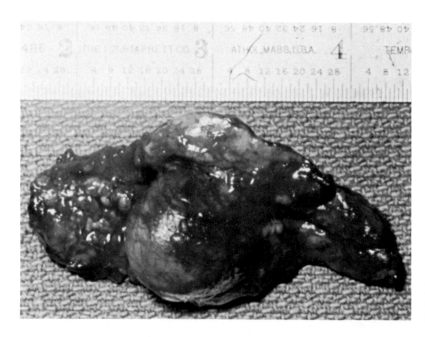

FIG. 1-22. In this aldosteronoma, areas of focal nodular hyperplasia are evident in addition to the primary tumor.

genous adrenal tissue offers a therapeutic potential. At the present time, supplementary corticosteroid therapy must be regarded as the only practical form of clinical management in patients undergoing extirpation of all or most of intrinsic functional adrenal tissue. Fortunately, such exogenous supplemental therapy has been facilitated by the introduction of a variety of corticosteroids, including prednisone, prednisolone, and fluorocortisone (Florinef).

Postoperative bleeding in patients undergoing adrenal surgery is and should be a rare occurrence, because adequate surgical attention to hemostasis is mandatory. Readjustment of extracellular fluid volume in patients with both cortical and medullary adrenal tumors may complicate postoperative evaluation, and immediate postoperative electrolyte and hematocrit determinations are essential. Serial evaluations accomplished daily at first and at 3-day intervals subsequently are of value in determining appropriate electrolyte and fluid volume replacement.

Surgical infections do not constitute a major problem in patients undergoing adrenal surgery. In patients who have received preliminary corticosteroid supplementation and who undergo total adrenalectomy demanding extensive postoperative supplementation, it may be prudent to use broad-spectrum antibiotics of the tetracycline variety during the first postoperative week to diminish the possibility of wound infection and to inhibit any potential pulmonary infections that might result from inadequate ventilation. Bronchodilators and

intermittent positive-pressure breathing may be beneficial to prevent or overcome atelectasis.

Surgical entry into the thoracic cavity usually does not demand the postoperative use of chest catheters. Adequate operative ventilation of the lung and thoracic closure under positive pressure effects satisfactory pulmonary expansion and obliteration of the pleural space in most cases. A postoperative chest film, obtained in the recovery room, is helpful in management. If lung collapse or accumulation of fluid in the thoracic cavity is evident, aspiration may be effected through the 10th intercostal space laterally, using a 50-ml syringe and an 18-gauge needle.

Convalescence of patients undergoing adrenal surgery by the posterior approach is surprisingly benign, and ambulation may be urged early in the postoperative period. The transthoracic, flank, and transabdominal approaches to adrenal surgery carry a higher incidence of postoperative morbidity and disability, and supplemental measures for early mobilization of the patient may include the use of abdominal supports such as the scultetus binder.

Postoperative complications of severe magnitude such as pulmonary embolism, pneumonia, thrombophlebitis, or cardiac difficulties constitute problems that are magnified in importance by the presence of relative adrenal insufficiency. Hypoadrenocorticism may be encountered in patients who have undergone total or partial adrenalectomy, and supplementary corticosteroid therapy becomes of paramount importance under such circumstances.

REFERENCES

1. ANDERSON EE: Nonfunctioning tumors of the adrenal gland. Urol Clin North Am 4:263, 1977
2. ANDERSON EE, GLENN JF: Cushing's syndrome associated with anaplastic carcinoma of the thyroid gland. J Urol 95:1, 1966
3. ATWILL WH, BOYARSKY S, GLENN JF: Effect of adrenalectomy on the course of experimental renovascular hypertension. Am J Surg 11:755, 1968
4. AYYAF F, FOSSLIN E, KENT R, HUDSON HC: Myelolipoma of the adrenal gland. Urology 16:415, 1980
5. BARRY JM, HODGES CV: The supracostal approach to the kidney and adrenal. J Urol 114:666, 1975
6. BENNETT AH, HARRISON JH, THORN GW: Neoplasms of the adrenal gland. J Urol 106:607, 1971
7. BIGLIERI EG, STOCKIGT JR, SCHAMBELAN M: Adrenal mineralocorticoids causing hypertension. Am J Med 52:623, 1972
8. BLACK J, WILLIAMS DI: Natural history of adrenal hemorrhage in the newborn. Arch Dis Child 48:183, 1973
9. BROWN, JJ, DAVIES DL, FERRISS JB et al: Comparison of surgery and prolonged spironolactone therapy in patients with hypertension, aldosterone excess, and low plasma renin. Br Med J 2:729, 1972
10. CAHILL GF: Adrenalectomy for adrenal tumors. J Urol 71:123, 1954
11. CERNY JC: Anatomy of the adrenal gland. Urol Clin North Am 4:169, 1977
12. CERNY JC, NESBIT RM, CONN JW et al: Preoperative tumor localization by adrenal venography in patients with primary aldosteronism: A comparison with operative findings. J Urol 103:521, 1970
13. CHUTE R, SOUTTER L, KERR WS: The value of the thoracoabdominal incision in the removal of kidney tumors. New Engl J Med 241:951, 1949
14. COLLETT A: Genito-suprarenal syndrome (suprarenal virilism) in a girl one and a half years old, with successful operation. Am J Dis Child 27:204, 1924
15. CONN JW: Primary aldosteronism: A new clinical syndrome. J Lab Clin Med 45:3, 1955
16. CONN JW, BEIERWALTES WH, LIEBERMAN LM et al: Primary aldosteronism: Preoperative tumor visualization by scintillation scanning. J Clin Endocrinol Metab 33:713, 1971
17. EGDAHL RH, KAHN PC, MELBY JC: Role of angiography in surgery of the adrenal. Am J Surg 117:480, 1969
18. FLINT FB, GORDON HE: Adrenal cysts. Am Surg 38:456, 1972
19. GLENN JF: Neonatal adrenal hemorrhage. J Urol 87:639, 1962
20. GLENN JF: Current concepts of adrenal surgery. Int Surg 48:121, 1967
21. GONZALEZ–SERVA L, GLENN JF: Adrenal surgical techniques. Urol Clin North Am 4:327, 1977
22. GUNNELLS JC JR, BATH NM, SODE J: Primary aldosteronism. Arch Intern Med 120:568, 1967
23. GUNNELLS JC JR, MCGUFFIN WL JR, ROBINSON RR et al: Hypertension, adrenal abnormalities, and alterations in plasma renin activity. Ann Intern Med 73:901, 1970
24. HOLMES G: A case of virilism associated with a suprarenal tumor: Recovery after its removal. J Med 18:143, 1925
25. HUGGINS C, SCOTT WW: Bilateral adrenalectomy in prostate cancer: Clinical features and urinary excretion of 17-ketosteroids and estrogen. Ann Surg 122:1031, 1945
26. KEARNEY GP, MAHONEY EM: Adrenal cysts. Urol Clin North Am 4:273, 1977
27. KHURI FJ, ALTON DJ, HARDY BE et al: Adrenal hemorrhage in neonates: Report of 5 cases and review of the literature. J Urol 124:684, 1980
28. LARAGH JH, BAER L, BRUNNER HR et al: Renin, angiotensin, and aldosterone system in pathogenesis and management of hypertensive vascular disease. Am J Med 52:633, 1972
29. LIDDLE GW: Management of aldosteronism. Am J Clin Pathol 54:331, 1970
30. MAYO CH: Paroxysmal hypertension with tumor of retroperitoneal nerve. JAMA 89:1047, 1927
31. MCGUFFIN WL JR, GUNNELLS JC JR: Primary aldosteronism. Urol Clin North Am 4:227, 1977
32. MENON M, MERSEY JH: Primary aldosteronism: A review. Urol Surv 30:95, 1980
33. OLDER RA: Radiologic approach to adrenal lesions. Urol Clin North Am 4:305, 1977
34. SCOTT WW, HUDSON PB: Surgery of the Adrenal Glands. Springfield, Charles C Thomas, 1954
35. TANK ES: Surgery of the adrenal glands in infancy and childhood. J Urol 106:280, 1971
36. TOCANTINS R, SMITH DR: The modified Garlock incision for adrenal surgery. J Urol 85:417, 1961
37. TURNER WARWICK RT: The supracostal approach to the renal area. Br J Urol 37:671, 1965
38. VARGAS AD: Adrenal hemangioma. Urology 16:389, 1980
39. WHITE EA, SCHAMBELAN M, ROST CR et al: Use of computed tomography in diagnosing the cause of primary aldosteronism. N Engl J Med 303:1503, 1980
40. WITHERINGTON R: Improving the supracostal lion incisions. J Urol 124:73, 1980
41. ZORNOZA J, BERNARDINO ME: Bilateral adrenal metastasis: "Head light" sign. Urology 15:91, 1980

Cushing's Syndrome

2

Robert K. Rhamy

Bartolommeo Eustachio was annoyed with the prevailing scientific writings of Rome in the mid-16th century. His discoveries impressed him with the multitude of inaccuracies in the anatomic dogmas of Galen, da Vinci, and Versalius. Rejecting their hegemony, he was outspoken in his criticism of the scientific writings endorsed as fact by his peers. Eustachio wrote, "I have judged it proper to write at this point concerning certain glands of the kidneys carelessly overlooked by other anatomists. I would have desired that this type of gland not have been overlooked by earlier anatomists and by those who today pursue this art and who have written quite long treatises on the parts of the human body, especially since they represent themselves as factual. They have, in fact, followed the errors of others and have done so, so painstakingly as to not uncommonly seem more contentious than interested in anatomical verity."[5]

The adrenal gland and its importance remained in obscurity until 1855, when Thomas Addison reported on 11 patients in whom a common clinical disorder existed. The syndrome consisted of wasting, weakness, vitiliginous rash, and bronzing of the skin. Therapy of these patients was to no avail, and all died. Autopsy demonstrated destruction of the adrenal glands in all 11 patients.[1]

The first successful removal of an adrenal tumor was in 1889. A large tumor (20 lb) of the left adrenal was excised *en bloc* with the left kidney in a 36-year-old female with hirsutism and virilization.[6]

The syndrome described by Cushing, in 1932, was based on his study of a series of patients who had manifestations of adiposity, amenorrhea, hypertrichosis, purplish striae, hypertension, polyphagia, polydipsia, polycythemia, and susceptibility to pulmonary infections.[4] In four of the eight patients, basophilic adenomas of the pituitary were found at autopsy, and Cushing ascribed this syndrome to pituitary basophilism.[3]

Twenty years later Plotz, Knowlton, and Ragan reviewed the results of therapy in 33 patients with Cushing's syndrome. Their report provides an interesting historical perspective because it constitutes a parting view of presteroid therapy in which residual adrenal function had to be preserved in order for the patient to survive. They concluded that more than half of the patients with Cushing's syndrome would die within 5 years of the onset of their disease if they were not treated.[18]

Etiology

Cushing's syndrome occurs whenever cortisol is chronically available in excessive quantities to peripheral tissues and, ultimately, to specific cytoplasmic receptors that complete the hormone's journey to nuclear deoxyribonucleic-acid (DNA) sites. Normally, cortisol secretion is governed solely by pituitary adrenocorticotropic hormone (ACTH), which declines as cortisol levels rise and increases in response to a hypothalamic corticotropin-releasing factor (CRF). CRF secretion by specific neurons is influenced, in turn, by at least three brain neurotransmitters and possibly by cortisol itself, which inhibits ACTH release by an action on hypothalamic or pituitary cells or both.[12]

Aside from the use of steroid hormones in medical therapy, hypercortisolism occurs spontaneously from three causes (Fig. 2-1): (1) bilateral adrenocortical hyperplasia under the stimulatory effect of increased secretion of ACTH by the pituitary, which may or may not contain an adenoma; (2) bilateral adrenocortical hyperplasia under the stimulus of ACTH or an ACTH-like polypeptide secreted by a nonendocrine tumor, such as certain carcinomas of the lung; and (3) adrenocortical tumor.[16]

Bilateral adrenal hyperplasia accounts for approximately 76% of all cases of Cushing's syndrome, with pituitary-dependent hyperplasia found in 63% and ectopic ACTH, in 13%. In adults 15% were found to have adrenal adenomas, and 9% had adrenocortical carcinoma. In contrast, carcinoma of the adrenal cortex in children represents 51% of all causes of Cushing's syndrome. As shown

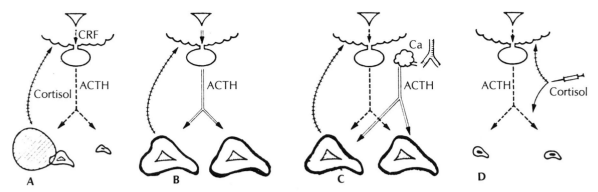

FIG. 2-1. Causes of Cushing's syndrome: **(A)** adrenocortical tumor; **(B)** adrenocortical hypertension of hypothalamic origin; **(C)** adrenocortical hyperplasia due to ectopic ACTH production; **(D)** exogenous cortisol administration

TABLE 2-1. Incidence of Adrenal Lesions in Cushing's Syndrome

	Incidence (%)	
Adrenal Lesion	ADULTS	CHILDREN*
Bilateral hyper-plasia	63	33
Pituitary tumor	40	
No tumor	23	
Adrenal cortical tumor	24	65
Adenoma	15	14
Carcinoma	9	51
Ectopic ACTH syndrome	13	2

*Gold EM: Cushing's syndrome: A tripartite entity. Hosp Pract 14: 67, 1979.

in Table 2-1, the incidence of ectopic ACTH production is much lower in children than in adults.

The age of patients with adrenocortical tumors ranges from 6 weeks to 72 years of age. In the age group below 20, and particularly before age 7, a heavy predominance of carcinoma is present. In 21 cases of children less than 1 year of age, 12 adrenal carcinomas, five adenomas, and four cases of bilateral hyperplasia were found.[15] The presence of hyperplasia before the age of 2 is unusual, and in those under 16 years of age, it represents only 33% of the causes of Cushing's syndrome. In adults the evidence of ectopic ACTH was six times greater (13% *vs* 2%) than that seen in children (Fig. 2-2).

Symptoms

The original description of the syndrome as characterized by adiposity, kyphosis, amenorrhea, polyphagia, and susceptibility to pulmonary infections is still the best.[3] The relative frequency of these symptoms is shown in Table 2-2.

Cushing's syndrome is a characteristic array of clinical features associated with prolonged overproduction of cortisol. The natural course is remarkably unpredictable. It can be rapidly progressive, disabling, and ultimately fatal in many cases, whereas in others it may be mild, intermittent, or periodic; or it may even undergo spontaneous remission, as in Cushing's first patient.[2,3,9,18]

The hormonal basis for the syndrome is obscure; only obesity and hypertension, of the most common features, are of equal frequency in patients given glucocorticoids. Excessive production of testosterone by the adrenal gland gives rise in women to hirsutism, menstrual disorders, and acne. In men, testosterone levels, as well as luteinizing hormone–follicle-stimulating hormone (LH–FSH) levels, are decreased. This accounts for the loss of libido, impotence, and oligospermia which are seen and which are returned to normal with correction of the hypercortisolism.[8]

Although the clinical symptoms alone may be sufficiently clear to establish the diagnosis of Cushing's syndrome, it is often necessary and certainly always desirable to confirm the clinical impression by precise studies of adrenocortical function and adrenal–pituitary relationships. These studies are of fundamental importance in differentiating Cushing's syndrome due to pituitary-dependent adrenocortical hyperplasia, extraendocrine tumor, and adrenocortical tumor. The level of urinary 17-ketosteroids and a more rapid clinical course may help preoperative differentiation of Cushing's syndrome due to adrenal adenoma from Cushing's syndrome caused by adrenocortical carcinoma (Table 2-3).

Endocrine Diagnosis

The full diagnosis of this condition falls into two parts: the diagnosis of Cushing's syndrome (demonstration of pathologically increased cortisol secretion) and the differential diagnosis (determination of its cause).[19]

Diagnosis

Although plasma ACTH or cortisol may remain within the normal range at 6 A.M., they are almost invariably elevated at 6 P.M. (Fig. 2-3). The loss of circadian rhythm in plasma cortisol remains one

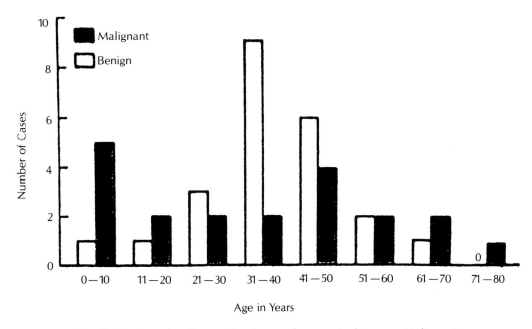

FIG. 2-2. Age distribution of patients with primary adrenocortical tumors. Malignant tumors show peaks in childhood and in middle age, whereas benign tumors have a maximum in middle life.

TABLE 2-2. Frequency of Clinical Features of Cushing's Syndrome

	Average (%)	Vanderbilt Series (%)	Range (11 Series, 601 Cases) (%)
Central obesity	88	93	50–100
Plethoric face	75	93	50–100
Hypertension	74	93	50–90
Hirsutism	64	79	28–93
Muscle weakness	61	82	18–96
Menstrual disorders	60	75	40–85
Acne	45	47	26–82
Bruising	42	57	23–62
Mental Aberrations	42	57	31–70
Osteoporosis	40	54	22–70
Edema		46	
Stria		36	

Gold EM: The Cushing syndromes: Changing views of diagnosis and treatment. Ann Intern Med 90: 235, 1975.

TABLE 2-3.   Features of Cushing's syndrome caused by adenoma and carcinoma of the adrenal

	Adrenal adenoma	Adrenal carcinoma
Age onset of symptoms	29.5 years	35.4 years
Duration of symptoms to diagnosis	3 years	6 months
Hypertension (diastolic > 100)	58%	82%
Muscle weakness	25%	42%
Osteoporosis	33%	39%
Pigmentation	0	0
Baseline 17-OHCS	37.2 mg	74.7 mg
Baseline 17 Ketosteroids	26.0 mg	64.2 mg
Hypokalemia < 3 mEq/liter	5%	15%

Jeffcoate WJ, Edwards CRW: Cushing's syndrome: Pathogenesis, diagnosis and treatment in comprehensive endocrinology. In James VHT (ed): The Adrenal Gland, pp 165–195. New York, Raven Press, 1979.

FIG. 2-3.   Plasma 17-OHCS and plasma ACTH concentrations of normal subjects and of patients with Cushing's disease at 6 a.m. and 6 p.m

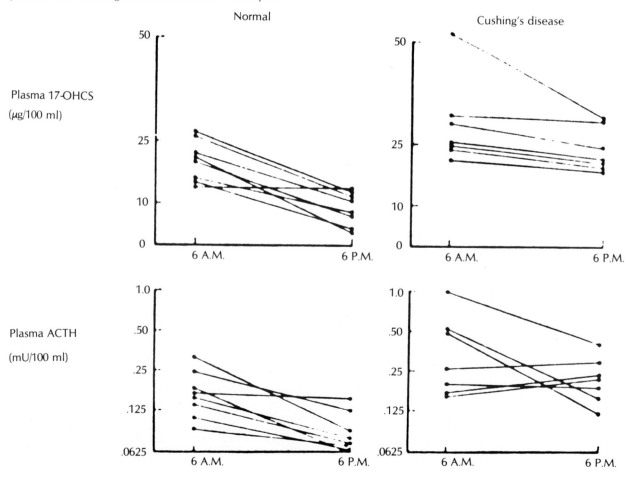

of the simplest and most suggestive pieces of evidence in support of the diagnosis.[13]

In addition to elevated plasma cortisol levels with loss of circadian rhythm, the urinary-free cortisol and its metabolites are elevated. The most commonly measured are 17-hydroxycorticosteroids (17-OHCS), which are elevated above the normal level of 3 mg to 7 mg to concentrations above 10 mg of 17-OHCS/g of creatinine.

Differential

Once the diagnosis of Cushing's syndrome has been established, it is necessary to determine the etiology of the adrenocortical hyperfunction.[7] A flow pattern of diagnostic tests for the differentiation of the etiology of the hypercortisolism is shown in Figure 2-4.[20]

The ACTH stimulation test will induce the bi-laterally hyperplastic adrenal glands' pituitary hypersecretion of ACTH to increase plasma cortisol and urinary 17-OHCS (Fig. 2-5). Ectopic ACTH syndrome will likewise respond, but adrenal tumors usually do not.[13]

Metyrapone inhibits 11β-hydroxylation to block the final step in the synthesis of cortisol; 11-deoxycortisol is secreted instead. In patients with pituitary-dependent Cushing's disease, there is an exaggerated response (elevation) of plasma 11-deoxycortisol and urinary 17-OHCS, whereas patients with adrenal tumors and ectopic ACTH syndrome have chronically suppressed pituitary function and, therefore, fail to release ACTH in response to metyrapone (Fig. 2-6).[13]

Other biochemical abnormalities are present in Cushing's syndrome and may help to confirm its presence in borderline cases (Table 2-4).

FIG. 2-4. Flow pattern of dexamethasone suppression tests for differentiation of the etiology of hypercortisolism

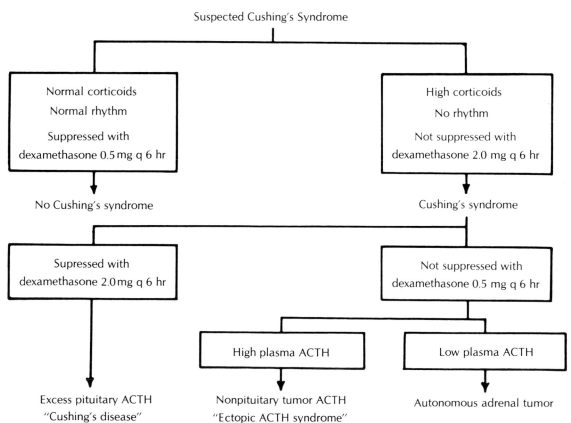

Localization

The techniques used to localize the tumor anatomically in a patient with Cushing's syndrome are indicated by the endocrinologic differentiation.

TABLE 2-4.   Other biochemical abnormalities in Cushing's syndrome

---
Glucose intolerance
Suppression of stress-induced growth hormone release
Suppression of TRH-induced thyrotropin (TSH) release
TRH-induced ACTH release
Suppression of basal levels of thyroxine, TSH, luteinizing hormone, and, especially in males, testosterone
Hyperprolactinemia

Neville AM, MacKay AM: The structure of the human adrenal cortex in health and disease. Clin Endocrinol Metab 1: 361, 1972.

ADRENAL CUSHING'S SYNDROME

1. Excretory urography is a relatively insensitive technique for the determination of adrenal enlargement. Bilateral hyperplasia is almost never detected by intravenous pyelogram (IVP); however, IVP combined with nephrotomography may show unilateral adrenal tumor with renal displacement, particularly in tumors 3 cm in diameter or larger. The presence of calcium in the mass is highly suggestive of carcinoma.

2. Retroperitoneal pneumography, although much more sensitive than the IVP, has been replaced by noninvasive techniques of lesser risk.

3. Arteriography of adrenal lesions is helpful only in highly vascular tumors, as manifested by

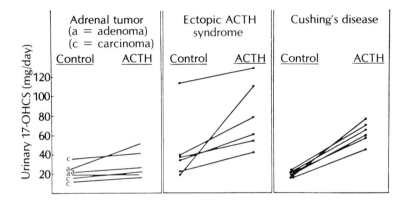

FIG. 2-5.   Urinary 17-OCHS under control conditions and in response to ACTH; 50 units administered as an 8-hr intravenous infusion in patients with Cushing's syndrome due to adrenocortical tumor, in patients with the ectopic ACTH syndrome, and in patients with Cushing's disease

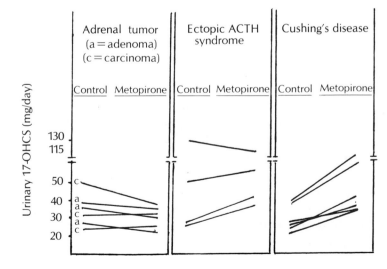

FIG. 2-6.   Urinary 17-OHCS under control conditions and in response to Metopirone, 500 mg or 750 mg every 4 hr for 6 doses in patients with Cushing's syndrome

tortuosity of vessels, vessel enlargement, and increase in density or "stain" during the capillary or venous phases.

4. Venography is another invasive technique that is more sensitive than arteriography, but complications of hemorrhage and infarction in 5% of patients have decreased its popularity.

5. Scintiscan (^{131}I-19-iodocholesterol) is a noninvasive technique, but it requires a millicurie dosage and a time lag of several days. A newer analog, NP-59, helps decrease dose and time, but both agents are best used for localizing adrenal adenomas and ectopic or residual adrenal tissue.

6. Computed tomography (CT) is an excellent technique for the localization of adrenal tumors that are 1.5 cm in diameter or larger.[14] In many instances, changes in adrenal size (hyperplasia) may be determined by this technique.

7. Adrenal-vein sampling with assay of the venous effluent for hormone concentrations may aid localization. Simultaneous adrenal-vein catheterization increases accuracy (Fig. 2-7).

ECTOPIC ACTH SYNDROME

1. Chest roentgenograms reveal a neoplasm responsible for this lesion in 50% of patients.

2. CT examinations help to demonstrate the presence of any one of a number of neoplasms to which this syndrome is ascribed.

PITUITARY CUSHING'S DISEASE

1. Skull films demonstrate an enlarged sella turcica in 15% of tumors of the pituitary causing this clinical picture.

2. Polytomography increases the accuracy of detection of pituitary tumors but does not show microadenomas.

Treatment

Ideally, treatment should fully restore the patient with Cushing's syndrome to normal, both clinically and in terms of ACTH and cortisol secretion without replacement needs.

PITUITARY CUSHING'S SYNDROME

In pituitary-dependent Cushing's syndrome, as in all other types of this disease, the options for medical, irradiation, or surgical management exist. The medical approach may be directed at either

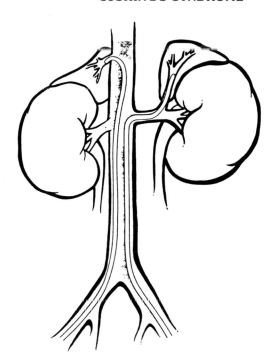

FIG. 2-7. Bilateral simultaneous adrenal-vein catheterization for collection of venous effluent. (Scott HW, Liddle GW, Mulherin JL *et al*: Surgical experience with Cushing's disease. Ann Surg 185:524, 1977)

the pituitary or the adrenal gland (Table 2-5).

Combinations of drugs may decrease toxicity. However, the major use of medical therapy is to prepare patients for surgery (Fig. 2-8).

Irradiation therapy may be used in conjunction with surgery, but cure rates are very low when it is used alone. Thus the use of this modality of treatment is decreasing (Table 2-6).

The use of surgery for pituitary-dependent Cushing's syndrome is the age-old standard. Adrenalectomy was the surgical procedure of choice until recent advances in surgical techniques with pituitary lesions (Table 2-7).

ECTOPIC ACTH SYNDROME

The tumors that cause ectopic ACTH syndrome are often highly undifferentiated and metastatic. In less than 10% of cases, the lesion is resectable. Medical therapy as described for pituitary-dependent hypercortisolism, as well as appropriate chemotherapy of the primary tumor, is most frequently the therapy of choice. Only a few tumors are resectable, and the cure rate is 2%. Life expectancy is usually a matter of a few months.

TABLE 2-5. Medical Management of Pituitary-Dependent Cushing's Syndrome

Drug	Effect
Pituitary Active	
CNS—active cyproheptadine (24 mg/day orally in 3–4 divided doses)	Remission 60%–65% after 6–8 weeks; rapid relapse with withdrawal; minor side-effects (increased appetite and weight gain)
CNS—active Bromocriptine (10 mg/day orally)	
Adrenal Active	
Adrenal—active o,p′ DDD (mitotane) (6.0 g/day)	Remission of hypercortisolism in 60%–90%; adrenocorticolytic; may require glucocorticoid or mineralocorticoid replacement; 6 months f,or remission; side-effects of sedation, depression, GI complaints, and rare convulsions
Metyrapone (1.0 g/day)	Remission of hypercortisolism in 60%–90%; relapse rapid with withdrawal, may require replacement of glucocorticoids or mineralocorticoids; side-effect of hirsutism
Aminoglutethimide (1.0 g/day)	Remission in 60%–90%; may require replacement therapy; relapse rapid with withdrawal; may produce goiters, somnolence, and skin rash in 20%–30%
Trilostane (1.0 g/day)	Remission in 60%–90%; may require replacement therapy; relapse rapid with withdrawal

Plotz CM, Knowlton AI, Ragan C: The natural history of Cushing's syndrome. Am J Med 13: 597, 1952.

TABLE 2-6. Irradiation of Pituitary

Type of therapy	Results
External high voltage x-ray (cobalt—60)	Children 80% remission; Adults 20% remission, 23% partial improvement: Long lag for results (up to 18 months)
Cyclotron (α-particle proton beam)	60% remission in adults, partial improvement 30%; 7%–8% morbidity (cranial-nerve palsy or permanent pituitary failure)
Internal yttrium—90	Requires surgery: results same as proton beam

Plotz CM, Knowlton AI, Ragan C: The natural history of Cushing's syndrome. Am J Med 13: 597, 1952.

ADRENAL CUSHING'S SYNDROME

The diagnosis of adrenal Cushing's syndrome almost always mandates adrenal surgery. Even in this era of microresection of pituitary adenomas, a few cases of pituitary-dependent Cushing's syndrome require bilateral adrenalectomy. When planning adrenal surgery, the nature of the lesion, its location, and the ravages of the hypercortisolism on the patient's metabolism must be considered. In severely debilitated persons preoperative blockage of cortisol production by medications decreases the mortality and morbidity of the surgical procedure (Table 2-5).

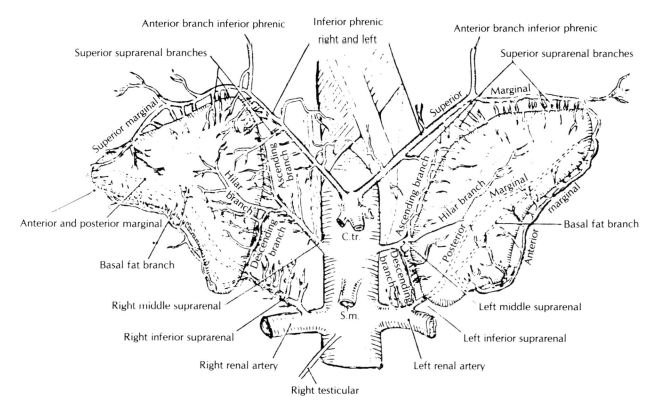

FIG. 2-8. Blood supply of the adrenal glands

TABLE 2-7. Surgery of Pituitary-Dependent Cushing's Syndrome

Procedure	Results
Trans-sphenoidal microresection	90%–95% remission rate after removal of microadenoma; temporary cortisol replacement may be necessary; morbidity low
Trans-frontal hypophysectomy	Panhypopituitarism; permanent replacement therapy; morbidity significant
Bilateral adrenalectomy (total or subtotal)	100% immediate remission rate; recurrence due to remnant or ectopic tissue 10%; mortality 4%–10%; permanent replacement therapy; Nelson's syndrome 10%–20%

Plotz CM, Knowlton AI, Ragan C: The natural history of Cushing's syndrome. Am J Med 13: 597, 1952.

BILATERAL ADRENALECTOMY

Bilateral adrenalectomy is less commonly performed since the advent of the trans-sphenoidal approach to the pituitary. When bilateral adrenalectomy is indicated, we strongly favor the posterior bilateral approach, which was first described by Young in 1936, over the transabdominal operation because of the markedly lower morbidity associated with this procedure.[23] The technique is shown in the following figures.

With the bilateral posterior approach, the patient is in the prone position and the table is flexed (Fig. 2-9). Compression of the abdomen (in a sandbag

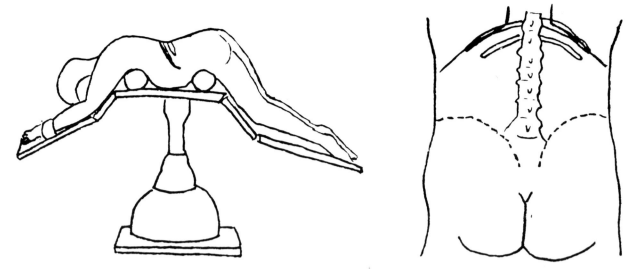

FIG. 2-9.   Posterior approach to the adrenals. Position of patient on operating table; bilateral incisions over 11th ribs

or kidney rest) pushes the abdominal viscera against the perirenal space and actually decreases exposure. The incision is made over either the 11th or the 12th rib bilaterally (Fig. 2-10). We prefer the 11th rib, particularly on the right, to ensure adequate exposure of the adrenal gland and the surrounding structures. The incision is made over and down to the rib in the standard fashion. Resection of the rib is done in the usual manner (Fig. 2-11). The pleura and lung can then be seen just beneath the fibers of the diaphragm. Incision of the diaphragm, starting laterally, usually allows retraction of the pleura cephalad, permitting an extrapleural exposure of the adrenal gland (Figs. 2-12 and 2-13).

The operative mortality of bilateral adrenalectomy by the simultaneous posterior approach in our series (28 cases) was 3.4%. The nonfatal complications are shown in Table 2-8.[21]

Cushing's syndrome was cured in 92% of patients, with persistent hypercortisolism in 8%. Nelson's syndrome developed in only 3% of those subjected to bilateral adrenalectomy and in none of those who had received prior pituitary irradiation.

UNILATERAL ADRENALECTOMY

Unilateral adrenalectomy is usually performed for tumors of the adrenal gland because bilateral adenomas of the adrenal glands have been reported in only 10% of cases. Adenomas are usually smaller

FIG. 2-10.   Operating surgeon's view of incision over left 11th rib; latissimus dorsi divided near its origin from lumbodorsal aponeurosis

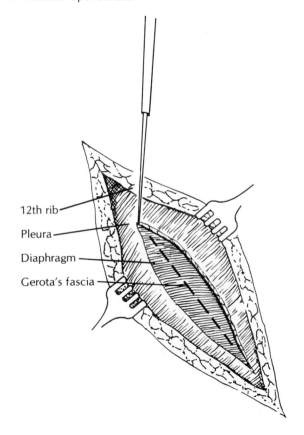

12th rib

Pleura

Diaphragm

Gerota's fascia

than carcinomas (mean weight 46 g *vs* 416 g) and are best approached by a unilateral flank incision with an extraperitoneal exposure of the adrenal gland. The adrenal adenomas with Cushing's syndrome were well encapsulated and ranged in size from 2.2 cm by 2 cm by 1.5 cm to 7 cm by 6.5 cm by 5 cm. The weight varied from 12.5 g to 126 g. Adrenocortical carcinomas tended to range from 3 cm or 4 cm to very large tumors invading adjacent structures. The weights of the carcinomas ranged from 39 g to 1800 g. The supra-11th rib or supracostal approach of Turner-Warwick has provided excellent exposure of the adrenal glands.[23] The standard flank incision (subcostal) may be too low and may require excessive mobilization and trauma to the kidney.

The major disadvantage of unilateral exposure is the inability to evaluate the status of the contralateral adrenal, thus the problem of whether to perform a total or subtotal adrenalectomy, or even, at times, surgical nonresection. The use of CT scans and selective adrenal-vein sampling reduces this problem to a minimum. Also, the ability to autotransplant adrenal tissue further decreases the risk of rendering the patient addisonian.[10]

SUPRACOSTAL FLANK APPROACH

For the supracostal flank approach, the patient is placed in the lateral position with the lumbar spine across the table break (Fig. 2-14). The leg is flexed at the hip and the knee is bent to 90 degrees with the upper leg straight. This lateral flexion opens the costo-iliac space to permit maximum exposure. In this position an incision can be made for a subcostal, transcostal, supracostal, or even thoracoabdominal approach (Fig. 2-15).

In the supracostal approach the skin incision extends over the 11th rib from just medial to the lateral edge of the paraspinal muscles to a short distance beyond the tip of the ribs. The intercostal muscle is detached from the upper edge of the rib. A finger is then inserted gently behind the rib but external to the insertions of the diaphragm. The release is then carried posteriorly so that the posterior supracostal ligament can be divided to allow mobilization of the rib inferiorly (Fig. 2-16). Release of the intercostal nerve and division of the extrapleural fascia expose the diaphragm readily. The diaphragm is now divided in the direction of the rib starting with the most anterior fibers (Fig. 2-17). This allows gentle retraction of the pleura cephalad and prevents entry into the pleural space.[22] Gerota's capsule is then entered, usually with

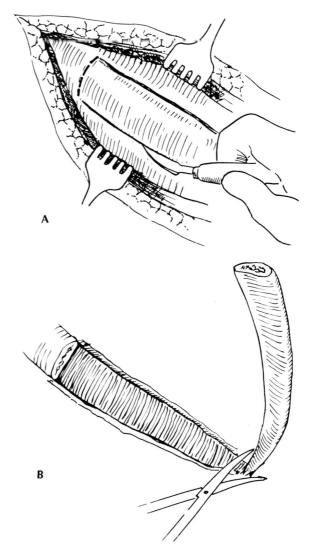

FIG. 2-11. Subperiosteal resection of 11th rib is done bilaterally. **(A)** Periosteum is stripped from the rib. **(B)** Rib is removed from the bed.

excellent exposure of the adrenal gland and the upper pole of the kidney. Even relatively large adrenal tumors may be removed through this incision.

When the kidney is drawn down in the operative field, the adrenal gland also is displaced downward into the vein. Although the adrenal is poorly encapsulated, its golden-yellow color and the consistency distinguish the gland from the pale, glistening perinephric fat. Tumors are usually readily palpable.

Hypercortisolism may produce severe catabolism and changes in all of the tissues commensurate

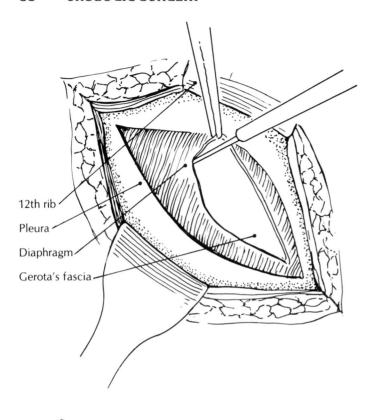

FIG. 2-12. Pleura is opened, diaphragm and Gerota's fascia are divided.

12th rib

Pleura

Diaphragm

Gerota's fascia

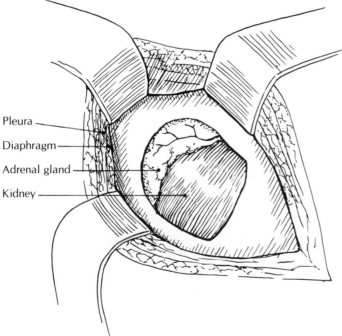

FIG. 2-13. Downward displacement of kidney facilitates exposure and dissection of adrenal gland.

Pleura

Diaphragm

Adrenal gland

Kidney

TABLE 2-8.   Nonfatal Complications of Bilateral Posterior Adrenalectomy

Complication	Frequency (%)
Wound infection (staphylococcal)	21
Laceration of vena cava	3
Pulmonary embolus	3
Renal failure	3
Pulmonary infusion	3
Acute cholecystitis	3
Total complications	39
No complications	57

with the level of 17-OHCS and the duration of the overproduction. The tissues exhibit a drab color, with poor strength and marked friability. Poor healing postoperatively is another manifestation of this deterioration.

The adrenal gland is then mobilized, and a myriad of unnamed small vessels are encountered. These are controlled by hemostatic clips. Caution, patience, and gentle dissection are required. At this stage, speed is no attribute. The entire adrenal gland with its pathology must be exposed before deciding whether total removal is necessary. The rich blood supply allows mobilization of the lateral, superior, inferior, anterior, and posterior surfaces without infarction. The hilar vessels should be preserved until last. Once the decision to remove the adrenal is made, the large hilar vessels must be dissected and clamped doubly, divided, and ligated with silk.

On the left side the dissection is somewhat easier, and the venous drainage is more readily controlled. However, on the right side the gland embraces the vena cava and curves around it posteriorly. The main venous drainage may be single or multiple but is always short and substantial. Great care is needed to control and ligate these veins adequately. The adrenal gland may then be removed.

The fossa should then be inspected for bleeding and controlled. Laceration of the upper pole of the kidney or, on the right side, of the liver may occur. Inspection will disclose these and allow proper repair and hemostasis.

The wound is closed in layers with interrupted silk or catgut sutures. Subcutaneous tissues are approximated with interrupted plain catgut. The skin is closed according to the surgeon's preference.

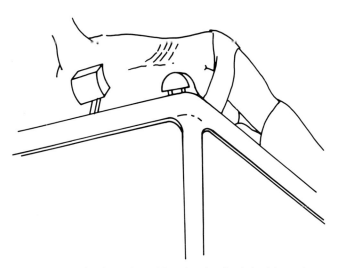

FIG. 2-14. The lateral position for the flank incision; the lower leg is flexed 90 degrees at the hip and knee, and the upper leg is kept straight.

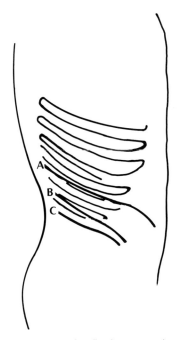

FIG. 2-15. Incisions in the flank approach: **(A)** supracostal, **(B)** transcostal, and **(C)** subcostal

THORACOABDOMINAL APPROACH

The anterior abdominal approach, whether through a midline incision or an upper abdominal, bilateral subcostal incision, is helpful in the resection of adrenal tumors, particularly with those extra-adrenal components; thus it is used with pheochromocytoma or neuroblastoma. However, in obese cushingoid patients with a large tumor, the thor-

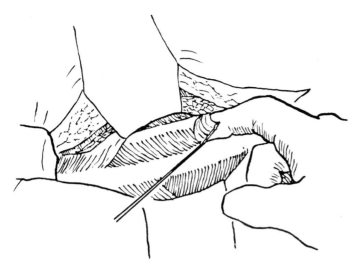

FIG. 2-16. Mobilization of the rib in the supracostal approach. The intercostal muscle is divided, with the finger behind to protect deep structures.

FIG. 2-17. Extrapleural fascia dissects away from the posterior surface of the rib with exposure of the insertion of the diaphragm and the pleura.

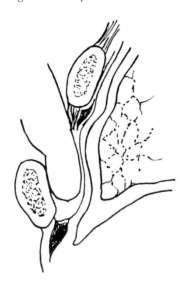

acoabdominal approach is preferred (Fig. 2-18). This incision allows adequate resection of extra-adrenal extension in adrenal carcinoma and major *en bloc* resection. In one case of adrenocortical carcinoma, the left adrenal, left kidney, retroperitoneal lymph nodes, tail of the pancreas, a portion of the greater curvature of the stomach, part of the left diaphragm, and the left lower lobe of the lung were removed through this incision.

The patient is supine on the table but is tilted with sandbags to a 45 degree angle into a modified lateral position, with the side to be operated being superior. Hyperextension of the table aids in the exposure.

One incision is made in the 9th- to 10th-rib interspace starting in the posterior axillary line and extending forward across the costochondral junction to the anterior abdominal wall. The abdominal component may extend directly across the abdomen, cutting one or both recti, or it may go to the midline of the abdomen and thence inferiorly along the midline.

The musculature of the ribcage and abdominal wall is divided in the direction of the incision and hemostasis is obtained (Fig. 2-19). This allows entry into the pleural space with exposure of the lung. The diaphragm is then opened in the direction of the chest-wall incision. The diaphragm's vascularity requires the ligation of numerous vessels with silk. Closing of these vessels allows entry with ease into the superior retroperitoneal space, as well as into the abdominal cavity anteriorly. Mobilization of the hepatic or splenic flexure of the colon allows wider exposure. On the right side, incision of the attachments of the liver laterally and superiorly allows mobilization of the liver and gives wider exposure (Fig. 2-20). Dissection of the adrenal mass is accomplished as described previously.

This incision provides both the opportunity to examine other abdominal organs and, more importantly, the ability to determine the size and shape of the contralateral adrenal gland. Resection of the adrenal tumor and any extra-adrenal extension can then be performed (Fig. 2-21).

Closure of the wound requires close adherence to detail. The diaphragm is closed in two layers with silk. A large-bore chest tube is placed through a stab wound in the interspace immediately above the incision and is positioned properly. The chest tube is then connected to closed-suction catheter

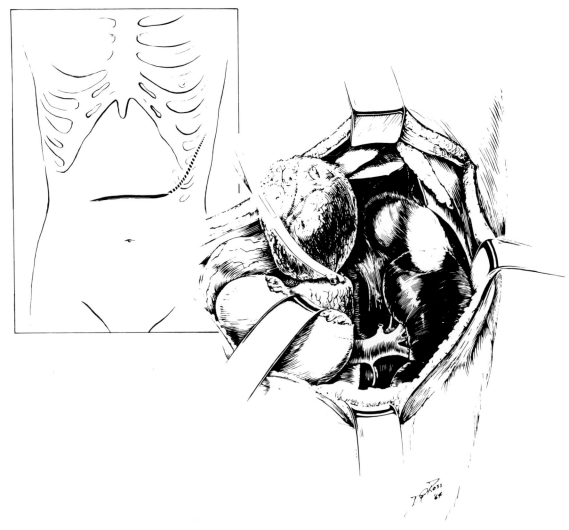

FIG. 2-18. Thoracoabdominal approach to the left adrenal with extension of the incision transversely across the midline, providing wide exposure of the retroperitoneal structures

FIG. 2-19. Division of the chest-wall muscles in the 9th- to 10th-rib interspace exposing the pleura. The incision extends through the costochondral junction.

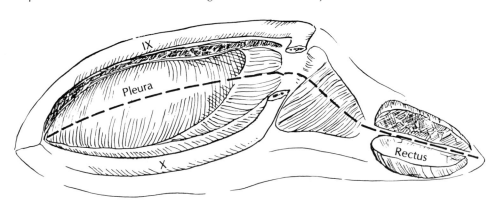

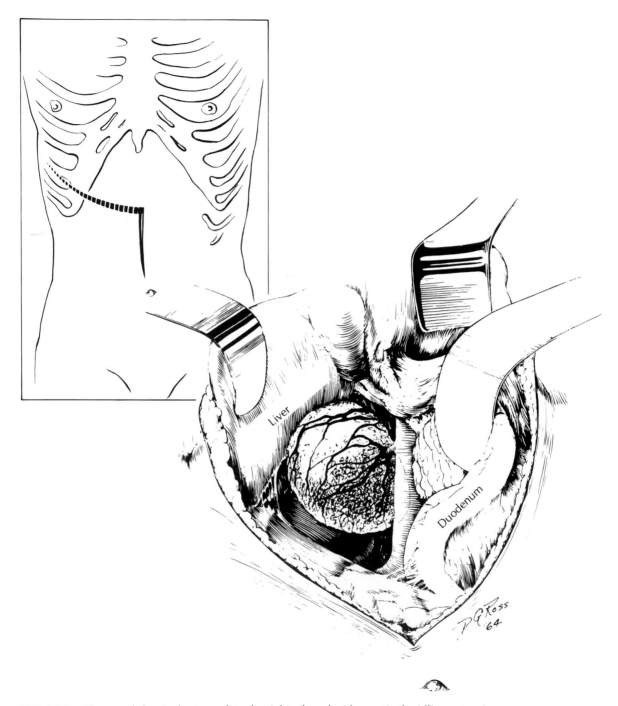

FIG. 2-20.   Thoracoabdominal approach to the right adrenal with a vertical midline extension of the incision, providing better mobilization of the liver

drainage for at least 24 hours. The pleura is then closed with fine silk or chromic catgut, with the lung expanded under positive pressure. The remainder of the incision is closed in the routine fashion.

Pre- and Postoperative Care

Many patients with severe Cushing's syndrome require extensive management prior to actual surgery. This may involve blockage of cortisol production by various medications and may require a significant period of time to accomplish (Table 2-5). In the absence of carcinoma this may be time well spent because significant reduction in morbidity will result.

In patients with adrenol cortical tumor, the opposite adrenal gland has undergone atrophy and initially is unable to handle significant levels of function. Thus, steroid substitution must begin prior to surgery. Table 2-9 shows the relative potency of these agents.[17]

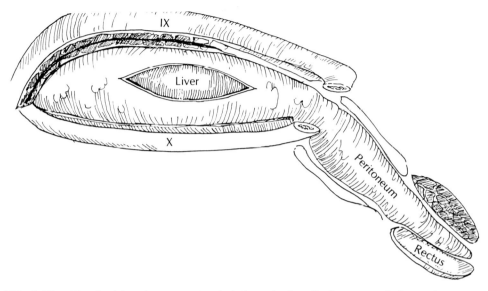

FIG. 2-21. The incision is now extended through the diaphragm and the peritoneum, exposing the intra-abdominal and the retroperitoneal structures.

TABLE 2-9. **Comparison of Orally Administered Adrenal Corticosteroids**

	Relative Anti-Inflamatory Potency	Equivalent Dose (mg.)	Sodium Retention	Brand
Hydrocortisone (same as cortisol)	1	20	2+	Cortef
Cortisone	0.8	25	2+	Hydro-cortone (Cortisone acetate)
Prednisone	3.5	5	1+	Deltasone Meticorten
Prednisolone	4	5	1+	Delta-Cortef
Methylprednisolone	5	4	0	Medrol
Triamcinolone	5	4	0	Aristocort Kenalog
Paramethasone	10	2	0	Haldrone Stemex
Betamethasone	25	0.6	0	Celestone
Dexamethasone	30	0.75	0	Decadron Hexadrol Decameth

TABLE 2-10.   Steroid Compounds Administered in Adrenocortical Surgery

	Cortisone acetate (intramuscular— in mg)	Hydrocortisone (intravenous)	Cortisone acetate (oral—in mg)	9α-Fluorohy-drocortisone (oral—in mg)
Preoperative day	100 b.i.d.			
Operative day	100 b.i.d.	50 mg in each 1000 ml IV fluids (total of 150–200 mg during 24 hr)		
Postoperative day 1	100 b.i.d.	25 mg in each 1000 ml IV fluids (total of 75 mg during 24 hr)		
Postoperative day 2	50 q 8 hr			
Postoperative day 3 (if oral intake is resumed)	25 q 8 hr		25 t.i.d.	
Postoperative day 4			25 t.i.d.	0.1 q.o.d.
Postoperative day 5			25 b.i.d.	0.1 q.o.d.
Maintenance			25–50 daily in divided doses	0–0.1 q.o.d.

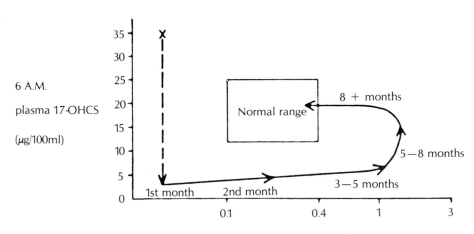

FIG. 2-22. Return of function of the contralateral adrenal gland following unilateral adrenalectomy for tumor

6 A.M. plasma 17-OHCS (μg/100ml)

6 A.M. plasma ACTH (mU/100ml.)

Immediately after the operation, adequate replacement therapy is essential. Insufficient treatment can be disastrous. A schedule of therapy is outlined in Table 2-10.

During the first few days the steroid dose is reduced to maintained levels. In the first month after supportive steroids are removed, plasma ACTH and urinary 17-OHCS are reduced. Response of the residual adrenal gland to ACTH is also subnormal (Fig. 2-22). During the second to the fifth months, plasma ACTH gradually rises and may even reach higher-than-normal levels. However, adrenal responsiveness lags and urinary 17-OCHS remains low (Fig. 2-23). By about the ninth month, responses of the pituitary and adrenal glands become normal.[13]

OUTCOME

Therapy of Cushing's disease/syndrome depends upon the fundamental etiology. Table 2-11 displays the usual causes of Cushing's syndrome and the medical and surgical treatment modalities that are available. The first, second, and third choices of therapy are indicated.

The surgical cure of adrenal adenomas is 100%. The operation mortality in adenoma is very low. With resection, the steroid levels promptly fall to normal, with return of elevated 17-OHCS.

The surgical results of adrenal carcinoma have been dismal. Twenty percent of those patients with adrenal carcinoma as the etiology of their Cushing's syndrome already had metastatic disease at the

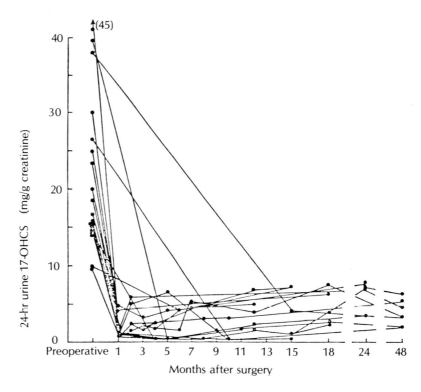

FIG. 2-23. Urinary levels of 17-OHCS in patients following removal of an adrenocortical tumor

TABLE 2-11. **Choice of Treatment in Cushing's Syndrome**

	Adrenal Tumor	Ectopic ACTH	Pituitary Cushing's disease
Unilateral adrenalectomy	1		
Remove ectopic ACTH tumor		1	
Pituitary irradiation			1 (children)
Metopirone (metyrapone)	3	2	
Bilateral adrenalectomy		2	2
Microresection pituitary adenoma			1 (adults)
o,p'DDD	2	3	3

time of diagnosis. The cure rate from surgical removal of the adrenal carcinoma is only 14%. Radiation offers little benefit. Medical therapy such as O,p'DDD offers temporary objective improvement. Occasionally patients with nonresected carcinoma enjoy long survival, but most patients die of recurrent or metastatic carcinoma within 7 years, many within 1 or 2 years.

REFERENCES

1. ADDISON T: On the constitutional and local effects of disease of the suprarenal capsules. Samaul Highly, 32 Fleet Street, London, 1855. Reprinted in facsimile by Dawson's, 16 Pall Mall, London, 1968

2. BROWN RD, VANHOON GR, ORTH DN, LIDDLE GW: Cushing's disease with periodic hormonogenesis: One exploration for paradoxical response to dexamethasone. J Clin Endocrinol Metab 36:445, 1973

3. CUSHING H: The basophil adenomas of the pituitary body and their clinical manifestations. Bull Johns Hopkins Hosp 50:137, 1932

4. EDIS AJ, AYALA LA, EGDAHL RH: Manual of Endocrine Surgery. New York, Springer-Verlag, 1975

5. EUSTACHI B: De glandulis quae rimbus incumbrent, opuscula anatomica. Printed by Vinceutius Huchinus, Venice, 1563

6. GLENN JF: Adrenal surgery. In Glenn JF (ed): Urologic Surgery, 2nd ed. Harper & Row, 1975

7. GOLD EM: Cushing's syndrome: A tripartite entity. Hosp Pract 14:67, 1979

8. GOLD EM: The Cushing syndromes: Changing views of diagnosis and treatment. Ann Intern Med 90:829, 1979

9. GREEN JRB, VAN'T HOFF W: Cushing's syndrome with fluctuation due to adrenal adenoma. J Clin Endocrinol Metab 41:235, 1975

10. HARDY JD: Surgical management of Cushing's syndrome with emphasis on adrenal autotransplantation. Ann Surg 186:290, 1978

11. JEFFCOATE WJ, EDWARDS CRW: Cushing's syndrome: Pathogenesis, diagnosis and treatment in comprehensive endocrinology. In James VHT (ed): The Adrenal Gland, pp 165–195. New York, Raven Press, 1979

12. KENDALL JW: Feedback control of adrenocorticotropic hormone secretions, pp 177–207. In Frontiers of Neuroendocrinology: New York, Oxford University Press, 1971

13. LIDDLE GW: Cushing's syndrome. In Eisenstein AB (ed): The Adrenal Cortex, pp 523–551. Boston, Little, Brown & Co, 1967

14. LINDE R, COULAM C, BATTINO R et al: Localization of aldosterone-producing adenomas by computed tomography. J Clin Endocrinol Metab 49:642, 1979

15. NEVILLE AM, MACKAY AM: The structure of the human adrenal cortex in health and disease. Clin Endocrinol Metab 1:361, 1972

16. O'NEAL LW: Cushing's Syndrome in Surgery of the Adrenal Glands, p 58. St. Louis, CV Mosby, 1968

17. PAULSON DF: Medical management of adrenal cortical disease. Symposium on adrenal diseases. Urol Clin North Am 4:297, 1977

18. PLOTZ CM, KNOWLTON AI, RAGAN C: The natural history of Cushing's syndrome. Am J Med 13:597, 1952

19. ROSS EJ, MARSHALL–JONES P, FREEDMAN M: Cushing's syndrome: Diagnostic criteria. Q J Med 35:149, 1966

20. SCOTT HW, FOSTER JH, RHAMY RK et al: Surgical management of adrenocortical tumors with Cushing's syndrome. Ann Surg 173:892, 1971

21. SCOTT HW, LIDDLE GW, MULHERIN JL et al: Surgical experience with Cushing's disease. Ann Surg 185:524, 1977

22. TURNER WARWICK RT: The supracostal approach to the renal area. Br J Urol 37:671, 1965

23. YOUNG HH: A technique for simultaneous exposure and operation on the adrenals. Surg Gynecol Obstet 54:179, 1936

Pheochromocytoma

3

Ruben F. Gittes

The diagnosis of pheochromocytoma is usually accomplished in an orderly sequence, and the preoperative studies permit the urologic surgeon the privilege of preparing both the patient and the surgical team for what is always a dramatic and usually a most gratifying surgical effort.

In two circumstances the urologist may be the first to encounter this unusual lesion in a patient. The first circumstance is that associated with pheochromocytoma of the bladder, which frequently presents as a bladder tumor identified on biopsy. The second circumstance is that of the exploration of a suprarenal tumor that had not been noted to be functional but that awakens with a vengeance during the surgical manipulation. Even in this case, the first diagnosis usually is made by the anesthetist taking the patient's blood pressure.

This chapter reviews and updates the current practice of the surgery of pheochromocytoma. It is clear that every urologist must be familiar with the condition, in the event of an unexpected encounter. However, most cases are referred to medical centers experienced in its management, where an experienced urologist is often the responsible surgeon.

Preoperative Localization

The diagnosis of the presence of a pheochromocytoma is clinical and biochemical.[17] Given a well-documented diagnosis, preoperative localization becomes a primary concern. Surgeons should direct their efforts at preoperative localization, using clinical experience to choose the optimal sequence and the minimum essential number of available sophisticated diagnostic tests.

Although 95% of the tumors are found below the diaphragm, chest x-ray films should include oblique films; these may show a chromaffin tumor in the paravertebral gutter adjacent to the thoracic spine. Suspicion about the possibility of metastasis to the lung from a malignant pheochromocytoma may first be raised by hilar adenopathy.

Computed tomography (CT) is clearly the procedure of choice now, replacing the previous sequence of intravenous pyelography followed by arteriography.[26] The CT scan is optimal for delineation of the normal and abnormal adrenal gland. Because symptomatic pheochromocytomas are usually large (90% weigh over 5 g when removed) and are usually within one or both adrenals (90% of cases), this still-improving technique settles the issue quickly in the vast majority of cases. When CT scanning shows normal adrenals, it also makes evident the cases of extra-adrenal pheochromocytoma that need further localization, as described below.

Arteriography, including bone subtraction films, is the next logical step when an extra-adrenal pheochromocytoma is suspected after the CT scan.[22] Of course, the extra-adrenal pheochromocytoma may be suspected on the scan because of its size and location in the prevertebral area along the large vessels, where it produces an image that might only be confused with an unsuspected second tumor or large lymph node. In the patient who is well prepared with α-adrenergic blockade, angiography now settles the issue by demonstrating the typical vascular tumor with a dense post-angiographic blush somewhere between the diaphragm and the sacral promontory.

In the truly rare case in which these radiologic procedures fail to demonstrate the tumor, persistent symptoms and confirmation of the diagnosis by plasma catecholamine assays lead back to the attempt to localize tumor by taking multiple venous samples with a catheter at different levels in the vena cava, taking care to collect the samples before any contrast is injected into the adrenals.[16] After multiple samples are taken from veins all the way from the neck to the pelvis, venography is performed. Some have claimed that venography is useful and might even be tried before arteriography, because 30% of pheochromocytomas are hypovascular and very difficult to locate by arteriography if they are small.[1,28]

The analysis of multiple venous samples has been greatly facilitated by the improvements in radioimmunoassay for catecholamines, providing levels of both epinephrine and norepinephrine in the plasma. It is a long-standing observation that plasma levels with a definitely elevated epinephrine fraction usually indicate an intra-adrenal pheochromocytoma. In contrast, tumors that only make norepinephrine are extra-adrenal. These findings probably result from the peculiar requirement of high corticosteroid concentrations, such as are obtained in the adrenal environment, for the induction of the enzyme that converts norepinephrine to epinephrine.[27] Exceptions are rarely noted.[8]

Pheochromocytomas may arise wherever chromaffin tissue exists, usually in the adrenal medulla or one of the sympathetic ganglia, including the celiac ganglion (Fig. 3-1). Much less commonly they may arise from chromaffin tissue in the wall of the bladder, the hilus of the liver or kidney, the chest, or even the neck. When a child is affected or whenever a residual or recurrent tumor has been demonstrated, the possibility of multiple tumors is enhanced and the use of multiple venous blood samples seems to be strongly indicated. These also can be useful in establishing the nature of possible metastases in malignant pheochromocytoma.

FIG. 3-1. Pheochromocytoma and paraganglioma may arise wherever chromaffin tissue occurs. The most common sites are indicated here.

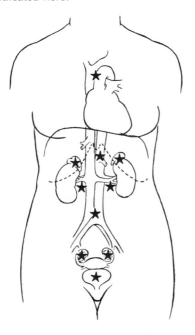

Pharmacologic Blockage

The danger and the symptoms of pheochromocytoma are due mostly to its alpha- and beta-adrenergic effects. These include hypertension, tachycardia with arrhythmias, vascular-bed constriction with decreased plasma volume, cardiomyopathy, and even urinary-bladder retention.[3] These certainly can be controlled and brought back to normal in most cases by the use of alpha blockade with or without beta blockers.

The use of alpha blockade with oral phenoxibenzamine is a relatively easy and reliable routine. Currently blockade is being used for at least a week before arteriography and surgery are contemplated. This allows normalization of the intravascular volume and total hemoglobin values. Some patients with very unstable cardiac disease, suggesting possible episodes of myocardial infarction or the presence of myocardiopathy, almost invariably have a remarkable response to the blockade, with resolution of their symptoms and reversal of abnormalities on electrocardiogram (EKG).[20]

The blockade reduces the possibility of cardiac or cerebral accidents during the preoperative evaluation period, lessens the chance of unmanageable swings in pressure or dangerous arrhythmias during surgery, and can forestall completely the syndrome of vascular collapse following the removal of the tumor. To all of these advantages there is counterposed a disadvantage: such blockade blunts the systemic response to manipulation of an unsuspected tumor during the surgical exploration. Several centers have arrived at the practice of incomplete blockade.[17] This is particularly defensible if there is uncertainty about the radiographic findings, if the procedure is a reexploration for a tumor, or if the patient is a child or a patient with familial pheochromocytoma such as Sipple's syndrome or von Recklinghausen's disease.[4] It is true that second or third pheochromocytomas of small size might be missed if there is no elevation of blood pressure or pulse during manipulation at surgery.

As a prerequisite for arteriography or surgery, our own practice is to establish sufficient blockade, both to eliminate the hypertension (if it is sustained) or the paroxysms (if they have been occurring frequently) and to indicate an increase in the vascular capacity and the blood volume by a drop of at least five points in the hematocrit. In our experience, this still leaves room for a hypertensive response to manipulation of the tumor while avoiding the risk of postoperative collapse of vascular tone. The alpha blockade may cause enough postural hypotension to require bed rest in order to achieve the other aims of a normotensive patient and an expanded blood volume. Benefit may be derived by treating the lower hematocrit preoperatively with elective transfusion.[6]

Although there are risks connected with pharmacologic blockade, it must be recognized that the absence of *any* blockade in the face of the known diagnosis of pheochromocytoma would be indefensible if the patient were to suffer from a cerebrovascular accident or fatal arrhythmia during localization studies or surgery. It is best to initiate some blockade, even if it is nominal. It should be stressed that beta blockade must never be started before the alpha blockade because it is likely to precipitate heart failure with severe cardiac complications.

Anesthesia for Pheochromocytoma

In the elective case, the anesthesiologist is an important and well-informed member of the treatment team. He is likely to order premedication with a tranquilizer and barbiturate, to avoid atropine and morphine, and to provide careful monitoring. After an initial small dose of a competitive neuromuscular blocking agent like curare to prevent fasciculations, the patient may be induced with thiopental and intubated using succinylcholine. The general anesthetic agent of choice is now enflurane (Ethrane), introduced in 1973, which has the advantage of superior muscular relaxation with minimal tendency to produce arrhythmia and with little nephrotoxicity.[14,18]

The anesthesia team is prepared to manage the hypertensive crisis, usually with a nitroprusside bolus (0.25 mg) or a drip (100 mg in 500 ml of 5 dextrose/water—D/W). This nonspecific and most effective relaxant of the vascular tree largely has replaced the intraoperative use of the specific short-acting alpha blockers like phentolamine. Arrhythmias that are apt to appear when sudden increases in blood pressure occur are managed by the intravenous bolus of lidocaine (50–100 mg) or propranolol (0.1–0.5 mg).[25]

The response of hypotension intraoperatively or in the recovery room after removal of a pheochromocytoma is best managed by volume replacement and norepinephrine. Prevention by vascular volume supplementation and preoperative α-adrenergic blockade had made such hypotension rare. Transfusion during surgery should be aggressive. It is an important precaution to have available a solution of norepinephrine (Levophed) in 5% dextrose for any hypotension that does not respond to volume replacement. These patients are particularly resistant to lesser pressor agents. Preoperative blood transfusion is particularly necessary when the alpha blockade is less than maximal as intentionally practiced in some centers.[6]

Choice of Incision

In spite of the advances in tumor localization, there is still a need for intraoperative palpation and exposure of both adrenals, the celiac ganglion and the paravertebral sympathetic ganglia, the organs of Zuckerkandl, and the pelvic brim. Either a "chevron" incision or a vertical midline incision is adequate in the presence of a small (<3 cm) adrenal adenoma or a demonstrated retroperitoneal tumor next to the major vessels (Fig. 3-2).

When the demonstrated tumor in one adrenal is large (>5 cm), a modified thoracoabdominal incision is helpful in providing the best exposure of the tumor from every direction (Fig. 3-3). This is important because retraction of the tumor itself is minimized. This procedure avoids both undue squeezing of catecholamines into the circulation with consequent hypertensive crises and arrhythmias and breakage and spillage of the friable tumor, which can leave local implants that could cause a later recurrence.[23,24] Such iatrogenic autotransplants may be incorrectly interpreted as evidence that the original tumor was in fact a malignant pheochromocytoma, and they can be very difficult to eradicate the next time.

It is imperative that wide exposure be ensured by the initial incision. This is no place for cosmetic considerations or posterior muscle-sparing incisions.

Intraoperative Maneuvers

Although a case can be made for proceeding first with the resection of the tumor to accomplish the primary purpose of the operation and to eliminate the main reservoir of dangerous catecholamines, we recommend assuming that there is a second tumor to be found prior to manipulation or exploration in the area of the known tumor. Careful transabdominal palpation of the opposite adrenal gland, the celiac ganglion, the sympathetic chains, and the preaortic tissue that makes up the organs of Zuckerkandl is best done first, because the patient may still respond with a rise in blood pressure that might be blocked later by nitroprusside bolus or drip required in dissection of the main tumor. The surgeon's patience and concentration in the search are also better before than after an extended resection of the known tumor.

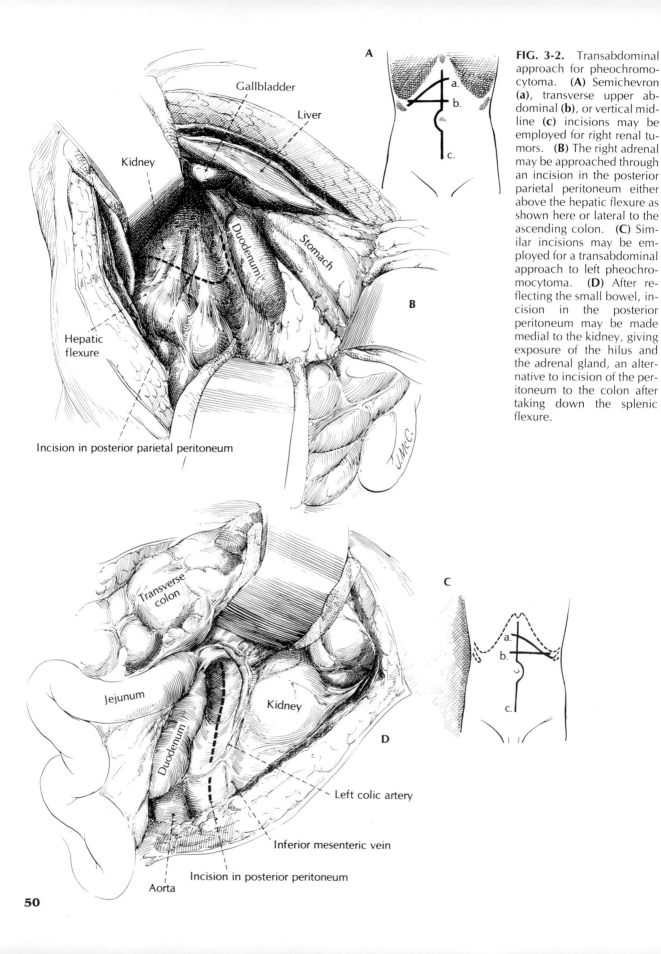

A

a.
b.
c.

Gallbladder

Liver

Kidney

Duodenum

Stomach

Hepatic
flexure

B

Incision in posterior parietal peritoneum

Transverse
colon

C

a.
b.
c.

Jejunum

Kidney

Duodenum

D

Left colic artery

Inferior mesenteric vein

Incision in posterior peritoneum

Aorta

FIG. 3-2. Transabdominal approach for pheochromocytoma. **(A)** Semichevron **(a)**, transverse upper abdominal **(b)**, or vertical midline **(c)** incisions may be employed for right renal tumors. **(B)** The right adrenal may be approached through an incision in the posterior parietal peritoneum either above the hepatic flexure as shown here or lateral to the ascending colon. **(C)** Similar incisions may be employed for a transabdominal approach to left pheochromocytoma. **(D)** After reflecting the small bowel, incision in the posterior peritoneum may be made medial to the kidney, giving exposure of the hilus and the adrenal gland, an alternative to incision of the peritoneum to the colon after taking down the splenic flexure.

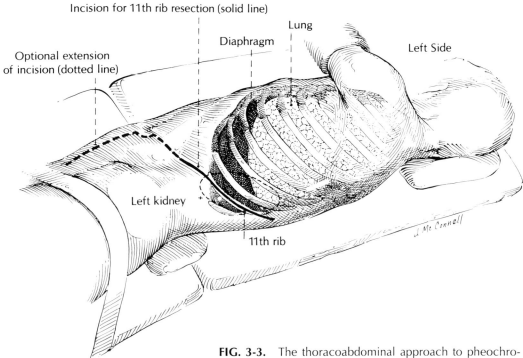

FIG. 3-3. The thoracoabdominal approach to pheochromocytoma is useful, particularly with large tumors or with suspected multiplicity or malignancy.

After the required exploration, the surgeon should "circle his quarry," anticipating exposure problems and ensuring alternate routes of dissection. The following are helpful maneuvers in specific locations:

1. For a right adrenal lesion, take down the hepatic flexure of the colon and divide the posterior peritoneum over the vena cava and to the right along the edge of the liver. Then, bluntly dissect the front of the cava from the liver for about 3 cm to 5 cm, double-tying and dividing the two to four lower hepatic veins. This maneuver yields a wide approach to the adrenal vein, allows the cava to be lifted away from the often retrocaval part of the adrenal, and avoids ill-timed tearing of the bridging hepatic veins by retraction of the liver.

2. If the right adrenal tumor is large or unusually cephalad, do not depend on exposure and dissection from below with upward retraction of the liver but add an initial dissection to free the liver laterally and superiorly from the diaphragm. With a thoracoabdominal incision, sharp division of the triangular and coronary ligaments and occasionally even of the medial ligamentum teres permits rotation of the liver to the left to give ample exposure of the entire subdiaphragmatic suprarenal area and control of the entire "intrahepatic" vena cava with direct access to the multiple short veins connecting the tumor and the cava.

3. For the left adrenal tumor, take down the splenic flexure of the colon and sharply divide the posterior peritoneum just below the spleen to avoid traction injury to its capsule.

4. For a large left adrenal tumor, add a careful division of the left omentum above the transverse colon to free up the stomach and expose the adrenal mass through the lesser sac. The inferior mesenteric vein crosses the field to join the splenic vein and is best divided to permit easier retraction of the tail of the pancreas and spleen.

5. For any apparent fixation of an adrenal pheochromocytoma to the upper pole of the kidney, start dissecting low on the kidney, include the perirenal fat, and creep upward along the renal capsule to expose the tip of the kidney. If it is still adherent, consider removing the kidney or its upper pole with the tumor rather than trying to separate the two and risking local spillage of the tumor.

Operative Mortality and Morbidity

Team experience and patient preparation have dropped operative mortality virtually to zero. Thus, no deaths occurred after surgery for pheochromocytoma in 46 patients operated upon at the Cleveland Clinic between 1952 and 1973.[6] In a series of 138 patients at the Mayo Clinic, four died before 1965, none after that.[21] Our only death in more than 30 patients in the last decade was a child with extensive malignant pheochromocytoma invading the head of the pancreas. However, in cases in which the diagnosis was unsuspected and operation was being performed for some other reason, the operative mortality has been estimated as high as 50%.[10]

Intraoperative hypertensive crises still occur commonly, and arrhythmias must also be anticipated. These occur with anesthesia induction and (especially with tumor manipulation) even if preoperative pharmacologic blockade has been used. Hypertension is now usually controlled by a nitroprusside drip from a solution of 0.20 mg/ml in 5% dextrose after an initial intravenous (IV) bolus of 0.20 mg to 0.25 mg. This drug has an almost immediate onset and a short duration of action of about 3 min.[13] Neither tachycardia nor tachyphylaxis occurs with nitroprusside. Some groups still use intravenous phentolamine by infusion to control pressure during surgery. It can be given as a bolus of 1 mg to 5 mg or as an infusion drip with variable concentrations between 5 mg and 80 mg of phentolamine in 500 ml of 5% dextrose.[19] This drug is shorter-acting than phenoxybenzamine but still may be expected to last 10 minutes.

In arrhythmias occur during the surgery in spite of control of the hypertension, the use of lidocaine or propranolol is indicated. The lidocaine is used for ventricular arrhythmia with the IV injection of 50 mg to 100 mg. Propranolol, (Inderal), 0.1 mg to 0.5 mg/min intravenously, is preferred by some for ventricular arrhythmias.[25] Cardioversion equipment should always be available in the operating room for immediate use.

Postoperative Complications

Special attention must be paid to the onset of hypotension in the immediate postoperative period or even intraoperatively after removal of the primary tumor. Prior volume replacement, as described in the section Anesthesia for Pheochromocytoma is the principal way of avoiding this complication. The occurrence of hypotension in spite of adequate preoperative blockade is probably due to bleeding, myocardial infarction, or (rarely)

steroid adrenal insufficiency. Central venous pressure and urine output are the easiest indices to follow for adequate volume replacement. It should be remembered that the vascular tree is probably hyporesponsive to most pressors. The objective in the postoperative period should be to maintain the systolic pressure above 90 torr with a good urine output and central venous pressure, but not necessarily to return to a normal pressure.

Postoperative bleeding is a possibility in any patient, but some have suggested that the adrenergic blockade increases venous oozing.[7] The usual techniques of the following the hematocrit and central venous pressure should be applied.

Hypertension in the recovery room is most uncommon. If present, it suggests that either a residual tumor has been left behind or a renal artery has been damaged in the course of surgery. If this persists in the postoperative period, careful repeat angiography and venous sampling for catecholamines must be carried out before reexploration.

The experience of most indicates that within a 1-year follow-up period, three quarters of the patients are normotensive after removal of their pheochromocytoma but that the remainder have either sustained or paroxysmal hypertension. Only some cases are due to another pheochromocytoma or metastases from the original tumor. In many, hypertension is established on another basis and should be so treated.

Malignant Pheochromocytoma

The incidence of malignant pheochromocytoma has been estimated to vary from 2.4% in children to 13% in adults.[11,21] Histology is a very poor determinant of malignancy, and many cases present with metastases long after a "benign" primary tumor was removed uneventfully. It generally has been agreed that before the diagnosis of malignancy is made, metastases should be present at a site where pheochromocytoma tissue is not normally found, and hormonal function of the metastases should be demonstrated.[5] Vena-cava sampling has been used for many years to demonstrate the function of metastases and to encourage palliative resection.[16]

Aggressive treatment is indicated pharmacologically for excellent palliation and surgically for excision of metastases. In our own series of malignant pheochromocytomas, seven cases had prolonged survival from 7 to 21 years, and some were apparently tumor free after removal of positive nodes. Our only two deaths in this group happened when recurrence was overlooked and had become inoperable.

Phenoxybenzamine has been given by chronic oral administration to patients who have unresectable malignant disease. Its use in malignant pheochromocytoma goes back at least 30 years.[2] In chronic use, it is recommended to be given orally twice a day; mild sedation has been reported as a side-effect in adults.[9] We noticed arrest of growth as a very disturbing side-effect of long-term therapy in an 8-year-old child treated for 4 years for a large, unresectable pheochromocytoma. It is accepted that management and palliation are more effective if the functioning tumor tissue is reduced surgically as much as possible.

Pheochromocytoma of the Bladder

Pheochromocytoma of the urinary bladder was first described by Zimmerman in 1953, and over 80 cases have been reported in the world literature.[17,29] Patients' ages have ranged from 10 to 79. It is unusual and startling to note that the tumors have occurred mostly in patients between 10 and 19 years of age. Also, about 10% of these patients have been reported to have malignant pheochromocytoma.[12]

The bladder tumors were usually submucosal and often bleed; painless hematuria was present in 58% of the cases. Some 80% were visible cystoscopically. Most were histologically intermingled with the muscle fibers, not because of invasion or malignancy but owing to their origin in chromaffin paraganglia that migrated into the bladder wall. The mean size of reviewed cases was 3 cm. Tumors were evenly distributed over the surface of the bladder, both in the dome and trigone. The combination of postmicturition hypertension and gross hematuria occurred in only one half of the reported cases. Some of these tumors were quite small and were found incidentally.[15]

Treatment of such tumors consists of transurethral biopsy followed by full-thickness partial cystectomy with a 2-cm to 3-cm margin of bladder. Neither transurethral biopsy nor segmental surgery in the suspected case should be done without systemic preparation and full cardiovascular precautions.

REFERENCES

1. AGEE OF, KAUDE J, LEPASOON J: Preoperative localization of pheochromocytoma. Acta Radiol [Diagn] 14:545, 1973
2. ALLEN EV, BANNON WG, UPSON M JR et al: A new sympatholytic and adrenolytic drug. Clinical studies on pheochromocytoma and essential hypertension. Trans Assoc Am Physicians 64:109, 1951
3. BAIRD IM, COHEN H: Pheochromocytoma: A case with hypotension, paroxysmal hypertension and urinary retention. Lancet 2:270, 1954
4. CATALONA WJ, ENGLEMAN K, KETCHAM AS, HAMMOND WG: Familial medullary thyroid carcinoma, pheochromocytoma, and parathyroid adenoma (Sipple's syndrome). Cancer 28:1245, 1971
5. DAVIS P, PEART WS, VAN'T HOFF W: Malignant phaeochromocytoma with functioning metastases. Lancet 2:274, 1955
6. DEOREO GA JR, STEWART BH, TARAZI RC, GIFFORD RW: Preoperative blood transfusion in the safe surgical management of pheochromocytoma: A review of 46 cases. J Urol 111:715, 1974
7. EDIS JA, AYALA LA, EGDAHL RH: Manual of Endocrine Surgery. New York, Springer–Verlag, 1975
8. ENGELMAN K, HAMMON WG: Adrenaline production by an intrathoracic pheochromocytoma. Lancet 1:609, 1968
9. ENGELMAN K, SJOERDSMA A: Chronic medical therapy for pheochromocytoma: A report of four cases. Ann Intern Med 61:229, 1964
10. GOLDFEIN A: Pheochromocytoma: Diagnosis and anesthetic and surgical management. Anesthesiology 24:462, 1963
11. HUME DM: Pheochromocytoma in the adult and in the child. Am J Surg 99:458, 1960
12. JAVAHERI P, RAAFAT J: Malignant phaeochromocytoma of the urinary bladder. Br J Urol 47:401, 1975
13. KATZ RL, WOLFE CE: Pheochromocytoma. In Mark CL, Ngai SH (eds): Highlights in Clinical Anesthesiology, pp 55–65. New York, Harper & Row, 1971
14. KOPRIVA CJ, ELTRINGHAM R: The use of enflurane during resection of a pheochromocytoma. Anesthesiology 41:399, 1974
15. LEESTMA JE, PRICE EB JR: Paraganglioma of the urinary bladder. Cancer 28:1063, 1971
16. MAHONEY EM, CROCKER DW, FRIEND DG et al: Adrenal and extra-adrenal pheochromocytomas: Localization by vena cava sampling and observations on renal juxtaglomerular apparatus. J Urol 108:4, 1972
17. MANGER WM, FROLICH ED, GIFFORD RW, DUSTAN HP: Norepinephrine infusion in normal subjects and patients with essential or renal hypertension: Effect on blood pressure, heart rate and plasma catecholamine concentration. J Clin Pharmacol 14:129, 1976
18. ORTIZ FT, DIAZ PM: Use of enflurane for pheochromocytoma removal. Anesthesiology 42:495, 1975
19. PERTSEMLIDID D, GITLOW SE, SIEGEL WC, KORK AE: Pheochromocytoma: 1. Specificity of laboratory diagnostic tests. 2. Safeguards during operative removal. Ann Surg 196:376, 1969
20. RADTKE WE, KAZMIER FJ, RUTHERFORD BD, SHEPS SG: Cardiovascular complications of pheochromocytoma crisis. Am J Cardiol 35:701, 1975

21. REMINE WH, CHONG GC, VAN HEERDEN JA et al: Current management of pheochromocytoma. Ann Surg 179:740, 1974

22. REUTER SR, TALNER LB, ATKIN T: The importance of subtraction in the angiographic evaluation of extra-adrenal pheochromocytomas. Am J Roentgenol Radium Ther Nucl Med 117:128, 1973

23. SELLWOOD RA, WAPNICK S, BRECKENRIDGE A et al: Recurrent phaeochromocytoma. Br J Surg 57:309, 1970

24. SIVULA A: Recurrence of benign phaeochromocytoma by intraoperative implantation. Acta Chir Scand 140:334, 1974

25. SJOERDSMA A, ENGELMAN K, WALDMANN TA et al: Pheochromocytoma: Current concepts of diagnosis and treatment. Ann Intern Med 65:1302, 1966

26. STEWART BH, BRAVO EL, HAAGA J et al: Localization of pheochromocytoma by computer tomography. N Engl J Med 299:460, 1978

27. WURTMAN RJ: Control of epinephrine synthesis in the adrenal medulla by the adrenal cortex: Hormonal specificity and dose-response characteristics. Endocrinology 79:608, 1966

28. ZELCH JV, MEANEY TF, BEKGIBEK GH: Radiologic approach to the patient with suspected pheochromocytoma. Radiology 111:279, 1974

29. ZIMMERMAN IJ, BIRON RE, MCMAHON HE: Pheochromocytoma of the urinary bladder. N Engl J Med 249:25, 1953

Neuroblastoma

4

John W. Duckett

Neuroblastoma is the most common solid tumor of infancy and childhood. More than one half of these tumors occur in children under the age of 2 years, with the peak incidence at the age of 18 months.[22] Unfortunately, the tumors are frequently not detected until dissemination has occurred; two thirds of the children over 2 years of age already have metastatic disease at diagnosis.[5] Despite the fact that some therapeutic agents induce a clinical response, the survival rate for patients with neuroblastomas has remained essentially unchanged over the past 20 years.[6,11,24]

Pathology

Neuroblastomas arise from primitive neural-crest cells associated with sympathetic ganglia or from wherever neuroblasts migrate from the mantle layer of the developing spinal cord. There is probably a continual process of "maturation" whereby malignant undifferentiated neuroblastomas may develop into benign ganglioneuromas.[14] Unfortunately, such maturation is a very rare occurrence clinically and histologic evidence of differentiation has not been found a useful sign for determining therapy or prognosis.

With the development of cell culture techniques, *in vitro* morphologic differentiation of neuroblastoma cells has been induced with nerve growth factor, vitamin B_{12}, and irradiation. These accomplishments have supported the rationale for vitamin B_{12} and radiation therapy of neuroblastomas, but so far there is no clinical evidence of effectiveness.[12] Attempts to estimate nerve growth factor levels in human sera and their correlation to histology and prognosis have been unsuccessful.

Neuroblastomas are diffusely cellular and consist of small cells predominantly composed of nuclear material with a minimal cystoplasm. The characteristic aggregation of the cells around central clear areas, which are unstained neurofibrils, produces the rosette or pseudorosette formation characteristic of neuroblastoma.

Grossly, the neuroblastoma is a purplish mass often confined by a pseudocapsule with areas of necrosis, making it feel cystic. The larger growths envelop and ensheathe surrounding structures. The tumor is extremely vascular, and a simple biopsy may produce significant bleeding. The firmer, more compact, and whiter in color the tumor is, the more likelihood there is of differentiation to ganglioneuroblastoma.

Neuroblastoma *in situ* have been found at autopsy in the adrenal gland in stillborn infants and infants dying under the age of 3 months.[27] This suggests that only a small portion of such lesions eventually develop into clinical neuroblastomas. There is a slight tendency for heredofamilial occurrence.[14] Neuroblastomas have been reported in four sets of twins.

Site of Origin

The majority (70%–75%) of neuroblastomas arise in the abdomen, and one half of these are adrenal in origin.[21] The next most common site of origin is the thorax (15%). Other sites include the pelvis (4%), the neck (4%), and unknown (2%). The adrenal site of origin carries a poorer prognosis than the periaortic ganglia, although pinpointing the origin in the abdomen is quite difficult at times. Patients with thoracic and pelvic neuroblastomas have a better prognosis than those with tumors within the abdomen. Their overall survival rate is 37%, whereas those with thoracic neuroblastomas have a 68% survival rate. However, most thoracic lesions are Stage 1. The survival of 36% for abdominal neuroblastoma reflects the fact that they are generally of higher stages.

The staging system proposed by Evans and coworkers in 1971 is generally accepted today.[7,8]

Stage 1–Tumor limited to organ of origin

Stage 2–Regional spread that does not cross the midline

Stage 3–Tumors extending across the midline

Stage 4–Distant metastases

Stage 4-S–Small primary metastases, limited to liver, skin, or bone marrow without radiographic evidence of bone metastasis.

Prognosis

Age has the most important influence on survival, with infants faring much better than older children. Our survival rate for children under 1 year of age is 67%; between 1 and 2 years of age, 26%; and over 2 years of age, 20%. These figures are affected considerably by the fact that Stage 4-S disease, which has a more favorable outcome than the other stages, is found primarily in infants.[25]

Besides age, other factors affecting prognosis are the stage or extent of disease, the pattern of metastatic spread, the primary site, the histology of the tumor in reference to differentiation, the absolute number of circulating lymphocytes, the percentage of bone marrow lymphoblasts, and the immune competence of the patient at diagnosis and during therapy.

The prognosis for ganglioneuroblastoma, which is closely related to neuroblastoma, is much better. Ganglioneuroblastoma may appear in the child, adolescent, or young adult, and has both malignant neuroblastoma elements and benign ganglioneuromas.[1]

Clinical Manifestations

MASS

The presence of an abdominal mass prompts the patient's presentation in about 75% of cases; either the mother notes the mass or the pediatrician finds it during a routine physical examination. The mass is usually fixed and nodular and often extends across the midline. In one third of the cases, it occupies more than one quadrant of the abdomen. Nearly one half of the masses are located on the left; one quarter are situated on the right; and widespread disease without a dominant large mass is noted in the remaining quarter. Sometimes sudden enlargement of the mass due to hemorrhage brings the tumor to the attention of the physician or parent.[28]

OTHER SYMPTOMS

Pain in the abdomen or bones is noted in about one half of the patients. Abdominal distention is present in about 25%. Disturbed gastrointestinal function, with nausea, vomiting, diarrhea, or constipation, is frequently present. The symptom complex may mimic arthritis, rheumatic fever, or poliomyelitis.

More than one quarter of the patients exhibit weight loss or failure to thrive. Fever in excess of 102° F (38.8° C) is found in about 10% of patients. Urinary tract symptoms are uncommon, as is hypertension.

METASTASIS

Metastasis occurs in retroperitoneal structures by direct extension. Distally it occurs first in the regional lymph nodes, liver, and bones; the lungs, subcutaneous tissue, and brain are affected later. Bone marrow biopsy reveals nonhemapoietic syncytial elements indicative of neuroblastoma.[10] When the metastatic lesion in bone has developed sufficiently to be demonstrable on x-ray films, it is well established and nearly always indicates a fatal outcome. The potential sites for bony metastases are the skull, femur, humerus, vertebrae, pelvis, ribs, and tibia. Skeletal metastases in neuroblastomas are often bilaterally symmetrical.

This invasive neoplasm may extend in a dumbbell fashion, with extradural and perivertebral lobules that may cause compression of the spinal cord and paralysis. Intrathecal spread and meningeal metastases are reported. Metastases not infrequently occur in the retro-orbit, causing proptosis, edema, and hemorrhage, and these symptoms may be the presenting signs of neuroblastoma.

Diagnosis

RADIOGRAPHIC STUDIES

Calcification is quite characteristic in neuroblastoma. Located centrally and finely stippled, it is five times more common in neuroblastoma than in Wilms' tumor. Central-type calcification occurs in about 50% of the cases, and a plaquelike or linear calcification is seen near the periphery in about 10% of the cases.

Usually the kidney outline is maintained, with any caliceal deformity created by extrinsic pressure, rather than intrinsic pressure as is found with Wilms' tumor. The kidney is usually displaced downward and outward as a "drooping lily" (Fig. 4-1), but neuroblastoma may displace the kidney in any direction. Lateral films are helpful in showing anterior displacement of the kidney, especially in relation to the calcific areas of the tumor. Neu-

FIG. 4-1. Intravenous pyelogram in a 4-year-old child with a right suprarenal neuroblastoma with a typical "drooping lily" sign

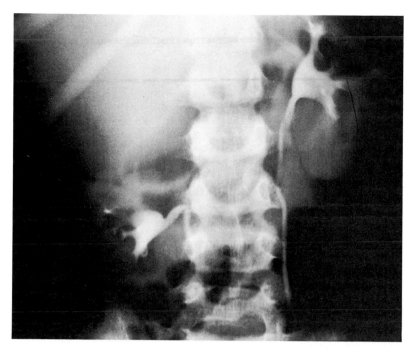

roblastomas rarely produce any considerable degree of hydronephrosis.[13]

Chest and skeletal surveys are mandatory. Special scrutiny for bony metastases is directed to the medial aspect of the distal metaphysis of the femur and a similar position of the proximal metaphysis of the humerus. The epiphysis is not involved.

Bone marrow aspiration of the ilium discloses neuroblast cells in a large percentage of cases.[10]

LABORATORY STUDIES

Anemia signals a poor prognosis. Hematuria is rare, occurring in only 5% of cases of abdominal neuroblastoma. Neuroblastoma cells of the sympathetic nerve tissue of the adrenal medulla produce excessive quantities of norepinephrine, dopa, and dopamine, which are tyrosine derivatives of amino acids. Vanillylmandelic acid (VMA), homovanillic acid (HVMA), and 3-methoxyl-4-hydroxyphenoglycol (MGPH) are the chemical derivatives detected in the urine in 80% to 90% of the cases.[23] These markers are useful in assessing the response to therapy, the recurrence of disease, and the need for a second look. Serum ferritin may prove to be a helpful guide to therapy.[15] It may even be that primary epidural neuroblastomas and those originating in dorsal ganglia do not secrete catecholamines.

Computed tomography, sonography, and selective arteriography are useful diagnostic tools in selected cases.

Treatment

SURGICAL MANAGEMENT

The goal of therapy is extirpation of the tumor, but there are many instances in which a neuroblastoma is wrapped around vital structures such as the celiac axis, making extirpation impossible. There seems to be little doubt that partial resection of the neuroblastoma when total extirpation is impossible is beneficial. Koop's early experience as Children's Hospital of Philadelphia, has led us to believe that cures were often associated with major surgical insults to the tumor without extirpation.[5,19,20,21,22] Perhaps partial excision contributed in some immunologic way to the patient's benefit; however, this has not been proven, nor has it been possible to show that metastases grow less rapidly after removal of the primary tumor.

It has not been our practice at Children's Hospital to do *en bloc* resections of other organs if they are contiguous with the tumor in an effort to remove the last cancer cell. Experience has indicated that such procedures do not improve survival. We have, however, been more aggressive in

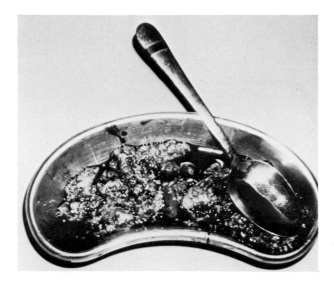

FIG. 4-2. Neuroblastoma tissue "spooned out" from a small capsulotomy in a Stage 3 tumor

dealing with the primary tumor if metastases were not demonstrated in bone.

Because neuroblastoma is a pseudoencapsulated tumor, it is possible at times to open the pseudocapsule to a limited extent and to "spoon out" the gelatinous contents within.[19] At no time should this endeavor be undertaken if the surgeon is not in a position to secure hemostasis, because bleeding may be brisk.

The technique for spooning out (Fig. 4-2) should be carefully controlled. A small incision is made through the pseudocapsule and carried down into the tumor through the relatively solid cortex and into the inner necrotic mass. If, at this point, bleeding becomes excessive, the pseudocapsule and the cortex may be sutured together to confine the hemorrhage. A long sweeping incision through the pseudocapsule could cause the patient to exsanguinate before controlling the bleeding.

Sometimes patients with neuroblastomas classified as Stage 4-S have a rapid expansion of the liver with metastases so that respiration is compromised. Schnaufer and Koop have had success in creating an artificial hernia for the abdominal contents by sewing a piece of Dacron faced with Silastic to the edges of the abdominal incision, similar to what is done for omphalocele.[26] This can be done without opening the peritoneum. Radiation may then be given both before and after the procedure, but we avoid using chemotherapy under these circumstances because of the danger of wound infection and sepsis.

There seems to be merit in reexploring the site of previous partial resection or biopsy if there is evidence that the tumor mass has decreased in size following irradiation or chemotherapy.[22]

RADIATION THERAPY

Postoperative irradiation has not been used routinely in the management of neuroblastoma at Children's Hospital of Philadelphia,[3] although many authors have relied heavily in its use in the management of their patients. Currently, we do not use irradiation for children under 1 year of age or for patients with Stage 1 or 2 disease. We use irradiation primarily to reduce the size of the large primary tumor in Stage 3 or 4 and to relieve pain from metastases. A comparison of the Children's Hospital experience with that of other published series strengthens the concept that irradiation does not improve survival in Stages 1 and 2 when the surgical management has been the same. Our experience with Stage 3, however, indicates that radiation therapy after operation increases the survival rate somewhat.[7]

CHEMOTHERAPY

Although we have tried many chemotherapeutic agents, we have not been able to prolong median survival time with chemotherapy. Our current use of chemotherapy involves participation in cooperative group studies according to study protocols.

Preliminary reports suggest that cyclophosphamide is of little benefit in decreasing the metastatic rate of States 1 and 2; therefore, we do not employ chemotherapy for these stages. This is not true for patients in Stage 3 disease, who apparently benefit from prophylactic therapy with cyclophosphamide, vincristine, and dimethyltriazenoimidazole carboxamide (DTIC).[7] Treatment of patients with Stage 4-S disease is individualized; decisions about treatment depend on the age, site of metastases, and evidence of active immune response.[4,9] Those infants who only have a small primary tumor and liver metastases receive no treatment other than removal of the primary tumor. On occasion, mechanical difficulties with respiration or renal function due to a very large liver may require treatment with small doses of radiation therapy or chemotherapy in order to speed tumor regression.

Patients with gross infiltration of the marrow, particularly those older than 1 year of age, probably require a course of chemotherapy similar to that employed in a child with Stage 4 disease.

Immunology

Neuroblastomas have been proven histologically to regress or mature spontaneously into benign ganglioneuromas with minimal or no therapy (1%–12% of the cases). Credit for this occurrence is given to host factors, which are most likely immunologic. Neuroblastomas are now known to be immunogenic tumors capable of evoking both cell-mediated and humoral-complement, independent immune responses.[16,17,18] This capability implies the presence of tumor-specific antigens or tumor-associated antigens. Patients with neuroblastomas have lymphocytes that are cytotoxic to cultivated tumor cells *in vitro;* however, these tumors manage to grow and metastasize *in vivo.* Sera blocking factors, considered important in this blocking of cytotoxicity *in vivo,* are thought to be antigen–antibody complexes. It may be postulated that as tumor cell lysis occurs, a hematogenous antibody is formed against intracellular antigens and the complex inadvertently functions as a blocking factor.

The relationship of sera blocking factors to disease status has been further clarified by identification of unblocking serum factors. These factors have been found only in patients in remission and are capable of abrogating the blocking effect *in vitro,* thus enhancing lymphocytotoxicity in tumor cell death. These factors have not been explained yet, although their specificity is thought to be mediated by antibodies. Monitoring unblocking serum titers may yield important information about the efficiency of a particular therapeutic procedure.

Evans and Hummeler have reported a probable survival advantage in patients with an increased number of bone marrow lymphoblasts.[10] This advantage in the immunology of neuroblastomas supports the following therapeutic principles: to remove the tumor mass completely or reduce it as much as possible, to increase tumor antigenicity, to augment a host antitumor immune response, to decrease or eliminate the presence of blocking factors, and to enhance the production of unblocking factors. Thus far, however, manipulation of the immune response (*e.g.*, bacillus Calmette-Guerin or BCG) has been unsuccessful.[7]

Results of Treatment

The results of the management of neuroblastoma at Children's Hospital of Philadelphia appear in Table 4-1. An analysis by age and stage is presented in Table 4-2.

The strong relationship between stage and age and survival must be considered when systems of therapy are chosen. A balance must be maintained between the dangers of the disease, their possible mitigation by treatment, and the hazards of therapy. The risk of major surgery is frequently overemphasized. In reality, the risk is quite small when performed in centers familiar with these problems. The risk of radiation therapy and chemotherapy is perhaps less well appreciated and may become evident only after years of treatment. Some of the known adverse effects of radiation therapy on normal structures may prove in time to be produced

TABLE 4-1. Number of Neuroblastoma Patients Surviving 2 Years by Primary Site and Stage at Diagnosis

Primary Site	Stage					%
	I	II	III	IV	IV-S	
Cervical	2/3	1/2		1/5		40
Thorax/Mediastinal	7/7	2/3	4/5	3/9	1/1	68
TOTAL	9/10	3/5	4/5	4/14	1/1	60
Abdominal	1/1	1/1	1/6	3/17	1/1	27
Adrenal	7/9	3/5	0/4	11/60	6/12	30
Paravertebral		0/1	1/2	1/2		40
Retroperitoneal	3/3	6/7	1/4	0/26	4/5	31
Pelvic	2/3	1/1	3/4	0/1		67
TOTAL	13/16	11/15	6/20	15/106	11/18	32
Other		1/1		1/1		100
Total %	85	71	40	16	63	37

The population is 212 patients diagnosed between February 1942 and December 1978. Eleven patients with unknown primary site are omitted from this table. Data are from the Tumor Registry, Children's Hospital of Philadelphia, March 1981.

TABLE 4-2. Number of Neuroblastoma Patients Surviving 2 Years by Age and Stage at Diagnosis

Age (Years)	Stage					%
	I	II	III	IV	IV-S	
<1	12/14	10/11	5/8	5/15	14/21	67
1–2	4/4	3/5	4/7	2/33	0/0	26
>2	6/8	2/5	0/10	12/81	1/1	20
Total %	85	71	36	15	68	

The population is 223 patients diagnosed between February 1942 and December 1978. Data are from the Tumor Registry, Children's Hospital of Philadelphia, March 1981.

also by chemical agents. These effects include impairment of somatic and gonadal growth and development, genetic changes, damage to growing organs, and oncogenesis. In addition, an unusual sensitivity to chemotherapeutic agents or inadvertent overdose might lead to profound bone marrow depression, which can be lethal. Another consequence of chemotherapy is decreased immunity, with the accompanying risk of overwhelming infection.

With these dangers in mind, Koop, at Children's Hospital of Philadelphia, evolved a therapeutic regimen many years ago that did not include irradiation or chemotherapy in Stages 1 and 2 of this disease. Comparison of our patients with those of the Children's Cooperative Study Group A supports this approach. Irradiation does not improve survival in Stages 1 and 2, whereas there is substantial evidence to support postoperative radiation therapy in Stage 3 as a means of increasing survival rates.

It is apparent that we must understand further those unknown intrinsic factors that seem to be adequate to control moderate amounts of tumor. The addition of radiation therapy does not improve the situation in Stage 2 patients regardless of whether the tumor is completely removed or appreciable amounts remain. Conversely, when large tumors remain (Stage 3 patients), radiation therapy seems to have distinct value. One may theorize that the irradiation reduces the tumor bulk to a level that allows host resistance to play a role. We must learn to enhance these intrinsic host factors to improve survival in patients with neuroblastoma.

REFERENCES

1. ADAM A, HOCHIHOLZER L: Ganglioneuroblastomas of the posterior mediastinum. Cancer 47:373, 1981
2. BRESLOW N, MCCANN B: Statistical estimation of prognosis for children with neuroblastoma. Cancer Res 31:2098, 1971
3. D'ANGIO GJ: Effects of radiation on neuroblastoma. J Pediatr Surg 3:110, 179, 1968
4. D'ANGIO GJ, LYSER KM, URUNAY G: Neuroblastoma, stage IV–S: A special entity? Memorial Sloan–Kettering Cancer Center Bulletin 2, No. 2, 61, 1971
5. DUCKETT JW, KOOP CE: Neuroblastoma. Urol Clin North Am 4:285, 1977
6. EVANS AE: Natural history of neuroblastoma. In Evans AE (ed): Advances in Neuroblastoma Research. New York, Raven Press, 1980
7. EVANS AE: Staging and treatment of neuroblastoma. Cancer 45:1799, 1980
8. EVANS AE, D'ANGIO GJ, RANDOLPH J: A proposed staging for children with neuroblastoma. Cancer 27:324, 1971
9. EVANS AE, GERSON J, SCHNAUFER L: Spontaneous regression of neuroblastoma. NCI Monographs 44:49, 1976
10. EVANS AE, HUMMELER K: The significance of primitive cells in marrow aspirates of children with neuroblastoma. Cancer 32:906, 1973
11. GERSON J, EVANS AE, ROSEN F: The prognostic value of acute phase reactants in patients with neuroblastoma. Cancer 40:1655, 1977
12. GERSON JM, KOOP CE: Neuroblastoma. Semin Oncol 1:35, 1974
13. GIBBONS MD, DUCKETT JW: Neuroblastoma masquerading as congenital ureteropelvic junction obstruction. J Pediatr Surg 14:420, 1979
14. GRIFFIN ME, BOLANDE RP: Familial neuroblastoma with regression and maturation to ganglioneurofibroma. Pediatrics 43:377, 1969

15. HANN HW, LEVY HM, EVANS AE: Serum ferritin as a guide to therapy in neuroblastoma. Cancer Res 40:1411, 1980

16. HELLSTROM I, HELLSTROM KE: Colony inhibition studies on blocking and non-blocking serum effects on cellular immunity to sarcomas. Int J Cancer 5:195, 1970

17. HELLSTROM KE, HELLSTROM I: Immunity to neuroblastoma and melanomas. Ann Rev Med 23:19, 1972

18. HELLSTROM I, SJOGREN HO, WARNER G et al: Blocking of cell-mediated tumor immunity by sera from patients with growing neoplasms. Int J Cancer 7:226, 1971

19. KOOP CE: The role of surgery in resectable, non-resectable, and metastatic neuroblastoma. JAMA 205:157, 1968

20. KOOP CE, JOHNSON DG: Neuroblastoma—An assessment of therapy in reference to staging. J Pediatr Surg 6:595, 1971

21. KOOP CE, SCHNAUFER L: The management of abdominal neuroblastoma. Cancer 35:905, 1975

22. KOOP CE, SCHNAUFER L: In Holden TM, Ashcraft KW (eds): Neuroblastoma in Pediatric Surgery. Philadelphia, W B Saunders, 1980

23. LABROSSE E: Catecholamines in neuroblastoma—A reappraisal and re-emphasis on assay of urinary metabolites. J Clin Endocrinol Metab 35:753, 1972

24. LINGLEY JF, SAGERMAN RH, SANTULLI TV, WOLFF JA: Neuroblastoma—Management and survival. N Engl J Med 277:1227, 1967

25. RANGECROFT L, LAUDER I, WAGGET J: Spontaneous maturation of stage IV–S neuroblastoma. Arch Dis Child 52:815, 1978

26. SCHNAUFER L, KOOP CE: Silastic abdominal patch for temporary hepatomegaly in stage IV–S neuroblastoma. J Pediatr Surg 10:73, 1975

27. SHANKLIN DR, SOTELO–AVILA C: In situ tumors in fetuses, newborns, and young infants. Biol Neonate 14:286, 1969

28. SNYDER HW, HASTINGS TN, POLLOCK WF: Neurogenic tissue tumors: Neuroblastomas. In Mustard WT (ed): Pediatric Surgery, 2nd ed. Chicago, Year Book Medical Publishers, 1969

This paper represents the joint efforts of the Children's Cancer Research Center, the Pediatric Surgery Department, and the Pediatric Urology Service at the Children's Hospital of Philadelphia, and the Radiotherapy Division of the University of Pennsylvania. The physicians involved include Audrey Evans, Gulio D'Angio, Beverly Raney, Anna Meadows, C. Everett Koop, Louise Schnaufer, Harry Bishop, and Howard Snyder. The updated tumor registry data were provided by Patricia Jarrett of the Tumor Registry of Children's Hospital of Philadelphia. We appreciate the secretarial assistance of Marolyn Buchanan. Supported in part by U.S.P.H.S. grant no. CA-14489.

Nephrectomy

5

John T. Grayhack

Renal surgery had its inception about a century ago. The courageous and enthusiastic contributions made by surgeons in several countries informed and stimulated their colleagues and led to rapid progress in renal surgery. The early surgeons operated on patients with overt disease but lacked complete diagnostic and physiologic information. Many of the operative and perioperative aids that are commonplace today were nonexistent. Under the circumstances the successful outcome of their endeavors seems remarkable.[18]

Although many credit the American surgeon Wolcott[57] with the first nephrectomy in 1861, Morris points out that Gustave Simon performed the first planned nephrectomy in 1869 and really initiated exploration of the feasibility of this procedure.[37] According to Morris, Simon practiced the technique in animals to confirm the reported survival following unilateral nephrectomy before proceeding with the operation in man. Of current interest is the apparent vigorous controversy among early renal surgeons about the advantages and disadvantages of the various operative approaches to the kidney.[53]

Embryology

Although the kidney is a frequent site of congenital anomaly and variations in anatomic configuration are common, review of the embryologic development of this organ makes its constancy of configuration and location seem remarkable.[6,40] In the first place, as Arey points out, the kidney and the gonad are unique in that they develop from a cellular mass that unites secondarily with its excretory system. Second, in its repetition of phylogeny, the human kidney develops two excretory organs, the pronephros and the mesonephros, which undergo degeneration except for the persistence of the wolffian duct. These two excretory organs and the final metanephros arise from the mesoderm of the nephrotome. The pronephros is located in a cephalad position; subsequent excretory units develop in a progressively more caudad location until, by the time the permanent kidney (metanephros) develops, it is initially far caudad (Fig. 5-1).

The metanephrogenic diverticulum, which gives rise to the ureter and pelvis, appears at about the fourth week of development as a bud of the wolffian duct. Mesoderm from the nephrogenic cord collects at its distal end. Then a process of development of collecting tubules and functioning nephrons begins. The process is completed except for an enlargement of the existing units by about 1 month before birth. As the development of the renal parenchyma is progressing, an upward migration of the kidney from the level of the fourth lumbar segment to the first occurs. This cephalic migration may be the result of straightening of the body curvature emphasized by the growth of the lumbar and sacral segments. With loss of its pelvic position, the kidney rotates 90 degrees so that the original dorsal border becomes the convex lateral border. The blood supply to the kidney is derived from a periaortic plexus with many branches. Bremer suggests that the vessel persisting as the renal artery is elected mechanically and that persistence of unusual vessels occurs if the usual vessels are occluded.[9]

Anatomy

The kidney is a parenchymatous organ lying retroperitoneally. Normally, its convex border is placed laterally. The medial border is marked by a notch— the hilum—containing the renal vessels. The lower poles of the kidney are farther from the midline (6 cm–9 cm) than the upper poles (4 cm–5 cm), thus the lines drawn through the long axis of the kidney tend to meet superiorly and diverge inferiorly.[35] The superior pole of the left kidney may normally lie as high as T10 and as low as L2.[3] The right kidney is usually (95% of the population) slightly lower than the left.[35]

SIZE

Review of the reports of renal size reveals some variation dependent apparently on the character and size of the population sampled and the techniques used.[35] Table 5-1 provides figures selected from various sources that seem likely to be representative of the middle-aged North American population. Throughout the reported studies the following observations seem to have been made with consistency: the right kidney is usually slightly smaller than the left; men's kidneys are on the average larger than those of women; and the average renal size tends to decrease in older age groups.

Symmetry between renal size is the rule; a difference in length of 1 cm to 1.5 cm on roentgen examination should cause consideration of an acquired abnormality.[20,25] In assessing relative size, the suggestion of the use of +2.0 cm and −1.5 cm as differences in length indicating significant variation from normal when right renal length is subtracted from left renal length seems reasonable.[8]

Attempts are being made to relate individual renal size to the size of other body structures. Simon has suggested that the normal renal size is 3 to 4.4 times the height of the second lumbar body.[49] Friedenberg and associates have used a renal index, utilizing a formula (length times width of the kidney/body surface area) to determine limits of normal renal size.[20] This complicated approach may be simplified with future effort.

BLOOD SUPPLY

The main renal arteries are branches of the aorta. The renal veins join the vena cava. The common configuration (47.6% of the population) is a single left renal artery lying dorsal to the renal vein and a longer right renal artery located dorsal to the vena cava and the right renal vein.[3] Almost as frequently (42% of the population), the dorsal cranially placed artery ascends to a ventral position with respect to the renal vein. Variations in this arrangement are common.[2,4]

Typically, the renal artery divides into anterior and posterior branches.[21,52] These branches give rise to five segmental arteries. The upper and lower poles are each supplied by a branch. Two of the remaining branches supply the anterior portion,

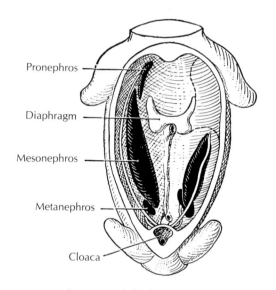

Pronephros

Diaphragm

Mesonephros

Metanephros

Cloaca

FIG. 5-1. Development of the kidney. Ventral dissection of embryo, showing locations and relations of the three kidney types in mammals. Left side shows later stage than right. (Arey LB: Developmental Anatomy, 7th ed. Philadelphia, WB Saunders, 1965)

TABLE 5-1. Representative Mean Measurements of Renal Size

Type of Measurement	Men		Women	
	RIGHT	LEFT	RIGHT	LEFT
Length (cm) Autopsy*	11.4	12	10.8	11.6
Radiograph†	12.9 ± .8	13.2 ± .8	12.3 ± .8	12.6 ± .8
Width (cm) Autopsy*	6.5	6.7	5.9	6.0
Radiograph†	6.2 ± .4	6.3 ± .5	5.7 ± .5	5.9 ± .4
Weight‡	320 g		260 g	

* Pourteyron cited by Moell H: Kidney size and its deviation from normal in acute renal failure. Acta Radiol (Suppl) 206:8, 1961.

† Moell H: Kidney size and its deviation from normal in acute renal failure. Acta Radiol (Suppl) 206:5, 1961.

‡ Wald H: The weight of normal adult human kidneys and its variability. Arch Pathol 23:493, 1937.

and one branch supplies the posterior portion of the kidneys between the poles. Variations in this pattern occur frequently. Each third of the kidney may have a separate artery. Accessory arteries may substitute for one or more branches of the main renal artery. Approximately 25% of kidneys have an accessory renal artery, and 1.5% have more than one accessory artery.[15] Accessory arteries supply the lower pole of the kidney more frequently than the upper. The renal artery and its polar accessory may be as close as 0.3 cm or as far apart as 6.5 cm.[52] When multiple renal arteries occur on the right side, they may be either dorsal or ventral to the inferior vena cava.

The right renal vein is usually less than half the length of the left. In one series, the right renal vein varied from 20 mm to 45 mm in length, with an average of 32 mm: the left renal vein varied from 60 mm to 110 mm, with an average of 84 mm.[3] In addition to being short, the right renal vein is relatively uncomplicated, usually being single. However, it may be double or even consist of three veins. Occasionally, the right renal vein receives a single tributary, the gonadal vein.[1] On the other hand, the long left renal vein, which is rarely duplicated, is characterized by receiving tributaries that may be both visceral and parietal in origin. In its course, it usually is joined by the adrenal and inferior phrenic veins superiorly and the gonadal vein inferiorly. A lumbar vein frequently joins the left renal vein, as do veins from the perirenal tissue. Division of the vein to form a venous ring surrounding the aorta is common.[21]

The arterial supply and venous drainage of anomalous kidneys is bizarre.[5,10] For this reason, preoperative arteriography is invaluable in patients with renal anomalies.

REGIONAL ANATOMY

The kidney capsule is surrounded by perirenal fat, which extends into the renal sinus. The kidney, perirenal fat, and adrenal gland are encompassed in a fascial envelope, Gerota's fascia.[54] The origin of Gerota's fascia is not definitely established, and anatomists disagree further on its extent and configuration. Last suggests that the inferior margins merge into the areolar tissue between the peritoneum and the posterior abdominal wall, pointing out that neither perinephric pus nor substances injected into the perinephric space tend to track downward.[30] However, carbon dioxide inserted presacrally does ascend into the perinephric space, supporting at least some failure of inferior closure or fusion.

Our experience agrees with that of Grossman, who did not observe diffusion from the perirenal space to the opposite side, although observations by others who report this phenomenon indicate that medial fusion is not invariably complete.[22] The concept that Gerota's fascia is closed superiorly, laterally, and usually medially in the regions of the vessels and the ureter but has some failure of approximation inferiorly seems to agree most nearly with clinical experience. The posterior or dorsal layer of perirenal fascia is a more definite structure than the anterior or ventral layer, which tends to adhere to the peritoneum. The pararenal fat lies outside Gerota's fascia, and it is continuous with the extraperitoneal fat of the abdominal walls.

The kidneys lie against the psoas and quadratus lumborum muscles. The crura of the diaphragm border the upper medial renal margins, and the leaves of the posterior diaphragm arch as a dome above the poles. The 11th and 12th ribs cross behind each kidney. The liver on the right and the spleen on the left lie against the upper poles, separated only by the peritoneum. The right kidney nestles in a hepatic fossa. The ascending and descending portions of the colon have retroperitoneal surfaces that border the convex surface of each kidney. The hepatic flexure often crosses the midsection, and the retroperitoneal second portion of the duodenum often touches the hilum of the right kidney. The pancreas extends retroperitoneally from the duodenum on the right to the medial edge of the left kidney. Its midportion or body lies just above the left renal vein.[27]

As the lumbar approach to the kidney demonstrates, the peritoneum reflects upward from the kidney at about its lateral margin. The plane of cleavage between it and the perinephric (Gerota's) fascia lies medially and posteriorly. As the peritoneum and Gerota's fascia are separated medially, the renal vessels are uncovered astride the vertebral column. In this dissection, the ureter often adheres to the peritoneum as it is lifted off the psoas. Continued medial dissection brings the vena cava into view on the right and the aorta on the left. The aorta with the celiac axis lying cephalad to the renal arteries is easily identified by palpation.

Indications for Nephrectomy

Accepted indications for nephrectomy include the following:

Calculus

Hemorrhage

Hydronephrosis

Hypertension
Infection
Neoplasm
Renal donation
Trauma
Vascular disease

Every reasonable effort is made to preserve renal tissue before resorting to nephrectomy. The surgical procedure chosen in a patient with a diseased kidney is influenced by many factors: the nature of the renal disease, the functional status of the diseased and contralateral kidneys, and the general condition of the patient are often of paramount importance. Technical considerations and the patient's prognosis also play a role in the choice of a therapeutic course.

Preoperative Evaluation

Nephrectomy and other operative procedures on the kidney must be considered major surgical undertakings and require thorough preoperative evaluation of the patient's general physical condition with correction of significant abnormalities, if possible. The history is particularly helpful in identifying systems that require further investigation. Valuable reassurance about the patient's cardiovascular status is provided by a history of engaging in physical activity without distress. Because pulmonary and cardiac disorders contribute significantly to the postoperative morbidity and mortality,[48] dyspnea, productive cough, and other cardiorespiratory symptoms require careful evaluation. A history suggesting a bleeding tendency is also of particular significance, and knowledge of medication that the patient is taking is extremely important. On physical examination, in addition to the careful assessment of the cardiorespiratory status, we take particular note of the status of the vascular system of the lower extremities. If varicosities are present, support and elevation are used to promote postoperative drainage.

A complete blood count, urinalysis, chest roentgenography, and electrocardiography are routinely done in adult patients in whom renal surgery is contemplated. A urine culture is also usually done. Since automated blood analysis techniques have become available, a battery of tests, including a fasting blood sugar, is usually carried out without specific indication. These are supplemented by studies indicated by the history and physical findings.

Before surgery, every effort should be made to establish the presence of an abnormality requiring surgical intervention, to assess the anatomic and functional status of the entire urinary tract, and to ascertain the functional status of the kidney that will be called on to support life if a nephrectomy is indicated.

The statement that renal exploration is often completed in the specimen pan, although far less true than in former years, continues to have merit. In general, the nature of a presumed renal lesion and its location should be determined preoperatively. The extent to which the etiology of a given lesion—for example, a mass—is explored preoperatively once its presence is recognized varies depending on the differential diagnosis, the patient, and the surgeon. With modern roentgenographic tools, it is possible to differentiate the causes of a renal mass with an accuracy exceeding 95%.

Exploration and tissue sampling to permit an accurate diagnosis continue to play an important role in patient management. However, therapeutic approaches based on acceptance of the preoperative diagnosis have become more commonplace as ultrasound, computed tomography, and angiography have provided increasingly accurate information.

A thorough evaluation of the entire urinary tract in the face of obvious pathology of one portion has become widely accepted as the ease of this evaluation has increased. Few experiences are more frustrating than to discover at operation that the surgical endeavor has been misdirected at a secondary site of pathology rather than at the unrecognized and unapproachable primary cause of the patient's genitourinary problem. Even more disheartening to the patient and physician is the prolonged convalescence sometimes occasioned by this type of error, undiscovered until the postoperative course causes a complete reevaluation of the patient's status.

Every reasonable effort should be made to determine the functional status of the renal tissue that is to be called on to support life postoperatively. Simple evidence of function on intravenous pyelography is no longer sufficient evidence of life-sustaining function except in unusual circumstances.[8] Prompt excretion of modern contrast media in concentrations exceeding or equaling the density of the 12th rib has been shown to occur in kidneys with significant renal functional impairment.[26,58] Increasing the amount of injected contrast medium provides visualization of some kidneys in severely azotemic patients. We would prefer individual clearance studies before every renal operation, but this is not without hazard.

Therefore, in the routine patient in whom no functional impairment is suspected, we use the following battery of tests: (1) serum creatinine or blood urea nitrogen, (2) intravenous pyelogram with standard amounts of contrast medium, (3) total creatinine clearance or suitable substitute, and (4) radioactive renogram and renal scan with calculation of relative function if available.[46] If the total renal function is normal and there is no indication on pyelography or renography that the diseased kidney is functioning more satisfactorily than the presumed normal kidney, we proceed on the basis of this evidence.[36] In case of doubt, individual renal clearance studies are carried out.

Operative Approaches to the Kidney

LATERAL INCISIONS

The traditional and most commonly used surgical approach to the kidney is retroperitoneal, using a lateral subcostal incision.[14] The lateral decubitus position (Fig. 5-2) used in this approach cannot be achieved in some patients because of spinal fusion or other deformity. In others, assumption of this position with the accompanying flexion routinely used to exaggerate the distance between the 12th rib and the iliac crest results in a decrease in vital capacity and may be accompanied by a drop in blood pressure, probably due to a decrease in the venous return to the heart.[11]

The most serious disadvantages of the subcostal incision are the difficulty in isolating the renal vessels before manipulation of a kidney containing a large renal mass and the compromised kidney exposure that may result if the fixed overhanging rib cage is respected as an inviolate boundary. The occasional muscular weakness that results from interruption or injury of the intercostal nerves if of less importance.

The subcostal incision is suitable for most surgical procedures performed on the kidney. It is relatively free of complications and has many advantages. The anatomic structures encountered are uncomplicated. Aside from the major vessels, which are essentially immobile, the retroperitoneal area is relatively free of other organs that complicate the exposure and the surgical procedure. The kidney is approached from its avascular posterior aspect with ease and safety. If inadequate exposure is a problem, the subcostal incision can easily be converted to a dorsolumbar flap procedure by resection or partial resection of the overlying ribs.

Once the kidney is mobilized, it can usually be delivered into the wound so that meticulous evaluation and correction of abnormalities can be carried out. In general, the pleural and peritoneal cavities need not be entered when the lateral approach is used. If they are, repair of the defect is readily accomplished. Dependent external drainage of the wound is easy to achieve. The incision provides an opportunity for a multiple layer closure that makes dehiscence uncommon.

Variations of this classic lumbar approach are innumerable;[7,28] they include incisions through the bed of the 12th or 11th rib, incisions through the 11th intercostal space,[43] and a more extensive dorsolumbar extrapleural flap.[38] These incisions share the advantage of enabling ready access to the subdiaphragmatic area. The 12th rib and 11th rib or interspace approaches are no more difficult to execute than the classic incision, although more care needs to be taken to avoid the pleura, which lies posteriorly. Closure and healing are satisfactory. The dorsolumbar flap (Nagamatsu) approach gives a wide exposure.[38,39] This is achieved by retracting the last two or three ribs upward after excising a posterior segment of each. The extrapleural, extraperitoneal field is especially favorable for large upper pole masses and compares well with a transthoracic transabdominal incision in exposure. However, the Nagamatsu incision is time consuming, both in its execution and closure. Entering the pleural cavity is unavoidable at times.

ANTERIOR INCISIONS

Renewed popularity of the anterior approaches to the kidney seemed to follow use of these incisions to correct vascular lesions[42] and a decreased fear of bacterial contamination of the peritoneum because of the antibiotics available. These approaches are performed with the patient lying supine or with the affected side partially elevated. Although it is possible to remain extraperitoneal,[31] a transperitoneal route is usually used. Maximum exposure can be achieved by extending the incision across the rib margin, enabling large upper pole renal masses to be managed without an excessive increase in morbidity. If a thoracic extension is used, the chest is usually entered, although it is possible to use an extrapleural approach.[33]

Once the abdomen has been entered, the kidney can be exposed by one of the following maneuvers: lateral dissection of the posterior peritoneum after incising longitudinally along the root of the mesentery, avoiding the inferior mesenteric vein; opening the posterior peritoneum over the kidney with care to avoid the colonic blood supply; and opening

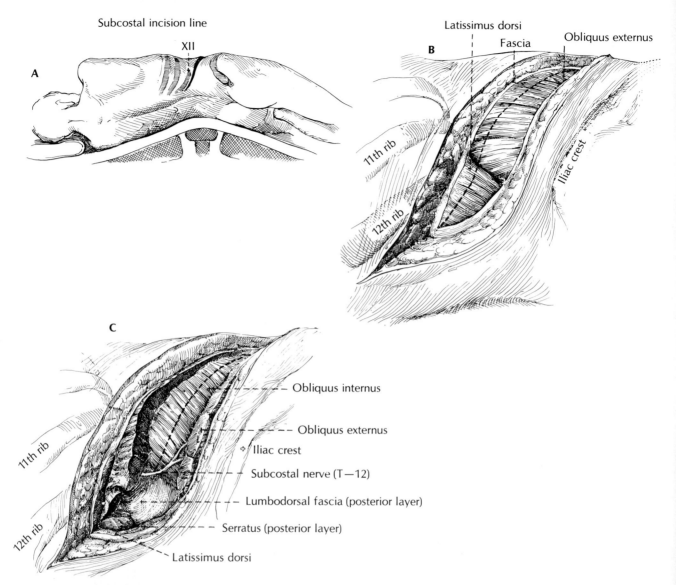

FIG. 5-2. **(A)** The subcostal incision begins below the tip of the 12th rib and extends toward the umbilicus, ending at the rectus and paralleling the rib. **(B)** The external oblique edge of the latissimus dorsi muscles are divided in the direction of the incision. Usually the 12th nerve is seen beneath this layer as it penetrates the lumbodorsal fascia. The nerve can be freed from its subcostal tunnel medially by sharp dissection until it is slack enough to be drawn out of the way (see **D**). **(C)** the internal oblique muscle is incised and can be seen to originate from the posterior layer of the lumbodorsal fascia. **(D)** The transversus abdominis muscle has the same origin and can be split in the direction of its fibers. Care is taken to separate the peritoneum bluntly from the transversalis fascia, which limits the transversus internally. **(E)** Retroperitoneal (paranephric) fat lies under the lumbodorsal fascia. Beneath is a smooth envelope of paranephric fascia (Gerota's). Paranephric fat is less lobular and lighter yellow. The kidney can be dissected with Gerota's fascia widely opened. If a tumor is present, fat and fascia are taken with the kidney. (*Illustration continues on facing page*)

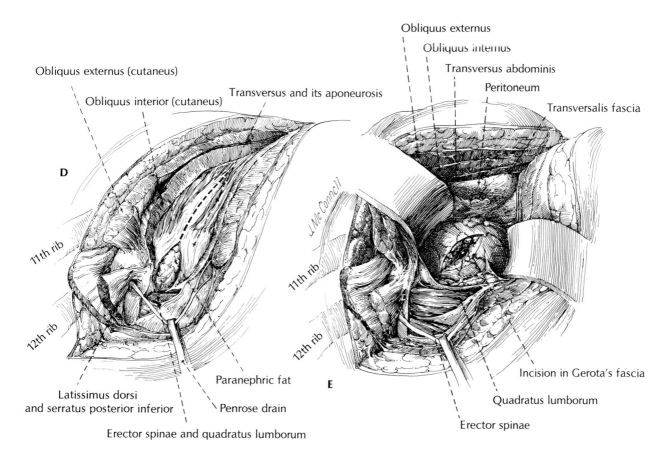

the lateral peritoneum along the paracolic gutters so that the right or left colon can be displaced medially. On the right, additional room is gained by freeing the hepatic flexure and the lateral margin of the duodenum. On the left, the splenic flexure can be mobilized by careful sharp dissection of its attachments.

Although anterior approaches require more anatomic and surgical skill than do the lateral routes to the kidney, they offer some definite advantages. The positioning required interferes less with vital functions than does the lateral decubitus position. A transperitoneal approach often provides more direct access to the major renal blood vessels than does a flank approach. This can be particularly advantageous in the removal of renal malignancies and in the control of unexpected bleeding. Exploration of the other kidney and abdominal contents is possible by this route; removal of adjacent bowel, viscera, and lymph nodes is facilitated. The transperitoneal route also enables the surgeon to elect to carry out unrelated surgical procedures with a single anesthetic. Some express the opinion that postoperative pain and ileus are lessened and

wound healing is superior to that seen following flank incisions.[42]

The transperitoneal approach is not without disadvantages. Manipulation of adjacent viscera increases the risk of their injury. If a thoracotomy is not used, the upper pole of the kidney may be very difficult to visualize and dissect. Although some help can be obtained by altering the patient's position with a kidney rest or a sandbag, the kidney lies farther away from the surgeon by this approach than it does when a flank incision is used. Furthermore, the anterior surface of the kidney presents to the surgeon, which can be an advantage if the blood supply is a primary target for surgical exposure; however, if a pyelotomy or a similar procedure is anticipated, a posterior approach is less hazardous. If the urine is infected, contamination of the peritoneal cavity is likely. Adequate drainage is more difficult to achieve and is less certain. Wound dehiscence is more likely with an abdominal incision than with a flank incision. Although reports today do not record the incidence of late complications such as bowel obstruction, there seems little doubt that the transperitoneal approach does carry a risk of this complication.

Operative Techniques

CHOICE OF INCISION

Factors that influence the choice of an incision include the nature of the renal disease, the general condition of the patient, anatomic considerations, and the surgeon's preference.

The nature of the renal disease is important because patients with kidney neoplasms and reparable renal artery lesions usually require an approach that will enable early isolation of major vessels. In the patient with a renal artery lesion, proximal control of the vessels, ability to attack associated arterial disease, and availability of adjacent arterial structures for use in correction of the defect are further considerations that usually favor an abdominal or thoracoabdominal approach. In general, other lesions in which functioning renal parenchyma is left in the renal fossa and the drainage of urine is probable or possible are preferably treated by a retroperitoneal approach. Occasionally, the desire to determine the nature of coexisting pulmonary and renal lesions dictates a thoracoabdominal approach.

The general condition of the patient also influences the choice of approach. If the patient has a severe deformity or disease of the spine, the decubitus position used in lateral approaches to the kidney may be unobtainable. Similarly, severe pulmonary disease may make this approach undesirable. Some patients develop severe hypotension in the lateral position, preventing its use. The presence of diffuse intraperitoneal disease, such as metastatic cancer or widespread adhesions from previous disease or surgery, weighs against the use of an anterior approach. On the other hand, unconfirmed suspicion of gastrointestinal disease may be an indication for simultaneous exploration of the abdomen and correction of a renal abnormality.

Anatomic considerations such as knowledge of the position of the kidneys in relation to the rib cage are essential in selecting an incision that provides adequate exposure. Similarly, awareness of previous surgical procedures is important in planning an approach to the kidney. In general, there is an advantage if the renal dissection can be started in a previously unoperated area, proceeding to a scarred region once major structures are identified.

The surgeon should evaluate his own capabilities and experience as objectively as possible. Lack of familiarity with a given approach should be a factor in making a decision about the ideal incision for a patient.

Subcostal Incision

With the patient in the lateral decubitus position (Fig. 5-2), an incision is made beneath and parallel to the 12th rib.[29,34,50,60] For a nephrectomy, it is advisable to begin the skin incision posterior to the angle of the rib and to extend it ventrally to the border of the rectus, erring if necessary on the generous side. The medial aspect of the incision is curved or extended in a straight line, depending on the position of the kidney and the operative procedure to be performed.

Division of the latissimus, the posterior aspect of the external oblique, and often a portion of the serratus posterior inferior (Fig. 5-2C) exposes the lumbodorsal fascia. If this is incised, a finger inserted and directed medially can sweep the peritoneum from the transversalis fascia. Division of the internal oblique and transversus abdominis muscles, avoiding the intercostal nerves, is thus facilitated (Fig. 5-2D). Once this is accomplished, blunt or sharp dissection hugging the quadrate and later the psoas muscles will expose Gerota's fascia over the posterior aspect of the kidney. A cleavage plane is then sought in the paranephric fat between anterior Gerota's fascia and the peritoneum. Variations in this approach are desirable, depending on the nature of the renal pathology, its location, and the previous surgical history of the kidney. At times the lower pole of the kidney may be completely mobilized and the renal vessels exposed and isolated before any manipulation of the upper pole. The surgeon may wish to enter the peritoneal cavity to explore it or facilitate removal of the kidney. In the absence of cancer, the posterior approach to the kidney and renal pelvis is preferred with the subcostal incision.

If the exposure is inadequate, division of the costovertebral ligament anchoring the 12th rib can increase it.[60] Usually this fibrous band is easily exposed by exerting pressure posteriorly on a sponge held in a clamp. Once exposed, it can be divided with scissors in its inferior aspect. This maneuver enables increased retraction of the 12th rib superiorly. Further exposure can be achieved by the use of a mechanical rib spreader of the Finochietto type, although we have tended to avoid this in recent years because its use seems to be associated with increased postoperative pain. If further exposure is necessary, the posterior aspect of the incision can be extended superiorly in a gentle curve to expose segments of the 12th, 11th, and 10th ribs. By resecting a segment of these, the exposure can be converted to a dorsolumbar flap (see Fig. 5-6).

Twelfth-Rib Resection Incision

With the patient placed in the same flexed lateral decubitus position used for a standard lumbar incision, an incision made over the 12th rib (or the 11th rib if the 12th rib is rudimentary) from its angle to its tip is usually continued medially and inferiorly. Muscle slips representing the origin of the external oblique muscle are divided from the rib margins as they pass over the 12th rib (see Fig. 5–6C). A subperiosteal resection is unnecessary. However, if it is elected, the periosteum of the exposed rib is incised for the entire length. The intercostal muscles are freed and separated from the bone with instruments such as the Alexander and Doyen periosteal elevators. Care is taken to avoid the neurovascular bundle along the lower margin of the rib. The exposed rib is severed posteriorly with a rib cutter. The tip of the rib is freed from its anterior muscular attachments with scissor dissection (Fig. 5-3).[24]

The incision is carried through the exposed periosteum into the retroperitoneal fat with care to avoid the pleura posteriorly. Anteriorly the three muscular layers of the abdomen are incised or separated, avoiding the peritoneum as in the standard lumbar incision. With the 11th rib retracted upward, the kidney is exposed as in the subcostal incision but at a somewhat higher level. The 11th and 12th intercostal neurovascular bundles are avoided without much difficulty during the incision, but they must be considered during closure because of their close relationship to the edges of the incision.

Eleventh-Rib or Intercostal-Space Incision

A retroperitoneal extrapleural incision involving partial resection of the 11th rib or entry through the 11th intercostal space is being employed with increasing frequency.[7,31] For either approach, the patient is placed in the standard flexed lateral decubitus (Fig. 5-4) or semirecumbent position. The incision extends from the angle of the rib forward and downward to the edge of the rectus muscle and is made over or below the 11th rib. If the rib is to be removed (Fig. 5-4), the latissimus dorsi and external oblique muscles are divided and subperiosteal resection of the rib is carried out. The retroperitoneal space is entered by dividing

(*Text continues on p. 75*)

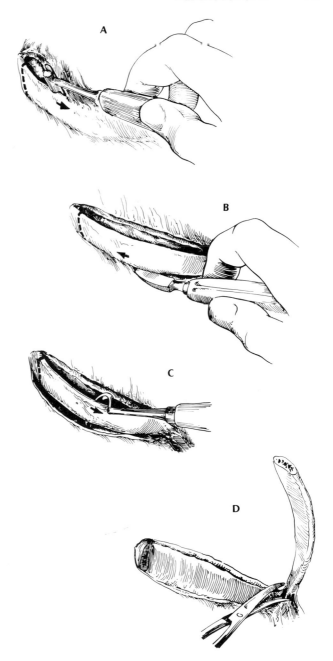

FIG. 5-3. Rib resection technique. **(A)** After exposure of the rib, the intercostal muscles are stripped from the upper and lower rib surfaces with an Alexander Farabeuf costal periosteotome. **(B)** The rib is freed from the periosteum by subperiosteal resection or from the pleura with a periosteum elevator. **(C)** A Doyen costal elevator is slipped beneath the rib to free it. The proximal and distal portions of the rib are immobilized with Kocher's clamps, and the rib is divided proximal to its angle with a right-angled rib cutter. **(D)** The costal cartilage is cut free with scissors. The cut surface of the rib is inspected for spicules, which are removed with a rongeur.

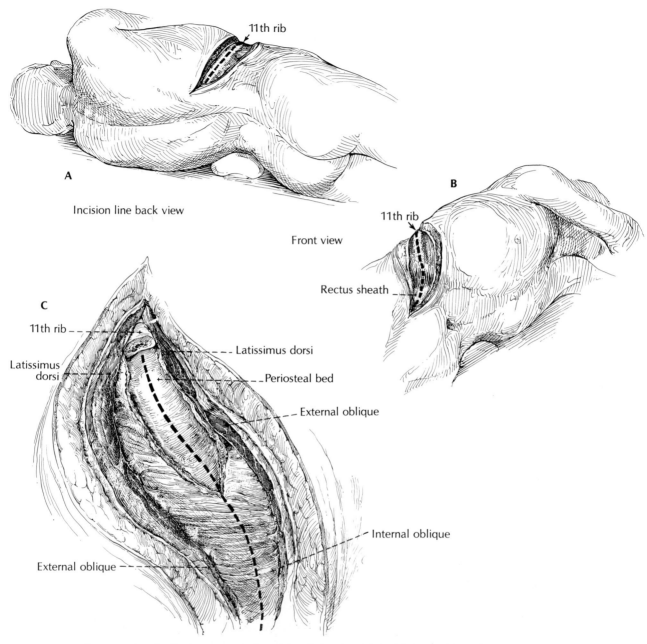

FIG. 5-4. Technique of 11th-rib resection. **(A and B)** The incision is made over the 11th rib. **(C)** After division of the latissimus and external oblique muscles, subperiosteal resection of the rib is performed. **(D)** The incision is carried through the periosteum posteriorly and the internal oblique and transversus muscles medially, exposing the paranephric space. A tongue of pleura lies in the upper portion of the wound. Diaphragmatic slips that come into view are divided, and the pleura can be retracted upward. **(E)** The paranephric fat is dissected bluntly. **(F)** Gerota's fascia is incised and entered. In nephrectomy for renal donation, a sharp technique is used to dissect the paranephric fat. **(G)** The renal vein is exposed to its entrance into the vena cava anteriorly. The tissue between the ureter laterally and the vena cava medially is dissected free, with care taken to preserve the periureteral blood supply. The hilar region of the kidney is avoided in dissection. **(H)** The kidney is rotated anteromedially, and the renal artery is isolated as far as possible. The ureter is divided as far inferiorly as possible. (*Illustration continues on pp. 73 and 74*)

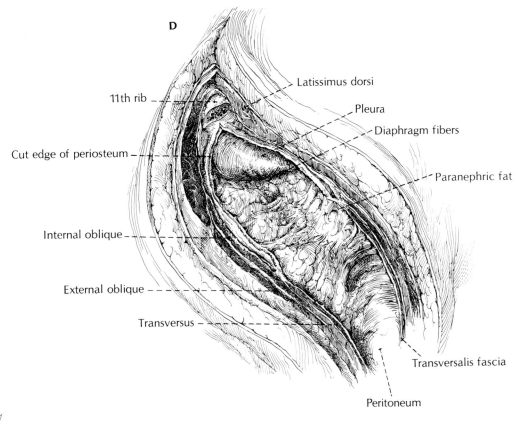

D

11th rib

Cut edge of periosteum

Internal oblique

External oblique

Transversus

Latissimus dorsi

Pleura

Diaphragm fibers

Paranephric fat

Transversalis fascia

Peritoneum

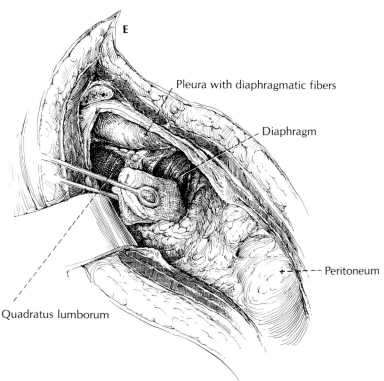

E

Pleura with diaphragmatic fibers

Diaphragm

Peritoneum

Quadratus lumborum

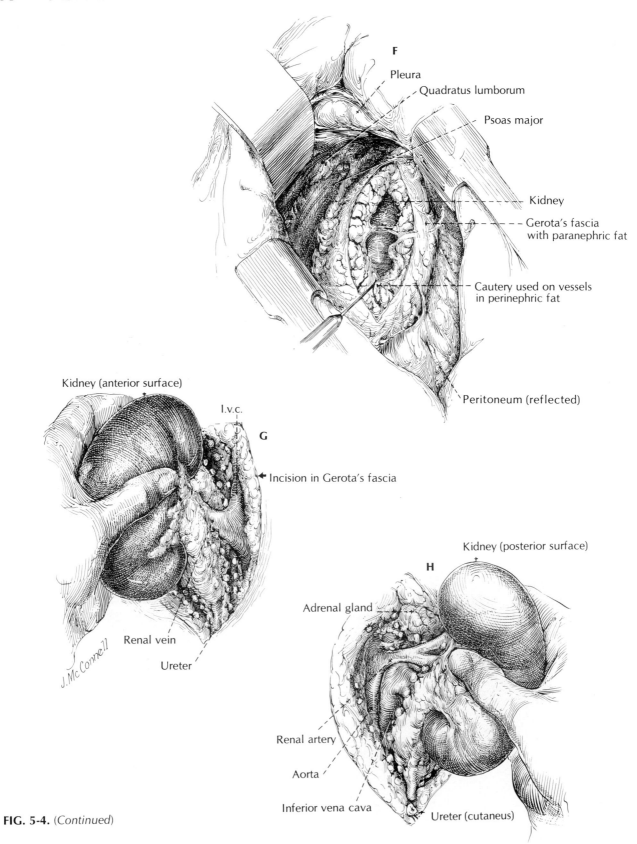

F

Pleura

Quadratus lumborum

Psoas major

Kidney

Gerota's fascia
with paranephric fat

Cautery used on vessels
in perinephric fat

Peritoneum (reflected)

Kidney (anterior surface)

I.v.c.

G

Incision in Gerota's fascia

Renal vein

Ureter

J. McConnell

Kidney (posterior surface)

H

Adrenal gland

Renal artery

Aorta

Inferior vena cava

Ureter (cutaneus)

FIG. 5-4. (*Continued*)

the internal oblique and transversalis muscles medially; the periosteum is incised, avoiding the tongue of pleura that extends beneath it. Diaphragmatic slips are visualized and divided, allowing retraction of the pleura upward and exposure of the retroperitoneum.

If the incision is to be carried through the 11th intercostal space, development of the medial aspect of the wound initially allows the index and second finger to be inserted through the transversalis fascia to assist in identifying and dissecting the structures of the interspace. Occasionally the posterior aspect of the skin incision is not made until the 11th interspace is identified by this method.[44] The interspace is entered in its anterior portion by dividing the intercostal muscles carefully until the muscular slips of the diaphragm can be seen. The neurovascular bundle at the under surface of the 11th rib is avoided. A purposeful expansion of the lungs helps to identify the pleura beneath the diaphragmatic attachments. After these are divided, the pleura can be retracted out of the operative field without injury and the 12th rib can be hinged downward, providing access to the retroperitoneum and kidney. On closing the wound, the drain, if used, is brought out through a stab wound beneath the 12th rib or the posterior angle of the incision.

Supracostal Incision

A supracostal flank approach described by Turner Warwick has gained in popularity.[55] The incision is made at the lower margin of the interspace adjacent to the superior margin of the 11th or 12th rib (Fig. 5-5). The anatomic dissection is similar to that described in the traditional interspace incision. To obtain full advantage from this approach, the rib must be freed superiorly to permit it to pivot downward. Turner Warwick suggests a two-layer closure of the wound with approximation of the detached diaphragm and inter-

costal muscle to the serratus posterior and the muscle immediately external to the rib as the first layer. The second layer approximates the edge of the latissimus dorsi and serratus above to the latissimus dorsi below. Drainage is accomplished with a stab wound below the 12th subcostal nerve.

Dorsolumbar Flap Incision

Efforts to increase exposure of the kidney by resection or partial resection of several ribs have been numerous and varied. The dorsolumbar flap described by Nagamatsu, not too dissimilar from the "barn door" incision of Kelly and Burnam,[28] is currently used most often. In this procedure, the patient is placed in the usual lateral decubitus position. A vertical incision is made from the 9th or 10th interspace inferiorly, paralleling the lateral border of the sacrospinalis muscles, to just above the upper border of the angle of the 12th rib (Fig. 5-6).[38,39]

At this point, the incision is curved medially to permit an extension along the 12th rib as far as is necessary to achieve adequate exposure. The latissimus dorsi and serratus muscles are divided to expose short segments of the 12th, 11th, and occasionally the 10th ribs. Subperiosteal resection of the ribs just medial to their angles is carried out; resection of a segment of sufficient length to ensure separation of the cut ends of the ribs reduces postoperative discomfort. Tendinous slips of the sacrospinalis muscle are freed from the lower border of the ribs; the costovertebral ligament of the 12th rib is divided. The posterior attachment of the diaphragm to the quadratus lumborum muscle is incised below the pleura. This enables easy retraction of the lower rib cage to the dome of the diaphragm. The medial aspect of the incision is similar to that used in the other lumbar incisions described.

Often it is advantageous to resect the entire 12th

FIG. 5-5. Supracostal incision. A modification of the interspace approach in which the incision is made along the superior margin of the rib. The rib should be freed to allow it to be hinged downward.

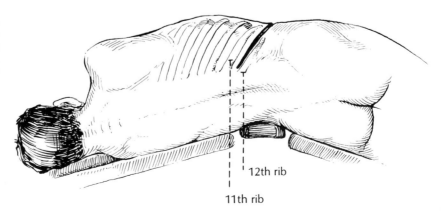

12th rib

11th rib

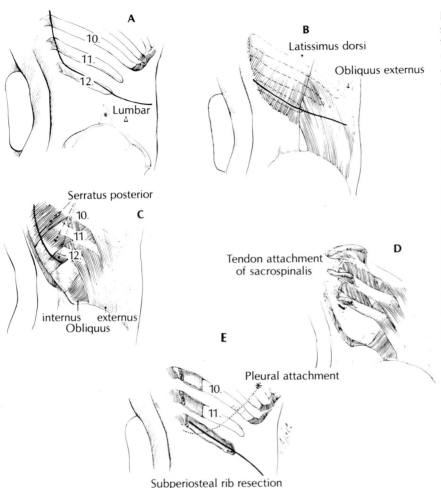

FIG. 5-6. Dorsolumbar flap incision. **(A)** The skin incision extends from the rectus muscle along the upper border of the 12th rib to its angle and then curves upward, paralleling the lateral border of the sacrospinalis muscles to the 10th or 9th interspace. **(B)** The latissimus dorsi muscle is divided along the upper margin to the 12th rib. **(C)** The serratus muscle is divided to expose segments of the 12th, 11th, and often 10th ribs. Portions of the muscle must be removed to allow resection of the ribs medial to their angles. **(D)** If the 12th rib remains in place, the costovertebral ligament must be divided to enable retraction of the flap to be created. Segments of the 12th, 11th, and often 10th ribs are resected to enable retraction of the overhanging rib cage. **(E)** We prefer to remove the 12th rib for exposure. The pleura often extends below the incision (*dotted line*).

rib. Conversion of a subcostal incision to a dorsolumbar flap is accomplished with little difficulty. Closure is accomplished by approximation of the muscle and fascial layers with interrupted sutures. Approximation of the divided costovertebral ligament and replacement of the divided lateral arcuate ligament of the diaphragm may be desirable but are not essential.

Subcostal Abdominal Incision

This incision, which gives excellent exposure, is carried out with the patient supine and the flank elevated. It usually starts just below and lateral to the tip of the 12th rib and is carried medially in an upward curve parallel to the costal margin and 1 cm to 2 cm medial to it. The exposure is increased by extending the incision across the linea alba 2 cm to 5 cm below the xiphoid and dividing at least a portion of the anterior sheath of the opposite rectus muscle.

The peritoneal cavity is entered carefully at or near the midline. This entry is extended laterally, dividing the rectus muscles and then the posterior rectus sheath. The ligamentum teres is clamped, divided, and ligated to enable the operator to place a hand in the peritoneal cavity. The hand lifts the abdominal wall and prevents bowel injury as the internal and external oblique and transversus abdominis muscles and fascia are divided or separated laterally. The peritoneal cavity should be explored before proceeding with surgery. All retractors should be padded and bowel manipulation minimized during the remainder of the operation. If necessary, the incision can be extended laterally or medially as a mirror image of the initial incision to obtain needed exposure.

Transverse Abdominal Incision

The transverse abdominal incision usually extends directly medial from its origin just beneath the tip of the 12th rib, although it may be made at any level, depending on the position of the kidney.

The technique used is essentially that used for the subcostal incision. This incision enables an extraperitoneal approach to the kidney if the transversalis muscle and fascia are split and the posterior rectus sheath is divided cautiously.[31] The peritoneal envelope can then be mobilized from the lateral aspect medially, just as in the lumbar approach. Usually the peritoneal cavity is entered, and the procedure carried out is similar to that used with a subcostal abdominal incision.

Vertical Abdominal Incision

Standard midline or paramedian incisions are the commonly used vertical abdominal incisions. In either instance, it is important to extend the incision near or above the xiphoid to ensure adequate exposure of the kidney. In the paramedian incision, which is approximately 2 cm lateral to the midline, the rectus muscle is mobilized medially and retracted laterally. Incising the anterior and posterior rectus sheaths permits a two-layer fascial closure. The peritoneal cavity is entered by using a technique similar to that used with the subcostal incision. Drainage of the renal fossa with an abdominal incision, if desired, is usually accomplished by using a stab wound in the flank for the rubber drains placed retroperitoneally or by using a sharp metal guide to lead plastic drainage tubing through the flank musculature.

Thoracoabdominal Incision

The transpleural transperitoneal approach to the kidney increased in popularity after its use in the removal of traumatized kidneys in World War II.[13,32] With endotracheal anesthesia, the patient is usually placed in a semirecumbent or modified lateral decubitus position. The 10th or 11th rib is usually selected for subperiosteal removal, although another rib or an interspace may be used (Fig. 5-7). The incision is extended into the abdomen and may then be carried inferiorly or medially, depending on the exposure required. The pleura is entered through the rib bed in a subperiosteal approach. Retraction of the ribs is assisted by a mechanical rib spreader, which should be padded generously. Similar care is required in retracting the lung. The diaphragm is split in the direction of the incision, avoiding the phrenic nerve. Some surgeons suggest crushing the nerve or infiltrating it with a local anesthetic.[12] This seems unnecessary.

Once the peritoneal cavity is entered, the spleen and liver are easily retracted superiorly. The kidney, particularly the superior pole, and the renal vessels are then exposed as in the transperitoneal approach. In closing the wound, the diaphragm is approximated with horizontal mattress sutures of 2-0 nonabsorbable material. The pleura and the muscular layers are closed with interrupted sutures. The lung should be reexpanded while closure is being accomplished. If desired, a catheter may be left in the pleural cavity to aspirate residual air after the wound is closed. It can be removed through an oblique tract. If the lung has been injured or bleeding is present, a chest tube should be left in place.

WOUND CLOSURE

Techniques of wound closure vary considerably, depending on the operative procedure, the pathology, and the patient's condition. If infection is present or urine drainage likely, absorbable sutures should be used for the deep layers. In other circumstances, nonabsorbable sutures may be chosen. If it is at all possible, we prefer to approximate each individual fascial layer with interrupted 0 chromic catgut, silk, wire, or braided polyester sutures. If infection, scarring, or loss of tissue prevents this, we use stay sutures through all fascial and muscle layers and the skin. For this purpose, we prefer heavy silver, stainless steel wire, or braided polyester suture material. In debilitated patients and those with neoplasms, it is advisable to use layer closure combined with the stay suture technique, particularly if a transperitoneal incision is used.

Specific Renal Operations

NEPHRECTOMY FOR NONMALIGNANT DISEASE

The common approach for nephrectomy for nonmalignant disease is through the flank. The peritoneum is separated from the lateral margin of the fibrous Gerota's fascia by blunt dissection (see Fig. 5-4E). Gerota's fascia is entered by sharp dissection posteriorly, well away from the margin of the peritoneum (see Fig. 5-4F). The posterior aspect of the kidney is then mobilized by blunt dissection. Next, the peritoneum is moved toward the midline, exposing the anterior aspect of Gerota's fascia and the ureter, which is identified, isolated bluntly, clamped, and divided. An obstructed, infected ureter should be excised. If this is impractical, the distal portion may be brought into the wound and drained temporarily through the flank. If the ureter is normal, the distal ureter is usually ligated with 2-0 chromic catgut. Traction on the proximal ureter

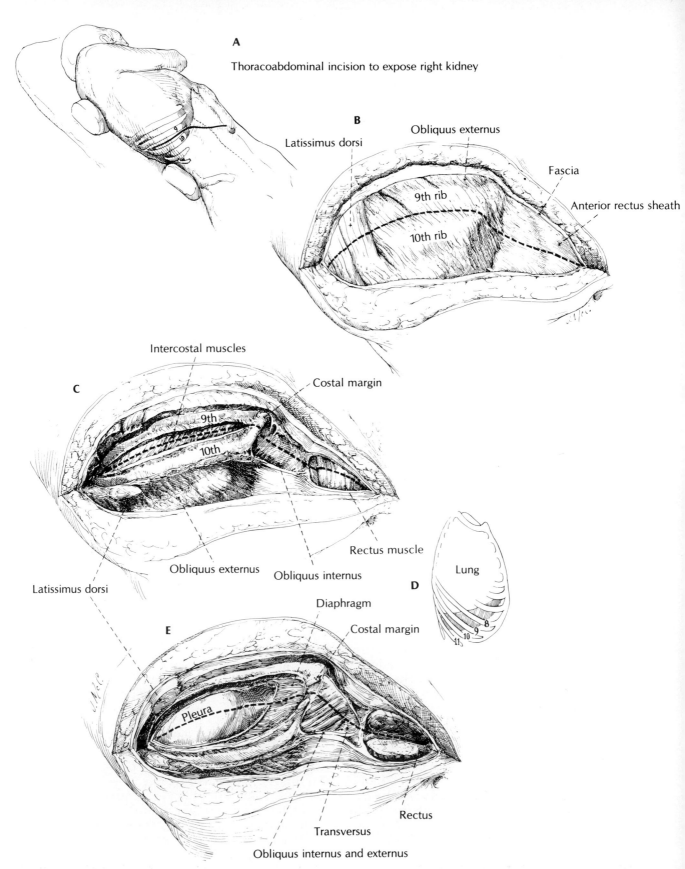

A

Thoracoabdominal incision to expose right kidney

B

Latissimus dorsi

Obliquus externus

Fascia

Anterior rectus sheath

9th rib

10th rib

Intercostal muscles

Costal margin

C

9th

10th

Latissimus dorsi

Obliquus externus

Obliquus internus

Rectus muscle

Lung

D

8

9

10

11

Diaphragm

Costal margin

E

Pleura

Rectus

Transversus

Obliquus internus and externus

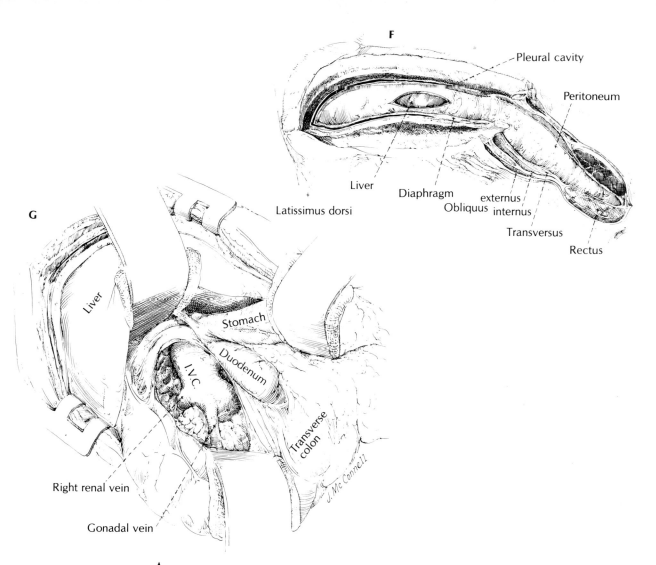

F

Pleural cavity

Peritoneum

Liver

Diaphragm

Obliquus externus

internus

Latissimus dorsi

Transversus

Rectus

G

Liver

Stomach

Duodenum

I.V.C.

Transverse colon

J. McConnell

Right renal vein

Gonadal vein

◄FIG. 5-7. Thoracoabdominal incision. **(A)** the patient is placed in a semirecumbent position using sandbags. If the chest is entered through the ninth intercostal space, the incision extends from the midaxillary line across the costal margin at the intercostal space to the midline or across it just above the umbilicus. **(B)** The anterior rectus sheath and the external oblique and latissimus dorsi muscles are divided. **(C)** The intercostal muscles parallel the direction of the three abdominal layers and are divided. The costal cartilage and the internal oblique and rectus muscles are incised. If more exposure is desired, the linea alba and opposite rectus can be divided. **(D)** The pleural reflection (*shaded areas*) lies progressively closer to the costal margin in the more cephalic intercostal spaces. **(E)** The pleura, reflecting as the costophrenic sinus near the costal margin, is exposed beneath the intercostal muscles. The diaphragm can be seen inferior and dorsal to the pleura. The pleura is opened with care to avoid injuring the lung, which comes into view with inspiration. After the lung is packed away gently, the diaphragmatic surface of the pleura is seen. The diaphragm is incised on its thoracic surface, avoiding the phrenic nerve. **(F)** The transversus abdominis muscle is divided, exposing the peritoneum with the liver lying beneath it. **(G)** The peritoneum is incised and a rib-spreading retractor (Finochietto) is inserted, enabling upward displacement of the liver (or the spleen on the left) into the thoracic cavity and giving wider access to the posterior peritoneum than in an anterior abdominal incision.

79

aids in manipulating the kidney and facilitates its removal.

The upper pole of the kidney is freed with blunt and sharp dissection. If a vessel is suspected or encountered as the upper pole is mobilized, clamping before division is desirable to avoid the difficult task of locating a vessel that has retracted. The small vessels communicating with the adrenal may cause bothersome oozing unless they are ligated, clipped, or fulgurated. The upper pole of the kidney may be rotated laterally and inferiorly as it is freed to help exposure the renal vessels. Next, the major renal artery and vein are identified. By this stage of the procedure, digital compression of these vessels should be possible if bleeding is encountered. Sharp scissor dissection combined with that achieved with a blunt clamp or a Kütner dissector usually enables the separate isolation of the artery and vein. Application of three clamps to each of these structures with division between the clamps near the kidney and the two on the side of the aorta or vena cava is a standard technique. The clamps should be inspected before use to be certain that the jaws meet properly and that

the box lock is satisfactory. Clamps with longitudinal serrations are preferable.

After division of the vessels and removal of the kidney, the clamps should be supported carefully until they are replaced by No. 1 chromic catgut or silk ligatures. Ligation of the individual vessels before division has become an increasingly popular alternate technique (Fig. 5-8). The risk of accidentally cutting the ligatures (Fig. 5-8C) can be minimized by protecting the proximal arterial and distal venous ligature with a clamp (Fig. 5-8B). After division, the vessel can be secured again by a second ligature or oversewing. *En masse* ligation of the vessels is rarely necessary, although it has been used commonly in the past. Many techniques have been described for securing the renal vessels.[23] If possible, the artery should be occluded before the vein is occluded. In concentrating on securing the portion of the vessels remaining in contact with the aorta and vena cava, the surgeon should be aware of the difficulty occasioned by bleeding from renal vessels torn at the junction with the great vessels.

Adequate exposure and a careful, thoughtful

FIG. 5-8. Technique of ligation of renal vessels prior to division. The vessel must be freed completely for an adequate length. The ligatures should be placed so that division of their posterior aspect or an inadequate arterial or venous cuff does not result when the vessel is divided.

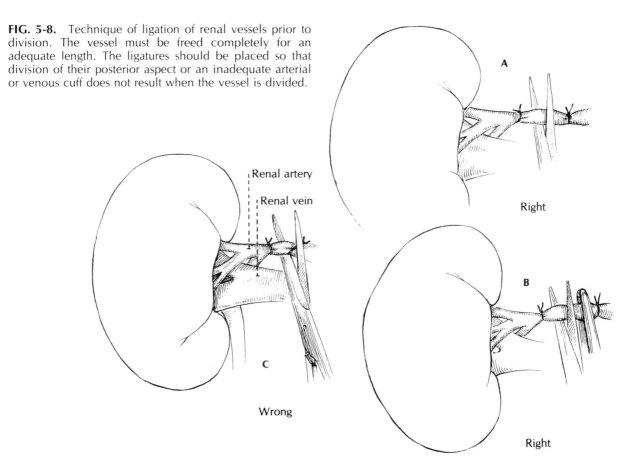

approach to the technical problems posed by nephrectomy are essential to reduce complications. In general, mobilization of the kidney should begin in an area where identification of structures is possible. The dissection should proceed from this region to the sites of previous surgery or pathology.

SUBCAPSULAR NEPHRECTOMY

When perinephric dissection of the kidney seems impossible because of a dense, markedly adherent fibrous reaction, a subcapsular plane of cleavage that will minimize risk of injury to important adjacent structures may be sought or entered inadvertently. As the dissection proceeds, the renal hilum will be covered by the inverted capsule as the tunica vaginalis covers the hilum and cord of the testis during eversion of a hydrocele.

To find and clamp the renal vessels requires that the dense apron of capsule be incised, usually on the anterior aspect. Control of bleeding can be difficult in these procedures. Frequently, all landmarks are obscured and progress in the dissection can only be made by cautious sharp dissection. Major vessels are often entered before they are recognized, but fortunately the dense fibrous tissue tends to prevent their retraction. Transfixion sutures are often invaluable aids to hemostasis in these patients.

To avoid injury to the duodenum or major blood vessels, pieces of capsule may be left behind. Prolonged drainage can ensue. The suggestion that the renal vessels by approached transabdominally or transthoracically before attempting removal of the fixed renal tissue seems to have merit.[12,17] Preoperative aortography is important in managing these problems.

Postoperative Care

A detailed discussion of the postoperative care of the patient subjected to renal surgery is beyond the scope of this text, but some general comments can be made. Management of the patient's convalescence should be carried out with a view to reducing factors that contribute to the development of postoperative complications. Little seems to be gained and much can be lost by initiating oral feeding before restoration of near-normal gastrointestinal motility; therefore, oral intake is usually avoided for a minimum of 48 hr and is instituted only when active bowel sounds or the passage of flatus is noted. Medication to ensure adequate pain relief, in order to reduce splinting of respiratory movements and thus allow coughing, is desirable.

Inhalation therapy to encourage deep respiratory movements and aid in expectoration of tracheobronchial secretions is advantageous. Early ambulation is encouraged. Adequate and appropriate fluid replacement is carried out through the veins of the upper extremities. Antibiotics are used if infection is known to be present or if the patient's general condition or a specific local condition makes infection seem highly probable, but their routine use is not of proven value. When possible, antibiotics or chemotherapeutic agents are prescribed on the basis of culture. Drains are removed as rapidly as possible.

Complications of Renal Surgery

The operative and postoperative complications of renal surgery depend on the pathology present, the procedure performed, and technique used (see Table 5-2).

OPERATIVE COMPLICATIONS

Bleeding from the renal parenchyma, a renal neoplasm, or the renal vessels is an ever-present threat during operation. **Hemorrhage** can be massive and life threatening, so precautionary steps to prevent or to manage such bleeding are essential. Adequate blood for replacement of loss should always be available. If a procedure associated with the risk

TABLE 5-2. Common Complications of Nephrectomy

Operative	Postoperative
Hemorrhage/shock	Wound
Pleural/pulmonary	Dehiscence
Cardiovascular	Infection
Visceral injury	Hernia
	Gastrointestinal
	Ileus
	Fistula
	Pulmonary
	Pneumothorax
	Pneumonia
	Atelectasis
	Cardiovascular
	Myocardial infarction
	Congestive failure
	Thrombophlebitis
	Pulmonary embolism
	Cerebrovascular accident
	Shock secondary to blood loss, septicemia
	Renal functional impairment

of significant bleeding is planned, the renal vessels should be identified and isolated initially. Bulldog and other vascular clamps, tourniquets, or digital compression may then be used to control bleeding. If securing the renal vessels is likely to be difficult, an approach should be chosen that would enable proximal control of the main vessels, if this becomes necessary.

Despite every precaution, surgeons operating on the kidney are occasionally faced with serious bleeding. Under these circumstances a rational approach is extremely important. Direct or proximal pressure with a finger, or a pack aided by manual compression, almost always enables the bleeding to be temporarily controlled. Once this is achieved, the surgeon should (1) mobilize ancillary help if necessary, (2) be certain that adequate blood and the means for its rapid administration are available, (3) reevaluate and adjust his exposure, and (4) ensure that the proper instruments are on hand. Next, if the site of bleeding is not known, it should be identified by judicious release of the bleeding site. Blind clamping should be avoided. Once identified, temporary control can be reinstituted while the necessary proximal control of the blood supply is carried out.

Direct compression of the major vessels while they are mobilized to enable placement of occluding arterial clamps (like those used in vascular reconstructive procedures on the renal vessels) is possible if an abdominal approach has been or can be used.[47,48] Deming and Ray used manual compression of the thoracic aorta to control bleeding from a renal artery in a patient in the lateral decubitus position.[16] Once the vessels on both sides of the vascular injury are controlled, divided arteries or veins can be identified, clamped, and ligated. Arteriotomies can be closed with 5-0 arterial silk or synthetic suture. Venous injuries can be identified, clamped with a Satinsky or similar vascular exlusion clamp, and sutured. With current techniques, the situation will rarely be such that direct and adequate control is impossible. If this should be the case, as might occur in parenchymal bleeding from a solitary kidney in which multiple procedures make anatomic identification of structures virtually impossible, use of hemostatic agents and gauze packing will enable vigorous bleeding to be controlled.

We have not used ligation of the vena cava to control bleeding from caval injury, but ligation below and even above the renals has been successfully used.[19] The technique of leaving clamps controlling bleeding vessels in the wound for several days has been used with frequent success in the past. Packs or instruments should be removed in the operating room with adequate preparation to follow a planned procedure if bleeding recurs.

Entering **the pleural cavity** during a renal operation is inconsequential if the patient's trachea is intubated and the entry is recognized. The opening may be closed at any time, but we usually prefer to ignore it until the wound is closed. Expansion of the lung accompanied by suction maintained on an intrathoracic catheter removed as the pleural rent is closed is usually adequate. If a pulmonary leak is suspected, a chest tube with water-seal drainage should be left in place. A chest roentgenogram should be obtained in the recovery room to confirm the pulmonary expansion evident on physical examination. Residual pleural air can be aspirated with a needle inserted into an upper anterior interspace.

Cardiovascular abnormalities, including cardiac arrest, myocardial infarction, and persistent hypotension secondary to drugs or abnormalities such as adrenal insufficiency or congestive failure, may occur. These complications can be minimized by careful preoperative evaluation and preparation.

Injury to the bowel or abdominal **viscera** such as the liver, the pancreas, and the spleen may also result from nephrectomy. In such instances, recognition of the abnormality is of primary concern. If the injury is recognized, it is usually readily dealt with by standard techniques. Although routine removal of the injured spleen is no longer invariably carried out, splenectomy deserves serious consideration as a treatment alternative when splenic injury is recognized. A rent in the bowel is usually readily closed in layers with interrupted sutures of 2-0 chromic catgut encompassing the mucosa, followed by one- or two-layer closure of the muscularis with interrupted silk sutures of the Lembert type.

POSTOPERATIVE COMPLICATIONS

Morbidity following renal operations is higher than most surgeons realize. Scott and Selzman reported an incidence of 19% complications in 450 patients subjected to nephrectomy.[48] Stanisic and associates reviewed 150 consecutive patients operated on for renal cyst at Northwestern from 1965 to 1975.[51] No deaths occurred; 9 patients had major complications and 13 had minor complications. Division of the complications according to site—gastrointestinal, pulmonary, and cardiovascular—seems reasonable. Some are related to surgical technique.[45,59]

Wound infection is the most common postoperative complication. This diagnosis must always be accorded primary consideration when a patient develops a temperature elevation after the first few days following operation. Because drains are commonly used after renal surgery, deep wound infection and abscess formation are uncommon. Usually the local findings of erythema, edema, and tenderness signal the presence of wound infection. Probing a suspicious wound in a febrile patient may disclose an accumulation of pus. The infecting organism should be identified by smear and culture.

Treatment with adequate drainage and antibiotics, indicated by culture, usually results in prompt control of the infection. Ineffective control suggests the presence of a systemic disease such as diabetes, an unusual organism, an abnormal wound condition such as the presence of a foreign body, or a communication with a hollow viscus.

Wound dehiscence after renal surgery has become uncommon since the popularization of the flank approach to the kidney, the correction and control of serious metabolic derangements, and the advent of measures to control abnormalities such as tuberculous infection. As the abdominal approach to the kidney is used with greater frequency, the risk of dehiscence may well increase. Hernia may follow any incision, particularly if infection has occurred. A protusion of the muscles often persists after healing of a flank incision, probably primarily because of interference with the nerve supply. Repeated difficulty with wound healing should stimulate revision of closure techniques.

Serious secondary bleeding, usually recognized by brisk blood loss from a drain site or the development of pain, tenderness, muscle spasm, ecchymosis, and at times a palpable mass, must be managed much as primary hemorrhage is. If the patient's condition permits, adequate preparation for blood replacement before exploration is essential. If the situation is catastrophic, blood volume can be restored temporarily with albumin or a substitute while the wound is rapidly reopened to enable temporary control of the bleeding. Control, identification of site, and logical approach to repair are carried out much as in primary hemorrhage. In either primary or secondary hemorrhage, multiple bleeding sites should raise the possibility of a clotting disorder, which may become manifest after multiple transfusions, complicating the initial cause of bleeding.

Postoperative gastrointestinal complications include ileus, obstruction, and hemorrhage. Ileus is not uncommon following renal surgery by any approach. Our routine practice is to resume oral feeding only when bowel sounds are unquestionably active and to discontinue it if there is any evidence of ileus. When in doubt, we tend to apply preventive measures such as nasogastric suction and feeding restrictions rather than risk development of serious ileus. Mechanical bowel obstruction is not usually a complication of a flank exposure of the kidney, but it may occur after a transperitoneal approach to the kidney.

Severe gastrointestinal bleeding, usually from a peptic ulcer, has been seen occasionally after nephrectomy. The source of the blood loss is rarely immediately apparent. Unless a routine postoperative hemoglobin determination has been obtained, recognition of active blood loss may be difficult. Preventive measures such as the use of antacids, cimetidine, or nasogastric suction, especially if oral feeding is delayed, should be considered in patients with a history of peptic ulcer or in those subjected to prolonged stressful surgery.

Pulmonary complications, including pneumothorax, pneumonia, and atelectasis, are seen frequently enough following renal surgery to warrant careful consideration if the postoperative course is complicated. Pneumothorax is usually the result of an unrecognized surgical complication. Needle aspiration of the pleural cavity or the insertion of a catheter into the pleural cavity corrects this abnormality and restores relatively normal respiration.

Pneumonia and atelectasis can be prevented to some degree by treatment of pulmonary infection and by measures to reduce mucous secretion and to induce drainage pre- and postoperatively. Adequate relief of pain in the operative site while avoiding excessive sedation helps to reduce the incidence of these complications. Stimulated coughing, postural drainage, and aspiration combined with use of a variety of physical devices may be necessary to keep the tracheobronchial tree free of excessive secretion; occasionally a tracheostomy is required.

Cardiovascular complications, such as cerebrovascular accident, coronary occlusion, congestive heart failure, dissecting or leaking aneurysm, pulmonary embolism, and thrombophlebitis, occur after renal surgery, as they do after other major surgery. It is our opinion that meticulous care in the pre- and postoperative period reduces the incidence of these complications. Several factors seem to be of importance. These factors include avoiding hypotension and prolonged ileus, maintenance of adequate hydration, use of elastic support and correct position to encourage drainage of extremities with varicosities, and early ambulation.

Constant suspicion of the possibility of a serious cardiovascular complication during the postoperative period enables its early recognition and prompt institution of therapeutic measures.

REFERENCES

1. AHLBERG NE, BARTLEY O, CHIDEKEL N: Right and left gonadal veins: An anatomical and statistical study. Acta Radiol 4:593, 1966
2. ANSON BJ, CAULDWELL EW, PICK JW et al: The blood supply of the kidney, suprarenal gland, and associated structures. Surg Gynecol Obstet 84:313, 1947
3. ANSON BJ, DASELER EH: Common variations in renal anatomy, affecting blood supply, form, and topography. Surg Gynecol Obstet 112:439, 1961
4. ANSON BJ, KURTH LE: Common variations in the renal blood supply. Surg Gynecol Obstet 100:157, 1955
5. ANSON BJ, PICK JW, CAULDWELL EW: The anatomy of the commoner renal anomalies: Ectopic and horseshoe kidneys. J Urol 47:112, 1942
6. AREY LB: Developmental Anatomy, 7th ed. Philadelphia, WB Saunders, 1965
7. BODNER H, BRISKIN HJ: Subdiaphragmatic renal exposure by resection of the eleventh rib. Urol Cut Rev 54:272, 1950
8. BOOKSTEIN JJ, ABRAMS HL, BUENGER RE et al: Radiologic aspects of renovascular hypertension. Part 2. The role of urography in unilateral renovascular disease. JAMA 220:1225, 1972
9. BREMER JL: The origin of the renal artery in mammals and its anomalies. Am J Anat 18:179, 1915
10. CAMPBELL MF: Renal ectopy. J Urol 24:187, 1930
11. CASE EH, STILES JA: The effect of various surgical positions in vital capacity. Anesthesiology 7:29, 1946
12. CHUTE R: The thoracoabdominal incision in urological surgery. J Urol 65:784, 1951
13. CHUTE R, SOUTTER L, KERR WS: The value of the thoracoabdominal incision in the removal of kidney tumors. N Engl J Med 241:951, 1949
14. CLARKE WB: Handbook of the Surgery of the Kidneys. London, Oxford University Press, 1911
15. DAVIES E, SUTTON D: Hypertension and multiple renal arteries. Lancet 1:341, 1965
16. DEMING CL, RAY TA: Aortic compression in the management of massive hemorrhage from the renal artery at nephrectomy: Report of a case. J Urol 77:348, 1957
17. DERRICK FC, JR, HUGHES JC, III, LYNCH KM, JR: Combined abdominolumbar nephrectomy. J Urol 96:635, 1966
18. ENGEL WJ: The expanding role of the urologist in diagnosis and surgical treatment of renal diseases. J Urol 84:594, 1960
19. FITZSIMONS LE, GARVEY FK: Inferior vena caval injury: Case report. J Urol 82:285, 1959
20. FRIEDENBERG MJ, WALZ BJ, MCALISTER WH, LOCKSMITH JP, GALLAGHER TL: Roentgen size of normal kidneys: Computer analysis of 1286 cases. Radiol 84:1022, 1965
21. GRAVES FT: The anatomy of the intrarenal arteries and its application to segmental resection of the kidney. Br J Surg 42:132, 1954
22. GROSSMAN J: A note on the radiological demonstration of the perirenal space. J Anat 88:407, 1954
23. HELLSTRÖM J, FRANKSSON C: Operations on the kidneys. In Alksen CE, Dix VW, Weyrauch HM et al (eds.): Encyclopedia of Urology. Vol 13, VII. Berlin, Gottingen, Heidelberg-Springer-Verlag, 1961
24. HESS E: Resection of the rib in renal operations. J Urol 42:943, 1939
25. HODSON CJ: Hypertension of renal origin. In McLaren JW (ed): Modern Trends in Diagnostic Radiology. New York, Hoeber, 1960
26. HOFFMAN WW, GRAYHACK JT: The limitations of the intravenous pyelogram as a test of renal function. Surg Gynecol Obstet 110:503, 1960
27. HOLLINGSHEAD WH: Anatomy for surgeons, Vol II, The Thorax, Abdomen, and Pelvis. New York, Hoeber 1956
28. KELLY HA, BURNAM CF: Diseases of the Kidneys, Ureters, and Bladder, Vol I, pp 375–406. New York, Appleton, 1914
29. KÜSTER E: Ueber einen Fall von Nierenextirpation. Berl Klin Wschr 20:604, 1883
30. LAST RJ: Anatomy, Regional and Applied. London, Churchill, 1949
31. LYON R: An anterior extraperitoneal incision for kidney surgery. J Urol 79:383, 1958
32. MARSHALL DF: Urogenital wounds in an evacuation hospital. J Urol 55:119, 1946
33. MARSHALL M JR, JOHNSON SH, III: A simple direct approach to the renal pedicle. J Urol 84:24, 1960
34. MAYO WJ: The incision for lumbar exposure of the kidney. Ann Surg 55:63, 1912
35. MOELL H: Kidney size and its deviation from normal in acute failure. Acta Radiol (Suppl)206:5, 1961
36. MORGENSEN P, ROSSING N, GIESE J: Glomerular filtration rate measurement and ¹³¹I-Hippuran renography before unilateral nephrectomy. Scand J Urol Nephrol 6:228, 1972
37. MORRIS H: On the Origin and Progress of Renal Surgery: The Hunterian Lectures for 1898. London, Caswell, 1898
38. NAGAMATSU GR: Dorsolumbar approach to the kidney and adrenal with osteoplastic flap. J Urol 63:569, 1950
39. NAGAMATSU GR, LERMAN PH, BERMAN MH: The dorsolumbar flap incision in urologic surgery. J Urol 67:787, 1952
40. PATTERN BM: Foundations of Embryology. New York, McGraw-Hill, 1958
41. POURTEYRON cited by Moell H: Kidney size and its deviation from normal in acute renal failure. Acta Radiol (Suppl)206:8, 1961
42. POUTASSE EF: Anterior approach to upper urinary tract. J Urol 85:199–205, 1961
43. PRESMAN D: Eleventh intercostal space incision for renal surgery. J Urol 74:578, 1955

44. ROLNICK HC: Nephrostomy: Some clinical and experimental observations. Surg Gynecol Obstet 67:224, 1938

45. SAKATI IA, MARSHALL VF: Postoperative fatalities in urology. J Urol 95:412, 1966

46. SCHLEGEL JU, HAMWAY SA: Individual Renal Plasma Flow Determination in 2 Minutes. J Urol 116:282, 1976

47. SCOTT HW JR, CANTRELL JR, BUNCE PL: The principle of aortic compression in the management of massive hemorrhage from the renal pedicle after nephrectomy. J Urol 69:26, 1953

48. SCOTT RF JR, SELZMAN HM: Complications of nephrectomy: Review of 450 patients and a description of a modification of the transperitoneal approach. J Urol 95:307, 1966

49. SIMON AL: Normal renal size: An absolute criterion. AM J Roentgenol 92:270, 1964

50. SMITH DR, SCHULTE JW, SMART WR: Surgery of the kidney. In Campbell M (ed): Urology, Vol III, p 2324. Philadelphia, WB Saunders, 1963

51. STANISIC T, BABCOCK JR, GRAYHACK JT: Morbidity and Mortality of Renal Exploration for Cyst. Surg Gynecol Obstet 145:733, 1977

52. SYKES D: The arterial supply of the human kidney, with special reference to accessory renal arteries. Br J Surg 50:368, 1963

53. THORNTON JK: The Surgery of the Kidneys. The Haverian Lectures. London, Charles Griffen, 1890

54. TOBIN CE: The renal fascia and its relation to the transversalis fascia. Anat Rec 89:295, 1944

55. TURNER WARWICK RT: The supracostal approach to the renal area. Br J Urol 37:671, 1965

56. WALD H: The weight of normal adult human kidneys and its variability. Arch Pathol 23:493, 1937

57. WATSON FS: Historical sketch of genito-urinary surgery in America. In Cabot H (ed): Modern Urology, Vol I. Philadelphia, Lea & Febiger, 1918

58. WINTER CC: The excretory urogram as a kidney function test. J Urol 83:313, 1960

59. YEATES WK: Postnephrectomy arteriovenous fistula. Proc R Soc Med 60:112, 1967

60. YOUNG HH, DAVIS DM: Practice of Urology, Vol II, p 261. Philadelphia, WB Saunders, 1926

Partial Nephrectomy

6

Sam D. Graham, Jr.

Partial nephrectomy is a technique which, until relatively recently, has not been highly favored. Early attempts, beginning with Czerny in 1887, were frequently complicated by severe hemorrhage, sepsis, and fistulas. A revival of this procedure began in the 1950s, notably in patients with either stones or tuberculosis. With the advent of isoniazid therapy, the number of partial nephrectomies done for renal tuberculosis drastically declined, but new indications have since evolved. The procedure is ideally suited for clinical situations of localized disease when preservation of maximum renal function is essential.

The actual technique of partial nephrectomy varies according to clinical preference, but all methods incorporate four basic principles: early control of the main renal vasculature, minimal renal ischemic time, meticulous hemostasis, and complete closure of the collecting system. As long as these four principles are observed, the incidence of complications will be minimal.

This chapter will be devoted to partial nephrectomy as performed *in situ*. Techniques such as bench surgery and autotransplantation, while having certain indications, are usually not necessary and require specialized expertise and equipment. Furthermore, they may be impossible in certain circumstances.[51,52] The potential of partial nephrectomy for maximal renal preservation may increase its popularity. The variety of available techniques, each with its own specific indications, makes this procedure a worthwhile compromise between no surgery and total nephrectomy.

Anatomy of the Intrarenal Vasculature

Graves, who used plastic postmortem injections of the renal vasculature, is credited with the classical description of the intrarenal vasculature.[13] There is usually one main renal vessel branching from the aorta, which divides into an anterior and a posterior branch. These two branches, in turn,

supply five main renal segments, which are constant (Table 6-1).

The anterior branch supplies the majority of the renal blood flow, with four of the five segmental arteries usually derived from this branch. The apical segmental artery supplies the medial anterior upper pole. The upper anterior segmental artery supplies the remaining upper pole and central anterior kidney. The other two branches supplying the lower kidney are the middle anterior segmental artery, supplying the lower anterior kidney, and the lower segmental artery, supplying the anterior and posterior portions of the lower pole. The posterior branch of the main renal artery chiefly supplies the remaining posterior portion of the kidney but may occasionally supply a branch to the apical segment.

Graves found no cases of collateral arterial flow between segments, and all segments were constant. Aberrant "polar" arteries were actually segmented vessels with a precocious origin. Disease states rarely affected the segmented arterial anatomy other than by passive displacement.[14]

The intrarenal venous system does not follow a segmental pattern but instead intercommunicates through a vast plexus of venules. Thus, it is the arterial and not the venous system that is surgically important in partial nephrectomy. Graves also found that the pooling seen in arteriograms of renal carcinomas was due to partial venous obstruction rather than to arterial aberrations.[14]

Indications for Partial Nephrectomy

The decision to perform a partial nephrectomy is usually based on the amount of impairment of the contralateral renal function and the concomitant desire to preserve as much total renal function as possible. Specific indications for the procedure are similar to the indications for total nephrectomy, namely, stones, tumors, infections, and congenital anomalies (Table 6-2). If there is concern that postoperative renal insufficiency may result from

TABLE 6-1. Intrarenal Vasculature

Major Branch	Segmental Branch	Segment Supplied
Anterior	Upper	Part of upper pole, central anterior
	Middle	Lower anterior
	Lower	Lower pole, anterior and posterior
	Apical	Medial anterior upper pole
Posterior	Posterior	Posterior and sometimes apical

Graves FT: The anatomy of the intrarenal arteries and its application to segmental resection of the kidney. Br J Surg 42: 132, 1954.

TABLE 6-2. Indications for Partial Nephrectomy

Tumors
Stones
Infections
  Bacterial
  Granulomatous, including tuberculosis
Congenital atrophy in duplicated system
Ischemia
  Atherosclerotic
  Ask-Upmark
Trauma

total nephrectomy, then partial nephrectomy is undoubtedly the procedure of choice. Somewhat less firm indications are a localized disease segment, usually either upper or lower pole, when removal of the affected portion would provide a good chance of a cure. As Semb states, "Total nephrectomy should be performed only when absolutely necessary; that in local diseases of the kidney, the operative intervention should, whenever possible, be limited to the diseased part only."[39]

The type of partial nephrectomy used is usually based on surgical preference. For upper or lower pole lesions, either the guillotine or wedge-type resection can be employed, but for midportion lesions either of these techniques may be difficult or may result in complete loss of the renal unit. The enucleation technique, although obviously limited to tumors, may be employed in all areas of the kidney with minimal loss of renal function.

STONES

The initial enthusiasm for the use of partial nephrectomy in calculus disease has been tempered by the subsequent long term follow-up which shows only slight, if any, advantage over pyelolithotomy in preventing stone recurrence. At present, indications for partial nephrectomy in stone disease are in those kidneys with single or multiple stones in a dilated calix. This may or may not include chronic pyelonephritis in the parenchyma drained by the calix. A somewhat less firm indication is the presence of multiple stones in a calix, usually the lower pole, or in patients with dendritic calculi when the arm of the stone intrudes into the calix.[1,34]

TUMORS

Perhaps the greatest recent increase in interest in partial nephrectomy is for patients with either a tumor in a solitary kidney or bilateral renal tumors. Data collected by Grabstald and Aviles, Graham and Glenn, and Wickham have shown the survival rate of patients with renal cell carcinoma treated by partial nephrectomy to be at least comparable to total nephrectomy with dialysis, and approaching the mean operative survival rate statistics for all patients with renal cell carcinoma.[11,12,51] Tumors of both the parenchyma and the collecting system can be treated by this method, foregoing the need for total nephrectomy, dialysis, and possible transplantation.[4,8] Furthermore, partial nephrectomy obviates the theoretical additional risks of the use of the immunosuppressive drugs required for renal transplantation in a cancer patient. These risks include the possible acceleration of occult metastatic disease and the increased incidence of *de novo* tumors.[3] In view of the complications inherent in dialysis and transplantation, some authors have been advocating doing no surgery if it is not possible to do a partial nephrectomy in this situation.[20,38]

INFECTIONS

Chronic pyelonephritis and granulomatous disease are becoming much less likely as indications for partial nephrectomy than in the past. In tuberculosis, for example, the advent of new chemotherapeutic regimens, especially isoniazid, has drastically reduced the incidence of renal tuberculosis.[19,24] Indications now for partial nephrectomy in tuberculosis are only after failure of adequate medical therapy, particularly when there is persistent bacilluria due to either an abscess that will not completely involute or drug-resistant bacteria.[1,39] Calcification of a tuberculoma may be a sign of an abscess requiring surgical intervention, because calcified tuberculous abscesses are usually quite difficult to sterilize.[39]

Chronic pyelonephritis has been an indication in the past for partial nephrectomy, especially if pain, hematuria, or uncontrollable infection is present.[29] However, the recurrence rates have been high and thus the indications, again, should be failure of adequate and intensive medical therapy in the presence of an anatomic deformity.

CONGENITAL ANOMALIES

The most common congenital lesion requiring partial nephrectomy is in duplex systems, usually associated with an ectopic ureterocele.[54] The upper pole segment in these patients is frequently atrophic and is excised along with the ureter to the affected segment. If, however, the upper pole segment does show function, then attempts should be made to preserve it either through reimplantation of the ureter into the bladder or by pyelopyelostomy to the lower segment.[17,26]

VASCULAR DISEASE

With the increased interest in renal vascular lesions, especially associated with hypertension, Poutasse and others have had good results with the use of partial nephrectomies for segmental vascular disease.[35] Specifically, isolated congenital or atherosclerotic arterial stenosis, arteriovenous malformations, and intrarenal arterial aneurysms are all amenable to partial nephrectomy.[6,15] Patients with segmental renin-induced hypertension due to these causes or due to embolization of a segment of the kidney frequently show marked and immediate improvement.

RENAL TRAUMA

Renal trauma is the other major indication for partial nephrectomy. All but the most massive blunt injuries are usually managed conservatively, but occasionally indications may arise for exploration and partial nephrectomy, such as morcellation of part of the kidney. Penetrating wounds, particularly due to high-velocity projectiles, are usually explored. The kidneys in these cases will exhibit late damage due to the concussion of the missile and will require wide débridement with the same techniques used in a formal partial nephrectomy.

MISCELLANEOUS

Localized polycystic renal disease, segmental medullary sponge kidney, benign renal cysts, localized hydronephrosis, and ureteropelvic junction (UPJ) obstruction are among the remaining indications for partial nephrectomy.[18,25,35] All of these cases are anecdotal and are mentioned only to show the potential applications of partial nephrectomy.

Preoperative Preparation

In most patients undergoing partial nephrectomy, the kidney requiring surgery maintains most, if not all, of the existing renal function. Therefore, it is imperative that all possible attempts be made to preserve as much renal function as possible. Preoperative renal function studies such as serum blood urea nitrogen (BUN) and creatinine are of particular interest if the patient has had iodinated contrast studies such as intravenous pyelograms or arteriograms 24 hr to 48 hr prior to surgery. Acute tubular necrosis may follow these studies, resulting in confusion about the cause of reduced function following surgery and adding to the postoperative morbidity. All patients should be well hydrated with intravenous fluid beginning the evening prior to surgery. The operating room personnel should be made aware of the need for ice-slush saline and vascular or other special instruments. Finally, it is important that the patient understand that there is some risk that the solitary kidney may not survive, rendering him anephric and requiring hemodialysis for the rest of his life.

Instruments

Other than vascular instruments, most of the necessary instruments for partial nephrectomy can be found in any standard abdominal tray. If a rib is to be taken, then periosteal elevators and rib cutters are obviously necessary. Vascular instruments that should be available include bulldog, DeBakey, and Satinsky vascular clamps, but other vascular clamps such as the Fogarty may be preferred by the operating surgeon. The renal parenchymal incisions can be made with a scalpel blade, the scalpel handle, or a neurosurgical spatula. Fine-tipped forceps and needle holders are useful for the collecting system and parenchymal closure.

Regional Hypothermia

With the advent of intraoperative regional hypothermia, the incidence of ischemia-related complications has fallen considerably. Experimental work reported by Semb showed that with warm ischemia, 11 minutes was the maximum time that could be taken to occlude the renal vessels and have only a minimum reaction. Eighteen minutes produced a medium reaction, and 50 minutes produced renal loss. By cooling the kidney with ice-slush saline, however, the safe occlusive time was increased to 26 minutes. This increase was primarily due to a marked slowing of the renal metabolism, as measured by a decrease in the oxygen consumption to 10% to 15%.[39] Novick and co-workers, by perfusing the *in situ* kidney through a preoperatively placed Swan–Ganz catheter, have been able to extend the safe ischemic time to 3 hours.[30]

The technique of local hypothermia is quite simple. After the kidney is dissected free, the vessels are isolated, and all other preparations are completed for the partial nephrectomy, a rubber dam, or plastic bag with a draw-string such as is used for intestinal surgery, is placed around the kidney. Sterile ice-slush saline, prepared before surgery, is then poured into the wound around and over the kidney and allowed to remain for 5 to 10 minutes prior to occluding the renal artery. Using this technique, rapid surface and core cooling are possible; the core temperature will drop to 20° C within 10 minutes and will remain at this level for another 30 minutes.[42] Additional ice-slush saline may be added as necessary.

Operative Approach and Techniques

APPROACH

The operative approach to a kidney for partial nephrectomy should ensure both adequate exposure of the segment to be excised and good control of the vessels. The standard 11th-rib flank approach with the patient in full or 45 degree modified flank position is usually adequate for this purpose. An alternative incision is the supracostal 11th-rib incision popularized by Richard Turner Warwick, especially for left-sided upper pole lesions.[44] The anterior transperitoneal approach offers good vascular exposure, but not as good exposure of upper pole lesions.

After Gerota's fascia is opened, the vascular pedicle is identified and the renal artery and renal vein are dissected free, with umbilical tapes being placed around them. Enough of each vessel must be isolated to ensure that vascular clamps can be easily placed. At this time, on left-sided lesions, the surgeon may elect to isolate, ligate, and divide the adrenal or gonadal branch veins to give better exposure of the renal artery as well as better control of the renal vein. If the procedure elected is either the wedge or the guillotine method, the ice-slush saline is usually used and a rubber dam is placed around the kidney. The anesthesiologist gives 25 g to 50 g of mannitol intravenously immediately prior to occluding the vascular pedicle. The vascular clamps are then applied, with the arterial clamp being applied first. The kidney should become pale and soft soon after the arterial clamp is applied. Failure of the kidney to do so indicates that there is a branch artery which has not been occluded. If a branch is suspected, the arterial clamp is removed and the branch isolated and occluded. After the clamps are applied and the kidney softens, the ice-slush saline is poured into the wound, and about 5 to 10 minutes are allowed for the kidney to cool.

An alternative method, advocated by Semb, involves meticulous dissection of the branch arteries to locate the branch supplying the segment to be resected.[39] An incision is made into the anterior parenchyma to expose the renal sinus, where the segmented vessels are dissected free. It is important that the dissection be done within the renal sinus because the vascular anatomy is most constant in this region. When the branch is located, temporary occlusion of the vessel should produce immediate paling and softening of the segment in question. Frequently, however, the demarcation line of the area supplied by the branch vessel and the line of proposed resection do not correspond, forcing the surgeon to resort to occlusion of the main renal artery. This approach, furthermore, is time consuming, thus adding to the possible hazards of the surgery.

SPECIFIC TECHNIQUES

The various surgical techniques all have several common traits. It is important that the surgeon move rapidly but skillfully through the procedure. Before occluding the vessels, the surgeon must make sure that all suture material and instruments needed are present on the instrument table to avoid unnecessary delays. During the surgery, care must be taken to avoid traumatizing more kidney than is absolutely necessary and especially to avoid traumatizing the major vessels. The closure of the collecting system should be as nearly watertight as possible. Hemostasis is obtained by figure-of-eight sutures of 4–0 Vicryl or chromic catgut, of the visible ends of vessels exposed during the incision. Arcuate vessels at the corticomedullary junction are tied on the medullary side because this tissue is firmer and holds sutures better. Interlobar vessels can be sutured by passing the needle into and then out of the adjacent infundibulum of the collecting system to catch the vessels below the cut parenchymal surface.[33] All smaller vessels can usually be controlled by closing the capsule and applying manual pressure for approximately 5 minutes.[35] Alternatively, large mattress sutures can be used to close the parenchyma, especially in the guillotine method, however, this destroys more nephrons and should be used only as a last resort in solitary kidneys.

Electrocoagulation of intrarenal vessels should never be used. Owing to the high electrolyte content of the renal parenchyma, the electrical current is widely dissipated. Murphy's studies showed extensive destruction of the parenchyma and delayed healing in kidneys in which electrocoagulation had been used, as compared to kidneys in which suture ligation of vessels had been performed.[27]

Most authors advocate complete resection of the caliceal neck to prevent a site of urinary stasis infection and subsequent stone formation, especially in partial nephrectomies for stones.[47] However, in cases in which complete resection of the caliceal neck would compromise the remaining renal tissue, as in crossed fused ectopia, it is better to leave some residual calix than to risk losing the entire kidney.[48]

Guillotine Method

The guillotine method is the oldest and most popular method of partial nephrectomy. It is simpler and quicker to perform than the wedge method, offers better exposure of the vessels and the collecting system, and is more amenable to intraoperative revisions. Its chief disadvantage is the obviously greater difficulty in closing the parenchyma.

After vascular occlusion and cooling of the kidney, the capsule is incised along the axis of the kidney and peeled back by sharp and blunt dissection to approximately 1 cm proximal to the intended line of excision (Fig. 6-1). This form of partial nephrectomy is presently practiced in two ways. The classical method involves deciding on a proximal line of excision, excising the tissue, and closure. A variation described by Oravisto and others involves serially slicing the kidney like a loaf of bread until the proximal border of the affected portion is found.[31] This variation is most frequently used for dendritic calculi, and the serial slicing is carried up to the calix containing the calculus. The calculus is removed and the collecting system is closed. Regardless of the technique, because of the renal vasculature patterns, all lines of excision should be done on a line radial from the hilum.

The necessity of obtaining a watertight closure of the collecting system cannot be overstressed, because a good parenchymal closure with the guillotine method is difficult to perform (Fig. 6-2). It is imperative that precise control of hemostasis be obtained by suture ligatures. Manual compression over the severed end, with or without Surgicel or Gelfoam, will usually control any venous ooze. Closure is easier if the vascular clamps are left in place until all sutures are placed. If the capsule cannot be closed over the defect, then a free peritoneal graft can be employed.[27,45]

Wedge Method

The wedge method was developed to aid in parenchymal closure, but it has the inherent disadvantage of possible ischemia of the bivalved edges, as well as limited access to the calices and severed vessels.[2] Revisions of the initial excision may also be somewhat more difficult.

The beginning of this technique, as in the guillotine method, involves excising the capsule along the axis of the kidney and peeling the capsule back (Fig. 6-3). The intended incision lines into the parenchyma should be planned to avoid damage to the hilar structures. The affected parenchyma is removed, and the visible vessels are suture ligated. Parenchymal closure may be performed with serial layers of absorbable suture in the parenchyma or just in the capsule, with manual pressure for a few minutes following vascular release. As in the guillotine method, the easiest closure is performed prior to release of vascular occlusion.

Modifications

Modifications of the guillotine and wedge methods are primarily directed at the more popular and

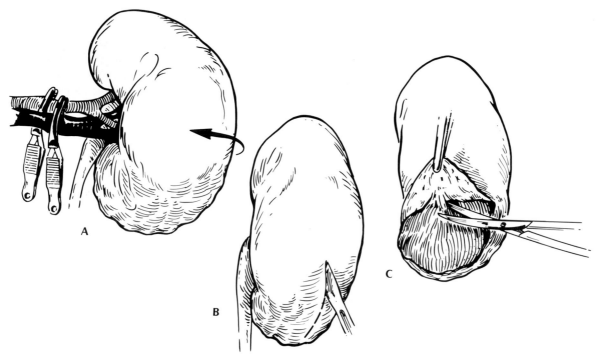

FIG. 6-1. General procedure prior to parenchymal resection: **(A)** once vascular control is attained, the lower pole lesion is visualized; **(B)** the renal capsule is incised; **(C)** the capsule is reflected by sharp and blunt dissection.

FIG. 6-2. **(A)** Shows the line of intended excision of the lesion with the guillotine method of partial nephrectomy. **(B)** Hemostasis is attained by suture ligation. **(C)** The collecting system is closed. **(D)** The capsule is closed over the severed parenchyma.

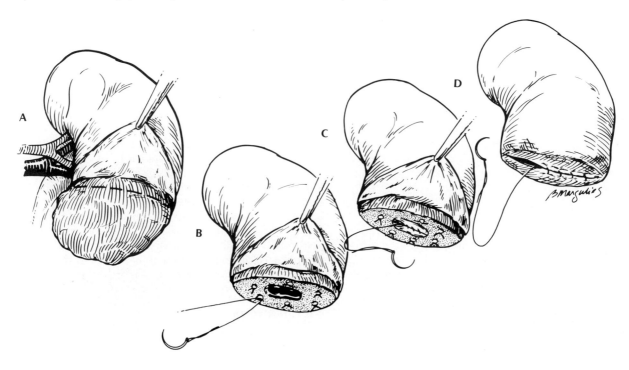

accepted guillotine method. Kim and Williams and co-workers describe similar techniques involving a circumferential No. 1 chromic ligature around the kidney proximal to the line of resection.[21,53] As the ligature is tightened, the relatively friable parenchyma is cut, while the more resistant vessels and collecting system are mass ligated. The resection is then carried out distal to this ligature with a knife. Attention to hemostasis and closure of the collecting system are the same as in all other techniques.

Modifications to reduce intraoperative blood loss have been described by Storm, Kauffman, and Longmire and Wein, Carpiniello, and Murphy.[41,50] Wein's technique involves using the assistant's hand to compress the parenchyma while the resection is performed, and then periodically releasing the pressure to locate several vessels. Storm's modification consists of a large clamp, capable of

surrounding the renal parenchyma and thus replacing the assistant's hand.

Additional modifications have been advocated to promote renal drainage. A few authors advocate the use of a nephrostomy tube, but this is not necessary and may in fact enhance fistula formation. Nephropexy is commonly performed. Occasionally a pyeloplasty is carried out in conjunction with a lower pole nephrectomy to promote emptying, but again this is rarely necessary.[18]

Finally, experimental modifications have been employed using CO_2 lasers for resection and various tissue glues such as 2-cyanoacrylate for closure,[43] but none of these newer modifications have gained widespread acceptance.[23]

Enucleation

The enucleation method as described by Colston, Graham and Glenn, and Vermooten is a form of

FIG. 6-3. In wedge resection, **(A)** the capsule is reflected proximal to the intended lines of excision; **(B)** hemostasis is attained by suture ligation; **(C)** the collecting system is closed; **(D)** the parenchyma is closed; **(E)** the capsule is closed.

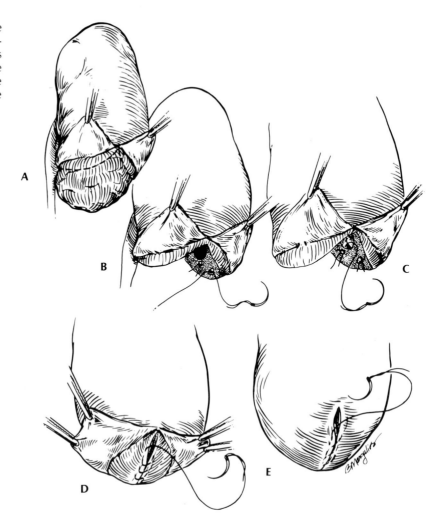

partial nephrectomy for renal tumors which, unlike the guillotine and wedge methods, is not limited to lesions of the upper or lower poles.[8,12,46] This method also has the advantages of rapidity, simplicity, and the possibility of removing multiple lesions. Complete vascular control is not necessary because simple compression of the vascular pedicle between the fingers or against the spinal column is usually sufficient. Finally, the method permits entry into the collecting system and thus results in a low incidence of urinary fistula. The major disadvantage of this method versus the other two methods is the risk of leaving residual malignancy. Furthermore, this technique is limited primarily to cortical tumors, which are usually surrounded by a fibrous pseudocapsule.

The technique first involves incision of the capsule over the lesion (Fig. 6-4). The butt end of the scalpel is then used to enucleate the tumor. Surface ligatures are used for hemostasis, and if an ooze persists, Gelfoam, Surgicel, or fat may be packed into the cavity.[12]

Miscellaneous

Other techniques of partial nephrectomy are dictated by the indication for the procedure. The most common of these cases have an ectopic ureterocele and a nonfunctioning, atrophic upper pole segment. In these cases, the ureter is traced to its juncture with the renal segment. By a combination of sharp and blunt dissection, the plane of cleavage between the upper and lower renal segments is defined and the upper segment is resected.[54] Watts notes that heminephrectomy in duplex or crossed fused ectopia can be performed by removing only the hydronephrotic sac, and that total excision of the collecting system is unnecessary. He reports good results, with no leaks, in six cases.[48]

Complications

The major complications following partial nephrectomy are of three types: bleeding, both immediate and delayed; fistula formation due to

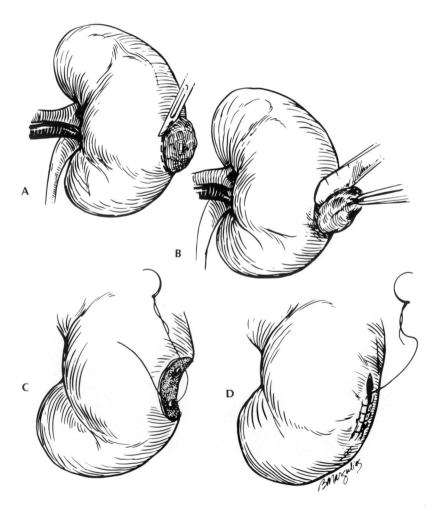

FIG. 6-4. Enucleation method: **(A)** incision of the capsule; **(B)** blunt enucleation of the tumor; **(C)** suture ligation of the parenchymal vessels; **(D)** closure of the capsule

inadequate closure of the collecting system; and loss of function, either spontaneously or because of other complications, leading to nephrectomy (Table 6-3). The overall morbidity rate in surgery on solitary kidneys has been reported to be as high as 37%, and the majority of these cases fall into the three major complications categories.[10] Less common complications include arteriovenous malformation and aneurysm formations in the resected parenchyma,[36,40] infection, and cardiopulmonary complications. The mortality rate in most series is approximately 0.5%.

The most commonly seen complication is bleeding. Intraoperative blood loss was measured in one series and averaged 906 ml.[49] Meticulous attention to hemostasis and the use of cold ischemia can reduce this complication rate considerably. Postoperative bleeding is the most common cause of secondary nephrectomy in most series.[16,34]

The second most common complication of partial nephrectomy is fistula formation. Usually this is due to inadequate closure of the collecting system, but fistulas due to infection have been reported. Most fistulas are temporary and close spontaneously with or without the aid of a ureteral catheter. Some, however, must be surgically corrected either by curettage or resection. In a few cases, the complication of a fistula necessitates a nephrectomy.

Perhaps the most disastrous complication of partial nephrectomies in solitary kidneys is the loss of the kidney, either spontaneously or surgically. The most commonly cited cause of complete spontaneous loss of function is an injury of the renal vasculature. Surgical removal of a kidney is most commonly the result of life-threatening hemorrhage. Partial loss of renal function is a more common complication and is usually related to either the ischemia time during surgery or the amount of resected tissue. In patients undergoing partial nephrectomies in the face of compromised or absent contralateral function, the serum BUN and creatinine will frequently show a small and transient elevation, which usually subsides within a week.

There is considerable controversy surrounding the recurrence rates in patients undergoing partial nephrectomy for stones. Several large series have shown a very low incidence of recurrence, especially when compared to either pyelolithotomy or nephrolithotomy.[22,49] Studies with longer followup, however, have shown the incidence to range from 37% to 54%.[28,37] This is further borne out by Williams's observations that the average time period between recurrences was 8.4 years.[55] Attempts have been made to distinguish between "true" stone recurrences and "false" recurrences due to residual stones, but the total incidence of recur-

TABLE 6-3. Complications of Partial Nephrectomy

Overall Morbidity	Percent Incidence	Reference
Bleeding		
Immediate (<48 hr)	37	10
Delayed	14	6
Fistula		
Urinary	0–6	6,9,16
Other	4	9
Loss of function—partial		
Spontaneous—complete	0.5–3	7,9,19,28,39
Nephrectomy due to complications	4–5	7,28
Stone recurrence		
<5 years followup	0–6.4–12	22,32
>5 years followup	34–57	28,37–55
Infection recurrence	8–30	6,7
Mortality	0–69	5,6,39
Repeat surgery	10	9,16
Other (anecdotal)		
Aneurysm formation		36
Arteriovenous fistula formation		40

rence is what is clinically important, and this remains high over the long term. Stone recurrences after partial nephrectomy were shown by Wald and co-workers to be positively correlated with residual stones and postoperative infections but not correlated with preoperative infection or kidney pathology.[47]

Postoperative Renal Function

Most patients undergoing partial nephrectomy in an actual or functionally solitary kidney will experience a brief decrease in renal function as measured by a rise in serum BUN and creatinine. The duration and degree of this elevation is usually directly proportional to the length of ischemic time and degree of trauma to the kidney.[39] The renal function, however, usually returns to levels comparable to the preoperative levels. Failure to do so, or a precipitous and progressive renal failure, should be aggressively studied for the etiology and managed appropriately; otherwise the rate of complications will increase and cause further loss of nephrons.

Long-term follow-up of patients undergoing partial nephrectomy shows that the degree of renal impairment correlates somewhat with the amount of parenchyma removed. Semb's studies of 28 patients who had 65% to 85% of their total parenchyma removed showed no patient suffering from severe renal insufficiency, with creatinine clearances ranging from 20 ml/min to 87 ml/min.[39] One patient with 85% of his parenchyma resected had a creatinine clearance of 72 ml/min. This also correlates with Hoeg's studies in dogs, in which the remaining parenchyma was found to have at least the same, and sometimes even a greater, percent of function as the percent of remaining renal mass, indicating some degree of compensatory hypertrophy.[19]

REFERENCES

1. ANDERSON CK: Partial nephrectomy: A pathological evaluation. Proc R Soc Med 67:459, 1974
2. BARZILAY BI, KEDEU SS: Surgical treatment of staghorn calculus by partial nephrectomy and pyelocalicotomy. J Urol 108:689, 1972
3. BELZER FO, SCHWEIZER RT, KOUNTZ SL et al: Malignancy and immunosuppression. Renal transplantation in patients with primary renal neoplasms. Transplantation 13:164, 1972
4. BERAHA D, BLOCK NL, POLITANO VA: Simultaneous surgical management of bilateral hypernephroma: An alternative therapy. J Urol 118:648, 1976
5. BISCHOFF PF: The surgical treatment of the solitary kidney. Urol Int 24:527, 1969
6. BUTARAZZI PJ, DEVINE PC, DEVINE CJ et al: The indications, complications, and results of partial nephrectomy. J Urol 99:376, 1968
7. COLEMAN CH, WITHERINGTON R: A review of 117 partial nephrectomies. J Urol 122:11, 1979
8. COLSTON JAC: Operation for tumor in a solitary kidney. Western Surg Gynecol Obstet 68:141, 1960
9. CULP OS, HENDRICKS ED: Potentialities of partial nephrectomy. Surg Clin North Am 39:887, 1959
10. DEES JE: Prognosis of the solitary kidney. J Urol 83:550, 1960
11. GRABSTALD H, AVILES E: Renal cell carcinoma in the solitary or sole functioning kidney. Cancer 22:973, 1968
12. GRAHAM SD, JR, GLENN JF: Enucleative surgery for renal malignancy. J Urol 122:546, 1979
13. GRAVES FT: The anatomy of the intrarenal arteries and its application to segmental resection of the kidney. Br J Surg 42:132, 1954
14. GRAVES FT: The anatomy of the intrarenal arteries in health and disease. Br J Surg 43:605, 1955
15. HALE RW, VIETA JO: Intrarenal aneurysm treated by partial nephrectomy: Report of a case. J Urol 91:137, 1964
16. HAMM FC, FINKELSTEIN P: Partial nephrectomy. J Urol 82:625, 1959
17. HENDREN WH, MONFROT GJ: Surgical correction of ureteroceles in children. J Pediatr Surg 6:235, 1971
18. HJORT EF: Partial resection of the renal pelvis and pole of the kidney for hydronephrosis. Br J Urol 43:406, 1971
19. HOEG K: The early forms of renal tuberculosis and the function of the resected kidney. Acta Chir Scand (Suppl)302:1, 1972
20. JOHNSON DE, VONESCHENBACH A, STERNBERG J: Bilateral renal cell carcinoma. J Urol 119:23, 1978
21. KIM SK: New techniques of partial nephrectomy. J Urol 102:165, 1969
22. MARSHALL VR, SINGH M, TRESIDDER GC et al: The place of partial nephrectomy in the management of renal calyceal calculi. Br J Urol 47:759, 1976
23. MEIRAZ D, PELED I, GASSNER S et al: The use of the CO$_2$ laser for partial nephrectomy: An experimental study. Invest Urol 15:262, 1977
24. MINAMI T: Partial nephrectomy in renal tuberculosis. Urol Int 5:358, 1957
25. MODARELLI RO, WETTLAUFER JN: Surgically documented segmental medullary sponge kidney: A case report. J Urol 117:244, 1977
26. MOGG RA: Some observations on the ectopic ureter and ureterocele. J Urol 97:1003, 1967
27. MURPHY JJ, GLANTZ W, SCHOENBERG HW: The healing of renal wounds. III. A comparison of electrocoagulation and suture ligation for hemostasis in partial nephrectomy. J Urol 85:882, 1961
28. MYRVOLD H, FRITJOFSSON A: Late results of partial nephrectomy for renal lithiasis. Scand J Urol Nephrol 5:57, 1971

29. MYRVOLD H, FRITJOFSSON A: Conservative renal surgery in pyelonephritis: A followup study. Scand J Urol Nephrol 6:116, 1972

30. NOVICK AC, STEWART BH, STRAFFON RA et al: Partial nephrectomy in the treatment of renal adenocarcinoma. J Urol 118:932, 1977

31. ORAVISTO KJ: Transverse partial nephrectomy. Acta Chir Scand 130:331, 1965

32. PAPATHANASSIADIS S, SWINNEY J: Results of partial nephrectomy compared with pyelolithotomy and nephrolithotomy. Br J Urol 38:403, 1966

33. PARRY WL, FINELLI JF: Some consideration in the technique of partial nephrectomy. J Urol 82:562, 1959

34. PEDERSON JF: Partial nephrectomy for nephrolithiasis. Scand J Urol Nephrol 5:171, 1971

35. POUTASSE EF: Partial nephrectomy: New techniques, approach, operative indications, and review of 51 cases. J Urol 88:153, 1962

36. REZVANI A, WARD JN, LAVENGOOD RW: Intrarenal aneurysm following partial nephrectomy. Urology 2:286, 1973

37. ROSE MB, FOLLOWS OJ: Partial nephrectomy for stone disease. Br J Urol 49:605, 1977

38. SCHIFF M, BAGLEY DH, LYTTON B: Treatment of solitary and bilateral renal carcinomas. J Urol 121:581, 1979

39. SEMB C: Conservative renal surgery. J R Coll Surg Edinb 10:9, 1964

40. SNODGRASS WT, ROBINSON MJ: Intrarenal arteriovenous fistula: A complication of partial nephrectomy. J Urol 91:135, 1964

41. STORM FIC, KAUFFMAN JJ, LONGMIRE WP: Kidney resection clamp: New instrument. Urology 6:494, 1975

42. TAYLOR JS: Evaluation of a technique of kidney cooling for partial nephrectomy. Br J Urol 47:230, 1975

43. TRUSS F, THIEL KH, RATHERT P et al: Improved technique of non-suture closure of renal wounds. J Urol 95:607, 1966

44. TURNER WARWICK RT: The supracostal approach to the renal area. Br J Urol 37:671, 1965

45. VANDEPUT JJ, TANNER JC, EBERHART C: Partial nephrectomy: Experimental closure with a free peritoneal graft. J Urol 93:364, 1967

46. VERMOOTEN V: Indications for conservative surgery in certain renal tumors: A study based on the growth pattern of the clear cell carcinoma. J Urol 64:200, 1950

47. WALD U, CAINE M, SOLOMON H: Partial nephrectomy in surgical treatment of calculous disease. Urology 11:343, 1978

48. WATTS HG: Heminephrectomy: A simplified technique. Aust NZ J Surg 37:256, 1968

49. WEIN AJ, CARPINIELLO VL, MULHOLLAND SG et al: Partial nephrectomy: Review of 80 cases emphasizing its role in management of localized renal stone disease. Urology 10:193, 1977

50. WEIN AJ, CARPINIELLO VL, MURPHY JJ: A simple technique for partial nephrectomy. Surg Gynecol Obstet 146:620, 1978

51. WICKHAM JEA: Conservative renal surgery for adenocarcinoma. Br J Urol 47:25, 1975

52. WIENER ES: Bilateral partial nephrectomy for large Wilm's tumors. J Pediatr Surg 11:867, 1976

53. WILLIAMS DF, SCHAPIRO AE, ARCONTI JS et al: A new technique of partial nephrectomy. J Urol 97:955, 1967

54. WILLIAMS DI, WOODARD JR: Problems in the management of ectopic ureteroceles. J Urol 92:635, 1964

55. WILLIAMS RE: Long term survey of 538 patients with upper urinary tract stone. Br J Urol 35:416, 1963

Radical Nephrectomy

7

Charles J. Robson

Radical nephrectomy is the removal *en bloc* of the kidney, perinephric fat, Gerota's fascia, overlying posterior parietal peritoneum, and the adrenal gland.[9] The lymph nodes from the crus of the diaphragm to the bifurcation of the great vessel on the ipsilateral side are also removed, together with the nodes behind, in front of, and medial to the great vessels. Whenever possible, this node dissection is done along with the nephrectomy, but frequently, as in the case of a very large tumor, the kidney has to be removed prior to lymph gland dissection in order to give better exposure.

Indications

The prime indication for radical nephrectomy is hypernephroma or adenocarcinoma of the kidney (nephrocarcinoma). It has been shown that the perinephric fat is involved in 42% of these cases, the adrenal in 6%, and the lymph nodes in 23%. This procedure also has been used in cases of carcinoma of the renal pelvis and in cases of Wilms' tumor, although with the advances in chemotherapy for the latter, dissection of the lymphatic drainage field is questionable.

There are a variety of ways in which renal carcinoma may present. The classic triad of pain, hematuria, and palpable mass is relatively rare and occurs late.[5] About 40% of the patients have hematuria or other urinary complaints, but just as many exhibit only systemic signs and symptoms—fever, anemia, erythrocythemia, hypercalcemia, and liver dysfunction.[1,4] The other 20% may show no evidence of a renal mass other than radiographic. When the diagnosis is made, 15% of the patients will already have symptomatic metastases such as chronic cough or bone pain. In these patients, a biopsy of the metastasis may lead to the primary diagnosis.[7]

Preoperative Assessment

Once a renal mass is found, there are a number of avenues to follow in making an accurate preoperative assessment. Intravenous and retrograde urography are seldom specific enough. Nephrotomography is a relatively safe and reliable way of differentiating renal cysts from tumors, with an accuracy rate of up to 85% when nephrotomograms are of excellent quality. Renal arteriography, venography, and venacavography all have their place in identifying and staging renal tumors. The degree to which they are used should be an individual consideration for each patient. These studies have considerable value in guiding the surgeon in the ultimate dissection of a renal tumor. It is our practice to explore most renal masses surgically for a final diagnosis, even when angiography suggests the lesion is cystic. A small percentage of avascular and cystic tumors exists, rendering the radiographic diagnosis imperfect by perhaps 5% to 10% false-negative results.[3]

We recommend percutaneous needle puncture and aspiration of apparent renal cysts in selected patients whose general physical condition makes exploration hazardous. Fluid from the cyst is characterized as to content of fat, blood, and malignant cells. The cyst space is studied radiographically by air and contrast instillations. It is difficult and potentially hazardous to attempt to puncture a cyst in the upper pole or peripelvic area.

Further staging of a tumor to determine its apparent operability involves a search for metastases. There is no convincing evidence that removing a primary renal tumor affects the secondary deposits. However, pain and bleeding sometimes require nephrectomy, even in the presence of spread beyond the kidney. Occasionally, removing a solitary metastasis seems justified, especially if it appears a considerable time after the nephrectomy.[13]

Metastases in the chest may be occult. Laminagraphy and mediastinoscopy have been recommended to detect them. Bone survey and isotope scanning may be used. An assessment of total and individual renal function by creatinine clearance and isotope renography, respectively, should accompany the general evaluation of a nephrectomy candidate.[11]

In addition to the preoperative assessment procedures already described, staging tools include a technetium skeletal scan with radiographic follow-up on any "hot spots," computed tomographic (CT) scans of the area, whole lung tomograms, angiograms, and liver function studies.

CT scans have been of great use in staging and show involvement of the liver by direct extension, the colon, the spleen, and the lymph nodes. Whole lung tomograms are important because in several cases multiple pulmonary secondaries have been seen by this technique when they were not apparent on a straight anteroposterior (AP) and lateral scan of the chest. CT chest scans may also be used but tend to be too sensitive for this purpose. They show small fibromas and other masses that may be interpreted as secondaries.

Angiography should include a "flush" aortogram to provide information on the position and numbers of renal arteries, thus allowing the surgeon to occlude them early in the procedure. Selective catheterization of the renal artery also should be performed, using epinephrine to demonstrate the presence of tumor vessels not only in the kidney but also in the perinephric fat and liver if these are involved. The celiac axis also should be catheterized in an attempt to ascertain the presence of liver metastases. The inferior vena cava should be catheterized in order to demonstrate the involvement by tumor thrombi of the renal vein and vena cava itself.

In about 10% of the cases, the results of certain liver function tests relate to prognosis. For example, if alpha-1 globulin levels, alkaline phosphatase levels, and prothrombin times are elevated, their return to normal following nephrectomy is a good prognostic sign, whereas their reelevation at a later date signifies a poor prognosis.

Surgical Approach

The surgical approach, by whatever route, should allow early occlusion of the renal vessels, preferably the artery prior to the vein; removal of the kidney, together with the overlying peritoneum, Gerota's fascia, and the perinephric fat capsule as an intact mass; and access to the lymphatics from the crus of the diaphragm to the pelvic brim.[10] We routinely use the thoracoabdominal approach through the bed of the 9th or 10th rib except in cases of previous chest disease or when respiratory reserve is low.[2,6,8] In such cases we use a supra-T10 extrapleural approach, as advocated by Turner Warwick.[12] For small tumors in the lower pole we use the transperitoneal route.

EXPOSURE OF THE RENAL VESSELS

After the peritoneal cavity has been opened and thoroughly palpated for presence of secondaries, the dissection begins on the lateral side of the ascending or descending colon where the posterior parietal peritoneum is opened along the "white" line (Fig. 7-1). The colon is then displaced toward the midline. On the right side the duodenum is also mobilized using the Kocher maneuver. Dissection is then carried out along the lateral aspect of the great vessel of the involved side until the renal vein and renal artery are located. On the left side the superior mesenteric artery must be carefully avoided; it may be displaced by a very large tumor and mistaken for the renal.

CLAMPING OF THE RENAL VESSELS

Whenever possible the renal artery should be occluded prior to the renal vein (Fig. 7-2). This minimizes the chance of tumor emboli due to either handling of the kidney or change of the hemodynamics, which may result from clamping the vein as a primary procedure. The renal artery usually lies behind the renal vein, which can usually be gently retracted by a long eyelid retractor, thus exposing the artery. The artery is then ligated using a nonabsorbable suture with two ligatures on the proximal end.

Figure 7-3 shows the left renal vein and the gonadal vein being occluded after the renal artery has been divided. On the right side is demonstrated one way of dealing with a thrombus which has involved the vena cava. After division of the renal artery a Satinsky clamp may be used to partially occlude the vena cava, thus allowing the renal vein and cava to be opened and the tumor thrombus to be removed. An alternative approach is to occlude the vena cava above and below and also to occlude the opposite renal vein and lumbar veins draining into that segment of the cava. The inferior vena cava may then be opened in a longitudinal fashion and the thrombus removed. The thrombus is usually found to lie freely in the cava and rarely invades the wall. The opening in the cava then should be closed using a running waxed silk 6-0 arterial suture.

DISSECTION AND LIGATION

The dissection proceeds, keeping Gerota's fascia intact, usually including posteriorly the fascia overlying the quadratus lumborum. Superiorly, the adrenal is included in the dissection and its blood

FIG. 7-1. The posterior peritoneum may be opened adjacent to the great vessels for exposure and isolation of renal vasculature.

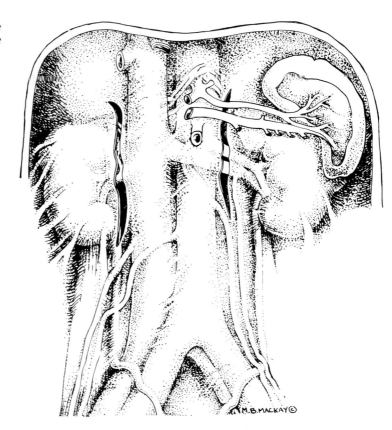

FIG. 7-2. The renal artery is clamped, ligated, and divided prior to occlusion of the renal vein.

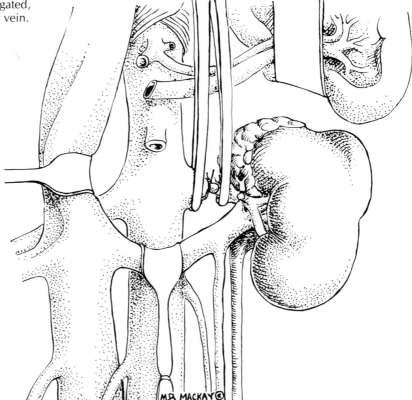

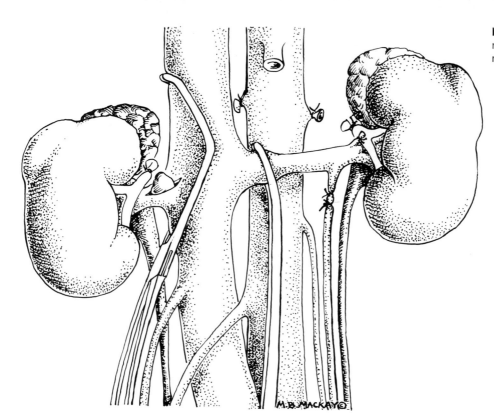

FIG. 7-3. On the left, both the renal vein and the gonadal vein must be secured and ligated.

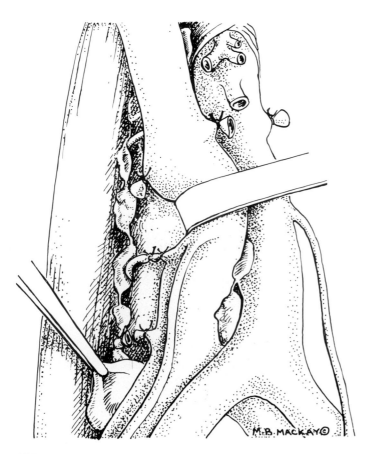

FIG. 7-4. Retroperitoneal node dissection should extend from the crus of the diaphragm to the lower extent of the aorta and vena cava.

supply is easily managed using small plastic clips. The ureter is divided in the usual manner and ligated.

NODE DISSECTION AND CLOSURE

Node dissection should extend from the crus of the diaphragm to the bifurcation of the aorta on the left and to the inferior end of the vena cava on the right (Fig. 7-4). Lymphatics should be removed in continuity from the lateral side of the great vessel, behind the involved great vessel, and between the two great vessels. Lumbar veins may be ligated with impunity, but it is wise not to divide more than three lumbar arteries in succession. Large retractors such as the type shown in Figure 7-4 are of great use in retracting the vessels, allowing as clean a dissection as possible. On the left side the inferior mesenteric artery may be divided without danger but should be interrupted as close to the aorta as possible in order to allow the collateral circulation to take over. We do not drain the operative site routinely, and, when the thoracoabdominal incision is used, the chest is not drained unless numerous pleural adhesions are divided in the dissection.

In the closure of the thoracoabdominal incision, the diaphragm is closed with a running suture of 2-0 chromic catgut, with interrupted silk sutures superimposed to minimize the chance of dehiscence of the diaphragm. This suture is then continued anteriorly, closing the peritoneum. The muscles of the chest wall and anterior abdominal wall are then approximated in two layers, again using chromic 2-0. Just prior to the complete closure of the pleural cavity, an 18Fr red rubber catheter is placed in the pleural space surrounded by a purse string suture. The anesthesiologist is asked to expand the lung fully, and the pursestring suture is tied after the catheter has been removed.

REFERENCES

1. CHISHOLM GD, ROY RR: The systemic effects of malignant renal tumors. Br J Urol 43:687, 1971
2. CHUTE R, SOUTTER L, KERR WS, JR: Value of thoracoabdominal incision in removal of kidney tumors. N Engl J Med 241:951, 1949
3. GLENN JF: Speculation on Genesis, Therapeusis and Prognosis of Nephrocarcinoma. In King JS Jr. (ed): Renal Neoplasia, pp 535–546. Boston, Little, Brown and Co, 1967
4. GLENN JF: Renal Tumors. In Harrison JH et al (eds): Campbell's Urology, 4th ed pp 967–1009. Philadelphia, WB Saunders, 1979a
5. GLENN JF: Tumors of the Kidney. In Beeson PB, McDermott W, Wyngaarden JB (eds): Cecil's Textbook of Medicine, 15th ed, pp 1458–1462. Philadelphia, WB Saunders, 1979b
6. MIDDLETON RG, PRESTO AJ: Radical thoracoabdominal nephrectomy for renal cell carcinoma. J Urol 110:36, 1973
7. MIMMS NM, CHRISTIANSON B, SCHLUMBERGER FC et al: A ten year evaluation of nephrectomy for extensive renal cell carcinoma. J Urol 95:10, 1966
8. MORTENSEN H: Transthoracic nephrectomy. J Urol 60:855, 1948
9. ROBSON CJ: Radical nephrectomy for renal cell carcinoma. J Urol 89:37, 1963
10. ROBSON CJ, CHURCHILL BM, ANDERSON W: The results of radical nephrectomy for renal cell carcinoma. Trans Am Assoc Genitourin Surg 60:122, 1968
11. SKINNER DG, VERMILLION CD, COLVIN D: The surgical management of renal cell carcinoma. J Urol 107:705, 1972
12. TURNER WARWICK RT: The supracostal approach to the renal area. Br J Urol 37:671, 1965
13. WHITMORE WF, JR, KRAUSE C: Survival Following Nephrectomy for Renal Cell Cancer. In King JS, Jr (ed): Renal Neoplasia, pp 447–459. Boston, Little, Brown and Co, 1967

Wilms' Tumor

8

John K. Woodard

With over 500 new cases in the United States each year, Wilms' tumor (nephroblastoma, renal embryoma) is one of the most frequently encountered intra-abdominal malignancies and unquestionably the most common cancer of the genitourinary tract in children.[42] It occurs once per 13,800 live births, with a peak incidence in the third year and a mean age at diagnosis of 3.6 years. There is neither a geographic nor a sexual predilection.[13] Composed of mixed embryonic elements and rarely occurring in adolescents or adults, the tumor does not appear to be an acquired lesion.[14,21,27,28,31]

Although true Wilms' tumor has been reported in the neonate, most renal tumors found at that age are congenital mesoblastic nephromas in which local complete excision constitutes definitive therapy. Accurate histologic identification in these cases will avoid unnecessary and possibly hazardous adjuvant therapy.[35]

Clinical Features

In patients with Wilms' tumor, the typical presenting manifestation is an abdominal mass. As the first symptom in approximately 80% of the patients, it is evident on physical examination in at least 90%. A parent is often the first to notice the mass, which seemingly appears rather suddenly. It is usually large, firm, and relatively immobile and may cross the midline.[29]

Abdominal pain may be a striking feature at presentation in as many as one third of the patients and on a number of occasions has led to the erroneous diagnosis of acute surgical abdomen.[32] Although microscopic hematuria is often present, unlike adult tumors, gross hematuria is not common, occuring in only 10% to 20% of the patients.[20]

Although it is difficult to determine the true incidence, hypertension even in severe degrees may occur in association with Wilms' tumor. On occasion, it may lead to congestive heart failure and constitute the presenting problem. Whether the hypertension is due to renin production by the tumor itself or to renal ischemia has been debated. Either mechanism may play a role, but renin production by the tumor has been well documented, and the hypertension can be expected to resolve with removal of the tumor.[2,12,25]

Other symptoms of Wilms' tumor include fever, which is relatively common, malaise, and weight loss, which may suggest metastatic disease.

Genetic Aspects

In 1964, a hospital chart survey of 440 children with Wilms' tumor revealed six patients with aniridia and three with congenital hemihypertrophy.[24] In 1969 when the National Wilms' Tumor Study (NWTS) began collecting such data from 68 cooperating institutions (547 patients), they found 6 with anirida and 16 with hemihypertrophy, plus 24 others with genitourinary abnormalities. In addition, three families demonstrated multiple cases of Wilms' tumor.[28]

For a child with nonfamilial aniridia, there is a one in three chance of subsequently developing a Wilms' tumor.[30] Because the true incidence of hemihypertrophy is unknown, it is difficult to estimate the risk of such a patient developing a Wilms' tumor. However, in patients with Beckwith's syndrome plus hemihypertrophy, there is a one in three or four chance of developing either a Wilms' or an adrenal tumor.[36]

Chromosomal abnormalities have been demonstrated in some Wilms' tumor patients. For instance, children with aniridia and Wilms' tumor have been found to have deletions in chromosome 11. From such genetic studies in propositi and parents, it might in the future be possible to define a carrier state for Wilms' tumor.[11,23,41,43]

In the 15% of Wilms' tumor patients having associated anomalies, many are of genitourinary origin.[28] These anomalies include horseshoe kidney, ectopic and solitary kidneys, ureteral duplication, cryptorchidism, and hypospadias.

105

Diagnostic Evaluation

Although the removal of a Wilms' tumor is no longer considered an emergency, the laboratory and clinical evaluation of such a patient should proceed rapidly to completion within 1 or 2 days. In addition to the routine urine and blood studies, liver function tests, serum electrolytes, creatinine, and uric acid should be obtained. When there is a suggestion that the mass might represent a neuroblastoma, bone marrow aspirate along with urinary homovanillic acid (HVA) or vanillylmandelic acid (VMA) should be included.

Historically, the excretory urogram (IVP) has been the single most useful diagnostic procedure in an infant or child with an abdominal mass, particularly one suspected of being a Wilms' tumor. In most instances, the diagnosis can be made and it can be distinguished from a neuroblastoma on this basis. Typically, there is excretion of contrast material demonstrating distortion of the architecture of the collecting systems (Fig. 8-1). Calcifications, common in neuroblastoma, are only occasionally seen in Wilms' tumor. Nonopacification is rare and may suggest vascular or ureteral occlusion.

A roentgenogram of the chest is essential because the lungs are the most common site of distant metastases. As many as 25% of the patients have pulmonary metastases at the time of diagnosis.[20] Although tomograms of the chest in infants may be difficult and computed tomographic (CT) scans may require anesthesia, both are more sensitive than the routine chest films in detecting metastatic lesions.

The liver, being the second most common site of distant metastatic disease, is evaluated both with liver function studies and radionuclide liver scan. Although osseous metastases are much less common, a metastatic bone survey or a radionuclide bone scan is commonly done.

Vena caval extension from a Wilms' tumor occurs only in approximately 5% of the patients, but its impact upon surgical management is such that thorough evaluation of the inferior vena cava is mandatory in the preoperative preparation of the patient. This may be accomplished by inferior vena cavography, abdominal CT scanning, or ultrasonography (Fig. 8-2).

Aortography or renal arteriography is not indicated in every instance, but there are times when it may either enhance diagnostic accuracy or facilitate the surgical management of Wilms' tumor (Figs. 8-3 and 8-4). This is particularly true with the unusually large or extensive tumor, with bilateral lesions, or with Wilms' occurring in horseshoe kidneys (Fig. 8-5). One might not wish to incur the morbidity of this procedure in the more routine cases or in an infant or small child.

The evaluation of abdominal masses, particularly in infants, by ultrasonography has become routine in most institutions and often proves to be both simple and useful. Particularly useful in distinguishing solid from cystic masses, it may also be instrumental in distinguishing renal from other retroperitoneal lesions. As already noted, it may effectively document the presence and extent of tumor protrusion in the vena cava (see Fig. 8-2F).

CT scanning for Wilms' tumor patients is often helpful but has not become a routine part of their evaluation. It requires a general anesthesia in infants and young children, and the information it produces is not usually essential to optimal management. However, in certain selected instances, particularly very extensive lesions (Fig. 8-6), it may prove helpful in demonstrating operability and caval involvement. Further, simultaneous CT scanning of the chest may detect small metastatic lesions not evident on a routine chest film.

Staging and Grading

The clinical staging (grouping) of Wilms' tumor patients has assumed utmost importance in relation to the NWTS. The staging system used during NWTS-2 is outlined in Table 8-1. At presentation, approximately 30% of the patients fall into Stage I, 30% into Stage II, and 30% into Stages III, IV, and V.

Some have suggested a numerical grading system that correlates with patient prognosis.[17] However, the data from NWTS-1 indicates that these tumors fall into two histologic categories—favorable and unfavorable—which have great prognostic significance. The favorable histology group, into which approximately 88% of the patients fall, includes nonanaplastic tumors composed predominantly of blastema, as well as those that are predominantly epithelial or mixed. Fortunately, only about 12% of Wilms' tumors have unfavorable histology. This group includes those with focal anaplasia, diffuse anaplasia, rhabdoid tumors, and clear-cell sarcomas. The rhabdoid type tends to be associated with cerebral metastases or independent small-cell brain tumors. Clear-cell sarcoma tends to metastasize to bone. While only 12% of the total patients in NWTS-1 had unfavorable histology, this group accounted for 52% of the tumor deaths.[3] Therefore, accurate determinations of the histologic pattern by the pathologist is crucial to the planning of adjunctive therapy. Those patients with unfa-

(Text continues on p. 110)

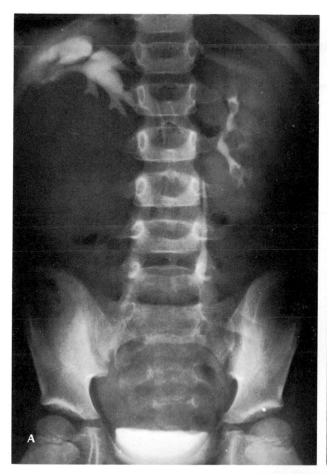

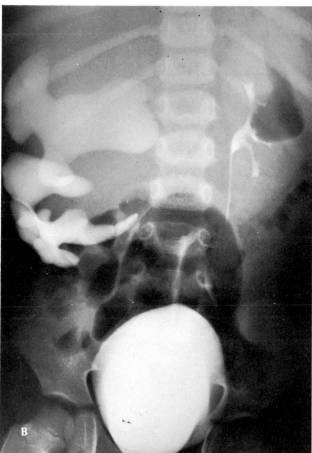

FIG. 8-1. Pyelograms of (**A**) a 5-year-old girl, (**B**) a 4-year-old boy, and (**C**) a 3-year-old boy demonstrate variations of the typical appearance of Wilms' tumors with distortion or displacement of the calices within the kidney.

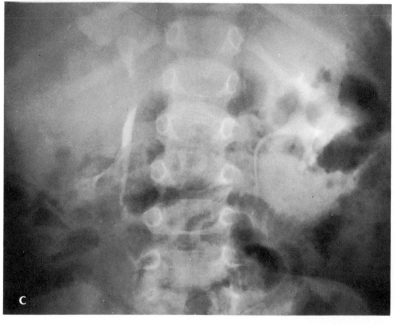

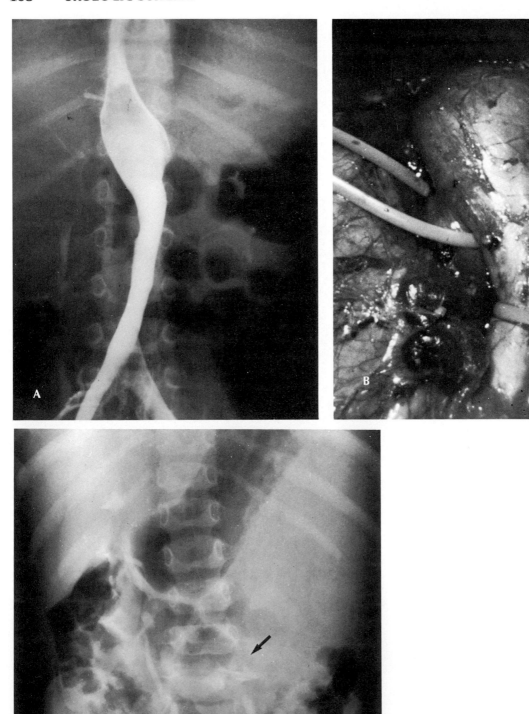

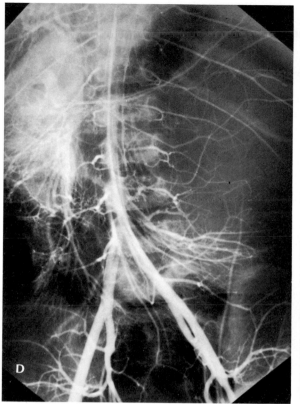

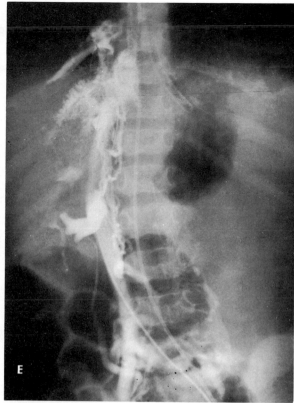

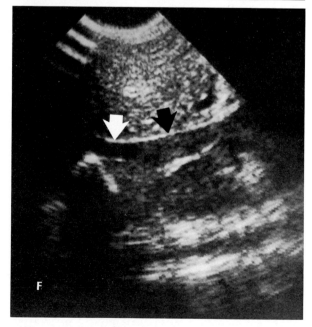

◄FIG. 8-2. **(A)** Inferior venacavogram of patient whose pyelogram (Fig. 8-1C) demonstrated right renal tumor. Cavogram demonstrates tumor thrombus filling the abdominal cava above the level of the renal veins. **(B)** Surgical photograph demonstrates vascular control of both renal veins and the cava below the level of the renal veins. Tumor thrombus is causing the cava to bulge above the level of the renal veins. **(C)** IVP in 2-year-old boy shows left renal mass with severe displacement downward and distortion of calices (*arrow*). **(D)** Aortogram in the same patient shows displacement of aorta toward the right with relative hypovascularity of the tumor. **(E)** Inferior vena cavogram of the same patient demonstrates filling defect in the suprarenal cava with filling of the azygos veins. **(F)** Abdominal ultrasonogram in the same patient shows the cephalad extent of the tumor thrombus (*black arrow*) with clear cava above (*white arrow*).

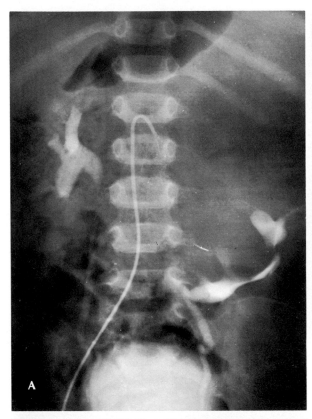

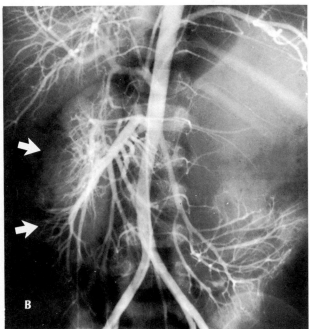

FIG. 8-3. This 3-year-old boy had a huge Wilms' tumor in the left kidney with typical pyelographic findings **(A).** The right pyelogram was unremarkable. His aortogram **(B)** confirms the large, relatively hypovascular tumor on the left but demonstrates two areas of probable tumor in the right kidney (*arrows*). On the nephrogram phase of the aortogram **(C)** these two tumor masses in the right kidney are nicely delineated.

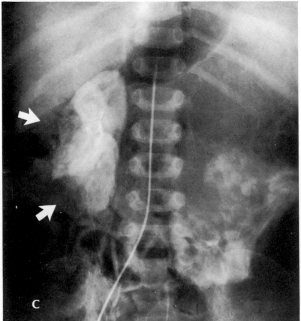

vorable histology require a much more aggressive therapeutic approach.

Surgical Excision

The goal of the surgeon is complete removal of the tumor. A generous, upper abdominal transverse transperitoneal approach provides adequate exposure in most infants and small children (Fig. 8-7*A*). For upper pole tumors in the slightly older patient, a thoracoabdominal approach (Fig. 8-7*B*) may occasionally be superior. The incision must allow complete abdominal exploration with inspection and palpation of the liver, exposure of the anterior and posterior surfaces of the contralateral kidney, and palpation of the periaortic lymph nodes. Because of the 5% likelihood of bilaterality, Gerota's fascia on the contralateral side should be opened and both surfaces of the kidney inspected. Suspicious lesions in the liver or the opposite kidney should be confirmed by biopsy.

The radical nephrectomy (Fig. 8-8) is begun by incising the peritoneum lateral to the colon, which,

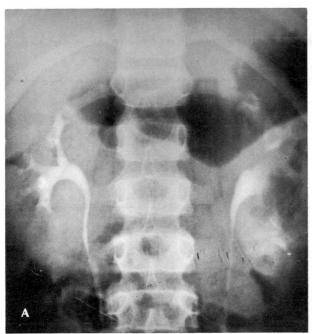

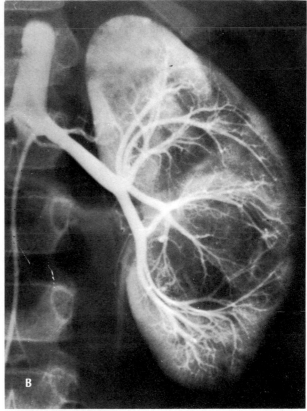

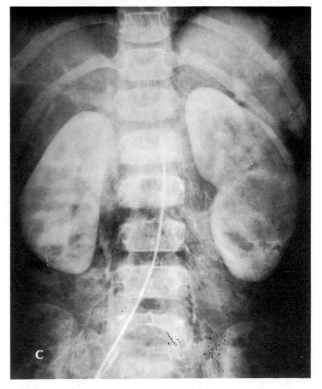

FIG. 8-4. This 7-year-old boy with hematuria resulting from minor trauma had an IVP (**A**) showing subtle caliceal distortion in the lower portion of the left kidney. However, his selective renal arteriogram (**B**) nicely delineated a lower-pole, intrarenal tumor mass that was also evident on his nephrogram (**C**).

with elevation of its mesentery, is reflected and retracted medially to expose the great vessels (Fig. 8-8*B*). The initial effort should be to locate and accurately identify the ipsilateral renal vein, which is often splayed and flattened over the medial portion of the tumor and not immediately recognizable. Working one's way up the vena cava from below may facilitate location of the vein. The corresponding renal artery should be found just posterior to the renal vein. There have been instances, particularly in large tumors, in which the contralateral renal vessels were mistakenly ligated. This serious error can be avoided by identifying the contralateral renal vessels or at least the aorta and vena cava prior to ligating and dividing the vessels to the involved kidney. Once the main vessels are ligated, the kidney, with Gerota's fascia still intact, is removed (Fig. 8-8*C–F*). In the lower pole lesions, the adrenal gland can often be spared. The ureter should be ligated and divided in its distal third, because extension to the ureter by the tumor is occasionally reported.[37] Once its blood supply is interrupted, the tumor tends to become quite soft and extreme care must be taken to prevent its rupture, because spillage leads to an

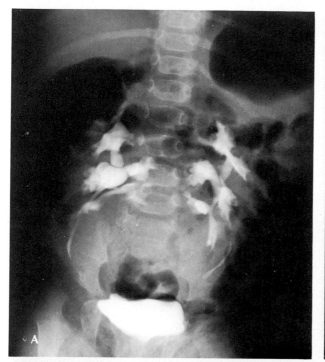

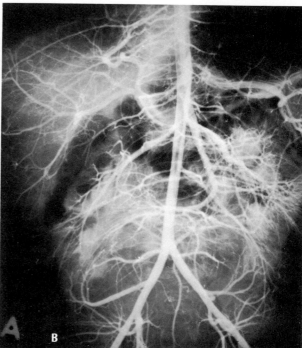

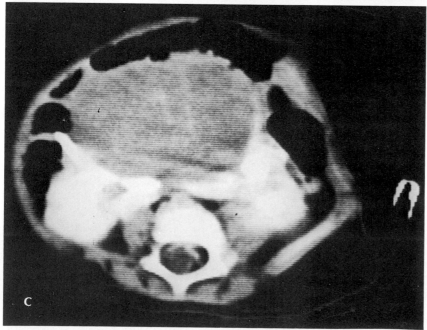

FIG. 8-5. The IVP (**A**) in this 1-year-old girl with a midabdominal mass demonstrates a bilateral rotational anomaly with lateral displacement of the upper ureters around the mass. Her aortogram (**B**) demonstrates multiple renal arteries to the kidney and the mass lesion with large vessels arising from the iliac arteries. Her CT scan (**C**) confirms the tumor mass to be arising from the right and left sides of what proved to be a horseshoe kidney.

increased abdominal recurrence rate and results in the need for additional postoperative therapy.[6,19]

Tumors in the left kidney may become densely adherent to or actually invade the pancreas, spleen, or descending colon. Resection of the tail of the pancreas to allow *en bloc* removal on several occa-sions has resulted in no complications. The cut end of the pancreas is carefully repaired with a silk running lock suture. Because of the resulting increased infection risk, particularly pneumococ-cal, an effort should be made to avoid removal of the spleen unless its sparing seriously compromises the operation. In several patients, a segment of colon, right or left, has been resected when there was invasion of its wall by tumor. When this possibility is suspected, a preoperative bowel preparation must be accomplished. Bowel resection, however, necessitates a delay in the institution of postoperative radiation therapy and, consequently, should be done only when necessary.

A tumor in the right kidney may extend into the liver. Often this is little more than invasion of the liver capsule and is usually removable. As in the case of large tumors, lymph node involvement, distant metastatic spread, and renal capsule infiltration, liver involvement carries a worse-than-average outcome. A Wilms' tumor of either kidney may invade the diaphragm. Fortunately, the portion of diaphragm involved is usually small enough to allow its resection and reapproximation of the diaphragm without the use of synthetic material.

Very rarely, the extent of the tumor will be such that an attempt at complete removal will clearly jeopardize the patient's chances of survival. This is particularly true when the root of the mesentery, the duodenum, or the head or body of the pancreas are invaded, or when there is encirclement of the great vessels. In such circumstances, it may be preferable to take biopsies, mark the extent of the tumor with silver clips, and close. Radiation and chemotherapy will, particularly with favorable histology, shrink the tumor to more manageable proportions, and successful excision can usually be accomplished later (see Fig. 8-6).[40] Given the importance of histology in judging the response to treatment, the need to biopsy in this circumstance should be evident.

Management of Special Conditions

METASTASIS TO REGIONAL LYMPH NODES

Metastases from Wilms' tumor to the regional lymph nodes occurs in approximately one third of the cases, with the hilar nodes being involved more often than the periaortic group.[16] Some advocate total periaortic (therapeutic) node dissection.[22] It is evident that the extent of lymph node involvement is clearly correlated with outcome, but the data available from NWTS provide no evidence that lymph node resection either does or does not alter the outcome.[19] It is, however, highly important to know the presence and extent of node involvement for accurate staging purposes so as to ensure adequate adjunctive therapy. Therefore, careful examination and selective surgical sampling

TABLE 8-1.   NWTS Clinical Groupings (Stages)

I   *Tumor limited to the kidney and completely resected:* The surface of the renal capsule is intact. The tumor was not ruptured before or during removal. There is no residual tumor apparent beyond the margins of resection.

II—*Tumor extended beyond the kidney but is completely resected:* There is local extension of the tumor; that is, penetration beyond the pseudocapsule into the perirenal soft tissues, or periaortic lymph node involvement. The renal vessels outside the kidney substance are infiltrated or contain tumor thrombus. There is no residual tumor apparent beyond the margins of resection.

III—*Residual nonhematogenous tumor confined to the abdomen:* Any one or more of the following occur:
1. The tumor has been biopsied or ruptured before or during surgery.
2. There are implants on peritoneal surfaces.
3. There are involved lymph nodes beyond the abdominal periaortic chains.
4. The tumor is not completely resectable because of local infiltration into vital structures.

IV—*Hematogenous metastases:* Deposits occur beyond Group III; for example, lung, liver, bone, and brain.

V—*Bilateral renal involvement either initially or subsequently*

Leap LL, Breslow NE, Bishop HC: The surgical treatment of Wilms' tumor: Results of the National Wilms' Tumor Study. Ann Surg 187:351, 1976.

of nodes is useful and may be essential to accurate staging.

INTRACAVAL EXTENSION

In NWTS-1, tumor was present in the renal vein or vena cava in 37 of 606 patients, but it was not associated with a poor outcome. That is, in Group (Stage) II or III patients the outcome was identical, whether or not there was tumor in the vein.[19] Because the outcome for these patients is potentially good, it is essential that intravascular extension be recognized and managed properly. There should be adequate preoperative evaluation of the inferior vena cava (see Fig. 8-2) by means of cavography, ultrasonography, or CT scanning. If the cava contains tumor, its upper extent must also be determined.

Unlike adult renal adenocarcinoma, in which such venous extension is more likely on the right side, left-sided Wilms' tumors appear equally vulnerable. Fortunately, most extensions are subdiaphragmatic and can be managed as described in

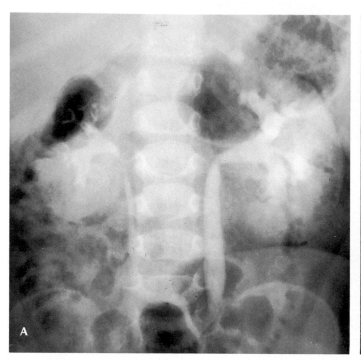

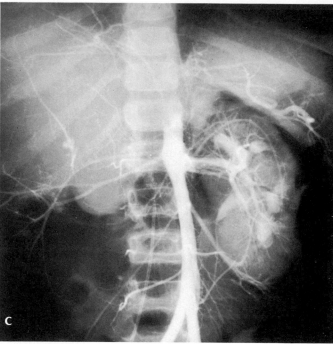

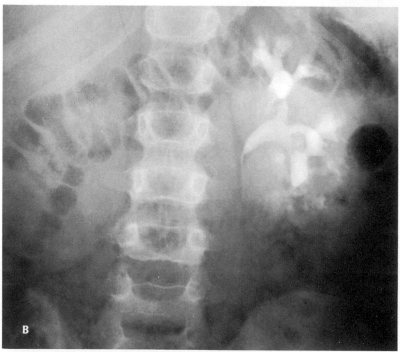

FIG. 8-6. The IVP in a 3-year-old girl with Beckwith syndrome and left-sided hemihypertrophy **(A)** demonstrates a normal right kidney. She developed a huge abdominal mass at the age of 6½ years; her IVP **(B)** demonstrated a right renal mass with "nonfunction." Her aortogram **(C)** showed a small right renal artery supplying the huge hypovascular tumor of the right kidney and her abdominal CT scan **(D)** demonstrated the extensive and diffuse nature of the neoplasm, with displacement and separation of the great vessels by tumor, which extended across the midline and lay in front of and intimate with the opposite kidney. At surgical exploration, it was found to be nonresectable because of its involvement with the great vessels (*white arrow* points to aorta), the superior mesenteric artery, and the root of the mesentery. However, after 6 weeks of chemotherapy and radiation, a repeat CT scan **(E)** demonstrated marked reduction in the tumor mass, which was then amenable to complete surgical resection. (*Illustration continues on facing page*)

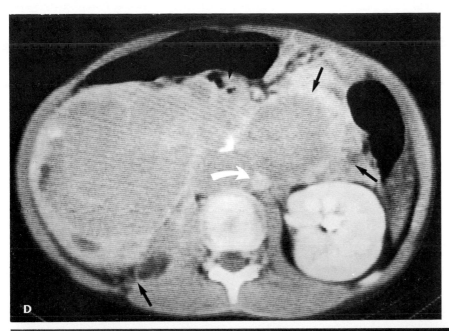

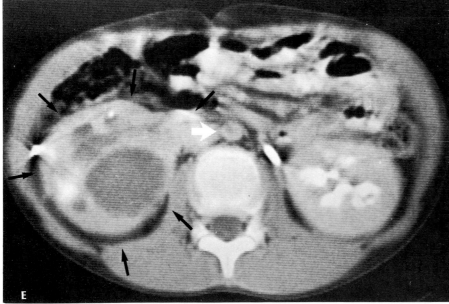

Figure 8-9. Because tumor embolism is a serious threat, proximal control is mandatory.

Cardiac murmur or even right heart failure may occur with tumor extension into the right atrium.[1,34,39] When the tumor does extend into the thoracic cava or the right atrium, a combined approach with a cardiovascular surgical team, possible with cardiopulmonary bypass, is necessary. The tumor usually does not invade the wall of the cava and can be extracted.

BILATERAL WILM'S TUMOR

In NWTS-1 and 2, 56 of 980 patients had bilateral lesions for an incidence of 5.7%.[7,26] The incidence of associated abnormalities in this bilateral group was also higher. Despite complete removal of tumor in only seven of these patients, there was an 87% 2-year survival for the bilateral group. Although all these patients received chemotherapy, it was not possible to standardize the surgical treatment. (*Text continues on p. 119*)

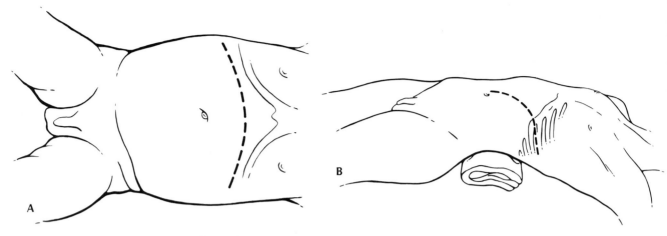

FIG. 8-7. An anterior transverse, subcostal incision **(A)** is used for most patients undergoing removal of Wilms' tumor. A thoracoabdominal incision **(B)** is useful in large upper-pole tumors, especially in older children.

FIG. 8-8. The surgical exposure of a Wilms' tumor of the left kidney **(A)** shows it to bulge through the mesocolon with lateral displacement of the left colon. After the posterior peritoneum has been incised along the left paracolic gutter **(B)** the colon is reflected medially, allowing exposure of the main renal vessels prior to manipulation of the tumor. With double nonabsorbable proximal ligatures, the renal artery is occluded and divided **(C)** prior to ligation of the renal vein. The renal vein is then similarly ligated and divided **(D).** After division of the main renal vessels, the tumor, Gerota's capsule, and the hilar nodes are removed. The ureter should be ligated in the distal third. The periaortic lymph nodes are then either removed or sampled selectively for staging purposes, leaving a clean renal fossa **(E).** (*Illustration continues on p. 117*)

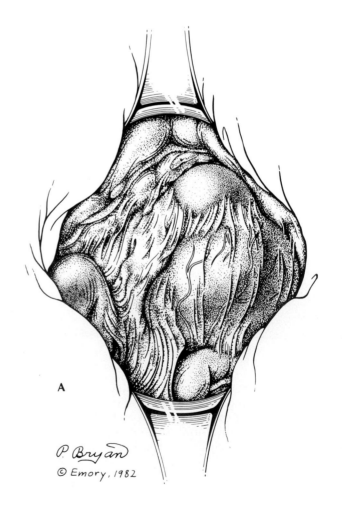

P. Bryan
© Emory, 1982

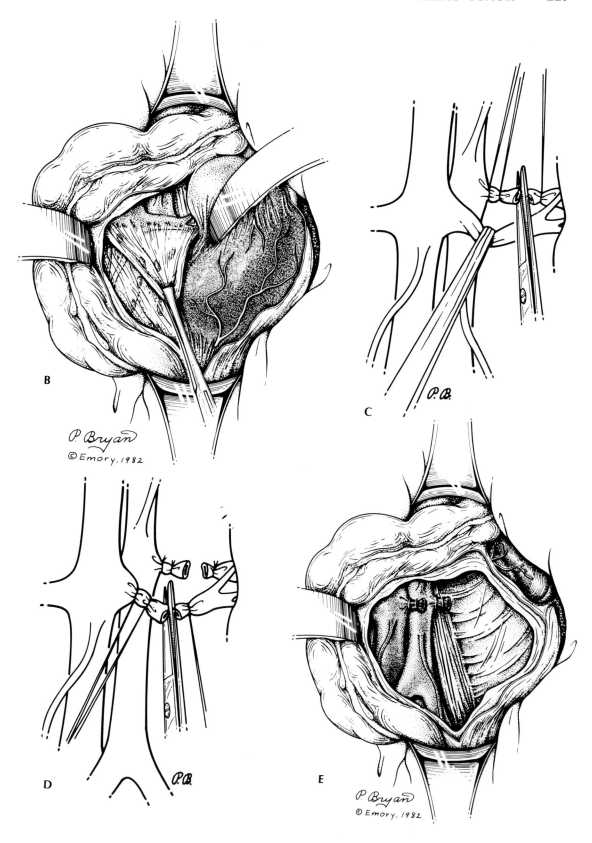

B

P. Bryan
© Emory, 1982

C

P. B.

D

P. B.

E

P Bryan
© Emory, 1982

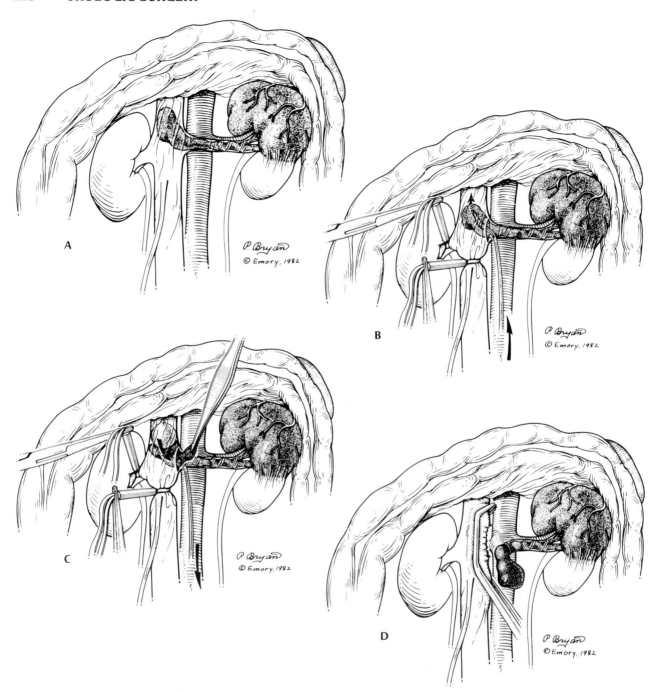

FIG. 8-9. When there is extension of the tumor through the renal vein into the inferior vena cava (**A**) and preoperative studies have demonstrated that the tumor is confined to the abdominal cava, the vessels are first exposed, the opposite renal vein and the cava below the level of the renal veins are controlled with vascular loops (**B**), and the cava is incised vertically at its junction with the involved renal vein. A Fogarty catheter is then passed beyond the tumor thrombus and the balloon is inflated (**C**). The thrombus is extracted from the vena cava, using gentle traction on the Fogarty catheter and forceps to manipulate the thrombus out of the cava; then a tangential occluding clamp is placed on the cava (**D**) and the involved renal vein is completely detached. The opening in the cava is closed with continuous 5-0 proline suture. The remainder of the operation is as shown in Fig. 8-8.

When one kidney contains a massive tumor and the other kidney contains one or more small tumors, it is advisable to remove the kidney containing the large tumor and to biopsy the contralateral lesions. Subsequent chemotherapy is followed by reoperation with an attempt at renal-sparing tumor excision. Because of the high success rate with lesser procedures, bilateral nephrectomy followed by "renal replacement therapy" should be considered rarely and as a last resort.[5]

NEPHROBLASTOMATOSIS AND NODULAR RENAL BLASTEMA

Nephroblastomatosis and nodular renal blastema appear to be a part of the Wilms' tumor disease spectrum. Nephroblastomatosis is a diffuse involvement of both kidneys with densely packed, rounded and elongated clumps of immature blastemalike cells resembling Wilms' tumor.[33] Nodular renal blastema (NRB) occurs as nests of primitive, undifferentiated cells similar to embryonic renal blastema just beneath the renal capsule.[18]

NRB is solely a microscopic diagnosis, but nephroblastomatosis may also be suggested radiographically and by the gross appearance of the kidney at operation (Fig. 8-10). When both kidneys are involved in a symmetrical fashion, treatment consists of biopsy followed by chemotherapy. When one kidney is much the more involved, nephrectomy may be the treatment of choice.

Radiation Therapy and Chemotherapy

Radiation therapy has played a major role in the evolution of modern treatment for Wilms' tumor, because most Wilms' tumors are radiosensitive. However, much of the early and delayed treatment morbidity, such as pneumonitis, nephritis, hepatitis, scoliosis, and secondary cancers, has been related to routine postoperative radiation therapy.[15] NWTS data have proved that Stage I patients do not benefit from postoperative irradiation.[8] Irradiation to the tumor bed does remain a part of the standard therapy for Stages II, III, and IV patients, as well as a means of treating metastatic and recurrent lesions.

Modern chemotherapy of Wilms' tumor had its beginning in 1954 when Farber observed the antitumor activity of actinomycin D.[9] Both actinomycin D and vincristine have subsequently been found to be highly effective against the tumor, and during NWTS-1 the two in combination proved more effective than either agent alone.[7,38] These two drugs in combination are now standard treatment.

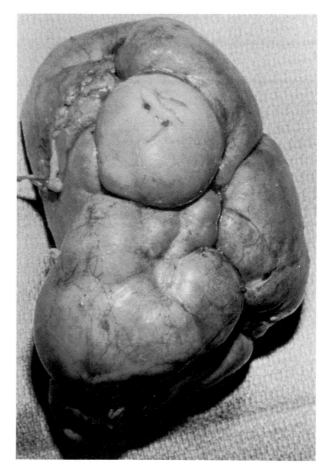

FIG. 8-10. The typical gross appearance of the kidney with nephroblastomatosis, showing diffuse enlargement and lobulation.

Doxorubicin hydrochloride (Adriamycin) and cyclophosphamide have also proved to be effective anti-Wilms' tumor agents.[4,10] Because of their toxicity, they are reserved for advanced stages, recurrent or metastatic disease, or unfavorable histology.

Surveillance for the High-Risk Patient

Several groups, notably those with hemihypertrophy and aniridia, have now been identified who are at greater risk than is the general population for the development of Wilms' tumor. Unfortunately, many of these patients still fail to have their tumors detected at a subclinical stage. The advent of ultrasound should greatly improve the surveillance of this population. Parents should be taught abdominal palpation, and renal ultrasound studies should be carried out every 2 to 3 months, thereby reducing the need for excretory urography to be done as frequently as previously suggested.[41] The age at which surveillance can be safely terminated remains vague. I recently had a patient with Beckwith's syndrome and hemihypertrophy who developed a Wilms' tumor (manifested by a huge abdominal mass) in her seventh year. Chromosomal studies currently underway may further define which patients with these associated anomalies are at greatest risk.[11,42]

The National Wilms' Tumor Study

The NWTS began in 1969 as a cooperative prospective study to compare treatment programs. Now, in its third phase, it represents an outstanding success story, not just in terms of meaningful data accumulated, but also in the impact it has had upon the management of Wilms' tumor nationwide. Not only have cure rates been improved upon, but the extent of treatment with its attendant morbidity has also been reduced.

NWTS-1 from 1969 to 1973 included 606 patients and demonstrated that double-agent therapy (actinomycin D plus vincristine) was superior to either agent alone, that Stage 1 patients under age 2 years did not benefit from radiation therapy, and that preoperative vincristine did not improve the survival of Stage IV patients.[7]

NWTS-2 demonstrated that Stage I patients of any age could be managed without radiation and that 6 months chemotherapy was as effective as 15 months. The relapse-free survival rate (RFS) was 90%. The addition of Adriamycin to actinomycin D and vincristine in Stage II, III, and IV patients has resulted in improvement to 85% RFS for these children.[8]

The data from NWTS regarding the effect of histology on patient outcome have already been alluded to and form the basis for the treatment arms of NWTS-3 presently well underway.

REFERENCES

1. ABDELSAYED MA, BISSADA NK, FINKBEINER AE et al: Renal tumors involving the inferior vena cava: Plan for management. J Urol 120:153, 1978
2. ARON BS: Wilms' tumor—a clinical study of eighty-one patients. Cancer 33:637, 1974
3. BECKWITH JB, PALMER NF: Histology and prognosis of Wilms' tumor: Report from the first NWTS. Cancer 41:1937, 1978
4. BELLANI FF: Adriamycin in Wilms' tumor previously treated with chemotherapy. Eur J Cancer 11:593, 1975
5. BISHOP HC, TEFFT M, EVANS AE et al: Survival in bilateral Wilms' tumor—review of 30 National Wilms' Tumor Study cases. J Pediatr Surg 12:631, 1977
6. D'ANGIO GJ, BECKWITH JB, BRESLOW NE et al: Wilms' tumor: An update. Cancer (Suppl) 45:1791, 1980
7. D'ANGIO GJ, EVANS AE, BRESLOW N et al: The treatment of Wilms' tumor: Results of the National Wilms' Tumor Study. Cancer 38:633, 1976
8. D'ANGIO GJ, EVANS A, BRESLOW N et al: The treatment of Wilms' tumor: Results of the Second National Wilms' Tumor Study. Cancer 47:2302, 1981
9. FARBER S, TOCH R, SEARS EM et al: Advances in chemotherapy of cancer in man. Adv Cancer Res 4:1, 1956
10. FINKELSTEIN JZ, HITTLE RF, HAMMOND GD: Evaluation of a high dose cyclophosphamide regimen in childhood tumors. Cancer 23:1239, 1969
11. FRANCKE U, HOLMES LB, ATKINS L et al: Aniridia–Wilms' tumor association: Evidence for specific deletion of 11p13. Cytogenet Cell Genet 24:185, 1979
12. GANGULY A, GRIBBLE J, TUNE B et al: Renin-secreting Wilms' tumor with severe hypertension. Ann Intern Med 79:835, 1973
13. GLENN JF, RHAME RC: Wilms' tumor: Epidemiological experience. J Urol 85:911, 1961
14. INNIS MD: Nephroblastoma: Index cancer of childhood. Med J Aus 2:322, 1973
15. JAFFE N, MCNEESE M, MAYFIELD JK et al: Childhood urologic cancer therapy related sequelae and their impact on management. Cancer 45:1815, 1980
16. JEREB B, TOURNADE MF, LEMERLE J et al: Lymph node invasion and prognosis in nephroblastoma. Cancer 45:1632, 1980
17. KHEIR S, PRITCHETT PS, MORENO H et al: Histologic grading of Wilms' tumor as a potential prognostic factor: Results of a retrospective study of 26 patients. Cancer 41:1199, 1978
18. KUMAR APM, PRATT CB, COBURN TP et al: Treatment strategy for nodular renal blastema and nephroblastomatosis associated with Wilms' tumor. J Pediatr Surg 13:281, 1978
19. LEAPE LL, BRESLOW NE, BISHOP HC: The surgical treatment of Wilms' tumor: Results of the National Wilms' Tumor Study. Ann Surg 187:351, 1976
20. LEDLIE EM, MYNORS LS, DRAPER GJ et al: Natural history and treatment of Wilms's tumour: An analysis of 335 cases occurring in England and Wales 1962–6. Br Med 4:195, 1970
21. LEMERLE J, TOURNADE M, GERARD–MARCHANT R et al: Wilms' tumor: Natural history and prognostic factors. Cancer 37:2557, 1976
22. MARTIN LW, SCHAFFNER DP, COX JA et al: Retroperitoneal lymph node dissection for Wilms' tumor. J Pediatr Surg 14:704, 1979
23. MILLER RW: Birth defects and cancer due to small chromosomal deletions. J Pediatr 96:1031, 1980
24. MILLER RW, FRAUMENI JF, MANNING MD: Association of Wilms's tumor with aniridia, hemihypertrophy

and other congenital malformations. N Engl J Med 270:922, 1964

25. MITCHELL JD, BAXTER TJ, BLAIR–WEST JR et al: Renin levels in nephroblastoma (Wilms' tumour). Arch Dis Child 45:376, 1970

26. National Wilms' Tumor Study Committee: The National Wilms' Tumor Study: A report from cancer cooperative study groups. Cancer Clin Trials: 61, Spring 1978

27. OLSEN BS, BISCHOFF AJ: Wilms' tumor in an adult. Cancer 25:21, 1970

28. PENDERGRASS TW: Congenital anomalies in children with Wilms tumor. Cancer 37:403, 1976

29. PEREZ CA, KAIMAN HA, KEITH J et al: Treatment of Wilms' tumor and factors affecting prognosis. Cancer 32:609, 1973

30. PILLING GP: Wilms' tumor in seven children with congenital aniridia. J Pediatr Surg 10:87, 1975

31. PRAT J, GRAY GF, STOLLEY PD et al: Wilms' tumor in an adult associated with androgen abuse. JAMA 237:2322, 1977

32. ROSENFELD M, RODGERS BM, TALBERT JL: Wilms' tumor with acute abdominal pain. Arch Surg 112:1080, 1977

33. ROUS SN, BAILIE MD, KAUFMAN DB et al: Nodular renal blastema, nephroblastomatosis and Wilms' tumor. Urology 8:599, 1976

34. SLOVIS TL, CUSHING B, REILLY BJ et al: Wilms' tumor to the heart: Clinical and radiographic evaluation. Am J Roentgenol 131:263, 1978

35. SNYDER HM, LACK EE, CHETTY–BAKTAVIZIAN A et al: Congenital mesoblastic nephroma: relationship to other renal tumors of infancy. J Urol 126:513, 1981

36. SOTELO–AVILA C, GONZALEZ–CRUSSI F, STARLING KA: Wilms' tumor in a patient with an incomplete form of Beckwith–Wiedemann syndrome. Pediatrics 66:121, 1980

37. STEVENS PS, ECKSTEIN HB: Ureteral metastasis from Wilms' tumor. J Urol 115:467, 1976

38. SUTOW WW, THURMAN WG, WINDMILLER J: Vincristine (Leurocristine) sulfate in the treatment of children with metastatic Wilms' tumor. Pediatrics 32:880, 1963

39. VAUGHAN ED, CROSBY IK, TEGTMEYER CJ: Nephroblastoma with right atrial extension: Preoperative diagnosis and management. J Urol 117:530, 1977

40. WAGGET J, KOOP CE: Wilms' tumor: preoperative radiotherapy and chemotherapy in the management of massive tumors. Cancer 26:338, 1970

41. WOODARD JR, GAY BB JR, RUTHERFORD CR JR: The incipient Wilms' tumor. Pediatr Radiol 3:81, 1975

42. YOUNG JL, MILLER R: Incidence of malignant tumors in United States children. J Pediatr 86:254, 1975

43. YUNIS JJ, RAMSEY NK: Familial occurrence of the aniridia–Wilms' tumor syndrome with deletion of 11p13–14.1. J Pediatr 96:1027, 1980

Nephroureterectomy

9

Harper D. Pearse

Tumors of the renal pelvis and ureter present a diagnostic and therapeutic challenge to the urologist. Complete nephroureterectomy is an appealing method of treatment because these tumors tend to be multiple and recur after incomplete nephroureterectomy.

In 1919, Judd recommended nephroureterectomy for transitional cell carcinoma of the renal pelvis.[19] Hunt, in 1929, suggested including the intramural ureter and a cuff of bladder as part of the *en bloc* procedure.[9] He noted that two thirds of his patients had involvement of the ureteral orifice and that stump recurrences were found following incomplete nephroureterectomy.

In 1960, Culp described a single anterior extraperitoneal incision for nephroureterectomy. He noted that it was neither new nor unique but had previously found little favor.[3] O'Conor and Logan later indicated their satisfaction with a single extended subcostal incision.[17]

Our incision of choice is a single supracostal incision with inferior extension to permit removal of a cuff of bladder under direct vision. According to Mouat, the supracostal approach to the kidney was first described nearly 60 years ago by Bernard Fey and was used extensively in France and Germany in the 1930s because of the excellent exposure of the upper pole of the kidney and renal vessels. Fey's basic procedure was popularized and modified in the Anglo-American surgical literature, first by Presman and then by Turner Warwick, when they changed the patient's position from supine to flank, extended the incision posteriorly to incise the costovertebral ligaments, and eliminated rib periosteal elevation. We have merely applied an old operation to a new surgical problem, extended the incision inferiorly to allow removal of the entire ureter, and modified the closure slightly. We have found this application of the operation to be very satisfactory.[1]

General Comments

About 10% of all neoplasms of the upper urinary tract occur in the renal pelvis and ureter, and 90% of these are transitional cell carcinomas. Squamous cell tumors are found in 8% of the cases and are likely to be associated with infection and stones. In contrast to many transitional cell tumors, they are usually asymptomatic in early stages and tend to be solitary, sessile, invasive, and associated with a poor prognosis.[14]

The ratio of urothelial tumors of the bladder to renal pelvis tumors to ureter tumors is approximately 50:3:1. Most of these neoplasms occur between the ages of 50 years and 70 years, with an average age of 65 years, and they are two to three times as common in men as in women.

The etiology of the majority of upper tract tumors is uncertain, although epidemiologic studies suggest that environmental factors are important. Two interesting associations with transitional cell carcinomas of the renal pelvis are phenacetin abuse and Balkan nephropathy.[6,8,18] Prolonged ingestion of phenacetin has been implicated in the etiology of transitional cell carcinoma of the renal pelvis, with a mean induction time of 19 years. These patients are predominantly female, present at a younger age, have the associated interstitial nephritis of analgesic abuse, and may present with chronic renal failure. Endemic Balkan nephropathy, a chronic tubular interstitial nephropathy, is unique because it is prevalent in geographically restricted areas of Bulgaria, Rumania, and Yugoslavia, where there also is a high frequency of papillary transitional cell carcinoma of the renal pelvis and ureter. The cause of Balkan nephropathy or its association with transitional cell tumors is unknown. Bilateral tumors occur in 5% to 10% of the cases, and 10% to 30% have multiple tumors.

Transitional cell carcinoma of the reval pelvis is often associated with other tumors in the renal pelvis, ipsilateral ureter, or urinary bladder. Approximately 30% of the patients with carcinoma of the renal pelvis or ureter have or will develop associated bladder carcinoma irrespective of initial treatment.[21–24] The contralateral renal pelvis and ureter are rarely involved (1%–3%).[15] At least 60% of the ureteral tumors occur in the lower one third of the ureter.[24]

We have no method of fully evaluating the neoplastic potential of the entire urothelium and therefore are limited in our ability to select proper treatment in all cases. The most widely accepted treatment for transitional cell carcinoma of the upper urinary tract is nephroureterectomy with removal of a cuff of urinary bladder adjacent to the ureteral orifice.[4,7,21] Failure to remove the ureteral stump has resulted in a 20% to 40% recurrence of carcinoma in the remaining portion of the ureter.[2,12,13,21] Because of this high rate of recurrence after incomplete nephroureterectomy and because of common ipsilateral multicentricity, we reserve local resection for carefully selected cases of benign tumors, bilateral tumors, tumors in a solitary kidney, and for situations in which preservation of functioning renal tissue is mandatory. It has been suggested that there is a place for conservative surgery in the patient with a solitary, low-grade, and noninvasive tumor; however, it is at times difficult to be assured that these criteria are met.[5,11,16] Local resection in such cases has given good results, although recurrences have been noted, so this approach may be used more often as our diagnostic, staging, and follow-up abilities develop and permit more precision.

Survival depends on the grade and stage of the disease at the time of treatment and is poor for patients with nodal metastases. Five-year survivals of 50% to 80% for patients with Grade 1 or 2 tumors is reported in contrast to the 15% 5-year survival in patients with Grade 3 or 4 tumors which are more likely to be invasive. Local extension or lymph node involvement is associated with 5-year survival of 5% to 10%. The treatment of choice for most transitional cell carcinomas of the upper urinary tract remains nephroureterectomy with a cuff of bladder. Effective adjuvant chemotherapy is currently not available, and the role of radiation therapy is undefined.

Preoperative Evaluation

Gross hematuria is the most common clinical manifestation of upper urinary tract transitional cell carcinoma. Flank pain, abdominal mass, frequency of urination, and dysuria are also common clinical presentations.

The classical urologic finding in transitional cell carcinoma of the renal pelvis is a negative filling defect in a more or less normal-appearing renal pelvis. Diagnostic accuracy for ureteral tumors is poor, and repeated examinations are usually required to demonstrate the negative filling defect. In our series, the intravenous urogram showed a filling defect in one third of the cases, hydronephrosis in one third, and nonvisualization of all or part of the collecting system and ureter in one third. Retrograde pyelography is the most dependable diagnostic study. Urinary cytologic examination by barbotage or at times brush biopsy is of great help in establishing the diagnosis preoperatively. Ultrasonography and computed tomography can be useful in differentiating a uric acid stone and transitional cell carcinoma. They can also be used effectively for estimating direct extension. Transitional cell carcinomas of the upper urinary tract are difficult to visualize angiographically; however, epinephrine-assisted arteriography and venography are sensitive indicators of direct extension. Neovascularity can be seen secondary to inflammatory disease; however, encasement of arteries and obliteration of veins is not seen in benign conditions.

Surgical Technique

The patient is placed in the modified flank position so that his torso forms a 45-degree angle with the flexed operating table rather than the usual 90-degrees. Depending on the relationship of the kidney to the lower ribs, an incision is made in either the 10th or 11th intercostal space from the lateral border of the erector spinae muscle to the midline just above the symphysis (Figure 9-1). The ensuing muscle and fascia layers are incised. Posteriorly, the costovertebral ligament is cut on the superior aspect of the lower rib, allowing this rib to hinge downward and the superior rib to hinge upward. This approach exposes the pleura and diaphragm fibers (Figure 9-2). The diaphragm fibers are then cut to allow the pleural cavity to be retracted superiorly (Figure 9-3). Inferiorly, the anterior rectus sheath is cut and the rectus muscle is retracted medially. With blunt dissection, the retroperitoneal fat surrounding the kidney and ureter is elevated superiorly over the aorta for a left nephrectomy and to the inferior vena cava for a right nephrectomy (Figure 9-4). Palpation of the aorta allows identification of the takeoff of the renal artery, which is isolated, ligated, and divided between ligatures. On the left, further dissection anterior to the aorta exposes the left renal vein proximal to the gonadal and adrenal vessels. The left renal vein is ligated and divided between ligatures. The perirenal fat and fascia are now freed from the abdominal surface of the diaphragm. Medially, adrenal vessels require division between hemostatic clips. The peritoneum is then dissected off the perirenal fat and fascia. Elevating the kid-

(*Text continues on p. 128*)

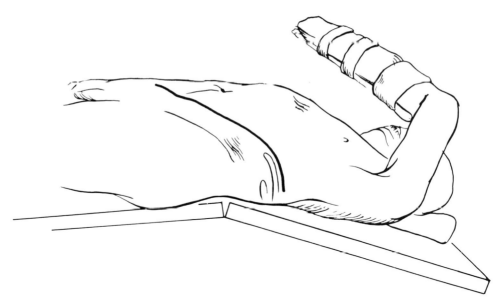

FIG. 9-1. The thorax forms a 45-degree angle with the flexed operating table. The pelvis remains relatively flat to permit better access to the bladder and lower ureter. The incision begins at the lateral border of the erector spinae muscle, continues between the ribs, and curves inferiorly toward the midline to end just above the symphysis. This extended supracostal incision provides excellent combined exposure from the level of the superior mesenteric artery to the ureterovesical junction.

FIG. 9-2. The external and internal oblique muscles have been incised anteriorly, and the latissimus, serratus posterior inferior, external intercostal, and outer layer of the internal intercostal muscles have been incised posteriorly. This exposes the 11th intercostal neuro-vascular bundle, which is preserved, and the costo-vertebral ligament, which is incised on the superior aspect of the 12th rib. If this ligament is not released, the inferior rib will not hinge downward and exposure will be compromised.

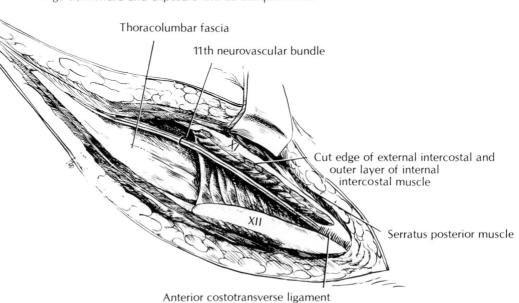

Thoracolumbar fascia

11th neurovascular bundle

XI

Cut edge of external intercostal and outer layer of internal intercostal muscle

XII

Serratus posterior muscle

Anterior costotransverse ligament

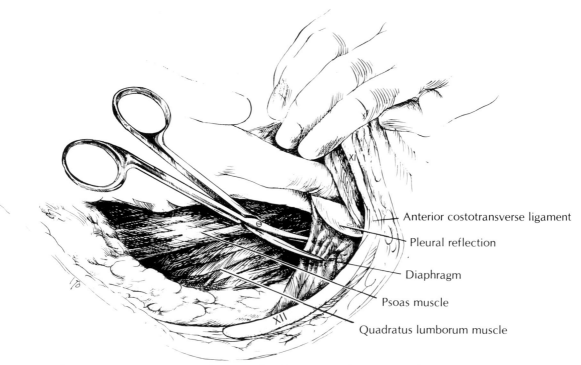

Labels in figure: Anterior costotransverse ligament — Pleural reflection — Diaphragm — Psoas muscle — Quadratus lumborum muscle

FIG. 9-3. The anterior costotransverse ligament has been incised, exposing the pleural reflection and diaphragm fibers. Releasing the posterior diaphragmatic attachment allows the pleural cavity to retract superiorly.

FIG. 9-4. The retroperitoneal fat surrounding the kidney and ureter is elevated over the aorta, allowing early vascular control and *en bloc* removal of the kidney and ureter with all fascial and fatty investments.

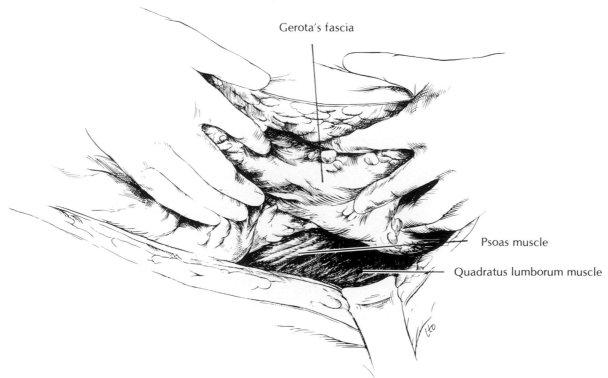

Labels in figure: Gerota's fascia — Psoas muscle — Quadratus lumborum muscle

126

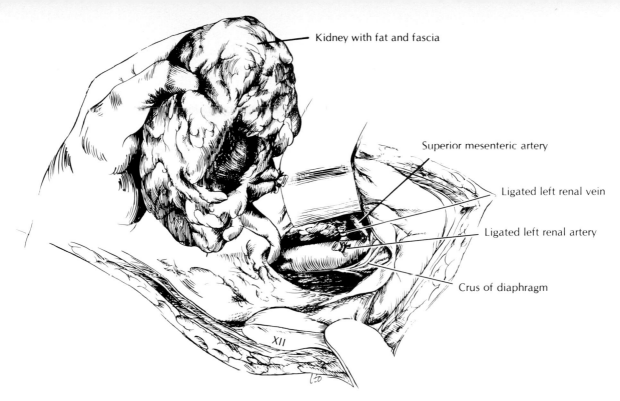

Kidney with fat and fascia

Superior mesenteric artery

Ligated left renal vein

Ligated left renal artery

Crus of diaphragm

XII

FIG. 9-5. The renal dissection is completed and the kidney, surrounding fat and fascia, adrenal gland, and lymph nodes have been lifted out of the wound, attached only by the ureter. Lymph nodes are routinely dissected to the medial side of the aorta for left-sided tumors, and to the medial aspect of the vena cava for right-sided tumors.

FIG. 9-6. Transvesical exposure of the left ureteral orifice in preparation for removal of the distal ureter and cuff of bladder

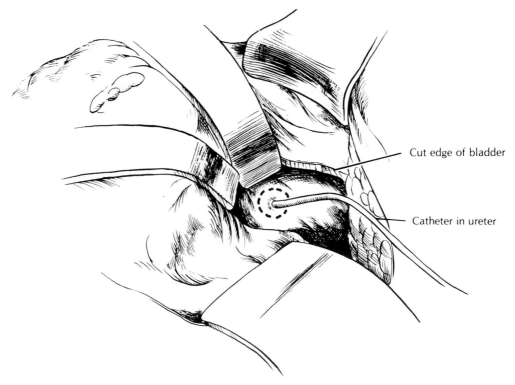

Cut edge of bladder

Catheter in ureter

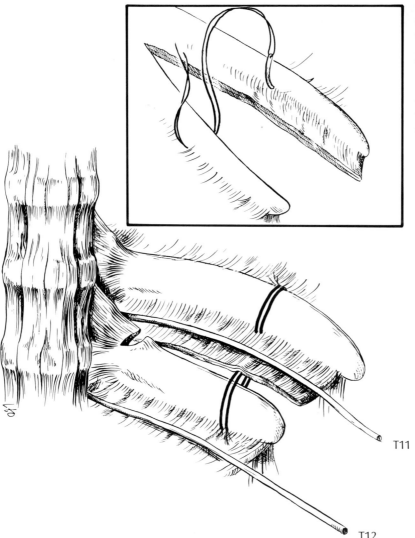

FIG. 9-7. The 11th intercostal nerve is blocked with a long-acting local anesthetic to provide pain relief in the early postoperative period, and closure is begun with a double pericostal suture of O-polyglycolic acid (*inset*). The diaphragm is not incorporated in the closure. Note that the intercostal bundle is excluded from the pericostal suture to avoid nerve entrapment.

T11

T12

ney, ureter, and its surrounding fat allows one to clean out the entire retroperitoneal space over the aorta. Dissection around the aorta removes the lymphatic tissue. The inferior vena cava is similarly dissected for a right radical nephroureterectomy. The spermatic cord is ligated and divided at the level of the external inguinal ring and taken with the specimen.

The kidney and surrounding fat, fascia, and lymph nodes can now be lifted out of the wound, attached only by the ureter (Figure 9-5). The urinary bladder is opened in the midline, the involved ureter is catheterized, and the ureteral orifice is circumscribed, sewn shut, and excised with a cuff of bladder (Figure 9-6). Removal of the distal ureter

and a cuff of bladder can be accomplished extravesically in selected cases; however, the uretero-vesical junction must be adequately exposed to ensure that a proper cuff is removed under direct vision. Inadequate visualization of the ureterovesical junction or removing the distal ureter by tenting up the ureter will result in inadequate removal of the distal ureter and cuff of bladder and will be associated with stump recurrences. The defect in the bladder is closed in two layers, and drainage is accomplished by a urethral catheter. A suprapubic tube and drains are not indicated. Intercostal nerve block is accomplished to provide early postoperative pain relief, and closure is begun with a doubled pericostal suture (Figure 9-7). A cystogram

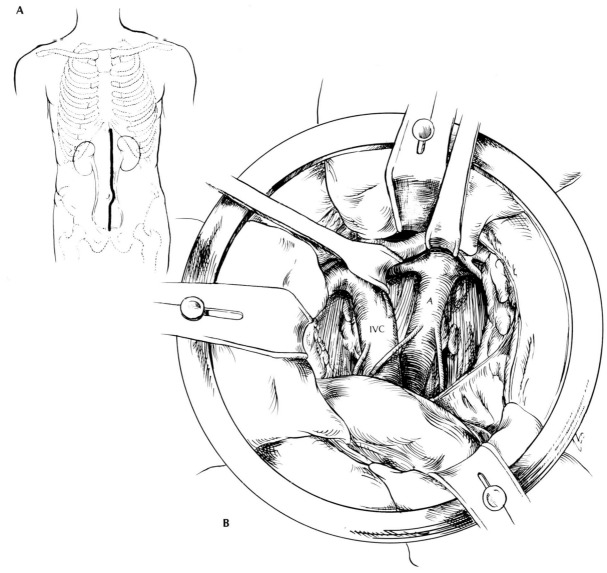

FIG. 9-8. **(A)** A midline incision is appropriate for bilateral tumors and some bulky tumors, and when a bilateral node dissection is contemplated. **(B)** We find the use of the ring retractor to be very helpful.

is performed on the 7th to 10th day after surgery and, if no extravasation is demonstrated, the urethral catheter is removed the following day.

A thoracoabdominal incision, which requires only slight modification of the supracostal, extrapleural incision, can be used for large tumors.[20]

An extended midline transperitoneal incision is useful for bilateral tumors, for bulky tumors with extension across the midline, and when an extended node dissection is indicated (Figure 9-8).

We find it useful to incise the posterior peritoneum around the right colon and along the small bowel mesentery, and to ligate the inferior mesenteric vein above the area of the left renal hilum. The right colon and small bowel are then placed in the protective bag in much the same way as is done for a suprahilar retroperitoneal lymph node dissection.

A complete nephroureterectomy can also be accomplished by using two separate incisions as shown in Figure 9-9.

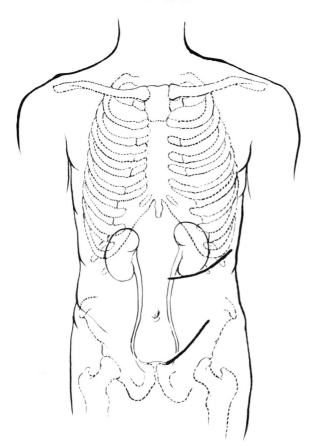

FIG. 9-9. Two incisions can be used for a complete nephroureterectomy. The flank incision is angled medially, and the pelvic incision is angled obliquely from the junction of the symphysis and rectal sheath.

REFERENCES

1. BARRY JM, HODGES CV: The supracostal approach for live donor nephrectomy. Arch Surg 109:448, 1974
2. BLOOM NA, VIDONE RA, LYTTON B: Primary carcinoma of the ureter—a report of 102 new cases. J Urol 103:590, 1970
3. CULP OS: Anterior nephroureterectomy; advantages and limitations of a single incision. J Urol 85:193, 1961
4. CUMMINGS KB: Nephroureterectomy: Rationale in the management of transitional cell carcinoma of the upper urinary tract. Urol Clin North Am 7:569, 1980
5. GITTES RF: Management of transitional cell carcinoma of the upper urinary tract: Case for conservative surgery. Urol Clin North Am 7:559, 1980
6. GONWA TA, CORBETT VMD, SCHEY HM et al: Analgesic associated nephropathy and transitional cell carcinoma of the urinary tract. Ann Intern Med 93:249, 1980
7. GRABSTALD H, WHITMORE WF, MELAMED MR: Renal pelvic tumors. JAMA 218:845, 1971
8. HALL, PW, DAMMIN GJ: Balkan nephropathy. Nephron 22:281, 1978
9. HUNT VC: Papillary epithelioma of the renal pelvis. Surg Clin North Am 9:853, 1929
10. JOHANNSON S, ANGERVALL L, BENGTSSON U et al: A clinical, pathologic and prognostic study of epithelial tumors of the renal pelvis. Cancer 37:1376, 1976
11. JOHNSON DE, BABAIAN RJ: Conservative surgical management for noninvasive distal ureteral carcinoma. Urology 13:365, 1979
12. KIMBALL FN, FERRIS HW: Papillomatous tumor of the renal pelvis associated with similar tumors of the ureter and bladder. J Urol 31:257, 1934
13. KINDER CH, WALLACE DM: Recurrent carcinoma of the ureteric stump. Br J Surg 50:202, 1962
14. KINN AC: Squamous cell carcinoma of the renal pelvis. Scand J Urol Nephrol 14:77, 1979
15. LATHAM HS, KAY S: Malignant tumors of the renal pelvis. Surg Gynecol and Obstet 138:613, 1974
16. MURPHY DM, ZINCKE H, FURLOW W: Primary Grade 1 transitional cell carcinoma of the renal pelvis and ureter. J Urol 123:629, 1980
17. O'CONOR VJ, LOGAN DJ: Nephroureterectomy. Surg Gynecol Obstet 122:601, 1966
18. PETKOVIC SD: Epidemiology and treatment of renal pelvis and ureteral tumors. J Urol 114:858, 1975
19. RUBENSTEIN MA, WALZ BJ, BUCY JG: Transitional cell carcinoma of the kidney: 25-year experience. J Urol 119:594, 1978
20. SKINNER DG: Considerations for management of large retroperitoneal tumors: Use of the modified thoracoabdominal approach. J Urol 117:605, 1977
21. STRONG DW, PEARSE HD: Recurrent urothelial tumors following surgery for transitional cell carcinoma of the upper urinary tract. Cancer 38:2178, 1976
22. WAGLE DG, MOORE RH, MURPHY GP: Primary carcinoma of the renal pelvis. Cancer 33:1642, 1974
23. WILLIAMS CB, MITCHELL JP: Carcinoma of the renal pelvis—a review of 43 cases. Br J Urol 45:370, 1973
24. WILLIAMS CB, MITCHELL JP: Carcinoma of the ureter—a review of 54 cases. Br J Urol 45:377, 1973

Nephrectomy With Cavotomy or Cavectomy

10

David L. McCullough

Etiology, Diagnosis, and Prognosis

Cavotomy associated with nephrectomy is occasionally necessary in renal cell carcinoma, Wilms' tumor, and some adrenal tumors. Most cases of caval involvement are associated with right-sided renal cell carcinoma because the right renal vein is much shorter than the left. The right renal vein also usually lacks collaterals, but the left renal vein has gonadal, adrenal, lumbar, and other collaterals. Ligation of the right renal vein at its caval junction almost always results in the loss of the kidney. Ligation of the left renal vein at its caval junction does not usually result in loss of the left kidney, although temporary renal dysfunction may occur (Fig. 10-1).

Approximately 25% of the renal cell carcinomas invade the renal vein, and 5% to 10% involve the vena cava. The ratio of incidence in men as compared to women is 4:1.[4] Patients with caval involvement may exhibit signs of caval obstruction such as unilateral or bilateral pedal edema, engorged superficial abdominal veins, proteinuria, a varicocele that fails to collapse in the supine position, the Budd–Chiari syndrome, or the nephrotic syndrome. The tumor thrombus may extend into the right atrium and even into the pulmonary artery and this occasionally results in right-sided congestive failure. It is also possible for patients with complete or partial caval obstruction to be completely asymptomatic.

Proper diagnosis of potential caval involvement is imperative. With arteriography one may be able to see the thrombus vascularized from the kidney side; a striated pattern may be seen. Epinephrine may enhance this pattern. If the renal vein is shown to be free of tumor following arteriography, cavography is unnecessary. If the renal vein is not visualized, either venography or cavography should be performed to evaluate the venous system. Some authors prefer a CT scan or ultrasound study when evaluating the venous system. Superior venacavography is occasionally necessary to evaluate the upper cava, especially when there is complete inferior caval obstruction.

If metastases are present in association with caval extension, surgery is absolutely contraindicated. The literature reports universally poor results when surgery is performed on such patients. Survival of more than 1 year is quite rare, and the operative mortality and morbidity are extremely high in such patients.[1,6] If caval extension is left undisturbed, nearly all patients will exhibit carcinomatosis, and most will die within a year.

Venacavotomy or cavectomy is indicated in patients with caval involvement who exhibit no other manifestation of extrarenal spread or metastases. Operative mortality and morbidity are quite acceptable. Survival of over 75% at 1 year has been reported, with an operative mortality of less than 10% from a number of cases reported in the literature since 1961.[2]

Operative Technique

If the tumor involves the atrium, a median sternotomy and a midline abdominal incision will be required, as will the services of the cardiac bypass team. If the subdiaphragmatic cava is involved, I use a thoracoabdominal incision, preferably at the 9th or 10th interspace. Others prefer a midline abdominal incision or a chevron incision.

A helpful adjunct in right-sided lesions is the division of the avascular attachments of the liver to the diaphragm (Fig. 10-2). The coronary ligament and right triangular ligament are sharply incised and the liver is rotated anteriorly like opening the pages of a book. This maneuver, which is easy to perform, exposes the intrahepatic cava and enables one to inspect and control the hepatic veins and gain control of the cava at a higher level than is otherwise feasible.

There are two or more main right hepatic veins and one left main hepatic vein draining into the intrahepatic cava at the most cephalad portion. At least two of these veins should be preserved. Small hepatic veins at about the level of the right adrenal vein caval junction can be divided with impunity to mobilize and control the cava.

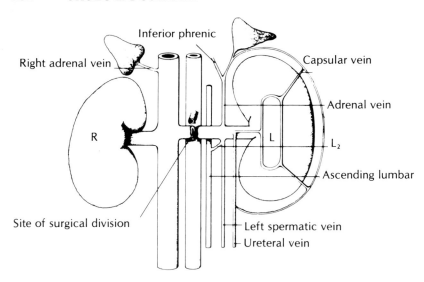

FIG. 10-1. Collateral venous drainage of left kidney and site of division close to cava (McCullough DL, Gittes RF: Vena cava resection for renal cell carcinoma. *J Urol* 112:162, 1974)

Some centers have reported angioinfarction of the involved kidney and subsequent renal and thrombus atrophy, which permits a less formidable procedure to be performed on the cava.

The renal artery should be ligated prior to mobilization of the kidney and the maneuvers described in the following paragraphs.

CAVOTOMY

Most tumor thrombi merely extend into the cava. If the extension is only 1 inch to 3 inches long and the thrombus is unattached to the lumen of the cava, then a cavotomy using a partial occluding clamp (such as a Satinsky clamp) may be performed. An ellipse of cava adjacent to the projecting thrombus is taken and the cava is resewn with a 3-0 vascular silk (Fig. 10-3).

Another method is to use vascular tapes to gain proximal, distal, and left renal vein control when performing a cavotomy. The cava may be partially closed, leaving a portion of the cavotomy open while the distal and left renal vein tapes are released to allow incoming venous blood to displace any air in the cava. The suture line is quickly completed while positive pressure ventilation is administered.

On occasion, a Foley catheter can be placed above the thrombus and the balloon inflated while the vascular tapes provide control of the cava. The catheter is slowly withdrawn and helps to retract the thrombus out through the cavotomy with a minimal amount of handling. Blind retraction of the thrombus with a Foley catheter without proximal and distal venous control can be dangerous because a fatal embolism could occur if the thrombus fragments.

CAVECTOMY

Figure 10-4A depicts cavectomy with ligation of the left renal vein and complete division of the cava above and below the thrombus, with *en bloc* removal of infradiaphragmatic vena cava below the hepatic veins. This procedure should be performed when it is thought that the entire caval circumference is invaded and extraction of the thrombus is not feasible.

Before this procedure is attempted, several tests should be performed to evaluate the ability of the left kidney to withstand ligation at the caval junction.[5] Five ml of Indigo Carmine given intravenously should appear in the bladder urine within 12 minutes of injection, which should be given after the renal artery to the right kidney has been clamped (assuming a right renal tumor). Pressure in the left renal vein of less than 40 mm Hg after occlusion is a favorable predictor of adequate collaterals in the left renal venous system. If the pressure is greater than 40 mm Hg, then edema, proteinuria, and possible renal failure may occur. If these tests suggest that there will be dysfunction of the kidney, then anastomosis of the renal vein to the portal vein or splenic vein, use of the saphenous vein bypass graft, or autotransplant of the kidney are possibilities; autotransplant is the least desirable method.

Figure 10-4B, C depicts partial cavectomy and includes leaving a strip of cava attached to the left renal vein. This strip can be rolled into a tube and closed with 3-0 vascular silk. This procedure is applicable when it is thought that a significant portion of the cava is actually invaded by the thrombus. The procedure works quite well and

FIG. 10-2. Posterior view of hepatic ligaments and relationship of vena cava to liver (McCullough DL, Gittes RF. Vena cava resection for renal cell carcinoma. *J Urol* 112:162, 1974)

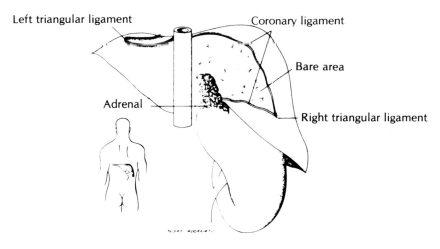

FIG. 10-3. **(A)** Extraction of caval thrombus with attached right renal vein.   **(B)** Closure of cavotomy after thrombus extraction

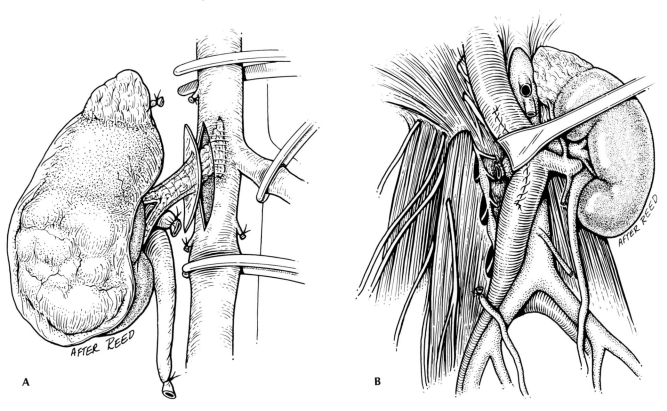

A

B

obviates the problem of left renal dysfunction that is sometimes seen when the left renal vein is ligated at the caval junction. When complete division of the cava is planned, the new vascular staples, which work well and are rapidly applied, can be used.

MANAGEMENT OF SUPRADIAPHRAGMATIC CAVAL EXTENSION

The problem of venous inflow from hepatic veins complicates the management of supradiaphragmatic caval extension. Use of the Pringle maneuver

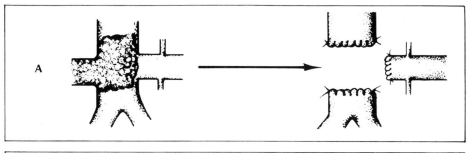

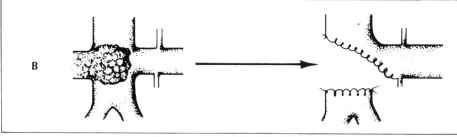

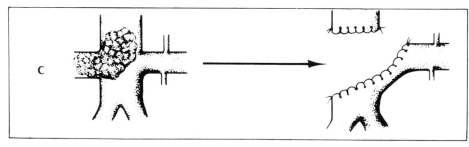

FIG. 10-4. Different methods of surgical management of vena cava invasion by renal carcinoma: **(A)** complete cavectomy and ligation of left renal vein; **(B)** partial cavectomy, strip of upper cava preserved; **(C)** partial cavectomy, strip of lower cava preserved. (McCullough, DL, Talner, LB: Inferior vena cava extension of renal carcinoma. Am J Roentgenol 121:825, 1974)

(clamping of the porta hepatis with a noncrushing vascular clamp) is quite helpful. However, one must work quickly because the safe warm ischemic time for the hepatic tissue is approximately 15 minutes. If the thrombus is nonadherent in the cava, then clamping the supradiaphramatic cava with infrarenal and left renal venous control may permit extraction of the thrombus from below. A Foley catheter may help. If the thrombus barely extends into the atrium, then it may be possible to use the same technique with partial occlusion of the atrium.[7]

If the cava is invaded at the level of the main hepatic venous inflow or higher, then the tumor is unresectable.

If the tumor extends well into the atrium but does not invade it, then cardiac bypass may be used to enable extraction of the thrombus while maintaining proper perfusion.

SPECIAL PROBLEMS

Several techniques may be tried if profound hypotension results when the cava is occluded because of inadequate venous return to the heart. The Trendelenburg position may help. Application of occlusive tapes quite slowly and progressively may prevent profound hypotension. One author cross clamped the aorta at the diaphragmatic level, to prevent pooling below the diaphragm, before cross clamping the cava.[3] Potential problems from this procedure include ischemic changes in bowel, legs, remaining kidney, liver, and spinal cord. Cross clamping the infrarenal aorta is less hazardous. Of course, cardiopulmonary bypass may be used if hypotension cannot be controlled in any other way.

When the left kidney, renal vein, and cava are associated with a caval thrombus, special consideration must be given to ensure proper venous drainage of the kidney. Most of the techniques described in the previous paragraph should be considered. In most cases simple ligation of the right renal vein results in loss of the kidney.

CONCLUSIONS

Cavotomy and cavectomy are complicated, tedious and demanding. A well-thought-out plan with several alternatives and contingencies must be made prior to surgery. Precise preoperative delineation of the extent of the thrombus is imperative. Familiarity with vascular instruments, staplers, and associated equipment is a prerequisite. If metastatic disease is found prior to nephrectomy, the procedure should be abandoned. Node dissection is often impossible because of numerous venous collaterals. The anatomy of the liver, heart, and venous system should be thoroughly reviewed. If these principles are observed, then the operation can be done with low morbidity and mortality and with gratifying results for the patient and the surgeon.

REFERENCES

1. ABDELSAYED MA, BISADDA NK, FINKBEINER AE et al: Renal tumors involving the inferior vena cava. Plan for management. J Urol 120:153, 1978

2. CLAYMAN RV, GONZALES R, FRALEY EE: Renal cell cancer invading vena cava. J Urol 123:157, 1980

3. CUMMINGS KB, LI W-I, RYAN JA et al: Intraoperative management of renal cell carcinoma with supradiaphragmatic caval extension. J Urol 122: 829, 1979

4. MCCULLOUGH DL, GITTES RF: Vena cava resection for renal cell carcinoma. J Urol 112:162, 1974

5. MCCULLOUGH DL, GITTES RF: Ligation of the renal vein in the solitary kidney: Effects on renal function. J Urol 113:295, 1975

6. SCHEFFT P, NOVICK AC, STRAFFON RA et al: Surgery for renal cell carcinoma extending into the inferior vena cava. J Urol 120:28, 1978

7. SKINNER DG, PFISTER RF, COLVIN R: Extension of renal cell carcinoma into the vena cava: The rationale for aggressive surgical management. J Urol 107:711, 1972

Renal Bench Surgery

11

Andrew C. Novick

Transferral of a kidney from one site to another in the same patient evolved as a logical extension of the field of renal allotransplantation. The first successful autotransplant was performed in 1962 by Hardy in a patient whose ureter had been severly damaged by previous aortic surgery; in 1963, Woodruff achieved the first successful autotransplant for renovascular hypertension.[6,29] Effective methods of renal presevation and microvascular surgical techniques subsequently resulted in the advent of extracorporeal renal surgery for complex renal disorders. In 1967, Ota reported the first successful extracorporeal renal arterial repair combined with autotransplantation in a patient with renovascular hypertension.[22] A wave of enthusiasm for this approach followed, and many other cases were reported employing varying methods of renal preservation and surgical repair. As experience was gained, more specific indications and contraindications were defined, and renal bench surgery with autotransplantation is now the treatment of choice for selected patients with complicated upper urinary tract disorders.[8,17]

In general, renal bench surgery should be considered when its use will improve the likelihood of a good result, or when *in situ* techniques cannot be safely performed. The current indications for this approach include complicated renovascular disorders, bilateral or solitary renal neoplasms, and advanced nephrolithiasis. The advantages of performing extracorporeal repair of the kidney include optimum exposure and illumination, a bloodless surgical field, greater protection of the kidney from ischemia, more facile employment of microvascular techniques and optimal magnification, and diminished risk of tumor spillage in cases of carcinoma.

PREOPERATIVE PREPARATION

In patients undergoing renal bench surgery, preoperative renal and pelvic arteriography should be performed to define renal arterial anatomy, to ensure relatively disease-free iliac vessels for auto-transplantation, and, in patients with branch renal artery disease, to evaluate the hypogastric artery and its branches as a reconstructive graft. Autotransplantation of kidneys involved with severe renal parenchymal or small vessel disease should be avoided. Such kidneys generally flush poorly following their removal, often leading to irreversible ischemic damage and nonfunction postoperatively. In patients with bacteriuria, organism-specific parenteral antibiotic therapy is initiated 48 hr preoperatively. In all cases, 200 ml/hr of intravenous fluids are ordered the evening prior to surgery to ensure optimal renal perfusion in the operating room.

Surgical Approach

Most extracorporeal renal operations are performed through an anterior subcostal transperitoneal incision to remove the kidney, combined with a separate lower quadrant transverse semilunar incision for autotransplantation. In nonobese patients, a single midline incision extending from the xiphoid to the symphysis pubis may be used. The technique for removing the kidney is identical to that employed in live donor nephrectomy for allotransplantation, and the same intraoperative measures are taken to ensure minimal renal ischemia and immediate function after revascularization. These measures include prevention of hypotension during the period of anesthesia, administration of mannitol, liberal hydration, and minimal surgical manipulation of the kidney. Systemic heparinization prior to nephrectomy is unnecessary.

Immediately following its removal, the kidney is flushed with 500 ml of chilled Collins Intracellular Electrolyte Solution and is then submerged in a basin of ice-slush saline to maintain hypothermia. Under these conditions, if there has been minimal warm renal ischemia, the kidney can safely be preserved for many more hours than are needed to perform even the most complex renal repair.[10] After completing the extracorporeal operation under ice-slush surface hypothermia, the reconstructed kidney may be placed on the pulsatile perfusion unit to assess pressure-flow relationships, to secure hemostasis, and to verify renal vascular patency and integrity.

In performing renal bench surgery, we have found it cumbersome to work on the abdominal wall with the ureter attached. It is preferable to divide the ureter and place the kidney on a separate workbench. This provides better exposure for the extracorporeal operation, facilitates the performance of radiography and nephroscopy, and allows a second surgical team to be simultaneously preparing the iliac fossa. This approach is also justified by the low incidence of complications following ureteroneocystostomy in renal allotransplantation.[15] However, in patients undergoing removal of large centrally located neoplasms in a solitary kidney, when complete tumor excision may unavoidably compromise renal pelvic or ureteral blood supply, it is best to leave the ureter attached for preservation of its distal collateral vascular supply. When this is done, the ureter must be temporarily occluded to prevent retrograde blood flow to the kidney and rewarming during the extracorporeal operation. Care must be taken not to rotate the kidney in moving it so as to produce an obstructive torsion of the ureter. Although the ureter may follow a redundant course to the bladder after autotransplantation, normal ureteral peristalsis will provide effective drainage of urine from the kidney. The vascular techniques for performing autotransplantation of the kidney are identical to those employed in renal allotransplantation, which is discussed in Chapter 33.

RENOVASCULAR DISEASE

The largest amount of experience in extracorporeal renal surgery has been gained in the management of complicated renovascular disorders, including preparation of donor kidneys for allotransplantation with anomalous vessels,[16] repair of extensive branch renal artery lesions that cannot be repaired *in situ*,[4,8,9,20,22,26] and repair of severely traumatized kidneys.[5,24] The various techniques for performing extracorporeal vascular reconstruction of the kidney are illustrated in Fig. 11-1.

Donor Arterial Repair Before Allotransplantation

The most common indication for renal bench surgery has been the preparation of donor kidneys for allotransplantation with diseased, damaged, or multiple arteries.[17] Multiple renal arteries occur unilaterally and bilaterally in 23% and 10% of the population, respectively, and comprise the most frequent indication for such vascular repairs when a Carrel aortic patch is unavailable. There are three basic techiques for extracorporeal donor arterial repair which, singly or combined, can be readily applied to most anatomic variants presented by kidneys with multiple arteries.

When two adjacent renal arteries of comparable size are present, a side-to-side (conjoined) anastomosis of the two vessels is performed to create a common ostium (Fig. 11-1A). This is done just prior to transplantation, with the kidney kept cool in iced saline solution. Continuous 6-0 or 7-0 vascular sutures are employed for the side-to-side anastomosis, with optical magnification provided by 3.5-power opthalmologic loupes. This method is simple technically and is also endowed with favorable hemodynamic characteristics. The union of two vessels in this manner forms a common ostium with a cross-sectional area greater than the sum of the cross-sectional area of the two separate vessels. Because resistance to flow in a vessel is inversely related to the vessel's radius, the coapted vessels have a lower resistance and, theoretically, a higher flow than a comparable length of either vessel prior to their union. The conjoined anastomosis may also be used to manage double renal veins of equal size.

The technique of choice for repairing kidneys supplied by two renal arteries of disparate caliber is extracorporeal microvascular end-to-side anastomosis of the smaller artery to the larger one (Fig. 11-1B). This procedure is also done with the kidney cooled in iced saline solution. To obviate narrowing of the arterial lumen, a short linear arteriotomy is made in the side of the main renal artery without excising any of the vessel wall. After the polar artery has been spatulated, an end-to-side anastomosis with the main renal artery is performed with interrupted 7-0 or 8-0 vascular sutures using microvascular instruments and 3.5-power opthalmologic loupes for magnification. A small catheter or probe may be placed through the suture line during its construction to prevent accidental entrapment of the back wall. For vessels less than 1.5 mm in diameter, 9-0 vascular suture material is used and the repair is done under the operating microscope. The completed anastomosis is tested for patency and integrity by gentle perfusion of the main renal artery. This technique is also readily applicable to the reconstruction of kidneys that are supplied by more than two renal arteries of varying diameters.

Another useful method for repairing donor kidneys with multiple arteries involves fashioning the

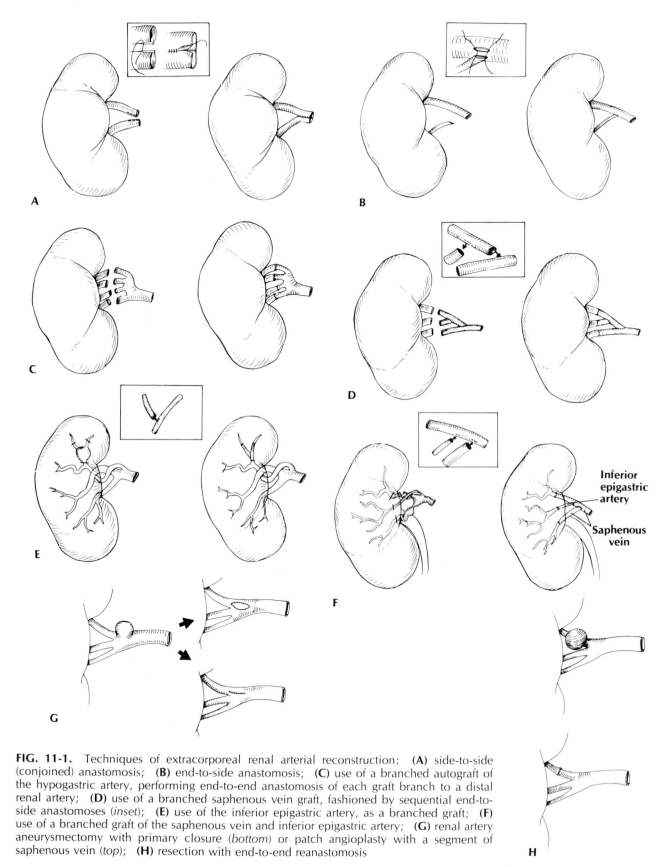

FIG. 11-1. Techniques of extracorporeal renal arterial reconstruction: **(A)** side-to-side (conjoined) anastomosis; **(B)** end-to-side anastomosis; **(C)** use of a branched autograft of the hypogastric artery, performing end-to-end anastomosis of each graft branch to a distal renal artery; **(D)** use of a branched saphenous vein graft, fashioned by sequential end-to-side anastomoses (*inset*); **(E)** use of the inferior epigastric artery, as a branched graft; **(F)** use of a branched graft of the saphenous vein and inferior epigastric artery; **(G)** renal artery aneurysmectomy with primary closure (*bottom*) or patch angioplasty with a segment of saphenous vein (*top*); **(H)** resection with end-to-end reanastomosis

arteries into a single renal artery by use of a branched autogenous vascular graft. The hypogastric artery can be removed intact with its branches and is the material of choice when it is free of disease (Fig. 11-1C). If extensive calcification of the hypogastric artery renders it unsuitable as a reconstructive graft, then a branched saphenous vein graft can be fashioned and employed (Fig. 11-1D). The extracorporeal vascular repair is performed under surface hypothermia, with end-to-end anastomosis of the graft branches to the distal renal arteries. This branched vascular graft technique is particularly useful for transplanting kidneys with more than two renal arteries or when insufficient arterial length prevents the use of either of the two methods previously described.

These three basic techniques for performing extracorporeal donor arterial repair are technically uncomplicated, are readily applicable to most anatomic situations, allow performance of a precise repair between arteries of similar thickness, and allow careful examination of the repair upon completion. In addition, because the kidney is kept cold throughout the extracorporeal procedure and transplantation is performed using the same method as with a single renal artery, there is no increase in revascularization time and ischemic allograft damage is minimized.

Branch Renal Artery Disease

Most branch renal artery lesions are caused by fibrous diseases that occur in young patients and often progress with nonoperative management. Hypertension in these cases is generally difficult to control, and revascularization is indicated both to preserve renal function and to minimize the need for long-term antihypertensive therapy.[19] Renal artery aneurysms are typically located at the bifur-cation of the main renal artery and therefore frequently involve arterial branches. Aneurysmectomy is indicated when the aneurysms cause significant hypertension or to obviate the risk of rupture associated with a lack of or incomplete calcification, size greater than 2 cm, or pregnancy.[25] Renal arteriovenous malformation provides a rare indication for revascularization. It is uncommon for atherosclerosis to involve branches of the renal artery.

Extracorporeal branch arterial repair and auto-transplantation are indicated primarily when preoperative arteriography with oblique views shows intrarenal extension of renovascular disease (Fig. 11-2).[20] Removing and flushing the kidney causes it to contract in size, thereby enabling more peripheral dissection in the renal sinus for mobilization of distal arterial branches. In patients with dissecting fibrous lesions, partially calcified aneurysms, or prior renovascular operations, the diseased renal vessels are also more difficult to mobilize *in situ* because of intense surrounding fibrotic reaction and adherence to adjacent hilar structures. Some of these cases are more safely and effectively managed with extracorporeal revascularization.

The most commonly employed method for extracorporeal branch renal artery reconstruction involves procurement or fashioning of a branched autogenous vascular graft. This technique permits separate end-to-end microvascular anastomosis of each graft branch to a distal renal arterial branch. A hypogastric arterial graft is the preferred material for vascular reconstruction because this vessel can be obtained intact with two or more of its branches (see Fig. 11-1C). When atherosclerotic degeneration precludes use of the hypogastric artery, a long segment of saphenous vein can be harvested, and, employing sequential end-to-side microvascular

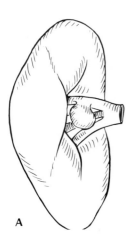 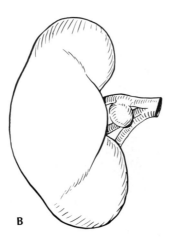

FIG. 11-2. **(A)** Branch renal artery lesions may appear intrarenal in location on standard anteroposterior radiographic view. **(B)** Proper oblique views will often demonstrate branch arterial involvement outside the renal hilus, making *in situ* vascular repair possible.

A

B

anastomoses, a branched graft can be fashioned from this vessel (see Fig. 11-1D).

Branched grafts of the hypogastric artery and saphenous vein may occasionally prove too large in caliber for anastomosis to small secondary or tertiary arterial branches. In these cases, the inferior epigastric artery provides an excellent alternate free graft for extracorporeal microvascular repair.[14] This artery measures 1.5 mm to 2 mm in diameter, is rarely diseased, and coapts well in caliber and thickness to smaller renal artery branches. The inferior epigastric artery can also be employed as a branched graft, either by itself (see (Fig. 11-1E) or in conjunction with a segment of saphenous vein (see (Fig. 11-1F). The branched graft is constructed so that its limbs will match the disease-free distal branches in caliber and thickness.

Although use of a branched autogenous vascular graft provides a simple, versatile, and effective method for branch arterial reconstruction, other techniques are occasionally preferable. In some patients with localized segmental intrarenal branch lesions, there may be other arterial branches that are either uninvolved or have more proximally located vascular disease. Such branches with longer disease-free distal segments may be anastomosed end-to-side either into a larger arterial branch or into the reconstructive vascular graft. Occasionally, two distal disease-free arterial branches of similar diameter are found adjacent to one another. When this occurs, the two adjacent branches can be conjoined and then anastomosed end-to-end to a single limb of the branched graft.

Renal artery aneurysms have a highly variable presentation, and the method of extracorporeal repair will be determined by whether renovascular involvement is focal or diffuse. If the renal artery wall at the base of an aneurysm is intact, aneurysmectomy with either primary closure or patch angioplasty can be performed (see Fig. 11-1G). Aneurysms with short focal involvement of renal artery branches may also be simply resected with end-to-end branch reanastomosis (see Fig. 11-1H). In other cases, with more diffuse vascular disease, aneurysmectomy and revascularization with a branched autogenous graft will be indicated.

Occasionally, multiple renal veins are encountered during the performance of bench surgery on the kidney. These veins are less common than multiple renal arteries and more frequently involve the right kidney. Small renal veins can simply be ligated without risk. When double renal veins of approximately equal size are present, both of these must be preserved to avoid increased intrarenal venous pressure after revascularization. In this situation, extracorporeal venous reconstruction is performed with either conjoined or end-to-side anastomosis of the two veins.

These extracorporeal renovascular operations are all performed with the kidney preserved by surface hypothermia in a basin of ice-slush saline and employing microvascular instruments, 7-0 to 9-0 suture material, and optical magnification. During dissection and mobilization of the renal vessels, care is taken not to interfere with the ureteral or pelvic blood supply. While revascularizing multiple arterial branches, the surgeon must anticipate the position that the various branches will assume in relation to one another upon completion of the repair. Individual branch anastomoses are then performed with careful attention to avoid subsequent malrotation, angulation, or tension.

When extracorporeal repair is completed, prior to autotransplantation, the kidney is placed on the hypothermic pulsatile perfusion unit. With the perfusion pressure set at the systolic pressure of the patient, any arterial anastomotic leaks can be readily identified and controlled. Another useful adjunct is to instill 2 ml of Indigo Carmine into the arterial cannula. If this dye is evenly distributed throughout the perfused kidney, then patency of all branch anastomoses can be verified.

These microvascular reconstructive methods are technically simple, allow for repair with autogenous tissue grafts, and involve anastomosis of vessels that are similar in caliber and thickness. In all cases, extracorporeal repair leads to fashioning of a single main renal artery so that autotransplantation may be performed with one arterial anastomosis *in situ* and no increase in the critical revascularization time. Postoperatively, urethral catheter drainage of the bladder is maintained; however, surgical drains are usually not employed in these cases.

Renal Trauma

There have been few reported cases of renal bench surgery in patients with extensive renal trauma involving the vascular pedicle.[5,24] This no doubt reflects the uncommon occurrence of such injuries and the requirement for early operative intervention to achieve successful renal salvage. One of our patients undergoing an extracorporeal renal operation for another indication developed cardiac arrhythmias during the bench procedure, requiring termination of the operation. The repaired kidney was maintained on pulsatile perfusion for 24 hr, and, when the patient's condition stabilized, autotransplantation was successfully performed. This approach might also be employed in the critically ill patient with multiple injuries and severe renal trauma, whose condition is too unstable to permit primary repair at the initial laparotomy, and in whom renal salvage is felt to be important. Extracorporeal vascular repair of the traumatized kidney can be accomplished with one or more of the techniques previously described according to the extent and location of renal vascular injury.

RENAL TUMORS

In patients with bilateral synchronous renal malignancies or carcinoma in a solitary kidney, partial nephrectomy represents the primary curative form of treatment.[7,18] In most cases, this operation can be satisfactorily performed *in situ*. Only those patients with large, centrally located renal cell carcinomas, Wilms' tumors, or transitional cell renal pelvic tumors will be candidates for extracorporeal partial nephrectomy and autotransplantation.[17,23] This approach is best reserved for patients with no metastatic disease wherein surgical therapy is undertaken with the aim of achieving complete tumor excision. Renal bench surgery offers the advantage of more accurate delineation and removal of the tumor-bearing portion of the kidney, with maximal conservation of the uninvolved parenchyma (Fig. 11-3). One study has also shown that postoperative local tumor recurrence is less common following extracorporeal partial nephrectomy than when this operation is done *in situ*.[7]

Extracorporeal excision of the tumor (Fig. 11-4) is performed following *en bloc* radical nephrectomy

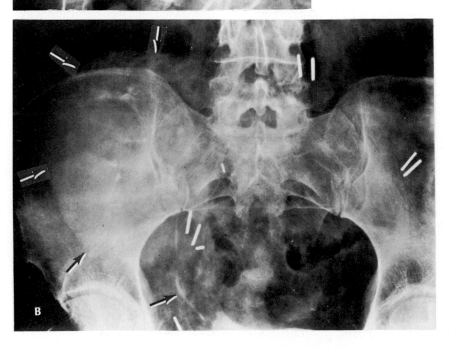

FIG. 11-3. **(A)** A selective renal arteriogram demonstrates a large carcinoma occupying the upper portion of a solitary right kidney, with tumor vessels involving the renal hilus. **(B)** An intravenous pyelogram following extracorporeal partial nephrectomy and autotransplantation demonstrates a large functioning renal remnant (outlined by *arrows*) and intact ureter (*lower arrow*).

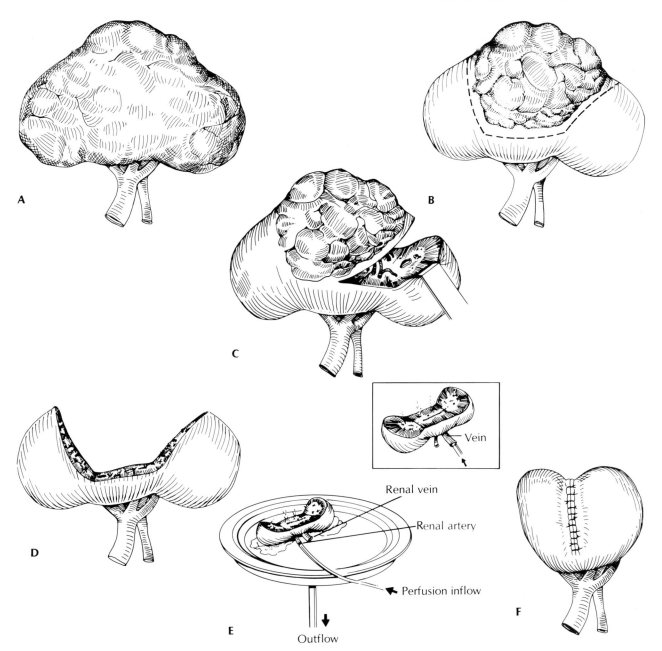

FIG. 11-4. Technique for extracorporeal resection of large central renal neoplasm: **(A)** The kidney is removed outside Gerota's fascia and is delivered to the workbench with its surrounding perinephric fat. **(B)** The flushed kidney is divested of all perinephric fat and the gross margins of the tumor in relation to uninvolved renal parenchyma are defined. The *dotted line* outlines the area of tumor to be excised with a margin of surrounding normal renal tissue. **(C)** The capsule and parenchyma are incised and vessels directed toward the neoplasm are secured and divided. **(D)** The renal remnant following extracorporeal excision of the tumor is shown. The collecting system is closed, and transected blood vessels are secured. **(E)** The renal remnant is placed on the pulsatile perfusion unit and is alternately perfused through the renal artery and vein (*inset*). This facilitates identification and ligation of remaining transected vessels and is important in ensuring complete hemostasis. **(F)** The defect created by the partial nephrectomy is closed by suturing the kidney upon itself to further ensure a water-tight repair.

and regional lymphadenectomy, with the flushed kidney in ice-slush saline. These operations may be particularly complicated, and, whenever possible, it is best to leave the ureter attached to preserve collateral ureteral vascular supply. The flushed kidney is first divested of all perinephric fat to appreciate the full extent of the neoplasm (Figs. 11-4A and 11-4B). Because such tumors are usually centrally located, dissection is begun in the renal hilus and carried out to the periphery of the kidney. Major arterial and venous channels directed toward the neoplasm are secured and divided, and those vessels supplying uninvolved renal parenchyma are preserved. The overlying capsule and parenchyma are progressively incised to preserve a 2-cm margin of normal renal tissue around the tumor (Figs. 11-4C and 11-4D). Microvascular techniques and optical magnification are invaluable aids to securing transected blood vessels and closing the collecting system, generally with interrupted 4-0 or 5-0 chromic sutures.

After completing the resection, tumor-free margins can be verified by frozen sections or extracorporeal arteriography. If arteriography is performed, iothalamate rather than diatrizoate contrast material should be employed, because the latter may crystallize at low temperatures. The kidney should also be immediately reflushed to further obviate toxicity of contrast agents or their cold-induced precipitation.[1] The renal remnant is then placed on the pulsatile perfusion unit to assess pressure-flow relationships and to facilitate identification and suture ligation of remaining potential bleeding points. At this stage, the kidney is alternately perfused through the renal artery and vein to ensure both arterial and venous hemostasis (Fig. 11-4E). Because the perfusate lacks clotting ability, there may continue to be some parenchymal oozing, which can safely be ignored. If possible, the defect created by the partial nephrectomy is closed by suturing the kidney upon itself to further ensure a watertight repair (Fig. 11-4F).

Following autotransplantation, a Penrose drain is positioned extraperitoneally in the iliac fossa away from the vascular anastomotic sites. When removal of the neoplasm has necessitated extensive hilar dissection of vessels supplying the renal pelvis or ureter, a nephrostomy tube is left indwelling for postoperative drainage.

ADVANCED NEPHROLITHIASIS

The vast majority of patients undergoing surgical therapy for renal calculus disease can be satisfactorily managed with *in situ* anatrophic nephrolith-

otomy or extended pyelolithotomy.[3,27] However, in selected patients with advanced nephrolithiasis and failed prior surgical therapy, renal bench surgery and autotransplantation provide the best method for achieving complete stone removal and unobstructed drainage from the upper urinary tract. The indications for this approach in patients with renal calculus disease are recurrent nephrolithiasis with stenosis of the renal pelvis or ureter, recurrent obstructing ureteral calculi and intractable colic, coexisting staghorn calculus and renovascular disease, and selected cases of recurrent staghorn calculi, particularly in a solitary kidney.[*†‡][2,4,17,21] For patients in the first two categories, it is often possible to remove the calculi with standard *in situ* methods. The rationale for removing the kidney in these cases is to perform autotransplantation and thereby ensure unobstructed drainage of urine or recurrent calculi from the upper urinary tract to the bladder.

Specific advantages of renal bench surgery in patients with stone disease include the superiority of extracorporeal radiography for detection of retained calculi, facilitation of nephroscopy, and the ability to extract difficult stones under direct fluoroscopic visualization. In reoperative cases with extensive perihilar fibrosis, the ureter and the renal pelvis can be meticulously dissected while preserving their blood supply and avoiding injury to major arterial or venous channels. Also, because the removed flushed kidney contracts in size, more peripheral intrasinusoidal exposure is possible for performing extended pyelolithotomy. This may obviate the need for nephrotomy incisions that would otherwise be required to achieve complete stone removal *in situ*.

Most patients will have undergone prior renal surgery, and mobilization of the kidney may be difficult because of perirenal scarring and obliteration of normal planes of dissection. In freeing the kidney, it is always preferable to include surrounding adherent fibromuscular tissue rather than to risk leaving behind some renal parenchyma attached to the retroperitoneum. The renal vessels are mobilized proximally, and dissection in the region of the hilus is scrupulously avoided. Preservation of the removed flushed kidney is achieved with surface hypothermia. Pulsatile perfusion in these cases is unnecessary and carries the risk of bacteria or tiny stone fragments entering the per-

---

* Faure AG: Personal communication, 1980
† Flatmark A: Personal communication, 1980
‡ Okada K: Personal communication, 1981

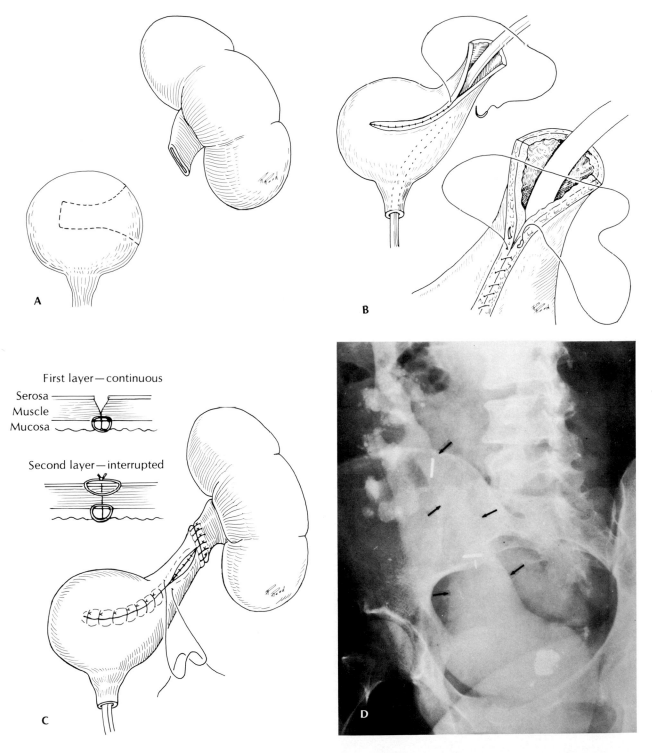

FIG. 11-5. **(A)** through **(C)** show the technique for fashioning a Boari bladder flap over a 22Fr catheter, which is then anastomosed directly to the renal pelvis; the bladder flap is closed in two separate layers. **(D)** shows an intravenous pyelogram following autotransplantation with a Boari flap pyelovesicostomy in a patient with renal tubular acidosis and recurrent renal colic, a wide-caliber bladder flap is outlined by *arrows*.

fusate and being disseminated into the renal circulation.

The extracorporeal operation begins with mobilization of the renal pelvis and infundibula posteriorly, extending well into the renal sinus. There may be considerable perihilar fibrosis, and meticulous microsurgical dissection is performed to avoid injury either to the collecting system or to the adjacent renal vessels. The exposure provided by this intrasinusoidal approach is excellent and allows most calculi to be removed with an extended pyelotomy incision. Nephroscopy is a valuable adjunct for locating and removing retained calculi. Direct extraction under fluoroscopy is also available for stones which are small and difficult to find. To preserve renal parenchyma, nephrotomy incisions are reserved for caliceal stones which cannot be removed through a pyelotomy because of either severe impaction or a stenotic infundibulum. In the latter case, repair of the intrarenal collecting system is performed as described by Smith and Boyce to ensure unobstructed drainage.[27] One can also inject several milliliters of Indigo Carmine into renal artery branches to demarcate clearly the most appropriate line for intersegmental incisions into the renal parenchyma. Plain radiographs of the kidney are essential to ensure complete removal of all calculi prior to autotransplantation.

Following the renal bench operation, there are several methods for restoring urinary continuity. Ureteroneocystostomy is the preferred technique when there is an adequate length of unobstructed proximal ureter. In patients with recurrent renal colic, the entire ureter is resected and pyelovesicostomy is performed by fashioning a Boari bladder flap over a 22F catheter for anastomosis to the renal pelvis (Fig. 11-5). In other cases, when fibrotic obstruction of the upper ureter and pelvis is present, the strictured areas are resected and the renal pelvis is anastomosed to the lower disease-free ureter.

Following autotransplantation, a Penrose drain is positioned in the iliac fossa and a urethral catheter is left in the bladder. Nephrostomy drainage is employed in selected cases when extensive upper urinary tract reconstruction has been performed.

Postoperative Care

Within the first 24 hr postoperatively, a technetium renal scan is obtained to verify perfusion of the autotransplanted kidney. Subsequent radioisotope monitoring is performed with ^{131}I orthoiodohippurate, which provides a functional assessment of the autograft. If there is no postoperative vaso-

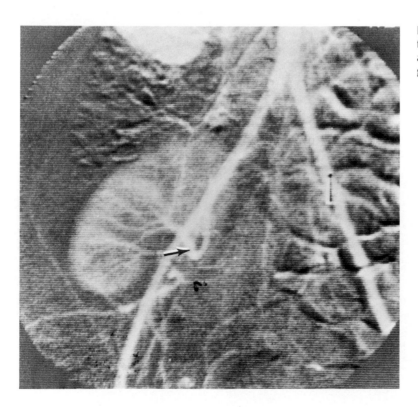

FIG. 11-6. Digital subtraction angiogram following autotransplantation shows patent anastomosis of the renal artery to the hypogastric artery (*arrow*).

motor nephropathy, this scan will show prompt uptake, early excretion, and complete clearance of the isotope from the graft. Urethral catheter drainage of the bladder is maintained for 1 week postoperatively. Patients are then instructed to void at least every 2 hr, and the Penrose drain, if present, is gradually removed over the next 48 hr. When a nephrostomy tube has been employed, a gravity nephrostogram is performed prior to its removal to document free flow into the bladder without extravasation.

Prior to discharge from the hospital, digital subtraction angiography of the pelvis is obtained following intravenous administration of 30 ml of contrast material.[11] This provides an excellent noninvasive method for evaluating main arterial patency of the autograft (Fig. 11-6). In patients undergoing extracorporeal branch renal artery reconstruction, conventional pelvic arteriography is performed to more accurately evaluate the intrarenal microvascular anastomoses. Six weeks postoperatively, a standard intravenous pyelogram is obtained to ensure unobstructed urinary drainage from the autograft.

REFERENCES

1. ALFIDI RJ, MAGNUSSON MO: Arteriography during perfusion preservation of kidneys. Am J Roentgenol Radiat Ther Nucl Med, 114:690, 1972
2. ANDERSEN OS, CLARK SS, MARLET MM et al: Treatment of extensive renal calculi with extracorporeal surgery and autotransplantation. Urology 7:465, 1976
3. GIL-VERNET J: New concepts in removing renal calculi. Urol Int 20:255, 1965
4. GIL-VERNET JM, CARALPS A, REVERT L et al: Extracorporeal renal surgery. Work bench surgery. Urology 5:444, 1975
5. GUTMAN FM, HOMSY Y, SCHMIDT E: Avulsion injury to the renal pedicle: Successful autotransplantation after bench surgery. J Trauma 184:469, 1978
6. HARDY JD: High ureteral injuries: Management by autotransplantation of the kidney. JAMA 184:97, 1963
7. JACOBS SC, BERG SI, LAWSON RK: Synchronous bilateral renal cancer: Total surgical excision. Cancer 46:2341, 1980
8. LAWSON RK, HODGES CV: Extracorporeal renal artery repair and autotransplantation. Urology 4:532, 1974
9. LIM RC et al: Renal autotransplantation. Adjunct to repair of renal vascular lesions. Arch Surg 105:847, 1972
10. MAGNUSSON M, STOWE N: Controversy in organ preservation. Urol Clin North Am 3:491, 1976
11. MEANEY TF et al: Digital subtraction angiography of the human cardiovascular system. Am J Roentgenol 135:1153, 1980
12. NOVICK AC: Management of intrarenal branch arterial lesions with extracorporeal microvascular reconstruction and autotransplantation. J Urol (in press)
13. NOVICK AC: Role of bench surgery and autotransplantation in renal calculous disease. Urol Clin North Am (in press)
14. NOVICK AC: Use of inferior epigastric artery for extracorporeal microvascular branch renal artery reconstruction. Surgery 89:513, 1981
15. NOVICK AC, BRAUN WE, MAGNUSSON MO et al: Current status of renal transplantation at the Cleveland Clinic. J Urol 122:433, 1979
16. NOVICK AC, MAGNUSSON M, BRAUN WE: Multiple-artery renal transplantation: Emphasis on extracorporeal methods of donor arterial reconstruction. J Urol 122:73, 1979
17. NOVICK AC, STEWART BH, STRAFFON RA: Extracorporeal renal surgery and autotransplantation: Indications, techniques and results. J Urol 123:806, 1980
18. NOVICK AC, STEWART BH, STRAFFON RA et al: Partial nephrectomy in the treatment of adenocarcinoma. J Urol 118:932, 1977
19. NOVICK AC, STEWART BH: Surgical treatment of renovascular hypertension. Curr Probl Surg 16:8, 1979
20. NOVICK AC, STRAFFON RA, STEWART BH: Surgical management of branch renal artery disease: In situ versus extracorporeal methods of repair. J Urol 123:311, 1979
21. OLSSON CA, IDELSON B: Renal autotransplantation for recurrent renal colic. J Urol 123:467, 1980
22. OTA K et al: Ex-vivo repair of renal artery for renovascular hypertension. Arch Surg 94:370, 1967
23. PETTERSSON S et al: Extracorporeal surgery and autotransplantation for carcinoma of the pelvis and ureter. Scand J Urol Nephrol 13:89, 1979
24. PFEFFERMANN RA et al: Successful repair of combined renal pedicle injury: A new application of the ex vivo "bench" technique. Isr J Med Sci 16:724, 1980
25. POUTASSE EF: Renal artery aneurysms. J Urol 113:433, 1975
26. SALVATIERRA O, OLCOTT C, STONEY RJ: Ex vivo renal artery reconstruction using perfusion preservation. J Urol 119:16, 1978
27. SMITH MJV, BOYCE WH: Anatrophic nephrolithotomy and plastic calyrhaphy, J Urol 99:52, 1978
28. SULLIVAN MJ et al: Extracorporeal renal parenchymal surgery with continuous perfusion. JAMA 229:1780, 1974
29. WOODRUFF MFA et al: Renal autotransplantation. Lancet 1:433, 1966

Regional Renal Hypothermia

12

John E. A. Wickham

Operations for removal of staghorn or multiple calculi in kidneys or for the excision of tumors in solitary kidneys frequently require that the renal circulation be arrested during the procedure to prevent excessive blood loss. Occlusion of the renal artery vein or whole pedicle depresses parenchymal function if the period of ischemia extends beyond 15 minutes and most surgery of this type requires a period of ischemia longer than 15 minutes—frequently 2 or more hr.

For many years the protective effect of cooling on cellular function has been well recognized.[1] Over the last 20 years, a number of proven techniques have been developed to achieve such protection by inducing renal hypothermia. Studies by Wickham, Ward, and others have demonstrated that the optimum temperature required for adequate functional protection is 15° C to 20° C, and that cooling to 0° C is not desirable and is perhaps damaging.[4,5] Most workers have attempted to maintain cooling in the 5° C to 20° C range.

Cooling of the kidney may be achieved by whole body hypothermia or by regional cooling. Whole body hypothermia is effective in protection of function and also has obvious cardiovascular implications. It has occasionally been used by peripheral vascular surgeons during aortic replacement surgery, but it has not been used by the urologist. Regional renal hypothermia has been used extensively, and the following techniques have been developed: external parenchymal cooling, intra-arterial cooling, and intrapelvic cooling.

External Parenchymal Cooling

It takes approximately 10 minutes to cool the adult human kidney to the 15° C to 20 ° C level by the application of a cold source to the surface of the organ. Three methods of achieving such cooling have been used widely: the ice-slush method, the plastic bag/ice water method, and the heat exchanger method. The method of choice depends on the operator's preference and the equipment available.

ICE-SLUSH METHOD

In the ice-slush method, the renal pedicle is displayed and the vessels are clamped. The kidney is then surrounded by approximately 1.5 kg of sterile crushed ice, prepared by placing bags of sterile physiological saline overnight in a domestic type of deep-freeze cabinet. The bags, when removed, are pummeled to break up the frozen mixture to an ice slush, which is then packed firmly around the kidney (Fig. 12-1). The wound margins and the renal fossa may be protected by insulated plastic sheeting or foil to prevent local cooling of surrounding tissues. In this way, very adequate hypothermia is achieved without recourse to complicated apparatus other than a telethermometer probe, which is placed in the parenchyma to monitor deep core temperature.

When the desired temperature is reached, the ice is removed and the operation may proceed. If reheating occurs, then a further application of crushed ice may be required. If the Boyce anatrophic method of nephrolithotomy is used, then there is no need to remove the ice, and the kidney can remain buried while the longitudinal nephrotomy is made above ice level.

There are certain inherent disadvantages to this method. First, it tends to be somewhat messy, because melting ice must be sucked out of the wound continually, and, unless the anatrophic method is used, ice must be removed and replaced from time to time. Second, if the ice is left in the renal fossa for periods of 2 hr to 3 hr, then general body cooling of the patient takes place with cardiovascular sequelae. Except for these criticisms, crushed ice provides a simple and effective way of cooling the kidney. The ice-slush method is probably the most universally useful of the cooling methods because it does not require sophisticated equipment.

149

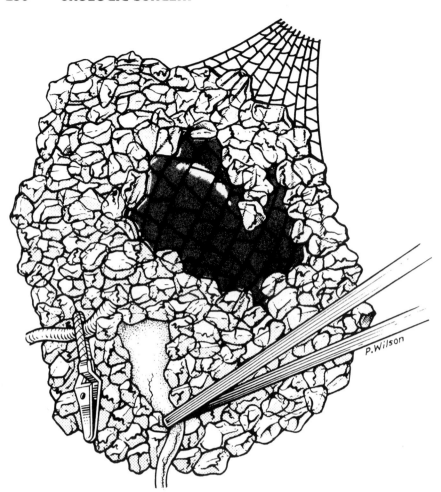

FIG. 12-1. Sterile saline "slush" is packed firmly around the kidney.

THE PLASTIC BAG/ICE WATER METHOD

In the plastic bag/ice water method, the mobilized kidney is enclosed in an invaginated plastic bag after occlusion of the renal vessels.[2] Cooled saline at about 1° C is poured from bottles (previously prepared overnight in a domestic refrigerator) into the trough formed by the bag around the kidney. A telethermometer probe is inserted into the parenchyma, and more saline is introduced until a core temperature of 15° C to 20° C has been achieved. The plastic bag is then removed and the operation proceeds.

This method of cooling is effective but slightly cumbersome in that the operation cannot proceed immediately after cooling has finished until the saline and the bag are removed. Reapplication of the bag and the saline for further cooling is not easy once the operative procedure has commenced.

HEAT EXCHANGER METHOD

In the heat exchanger method, a cold irrigant of one third ethyl alcohol and two thirds water is circulated from an external reservoir at 1 liter/min, through two small plastic heat exchanger coils (Fig. 12-2) placed on either side of the mobilized kidney.[5] The irrigant, of approximately 30 liters volume, is maintained at 1° C at the reservoir by the addition of approximately 5 kg of ice cubes, and reaches the cooling coils at about 4° C. Cooling takes approximately 10 minutes, and a telethermometer is used.

When the correct temperature is achieved, the coils are removed and the operative procedure can start. As rewarming to 25° C occurs, the coils can be replaced and further cooling produced as necessary. The coils slip in and out of the wound easily, and there is no messy fluid to inhibit the dry operative field. The apparatus required for

FIG. 12-2. Plastic heat-exchanger coils are placed on either side of the kidney.

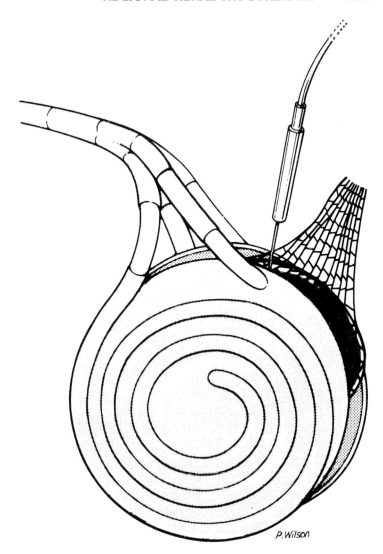

P. Wilson

this technique is commercially available and not costly.

For those with equipment available, the coil perfusion method is probably the neatest and best controlled of the cooling methods. The method can be approximated in most hospitals by using a roller pump, ice reservoir, and Silastic tubing wound in the nature of the heat exchanger coils. The roller pump must have an output of at least 1 liter/min.

Intra-Arterial Cooling

The kidney can be cooled most rapidly by direct intra-arterial perfusion with a cooled physiological saline medium.[3] In this way a deep core temperature of 15° C to 20° C can be achieved in approximately 1 minute. The renal artery can be accessed by direct needle puncture, a slightly hazardous maneuver, or by indirect intubation by Seldinger puncture of the femoral artery and the negotiation of a Swan–Ganz catheter up the aorta into the renal artery. Here vascular occlusion can be achieved by inflation of the balloon of the catheter (*channel a*, Fig. 12-3). Cold perfusion of the kidney can then be carried out through a second catheter lumen opening distal to the occluding balloon (*channel b*, Fig. 12-3). Cooled physiological saline is infused at approximately 1 liter/min to 1.5 liters min and vented through a small venotomy in the renal vein. After the initial cooling period, the perfusate is switched off and the operation can proceed in a dry field. As rewarming occurs, further perfusate can be reinjected to produce the required lowering of the parenchymal core temperature.

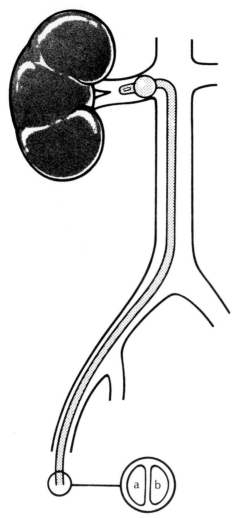

FIG. 12-3. A Swan-Ganz catheter is introduced through the aorta into the renal artery. *Channel a* shows vascular occlusion by inflation of the catheter balloon; *channel b* indicates a second lumen opening distal to the occluding balloon.

Intra-arterial cooling is a very elegant method of achieving hypothermia but is somewhat complicated, requiring a preoperative intubation in a radiologic department and transfer of the patient to the operating room, with the occasional risk of catheter dislodgement. The logistics required probably place it beyond the capabilities of most urologic departments. The method has the advantage that detailed dissection of the renal pedicle is not required but is limited to kidneys with a single arterial supply. If tumors in solitary kidneys are being tackled, then the ability to considerably reduce the vascularity of the tumor without prior dissection of the pedicle is an added bonus.

Intrapelvic Cooling

Cooling of the kidney may also be achieved by perfusion of the renal pelvis with cooled physiological saline, either by way of the ureter with a relieving nephrostomy or through a simple pyelostomy allowing the irrigant to escape into the wound. Cooling is adequate with this method, but an adjuvant method of cooling, either by using ice slush or by pouring cold saline over the kidney, is required. The wound edges are protected by plastic sheeting, and the excess irrigant is removed by suction. This method if simple but has the disadvantage of being messy. It does not appear to have any advantages over the ice-slush technique.

REFERENCES

1. FUHRMAN FA, FIELD J: The reversibility of the inhibition of rat brain and kidney metabolism by cold. Am J Physiol 139:193, 1943
2. GRAVES FT: Renal hypothermia an aid to partial nephrectomy. Br J Surg 50:362, 1968
3. MARBERGER M, GEORGI M: Balloon occlusion of the renal artery in tumour nephrectomy. J Urol 114:360, 1975
4. WARD JP: Determination of the optimum temperature for regional renal hypothermia during temporary ischaemia. Br J Urol 47:17, 1975
5. WICKHAM JEA: A simple method for regional renal hypothermia. J Urol 99:246, 1968
6. WICKHAM JEA, HANLEY HG, JOEKES AM: Regional renal hypothermia. Br J Urol 39:727, 1967

Nephroscopy and Other Localization Techniques

13

Donald E. Novicki

Modern surgical techniques enable the urologic surgeon to remove large amounts of diseased renal tissue while preserving adequate renal function to maintain life. *In vivo* renal hypothermia, microvascular renal surgery, renal autotransplantation with bench surgery, and intraoperative nephroscopy represent but a few of these current techniques. Accurate preoperative localization of renal lesions and the ability to assess rapidly the thoroughness of renal surgery in the operating theater are prerequisites to performing a nephron-conserving procedure. There are a variety of sophisticated imaging techniques that allow accurate and complete localization of abnormalities prior to and during surgery. The localization of lesions in the ureters and more distal urinary system is readily accomplished with traditional radiographic techniques or by endoscopic visualization. Localizing pathologic changes in the renal parenchyma and upper collecting system is more difficult and requires some or all of the techniques described in this chapter.

Most imaging techniques provide information in two dimensions which must be applied to a three-dimensional organ. Models should be used to aid in conceptualizing information in three dimensions (Fig. 13-1). Experience is vital to apply the information obtained from these diagnostic methods.

Preoperative Localization

RADIOGRAPHIC TECHNIQUES

Plain radiographs visualize radiopaque densities in the renal parenchyma and collecting system. By combining anterior–posterior projections with lateral and oblique views, general localization in the kidney can be achieved (Fig. 13-2). Accurate information can be obtained by rotating the kidney under the fluoroscopic beam, but many small lesions are beyond the resolution of the fluoroscope. Radiolucent filling defects in the collecting system can be localized in a similar fashion when they are outlined with contrast material. An appreciation of the anatomy of the collecting system can be gained with simple rotation during opacification.

When contrast material is administered, small radiopaque calculi can be totally obscured and are difficult to localize. This problem can be resolved with the following technique of overlapping films:

1. Obtain a nonenhanced anterior–posterior radiograph on which the renal parenchymal outline is well visualized. Outline the renal parenchyma and highlight the calculus with a grease pencil.
2. Obtain an enhanced film with the patient in the same postion and the collecting system well opacified. Outline the renal parenchyma with a grease pencil.
3. Place the films on a viewbox or in front of a hot light with the plain film behind the contrast study. Align the renal margins, and the highlighted calculus will be localized in the collecting system.

Renal tomography with or without contrast enhancement can be used to gauge the depth of lesions in the kidney. Small abnormalities can be missed if they lie between the layers of tomographic slices. Tomographic cuts less than the standard 1-cm interval should be obtained when small lesions are suspected.

COMPUTED TOMOGRAPHIC SCANNING

Computed tomographic (CT) scanning of the kidneys represents a spectacular advance in imaging.[5] Localization of parenchymal and collecting system abnormalities is accurate and rapid. This procedure can be used safely and efficiently in individuals with sensitivity to contrast material and in those with poorly functioning kidneys. Nonopaque calculi can be readily distinguished from other lesions in the collecting system because of their dense appearance by CT scanning. Visualization of the

153

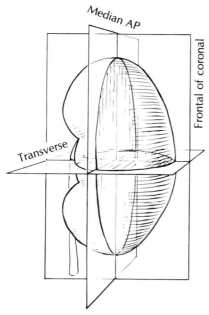

FIG. 13-1. Three-dimensional anatomic model of the kidney

FIG. 13-2. When the sphere is rotated in a counterclockwise direction, objects posterior to the midplane (**A**) will rotate laterally and anterior objects (**B**) will rotate medially. The converse is true with clockwise rotation.

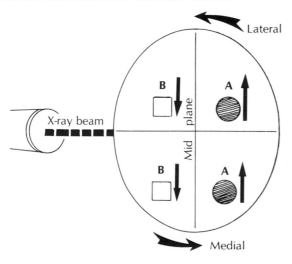

retroperitoneal lymph nodes and major abdominal vessels is easily accomplished and is helpful in staging malignancies.

A disadvantage of this procedure is that small lesions can be missed or misinterpreted unless plain radiographs or urograms are available to the scanner. Preliminary scout films with the CT scanner, adjustment of scan intervals, and overlapping

scans can be performed to preclude misdiagnosing these small lesions. Volume averaging may lead to misinterpretation of masses less than 2 cm in diameter. A lack of sufficient fat to separate contiguous structures adequately, artifacts from metallic hemostatic devices used in surgery, and the necessity to suspend respiration during scanning limits this procedure's application in some individuals. If these limitations are considered, CT scanning can provide an abundance of valuable localizing information.

ULTRASONOGRAPHY

Ultrasonic examination of the kidneys and surrounding structures requires a skilled operator who is experienced in interpreting the complex data displays. Graphic information with the A-mode, static anatomic cross sections with the B-mode, and true-life images with the real-time mode can be provided with modern equipment. Rapid, repeated, low-cost examinations with portable instruments are attractive features of this procedure. The ability to obtain useful data without suspending respiration makes ultrasonography useful in children and uncooperative adults. Poor resolution of small mass lesions and of calculi smaller than 1 cm are inherent limitations.[6,11,13]

Renal imaging using the B-mode is best accomplished by obtaining transverse and longitudinal scans with the patient in the prone position. When lesions are in unusual locations, scans can readily be performed in other planes. Overlapping anatomic structures often obviate clear visualization of the upper renal poles, but suspending respiration in deep inspiration can overcome this problem. Real-time imaging enables renal visualization during respiration. Renal mobility can easily be determined, and the kidney can often be separated from extrinsic lesions.

ANGIOGRAPHY

Renal arteriography provides direct and clear visualization of the renal vasculature and parenchyma. Selective catheterization of the renal arteries and their major branches can aid in localizing renal lesions and aids in defining their nature. This information is sometimes vital when planning to remove large volumes of renal tissue. Knowledge of the normal arterial supply of the kidney (Fig. 13-3) and an understanding of the wide variations that may occur are necessary to use these studies efficiently. Commonly occurring accessory vessels and early branch vessels from the main renal artery should be selectively injected to opacify the entire kidney. Rotational views should be obtained when abnormalities are poorly seen on anterior–posterior projections. Vigorous hydration for at least 12 hr prior to the study will preclude renal failure induced by the contrast media. One should strictly adhere to the volume limits of the contrast material.[3]

Venography with sampling of blood from various intra-abdominal locations or from renal segments can be a useful localizing technique. When planning retroperitoneal surgery for pheochromocytomas and hormonally active adrenal cortical tumors, this method can be used to localize small tumors not found with other techniques.[8,10] Occult retroperitoneal metastases from tumors that produce marker substances can sometimes be located,[9] and renovascular hypertension originating from a renal segment can be documented by segmental vein catheterization with renin sampling.[15]

URETEROPYELOSCOPY

Direct visualization of the urothelium of the ureter, renal pelvis, and more proximal collecting system may be accomplished with the ureteropyeloscope. This instrument is passed cystoscopically and provides information not previously available in a nonoperative situation. Visual biopsy of lesions in the collecting system, manipulation or disintegration of calculi, and direct visualization and fulguration of renal bleeding sites will be possible when this instrument is perfected. Current limitations due to the size of the instrument and its fragility preclude routine clinical use. Refinements in optics and miniaturization techniques will allow widespread application of this innovative instrument in the future.

Intraoperative Localization

Confirmation that renal lesions have been completely excised can sometimes be obtained only in the operative setting. Rapid assessment is essential, and any surgeon performing complex renal surgery should master intraoperative localizing techniques. Time and space limitations in the operating theater preclude the use of some of the previously outlined procedures, but operative exposure of the kidney permits the application of more direct methods. Judicious use of pathologic frozen sections is indicated when dealing with malignancies. Intraoperative radiography, direct sonography, and nephroscopy are applicable in a variety of intraoperative situations.

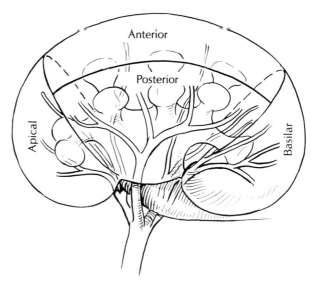

FIG. 13-3. Usual distribution of major segmental branches of the renal artery

RADIOGRAPHIC TECHNIQUES

Failure to remove all fragments of calculi during renal stone surgery is a common error and uniformly heralds recurrent calculus formation. Modern radiographic techniques provide the surgeon ample opportunity to avoid this error. No kidney should be considered free of stones unless this is proven radiographically.[2] Commercially prepared film, appropriately sized and shaped and suitable for cold sterilization, is available for intraoperative use. One such preparation contains two sheets of film of different sensitivity to permit relatively soft and hard radiographs to be obtained during a single exposure. Mammography film has been used recently and has been found to be of superb resolution in visualizing very small and relatively lucent stone fragments.

Complete renal mobilization for direct contact of the kidney with the film and precise centering of the x-ray beam are prerequisites for quality organ films. An x-ray film of the kidney before attempting stone removal should be routinely obtained for later comparison.[2] Prepared radiopaque grids are available for orientation,[14] but more commonly simple parenchymal puncture with fine needles is employed. This technique involves placing two needles at right angles to each other prior to taking a radiograph of the kidney for stone fragments. Other needles can be placed after the first exposure if localization is not accurate. Multiple exposures with the kidney in various positions relative to the x-ray beam should be employed if other techniques fail. Operative pyelography before opening the collecting system will clearly separate caliceal from parenchymal stones. Intraoperative fluoroscopy is less sensitive, more cumbersome, and of limited use.

SONOGRAPHY

Successful intraoperative localization of calculi has been accomplished with A-mode, B-mode, and real-time sonography.[1,4] Rapid, three-dimensional information can be obtained in a noninvasive fashion, and examinations can be repeated as often as necessary. This technique can detect stone fragments as small as 1 mm to 2 mm, and fine needles can be guided directly to the stone under ultrasonic visualization. However, the infrequent availability of this equipment in the operating room and the inexperience of most surgeons in performing this procedure render ultrasonography impractical in most situations.

NEPHROSCOPY

Nephroscopy provides the most direct means of inspecting the renal collecting systems and enables removal of residual lesions under visual control. The right-angled, rigid nephroscope with irrigation and manipulation sheaths can be used to remove very small fragments of stone or tissue. Complete mobilization of the kidney is usually necessary to maneuver the instrument into all portions of the collecting system. Familiarity with the appearance of the collecting system as viewed through the nephroscope requires experience and can be best achieved by practicing on cadaver kidneys.

Significant renal bleeding can obscure vision with the nephroscope. Delicate tissue techniques and planned use of the instrument prior to blind intrarenal probing are necessary to ensure success. Systematic, planned visualization of all calices is required and is best accomplished by rolling the kidney and tipping and rotating the nephroscope. Mucosal flaps or blood clots that obscure vision should be gently washed with pulsatile irrigation using a syringe attached to the input line. Small stone fragments can often be irrigated free in the same manner.[7]

The flexible fiberoptic nephroscope (Fig. 13-4) can be rotated 90 degrees with a remote control. More complete visualization of the collecting system with less renal mobilization can be achieved, and insertion through a nephrostomy tract is possible.[12] Optical limitations and small working channels limit the use of this instrument, but improvements are forthcoming.

FIG. 13-4. Model G960 Rigi-Flex nephroscope (Courtesy of American Cystoscope Manufacturers, 300 Stillwater Avenue, Stamford, Ct)

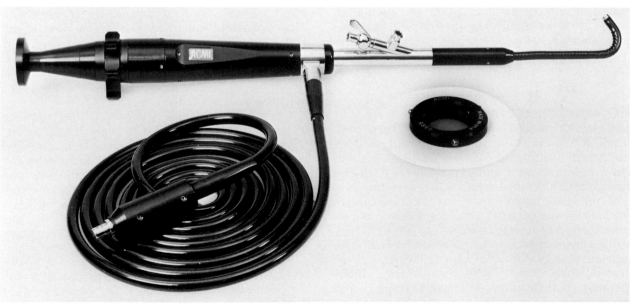

REFERENCES

1. ANDALURO VA JR, SCHOR M, MARANGOLA JP: Intraoperative localization of a renal calculus using ultrasound. J Urol 116:92, 1976
2. BOYCE WH: The localization of intrarenal calculi during surgery. J Urol 118:152, 1977
3. BYRD L, SHERMAN RL: Radiocontrast-induced acute renal failure: A clinical and pathophysiologic review. Medicine 58:270, 1979
4. COOK JH, III, LYTTON B: Intraoperative localization of renal calculi during nephrolithotomy by ultrasound scanning. J Urol 117:543, 1977
5. CURTIS JA, BRENNAN RE, RUBIN C et al: Computed tomography of the kidneys. Comput Tomogr 4:17, 1980
6. EDELL S, ZEGEL II: Ultrasonic evaluation of renal calculi. Am J Roentgenol 130:261, 1978
7. GITTES RH: Nephroscopy. Urol Clin North Am 6:3, 555, 1979
8. HORTON R, FINCK E: Diagnosis and localization in primary aldosteronism. Ann Intern Med 76:885, 1972
9. JAVADPOUR N, MCINTIRE KR, WALDMANN TA et al: The role of the radioimmunoassay of serum alpha-fetoprotein and human chorionic gonadotropin in the intensive chemotherapy and surgery of metastatic testicular tumors. J Urol 119:759, 1978
10. JONES DH, ALLISON DJ, HAMILTON CA, REID JL: Selective venous sampling in the diagnosis and localization of phaeochromocytoma. Clin Endocrinol 10:179, 1979
11. LINGARD DA, LAWSON TL: Accuracy of ultrasound in predicting the nature of renal masses. J Urol 122:724, 1979
12. MIKI M, INABA Y, MACHIDA T: Operative nephroscopy with fiberoptic scope: Preliminary report. J Urol 119:166, 1978
13. POLLACK HM, ARGER PH, GOLDBERG BB, MULHOLLAND SG: Ultrasonic detection of nonopaque renal calculi. Radiology 127:233, 1978
14. ROTH RA: Two aids for removal of renal calculi. J Urol 120:666, 1978
15. SCHAMBELAN M, GLICKMAN M, STOCKIGT JR, BIGLIERI EG: Selective renal vein sampling in hypertensive patients with segmental renal lesions. N Engl J Med 290:1153, 1974

Pyelolithotomy

14

José-María Gil-Vernet

Conceptual and technologic advances of the past 20 years have greatly benefited the surgery of renal lithiasis.[1,3] These advances have included an approach to the renal sinus with the development of intrasinusal surgery, which permits removal of calculi without incisions into the renal parenchyma or its vessels. The development of the transverse or "spiral" pyelotomy to be used instead of the classic longitudinal pyelotomy has provided a more anatomic and physiologic approach to the pelvis, thus greatly reducing the complications of injury to the ureteropelvic junction, postoperative drainage of urine, and delayed scarring with urinary obstruction. Regional renal hypothermia allows us to operate on the ischemic organ for hours, with preservation of its function and repair of the pathology. Autotransplantation with extracorporeal surgery of the kidney permits the conservation of functional kidneys which under other circumstances would be unsalvageable. The advances in intraoperative renal radiography have included addition of a third dimension to the kidney, as well as a more precise definition and visualization of small calculi and their relation to the renal structures, and have thus greatly reduced the serious problem of residual postoperative calculi.

History

The first pyelotomy was performed by Czerny in 1880, and the first removal of a calculus by nephrotomy was by Morris in the same year. The advantages and disadvantages of each approach have subsequently been debated by surgeons to the present time. In the remainder of the 19th century nephrolithomy was favored by the majority of surgeons in Europe. Radiographic methods were nonexistent, and visualization of stones within the kidney was more easily accomplished through a large nephrotomy. The healing of many wounds by secondary intention permitted the nephrotomy to heal more readily than the pyelotomy, which was frequently accompanied by persistent urinary fistulas and ultimately by secondary nephrectomy. At the turn of the century pyelotomy was in use only in England. Morris, Israel, Kuster, Guyon, Kelly, and Zondek were pioneers in establishing the technique of nephrolithomy.

With the technologic advances that occurred in the first quarter of this century, pyelolithomy became the surgical procedure of choice for removal of the vast majority of renal calculi. With the development of both retrograde and excretory urography, surgeons were able to define the pathologic changes in the kidney and to localize stones precisely. Pyelotomy for the majority of calculi provides a technically simple approach to the calices; it carries little danger of immediate or delayed hemorrhage, which had been the most serious complication of nephrotomy; and, when properly performed, it greatly reduces the incidence of ureteropelvic injury with resultant fistulas or secondary stenosis. The controversy over the choice of pyelotomy or nephrotomy applies to a minority of renal calculi, especially the staghorn or equivalent calculus with their peculiar features of pathologic change within the kidney, cicatrization from prior surgery, or perinephric abscess.

Historically, the renal pelvis has been approached from its posterior, anterior, and inferior aspects. Direct surgical approach to the anterior and inferior aspects endangers major renal vessels or provides poor exposure of the calices, requiring extension by nephrotomy. The techniques of Marion, Papin, and Prather are examples of extended pyelolithotomies. These incisions may involve either vascular injury to the major branches of the renal artery and consequently a significant decrease in renal function or the development of serious immediate or delayed hemorrhage. In the first half of this century, technical difficulties and imperfect results of operative methods led many physicians and surgeons to adopt a noninterventionist attitude toward complex renal lithiasis, even though it was known that presence of a staghorn calculus sooner

159

or later would result in loss of the kidney. Nephrectomy thus became an acceptable operation for renal calculi.

In 1960, an approach to the renal sinus was found which allows visualization of the intrasinusal portion of the pelvis and calices with minimal damage to the renal parenchyma or the vessels and which is applicable even in the presence of advanced peripyelic inflammation or scarring.[4] This approach, together with transverse pyelotomy and posterior vertical lumbotomy, provides the basis of modern pyelolithotomy, a procedure that is less traumatic, involves less mortality, is more efficient, and is safer than traditional calculus surgery. By 1974, methods of radiographic exploration of the kidney during surgery had been developed. These methods represent a decisive aid in detection and localization of the smallest calculi.

Postulates and Guidelines

Present-day surgery for renal lithiasis should be subject to the following postulates:[12]

It is conservative. It is necessary to avoid nephrectomy and even resection of a part of the parenchyma that has been condemned under the pretext of the "lithogenic focus."

It is complete. The extraction must be total because recurrence is certain when there is infection. If the surgeon is unable to extract all the calculi, it is preferable not to operate because the next operation will be more difficult.

It is atraumatic. An effort must be made to avoid a nephrotomy, a lesion of the renal parenchyma. If this is unavoidable it should be a minimal, radial, controlled, and directed nephrotomy.

The guidelines for lithiasis surgery are as follows:[3]

Be thorough and exhaustive in the preoperative radiographic exploration, particularly with staghorn calculi.

Use the posterior vertical lumbotomy as a surgical approach to the kidney for simple lithiasis and the posterior lateral incision for complex lithiasis.

Use the extracapsular surgical approach to the renal sinus.

Use the transverse pyelotomy, intrasinusal enlarged pyelotomy, and infundibulotomy.

Remove staghorn calculi completely and intact whenever possible.

Use three-dimensional intraoperative radiography for localization of residual calculi.

Use complementary minimal radial nephrotomy.

Use atraumatic axial nephrostomy if one is required.

Use renal hypothermia *in situ* in exceptional cases.

Use extracorporeal renal surgery when recurrent lithiasis is associated with an important lesion of the excretory tract that is not repairable by conventional surgery.

In addition to conventional anteroposterior exposures of the kidney, preoperative radiographic evaluation should include oblique films from different angles, tomography, and the internal profile by photofluorography. These methods are helpful in determining the number, orientation, and branches of the staghorn calculus. Identification of the articular surfaces and localization of accessory calculi will assist in planning an operation that will remove all fragments. In combination with pyelography it is possible to plan the axis and direction in which traction is to be applied to the stone and to relate these to the characteristics of the cavities where the calculi are lodged.

Surgical Approaches to the Kidney

Surgical approaches to the kidney may be posterior through the flank or lumbar areas, permitting extraperitoneal exposure, anterior through the abdominal incisions, which may be either transperitoneal or extraperitoneal, and transthoracic through the diaphragm. More than 40 incisions for these approaches have been devised since Gustav Simon initiated renal surgery in 1869.

Most renal surgery is accomplished through the posterior approach by some modification of the lumbotomy incision. **Simon's incisions** consisted of making a vertical approach three fingers from the spinous processes extending from the posterior superior iliac process to the 11th rib. The exposure is developed by a vertical incision of the latissimus dorsi aponeurosis, reflecting the sacrol lumbar muscle toward the spine, sectioning the transverse aponeurosis, and releasing the quadratus lumborum muscle. **Pean and Ollier's** incision is longer and more complicated because it includes the disinsertion of the quadrous lumborum muscle from the iliac crest. **Riche's incision** resects the 12th rib and divides the quadratus lumborum muscle.

TECHNIQUE OF THE GIL–VERNET INCISION

When the **Gil–Vernet incision**[2] is used, the patient is placed in the lateral position without lumbar support (Fig. 14-1*A*), and the knees are flexed to

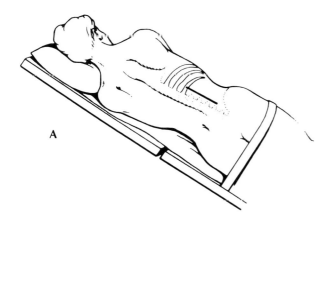

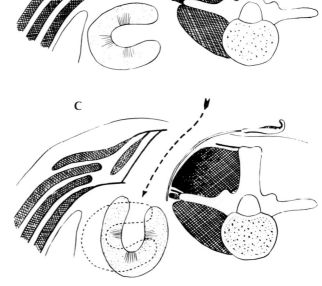

FIG. 14-1. Gil–Vernet incision. **(A)** Line of posterior vertical lumbotomy with patient in Murphy's position. **(B)** Plane of dissection. **(C)** With sacrolumbar and quadratus lumborum muscles retracted, the kidney is rotated to present the hilar surface.

the point of obliterating or maximally suppressing the physiologic lordosis. The operation may also be performed with the patient in a prone position provided there are no problems with pulmonary ventilation.[7] The vertical incision is performed in the middle of the mass of the sacrolumbar muscle and extends from the 12th rib to the posterosuperior iliac crest. The latissimus dorsi aponeurosis is sectioned and detached from the posterior surface of the sacrolumbar muscle. The external edge and the anterior surface of this muscle are freed until contact is made with the transverse spinous processes (Fig. 14-1B). At this point the posterior leaflet of the transverse aponeurosis presents as a thin fascia, having the appearance of mother-of-pearl. The leaflet covers the quadrous lumborum muscle and is crossed by the abdominogenital nerve, which is carefully preserved. This aponeurosis is sectioned very close to the transverse processes in a longitudinal fashion, extending from the iliac crest to the inferior margin of the 12th rib. Henle's ligament is sectioned by the 12th intercostal musculature, which is carefully preserved. The superior edge of the transverse aponeurosis is lifted, exposing the margin of the quadratus lumborum muscle, which is reflected toward the spine. Access to the kidney is achieved through the anterior leaflet of the transverse aponeurosis, which

is poorly developed and intimately related to the perinephric fascia. Incision of the perinephric fascia at this point express the kidney (Fig. 14-1C).

At this stage a special autostatic retractor (Fig. 14-2) with asymmetric blades is placed in position and the perinephric fat is separated from the posterior surface of the kidney. The patient is placed in Murphy's position (reverse Trendelenburg) and the kidney descends a few centimeters. When greater exposure is required, a requisite length of the 12th rib is removed. The removal of this rib facilitates the introduction of the contact minichassis and film for intraoperative radiography. In very complex renal lithiasis, more extensive exposure is achieved with posterolateral lumbotomy, which includes resection of the 12th rib near its articulation, detachment of the pleural cul-de-sac, and division of the posterior leaf of the diaphragm.

After completion of the renal surgery, closure of the incision is performed in only two layers, that of the transverse muscle aponeurosis and that of the latissimus dorsi. This simplicity of closure reflects the atramatic nature of the incicion, which is achieved primarily by division of aponeurotic planes rather than muscles. Because few, if any, muscles and no nerves are divided, postoperative pain and other complications are reduced to the

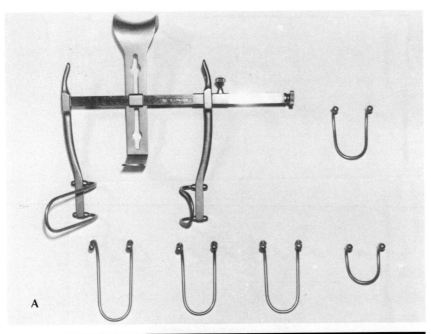

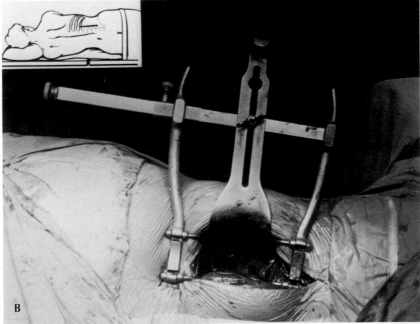

FIG. 14-2. Autostatic retractor. (A) Interchangeable asymmetric blades. (B) Retractor is in place with auxiliary blade elevating the superior margin of the incision.

point where the patient may be discharged from the hospital on the fourth postoperative day. Because of the minimal postoperative morbidity, a double operation for bilateral lithiasis is frequently performed as one surgical procedure. Drainage of this incision is attained by using the Redon aspiration system (a low-pressure mechanical suction system).

EXTRACAPSULAR APPROACH TO THE RENAL SINUS

Anatomic and Surgical Considerations

The term *sinus renalis* was introduced in 1866 by Henle, who described it as a rectangular cavity within the kidney. Its external edge borders on the medulla in the parenchyma and its internal edge on the hilus (Fig. 14-3). This sinusal cavity has two prolongations, one superior and one inferior, each containing the major infundibulum of the corresponding calices. The hilus is lined by the internal sheet of the fibrous capsule of the kidney, which melds with the pericaliceal connective tissue. The average dimensions of this sinus are 5 cm vertically, 3 cm from outside to inside, and 2 cm from front to back. Surgical access to the hilar space is through the hilar recess, which has the shape of an oval fissure vertically elongated, 3.5 cm in length and 1.5 cm in width. In elongated kidneys these dimensions may be as large as 7 cm in length by 2.5 cm in width. The configuration of this opening or hilus may vary from angular to semicircular, with variations produced by the embryologic process of fusion. In the surgically exposed kidney the anterior left of the renal hilus appears retracted, the posterior protruding. In general, the more recessed the sinus and the more open the hilus, the easier the intrarenal surgery.

In the normal kidney the sinus is occupied by the intrarenal portion of the pelvis, the infundibula, the calices, the vessels, the lymphatics, and the nerves that supply the parenchyma.[5] The space between these structures is filled with a loose areolar fatty tissue which facilitates the free movement of the collecting system (Fig. 14-4). The elasticity of the sinus permits distention of these structures and accommodates various pathologic processes such as the formation of cysts. In 1891, Disc demonstrated that at the hilar margin an extension of the fibrous capsule of the kidney forms a sheath of dense fibers which surrounds and adheres to the extrarenal portion of the pelvis. This capsular diaphragm closes the entrance to the sinus and isolates it from the retroperitoneal space. It is a misconception that the lithiasic kidney always presents a sinus "closed by perinephritis with agglomeration of vessels which goes against all attempts of intrasinusal pyelotomy."[10] When inflammation is present a plane of dissection may be developed between the adventitia of the renal pelvis and the diaphragm that encloses it (Fig. 14-5). This diaphragm is cleared and perfectly defined by blunt dissection without damaging any hilar or parenchymal structures, even in those kidneys with severe sclerolipomatous inflammatory reaction. Once this diaphragm has been cleared, the surgeon may penetrate the intrasinusal space and totally explore the area without damaging the vessels or other structures because the internal sheath of the fibrous capsule of the kidney and the intrasinusal fatty tissue are interposed between these structures and the collecting system. In sum-

mary, the approach into the sinus is extracapsular.[10]

Although the vascular relationships of the pelvis are not of paramount importance in intrasinusal surgery, one should know the variations of the retropelvic (posterior segmental) artery in order to

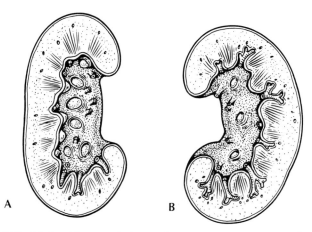

FIG. 14-3. The renal sinus after contents are removed. **(A)** Anterior surface. **(B)** Posterior surface

FIG. 14-4. Schematic representation of the renal sinus shows relationship of calices **(a)** to vessels and capsular extension and adherence **(b)** which effectively blocks entry into the sinus, necessitating surgical incision. (After Narath et al: The Renal Pelvis and Ureter. New York, Grune & Stratton, 1951)

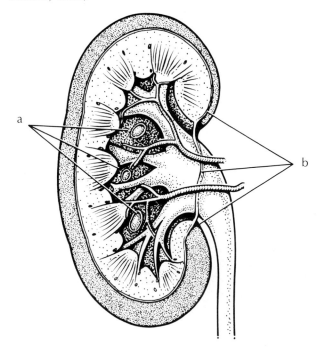

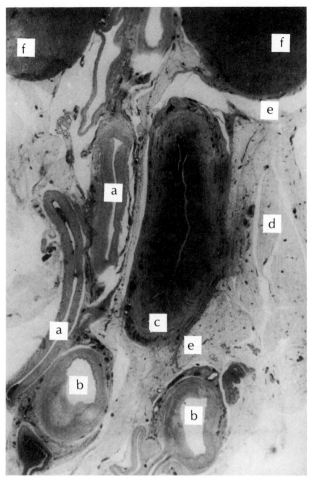

FIG. 14-5. Photomicrograph of sagittal section of the renal hilus displays veins (**a**), arteries (**b**), renal pelvis (**c**), adipose (**d**), capsular diaphragm enclosing the pelvis (**e**), and renal parenchyma (**f**).

FIG. 14-6. Usual position of the retropelvic renal artery within the renal sinus, well removed from the posterior lip of the hilus

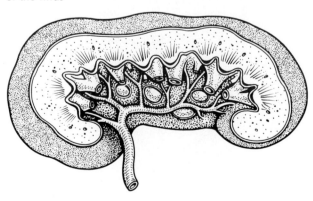

avoid damage or prolonged compression by the sinus retractors. The retropelvic artery arises from the main renal at an acute angle and passes along the superior edge of the pelvis on either its extra-hilar or its intrasinusal surface. When the artery passes outside the posterior edge of the hilus, it may be identified by palpation when freeing the pelvis. In the more frequent variations in which the retropelvic artery passes inferior to the renal sinus, there is little danger in sectioning it (Fig. 14-6). We have performed more than 6000 intra-sinusal pyelotomies with only one section of the retropelvic artery; this was corrected by microsurgical end-to-end anastomosis and the operation for lithiasis was completed.

Technique of Sinusotomy

The approach to a normal sinus is quite simple (Fig. 14-7A). The ureteropelvic junction is identified and the peripelvic fat is retracted toward the parenchyma by means of curved scissors with blunt points. The pelvic adventitia is separated from the pelvic fat by continuing blunt dissections, with the scissors progressing in close contact with the adventitia (Fig. 14-8A). When passing beneath the capsular diaphragm, the scissors are opened vigorously, breaking the diaphragm circle. At this point, a retractor is passed into the entrance of the sinus, carrying the whole mass of peripelvic fat, the interior lip of the posterior edge of the kidney, and the retropelvic vessels away from the collecting system (Fig. 14-8B). Retraction may be quite vigorous with no danger of tearing the parenchyma, which is protected by the capsule and peripelvic fat. At this point an open wet gauze is introduced into the sinus until it is totally filled, then the gauze is removed and a smaller retractor is inserted. With two retractors, the posterior half of the kidney is firmly lifted, thus tilting the organ and making visible the entire pelvis, the major infundibula, and the calices. When the maneuver is performed correctly it is completely bloodless, and the pelvis and calices are free within the sinus.

The chronic inflammatory reaction in the peripelvic structures associated with pelvic lithiasis and especially with staghorn calculi increases the difficulty of this exposure. This is particularly true at the hilus, where the chronic inflammatory reaction of the perirenal fat is particularly intense. In these circmstances, the sinus fat may be very little changed, even when a dense shell of sclerolipomatous tissue blocks the entrance to the hilus. In these circumstances, the most advisable procedure is to identify the adjacent ureter which is free from inflammatory reaction and to follow a retrograde dissection with blunt scissors to the detachment plane, which is always present between the adventitia of the pelvis and the surrounding tissue at the hilus. (Figs. 14-9*A* and *B*). The posterior surface of the pelvis is freed from the sclerosing shell that encloses it (Fig. 14-9*C*). This may not only facilitate the operation but also free the ureteropelvic peristalsis following the operation. Resection of the sclerosed tissue is continued toward the hilar margin of the posterior lip of the kidney with care to avoid sectioning of the retroplevic vein and artery. A small strip of sclerolipomatous tissue left along the posterior lip protects the artery and is used as support by the retractors, which vigorously lift the renal edge (Fig. 14-9*D*). Two small retractors, one at the superior commissure, the other at the inferior, are preferable to a single large retractor (Fig. 14-9*E*). In any type of lithiasis, access to the renal sinus is always possible by following the free ureter as a guideline and dissecting the pelvis and the entrance to the sinus.

TRANSVERSE PYELOTOMY, INFUNDIBULOTOMY, AND ENLARGED PYELOTOMY

When Czerny performed the first pyelotomy, he used a vertical incision. In 1960, we rejected the vertical pyelotomy in favor of a transverse pyelotomy.[3] This decision was based on studies of the functional anatomy of the ureteral musculature, which show that the pelvis is a system of spiral funnels of smooth muscle which stretch by gentle inclination from the infundibula to the ureteropelvic junction. A transverse pyelotomy that follows the direction of these spirals is the most logical and anatomic incision. The incision should be performed as far as the ureteropelvic junction as the anatomy permits (Fig. 14-10*A*). An incision at this point minimizes the possibilty of a tear into the ureteropelvic junction and facilitates exploration of the calices under visual control. If the pelvis is of the extrahilar type, the pyelotomy incision must not violate the sinal space (Fig. 14-10*C*). When it becomes necessary to remove a caliceal calculus, we perform the longitudinal incision along the axis of the caliceal infundibulum (Fig. 14-14*D*). This infundibulotomy incision does not adversely affect infundibula motility and indeed may relieve the obstructive action of a hypertonic or strictured "musculus sphincter calycis."

When the infundibulum is of small caliber it may not be sutured in anticipation of the possibility that secondary epithelialization from its edges will give a greater caliber to the infundibulum.

In the presence of staghorn calculi and in some pelvicaliceal lithiasis, the ends of the transverse incision are prolonged toward the superior and inferior calices (Fig. 14-11*A*). This enlarged intrasinusal pyelotomy is longitudinal along the calices

FIG. 14-7. Gil–Vernet approach to the renal sinus. **(A)** In the absence of inflammation, direct dissection between the capsular diaphragm and the renal pelvis is possible. **(B)** In the presence of peripyelitis, dissection should begin along the upper ureter.

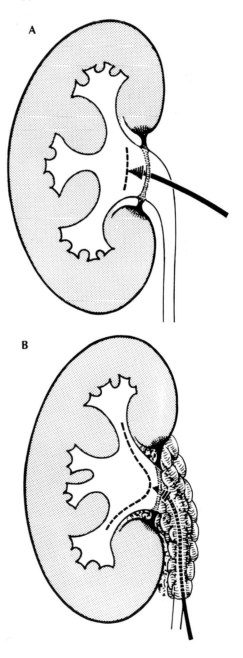

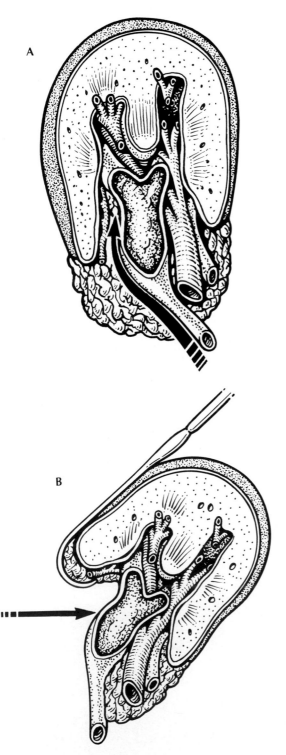

FIG. 14-8. Horizontal view of kidney with pelvic calculus and peripyelitis. **(A)** Plane of dissection along upper ureter and pelvis. **(B)** With retractor elevating the posterior lip of the hilus, the *arrow* indicates the point of transverse pyelotomy.

and transverse over the pelvis.[5] This arched incision may undergo considerable variation depending upon the morphology of the pelvis and the calculus. (Figs. 14-11*B* and *C*).[9] The convex portion of the incision should be performed near the vertex of the calculus but as far as possible from the ureteropelvic junction.

The incision into the pelvis and infundibula is performed within the sinus with a small scalpel (Fig. 14-12). The incision must not "feather" the margins of the tissue, and the edges of the incision must not be clamped or used for placing traction or reference sutures. These edges are manipulated during suturing with very fine atraumatic forceps. The incisions in the pelvis and infundibula are closed with absorbable catgut sutures not larger than 6-0 in size.

Removal of Calculi

REMOVAL OF THE STAGHORN CALCULI

Both preoperative and intraoperative radiographs are consulted to localize free culculi, to study the lines of force within the calculus, the branches, axis, and direction to which the traction maneuvers for removal must be applied, and to detect lines of nonunion of branches of calculus. *Staghorn calculi must never be wrenched out.* These calculi must be mobilized gently from their points of fixation and from all the obstacles to their removal by gentle traction. After this appraisal, the first consideration is to perform a pelvic and infundibulocaliceal incision which will allow one to obtain the greatest possible access to the internal branches of the lithiasic traingle, to luxate the pelvic angle, and to remove all calculi.

The second consideration is to avoid any damage caused by instruments to the excretory ducts. Insofar as possible, the operation is conducted under visual control with blunt instruments. The introduction of fingers into the infundibula must be avoided, and if they require dilatation this is done gently with forceps.

The third consideration is to avoid damage to the renal parenchyma. Once the pyelotomy incision has been established, the vertex of the triangle formed by the stone is gently freed (Fig. 14-12*B*). This easy maneuver must be done by means of a malleable stylet, mobilizing the lateral and inferior surfaces of the vertex of the calculus. In many instances this maneuver will expose 60% to 70% of the calculus (Fig. 14-12*C*). The next step is usually to remove the branch which seems shortest and

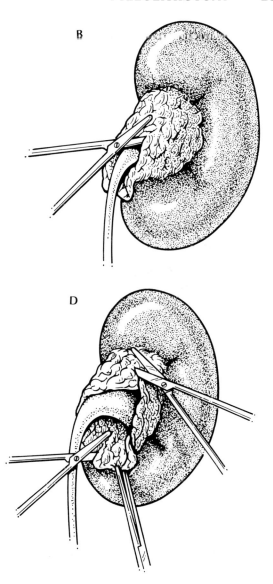
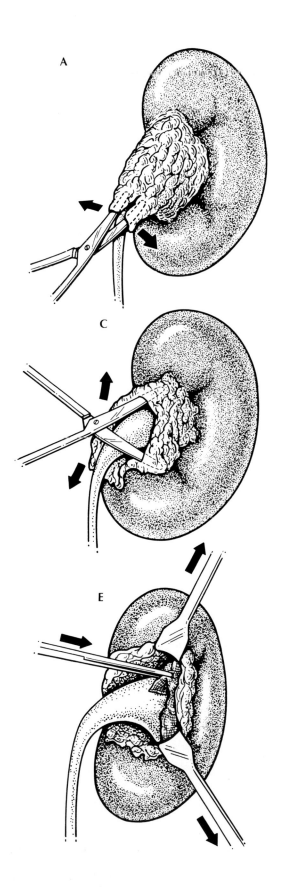

FIG. 14-9. Exposure of the renal sinus in the presence of severe inflammatory reaction. **(A)** Dissection begins along the upper ureter and proceeds superior. **(B)** Peripelvic fat is mobilized, then incised. **(C)** Near the hilus, peripelvic tissue is dissected bluntly. **(D)** Excessive adipose tissue may be excised. **(E)** With hilar retractors in place, intrasinusal fat is dissected away by blunt dissectioning using surgical gauze.

most mobile (Fig. 14-12*D*). If the exteriorization of the second branch is particularly difficult, the neck of the caliceal infundibulum must be dilated. This is done by using a very fine, long mosquito forceps of adequate curvature and opening them gently. After mobilization of the second branch, the remaining calculus follows easily. It is important to take into consideration the "free spaces," that is to say, those calicoinfundibular cavities that allow partial mobilization of the calculus and exteriorization of one of its embedded branches. When it is impossible to remove the calculus by these maneuvers, damage to the intrarenal excretory tracts is prevented by breaking the calculus. This

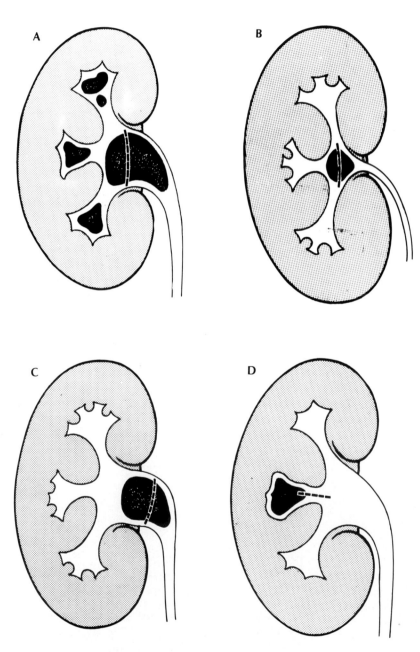

FIG. 14-10. Choice of incisions of the renal pelvis. **(A)** Transverse pyelotomy involves incision in the midportion of the pelvis, well away from the ureteropelvic junction. **(B)** Intrarenal pelvis also requires incision in the midportion. **(C)** Extrarenal pelvis should not be incised within the sinus. **(D)** Infundibulotomy incision should be longitudinal.

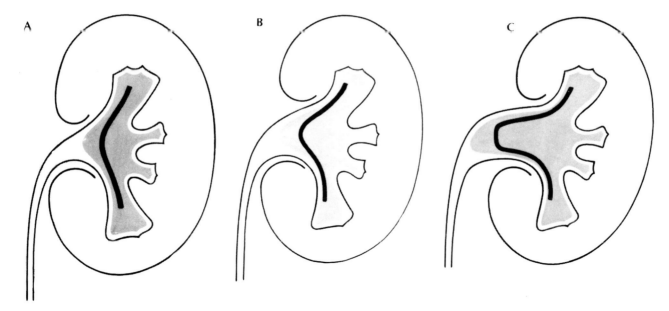

FIG. 14-11. A variation of the extended pyelotomy incision based upon morphological characteristics of the renal pelvis

must be done without violence and by breaking the branch that is most intractable to removal by the maneuvers previously described. The residual calculus is removed by dilatation of the infundibular neck or by prolongation of the incision, even to the entire length of the infundibulum.

REMAINING CALICEAL CALCULI

After removal of the body and principal branches of the staghorn, we make a three-dimensional x-ray study. Unless this done, the surgeon cannot be sure of the complete removal of the calculus. Any residual calculi illustrated on the film are localized by a malleable stylet with a small rounded end (Fig. 14-13A). Visual exploration is frequently possible, particularly in the middle group of calices. Once the existence of calculi is determined, they are removed with blunt forceps which may also be used to dilate the infundibulum (Fig. 14-13B). Successive intraoperative radiographs are made until total removal of all calculi and fragments is achieved.

The pyelotomy is sutured with chromic 6-0 catgut, but no sutures are placed in the caliceal portion of the incision (Fig. 14-14A). Once the retractors are removed, the posterior lip of the kidney covers the enlarged pyelotomy (Fig. 14-14B).

Related Procedures

COMPLEMENTARY NEPHROTOMIES

In approximately 25% of patients with staghorn calculi, the enlarged pyelotomy must be completed by one or more small radial nephrotomies. Such nephrotomies are required under the following circumstances:

A very big caliceal cavity, full of calculi with a thin parenchyma
A big calculus localized within the calix with long and narrow infundibulum
A calculus localized in an ectopic calix

The radial nephrotomy must be as small as possible, placed where the parenchyma is thinnest and where sectioning of interlobar arteries is avoided. If the calculus is large it is preferable to fragment it rather than to enlarge a small nephrotomy.

If the parenchyma is of normal thickness, prior to each nephrotomy the renal artery is occluded with a small, very soft, rubber-shod bulldog clamp to avoid damaging the artery. Clamping must not exceed 7 to 9 minutes, which is sufficient time to remove the calculus, explore and wash out the caliceal cavity, and resuture the nephrotomy. Clamping may be repeated as many times as

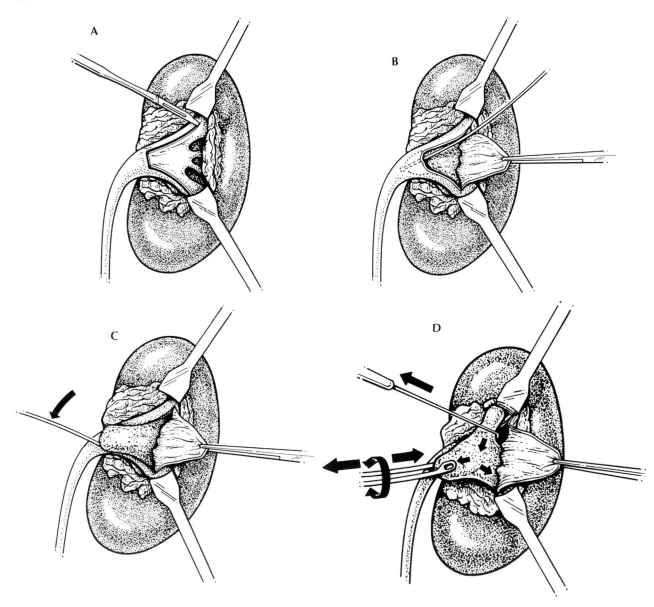

FIG. 14-12. Removal of large branched calculus. **(A)** With the sinus exposed, extended incision is made into the pelvis and the upper and lower infundibula. **(B)** With the pelvic flap elevated, the calculus is mobilized using a malleable probe. **(C)** The distal extent of the stone is subluxated out of the pelvis by rotating the probe. **(D)** Gentle rotation of the calculus, removing the least adherent branch first, permits extraction of the stone intact.

necessary if the intervals between clamping are the same as the ischemia time (7 to 9 minutes). In order to prevent vasospasm from producing renal ischemia,[11] the patient's blood volume must be maintained and traction of the pedicle avoided. This may be difficult when the kidney is exteriorized to obtain radiographs. However, the mini-chassis film cassette will reduce the need to exteriorize the kidney.

If multiple nephrotomies through a thick parenchyma are necessary, it is advisable to give mannitol or furosemide 30 minutes prior to the ischemia.[8] The osmotic diuresis may have some protective effect from the renal ischemia, but hypothermia is unquestionably the safest way to preserve renal function when the kidney must be ischemic for hours. In our experience, this occurs in 3% to 4% of patients with staghorn calculi.

In patients with complicated lithiasis and renal insufficiency, the parenchyma is usually very thin and we do not clamp the renal artery because the nephrotomy bleeds only slightly and does not interfere with the view of the cavity. Also, the pyelonephritic kidney is very sensitive to anoxia and thus tolerates ischemia poorly.

CAVITY WASHOUTS

In all renal surgery, it is useful to wash the renal cavities with normal saline at body temperature. The washing must be atraumatic and should in-

clude all calices, including those in which no stone was demonstrable. Mucoprotein material and similar debris are not detectable by radiography. At the end of the washout, a final radiograph must be done. A lumbotomy should never be closed without making sure that the removal of the calculus has been completed.

NEPHROSTOMY

As a general principle we do not use urinary diversion either by ureteral tubes or by nephrostomy. However, in the large sclerosed intrarenal

FIG. 14-13. Removal of residual calculi. **(A)** Calices are explored with a malleable probe. **(B)** Identified fragments are extracted, dilating the infundibula with the forceps.

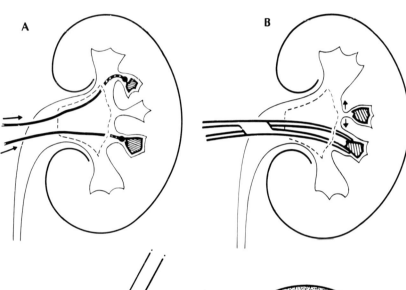

FIG. 14-14. Closure of the renal pelvis with interrupted sutures (**A**) leaving the infundibular portions of the incision open, to be covered by posterior hilar tissue and kidney parenchyma (**B**)

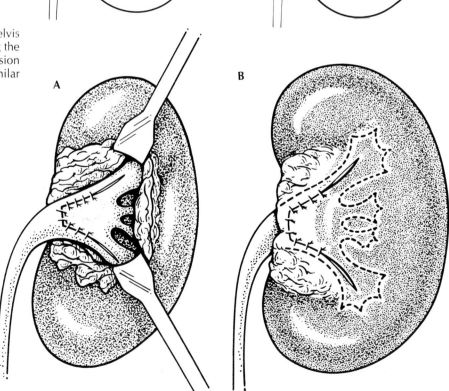

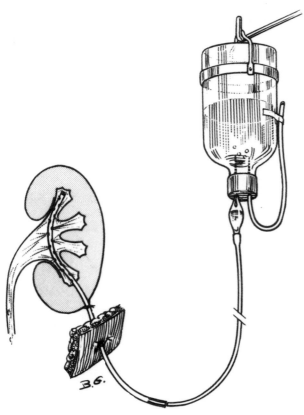

FIG. 14-15. Axial nephrostomy irrigation with a multi-perforated tube

cavities which may contain viable calculi and mucoprotein matter with persistent infection, especially *Bacillus* and *Proteus*, we perform an *axial minimal nephrostomy*.[6] A small multiperforated Silastic tube is placed in an inferior calix and after the sixth postoperative day, an intravenous pyelogram is made to check the patency and function of the ureter (Fig. 14-15). In the absence of leakage, a chemotherapeutic solution drip is begun through the nephrostomy tube and continued for 2 to 3 days. The pressure should not exceed 30 cm of water regulated by the height of the irrigation reservoir. This is very efficient as a local treatment of infection and to wash out cellular detritus, fibrin, and so forth. It would be dangerous and absurd to use the nephrostomy to attempt a dissolution of residual calculi.

In summary, we perform axial minimal nephrostomy in most of the different forms of lithiasis and particularly in all staghorns, with the exception of patients with systemic infections and a nonfunctioning kidney as seen by gammagram. The absence of contrast elimination on intravenous pyelography is not a contraindication to conservative surgery. Even in renal insufficiency with urolithiasis our position is interventionist for the following reasons:

This technique produces relatively little or no damage to the renal parenchyma.

Renal disease resulting from urinary obstruction is much more stable and subject to recuperation than a primary nephropathy provided one has been able to relieve the urologic obstruction.

The patient can be adequately prepared and if necessary kept on dialysis during the time required for recovery of renal function.

Modern supportive measures including fluid and electrolyte regulation permit us to operate on patients with a very poor renal function with minimal mortality and morbidity.

It is also important to operate in nonobstructive cases of lithiasis because the infection cannot be eradicated unless all stones are removed. If the renal insufficiency is irreversible, the patient may be a candidate for chronic dialysis or renal transplantation after all foci of infection have been removed.

The instruments required for this type of surgery are illustrated in Figure 14-16. These renal sinus retractors have an amplitude, a curvature, and a depth of blade which adapt to the thickness of the posterior lip of the renal hilus. The edges are blunt, and the handles are long and rigid. Different sizes are required to accommodate the morphological variations of the hilus for the adult as well as for the child. For the enlarged pyelotomy, two narrow retractors are placed, one on the superior and the other on the inferior commissure. For the simple transverse pyelotomy a single wider retractor is used. If the operation is prolonged, it is advisable to periodically loosen the retractors, which may compress the retropelvic vessels.

REOPERATIONS

The presence of residual or recurrent calculi may require reoperation, in which instance the mobilization of the kidney must be very carefully accomplished. How to perform the pyelotomy depends upon whether the sinus space was entered at the time of the former operation. There will be no problem if the pyelotomy was extrahilar, but it may be very difficult or almost impossible to develop the intrasinal planes if adhesions have occurred between the posterior wall of the pelvis and the internal sheath of the fibrous capsule of the kidney. Sometimes the sinus may be reached

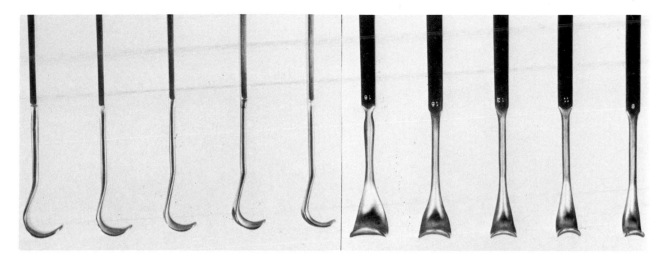

FIG. 14-16. Gil–Vernet sinus retractors of various sizes

by entering through the anterior and inferior surface of the pelvis, thereby developing a virgin plane into the sinus. By contouring this surface, one may reach the posterior surface of the pelvis by proper use of scissors.

RENAL HYPOTHERMIA IN LITHIASIS

In approximately 2% to 4% of our patients hypothermia is an important means of preservation of renal function. This is true in those patients whose residual calculi are exceptionally difficult to remove and who have moderate renal insufficiency and pyelonephritis, when a large number of small nephrotomies would otherwise be required. There are two different methods to produce hypothermia in the lithiasic kidney: the superficial method using external cooling or the intrarenal method by intravascular perfusion with cold solution. A third method is a combination of both: initial reduction of the renal temperature by perfusion and subsequent maintenance of hypothermia by surface cooling. We prefer the third method.

To avoid damage to the artery we have designed an "atraumatic needle" with an exaggerated curve, a very short bevel, and a stop 5 mm from the point (Fig. 14-17). Once the kidney is freed and its pedicle dissected, a clamp covered with foam rubber is placed at the level of the ureter (Fig. 14-18A). Once the artery has been punctured, a soft bulldog clamp is placed proximally beneath the needle. A second bulldog clamp is placed on the vein on whose superior edge a small incision is performed to

FIG. 14-17. Needle for renal arterial perfusion *in situ*

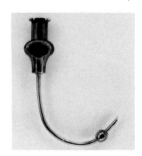

permit efflux of the perfusate (Fig. 14-18B). After perfusion with 300 ml of Eurocollins solution at 4° C the needle is removed, the phlebotomy is closed, and hypothermia is maintained by continuous surface irrigation with normal saline at 4° C. Perfusion avoids the danger of renal venous thrombosis and sludging of blood within the kidney. The kidney thus freed of blood is of lesser thickness and more pliable, which facilitates the entrance to the sinus cavity as well as the localization of the calculi by palpation.

Preoperative and Postoperative Care

Regulation of fluids and electrolytes requires complete evaluation of the patient, including blood pressure, diuresis, acid base balance, creatinine clearance, plasma ionogram, and urinary cultures.

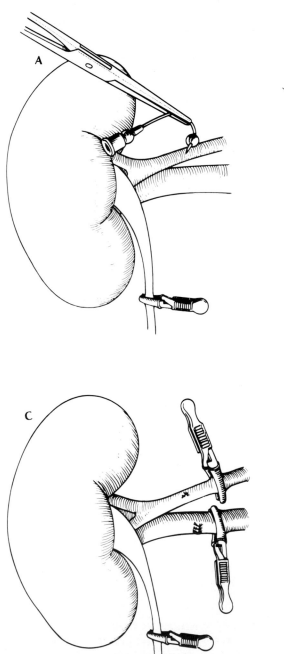

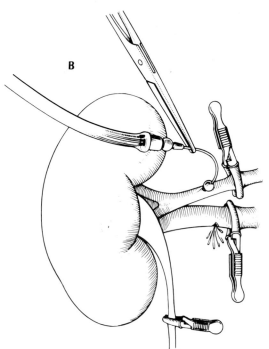

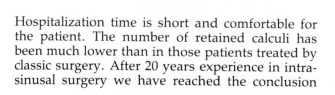

FIG. 14-18. Technique of renal perfusion. **(A)** Artery is punctured prior to clamping. **(B)** Artery, vein, and ureter are secured and a venting venotomy is accomplished. **(C)** Following perfusion, the needle puncture site and the venotomy are closed with arterial silk and hypothermia is maintained by irrigating the kidney with normal saline at 4°C.

Hospitalization time is short and comfortable for the patient. The number of retained calculi has been much lower than in those patients treated by classic surgery. After 20 years experience in intra-sinusal surgery we have reached the conclusion that intrasinusal surgery is the least aggressive of all the recommended operations for removal of renal calculi. The latest advances obtained in the intraoperative radiographic control greatly improve the efficacy of this method.

REFERENCES

1. FEY B, DOSSET R, QUÉNU L et al: Traite de Technique Chirurgicale, T. VIII. Paris, Masson et Cie, 1956
2. GIL–VERNET J: La lombotomie verticale posterieure; considerations a propos de 366 cas. Acta Urol Belg 32:391, 1964
3. GIL–VERNET J: New surgical concepts in removing renal calculi. Urol Int 20:255, 1965
4. GIL–VERNET J: La cirugia intrasinusal de los calculos coraliformes, Vol. 1. Tokyo, Rapport XVᵉ Congr Soc Inter Urologia, 1970
5. GIL–VERNET J: Las voies d'abord du bassinet et des calices dans la chirurgie de la lithiase renale. Progres de la Medicine, 479 Editions Medicales. Paris, Flammarion, 1967
6. GIL–VERNET J: Minimum nephrostomy. Urology 6:620, 1977
7. GIL–VERNET J, CARRETHERO P, BALLESTEROS JJ et al: New approach to the kidney in kyphoscoliosis. Eur Urol 2:105, 1976
8. LEAF A: Regulation of intracellular fluid volume and disease. Am J Med 49:291, 1970
9. MARSHALL VF: Complete longitudinal nephrolithotomy. Surgical procedures (Warner–Chilcott). 9:5, 1966
10. PIATRE F, GIRAUD D, DUPRET J: Prac. Anatomoquirurgica Ilustrada. Los Elementos del Pediculo in Fasc. 3, Barcelona, Salvat, 1941
11. SUMMERS WK, JAMISON RL: The no reflow phenomenon in renal ischemia. Lab Invest 25:635, 1971
12. TRUC E, GRASSET D: Lithiase renal. Encyclop, Med Cir, 9:5, 1960

Coagulum Pyelolithotomy

15

F. Everett Anderson

In 1943, Dees first published his concept and technique for the injection of a coagulable material into the renal pelvis to entrap renal calculi and to aid in their operative removal.[1] Coagulum formed from the action of thrombin on human fibrinogen satisfied most closely the requirements for a material to be used for this purpose.[2,3,4,6,7,9,10] Coagulum pyelolithotomy did not become popular at that time because no suitable commercial fibrinogen was available.[7,8,12] The Food and Drug Administration prohibited the use of pooled human fibrinogen because of the potential danger of transmission of serum hepatitis, and there was too little demand for bovine fibrinogen for its production to be profitable. Cryoprecipitate prepared from single-donor fresh-frozen plasma is currently the source of human fibrinogen.[10,11,14] There is still a minimal risk for transmission of serum hepatitis, but it is small because a single donor source is used.[9,15]

Indications and Contraindications

Coagulum pyelolithotomy is indicated for the removal of multiple stones, soft stones, or small mobile stones. It can also be used to entrap caliceal calculi prior to partial nephrectomy. An advantage offered by coagulum pyelolithotomy over standard pyelolithotomy is that all free stones, regardless of size, number, or position within the renal pelvis, can be removed. Fragmentation of calculi during removal is avoided, and trauma to the kidney is reduced to a minimum. Complete surgical mobilization of the kidney is unnecessary because access to the renal pelvis alone provides adequate exposure for the procedure.

The coagulum cannot remove a caliceal calculus of larger diameter than that of the infundibulum through which it must pass, nor can it remove a calculus embedded in or adherent to the walls of the renal pelvis. Significant hemorrhage into the renal pelvis from the renal parenchyma (e.g., hemorrhage that occurs after prolonged probing of the renal pelvis with stone forceps) is a definite contraindication.

Current Operative Technique

MATERIALS

Cryoprecipitate prepared easily and inexpensively in blood-bank laboratories from fresh-frozen plasma is used as a source for human fibrinogen.

Topical Thrombin (Parke, Davis) is supplied in 1,000-unit, 5,000-unit, or 10,000-unit vials of freeze-dried thrombin. It is mixed with normal saline to produce a concentration of 50 units/ml.

Calcium Chloride 10% solution (Cutter Laboratories) is supplied in vials of 10 ml of 10% solution. Calcium chloride is used if the cryoprecipitate is preserved with EDTA (usual case). Protamine is used if the cryoprecipitate is preserved with heparin.

Indigo Carmine (Hynson, Westcott & Dunning) is supplied in 5-ml ampules. This material is optional. It stains the coagulum a dark blue color, enhancing its identification during the operation.

RATIO OF MATERIALS

Cryoprecipitate	25 ml
Thrombin	4 ml (50 units/ml)
Calcium Chloride	1 ml
Indigo Carmine	1 ml

All materials are used at room temperature. Cryoprecipitate is stored as a frozen preparation and should be thawed by exposure to room temperature for several hours prior to surgery. A less desirable alternative is to thaw the cryoprecipitate by placing it in warm water.

SURGICAL TECHNIQUE

The preoperative intravenous pyelogram is examined to estimate the volume of the renal pelvis. The renal pelvis and the upper ureter are exposed through a standard lumbar incision.[5,8,11,12,14,15] Following preparation of the materials, a rubber-shod clamp is placed across the ureter just below the ureteropelvic junction. Two No. 19 butterfly needles (Abbott) are inserted into the renal pelvis, and the

177

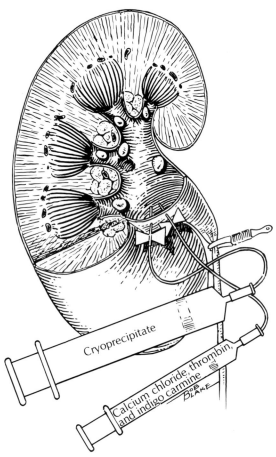

FIG. 15-1. Operative technique: simultaneous injection of solutions

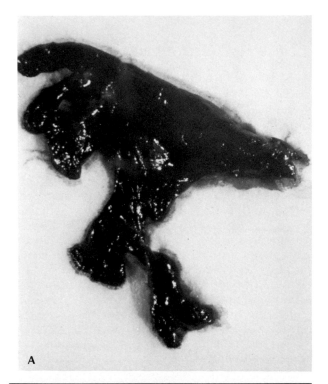

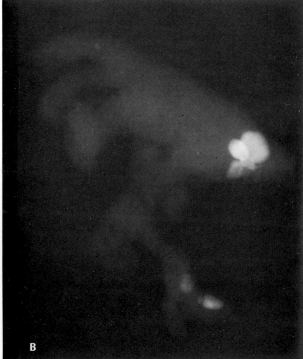

FIG. 15-2. **(A)** Coagulum extracted with indwelling calculi; **(B)** radiograph of coagulum delineating calculi

indwelling urine is aspirated through one needle. A 10-ml syringe containing calcium chloride mixed with thrombin and Indigo Carmine is attached to one infusion set, and a 30-ml syringe containing cryoprecipitate is attached to the other. The solutions are injected simultaneously until the renal pelvis is filled to maximum capacity (Fig. 15-1).

After 10 minutes, the renal pelvis is opened through a high transverse incision, and the protruding coagulum is grasped with ring forceps. The cast of the lower calices is first extracted by pulling the clot toward the upper pole of the kidney.[13] The cast of the upper calices is then delivered by pulling the clot toward the lower pole of the kidney. The coagulum filling the upper calices is removed last because these calices are usually larger and contain more clot (Fig. 15-2A). The renal pelvis is irrigated with sterile saline, and an x-ray film of the kidney is obtained to ensure complete evacuation of the calculi. If necessary, a radiograph of the coagulum can be obtained to identify the indwelling calculi (Fig. 15-2*B*). Any remaining stones are removed with stone forceps. The renal pelvis is irrigated with sterile saline, and the rubber-shod clamp is removed from the ureter. A ureteral catheter is passed to the bladder and then removed. The renal pelvis is closed with interrupted fine absorbable sutures.

If there are large calculi within the renal pelvis that might obstruct the free flow of solutions, they should be removed by standard pyelolithotomy technique, with watertight closure of the pyelotomy incision using a continuous suture, prior to introduction of the coagulum.

REFERENCES

1. DEES JE: The use of intrapelvic coagulum in pyelolithotomy. South Med J 36:167, 1943
2. DEES JE: Fibrinogen coagulum as an aid in the operative removal of renal calculi. J Clin Invest 23:576, 1944
3. DEES JE: The use of fibrinogen coagulum in pyelolithotomy. J Urol 56:271, 1946
4. DEES JE: Coagulum pyelolithotomy. J Urol 73:445, 1955
5. DEES JE, ANDERSON EE: Coagulum pyelolithotomy. Urol Clin North Am 8:313, 1981
6. DEES JE, FOX H: The properties of human fibrinogen coagulum: Preliminary report. J Urol 49:503, 1943
7. HARRISON JH, TRICHEL BE: Fibrin coagulum in pyelolithotomy. J Urol 62:1, 1949
8. HOFFMAN, HA: Coagulum pyelolithotomy. Am J Surg 79:598, 1950
9. KLOSTERHALFEN H: Experimentalle untersuchungen zur fibrinpyelotomie. Urologe 8:167, 1969
10. MARSHALL S: Commercial fibrinogen, autogenous plasma, whole blood and cryoprecipitate for coagulum pyelolithotomy: A comparative study. J Urol 119:310, 1978
11. MARSHALL S, LYON RP, SCOTT MP, JR: Further simplifications for coagulum pyelolithotomy. J Urol 119:588, 1978
12. MOORE TD, SWEETSER TH, JR: Coagulum pelviolithotomy. J Urol 67:579, 1952
13. PATEL VJ: The coagulum pyelolithotomy. Br J Surg 60:230, 1973
14. RATHORE A, HARRISON JH: Coagulum pyelolithotomy using autogenous plasma and bovine thrombin. J Urol 116:8, 1976
15. STOLL HG: Koagulum-pyelolithotomie. Z Urol 52:610, 1959

Nephrolithotomy

16

William H. Boyce

Nephrolithotomy is the most common type of intrarenal surgery. The term encompasses all those surgical procedures that conserve renal function by removing intrarenal pathologic processes and reconstructing the renal parenchyma and collecting system. In addition to the removal of stones, intrarenal surgery permits the precise removal of benign and malignant tumors and arteriovenous fistulas with minimal sacrifice of functional renal tissue.

Intrarenal surgery qualifies as a subspecialty of urologic surgery because it requires a profound knowledge of renal anatomy and physiology; skill and versatility in microsurgical techniques; special tools and materials, including absorbable sutures of microdimensions; instruments for quantitating blood flow and velocity; thermocouples and regional hypothermia; intraoperative radiography; and facilities for intensive postoperative care. This list of essential elements of intrarenal surgery does not include a vast array of ancillary skills, services, and instruments that are desirable and that may, on occasion, also be essential.

Renal Anatomy

The surgical anatomy of the kidney has been reviewed in numerous recent publications.[11,12,13,14] The compound human kidney is formed by fusion of individual reniculi, which are embryologically basic units, each with a single papilla and calix and its own cortex, medulla, and blood supply. The process of fusion melds the cortical medullary and papillary components into grossly confluent structures with some degree of shared venous and lymphatic circulations. The arterial circulation, on the other hand, retains its original relationship to each reniculus, and thus, at every level of renal arterial bifurcation, each division becomes an end-artery devoid of collateral circulation from other divisions. The interface between these arterial segments provides a number of relatively avascular planes, the proper selection of which permits access to the internal structures with minimal blood loss, minimal loss of renal tissue, and minimal scarring (Figs. 16-1, 16-2, 16-3, and 16-4). Thus, the precise delineation of the parenchymal distribution of one or more of the major arterial segments of the kidney is a prerequisite to every intrarenal operation.

Delineation of Intersegmental Planes

After the kidney is mobilized, all but one of the first-order (segmental) branches are isolated and temporarily occluded. The choice of which segment to exclude depends on the intrarenal disease. In general the plane between the posterior and anterior segments will provide access to the majority of calices as well as to the pelvis, and is the one defined most often.

The intravascular administration of a bolus of 10 ml to 20 ml of methylene blue defines two intersegmental planes by imparting a dark blue color only to the parenchymal area between them that is supplied by the nonoccluded arterial branch. The intersegmental planes are generally convoluted and angular where two or three arterial segments join. The segments are mapped on the capsular surface with a methylene blue marker. It is possible to outline two or three arterial segments with a single injection of methylene blue by removing the clamps from each artery in succession.

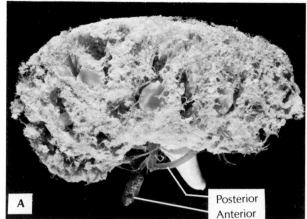

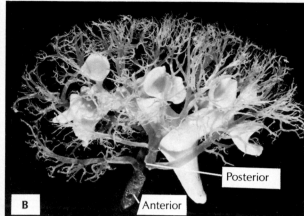

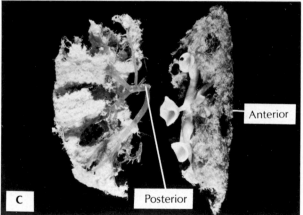

FIG. 16-1. In this corrosion cast of a right kidney, the anterior and posterior divisions of the main renal artery have been injected separately with plastic of different colors; the pelvis has been filled with white plastic. **(A)** On the posterior surface, note the arterial variation whereby the posterior half of the basilar segment is supplied by an artery arising from the posterior division and crossing the posterior surface of the renal pelvis. **(B)** This is the same specimen after the glomeruli have been removed with an airbrush. The anterior division of the renal artery supplies the apical segment, the anterior segment, and the anterior half of the basilar segment. **(C)** The anterior and posterior divisions of the renal artery have been separated, and the renal pelvis remains with the anterior division. The anterior division supplies the major portion of the apical and basilar segments. This illustrates the obvious necessity for identifying the distribution of the major arterial segments at the time of operation.

Before the methylene blue study is done, renal blood flow should be measured and, if possible, should be increased to a maximum. Surgical manipulation, muscle relaxants (d-tubocurarine), antihypertensive agents (sodium nitroprusside), and vasopressor agents may greatly reduce renal blood flow;[1] local anesthetic agents infiltrated about the renal artery, intravenous procaine, and warm saline in the wound with relaxation of any tension on the renal pedicle may improve renal blood flow. Because methylene blue administered as a bolus usually temporarily reduces renal blood flow,[2] we commonly administer mannitol before the methylene blue, the assumption being that an expanding blood volume will increase renal blood flow.

The injection of methylene blue may be made directly into the aorta, but it should not be made into the renal artery because of technical difficulties and the danger of dissection beneath the arterial endothelium or intima. Following the procedure as just described, we have observed no complications from its use in the *in situ* kidney. The patient

should be well oxygenated during the test, because methylene blue assumes a colorless leuco form in solutions of low oxygen content.

Measuring the temperature gradient between the ischemic and perfused renal segments may be used to define the intersegmental planes, but the technique is laborious and is less exact than using an intravascular dye.

The all-important dictum is that, once these planes have been established, the nephrotomy should follow the selected plane (or planes) through all its convolutions and angles. If that is done, the renal parenchyma will heal with hairline cicatrization regardless of the configuration of the wound.

In some kidneys in which cortical atrophy has brought the atrophic papilla very near the capsule and the stone is readily palpable, the inexperienced surgeon may want to abandon the intersegmental plane and plunge directly into the palpable calix, because he is not cutting through much cortex. This should *not* be done. The immediate cortical damage may well be of little consequence, but the

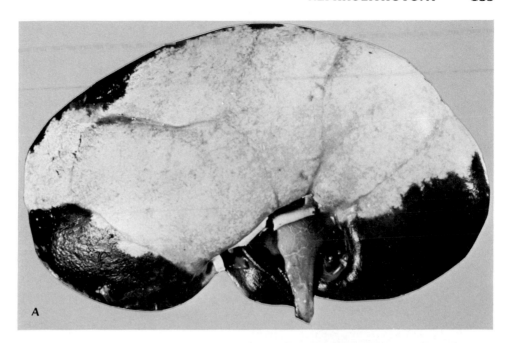

FIG. 16-2. **(A)** Microfil (Canton Bio-Medical Products, Inc., P. O. Box 2017, Boulder, CO 80302) injection of the posterior (*white*) and anterior (*black*) divisions of the renal artery of a right kidney. **(B)** Section through midtransverse plane of specimen in **A.** Hilar fat and other structures have been removed. Note the relative size of the anterior and posterior arterial segments. Renal surface lobulations result from the fusion process, which bears no relationship to the segmental arterial blood supply. Any anatomic correlation between surface markings and arterial intersegmental planes is entirely coincidental, thus the surgeon can not rely upon surface lobulations as a guide to nephrotomy sites. Rather, the intersegmental planes must be defined by selective arterial occlusion for each kidney. Note that the papilla in the posterior segment (*arrow*) includes a reniculus from the anterior segment. (Preparation courtesy of Dr. William Taylor)

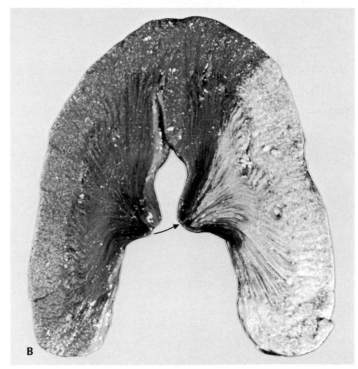

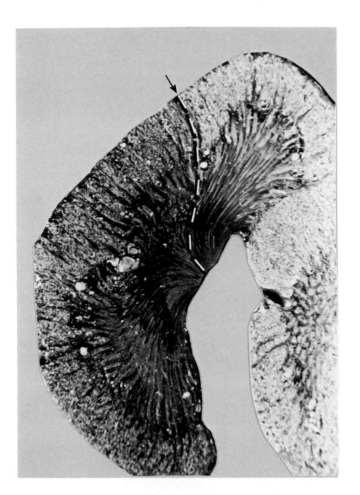

FIG. 16-3. Midtransverse section of a kidney arterially injected with Microfil; the anterior segment is *white*, the posterior segment is *black*. The dotted line (*arrow*) outlines the junction of these segments, which is the path of the most frequently employed nephrotomy for staghorn calculi. Note the close proximity of the cortico medullary veins (*empty circles*) to the line of the nephrotomy, hence the need for blunt dissection of the renal parenchyma. The papilla in the posterior segment contains, by fusion, a reniculus from the anterior segment. A proper nephrotomy in this area will split the papilla and enter the calyx of this kidney. (Preparation courtesy of Dr. William Taylor)

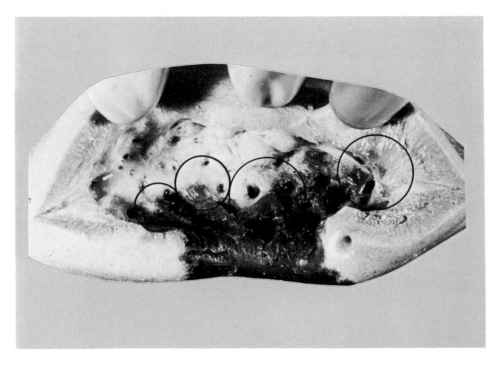

FIG. 16-4. View through the hilum of a right kidney arterially injected with Microfil; the posterior segment is *black*, the anterior segment is *white*. The apical segment is to the viewer's right. The hilar structures have been removed to demonstrate papillae. Those papillae that, by fusion, contain reniculi from both the anterior and posterior arterial divisions are *encircled*. Access to the hilar structures afforded by a nephrotomy along any margin of the posterior segment may be visualized from this preparation. (Preparation courtesy of Dr. William Taylor)

necessary extension of the dissection into the pelvis and other calices in a plane outside the intersegmental line seriously jeopardizes the arterial supply of the cortical and medullary tissues between the infundibula. It is the latter tissues specifically that are responsible for the remaining function in such kidneys.

Preservation of Renal Viability During Ischemia

Blood flow in the surgically exposed diseased kidney is rarely less than 300 ml/min, but it may exceed 1400 ml/min. The total blood flow to the kidney must be interrupted by atraumatic occlusion of the renal artery for the duration of the surgical procedure. The kidney must be drained of blood to achieve pliability—and thus to allow manipulation—and to reduce complications such as intravascular thrombosis.

The renal artery is particularly susceptible to injury, and only spring-loaded plastic clamps that are rubber shod or free of sharp teeth should be used. The arterial clamp should be placed just distal to the origin of the adrenal artery or as near the aorta as is feasible. Aberrant renal arteries, aberrant origins of the segmental arteries, or some contribution to medullary flow by the pelvic artery occurs in approximately 30% of the cases. The sterile ultrasonic Doppler probe is an invaluable aid at this step in the intrarenal operation. When applied to the surface of the kidney, it is capable of detecting flow in arcuate arteries and thus of detecting an aberrant blood supply after the artery is clamped and before the nephrotomy is made.

Cross clamping of the renal pedicle and the renal vein should be avoided because both create renal suffusion.

Preservation of renal function during the ischemic period, followed by rapid postoperative recovery, may be facilitated by hypothermia, inhibition of renal enzymatic systems, provision of certain metabolites preoperatively, avoidance of any potentially nephrotoxic substance or therapy preoperatively, and prevention of renovascular thrombosis with heparinization and administration of methylprednisolone.

The single most important adjunct to renal preservation during prolonged ischemia is local hypothermia (see Chap. 12). We have found the most satisfactory technique to be immersion of the ischemic kidney in a bath of ice-slush formed from physiologic solutions such as Ringer's lactate solution. The core temperature in the kidney is monitored with a needle thermocouple and main-

tained at approximately 14° C. Judging by immediate renal biopsy and the rate of recovery of renal function, we have not found that adding to the bath such enzyme inhibitors as phenoxybenzamine or chlorpromazine significantly improves the results.

The majority of patients receive a single dose of methylprednisolone, 13 mg/kg, approximately 2 hr before the renal artery is clamped, and mannitol diuresis is established immediately before clamping. The objective of the latter procedure is to increase the osmolarity of the intratubular glomerular filtrate and thus to reduce ice crystallization. The preservation of lysosomal integrity and the prevention of sludging of blood components in the renal capillaries by these measures is well documented.[15]

Several additional procedures are followed to protect the kidney from ischemia. All patients are brought to as near a normal state of electrolyte balance before operation as is feasible. Blood volume deficits are corrected by transfusion. In addition to dietary and intravenous corrections of electrolyte and nitrogenous abnormalities, the azotemic patient may receive an essential amino acid supplementation (Nephramine, McGraw Laboratories) to his low-protein diet and peritoneal or vascular dialysis. Amino-glycosides and all other potentially nephrotoxic agents are withheld before operation and until the kidney has recovered. After completion of the operation, a sterile ultrasonic Doppler probe is used to check returning blood flow in the unclamped renal artery and subsequent perfusion throughout the renal parenchyma, segment by segment.[6]

Hemostasis

Intraoperative blood loss from capillary oozing is prevented by the cross clamping of the main renal artery and any accessory arteries. If the intersegmental (arterial) planes are accurately determined and meticulously followed during nephrotomy, few, if any, arterioles large enough to require suture ligation will be divided. Large veins near the calices and infundibula may be injured, even by blunt dissection, because they are very thin walled and their locations are unpredictable. The venous injury is usually a rent or a slit rather than a transection. Therefore, the vein should not be ligated, but should be repaired with a running stitch of microsuture material.

Temporary release of the arterial clamp just before closure of the nephrotomy should identify any injured vessel of significant size that has

(Text continues on p. 188)

escaped the surgeon's inspection. Properly placed and executed nephrotomy wounds closed only by suture of the collecting system and capsule will not bleed when full-volume blood flow is returned to the kidney.

Preoperative Preparation

The complete preoperative preparation of the patient with intrarenal disease for prolonged anesthesia and operation is vitally important in reducing morbidity of intrarenal surgery. In addition to the measures already discussed, antibiotic prophylaxis is important. Infection is a usual accompaniment of large renal calculi, and intensive antimicrobial therapy with the most potentially effective antibiotic is begun 12 hr to 24 hr preoperatively and continued throughout the procedure.

Microsurgical Techniques and Instruments

The surgeon attempting intrarenal surgery should have completed a formal course in microsurgical technique, at least to the level of successful suturing of the divided rat aorta. Proficiency in the use of 2- to 4-power magnifying glasses (loupes) and the microinstruments is a skill not easily acquired.

Intrarenal surgery differs from the majority of microsurgical procedures in many particulars. All sutures in contact with urine must be rapidly absorbable (within 8 to 12 days) and yet initially strong. Suture lines must be watertight, because leakage is the source of many postoperative complications. Catgut remains the most predictably absorbable suture for use in the urinary system. Strength, a minimum of knots, and watertightness are achieved with a running cross-stitch of 6-0 catgut, hence the need for double-armed sutures. The needles must be taper-point and semicircular.

In addition to the standard set of microinstruments, the surgeon should have malleable microspatulas (chemists' models), elongated nerve hooks, microretractors, and blunt, angular drum elevators.

Intraoperative Radiography

Renal roentgenograms of excellent quality are readily attainable and are indispensable during nephrolithotomy.[4] A prenephrotomy renogram with markers outlining the arterial segments aids in the selection of the site of the nephrotomy and in the determination of its length (Fig. 16-5E). The sur-

geon should demand a fine-grained film with exposure of such quality that the warp and the woof in a cotton umbilical tape can be demonstrated.

Surgical Approach and Techniques

Which kidney to operate on first is always a question in bilateral renal disease. When stones are the problem, there should be no consideration of nephrectomy or partial nephrectomy of viable parenchyma that could be preserved by reconstructive intrarenal surgery. The kidney in greatest jeopardy (*i.e.*, the kidney losing nephrons at the greatest rate) is always the kidney to be repaired first, regardless of its total function. Pain in the less-jeopardized kidney should not sway this decision, because pain can usually be controlled temporarily by stents or simultaneous ureterolithotomy.

Whether to use a flank or an abdominal approach is rarely a question in nephrolithotomy requiring ice-slush hypothermia and renal roentgenography. Neither is it a question in patients with obstructed calices and virulent infection who may have intracaliceal pus and unsuspected perinephric abscesses, nor in azotemic patients who are on peritoneal dialysis or who may require it postoperatively. In all those situations, the extraperitoneal flank incision is preferred because it reduces total body hypothermia from ice water in the peritoneum, facilitates adequate roentgenography, and prevents inoculation of the peritoneal cavity. The postoperative pain of flank incisions can be reduced by infiltration of the nerve roots with long-acting local anesthetics. Postoperative hernias are prevented by meticulous closure of the incision in layers.

The congenitally deformed kidney (horseshoe, pancake, or "J" deformity) presents the most technically difficult problems in intrarenal surgery. The presence of multiple major arteries, renal fixation, and ureteral and caliceal inaccessibility hamper the procedure. Nevertheless, the flank approach is generally the most satisfactory in these situations.

BASIC TECHNIQUE

The basic technique of the anatrophic nephrolithotomy is illustrated in Figure 16-6. The nephrotomy is begun by sharp incision of just the capsule along the entire length of the proposed incision.[3,5] The capsule must not be torn or separated from the cortex. The underlying parenchyma is separated by blunt dissection with a thin spatula following the intersegmental plane in all its convolutions. If the transfer of arterial clamps from segmental to main renal artery has been properly timed with administration of methylene blue, the plane will be clearly defined from capsule to pelvis by the junction of blue and pink tissue. This dissection is continued evenly along the entire length of the nephrotomy until the surgeon either enters a calix, in which case he has split a compound papilla, or encounters the renal pelvis. In either case, he stops the forward dissection at that point until he has developed the rest of the nephrotomy down to the pelvis. This step usually permits a more precise development of the pyelotomy and infundibulo-calicotomies. The surgeon must remain completely oriented to the patient's pyelograms so that he knows where each calix and infundibulum is located.

If the nephrotomy is being done for nephrolith-otomy, no attempt is made to remove the stone(s), other than loose fragments, until the entire neph-rotomy has been completed. Injury to the renal parenchyma, tears of the collecting system, and loose fragments or retained caliceal stone are all hazards of attempts to fracture or wrest large stones from inadequately opened infundibula. The neph-rotomy is complete when all involved calices, all involved infundibula, and the pelvis have been opened in a single incision. Even then, the calcu-lus is usually densely adherent to the epithelium in many places. It is freed gently with a blunt drum elevator and is lifted from the incision only when there is no longer any resistance to the ma-neuver.

A Silastic tube or stent is passed from the pelvis into the bladder to be left indwelling and removed cystoscopically at a later date.[7] Any retained frag-ments are removed by microsuction and gentle irrigation. A roentgenogram of the kidney is es-sential to confirm the removal of all fragments.

Closure of the nephrotomy is begun by the suturing of all opened infundibula and calices. Very large infundibula may be reclosed along the infundibulotomy to the cusp of the calix. More commonly, cicatrization has narrowed the infun-dibular lumen and the margins of adjacent infun-dibula are sutured to one another. If there is no adjacent infundibulum, the margins are approxi-mated to the adjacent pelvis. Temporary stay su-tures placed to define all these suture lines greatly facilitate complete closure and reepithelialization

of the collecting system. The sutures should not be larger than 6-0 and should be rapidly absorbable; the knots should be placed outside the collecting system; and the whole should be watertight. A running cross-stitch with a double-armed suture eliminates one knot in each suture line.

When all infundibula and calices have been closed, the reconstituted pelvis is closed by the same technique; the suture is interrupted at points of stress. Where papillae have been split, the pelvic closure is interrupted at the margin of the caliceal cusp, where a reinforcing pocket stitch may be used. No suture line should cross a papilla. The closure of the nephrotomy is completed by su-ture of the capsule after the arterial clamp has been released temporarily so that any injured vessel of significant size can be identified and repaired.

The return of blood flow is checked with the Doppler probe, and the flank incision is closed with only a temporary Penrose drain in place. Nephrostomy and pyelostomy tubes are permis-sible only in the exceedingly rare instance when there is a ureteral defect that cannot be repaired or bypassed during the same operation, and there is thus a more than reasonable doubt that the ureter is functional. Postoperative renal irrigations are unnecessary, hazardous, and frequently coun-terproductive.[8]

SPECIAL TECHNIQUES

Calicorrhaphy

Closure by simple suture of an open calix, an open infundibulum, or both is an extremely rare pro-cedure, because the majority of calices requiring operative repair have obstructive or other indica-tions for surgical modification of their structure. Only the margins of the infundibulocaliceal walls should be included in the suture, hence the need for microsurgical techniques. Passage of the needle through adjacent parenchyma endangers paracal-iceal (interlobar) vessels by either occlusion or perforation. Postoperative arteriovenous fistulas and hemorrhage may result from such vascular perforation.

Calicoplasty

The pelvis and infundibula, especially the first divisions of the pelvis, are remarkably mobile within the hilar fat. This mobility permits the application of virtually all the techniques of plastic surgery for enlarging lumens. The combination of

(*Text continues on p. 192.*)

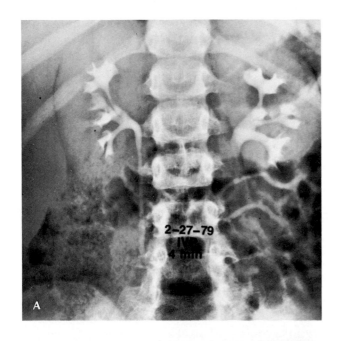

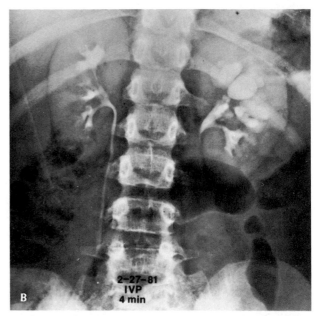

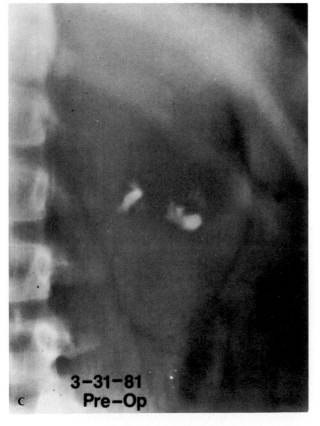

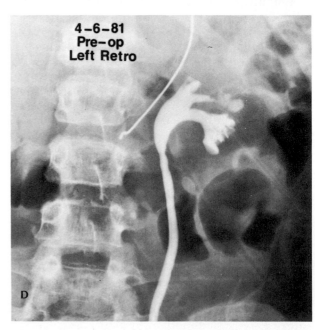

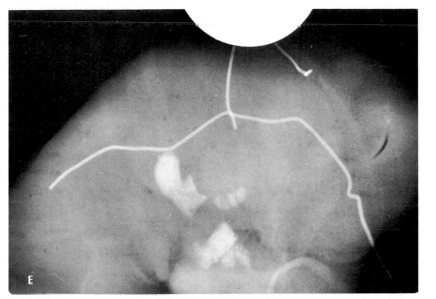

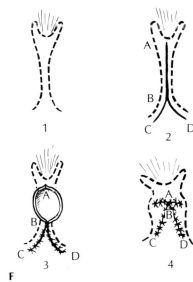

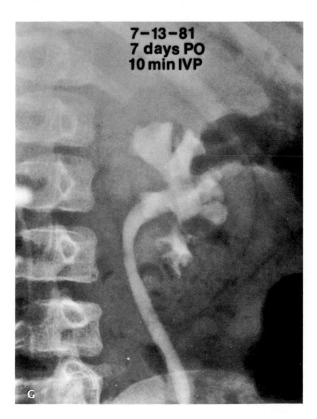

7-13-81
7 days PO
10 min IVP

FIG. 16-5. Calycoplasty by combined Y–V and sliding pelvic flap. **(A)** Excretory urogram obtained 2 years before operation illustrates elongated apical infundibula. **(B)** Excretory urogram obtained 2 months before operation illustrates hydrocalyces in left kidney. **(C)** KUB was obtained 1 week before operation. **(D)** Retrograde urogram obtained on day of operation illustrates virtual occlusion of infundibula. Nasogastric tube is visible within the stomach. *(Illustration continues on p. 192)* **(E)** Renal roentgenogram obtained intraoperatively demonstrates multiple calculi and radiopaque thread outlining the cortical configuration of planes between the posterior apical and anterior arterial segments. **(F)** Method of repair of strictured infundibula: **(1)** Infundibulum is elongated. **(2)** Incision from bell of calyx forms an inverted Y in the renal pelvis. **(3)** Pelvic flap is advanced as far as possible into the infundibulotomy. **(4)** Incision in the dilated calyx is closed transversely. **(G)** Oblique excretory urogram was obtained 7 days after operation immediately following removal of ureteral stent.

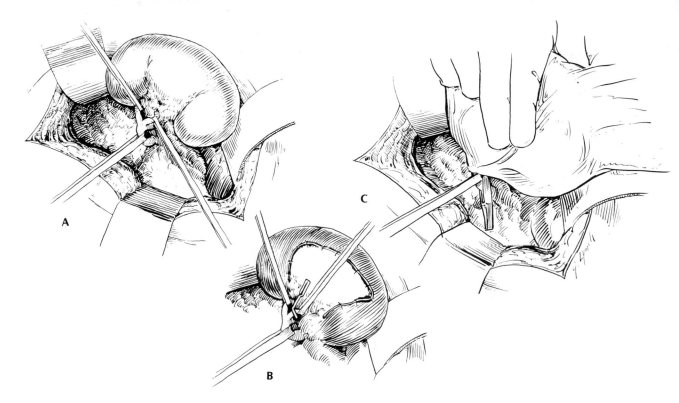

FIG. 16-6. Anatrophic nephrolithotomy. **(A)** The renal artery of a right kidney is exposed, and selected branches (here the apical, posterior, and main) are secured by vessel loops. **(B)** Occlusion of the posterior segmental artery produces blanching of the cortex supplied by this segment. An intravenous bolus of methylene blue (10–20 ml) enhances the contrast between ischemic segments and those with blood flow. The occlusive clamps will be removed as soon as the desired arterial segments are outlined. A radiopaque thread removed from a gauze sponge has been fixed along the margins of the posterior arterial segment. Renal roentgenograms will then be made to plan more precisely the position and extent of the nephrotomy (see Fig. 16-8*E*). **(C)** The kidney with all arteries occluded by gauze-shod atraumatic clamps is surrounded by a sheet of rubber dam and immersed in ice-slush. Dry gauze packs protect the adjacent peritoneum and peritoneal contents from prolonged hypothermia. **(D)** Only the capsule along an intersegmental plane is incised with a microblade. Here the place between the posterior segment and adjacent portions of both apical (cephalad) and anterior segments is used. **(E)** The parenchymal incision is developed carefully with a blunt spatula to expose the pelvis and calyces along the entire length of the proposed pyelocalycotomy. **(F)** The parenchyma has been separated from the collecting system sufficiently to permit incision and subsequent suturing of the latter structures without parenchymal injury. **(G)** The stone is lifted out only after all involved infundibula and calyces have been opened. Calculi are frequently adherent to pelvic mucosa and must then be gently freed with drum elevators. Fracture of stones to facilitate removal is unnecessary, creates fragments, and may injure the parenchyma. **(H)** All stones and fragments have been removed, as confirmed by inspection and renal roentgenography. A Silastic stent has been inserted through the pelvis into the bladder. Traction stay sutures mark the points to which the walls of adjacent calyces will be approximated by continuous sutures begun in the renal pelvis. Note peripelvic fat protruding between the open infundibula. **(I)** A running cross-stitch of 6-0 chromic suture is begun in the renal pelvis to approximate adjacent infundibula and calyces. The angular drum elevator depresses hilar fat and brings infundibula into approximation for ease of suturing. **(J)** All opened calyces have been resutured by approximation to adjacent calyces, approximation to adjacent pelvis, or simple reclosure. **(K)** The reconstituted renal pelvis is closed with a running cross-stitch of 6-0 chromic catgut. This stitch is interrupted at any calyceal cusps encountered during the closure. All knots are tied outside of the calyces and pelvis. **(L)** The nephrotomy repair is completed by a running lockstitch of 4-0 catgut in the capsule only. No parenchymal or mattress sutures are used. No tubes, drains, or foreign bodies are left in the nephrotomy closure.

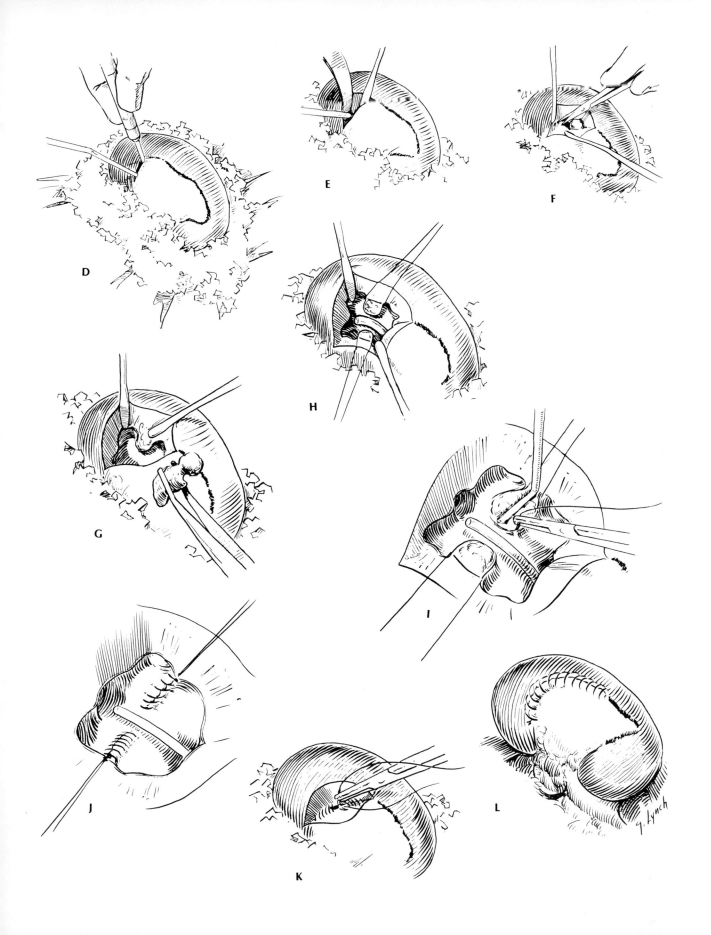

D

E

F

H

G

I

J

K

L

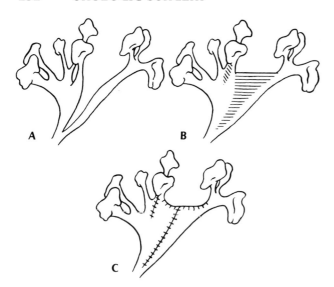

FIG. 16-7. Calycoplasty through a nephrotomy. **(A)** The original configuration. **(B)** Pelvic and infundibular incisions. A large silk suture passed through the two arms of the bifid pelvis as a tractor will facilitate development of the infundibulotomies without vascular injury. **(C)** Closure

two or more infundibula into a single unit is illustrated in Figures 16-7 and 16-8. The use of sliding flaps from both a dilated calix and the renal pelvis to enlarge a single infundibulum is illustrated in Figure 16-8. The Y–V plasty is an integral part of such procedures, and it is often used alone.

Calicocalicostomy

Developmental anomalies of the pyelocaliceal system may result in a virtual absence of the renal pelvis, with multiple dilated calices.[10] Side-to-side anastomosis of the dilated calices with subsequent anastomosis of one or more of the calices to the rudimentary pelvis, to the ureter, or to both structures may result in a most satisfactory preservation of renal function.

Diverticulectomy

It is frequently impossible to determine intraoperatively whether a dilated calix is a true diverticulum or a strictured calix with papillary atrophy. The thickness of the overlying cortical tissue, the identification of the papilla within the open calix, the identity of the infecting organism, and the technical feasibility of repair by anastomosis to a large conduit rather than a small infundibulum are the considerations that determine whether excision or repair should be done. When excision is the proper treatment, the thick-walled diverticulum is shelled

FIG. 16-8. Calycoplasty of adjacent minor calyces. **(A)** The infundibular walls are incised from the pelvic orifice to the calyceal bell. **(B)** The intervening peripelvic tissue is separated by blunt dissection. **(C)** The V incision thus produced in each infundibulum is joined by a double-armed suture beginning at the point of the two Vs and **(D)** is run as a single suture out each arm to join the two infundibula.

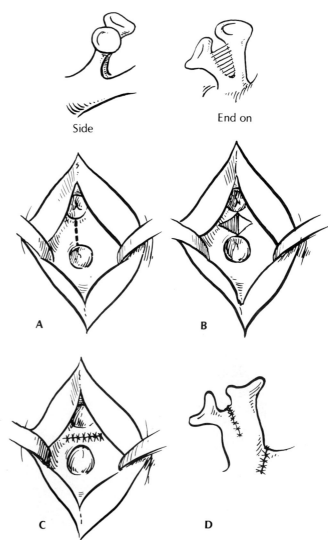

Side   End on

A   B

C   D

out of the parenchyma by blunt dissection. The stoma is sutured shut and the capsular incision is closed. No filler is required for the empty space in the parenchyma, because that space may be reduced by excision of small amounts of subcapsular cortex.

Papillary Transection

When the single reniculi of the embryologic human kidney fuse into a compound kidney containing a continuum of cortical and medullary layers, two or more papillae may join to form a single unit surrounded by a single calix. If the reniculi that fuse into a single papilla all derive their blood supply from a single segmental artery, the compound papilla will lie entirely within that arterial segment of the kidney. However, in virtually all kidneys, there are some compound papillae that contain embryonic papillae from two different arterial segments. Such papillae lie directly within the arterial intersegmental plane.

If the surgeon opens all kidneys precisely along the planes between arterial segments, he may not encounter a papilla, but, if the nephrotomy is long, the probability is that he will split one or more papillae. The pyramidal or conical structure of the parenchyma warns him of an impending papillary split. Both clinical and laboratory observations suggest that less damage to functional renal tissue results from a precise and deliberate split of the structure than from efforts to circumvent the papilla.[9] It is most important that the surgeon stop the dissection as soon as he opens the calix, lest he completely sever it from its infundibulum. He then separates the infundibulum from the adjacent parenchyma and opens it by a single linear incision into the renal pelvis.

The repair of such split papillae consists of a resuturing of the calices, with the suture line ending at the cusp of the calix. This brings the papillary surfaces into apposition, and no sutures are required to cross the papillary tubules. A reinforcing pocket stitch may be placed in the cusps of calices that are unusually large. Postoperative hemorrhage from such papillary repair is uncommon.[16]

Papillary Resection

The papillary tips may be the source of progressive stone formation and persistent infection due to massive intraluminal calcification and ulceration. If only one or two intraductal calculi are visible, they may be removed by incision of the overlying urothelium in line with Bellini's papillary ducts.

More extensive calcification may be removed by resection of the entire papilla at the level of the caliceal cusps. Such transected ducts appear to heal with patent lumens and a minimum of cicatrization.[16]

REFERENCES

1. BIRCH AA, BOYCE WH: Changing renal blood flow following sodium nitroprusside in patients undergoing nephrolithotomy. Anesth Anal (Cleve) 56:102, 1977
2. BIRCH AA, BOYCE WH: Hypertension and decreased renal blood flow following methylene blue injection. Anesth Analg (Cleve) 55:674, 1976
3. BOYCE WH: Reconstructive renal surgery for infectious staghorn stones. Topics in Urology, pp 4–13. Kenilworth, Schering Corp, 1979
4. BOYCE WH: The localization of intrarenal calculi during surgery. J Urol 118:152, 1977
5. BOYCE WH: Three key methods. Advanced renal repair. Contemporary Surgery III, No 3, pp 15–21. New York, McGraw-Hill, 1973
6. BOYCE WH: Ultrasonic velocimetry in resection of renal arteriovenous fistulas and other intrarenal surgical procedures. J Urol 125:610, 1981
7. BOYCE WH: Use of the internal ureteral stent in surgery of the kidney and ureter. In Boyarsky S (ed): Urodynamics. New York, Academic Press, 1971
8. BOYCE WH, HARRISON LH: Complications of renal stone surgery. In Smith RB, Skinner DG (eds): Complications of Urologic Surgery: Prevention and Management, pp 87–105. Philadelphia, WB Saunders, 1976
9. BOYCE WH, RUSSELL JM, WEBB R: Management of the papillae during intrarenal surgery. Trans Am Assoc Genitourin Surg 71:76, 1979
10. BOYCE WH, WHITEHURST AW: Hypoplasia of the major renal conduits. J Urol 116:352, 1976
11. DOUVILLE E, HOLLINSHEAD WH: The blood supply of the normal renal pelvis. J Urol 73:906, 1955
12. GRAVES FT: The Arterial Anatomy of the Kidney. Baltimore, Williams & Wilkins, 1971
13. HODSON J: The lobar structure of the kidney. Br J Urol 44:246, 1972
14. RESNICK MI, BOYCE WH: Surgical Anatomy of the Human Kidney and its Clinical Application. New York, Motion Picture, Aegis Productions, 1979
15. TOLEDO-PEREYRA LH, RAMAKRISHMAN VR, ZAMMIT M: Study of the protective effect of methylprednisolone, furosemide, and mannitol on ischemically damaged kidneys. Eur Surg Res 11:179, 1979
16. WEBB R, RUSSELL JM, BOYCE WH: Healing properties of the renal papilla: Animal model II. Invest Urol September 1981

Renal Cysts

17

Kenneth N. Walton

The term *renal cyst* refers to a variety of renal disorders characterized by one or more fluid-filled cavities.[33] In general, cystic disorders that involve both kidneys diffusely are less commonly of surgical interest than those lesions that involve a portion of one kidney. This chapter will emphasize the latter group.

Cystic intrarenal lesions may be classified according to whether or not they are commonly of surgical interest, and whether they are true cysts or pseudocysts. Table 17-1 presents a modification of such a surgically useful classification.

True renal cysts, whether single, multilocular, or multiple, by definition are benign, thin walled, and epithelium lined and contain clear or straw-colored fluid.[4] Their clinical importance is often in distinguishing them from renal carcinoma, a lesion which may also be round, cystic, and relatively avascular. Proper evaluation through a variety of techniques affords accurate diagnosis in most cases.[24] Other cases may require surgery for resolution of the diagnosis and proper management.[16] Benign intrarenal cystic lesions may require surgery in order: to preserve critical renal parenchyma when, with compromised renal function, intrarenal expansion of the cyst produces atrophy; to relieve obstruction of the collecting system; to drain infected cysts (essentially abscesses); or to arrest hemorrhage into an intact or ruptured cyst. Appropriate surgery should relieve symptoms and preserve renal function.[16, 28]

True Cysts

Simple and multilocular cysts present similar problems in diagnosis and indications for surgical management. These are the cystic lesions that must be distinguished from renal carcinoma. Certain special features of multilocular cysts require separate discussion, although the radiographic evaluation is similar to that of a simple cyst.

SIMPLE CYSTS

Simple cysts are the most common space-occupying lesions of the kidney.[4,8] Computed tomography (CT scan) of the abdomen commonly demonstrates small, clinically insignificant cysts in one or both kidneys in older adult patients. In 426 clinical cases of cystic renal disease, Emmett and associates found 314 to be solitary, 54 to be multiple, and 58 to be hilar or parapelvic.[8] The appearance of these cysts as incidental findings on a CT scan increases with age, as does the clinical incidence of a cyst presenting as a renal mass. Simple cysts are rare in children but when seen are often large.

Simple cysts are generally problems of diagnosis in asymptomatic patients and are often incidental findings in routine abdominal or urinary radiographic studies. A vague flank fullness may be present in uncomplicated large cysts. Infection occurs less commonly than in polycystic disease; when it does occur, it is as a consequence of urinary infection. It is therefore more common in women and is usually due to *Escherichia coli* or other gram-negative rods. The presenting features are abscesslike chills, fever, and flank pain with exquisite tenderness. The urine is infected, and the pyelogram is deformed by an intrarenal mass.

TABLE 17-1.   Surgical Classification of Renal Cysts

Intrarenal Cystic Diseases of Surgical Interest
   True Cysts
   Simple cysts
   Multilocular cysts
   Parapelvic cysts
   Cystic dysplasia, including multicystic kidney
   Adult polycystic disease
   Cystic hamartoma

   Pseudocysts
   Caliceal diverticula
   Hydrocalices
   Parasitic cysts
   Neoplastic cysts

Intrarenal Cystic Diseases of Little Surgical Interest
   Infantile polycystic disease
   Medullary cystic disease
   Medullary sponge kidney

Pararenal Cysts
   Renal or ureteral origin
   Nonrenal origin—pancreatic pseudocyst

Studies must be done to distinguish this infection from pyelonephritis in a kidney with tumor so that treatment will be appropriate. Hemorrhage into a simple cyst may be a very serious situation, because the cyst is large and thin walled and may rupture into the retroperitoneal space. Sudden severe pain may be followed by shock and even death.[34] Only a high level of suspicion, especially with patients on anticoagulants, will lead to the swift care required to prevent catastrophe.

Rare but definite complications of simple cyst include intrarenal cyst expansion producing renal parenchymal atrophy in a patient with compromised kidney function, ureteral or pelvic obstruction from a large cyst, erythrocythemia, and hypertension.[12,23] Hypertension in a child with elevated lateralizing renal vein renins has reversed following unroofing of a large cyst compressing the parenchyma.[12] In the case of cyst compression in a patient with borderline function, unroofing may not improve function but may prevent further atrophy and loss of function.

Diagnosis

Most simple cysts are not a problem except to distinguish them from renal neoplasms.[17] This is currently accomplished short of surgical exploration with an accuracy exceeding 95%.[16] Neverthe-

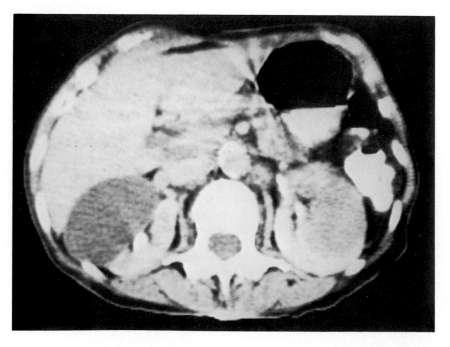

FIG. 17-1.   The CT scan of a typical cyst of the right kidney shows a smooth-walled, homogeneous lesion of water density. This contrasts with the co-existing carcinoma of the left kidney featuring a nonhomogeneous, irregular mass whose density is that of soft tissue.

less, there is considerable controversy about which tests are required to make this distinction and in what sequence they should be performed.[24]

In the evaluation of a space-occupying lesion, one should proceed from the most benign test to the most hazardous until the diagnosis is firmly established. Availability of studies and costs will influence this sequence, but the reward for performing these tests is the high accuracy level (>95%) in identifying benign and malignant disease, sparing unnecessary surgery for the former and offering curative treatment for the latter.

Calcification is more commonly seen in tumors than in cysts. Mottled calcification is typical of tumors and curvilinear calcification is typical of simple cysts, but these signs are not reliable. Many authors have reported curvilinear calcification in renal carcinoma.[6]

Nephrotomography is routinely a part of intravenous urography at some institutions. It delineates the renal outline more precisely, picking up masses missed otherwise for technical reasons. It also defines the discreteness of the rim of the parenchyma adjacent to the mass, and where the cyst protrudes from the cortex a smooth crescent or beaklike deformity is seen.

Sonography, when performed in a technically competent manner with sophisticated equipment, is an inexpensive, noninvasive technique used to establish whether a lesion is homogeneous in sound density with smooth margins and therefore likely a cyst.[20,24] Confidence in this study is often related to the previous experience of the surgeon and the sonographer as a team.

Selective renal arteriography provides a diagnosis for all cysts and 95% of tumors, because all cysts and only 5% to 10% of renal tumors are avascular. Neovascularity and tumor staining are as convincing to the surgeon as to the radiologist. The number and distribution of vessels may be valuable at surgery for tumor. Classically arteriography should follow sonography in all solid or questionable lesions and when for any reason sonography is not reliable.

Those lesions that are cystic on sonography have in many institutions been confirmed by cyst puncture. As described by Lang the patient is placed in the prone position, the collecting system is visualized by the intravenous or retrograde injection of contrast material, and a marker is placed on the skin to help localize the cyst relative to the surface.[18] Under local anesthesia and fluoroscopic control, a thin-walled, 20-gauge spinal needle is advanced into the mass as the patient holds his breath. With the needle in the mass attached to flexible tubing, fluid is aspirated for a Pap smear and fat analysis and an equal volume of contrast material replaces the fluid. The needle is withdrawn and films are obtained in several projections, rotating the patient to determine if there are any irregularities of the cyst cavity that might indicate the presence of cancer.

Lingard and Lawson have described the use of sonography to identify a cyst and locate it with a needle.[20] Recently developed equipment allows television screen monitoring in several planes. This technique eliminates radiation exposure. Although it has been pointed out that aspiration of a cyst or merely puncturing it may be followed by disappearance of the cyst in one third of the cases,[36] this is not really an argument for managing simple cysts by cyst puncture, because simple cysts are harmless and asymptomatic. Cyst puncture has no place in the management of complicated cysts.

The need for cyst puncture in any case as well as the sequence of studies is a matter of current controversy since the advent of CT scanning.[24,35] The CT scan is now competitively priced and can logically follow sonography. It provides a three-dimensional view of the mass, an assessment of the uniformity of internal structure, and, uniquely, a measure of the density of the mass (Fig. 17-1).[35] Cysts are smooth walled and have a uniform density of water or slightly greater, 0 to 9 Houndsfield units; tumors have a density that is often not homogeneous and is of 15 units or more. Lesions 10 to 15 units in density are uncommon and, if the test is not diagnostic, should be explored. Whenever the original density scale of −500 to +500 has been expanded to −1000 to +1000, the above units should be multiplied by two.

CT scanning has its limitations, but as long as equivocal lesions as well as tumors are explored and any combination of tests exceeds 95% accuracy, only a small number of patients will be explored for diagnostic reasons. This is acceptable, just as a certain number of normal appendixes will be operated on to ensure that no cases of appendicitis are missed.

CT scanning, when it follows arteriography, will diagnose as solid tumors many avascular cancers. Thus the combination has a diagnostic accuracy greater than arteriography alone. Currently it is logical to proceed from sonography to CT scanning directly.

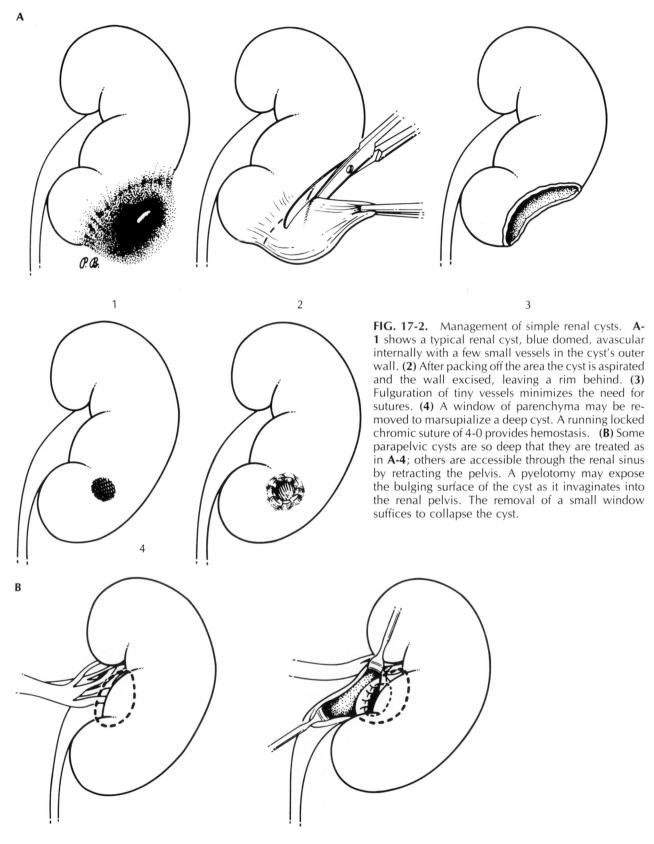

A

1

2

3

FIG. 17-2. Management of simple renal cysts. **A-1** shows a typical renal cyst, blue domed, avascular internally with a few small vessels in the cyst's outer wall. **(2)** After packing off the area the cyst is aspirated and the wall excised, leaving a rim behind. **(3)** Fulguration of tiny vessels minimizes the need for sutures. **(4)** A window of parenchyma may be removed to marsupialize a deep cyst. A running locked chromic suture of 4-0 provides hemostasis. **(B)** Some parapelvic cysts are so deep that they are treated as in **A-4**; others are accessible through the renal sinus by retracting the pelvis. A pyelotomy may expose the bulging surface of the cyst as it invaginates into the renal pelvis. The removal of a small window suffices to collapse the cyst.

4

B

1

2

Treatment

The treatment of renal cysts complicated by infection is surgical exploration, unroofing of the cyst, and drainage. When hemorrhage into a cyst has occurred, hemostatic suturing is required. If there is massive retroperitoneal and intrarenal hemorrhage associated with cyst rupture, then a rapid nephrectomy may be lifesaving and is indicated if the contralateral kidney functions satisfactorily.

Uncertainty over the diagnosis occasionally necessitates exploration.[2,24] A small subcostal incision is suitable for lower pole lesions, but an intercostal one is preferable for upper pole lesions. Either incision may be extended if tumor is encountered.

Most cysts present on the renal surface and typically have a blue dome with a margin of attenuated parenchyma (Fig. 17-2). Unroofing the cyst is accomplished by excising the thin blue dome and fulgurating the margins.[28] With deeper cuts the parenchymal margins may be thick enough to require a running chromic suture for hemostasis. The cyst should be inspected, and suspicious areas of the wall should be biopsied and frozen sections obtained. Occasionally a cyst with clear contents will have tumor within the wall, but this is rare.[2,24] Otherwise it is ill advised and unnecessary to remove the inner lining of the cyst. Care should be taken not to enter the collecting system, because such calix fistulas with no overlying parenchyma tend to drain for a long time. A bit of perinephric fat may be placed inside. A small drain may be removed in 48 hr if nonproductive.

Cysts deep within the substance of the kidney are not common but are difficult to localize and at surgery present an increased risk of bleeding because of the highly vascular parenchyma overlying the cyst. A deep cyst may not be visible but may be rendered more palpable by temporarily occluding the renal artery to soften the kidney. This maneuver assists in minimizing blood loss if parenchymal suturing is difficult, and is also helpful when dealing with a cyst into which hemorrhage has occurred.

One cannot be too careful in exposing "parapelvic" cysts, which often produce a compression-filling defect of the renal pelvis on urography, indicating their location within the renal hilum. Indeed, renal artery aneurysms have produced similar indenting deformities of the pelvis. Care must be taken to avoid injury to overlying renal vessels. Often the cyst is exposed by elevating the operculum of the renal parenchyma, which overlies cyst located within the renal sinus. The collecting system can generally be retracted from the cyst's surface, but occasionally the cyst is best exposed through a pyelotomy. Decompression is accomplished by safely excising a small window of the cyst wall once it has been adequately exposed. A simple cyst in a child may be very large.[13] Treatment is similar to that in an adult, but care must be taken to distinguish it from Wilms' tumor and to avoid vascular structures by creating the window away from the hilum.

MULTILOCULAR CYSTS

A multilocular renal cyst is a unilateral localized lesion composed of several noncommunicating cystic spaces separated by thin septa which contain no renal elements.[14,27] There is no communication with the collecting system. Internal echoes on sonography are a result of the septa. The precise septal structure is clearly seen on a CT scan. Osathanondh and Potter regarded multilocular cysts as variants of dysplasia;[25] Spence and Singleton considered them neoplastic.[33]

Multilocular cysts are uncommon: Emmett and associates reported only 2 multilocular cysts among 428 true cysts of the kidney.[8] Unlike simple cysts they are encountered fairly equally throughout all ages. In young adults they may be part of a hamartomatous lesion with smooth muscle in the stroma. There may be many tiny cysts at the periphery which, if not removed with the larger cysts, may grow and lead to recurrence of a large multicystic lesion.[10] Some multilocular cysts are large and cause the renal axis to be altered; when such a lesion is removed the remaining space may predispose to nephroptosis. In infancy and childhood the lesion may virtually replace the kidney, greatly enlarging it.[14] Distinguishing this lesion from Wilms' tumor is difficult, and nephrectomy is often required.[1,15] To complicate matters this lesion and Wilms' tumor have been reported to coexist.[29]

Treatment of those multilocular cysts reported in the literature has often been nephrectomy. This represents skewed incidence because the need for extensive replacement, although commonly reported, is actually less common than the involvement of a portion or pole of the kidney. The presentation varies from a cystic structure with internal septa and fairly well-defined peripheral margins to a conglomeration of cysts of varying sizes with many small cysts at the periphery. The latter are perhaps more realistically viewed as hamartomas, and a partial nephrectomy should include a wide margin; otherwise, the small peripheral cysts may grow and the patient may again present with a renal mass.[10] Intraoperative frozen section evaluation of such lesions, especially those with thick walls, occasionally shows a carcinoma involving the wall.[2] Appropriate treatment makes a second operation unnecessary in such cases (Fig. 17-3).

CYSTIC RENAL DYSPLASIA AND MULTICYSTIC KIDNEY

Cystic renal dysplasia includes a spectrum of renal disorders ranging from tiny cortical cysts to total replacement of the kidney by cystic clusters. It seems well established that obstruction during early gestation produces cystic dysplastic changes.[3] Obstruction during later gestation produces hydronephrosis. These latter obstructions are often partial, and may most commonly obstruct urethral valves. When the obstruction is partial but significant during both early and late gestation, one may see a combination of hydronephrosis and relatively minor cystic dysplasia in the form of multiple small cortical cysts.[22] Beck found that in sheep the pivotal gestation time was 80 days; obstructions occurring earlier than 80 days produced cystic change and obstructions occurring later than 80 days produced hydronephrosis.[3]

A practical clinical classification has been offered by Pathak and Williams, who divided multicystic and cystic dysplastic lesions into three categories: cystic changes associated with hydronephrosis, dysplasia with hypoplasia, and multicystic kidney.[26]

Diagnosis

Cystic changes associated with hydronephrosis appear as multiple cysts over the surface of a hydronephrotic kidney. Presumably there is obstruction in the early and late fetal period, with the former responsible for the cysts.

Dysplasia associated with hypoplasia is often associated with a degree of ureteral obstruction. Williams and Woodard noted that, in ectopic ureterocele, the obstruction involving the upper segment is associated with dysplastic changes varying from moderate to severe.[39] The lower segment may

reflux, but without obstruction there is no dysplastic change.

With total ureteral obstruction, also termed ureteral atresia, the kidney is completely cystic with virtually no functional elements.[26] It clinically presents as an abdominal mass in a child with nonfunction on excretory urography, and it must be distinguished from hydronephrosis and Wilms' tumor.[7] The mass transilluminates and is associated with an atretic ureter. Ultrasonography and CT scan studies show the mass to be a series of smooth-walled cysts filled with material of water density.

Treatment

The small peripheral cysts associated with hydronephrosis require no treatment. The degree of dysplasia must be considered in determining whether to preserve a partially obstructed renal unit or the upper segment of a duplex kidney obstructed by an ectopic ureterocele.[39] Biopsy and gross appearance indicate whether to reconstruct or to simply remove the segment.

With increasing precision in the diagnosis of multicystic kidney, it is questionable whether surgical intervention is justified except in unusual cases when the diagnosis is not clear or the mass is problematic because of its size. The cysts tend to acquire calcium in their walls with the passage of time. Flank pain or diagnostic considerations may lead to surgical removal in adult life, but these indications for late surgery occur so infrequently that it does not seem justified to routinely remove the kidneys in childhood.

Bilateral multicystic kidney, although rare, is followed by neonatal death. In unilateral cases it is important to evaluate the remainder of the urinary tract and to preserve the function of the remaining kidney.

ADULT POLYCYSTIC DISEASE

Polycystic renal disease is a hereditary familial disease transmitted by a dominant gene. It is characterized by the appearance and progressive enlargement of cysts throughout the parenchyma involving and replacing tissue in both the renal cortex and medulla.

The kidneys are not abnormal at birth. Cysts develop in adult life with considerable variation in the time of presentation and the rate of progression. The disease becomes manifest most commonly in the third or fourth decade of life. Although it is a bilateral disease, it may develop asymmetrically

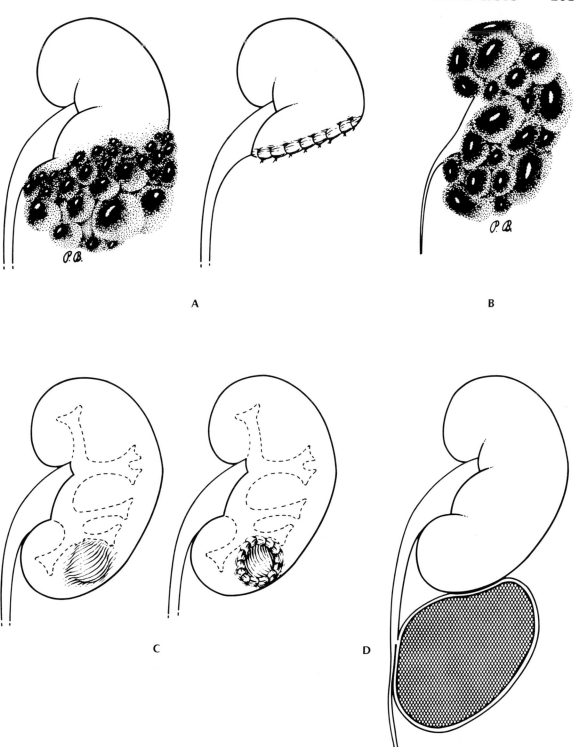

FIG. 17-3.   **(A)** Multilocular cyst is treated by partial nephrectomy.   **(B)** Multicystic kidney with ureteral atresia.   **(C)** Calyceal diverticulum. Marsupialization is accomplished similar to that of simple cyst.   **(D)** Pararenal pseudocyst. The capsule is entirely extrarenal, and the ureter is embedded in the fibrous capsule.

and thus present unilaterally. It is important to consider this condition and evaluate the opposite kidney when multiple cysts are found in one kidney in a middle-aged patient. More sophisticated studies such as arteriography and CT scanning often show cysts in the seemingly uninvolved kidney. With the passage of time the other kidney shows clinical evidence of cyst formation in true polycystic disease.

Diagnosis

Polycystic renal disease may come to light when physical examination reveals renal masses or radiographic studies of the abdomen reveal unsuspected renal enlargement. Routine medical evaluation may discover hypertension, proteinuria, hematuria, or decreased renal function. Flank pain may result from hemorrhage into a cyst, and such rapid expansion may lead to gross hematuria. More dramatically, the hectic sepsis of an abscess follows the infection of one or more cysts, usually secondary to urinary tract infection. The diagnosis is established by the characteristically large and deformed collecting systems in large kidneys.

Excretory urography alone is often diagnostic. In unclear cases a CT scan with contrast will firmly establish the diagnosis. Since the advent of the CT study, arteriography is rarely indicated and retrograde studies are unnecessary other than to evaluate associated obstruction from stones, clots, or other pathology.

Treatment

There is no effective treatment of the primary condition of polycystic renal disease. It is important to note that Rovsing's recommendation that multiple cysts be punctured to relieve compression of the remaining parenchyma has been shown by subsequent investigators and general experience not to improve renal function or to slow the rate of its deterioration.[11,21,30] Considering that surgery now is confined to treating complications, it is important that invasive procedures predisposing to complications be minimized. Polycystic kidneys are subject to the usual surgical kidney diseases; therefore, flank pain, hematuria, or fever must be evaluated. Calculi, ureteropelvic junction obstruction, and transitional cell carcinoma occurring in polycystic kidneys require surgery appropriate to the condition. Because the primary condition may progress to renal failure, it is important that associated pathology be diagnosed early and that treatment preserve as much renal function as possible.

Bleeding is common in polycystic disease, but it is occasionally due to a coexisting neoplasm. Arteriography should be considered when there is a significant index of suspicion of tumor. Well-defined tumors may be located by CT scan or arteriography, but atypical tumors may be obscured by parenchymal distortion due to the innumerable cysts of varying size and the presence of hemorrhage in some cysts.

The most difficult problem to deal with is that of one or more infected cysts.[37] The clinical course is the same as that for abscess. Antibiotics do not penetrate well into cyst fluid, and the patient may be seriously septic. Cyst drainage is the treatment, but finding the cyst which is infected is very difficult. A CT scan may show gas formation. It is important to preserve parenchyma by providing drainage, but when multiple cysts are infected nephrectomy may be required as a lifesaving procedure. A very extended subcostal incision reaching to the lower abdomen may be required, because these kidneys can be the size of watermelons. A long midline incision is an alternative and is preferred when bilateral nephrectomy is carried out prior to transplantation. Bilateral nephrectomy is often recommended prior to administering immunosuppressive agents because of the risk of an uncontrolled infection in these cysts following transplantation. Removal of at least one polycystic kidney is often required merely to make room for a transplant.

Pseudocysts

Cystadenoma, cystadenocarcinoma, and cystic degeneration of renal cell carcinomas are more properly discussed in the chapters dealing with renal tumors. It is important to point out here that lesions appearing cystic may in fact be tumors.[2,7,24] Such lesions may be avascular on angiography. Cystadenocarcinomas may have cystic portions containing clear fluid. Occasionally renal cell carcinoma is found in the wall of a cyst containing clear fluid;[7] this is a different and less common problem than cystic degeneration within a tumor. Percutaneous aspiration may be misleading in these lesions. CT scan studies are most helpful, and surgery may be required to discriminate these lesions.[2,35]

CALICEAL DIVERTICULA

Caliceal diverticula are cystlike in that they are filled with fluid and expand within the renal parenchyma. Unlike other cysts, they communicate with the collecting system and their lining is transitional cell. This latter point of differentiation is important when the communication is sealed by inspissated debris, stones, or scar tissue. Some diverticula, which are large, solitary, and not associated with obstruction, are probably congenital. There is good evidence that others are acquired, either representing the remains of a parenchymal abscess that drained into a calix or the result of a calculus forming within a papilla and eroding into the collecting system. With passage of the calculus into the collecting system, the original site remains as a diverticulum.

Obstruction of the ostium leads to enlargement and poor drainage of the diverticulum. Not surprisingly, these diverticula are commonly infected and filled with debris or milk of calcium stones which may appear in the urine as sand.[5] Smaller diverticula usually fill on excretory urography, but the larger ones, which are of surgical significance, often do not because of the small ostium. Retrograde pyelography may fill the diverticula but we have seen this fail too.

Small diverticula rarely require surgery, but large ones complicated by intractable infection and stones require surgical drainage and marsupialization.[5] Perinephric fat may be used to fill the space. Rarely is the ostium to the collecting system visible at surgery, and it is not necessary to deal with it then. As with the unroofing procedure for a cyst, care must be taken not to enter the collecting system inadvertently. If such openings are not properly closed, they may drain for a prolonged period because there is essentially no parenchyma to seal the leak.

HYDROCALYX

Obstruction of an infundibulum may lead to a cystlike dilatation of the calix supplied by it. This is an uncommon lesion and not likely to be confused with true cysts or the other pseudocysts. The upper pole calix is most often involved. In children the caliceal expansion may be so great as to produce an abdominal mass.[38] Partial nephrectomy is appropriate because little functioning tissue surrounds the expanded calix. A lesion of lesser degree has been described in adults, with intermittent pain being the presenting symptom. Infundibuloplasty has been recommended in these cases.[9]

It is important to distinguish significant obstruction from a mild form, seen more frequently, in which the vascular pedicle compresses the upper pole infundibulum. We believe that a surgically significant lesion in the adult patient is rather rare.

PARASITIC CYSTS

The only truly significant parasitic lesion that involves the kidney is the cystic disease associated with echinococcal infestation. Although rare in the continental United States, except Alaska, it is still observed with some frequency in other areas of the world, notably Australia and the Middle East. As the world's population travels more, the likelihood increases that physicians will encounter this disease. It is important that it not be mismanaged, because the results of mismanagement may be disastrous.

Silber and Mayad described three forms of the disease: (1) a benign sylvatic form of *Echinococcus granulosus* endemic to Alaska in which the renal lesion is a calcified unilocular cyst, (2) a pastoral form of *E. granulosus* in which the cystic lesion expands more rapidly and carries the risk of rupture, and (3) a less common *E. multilocularis* form that is invasive and has a high mortality rate.[32]

The disease is often asymptomatic but may cause flank pain. Laboratory findings include eosinophilia in about one half of the patients and occasionally daughter cysts in the urine. The Casoni test is meaningful when positive but is often negative, especially in the sylvatic form of the disease. The plain abdominal radiograph shows one or more calcified cystic masses. The kidney is often nonfunctioning on excretory urography.

Care must be taken to avoid spillage of cyst contents, because the daughter cysts will implant in the surgical bed. It is better to avoid surgery in nonprogressive cases in which the cyst walls are calcified and spontaneous rupture is unlikely than to risk seeding the wound. For this reason, and because the kidney often functions poorly, nephrectomy is preferred to a parenchyma-sparing procedure such as partial nephrectomy or cyst drainage.

Other Cystic Diseases

Medullary sponge kidney in its mild form is characterized by a blush of contrast in each papilla on excretory urography. The prominence of this blush is related to how dilated the collecting ducts are. The cysts, dilated distal collecting ducts, are small, as are the calculi that may develop. The calculi rarely enter the collecting system to cause obstruction. For these reasons neither the cysts nor the stones are commonly surgical problems. Occasionally, when they are associated with chronic infection and the stones are sufficiently localized, partial nephrectomy or papillectomy may be justified.

Medullary cystic disease and infantile polycystic renal disease are not surgical problems. The former may lead to renal failure at an age when dialysis or transplantation is feasible, and bilateral nephrectomy may be required if there is associated chronic infection or hypertension.

Pararenal Pseudocysts

A pararenal pseudocyst is formed when a sizable amount of extravasated urine becomes encapsulated.[31] It is usually intimately related to the site of urinary extravasation that formed it. Penetrating or nonpenetrating trauma may produce parenchymal fracture or perforation of the renal pelvis or ureter, resulting in extravasation.

Occasionally distal ureteral obstruction with a calculus may result in extravasation from thinned areas of the caliceal fornices. Inadequate drainage following surgery involving the opening of any portion of the upper urinary tract or removal of the drain before urinary leakage has permanently ceased may lead to an iatrogenic pseudocyst. Unrecognized ureteral perforation with a ureteral catheter or stone basket may also be followed by urinary extravasation. Early diagnosis and prompt drainage usually lead to complete recovery, but delayed treatment is associated with significant complications. In particular, those pseudocysts associated with the ureter develop associated obstruction, and careful ureterolysis and repair are required.

Because of the proximity of the tail of the pancreas to the left kidney, a pancreatic pseudocyst may compress and displace the kidney.[19] The possibility of pancreatic origin must be kept in mind and strongly considered when there is no associated renal or ureteral pathology. We have observed one pancreatic pseudocyst that was perinephric following blunt trauma to the left upper abdomen in a child. A brown discoloration to the cyst wall provided a clue to the origin. Clearly pararenal pseudocysts are a heterogeneous group, and management must be individualized. Delayed diagnosis and associated ureteral obstruction due to encasement with fibrous tissue increase the complexity and the likelihood of significant hydronephrosis. The degree of renal damage at the time of diagnosis and the ability to correct obstruction determine the outcome.

REFERENCES

1. AKHTAR M, QADEER A: Multilocular cyst of kidney with embryonic tissue. Urology 16:90, 1980

2. AMBROSE SS, LEWIS EL, O'BRIEN DP et al: Unsuspected renal tumors associated with renal cysts. J Urol 117:704, 1977

3. BECK AD: The effect of intra-uterine urinary obstruction upon the development of the fetal kidney. J Urol 105:784, 1971

4. BRAASCH WF, HENDRICK JA: Renal cysts, simple and otherwise. J Urol 51:1, 1944

5. BURNETT BB: Multiple renal calculi within non-communicating pyelogenic renal cyst. Urology 16:496, 1980

6. CANNON AH, ZANON B, KARRAS BG: Cystic calcification in the kidney; its occurrence in malignant renal tumors. Am J Roentgenol 84:837, 1960

7. DEKLERK DP, MARSHALL FF, JEFFS RD: Multicystic dysplastic kidney. J Urol 118:306, 1977

8. EMMETT JL, LEVINE SR, WOOLNER LB: Co-existence of renal cyst and tumor: Incidence in 1007 cases. Br J Urol 35:403, 1965

9. FRALEY EE: Surgical correction of intra-renal disease: Obstructions of the superior infundibulum. J Urol 98:54, 1967

10. GELLER RA, PATAKI KI, FINEGOLD RA: Bilateral multilocular renal cysts with recurrence. J Urol 121:808, 1979

11. GOLDSTEIN AE: A new procedure for treatment of polycystic kidneys. J Urol 34:536, 1935

12. HOARD TD, O'BRIEN DP: Simple renal cyst and high renin hypertension cured by cyst decompression. J Urol 115:326, 1976

13. HOLL WH, DELPORTO GB, KEEGAN GT et al: Simple renal cyst in child. J Urol 115:465, 1976

14. JOHNSON DE, AYALA AG, MEDELLIN H et al: Multilocular renal cystic disease in children. J Urol 109:101, 1973

15. KEEGAN GT, PETERSON RF, STUCKI WJ et al: Cystic partially differentiated nephroblastoma (Wilms' tumor). J Urol 121:362, 1979

16. KROPP KA, GRAYHACK JT, WENDELL RM et al: Morbidity and mortality of renal exploration for cyst. Surg Gnyecol Obstet 125:803, 1967

17. LANG EK: The differential diagnosos of renal cysts and tumors. Radiology 87:883, 1966

18. LANG EK: The Roentgenographic Diagnosis of Renal Mass Lesions. St Louis, Green, 1971

19. LILIENFELD RM, LANDE A: Pancreatic pseudocysts presenting as thick-walled renal and perinephric cysts. J Urol 115:123, 1976

20. LINGARD DA, LAWSON TL: Accuracy of ultrasound in predicting the nature of renal masses. J Urol 122:724, 1979

21. MILAM JH, MAGEE JH, BURUNTS RC: Evaluation of surgical decompression of polycystic kidneys by differential renal clearances. J Urol 90:144, 1963

22. MILLIKEN LD, JR, HODGSON NB: Renal dysplasia and urethral valves. J Urol 108:960, 1972

23. MURPHY GP, MIRAND EA, JOHNSTON GS et al: Erythropoietin alterations in human genitourinary disease states: Correlation with experimental observations. J Urol 99:802, 1968

24. MURPHY JB, MARSHALL FF: Renal cyst versus tumor: A continuing dilemma. J Urol 123:566, 1980

25. OSATHANONDH V, POTTER EL: Pathogenesis of polycystic kidneys. Arch Pathol 77:459, 1964

26. PATHAK IG, WILLIAMS DI: Multicystic and cystic dysplastic kidneys. Br J Urol 36:318, 1964

27. POWELL T, SHACKMAN R, JOHNSON HD: Multilocular cysts of the kidney. Br J Urol 23:142, 1951

28. PRATHER GC: Surgical treatment of serous cyst of the kidney. J Urol 77:14, 1957

29. REDMAN JF, HARPER DL: Nephroblastoma occurring in a multilocular cystic kidney. J Urol 120:356, 1978

30. ROVSING T: Treatment of the multilocular renal cyst with multiple punctures. Hospitalstid 4:105, 1911

31. SAULS CL, NESBIT RM: Pararenal pseudocysts: A report of four cases. J Urol 87:288, 1962

32. SILBER SJ, MAYAD RA: Renal echinococcus. J Urol 108:669, 1972

33. SPENCE HM, SINGLETON R: Cysts and cystic disorders of the kidney: Types, diagnosis, treatment. Urol Survey 22:131, 1972

34. SPIRES MS, GAEDE JT, GLENN JF: Death from renal cyst. Urology 16:606, 1980

35. STEWARD BH, JAMES R, HAAGA J et al: Urological applications of computerized axial tomography: A preliminary report. J Urol 120:198, 1978

36. WAHLQUIST L, GRUMSTEDT B: therapeutic effect of percutaneous puncture of simple renal cyst: Follow-up investigation of 50 patients. Acta Chir Scand 132:340, 1966

37. WATERS WB, HERSHMAN H, KLEIN LA: Management of infected polycystic kidneys. J Urol 122:383, 1979

38. WILLIAMS DI, MININBERG DT: Hydrocalycosis: Report of three cases in children. Br J Urol 40:541, 1968

39. WILLIAMS DI, WOODARD JR: Problems in the management of ectopic ureteroceles. J Urol 92:635, 1964

Renal Carbuncle and Perinephric Abscess

18

Culley C. Carson III

Abscess formation in the kidney and its surrounding tissues has been uncommon since the advent of effective antibiotics. Abscesses are most likely to occur in young adults and are rare in childhood. Gram-negative abscesses are usually associated with ascending infection; those due to gram-positive organisms are most commonly hematogenously seeded. In all cases, diagnosis is by physical examination, urine culture, and urography. Appropriate therapy is, as with all purulent collections, complete surgical drainage.

Anatomy

The understanding of anatomic relationships in the retroperitoneum and kidney is an integral part of the appropriate treatment of renal and perinephric infections. To better understand these relationships, surrounding anatomic landmarks must be familiar to the operating surgeon. The renal fossa is formed by the quadratus lumborum muscle posteriorly, the psoas muscle medially, the muscular layers of the abdomen laterally, and the posterior parietal peritoneum anteriorly (Fig. 18-1). Superiorly, the adrenal glands and diaphragm provide a roof for the fossa. The extension of the pleura to the 12th rib, where the diaphragm inserts, is important in abscess drainage because high incisions in these drainage procedures risk pleural entry and contamination of the chest cavity.

The renal parenchyma is surrounded by a thin, fibrous, true capsule. Renal capillary vessels penetrate this capsule, which is loosely adherent to the renal surface. Surrounding the kidney itself is a lemon yellow layer of perirenal fat which is thickest posteriorly and laterally. This adipose tissue is contained within the anterior and posterior layers of renal fascia known as Gerota's fascia. Superiority, the anterior and posterior leaves of this renal fascia fuse above the adrenal gland, becoming continuous with the diaphragmatic fascia.[8] A thinner, more variable layer meets between the adrenal gland and the kidney. Laterally, the fascial layers join to form the lateroconal fascia,

which becomes continuous with the posterior parietal peritoneum. Between the posterior renal fascia and the transversalis fascia is the pararenal fat, a thinner, paler-colored adipose layer which fills much of the retroperitoneal space.

Medially, the renal fascia has no continuity between its anterior and posterior leaves.[1] The posterior layer fuses with the psoas muscle fascia, and the anterior layer of the renal fascia disappears into the connective tissue surrounding the great vessels and organs of the anterior retroperitoneum (*i.e.,* the pancreas, duodenum, and colon). Thus, the fascial envelopes surrounding each kidney do not usually have any established communication across midline.

The inferior extension of the renal fascia is quite important in understanding the behavior of perirenal infections. The renal fascial layers do not close inferiorly, but rather become continuous with the psoas and ureteral coverings.[1,8] This opening inferiorly allows spread of retroperitoneal infections to the pelvis, to the psoas muscle, and, in some cases, to the contralateral retroperitoneum (Fig. 18-2).

Abscess location is variable and is determined by the etiology and associated pathology. Paranephric abscesses are located in the adipose tissue outside Gerota's fascia and are generally the result of blood-borne staphylococci from skin or bone. Occasionally gram-negative organisms may cause these infections as a result of generalized bacteremia. Drainage of the abscesses without disturbing the renal fascia is essential in preventing perinephric spread and possible renal damage (Fig. 18-3).

Abscesses resulting from primary renal infection usually begin by retrograde infection of the renal parenchyma with subsequent microabscess formation. These abscesses have a predilection for the corticomedullary region and may drain spontaneously through the renal collecting system. When formed from hematogenous spread, these collections are called carbuncles and may resolve with aggressive antibiotic therapy if treated prior

207

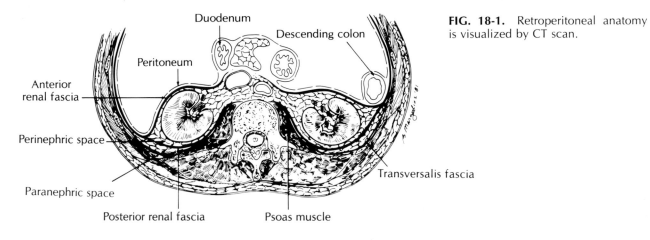

Duodenum

Descending colon

Peritoneum

Anterior
renal fascia

Perinephric space

Paranephric space

Posterior renal fascia

Psoas muscle

Transversalis fascia

FIG. 18-1. Retroperitoneal anatomy
is visualized by CT scan.

FIG. 18-2. Retroperitoneal anatomy and relationships are
shown in sagittal section.

FIG. 18-3. Illustration gives names and locations of abscesses associated with the kidney.

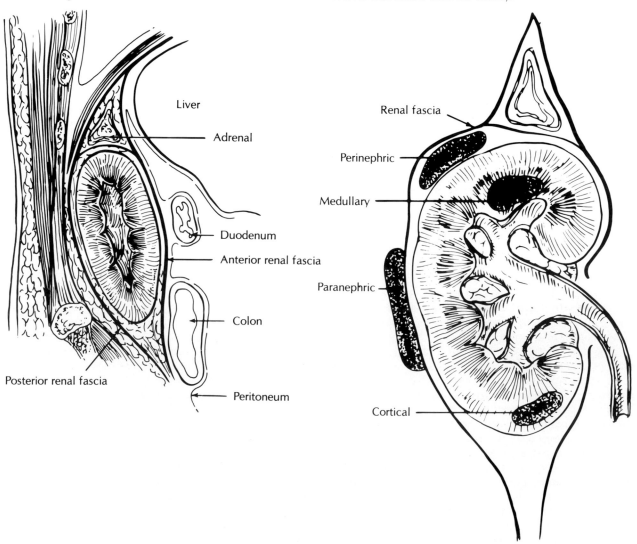

Liver

Adrenal

Duodenum

Anterior renal fascia

Colon

Posterior renal fascia

Peritoneum

Renal fascia

Perinephric

Medullary

Paranephric

Cortical

to frank suppuration. Once an abscess has formed, the extension of bacteria and suppuration through the renal capsule into the perirenal space forms a perinephric abscess. Occasionally, there is no preceding renal abscess, but instead bacteria extend through the renal capsule during severe pyelonephritis. In most cases, however, preceding renal damage is present.

Surgical Treatment of Retroperitoneal Abscess

DRAINAGE

Once the diagnosis and location of a renal or perinephric abscess has been established, appropriate surgical therapy should be undertaken immediately. The basic approach for surgical treatment of any abscess is incision and drainage of the localized collection of pus. Complete decompression of the purulent area and evacuation of all debris is essential to this approach.

If urine and blood culture information is available prior to surgery, an appropriate preoperative antibiotic choice may be made. In all cases, however, premedication with intravenous, broad-spectrum antibiotics is essential before and during drainage procedures to achieve antibiotic blood levels adequate to eradicate associated bacteremia.[9] The best choice for these agents is based on knowledge of the probable etiologic agent and underlying renal pathology. In most cases, however, coverage of gram-negative bacilli and beta-lactamase–producing gram-positive cocci is effective. An aminoglycoside and a beta-lactamase–resistant cephalosporin is a good combination for these patients. Coverage of anaerobic bacteria is also desirable, especially if gastrointestinal communication or spillage is suspected as the cause of abscess formation. The addition of clindamycin or cefoxitin to the antibiotic program is essential in these cases.

As with any surgical procedure, abscess drainage should be performed under controlled, sterile conditions in order to avoid the introduction of additional bacterial species into the wound. While needle aspiration under ultrasound or computed tomographic control may aid in the diagnosis of an abscess in cases of diagnostic dilemma, percutaneous abscess drainage is inadequate for definitive therapy.

Because transabdominal exploration risks intraperitoneal contamination and a high flank incision risks intrapleural spread, the patient is placed in a full flank position and a 10-cm to 12-cm posterolumbar incision is made below the 12th rib. The oblique muscles of the abdominal wall are separated in the direction of their fibers and the retroperitoneum is entered. The tissues surrounding the abscess are frequently edematous and indurated, but palpation of the abscess is usually possible. If the exact position is in doubt, needle aspiration will confirm the location of the cavity.

After the abscess has been opened, samples should be obtained for both anaerobic and aerobic cultures. Simultaneously, a Gram stain can be obtained for immediate information about the causative organism. Thorough digital exploration of the abscess cavity must be performed to completely eliminate all loculations and remote abscess cavities. Biopsy of areas of the wall of the abscess cavity should be encouraged; we have encountered several abscesses associated with malignancy.

Copious saline irrigation of the cavity an entire wound is essential following drainage. Additional irrigation with 1% neomycin solution is also desirable. Several large Penrose drains are carefully inserted into all areas of the cavity and brought to the skin through a separate stab wound in the lateral abdominal wall in such a way that dependent drainage is ensured. The ends of the drains should be sutured to the skin and tagged with a large sterile safety pin. Fascial and muscular closure may be performed with chromic catgut suture, but skin and subcutaneous tissue are left open to prevent the formation of a secondary body wall abscess. This wound can be left to heal from within, or skin sutures may be placed and left untied for dermal approximation 5 to 7 days postoperatively, once drainage has ceased. I prefer loosely packing these open wounds with iodophor gauze and changing the packs daily. The Penrose drains are left in place until purulent drainage has decreased. Drains are then advanced slowly over several days until completely removed. Documentation of each drain removed in the hospital chart is essential. Continued, prolonged purulent drainage may indicate a retained foreign body, renal calculus, fistulous tract, or persistent abscess cavity and should be thoroughly evaluated before removal of the Penrose drains.

Drainage of a perinephric abscess should usually be done as a primary procedure, with nephrectomy performed at a later date if necessary. Patients are frequently septic and too ill for prolonged general anesthesia and surgical manipulation. At Duke University Medical Center the mortality rate for primary nephrectomy with perinephric abscess drainage is fivefold higher than that for drainage

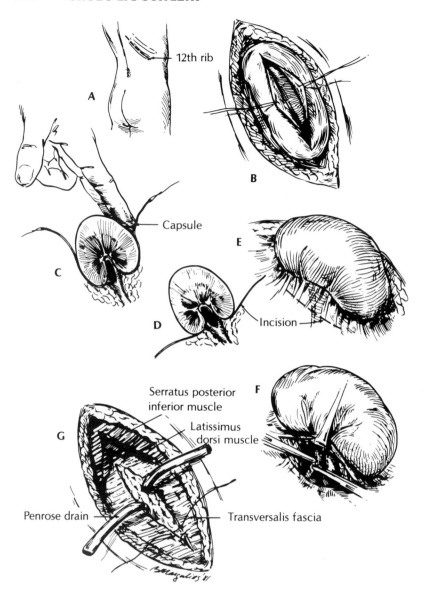

FIG. 18-4. Subcapsular nephrectomy by twelfth rib flank approach: **(A)** twelfth-rib incision; **(B)** lateral renal border exposed and renal capsule incised; **(C)** subcapsular dissection; **(D)** level of transcapsular incision; **(E)** incision exposes hilar structures; **(F)** vessels are clamped and tied; **(G)** closure is performed around multiple Penrose drains.

alone.[3] Furthermore, with removal of obstruction and abscess drainage combined with an appropriate antibiotic regimen, some kidneys will again begin to function and can be salvaged.[7] If secondary nephrectomy is unavoidable, the subcapsular technique is usually imperative because of extreme perinephric reaction and adhesion formation.

SUBCAPSULAR NEPHRECTOMY

After a retroperitoneal infection and abscess, the kidney is frequently densely adherent to the perinephric fat and fascia, and dissection of the kidney from its bed is impossible. In this event, nephrectomy by the subcapsular technique is preferred.

This technique is inadequate, however, for patients with renal malignancy or tuberculosis.

A classic flank approach is used for best exposure with an incision through the bed of the 11th or 12th ribs (Fig. 18-4). A subcostal approach is usually too low for adequate exposure because the mobility of these kidneys is minimal. As with abscess drainage, pleural entry should be avoided to maintain sterility of the pleural cavity. Sharp dissection is frequently necessary to reach the kidney, but once its lateral border is identified, the renal capsule is incised sharply (Fig. 18-4B). The capsule is bluntly freed from the renal parenchyma to the hilum, and the kidney is delivered into the wound. This natural cleavage plane greatly facilitates dissection. The decapsulated kidney is now free, but the renal pedicle is shrouded by the reflected renal capsule (Fig. 18 1E). An incision is carefully created in the capsule at the renal hilum anteriorly to expose the renal vessels. Hilar reaction may prevent isolation of each vessel and its individual ligation. The pedicle, once exposed, can be claimed and suture ligated in the renal hilum with only minimal dissection. Heavy chromic catgut ligatures of doubled No. 1 suture can be applied prior to specimen removal if individual vessel ligation is impossible. The kidney is delivered into the wound, and the ureter is identified and traced distally as far as possible, ligated with a 2-0 chromic catgut ligature, and excised.

In difficult cases, morcellation may be required to remove the kidney prior to pedicle ligation. In all cases, the remaining perinephric tissue may produce a persistent draining sinus. This drainage can be avoided by wide excision of reactive perirenal tissue after nephrectomy. Closure is as described for abscess drainage with multiple Penrose drains, chromic catgut fascial closure, and subcutaneous iodophor wound packing. Delayed reaproximation of the wound edges is also desirable. With carefully placed drains, meticulous attention to wound care, and appropriate perioperative antibiotics, postabscess nephrectomy can be a safe, effective procedure.

TREATMENT OF TUBERCULOUS ABSCESSES

Renal involvement by blood-borne tuberculosis is bilateral initially and usually resolves with medical therapy. If healing of the glomerular lesion does not occur, caseation necrosis may ensue with formation of a renal parenchymal abscess. These abscesses usually form in the renal poles in calices which have been isolated from the renal collecting system by severe infundibular scarring.[2] If segmental renal damage is obvious and salvage of the kidney is possible, a drainage procedure or cavernotomy can be performed.[5] This is a safe, conservative method to save a maximum of renal parenchyma. Any surgical procedure performed on patients with active or possibly active tuberculosis requires a minimum of 3 weeks of triple antituberculous drug therapy.[10] The use of 300 mg/day of isoniazid (INH) with 100 mg/day of pyridoxine, 600 mg/day of rifampin, and 1200 mg/day of ethambutol is recommended. Gow has used only INH and rifampin with equally good results.[4]

After exposure through the flank, the kidney is mobilized and the area of tuberculous abscess is identified. To minimize wound contamination and tuberculous spread, thorough needle aspiration of purulent material and saline lavage of the abscess cavity should be performed using a large bore needle and syringe. The roof of the cavity is then excised and its interior completely examined. Any connection with the renal pelvis by an open infundibulum must be closed using 5-0 chromic catgut to prevent fistula or urinoma formation. The roof of the calix is resected and its edges oversewn with a running suture of 3-0 chromic catgut. Closure with multiple drains after thorough wound irrigation is then undertaken. Drains are managed as previously described for perinephric abscess.

In cases of unilateral tuberculous with massive parenchymal destruction or nonfunction, a partial or total nephrectomy should be performed. Simple and partial nephrectomy are described in Chapters 5 and 6, respectively. In cases of total nephrectomy, management of the ureteral remnant differs from routine nephrectomy procedures. Because pyoureter or psoas abscess may follow ureteral transection, the ureter should only be transected while securely cross clamped. The residual ureteral stump should be brought out to the skin to ensure adequate drainage. In these cases, subsequent ureteral stump removal may be necessary. Wechsler and Lattimer state that if nephrectomy is associated with severe tuberculous cystitis, ureteral catheterization for 7 days postoperatively to minimize subsequent ureteral stump abscess formation should accompany the primary nephrectomy.[10]

TREATMENT OF ECHINOCOCCOSIS

Echinococcal or hydatid cysts are formed in humans from exposure to the canine tapeworm *Echinococcus granulosus*. Hydatid cysts occur in the kidney in less than 5% of the patients who develop cysts. These cysts develop from the larval form of the parasite and are most common in sheep-raising areas such as Greece, Lebanon, and Australia. The cysts are usually slow growing, increasing 2 to 3 cm/yr. Symptoms, if present, are due to compression of the host organ or adjacent organs by an enlarging mass. Diagnosis is by excretory urogram revealing single or multiple cystic masses lined usually by peripheral calcification. Diagnosis is best made by indirect hemagglutination and serum latex antibody determinations. Diagnostic needle puncture is associated with a significant risk of anaphylaxis due to leakage of toxic cyst contents.[6] Cyst removal is indicated when an enlarging cyst threatens kidney function or produces obstruction.

Surgical treatment of hydatid cysts is best accomplished by total removal of the intact cyst. This may involve partial or simple nephrectomy if large amounts of renal tissue have been damaged. In some cases, when cyst removal is impossible owing to size and adjacent organ involvement, careful opening of the cyst after complete aspiration of cyst contents may be considered. Sterilization of cyst contents with 2% formalin, hypertonic solutions of 30% sodium chloride, or 1% iodine prior to marsupialization aids in the prevention of anaphylaxis and systemic effects of cyst contents contacting surrounding tissue.[6] Complete evacuation of all hydatid tissue and thorough postmarsupialization irrigation is critical in preventing these systemic effects. Penrose drains are left in the cyst cavity until drainage ceases.

REFERENCES

1. AMIN M, BLANDFORD AT, POLK HC: Renal fascia of Gerota. Urology 7:1, 1976

2. BRUCE AW, ARWAD SA, CHALLIS TW: The recognition and treatment of tuberculous pyocalyx of the kidney. J Urol 101:127, 1969

3. GONZALES-SERVA L, WEINERTH JL, GLENN JF: Minimal mortality of renal surgery. Urology 9:253, 1977

4. GOW JG: The surgery of genitourinary tuberculosis. Br J Surg 53:210, 1966

5. HANLEY HG: Cavernotomy and partial nephrectomy in renal tuberculosis. Br J Urol 42:661, 1970

6. KIRKLAND K: Urologic aspects of hydatid disease. Br J Urol 38:241, 1966

7. MALIGIERI JJ, KURSH ED, PERSLEY L: The changing clinicopathologic pattern of abscesses in or adjacent to the kidney. J Urol 118:230, 1977

8. MITCHELL GAG: The renal fascia. Br J Surg 37:257, 1950

9. THOMLEY JD, JONES SR, SANFORD JP: Perinephric abscess. Medicine 53:441, 1974

10. WECHSLER M, LATTIMER JK: An evaluation of the current therapeutic regimen for renal tuberculosis. J Urol 113:760, 1975

Nephrostomy

19

Geoffrey D. Chisholm

Attitudes toward nephrostomy vary: it is common in some countries, rare in others. The question of indications for the procedure often leads to much debate, especially over those patients with obstructive uropathy due to advanced malignant disease. Improvements in techniques of radiotherapy, chemotherapy, and even surgical procedures have all resulted in a more positive approach to the patient with obstructive uremia, and relief of the obstruction is only part of the program of management.

A nephrostomy as a permanent procedure is uncommon and is rarely done with enthusiasm. Usually either the patient is too ill for a definitive procedure or the underlying pathology precludes other surgical procedures that would allow the normal passage of urine to the urethra. Fortunately, the technique of percutaneous nephrostomy has now given the urologist a relatively straightforward method for the emergency drainage of the upper urinary tract (see Chap. 20); this technique has almost entirely replaced the more traditional formal nephrostomy. The advantage of a percutaneous nephrostomy is not only that it spares the patient from an operative procedure but also that radiologic and functional investigations can be carried out as soon as the drainage is established.

Types of Formal Nephrostomy

There are three types of formal nephrostomy: peroperative nephrostomy, temporary nephrostomy, and permanent nephrostomy.

PEROPERATIVE NEPHROSTOMY

It is not possible to list the indications for peroperative nephrostomy, because most are relative and depend on the surgeon's judgement of the need for this type of temporary drainage. Some surgeons believe that a nephrostomy reduces the incidence of immediate postoperative complications such as a urinary leak, wound infection, and hemorrhage, and they will use a nephrostomy in most renal operations. Other surgeons are more selective and reserve a nephrostomy for those situations in which there has been a difficult operative procedure and the tissues are less healthy.

Pyeloplasty

A common example of the differing attitudes toward peroperative nephrostomy is found in the use of tubes or stents for a pyeloplasty. Rickwood and Phadke studied the postoperative course in a series of children who underwent a pyeloplasty. They compared pyeloplasty (de Pezzer catheter) drainage with tissue drainage only and concluded that there were fewer complications in the latter group.[7]

Anderson did not drain the renal pelvis or use a transanastomotic splint for his pyeloplasty, because he believed that encouraging urine to pass through the anastomosis was the best way to keep the anastomosis patent.[1]

The techniques for pyeloplasty are discussed in Chapter 21. In general, when the reconstruction has been carried out with a technique that aims to be watertight, a peroperative nephrostomy is unnecessary. If, however, the anastomosis is not secure or the state of the tissues prevents a confident reconstruction, then either a simple nephrostomy or a transanastomotic stent/nephrostomy (Cummings tube) may be used. A wound drain is also placed and then removed after 3 days. A nephrostogram is carried out on approximately the sixth postoperative day. If there is free drainage down the ureter and no leakage, the nephrostomy tube is usually removed on the seventh or eighth postoperative day, but it may be left for at least another week if there is any doubt about the healing of the reconstruction.

Stone Surgery

A simple pyelolithotomy requires only a temporary wound drain through a separate stab incision. However, a combined pyelolithotomy and multiple nephrolithotomy will heal more rapidly and reliably if nephrostomy drainage is established as part of the operative procedure. Occasionally, as with a reexploration for recurrent stones, the pelvis may be scarred and the tissues so poor that reconstruction of the pelvis and ureter is difficult. In this situation a stent/nephrostomy of the Cummings type is of considerable advantage. The sequence of removal of the drain and the nephrostomy tube is the same as for a pyeloplasty.

Upper Urinary Tract Reconstruction

Reconstructive procedures such as ileal replacement of the ureter or calicoureterostomy are best drained by a nephrostomy or splinting tube as well as a separate wound drain. It is particularly im-

FIG. 19-1. Nephrostomy forceps (Martin)

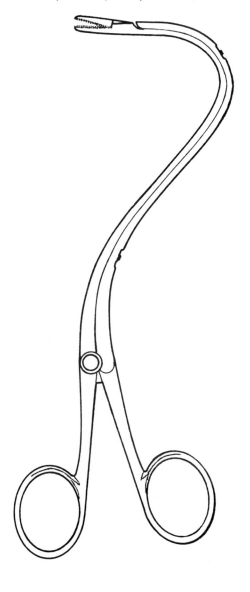

portant to be able to monitor the urine output if the patient has some degree of renal failure. The removal of the tubes and drains should again follow an orderly sequence, in which the wound drains are removed and the wounds are healed before the nephrostomy tube is removed.

TEMPORARY NEPHROSTOMY

A temporary nephrostomy is one that is carried out not as part of another operative procedure but specifically to allow drainage of the kidney for a limited period. A percutaneous nephrostomy can fulfill these requirements, but if the drainage is required for more than approximately 1 week, formal nephrostomy drainage may be preferred.

The use of a temporary nephrostomy implies that the clinician requires free urine drainage while the kidney recovers and often while other treatment is given to the patient. It also implies that the patient is not fit enough for other definitive surgical procedures or that the temporary delay is being used to assess other aspects of the patient's medical problem. Sometimes the progress of the patient does not fulfill expectations and the nephrostomy becomes permanent.

It is important to recognize that a nephrostomy is not a form of urinary diversion. If the purpose of the procedure is to keep urine away from the lower urinary tract (*e.g.,* in trauma, sepsis, or malignant fistula), then a nephrostomy is the wrong procedure and a ureterostomy (see Chap. 48) or ileal diversion (see Chap. 49) is necessary. A ureterostomy *in situ,* described by Walsh in 1967, is not a good choice, because urine can leak around the tube and down to the bladder.[10]

The indications for a temporary nephrostomy are therefore mainly to allow recovery of renal function prior to a definitive operative procedure. The so-called salvaging of such a patient usually applies to a person with pelvic malignancy. For example, a transitional cell carcinoma of the bladder may involve both ureters and cause uremia; a possible course of management begins with nephrostomy drainage, then provides radiotherapy to the tumor, with subsequent cystectomy and ileal diversion of urine.

The subject of temporary urinary drainage in malignant disease cannot be fully presented in this chapter, and the reader is directed to some of the published reports on this difficult urologic and even ethical problem.[2,4,5,9] There is consensus that nephrostomy drainage should be strongly considered when malignant disease was previously undiagnosed and therefore untreated. Alternative

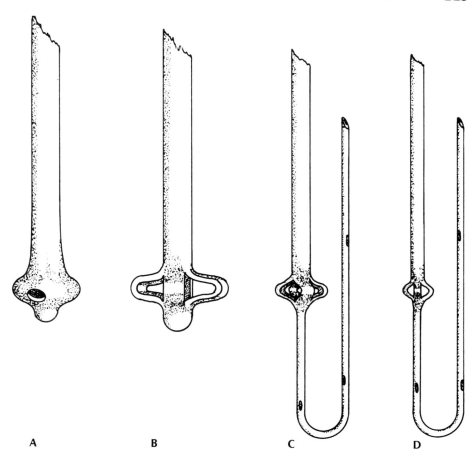

FIG. 19-2. Nephrostomy catheters: **(A)** Malecot, **(B)** de Pezzer, **(C)** Cummings tube, **(D)** Gil-Vernet modification of Cummings tube

A   B   C   D

techniques for relieving obstruction use silicone rubber stents of the type devised by Gibbons, Mason, and Correa.[6]

PERMANENT NEPHROSTOMY

Irreparable damage to the ureters is not an absolute indication for a permanent nephrostomy, but it may be concluded that this is the best form of treatment for a patient when all other factors, including the state of the patient and the state of the lower urinary tract, are taken into account. Before reaching this decision, the possibility of an ileal replacement of the ureter or a ureterointestinal conduit should be considered. It should not be forgotten that the contralateral ureter may be available to provide a "spare" ureter for a ureteroureterostomy (see Chap. 39).

Surgical Techniques

SPECIAL EQUIPMENT

Various instruments have been developed to aid the technique of nephrostomy, but in practice they rarely offer any advantage. Two factors govern the ease of inserting a nephrostomy tube: the access to the renal pelvis and the thickness of the cortex. If the pelvis is extrarenal and dilated and the cortex is thinned, then a simple curved artery forceps may be passed easily through a calix to draw the catheter into the pelvis. If access to the pelvis is difficult and the cortex is thick, then a special curved forceps designed for the purpose is useful (Fig. 19-1). Alternatively, a malleable probe with an eye is passed from within the outside and the catheter is firmly sutured and drawn into the pelvis.

Traditionally a de Pezzer or Malecot catheter (Fig. 19-2) was used, but now a Foley-type catheter with a small (5 ml) balloon is often preferred. Either of the other catheters is a reasonable second choice, but in any case the catheter must be sutured carefully to the skin and little reliance should be placed on the self-retaining characteristics of the tube to hold it in position.

An ingenious catheter, the Cummings nephrostomy tube, is a de Pezzer-type catheter with a tail (6 inches–8 inches) that is sufficiently narrow to pass down the upper ureter; for example, a 14Fr

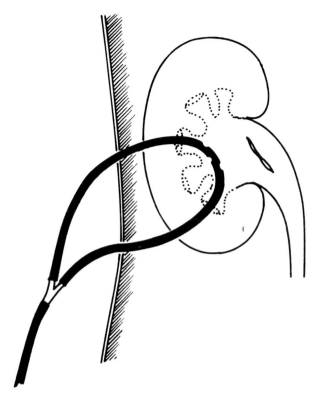

FIG. 19-3. Tresidder loop nephrostomy tube

Cummings tube has a 8Fr tail (Fig. 19-2). This tube combines the adantages of a simple nephrostomy tube with an extension for stenting an anastomosis or damaged upper tract. A recent modification of this tube, designed by Gil–Vernet, uses a Foley-type balloon to retain the catheter.

For a permanent nephrostomy, a ring or through-and-through-type catheter (Tresidder) should be considered.[8] A piece of Silastic tube may be fashioned to fulfill these needs, but it is much easier to use the loop catheter manufactured specially for this procedure (Fig. 19-3).

PREOPERATIVE PREPARATION

If a percutaneous nephrostomy can be performed, it is always the preferred procedure of choice in an emergency. If not, the patient must be prepared for general anesthesia. If the patient is uremic or hyperkalemic, then these conditions must be corrected sufficiently to allow a safe operative procedure. Treatment for a urinary infection must be started. Good general anesthesia and optimum operating conditions are essential for the insertion of either a temporary or permanent nephrostomy

tube; it is a mistake to regard this as a minor procedure.

When the nephrostomy is placed as part of a peroperative procedure, the additional dissection and placing of the tube is relatively minor and adds only minutes to the operating time.

OPERATIVE APPROACH

The surgical approach for either a temporary or a permanent (ring) nephrostomy is the same. The patient is placed in the full lateral position, with the 12th rib over the center break of the operating table (or over an adjustable bridge); the leg that lies underneath is flexed and the superior leg is extended. The hips and shoulders are secured with strapping or belts to stop any movement of the patient. Ideally the upper shoulder and buttock should tilt slightly backward toward the surgeon.

A routine subcostal or 12th rib incision is made. Depending on the nature of the disease and extent of the obstruction, the posterior aspect of the kidney is dissected to allow access to the pelvis. If the pelvis is grossly distended, then access may be easy and require little mobilization of the kidney.

The pelvis is opened between fine chromic catgut stay sutures. It may be possible to slip the index finger easily into the pelvis and the calix so that a suitable middle or lower calix can be selected for the tube. It may be easier to pass an artery forceps through the cortex onto the finger and then grasp the end of the catheter and draw it through the pelvis and out of the kidney. The end of the catheter should be rolled up to enable a smooth passage through the cortex. Usually the forceps is passed through the pelvis, the calix, and the cortex (cutting with a scalpel on the tip of the forceps to help it through), and then the end of the catheter is grasped and drawn into the pelvis (Fig. 19-4). A third choice is available if the access is difficult and a malleable probe is available: a strong suture is passed through the eye of the probe and secured to the end of the catheter. The probe is then passed through the pelvis, the calix, and the cortex, drawing the tube through until the drainage end of the tube lies within the pelvis.

Placing a Cummings tube requires the same basic approach as a nephrostomy: a suitable calix is selected and the tube is passed through the cortex. The drainage part of the tube is placed centrally in the renal pelvis and then the tail of the Cummings tube must be slipped down the upper ureter. This can be an awkward maneuver; if the tail seems too long and will not pass down easily, then it can be shortened without disadvantage.

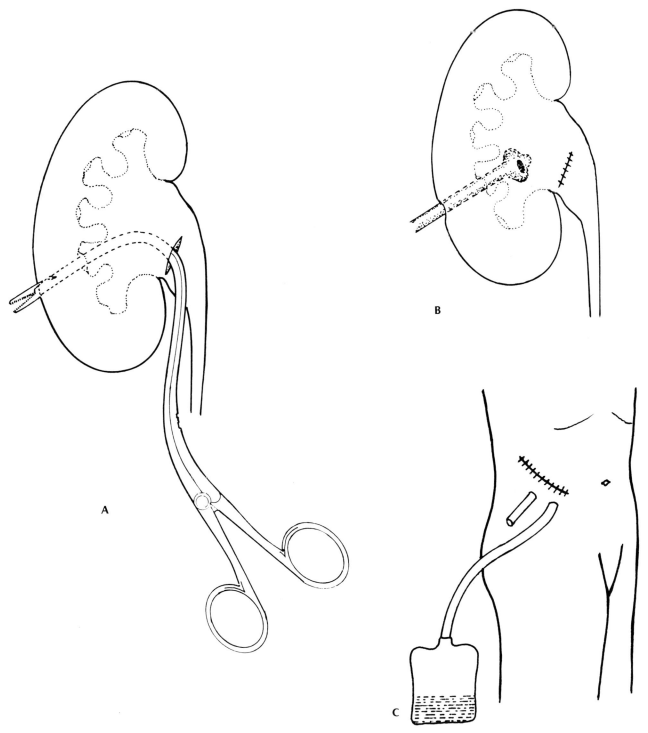

FIG. 19-4. Temporary or peroperative nephrostomy technique: **(A)** forceps passing through pyelotomy and cortex; **(B)** de Pezzer tube in position; **(C)** abdominal wall with position of tube and drain

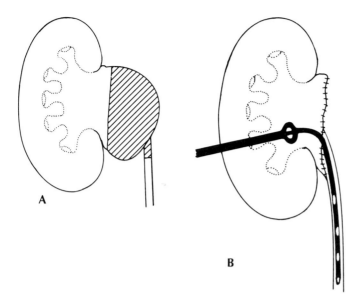

A

B

FIG. 19-5. Peroperative nephrostomy with pyeloplasty: **(A)** Anderson–Hynes pyeloplasty before excision; **(B)** Anderson–Hynes pyeloplasty after excision and with Cummings tube in position

When the Cummings tube is used as part of a pyeloplasty, the tail is passed into the upper ureter before the ureteric anastomosis is completed. It then acts as a useful guide for the correct positioning of the anastomosis (Fig. 19-5).

The position of the nephrostomy tube as it leaves the kidney and passes through the abdominal wall is critical for free drainage and patient comfort. All nephrostomy tubes should come through an anterolateral calix; it does not matter whether it is a middle or lower calix provided that it lies anteriorly when the kidney is replaced in the loin. If this position is correct, then it will be easy to bring the nephrostomy tube through a separate stab incision in the anterior part of the loin. A tube placed too posteriorly will be a nuisance because the patient will lie on it and it will tend to buckle and generally prove inconvenient.

The pyelotomy is closed with fine chromic catgut, and the wound is closed in the usual way. A Penrose or tube (nonsuction) drain is placed through a separate stab incision for approximately 48 hr.

The only additional point to remember when placing a loop nephrostomy tube is that the tube must lie in a gentle curve (Fig. 19-3). The loop into the kidney and then through the anterior loin must be a smooth curve so that the tube can be changed without undue difficulty. Only moderate analgesia is required after the nephrostomy track has formed, usually in 3 to 4 weeks.

The use of a nephrostomy tube in association with more complicated procedures such as ureteric replacement or calicoureterostomy depends on personal preference. A nephrostomy of the Cummings type may be sufficient; alternatively, a simple Foley or de Pezzer nephrostomy plus a longer stent with side holes passing down to the bladder may be desirable (Fig. 19-6). One or even two wound drains may be needed for an extensive operative procedure.

POSTOPERATIVE CARE

The relief of a urinary obstruction may be associated with excessive losses of solute and water.[3] Measuring both nephrostomy drainage and wound drainage is an essential guide to the fluid balance of the patient.

Perhaps of more immediate concern to the urologist is that the nephrostomy tube remains in the optimum position in which it was placed at the operation. In addition to a careful skin/tube suture, the surgeon must ensure that the wound dressings are fixed to protect the tube from unnecessary traction; he must supervise the transfer of the patient from the operating room to the recovery room and instruct the staff about the tubes and drains.

The type of wound drain is also a matter of preference. This author is opposed to suction drainage when there is a risk of a urinary leak and prefer to use a Silastic tube drain (20Fr). The advantage of this type of tube drainage is that it can be connected to a urinary drainage bag, thus avoiding the leakage of urine into the dressings. There is a disadvantage: the wound tube drain may be mistaken for the nephrostomy tube. If there is any risk of this confusion, each tube should be labeled.

If the nephrostomy tube has been placed in the

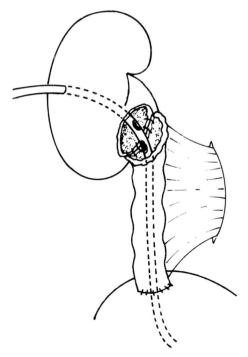

FIG. 19-6. Nephrostomy plus tube drainage with ileal replacement of ureter

anterior loin, then the patient should be able to avoid accidentally pulling or lying on the tube. The end of the nephrostomy tube will have been connected to a urinary drainage bag in the operating room, and aseptic techniques must be used thereafter when the connection is opened or when urine samples are taken.

The wound drain is usually removed by the third to fifth postoperative day, and the track closes quickly. In a simple operative procedure, a nephrostogram can be done at 7 days postoperatively; in a more complicated procedure the nephrosto-

gram may be done at about 14 days. If there is no extravasation and free drainage of contrast to the bladder, then the tube is removed. Valium (5 mg intramuscularly) is a useful sedative prior to the removal of the tube.

There may be a leakage of urine from the nephrostomy site for 2 to 4 days; if the leakage is more prolonged and the nephrostogram was satisfactory, then there is no urgency to intervene. If there is doubt about the patency of the ureter, then a retrograde ureteric catheter and ureteropyelogram under radiographic screening should be carried out to ensure that there is no unsuspected obstruction.

REFERENCES

1. ANDERSON JC: Hydronephrosis, p. 41. London, Heinemann Medical Books Ltd, 1963
2. BRIN EN, SCHIFF M, JR, WEISS RM: Palliative urinary diversion for pelvic malignancy. J Urol 113:619, 1975
3. CHISHOLM GD, OSBORN DE: Pathophysiology of obstructive uropathy. In Williams DI, Chisholm GD (eds): Scientific Foundations of Urology, Vol. I. London, Heinemann Medical Book Ltd, 1976
4. CHISHOLM GD, SHACKMAN R: Malignant obstructive uraemia. Br J Urol 40:720, 1968
5. FALLON B, OLNEY L, CULP DA: Nephrostomy in cancer patients: To do or not to do. Br J Urol 52:237, 1980
6. GIBBONS RP, MASON JT, CORREA RJ, JR: Experience with indwelling silicone rubber ureteral catheters. J Urol 111:594, 1974
7. RICKWOOD AMK, PHADKE D: Pyeloplasty in infants and children with particular reference to the method of drainage post-operatively. Br J Urol 50:217, 1978
8. TRESIDDER G: Nephrostomy. Br J Urol 29:130, 1957
9. VAN DYKE AH, VAN NAGELL JR, JR: The prognostic significance of ureteral obstruction in patients with recurrent carcinoma of the cervix uteri. Surg Gynecol Obstet 141:371, 1975
10. WALSH A: Ureterostomy *in situ.* Br J Urol 39:744, 1967

Percutaneous Nephrostomy

20

Zoran L. Barbaric

Ever since Goodwin in 1955 described a trocar-nephrostomy technique,[7] percutaneous nephrostomy has been gradually but surely replacing operative nephrostomy tube placement done solely for supravesical drainage. The technique has undergone several stages of evolution. Presently, the most commonly used modification employs the angiographic method of percutaneous nephrostomy tube (PNT) introduction.[8,13,16] The single most important factor contributing to the success of the PNT method was the employment of fluoroscopy, which made it possible to position the draining tube in the most desirable place in the renal pelvis and thus to minimize the number of complications. Occasionally, ultrasonic assistance may be helpful in determining the depth and the angle of approach. Others have used ultrasound without fluoroscopic assistance.[11]

Surgical Approach

Preprocedural planning contributes significantly to the success of percutaneous nephrostomy. Previous and current excretory urograms, retrograde pyelograms, computed tomographic scans, and ultrasonographic examinations should be analyzed. Most patients will have had at least one of these studies, and the degree of hydronephrosis, anatomic variance of the pelvicaliceal system, and relative position of the kidney should all be assessed. Choosing the optimal point of entry will influence the final position of the PNT within the pelvicaliceal system. One should anticipate a potential need for subsequent manipulation of intraureteral calculi or antegrade placement of a ureteral stent. Choosing the optimal entry site will aid greatly in any such manipulation.

Most patients undergo the procedure in the prone position. Very thin patients may require some support under the abdomen. Occasionally it will be impossible to place a seriously ill patient in the prone position. Patients with endotracheal tubes, patients with complicated fractures, patients on respirators, patients in congestive heart failure, and patients who have undergone a major surgical procedure may not tolerate the prone position well. Because these patients are at high surgical risk, they will particularly benefit from PNT placement as opposed to operative nephrostomy. Such patients can be placed in the supine oblique position, with the affected side elevated from the table. Placement may be somewhat more difficult because the entering needle is parallel to the tabletop and thus the operator has no depth perception, but at least two series of patients demonstrate that PNT placement in this position is highly successful.[1,3]

Premedication may include atropine and Demerol HCl, but most patients will need only local anesthesia. It is particularly important to sedate uncooperative pediatric patients adequately. Once the skin is prepped and draped, if the collecting system is not visible under fluoroscopy, a 22-gauge needle is introduced under local anesthesia toward the expected site of the renal pelvis (Fig. 20-1A). This may be facilitated by the use of a portable real time ultrasound. Urine is aspirated and an equal amount of contrast material is injected into the renal pelvis. The volume of injected contrast material should never exceed the volume of aspirated urine, particularly in the presence of infection.

As the PNT is placed under fluoroscopic control, it is most desirable that the pelvicaliceal system be made visible. This can be done by intravenous administration of contrast material if renal function is not severely depressed. Alternatively, the renal pelvis may be opacified by percutaneous placement of a thin, 22-gauge aspirating needle under either fluoroscopic or ultrasonic guidance.

Once the pelvicaliceal system is clearly visible on the fluoroscopic screen, a more lateral point of entry for PNT placement is chosen.[4] This point is usually along the posterior axillary line under the 12th rib. The more lateral approach offers these advantages: entry through the bulky paraspinal muscles is avoided, placement through the renal parenchyma is ensured, and there is less chance of damaging a major vessel as the PNT passes through the most lateral aspect of the kidney. After

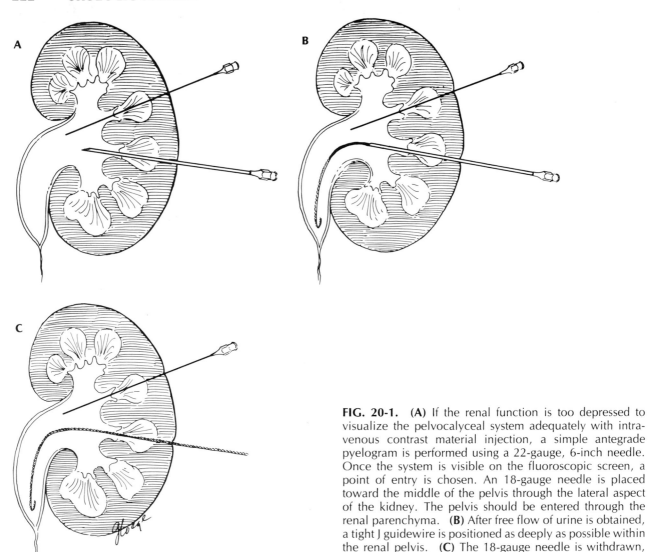

FIG. 20-1. **(A)** If the renal function is too depressed to visualize the pelvocalyceal system adequately with intravenous contrast material injection, a simple antegrade pyelogram is performed using a 22-gauge, 6-inch needle. Once the system is visible on the fluoroscopic screen, a point of entry is chosen. An 18-gauge needle is placed toward the middle of the pelvis through the lateral aspect of the kidney. The pelvis should be entered through the renal parenchyma. **(B)** After free flow of urine is obtained, a tight J guidewire is positioned as deeply as possible within the renal pelvis. **(C)** The 18-gauge needle is withdrawn, leaving the guidewire in place.

choosing the point of entry, local anesthesia is administered and a small cutaneous incision is made to facilitate cutaneous passage of the catheter. The patient may be kept in the prone position or may be turned obliquely enough so that the point of entry is superimposed on the renal pelvis on the fluoroscopic monitor.

A 6-inch, 18-gauge needle is introduced into the collecting system. Once the urine flow is obtained, a tight J .038 angiographic guidewire is introduced into the collecting system and placed as deeply as possible within it (Fig. 20-1B). The 18-gauge needle is then removed (Fig. 20-1C), and progressively larger (6, 7, or 8 French) stiff Teflon dilators are introduced over the guidewire to dilate the fascial planes (Fig. 20-2). This greatly facilitates further

placement of the PNT and should be done conscientiously. Some prefer not to dilate the renal capsule and renal parenchyma. Others find it more useful to dilate the entire tract. Once the dilatation is accomplished, an appropriately sized (usually 8.3Fr pigtail) PNT is introduced over the guidewire (Fig. 20-2B) and positioned in an optimal place within the collecting system. The guidewire is withdrawn, and the catheter is secured to the skin with the help of a plastic disc (Fig. 20-2C) or with a nonabsorbable suture and sterile tape. Because one of the more common complications is dislodgement of the nephrostomy catheter, it is of the utmost importance that it be properly secured. With the help of a connecting tube, the nephrostomy is connected to an appropriate drainage bag.

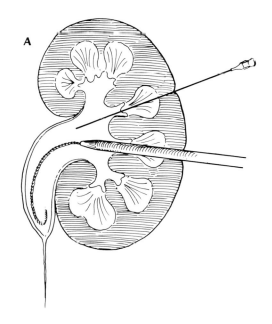

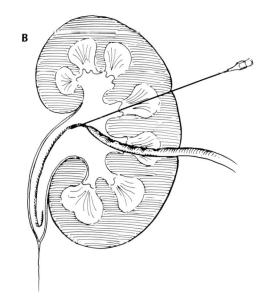

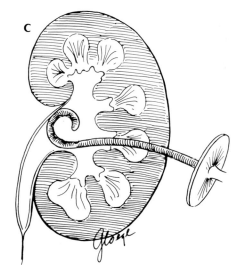

FIG. 20-2. **(A)** Using Teflon dilators, the fascial layers and the renal capsule are dilated up to 8Fr to accommodate subsequent placement of the PNT.   **(B)** A specially made PNT 8.3Fr Pigtail Catheter is threaded over the guidewire and positioned well within the renal pelvis. (Any other shortened 8Fr angiographic catheter may be used if the PNT catheter is unavailable.) During this manipulation, care should be taken to avoid dislodging the guidewire from the renal pelvis.   **(C)** The PNT is secured to the skin using a plastic disc to prevent it from dislodging from the renal pelvis.

In uncomplicated cases, experienced radiologists can complete the entire procedure within 20 minutes.

A special PNT kit is commercially available. It contains a 22-gauge needle, an 18-gauge needle, tight "J" guidewire Teflon dilators, a percutaneous nephrostomy pigtail catheter, a plastic disc, and connecting tubing. Should a kit be unavailable, percutaneous nephrostomy can readily be accomplished using a standard straight or pigtail angiographic catheter cut down to a length of 30 cm.

The angiographic method that has been described here is preferable to the trocar technique primarily because the latter can be dangerous if the collecting system is not entered in the first pass. The trocar technique uses an 8Fr trocar with an outside metal sleeve. The trocar is positioned into the collecting system and then withdrawn, leaving the sleeve behind as a passageway for introduction of the catheter. A trocar set developed specifically for PNT is not yet commercially available.[12] The instruments of the commonly used suprapubic cystotomy set are too short to reach the renal pelvis in a moderate-sized patient.

Applications

Once in place, the PNT can be used for various purposes other than drainage, including conversion to a permanent nephrostomy, dissolution of urinary calculi, extraction of urinary tract calculi,

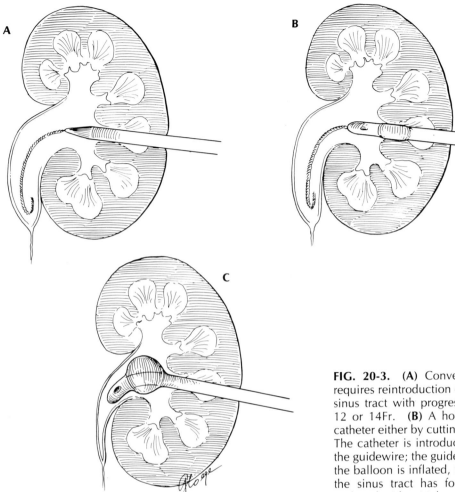

FIG. 20-3. **(A)** Conversion to permanent nephrostomy requires reintroduction of the guidewire and dilation of the sinus tract with progressively larger Teflon dilators up to 12 or 14Fr. **(B)** A hole is made at the tip of the Foley catheter either by cutting it or piercing it with a hot needle. The catheter is introduced into the collecting system over the guidewire; the guidewire is then withdrawn. **(C)** Once the balloon is inflated, the catheter is well anchored. After the sinus tract has formed, the Foley catheter can be replaced with a Malecot catheter.

brush biopsy and nephroscopy, ureteral stenting, and intraureteral balloon placement.

Percutaneous nephrostomy is usually performed for temporary supravesical urinary diversion. If it becomes obvious during the course of the illness that permanent nephrostomy is the only possible method for urinary diversion, a temporary percutaneous nephrostomy can be easily converted into a permanent one.[1] This requires dilatation of the sinus tract over angiographic guidewire with larger and larger Teflon dilators up to 12Fr or 14Fr (Fig. 20-3). Once this is accomplished, an appropriately sized Foley catheter is introduced over the guidewire (Fig. 20-3B) (the tip may be cut off or pierced with a hot needle) and anchored in the renal pelvis (Figs. 20-3C and 20-4). Several weeks later, after the sinus tract has formed, the Foley catheter can be replaced with a Malecot catheter.

It is possible to dissolve struvite or uric acid calculi in patients who cannot tolerate oral or parenteral alkalinization of urine.[5,14] In both instances, it is imperative to have an input and output catheter. This is accomplished by placing either two PNTs or one PNT and one ureteral catheter. Precautionary measures should be taken to ensure that the perfusion pressure within the collecting system never exceeds 20 ml of water; particularly in patients with struvite calculi, one must try to prevent complications such as hypermagnesemia and sepsis.

Several radiologists have already gained considerable experience in extracting renal calculi with the use of a basket through a large nephrostomy sinus tract. This technique is still considered experimental, but it certainly has potential.

Brush biopsy and nephroscopy are seldom used to diagnose intrapelvic or intraureteral abnormalities, but in rare instances they may be beneficial.[2,9]

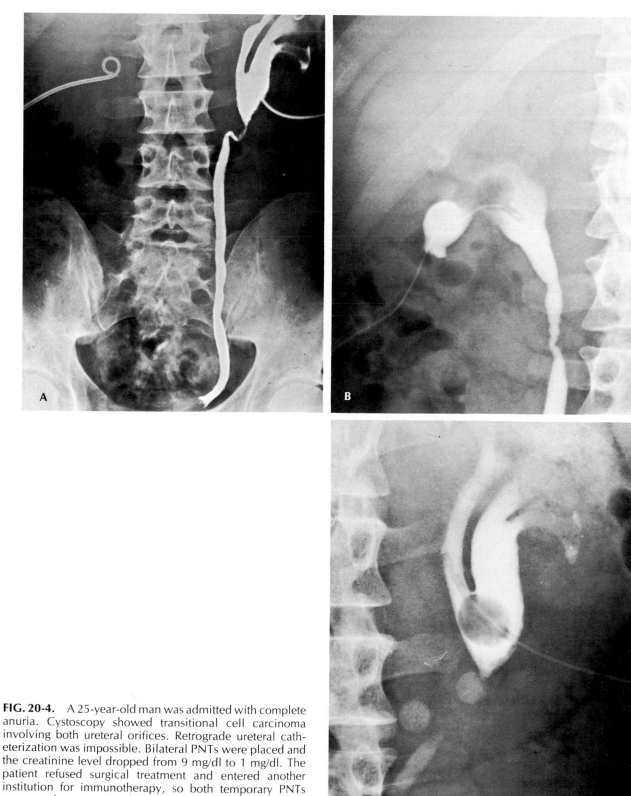

FIG. 20-4. A 25-year-old man was admitted with complete anuria. Cystoscopy showed transitional cell carcinoma involving both ureteral orifices. Retrograde ureteral catheterization was impossible. Bilateral PNTs were placed and the creatinine level dropped from 9 mg/dl to 1 mg/dl. The patient refused surgical treatment and entered another institution for immunotherapy, so both temporary PNTs were made permanent by enlarging the sinus tract and placing Foley catheters into the renal pelvis.

It is frequently impossible, using standard retrograde approach, to negotiate ureteral narrowing responsible for the obstruction. In many cases it is possible to negotiate the obstructed ureter with the guidewire or catheter from above by manipulating the nephrostomy tube or other types of angiographic catheters. Once that is accomplished, it is possible to slip the internal stent either by pushing it over the guidewire from above[6] or by extracting the guidewire with a cystoscope, bringing it out through the urethra and placing the stent from below. The former method is preferable when the obstructed lesion is high in the ureter; the latter method is preferable if the ureteral lesion is distal. Both methods have been used to internalize drainage in patients with ureteral strictures, periureteric neoplasms, inadvertent ureteral ligation with reabsorbable sutures, and ureteral fistulas.[10]

On rare occasions, it may be desirable to occlude the ureter above a ureteral fistula after PNT drainage has been established. Detachable balloons, developed for intervascular use, can be employed for this purpose.[17] The balloon-carrying catheter is negotiated into the ureter from above and placed proximal to the fistula site. Once inflated and anchored, it is detached from the catheter and left as a permanent occlusive device, allowing the fistula to dry out.

Complications

Considering the poor general condition of patients who receive the PNT, the complication rate is rather low, approaching 4%.[15] It is almost equally divided between significant hemorrhage, introduction or exacerbation of infection, and the consequences of improper catheter placement, which is most commonly associated with a PNT dislodging after initial proper placement. It is of utmost importance to properly secure the tube to the skin. Patients with suspected upper urinary tract infection, pyonephrosis, or struvite calculi should be given antibiotics during and after the procedure. There have been two deaths reported from percutaneous nephrostomy, both due to uncontrollable hemorrhage.

Although percutaneous nephrostomy was described some three decades ago, use of the technique has really gained momentum only in the last 10 years. I believe that this important endouroradiologic procedure and its numerous ramifications can be successfully practiced only in those institutions where a spirit of cooperation between the two specialties exists.

REFERENCES

1. ALMGARD LE, FERSTROM I: Percutaneous nephrostomy. Acta Radiol (Diagn), 15:288, 1974
2. BARBARIC ZL: Interventional uroradiology. Radiol Clin North Am 17:413, 1979
3. BARBARIC ZL, WOOD BP: Emergency percutaneous nephrostomy: experience with 34 patients and review of the literature. Am J Roentgenol 128:453, 1977
4. BURNETT LL, CORREA RJ, BUSH WH: A new method for percutaneous nephrostomy. Radiology 120:557, 1976
5. DRETLER SP, PFISTER RC, NEWHOUSE JH: Renal-stone dissolution via percutaneous nephrostomy. N Engl J Med 300:341, 1979
6. GOLDIN AR: Percutaneous ureteral splinting. Urology 10:165, 1977
7. GOODWIN WE, CASEY WC, WOOLF W: Percutaneous trocar (needle) nephrostomy in hydrocephrosis. JAMA 157:891 1955
8. HARRIS RD, MCCULLOUGH DL, TALNER LB: Percutaneous nephrostomy. J Urol 115:628, 1976
9. LANG EK: Brush biopsy of pelvocalyceal lesions via a percutaneous translumbar approach. Radiology 129:623, 1978
10. LANG EK: Diagnosis and management of ureteral fistulas by percutaneous nephrostomy and antegrade stent catheter. Radiology 138:311, 1981
11. PEDERSEN JF: Percutaneous nephrostomy guided by ultrasound. J Urol 112:157, 1976
12. PFISTER CR, NEWHOUSE CH, YODER IC: A new system for percutaneous nephrostomy: Use of a trocar-cannula unit in 100 kidneys. Presentation, Radiological Society of North America, Chicago, December 1977
13. RUTNER AB, FUCILLA I: Percutaneous pigtail nephrostomy. Presented at the Western Section, American Urologic Association, Tucson, Arizona, March 1973
14. SPATARO RF, LINKE CA, BARBARIC ZL: The use of percutaneous nephrostomy and urinary alkalinization in dissolution of obstructing uric acid stones. Radiology 12:623, 1978
15. STABLES DP: Percutaneous nephrostomy. In Syllabus for Categorical Course on Genito-Urinary Radiology. Radiological Society of North America, Syracuse, New York, 1978
16. STABLES DP, GINSBERG NJ, JOHNSON ML: Percutaneous nephrostomy: A series and review of the literature. Am J Roentgenol 130:75, 1978
17. WHITE RI, USIC TA, KAUFMAN SL et al: Therapeutic embolization with detachable balloons. Radiology 126:521, 1978

Ureteropelvioplasty

21

James H. DeWeerd

A significant portion of all urologic operations entails surgical correction of problems related to the urine transport system. The renal pelvis is the first, or upper, segment of this transport system formed by a coalition of minor calices to form major caliceal groups or subdivisions of the pelvis (Fig. 21-1). The renal pelvis, then, lies largely within the renal sinus. Normally it is funnel shaped and flattened in its dorsoventral axis to conform to the elliptic contour of the renal sinus and the renal hilus through which it passes.

There is considerable variation in the proportion of renal pelvis that projects beyond the renal hilus as extrarenal pelvis. Beyond the hilus, the elliptic conformation of the pelvis changes to a conical one and becomes tubular, contiguous with the ureter at an often ill-defined site called the ureteropelvic juncture.

HISTORICAL NOTES

Definitive surgical procedures performed on the renal pelvis were first described just before the turn of the 20th century. Küster in 1891 (10 years after the first successful partial gastrectomy) described end-to-side ureteropelviostomy (Fig. 21-2A), and Fenger in 1892 applied the Heineke–Mikulicz principle of transverse closure of a vertical incision to the ureteropelvic juncture (Fig. 21-2B). Natural evolution of this procedure is seen in the Finney pyeloureteroplasty (Fig. 21-2C).

The Durante pyloroplasty was a natural forerunner of the Schwyzer (1923) pyeloureteroplasty (Fig. 21-2D). This was the first of the flap pyeloureteroplasties, and as such it inaugurated a new era, in which significant strides have been made in surgical technique and control of infection to greatly enhance the urologist's ambition for conservation of renal tissue. Modifications and refinements of the basic principles embodied in these largely outmoded historic procedures will be self-evident in the detailed considerations of operations currently accepted as producing the most satisfactory results.

ANATOMIC CONSIDERATIONS

The renal pelvis is ordinarily a single structure, but the bifid or partially divided pelvis and the completely reduplicated pelvis are variants. In any event, the pelvis, as the first common segment of the transport system, is formed by coalition of infundibula leading from an individual calix or a composite of calices. When complete reduplication of the renal pelvis and variable lengths of the ureter occur, the upper part of the pelvis is ordinarily the smallest, draining a single calix or a combination of calices.

The wall of the renal pelvis, like other portions of the urine transport system, is composed of an outer fibrous coat, a muscular layer, and a transitional cell mucous membrane.[20] The smooth muscle layer, disposed chiefly in a circular fashion with fewer internal and external bundles, is significantly reduced in the proximal components of the pelvis. The wall may be markedly thickened by pathologic conditions including work hypertrophy and inflammation. Normally, one cannot discern any gross difference in the appearance of the incised pelvic wall and the adjacent ureter; but when obstruction is present, the transition may be evident to the naked eye.

Peripelvic fat enmeshed in a loose connective tissue is present in varying amounts and ordinarily provides a plane of cleavage between important structures that may be closely associated with the renal pelvis, particularly when the pelvis is dilated. The main renal vessels usually cross the superior ventral surface along with branches or accessory vessels coursing to the inferior aspect of the renal hilus in a significant number of cases.[2] The proximity of the duodenum and the vena cava on the right side and the aorta and the tail of the pancreas on the left is familiar to all.

The rich arterial and venous anastomosis of blood vessels entering the fibrous coat of the renal pelvis and adjacent ureter from several levels of the renal artery and its branches suggests that dangerous interruption of the blood supply by

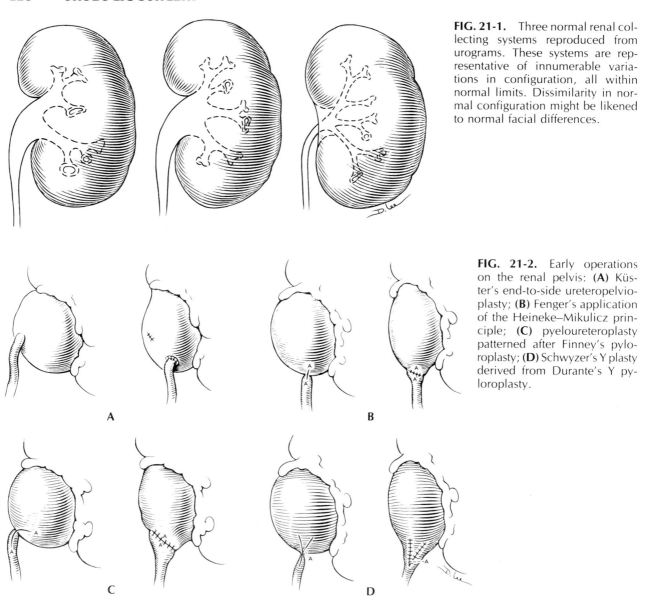

FIG. 21-1. Three normal renal collecting systems reproduced from urograms. These systems are representative of innumerable variations in configuration, all within normal limits. Dissimilarity in normal configuration might be likened to normal facial differences.

FIG. 21-2. Early operations on the renal pelvis: (**A**) Küster's end-to-side ureteropelvioplasty; (**B**) Fenger's application of the Heineke–Mikulicz principle; (**C**) pyeloureteroplasty patterned after Finney's pyloroplasty; (**D**) Schwyzer's Y plasty derived from Durante's Y pyloroplasty.

incision is unlikely.[12] However, close scrutiny of these vessels, careful planning, and judicious placement of incisions are necessary, particularly if the incisions are parallel or approximately so.

Indications for Operation

Surgical procedures on the renal pelvis, ureteropelvic juncture, and adjacent ureter are guided by well-defined pathologic states incorporated under the broad classifications of hydronephrosis and filling defects within the pelvis. These pathologic states include opaque or nonopaque stones, blood clot, primary urothelial carcinoma, primary sar-

coma, benign fibromuscular polypoid lesions, and local intrinsic and extrinsic obstructing lesions.

Obstructing lesions at the ureteropelvic juncture are relatively common and are an indication for surgical intervention in most cases.[19] *Hydronephrosis* (Fig. 21-3A), which is defined as a distention of the pelvis and calices by urine due to obstruction of the ureter, actually may be associated with or due to various pathologic, anatomic, or physiologic conditions, some of which are situated at the site under consideration.[27,28] All too commonly the term or diagnosis "hydronephrosis" is used loosely. For example, pyelectasis (dilatation of the renal pelvis) is often improperly called hydronephrosis (Fig.

FIG. 21-3. **(A)** Typical hydronephrosis with dilation of all collecting system elements down to the obstructed ureteropelvic juncture. **(B)** Pyelectasis, a congenital variation that does not embarrass renal cortical substance; surgical relief is not indicated. **(C)** Calicectasis without pyelectasis, usually due to a long-standing inflammatory process; the condition is not improved by surgical attempts to improve drainage.

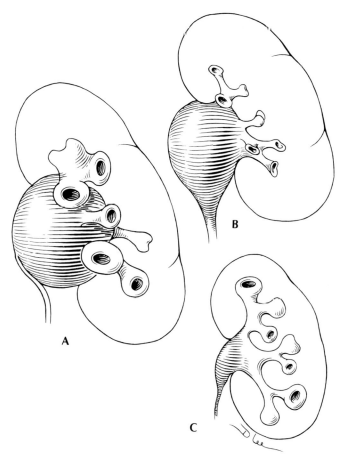

21-3*B*). Pyelectasis without calicectasis is frequently an asymptomatic, nonprogressive process and may well be considered a variation of normal. Reparative surgery is contraindicated because it accomplishes nothing for the patient and may actually be deleterious. Calicectasis (dilatation of one or more of the calices), which is often due to chronic inflammatory disease, should also be differentiated from hydronephrosis (Fig. 21-3*C*). Calicectasis without pyelectasis or with intrarenal pyelectasis (intrarenal hydronephrosis) is usually the result of chronic pyelonephritis or may represent a poorly understood congenital anomaly in which the obstructive features are more apparent than real.[16] These conditions that resemble hydronephrosis must be approached with caution, because the opportunity for improvement is small and the chance of failure is great.

Classic obstruction of the ureteropelvic juncture is often an ill-defined lesion affecting the pelvic outlet and adjacent ureter. It is generally conceded to be on a congenital basis and seemingly is due to an anomalous arrangement of normal tissues including blood vessels, to abnormal physiologic

function of apparently normal tissues, or to a combination of both.[14,31] A small but definite percentage of patients with borderline, asymptomatic hydronephrosis, positively including those with pyelectasis, are not candidates for surgical intervention; but the current, well-founded concepts of conservation of renal function strongly indicate the need to relieve the obstruction, whether intrinsic or extrinsic, in most circumstances.[15] This indication is particularly valid when the disease is bilateral or involves a solitary kidney in all except perhaps the aged. Unilateral obstruction of a salvageable kidney demands correction when progressive or symptomatic disease (pain, infection, or calculus) is found in patients up to late middle age, except occasionally when a bizarre congenital anomaly defies surgical skill.

Reparative surgery is not always the most conservative surgery. When preliminary urograms and isotope renograms reveal a nonfunctioning kidney and exploration discloses marked reduction of renal cortical substance, or when long-standing chronic infection with or without cortical abscesses or parenchymal scarring is encountered, it is more prudent to do a nephrectomy if the contralateral kidney is normal or adequate to sustain life. Likewise one is inclined to be cautious about deciding to do a repair for a unilateral obstructive lesion in a patient whose physiologic age appears to be greater than 55 or 60 years. Minimal, asymptomatic, uninfected pyelocalicectasis in the adult is best observed periodically for evidence of progression despite what may appear to be good urographic evidence of obstruction at the ureteropelvic juncture.

Bilateral disease often present in a variety of interrelated circumstances. If the bilateral processes are urographically equal, either side may be repaired first; usually the patient will indicate which side is most symptomatic. If both kidneys are considered salvageable in unequal disease processes, the more severely damaged kidney should be operated on first unless the contralateral side is severely symptomatic.

When there is real concern regarding the salvage of one kidney, the better kidney should be repaired first; then, after a sufficient interval to ascertain the result and adequacy of function of the operated kidney, one may proceed with operation on and possible removal of the questionable kidney. Under optimal conditions, simultaneous bilateral repair may be a reasonable procedure for the seasoned surgeon who prefers the anterior approach for ureteropelvioplasty.[24] Likewise it is not unreasonable, under optimal or urgent conditions, to operate on the second kidney after an interval of a week. Generally, however, it is more prudent to allow an interval of approximately 4 weeks between operations, and usually an even longer interval is desirable and not deleterious.

Renal fusion, particularly of the lower poles, commonly referred to as horseshoe kidney, is a fairly common congenital anomaly. Approximately 25% of horseshoe kidneys have abnormalities that require surgical correction. Crossed renal ectopia in the form of unilateral fused kidney, sigmoid- or S-shaped kidney, or pancake kidney may likewise present developmental problems that can only be resolved surgically.

Hydronephrosis and the presence of calculi, frequently the two in combination, are the chief indications for surgery. Outlet obstruction must be considered in each instance, and the need for ureteropelvic revision or for adjustment or alteration of the course of the ureter to relive stasis must be carefully evaluated. Less prominent indications are persistent pain (usually periumbilical) and expanding parenchymal lesions or those originating in the renal pelvis.

Diagnostic Maneuvers

The diagnosis of hydronephrosis is ordinarily a straightforward one, the possibility being suggested by a variety of symptoms and signs. Prominent complaints include continuous or episodic aching or pain in the flank, at times associated with nausea (and vomiting), fever and dysuria (if infection is present), and rarely hematuria. Tenderness is usually present in the costovertebral angle but is of variable intensity. Occasionally, the diagnosis is more elusive, because the symptoms may mimic those common to gastrointestinal disease.

Children frequently refer to the abdominal (periumbilical) region as the site of pain. It is not uncommon for hydronephrosis to be entirely asymptomatic and to become suspected because of the finding of a mass in the flank (particularly in the newborn), abnormalities of the urinary sediment, or unsuspected azotemia (bilateral hydronephrosis particularly in the newborn or young child). A severely hydronephrotic kidney presenting as an abdominal mass in the thin newborn child or young infant may be transilluminated by an appropriate light source placed on the flank.[33]

A complete urographic survey is mandatory. Excretory urography is obviously the basic roentgenographic study to be used initially. A marked reduction or lack of opacification of the collecting system at ordinary intervals suggests the need to make exposures at intervals up to 3 hr or 4 hr after injection of medium. Late films often aid in evaluating the amount of retention and therefore indicate the degree of obstruction.

Infusion urograms made after hydration of the patient occasionally accentuate the hydronephrosis and thus facilitate diagnosis. Intermittent hydronephrosis (Fig. 21-4) can be best demonstrated by obtaining an excretory urogram as an emergency without preparation during an acute attack of flank pain.[4,22] Retrograde filling of the pelvis and calices is indicated *only* if the late films prove to be inadequate.

Retrograde pyelography is performed at the definite risk of infecting a heretofore sterile hydronephrotic pelvis and precipitating acute pain by overdistending the kidney; it cannot be recommended as a routine procedure. If the test is necessary, antibiotic coverage and catheter drainage of the pelvis may obviate the risks incurred. Study of retention of medium for various intervals cannot be considered a valid reason for retrograde injection.

Retrograde ureterography performed with an acorn- or bulb-type catheter at the ureteral meatus

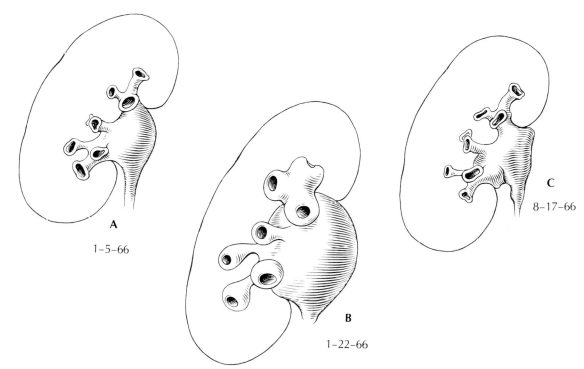

FIG. 21-4.   Intermittent hydronephrosis is demonstrated by reproductions of urograms of a 26-year-old woman.   **(A)** A normal right kidney was demonstrated during investigation for the cause of episodic right abdominal pain.   **(B)** Acute exacerbation of the pain 2 weeks later was considered due to acute (surgical) cholecystitis. Immediate urography revealed the actual cause of the attacks.   **(C)** The right renal collecting system was viewed 8 months after surgical reconstruction of the ureteropelvic juncture by the Foley Y–V operation.

is necessary if the ureter is not satisfactorily outlined, because one must have adequate evidence that the obstruction is at the ureteropelvic juncture or adjacent ureter before proceeding with surgical intervention. In most circumstances a convenient and appropriate time for retrograde study is during anesthesia immediately before operation.

Determination of total creatinine clearance, isotope renography, renal scans, and, under very special circumstances, renal arteriography often provide valuable supplemental information regarding total and unilateral renal function and the remaining renal cortex to assist in decisions to be made at operation about the feasibility of conservative surgery.

Preoperative Preparation

Preparation of the patient for operation on the renal pelvis can follow generally accepted patterns in most instances. Important specific measures, however, may be indicated by the presence of urinary tract infection, severely symptomatic acute obstruction at the pelvic outlet (often intermittent hydronephrosis), or seriously impaired total renal function. If prophylactic anti-infection measures are to be used (see Postoperative Care), it seems feasible and prudent to establish a therapeutic blood level of the drug of choice by giving the initial dosage the day before operation. Selection of a drug that can be given parenterally enables one to continue its use during the early postoperative period.

A concerted effort should be made to eradicate bacterial infection or, if this is impossible, to effect a beneficial suppression of bacterial growth by adequate dosage of the appropriate antibiotic, chemotherapeutic agent, or both. Fever, pain, and flank tenderness accompanying infection of a hydronephrotic renal pelvis may not respond to drug therapy alone. Ureteral catheter drainage for 3 to 6 days can be important in making conservation of the kidney feasible.

Severe, unrelenting flank pain associated with sudden complete obstruction of the ureteropelvic juncture may indicate a need for drainage—that is, placement of a ureteral catheter to decompress the kidney while necessary preoperative investigations are being completed.

Bilateral obstructive disease or that affecting a

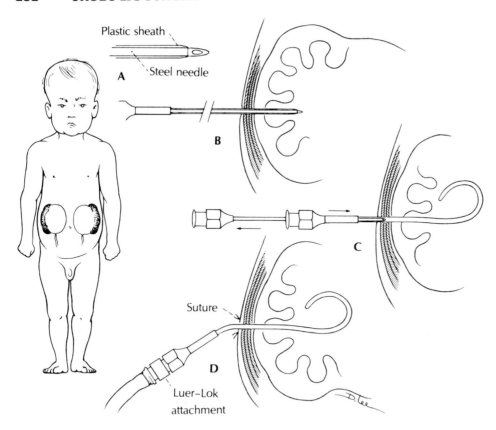

FIG. 21-5. Percutaneous needle nephrostomy in an infant with bilateral hydronephrosis. The infant is placed in a prone position to make both flanks accessible. **(A)** A 15-gauge, 6-inch plastic intravenous needle is used. **(B)** A 2-mm stab skin incision is made, and the needle is thrust through the flank wall into the hydronephrotic kidney. Urine will flow freely from the needle. **(C)** A plastic sheath is advanced to within 1 cm of the hub, and the steel needle obturator is withdrawn. **(D)** A silk suture is placed to secure the tube, and dependent drainage tubing is attached.

solitary kidney may produce a total renal deficit of such a degree that preliminary nephrostomy diversion is advisable. This sort of problem is much more prevalent in the infant or child than in the adult.[30] Protracted ureteral catheter drainage is not feasible and is generally ineffective in all age groups, but particularly in the young. In two instances I have successfully used percutaneous needle nephrostomy in infants with bilateral hydronephrosis to provide unimpaired drainage from one kidney as the ureteropelvic juncture of the other was repaired (Fig. 21-5). A 15-gauge, long, plastic, sheathed needle can be introduced easily through the renal cortex and coiled in the collecting system. Little or no reaction occurs and the procedure is not likely to interfere with the definitive operation 1 to 3 weeks later.

Surgical Approach and Techniques

Obstructive phenomena at the ureteropelvic juncture and the resulting hydronephrosis are associated with various and often complex abnormalities. It is therefore imperative that the surgeon be equipped to evaluate the findings correctly, to select the appropriate procedure, and to perform

that procedure with necessary adaptations in order to achieve the optimal functional result.[6] The wrong operation, even though skillfully performed, invites disaster.

Operation on the renal pelvis and ureteropelvic juncture is best accomplished through a classic flank incision. There can be no compromise with adequate exposure. The incision, therefore, must be carefully planned and placed to conform with the position of the kidney and the habitus of the patient, and it must be of adequate length. One should not hesitate to remove part or all of the 12th or 11th rib subperiosteally, or segments of the neck and angles of these ribs as necessary to provide adequate exposure.

A transverse abdominal incision in the upper quadrant with extension to the midaxillary line is often preferable in the infant or small child presenting a large low-lying kidney, particularly when the diagnosis remains uncertain.

Proponents of the midline or subcostal transperitoneal approach[24] to renal lesions indicate that operation on the renal collecting system may be facilitated by the opportunity to visualize the undisturbed anatomic features, to operate on the pelvis or ureteropelvic juncture without mobilization of the kidney, and to position more properly the involved structures at the conclusion of the procedure. These advantages may be lost in the face of obesity and peritoneal adhesions from a previous operation.[26]

Extraperitoneal exposure of either half and the isthmus of a horseshoe kidney is readily accomplished through a flank incision, if it is placed lower and extended medially rather than into the costovertebral angle. Both pelves of a fused kidney, particularly the horseshoe deformity, are best exposed through a long midline transperitoneal incision.

The degree to which the kidney is mobilized for operation on the pelvis and its juncture with the ureter varies considerably; excessive mobilization is to be avoided. Gerota's fascia is lifted away from its loose attachment to the psoas and quadratus lumborum muscles. An incision through this definitive layer of fascia may be made opposite the midposterior surface of the kidney, revealing a variable layer of perirenal fat. Once incised, Gerota's fascia is readily divided in the cephalocaudad direction. The posterior surface of the renal pelvis is the most accessible, and exposure for pyelotomy requires little or no mobilization beyond that described.

Exploration and surgical revision of the pelvis and ureteropelvic juncture require complete mobilization of the lower two thirds of the kidney, its pelvis, and the upper part of the ureter. The envelope of perirenal fat is stripped back and removed, and Gerota's fascia is lifted away from the anterior and medial aspects of the renal pelvis and ureter. The renal artery and vein are carefully exposed by blunt dissection and lifted from their loose attachment to the dilated pelvis. The upper pole need not be mobilized under ordinary circumstances. In fact, in most instances it is best left undisturbed because it gives a point of fixation or fulcrum about which to move the remainder of the kidney for exposure to facilitate operative maneuvers.

Plastic Reconstruction of the Ureteropelvic Juncture

Plastic reconstruction of the ureteropelvic juncture is a term used to embrace the various surgical techniques designed to relieve hydronephrosis by removing or nullifying the obstructive process, whether it be purely mechanical, physiologic, or both. Transportation of urine through the normal renal pelvis into and down the ureter is undeniably a function of peristaltic muscular activity. Gravity can scarcely be a significant factor. Normal anatomy (see Anatomic Considerations) is plainly one in which the conical or funnel-shaped pelvis is directed caudad (dependent, in terms of erect position) for uninterrupted or unobstructed contiguity with the ureter. When extrarenal hydronephrosis exists, one or more of these features are lost. Reconstruction efforts must necessarily embody features that reestablish as nearly as possible a conical or funnel-shaped ureteropelvic juncture of adequate caliber that is directed and positioned in a caudal or dependent fashion. If these goals can be achieved surgically, funneled peristaltic activity can effectively discharge the pelvic contents into the ureter for transportation to the bladder.

The need for careful study of the problem presented, circumspect deliberation in most instances, and sound surgical judgment in all cases is self-evident. An accurate comprehension of proved methods greatly complements surgical skill and ingenuity, and it reduces the risk of disappointing failures.

One cannot overemphasize the need for meticulous care in handling the tissues of the renal pelvis and ureter. Small, sharp, straight scissors should be used to provide straight, clean margins. Fine vascular thumb forceps minimize crush damage to the tissues. Bleeding from minute vessels is ordinarily self-limited and may be disregarded. Occasionally a larger surface vessel will require a carefully placed, superficial, fine-suture ligature. Tissues must be accurately approximated with interrupted sutures of fine catgut (chronic 4-0 or 5-0) swedged on an atraumatic needle. Delicate "bites," avoiding the mucosa, approximating the tissues without crushing are desirable.[1] Sutures placed at intervals of 3 mm to 6 mm should have the knots tied on the exterior surface. Some surgeons prefer a fine running suture for rapid closure of residual pelvic defects.

PELVIC FLAP OPERATIONS

When properly applied, pelvic flap operations achieve the conditions established for satisfactory reconstruction without loss of ureteropelvic tissue continuity.

Y–V Operation

The Y–V operation (Fig. 21-6), described by Foley in 1937,[13] continues to pace the field as the classic procedure that is properly applied in a greater percentage of cases than any other single operation. The Y–V principle embodies important features, including minimal incisions (hence less interfer-

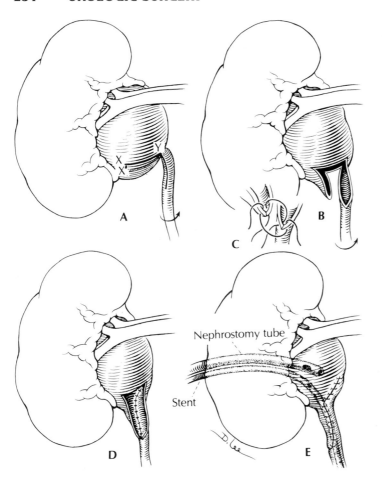

FIG. 21-6. A high ureteropelvic insertion is corrected by a Y–V flap operation. **(A)** Converging incisions X–Y and X'–Y are placed on the anterior and posterior surfaces of the pelvis and are continued down the lateral surface of the ureter. **(B)** The broad-based flap tends to fall into its new position. **(C)** The apical sutures are placed and secured. **(D)** The posterior side of the incision is closed. **(E)** The reconstruction is completed, producing a conical, dependent juncture (see Fig. 21-24). Note that the size of the pelvis remains unaltered.

ence with blood supply) for maximal alteration of contour with less resultant distortion than other operations.

A clear comprehension of the basic principles involved makes it the obvious solution for correction of hydronephrosis with a high insertion of the ureter. A high insertion in itself ordinarily implies adequate pelvic tissue between the juncture and the renal hilus to enable construction of a lengthy flap. An insertion at the level of the inferior margin of the pelvis may fall within the scope of the procedure, if adequate pelvic tissue is available.

Cautious mobilization, discussed in a preceding paragraph, includes incision of connective tissue folds to liberate the upper part of the ureter from the pelvis up to the point of actual juncture. Careful planning of the length and position of pelvic incision must include an estimation of the length of ureteral incision required to reach the portion of ureter having a normal caliber and to provide the desired dependency.

Incisions are made in the same plane on the anterior and posterior surfaces of the pelvis, each directed at the inferior margin of the juncture of the ureter with the pelvis. The converging incisions meet at this point and continue as a single vertical incision down the lateral aspect of the ureter. The limbs of the Y incision may be extended toward the hilus to provide an adequate, broad-based flap that falls naturally into position to provide the desired conical funneling. The stem of the Y is lengthened to correct narrowed ureter and to enable proper dependency of the new juncture.

The reconstruction is started by placing sutures so that they accurately position the tip of the flap at the apex of the incision in the ureter. Two sutures, each about 1 mm from the rounded tip of the flap engaging the ureteral wall similar distances from the apex of the incision, accomplish this nicely. Sutures at the tip and apex are undesirable because unnecessary reaction there may jeopardize the lumen. A stent of appropriate size will assist in the accurate placement of these and subsequent sutures as the edges of the pelvis are carefully sutured to the edges of the ureter (see Adjuvants to Reconstructive Procedures).

Closure of the remaining defects in the anterior and posterior surfaces of the pelvis is accomplished. Any discrepancy in the length of the edges can be adjusted In this area where the puckering or distortion is of little or no significance. Excision of pelvic tissue to overcome this distortion is condemned, because even greater distortion or serious embarrassment of the blood supply may occur. If the surgeon believes that the size of the pelvis must be reduced, a procedure other than the Foley Y–V plasty should be used.

Spiral Flap Operation

The spiral flap operation was proposed by Culp and DeWeerd in 1951 to correct the already dependent, obstructed juncture, and when necessary, to provide a flap of pelvic tissue of adequate length to bridge unusually long segments of narrowed upper ureter.[7] Figure 21-7 illustrates how the spherical contour of the dilated pelvis provides a broad-based tongue that falls into position and is readily sutured to the margins of the incised ureter. The pliable fibromuscular character of the pelvic wall facilitates deployment of the tissue flap and subsequent molding into a conical form. Like the Y–V plasty, the technique calls for a flap the base of which opens to the renal cortical substance and the origin of nutrient vessels. Lines drawn through the base of the flap and the margin of the

hilus may vary from nearly parallel to nearly perpendicular to each other. The operation is not applicable to a high insertion of the ureter.

When preliminary exposure and mobilization of the pelvis and upper part of the ureter have demonstrated that a spiral flap repair is the operation of choice, either the anterior or the posterior surface of the pelvis is selected for the base of the flap. This is determined by several factors, including the symmetry of the pelvis, the particular anatomic position of the kidney in its fossa and its relation to the exposure achieved, and the presence of accessory vessels entering the lower aspect of the hilus or the lower pole of the kidney.[3]

If the pelvis is asymmetric, the body and the tip of the flap are properly constructed from the largest portions. The base of the flap should be planned on the posterior surface when accessory vessels cross anteriorly. These vessels will, when the revision is completed, cross intact pelvic wall rather than suture lines. The projected flap may be outlined with Indigo Carmine markings or fine temporary stay sutures to serve as guides for accurate incision in the collapsed pelvis. The surgeon should plan and create a flap that is longer than his anticipated needs. Excess length can be sacrificed if natural muscular contraction does not reduce it to the proper length.

The pelvic portions of the incision are completed

FIG. 21-7. Spiral flap reconstruction of the dependent ureteropelvic juncture. The kidney is shown in three fourths anteromedial projection. **(A)** The outlined projected flap is planned, and the initial incision is made along one of the lines, preferably the more medial one. **(a)** Application of the method to a short dependent structure is shown in anterior projection. Note the desirable sweeping, curved continuation of the medial incision into the juncture and the upper part of the ureter. **(B)** The apical sutures are placed and secured. **(C)** The flap margin is sutured to the ureteral wall. **(D)** Closure is completed; the ureteral stent and nephrostomy tube may be used (see Fig. 21-24). Pelvis size is not materially altered, but the dependent pelvis is now conical, funneling down to a new ureteropelvic juncture.

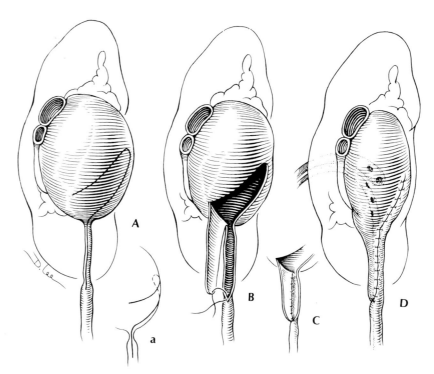

first, after which the medial limb of the gradually diverging incisions is continued in a sweeping curve down the anterolateral or posterolateral aspect of the ureter. Reconstruction follows the same principles and techniques described for Y–V plasty. The flap should fit the ureteral defect exactly. Tension must be scrupulously avoided, and excess length must be trimmed away to prevent the formation of redundant folds at the upper end of the line of closure. Fine sutures of 4-0 or 5-0 chromic catgut, placed 1 mm to each side of the center of the rounded flap tip, also engage the ureteral wall 1 mm from each side of the apex of the ureteral incision. A stent facilitates the placement of sutures in this most critical area.

Closure of the shorter posterolateral incision is simplified by cautiously elevating and rotating the ureter and pelvis by traction on the apical sutures and a suture through the pelvis at the vertex of the incision. Placement of individual sutures in both the posterior and the anterior closure must

start adjacent to the apical sutures, progressing cephalad. Attempts to excise portions of the renal pelvis to reduce its size or to eliminate dog ears are ill-advised and generally unnecessary.

Vertical Flap Ureteropelvioplasty

The vertical flap ureteropelvioplasty described by Scardino and Prince in 1953, embodies many principles that are identical with those of the spiral flap operation (Fig. 21-8).[25] The only difference is that the flap is formed by straight converging incisions from a broad base that is directed toward the opposite (posterior or anterior) pelvic wall and is therefore at an approximate angle of 90 degrees with the vertical axis of the kidney. It is appropriately used when the dependent ureteropelvic juncture is situated at the medial margin of the large, square, extrarenal pelvis. The operation cannot be classically applied unless there is adequate pelvic wall between the ureteropelvic juncture and the renal hilus. Stenotic areas of average length are

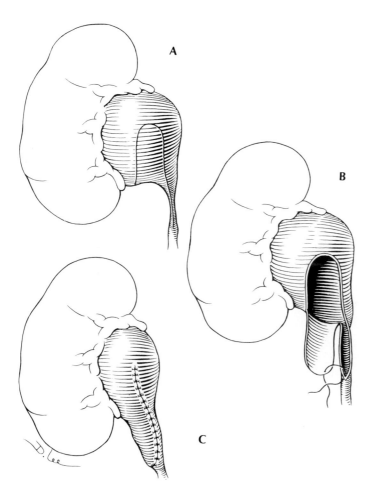

FIG. 21-8. Vertical flap ureteropelvioplasty. The kidney is shown in anterior projection. Note the "square" pelvis and the adequacy of pelvic tissue between the medially placed ureter and renal cortex. **(A)** The broad base of the flap is directed inferiorly (rather than toward the renal cortex as in the spiral flap). **(B)** The flap tip is sutured to the ureteral wall at the vertex of the ureteral incision. **(C)** Closure is completed.

readily bridged, but the procedure is not designed to produce a long flap. Like the spiral flap, it has no place in repair of the high insertion.

The vertical flap should be mapped out on either the anterior or the posterior wall of the pelvis. After fashioning the flap, the medial incision is carried down the anterolateral or the posterolateral surface of the ureter. The tongue of pelvic tissue is sutured into the ureteral defect beginning with two sutures just off the center of the rounded tip and continuing as described for the Y–V and spiral flap reconstructions.

PYELOSTOMY AND URETEROTOMY

The operation of longitudinal incision through all layers of the ureter, ureterotomy (Fig. 21-9), and placement of a stent or mold about which ureteral generation could occur was introduced by Davis in 1943 as a method of correcting obstruction at the ureteropelvic juncture.[9,10] A silver probe is passed through a pyelostomy incision into and down the ureter. Knife incision over the probe enables the insertion of the tip of a pair of fine scissors so that stenotic area can be accurately incised. Davis advocated the use of a large-caliber tube inserted through the pyelostomy incision and passed down into the bladder. Nephrostomy drainage is established and maintained during the 6- to 8-week period of intubation. If necessary, fine catgut sutures are placed to maintain the open ureter in apposition to the stent.

Intubated ureterotomy is a recommended, well-recognized, successful procedure for treating single or multiple areas of ureteral stenosis. Its use in obstruction of the ureteropelvic juncture should be in conjunction with flap operations that incorporate deployment of tissue to create the desired funneling and dependency of the juncture. Obviously, it is used when the length of the structured ureter precludes bridging by available pelvic tissue.

Intubated ureterotomy and the Y–V spiral flap (Fig. 21-10) or vertical flap operations are logically combined to produce the desired correction of long stenosis beginning at the ureteropelvic juncture. In each instance, the flap procedure is accomplished as previously described. The tip of the pelvic flap is secured at a position reached without tension. The length of the residual defect has no bearing on the result, because regeneration of the ureter is circumferential, not longitudinal.

DISMEMBERED URETEROPYELONEOSTOMY

Dismembered ureteropyeloneostomy (Fig. 21-11), one of the earliest if not the first operation for

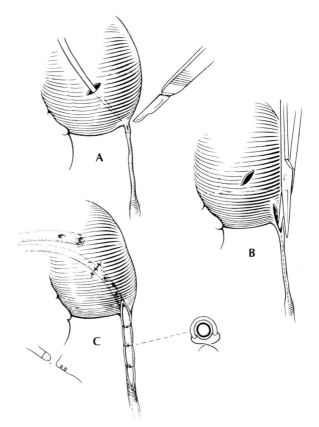

FIG. 21-9. Davis intubated ureterotomy. **(A)** A silver probe, inserted through a pyelotomy incision, is used to explore the ureteropelvic juncture and to aid in the initial ureterotomy incision. **(B)** The ureteropelvic juncture and the ureter are opened with scissors. Two catheters drawn through the renal cortex are used as a nephrostomy tube and a ureteral stent (see Fig. 21-24). **(C)** Fine chromic catgut sutures are placed at intervals to maintain the ureter in accurate relation to the stent. The pyelotomy incision is closed with interrupted sutures.

outlet obstruction, continues to be the operation of choice of some urologic surgeons.[11] This operation implies exclusion of the constricted or obstructed site by excision. Successful application of this principle of repair seems to refute the argument that continuity of tissue at the reconstructed ureteropelvic juncture is necessary or desirable. True end-to-end ureteropyeloneostomy should be avoided because of increased risk of stricture associated with suture of a tubular structure of small caliber. A modified side-to-side anastomosis can be accomplished after spatulating the end of the ureter or after an oblique transection if the ureter is of adequate caliber.[21]

Ureteropyeloneostomy may be used in almost any circumstance in which a ureter of normal

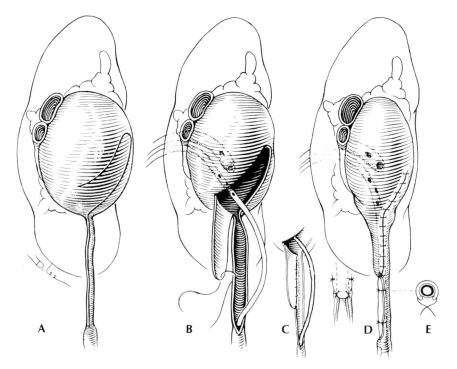

FIG. 21-10. Intubated ureterotomy combined with spiral flap operation. **(A)** The projected incisions are shown in a three fourths anteromedial projection. **(B)** Whistle-tip catheters have been placed to serve as a stent and a nephrostomy tube (see Fig. 21-24). The first apical suture has been placed to position the tip of the flap without tension. **(C)** Posterior approximation is completed. **(D)** Anterior closure is completed beginning with the apical suture. Note the funnel-shaped transition of the pelvis to the ureter. **(E)** Ureteral regeneration about the stent is ensured by spaced sutures to maintain proper apposition.

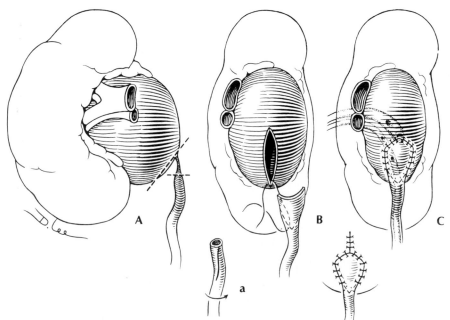

FIG. 21-11. Dismembered ureteropyeloneostomy. **(A)** Transection of the ureter and excision of the ureteropelvic juncture; such excision should provide an appropriate aperture for reanastomosis. **(a)** A vertical incision is made in the lateral margin of the ureter to spatulate it. **(B)** The apical sutures are placed first. **(C)** Methods of completing approximation of the edge of the ureter to the margins of the pelvis are shown (see Fig. 21-24).

caliber can be brought without tension to a level at least 1 cm above the lower aspect of the pelvis. Thus, the circumstance in which a high insertion or redundancy or tortuosity of the upper part of the ureter is encountered seems to be ideal. Partial resection of the renal pelvis is not necessarily a part of ureteropyeloneostomy. However, it seems that the most evident indication for its choice is the need to reduce the size of an unusually redundant extrarenal pelvis by subtotal pelvectomy. The operation is obviously unsuited for most dependent stenoses and lenghty upper ureteral strictures.

FIG. 21-12. Ureteropyeloneostomy after subtotal resection of an excessively large renal pelvis. **(A)** The line of excision provides an adequate margin of pelvis to enable closure without tension. **(a)** A vertical incision is made in the lateral aspect of the ureter to spatulate it. **(B)** The apical sutures are carefully placed. **(C)** Approximation and closure of the pelvis are completed (see Fig. 21-24).

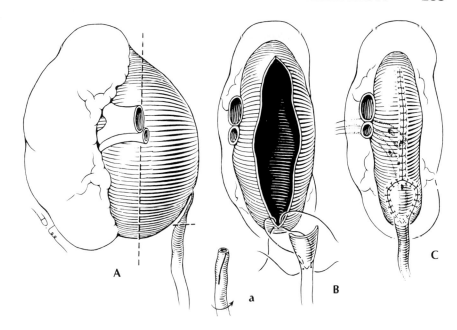

Preliminary exposure and mobilization follow the procedures discussed in preceding paragraphs except that when partial excision of the pelvis is contemplated, complete mobilization of the pelvis is necessary. The redundant portion of the pelvis is excised along a projected line that leaves an adequate margin for closure without tension (Fig. 21-12). One should remember that additional margin can be excised, but it cannot be restored. Rather vigorous bleeding is apt to occur because the excessively large pelvis has correspondingly larger vessels. Brisk arterial bleeding is controlled by delicate suture ligature. Electrocoagulation should not be used.

The ureter is transected immediately below the strictured site, and a vertical incision 1 cm long is made in its lateral aspect to spatulate it. Interrupted sutures of 4-0 or 5-0 chromic catgut approximate the lower aspect of the pelvis to the ureteral wall immediately adjacent to the apex of the incision. Additional sutures secure the margin of the ureter to the pelvis, and the pelvic margins are sutured to complete the closure. The eliptically transected ureter is anastomosed in the same fashion.

The dismembered Y plasty (Fig. 21-13) is a refinement of the operations described in the preceding paragraphs. The distinct advantage of providing a funneled or conical transition is apparent, and its application is particularly useful when a high insertion is to be corrected without need to excise redundant pelvis. When excess pelvis is to be excised (Fig. 21-14), the line of incision varies to provide a lip inferiorly instead of being uniformly circumferential.

SPECIAL AND SECONDARY PROCEDURES

Management of Accessory Blood Vessels

Accessory blood vessels (Fig. 21-15) to the lower aspect of the renal hilus are often found in close relation to the ureteropelvic juncture or upper part of the ureter.[23] Their causal relation to the obstructive process at its inception is a matter of debate. We must at least recognize that frequently their presence accentuates the hydronephrotic process at the stage at which they are exposed surgically; hence, they cannot ordinarily be ignored. The ligation and division of accessory vessels without concomitant resection of the resultant ischemic renal tissue are mentioned only to be condemned, despite published opinions that accessory vessels can and should be divided without concern.

One can scarcely ignore the very significant incidence of hypertension that develops secondary to local renal ischemia.[3] These vessels can be preserved in most instances. Each of the pelvic flap reconstruction procedures (Fig. 21-16) described will relocate the ureteropelvic juncture beyond (below) the accessory vessels, thus neutralizing any possible compression effect that they may have had. Dismembered ureteropyeloneostomy may also be applicable in certain instances. It may actually be preferable to perform such a dismembered operation to enable the relocation of

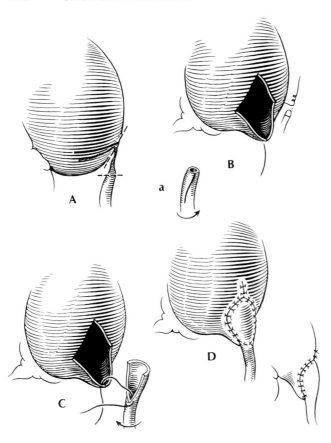

FIG. 21-13. The dismembered Y plasty very closely approximates the reconstruction achieved by the Foley Y–V operation. **(A** and **B)** Excision of the ureteropelvic juncture and the strictured ureter provides an aperture from which incisions are made in the anterior and posterior walls to form V-shaped structures. **(a)** The ureter is spatulated along its lateral margin. **(C)** Anastomosis of the ureter to the pelvis is started with apical sutures. **(D)** Anastomosis is completed to provide a dependent conical transition from the pelvis to the ureter.

the ureter on the opposite side of unusually situated vessels.

Pyelopyelostomy is rarely used, but the procedure must be kept in mind when hydronephrosis is encountered in a kidney with reduplication of the pelvis and the ureteropelvic juncture. In most instances, a diminutive upper segment is hydronephrotic because of an abnormality in the distal portion of a ureter such as ureterocele or ectopia, and the treatment of choice becomes resection of the segment or partial nephrectomy. In rare instances, obstruction at the outlet of one or both pelves requires, and lends itself to, surgical correction. Endless varieties of situations are conceivable, but Figure 21-17 reduces these to a simple illustration. Incisions are made in adjoining surfaces of the dilated and normal pelves, and edges are joined with interrupted sutures of fine chromic catgut to create a permanent window between the two. The ureter need not be interrupted, but it may be if an end-to-side anastomosis seems more appropriate.

Dismembered ureteropelvioplasty may be appropriate for surgical correction of hydronephrosis of both segments. The spatulated ends of the

ureters are joined to form a single unit and sutured to the pelvis, which results from similar consolidation (Fig. 21-18).

Dismembered pyelopyelostomy (Fig. 21-19) should be considered in the isolated instance in which the upper part of the ureter is obstructed by accessory vessels. This situation is apt to occur in the hypermobile (ptotic) kidney that is intermittently hydronephrotic. If mobilization of the pelvis and ureter demonstrates a dependent, funneled ureteropelvic juncture without evidence of intrinsic obstruction, this normal juncture may be preserved by a circular incision leaving a cuff of pelvic wall attached to the juncture and ureter. Excess pelvis is excised and pyelopyelostomy is accomplished with interrupted fine chromic sutures, after which closure of the residual pelvic defect is completed. The kidney must then be stabilized in optimal position by fixation of its capsule to the fascia of the psoas and quadratus lumborum muscles.

Dismembered pyelopyelostomy can be effectively applied for correction of the retrocaval ureter. After identification of the anomalous relation, the vena cava is locally mobilized and the ureter is

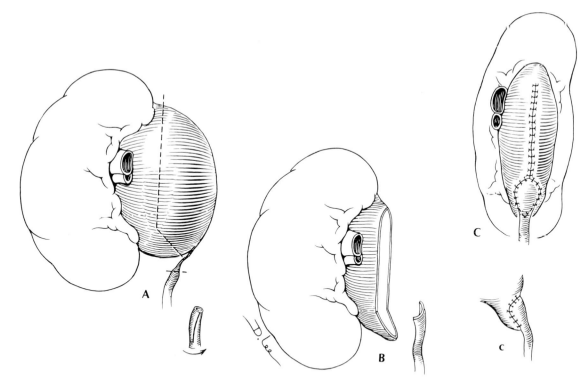

FIG. 21-14. Dismembered Y plasty with excision of excess renal pelvis. **(A)** Compare the line of incision with that shown in Figure 21-12. **(B, C,** and **c)** The dependent lip provides a funnel-shaped ureteropelvic juncture, where the spatulated ureter is sutured into place.

carefully released. If on careful inspection the portion of the ureter situated behind and medial to the vena cava appears normal, the proximal part of the ureter and the pelvis are mobilized and the pelvis is transected. The ureter and cuff of pelvis are then drawn from the abnormal position, and pyelopyelostomy is performed.

Personal experience includes only one case in which **Hellstrom's procedure** (Fig. 21-20) for relocation of accessory vessels was considered applicable. One must be satisfied after lysis of adhesions between the dilated upper ureter and the obstructing accessory vessels that no other obscure obstructive process exists. Normal saline solution injected slowly into the pelvis through a 24-gauge needle simulates urine collecting within the pelvis and reveals the capacity of the pelvis to discharge its contents into the ureter. Chromic catgut sutures (3-0) are placed to fix the perivascular connective tissue to the pelvic wall. If such fixation seems insecure, a tubular support for the vessels may be created by suturing a fold of the redundant wall about the vessels.

Management of Horseshoe Kidney

Horseshoe deformity of the kidney is a congenital fusion anomaly that requires special consideration because of the significant incidence of secondary hydronephrosis associated with it.[8,16] In most in-

stances, the fusion involves the lower poles, and generally the resulting isthmus rests at the level of the third lumbar interspace. The renal masses are usually symmetrically situated close to either side of the midline; however, considerable variation, with the body of one kidney extending over the midline, may be seen. Both kidneys are malrotated on all axes, with rotation about the vertical axis placing the pelvis in a more or less ventral position. The ureter normally crosses the ventral surface of the isthmus.

Correction of coexistent hydronephrosis (Fig. 21-21) requires preliminary division of the isthmus (symphysiotomy). The midline transperitoneal approach provides uniformly excellent exposure. It is the recommended approach for some unilateral problems and must be used if simultaneous bilateral operations are contemplated. Unilateral disease can be managed nicely through the anteriorly placed flank incision.

Preliminary mobilization of the kidney must be complete, extreme caution being exercised in dissecting the vascular elements. Accessory vessels

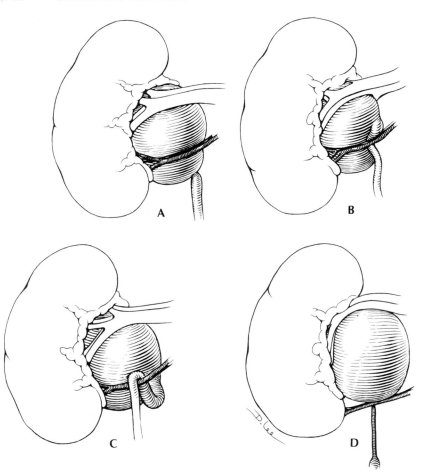

FIG. 21-15. Accessory blood vessels. **(A)** The vessels crossing the dilated pelvis are not related to hydronephrosis. **(B)** Ureteral compression is suggested. **(C)** The accessory vessels are actually aberrant because the ureter is ventral or anterior to the vessels. **(D)** The polar vessels are associated with a lengthy dependent structure.

are common and must be preserved until final decisions regarding management are made. Anomalous vessels sometimes only 1 cm to 2 cm long may enter the isthmus, and vessels to the lower margin of the hilus may likewise be too short to enable the proper correction of malrotation. These vessels should be preliminarily occluded with small bulldog clamps to define the ischemic cortical tissue to be excised after division of the vessels.

Symphysiotomy is a matter of simple incision in the occasional case in which a purely fibrous isthmus is encountered. In most instances, however, an isthmus composed of normal renal tissue requires the placement of two rows of vertical mattress sutures of 1-0 chromic catgut to provide a narrow avascular area through which the incision can be made. Residual bleeding points on each surface are controlled with 4-0 suture ligatures. If the isthmus is broad and thin (less than 1 cm), bleeding can be controlled by digital compression or use of a Doyen clamp while suture ligature of bleeding points is being accomplished. Stay sutures

at the superior and inferior margins are recommended. I make no effort to close the capsule over the cut surface.

The ureteropelvic juncture is reconstructed according to the principles just outlined. Devitalized cortical tissue resulting from ligation of accessory vessels is excised (Fig. 21-22). The segment of isthmus attached to the lower pole may likewise be excised if it seems to encroach on the revised ureteropelvic juncture or ureter. The kidney is positioned and nephropexy is performed.

Management of Ectopic or Unilateral Fused Kidney

The ectopic or unilateral fused kidney (crossed renal ectopia) may on rare occasion be seen first as a hydronephrotic organ. An attempt to describe or illustrate the variety of conditions presented or their correction serves no useful purpose. The surgeon must rely on his ingenuity in applying established principles of ureteropelvioplasty to these unusual and difficult circumstances.

FIG. 21-16. Management of accessory blood vessels by Foley Y–V reconstruction. **(A)** Vessels cross a high insertion of the ureter into the renal pelvis. **(B)** Careful dissection enables displacement with a vein retractor so that dissection of the ureteropelvic juncture can be completed. **(C)** Foley Y–V reconstruction is applicable in this instance, and appropriate incisions create a V defect. **(D)** The reconstructed outlet corrects the relation and removes any possible influence exerted by the accessory vessels. The spiral flap operation is similarly applied when the inferior hilar or polar vessels are related to the dependent juncture.

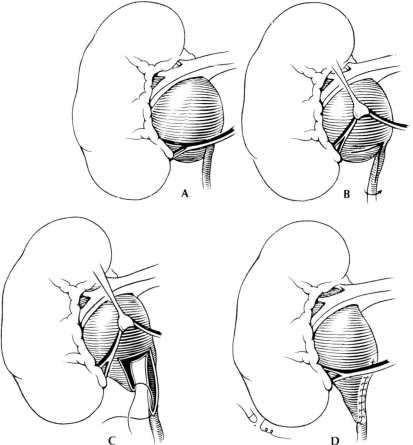

Secondary Procedures

Secondary operative procedures made necessary by the failure of previous surgical attempts to improve drainage are invariably a major challenge. If the contralateral kidney is normal, it is often more prudent to do a nephrectomy. If only one kidney is present or the disease is bilateral, further surgical effort is required. The time interval between operations is important. Early secondary reparative surgery should be avoided. An interval of 4 to 6 months to enable the operative reaction to resolve is desirable. A nephrostomy tube should be used to divert the urine for a 6-month period if the kidney is being further (seriously) jeopardized by obstruction and infection.

Identification of structures and mobilization of the upper part of the ureter and the pelvis are invariably tedious and difficult. Extreme caution must be taken to avoid inadvertently injuring these structures. A ureteral catheter or catheters placed cystoscopically immediately before operation greatly facilitate the dissection.

Some variations of flap ureteropelvioplasty should be considered, whenever possible to bridge what frequently amounts to cicatricial stenosis of the upper part of the ureter. If extensive incision into or excision of the pelvic wall was done in previous operations or is necessary during the secondary operation, dismembered ureteropyeloneostomy is the only recourse (Fig. 21-23). The success of secondary dismembered ureteropyeloneostomy depends to a large extent on the availability of normal ureter to reach the pelvis without tension. A long vascular pedicle may enable the downward displacement of the mobilized kidney in order to make such anastomosis possible. Anastomosis of the ureter to a lower pole calix may be considered, but it is not a practical solution and offers limited chance of success.

Some situations defy the ingenuity of the most experienced and skilled surgeon, and in these circumstances pelvioileovesicostomy (ureteral replacement) or autotransplantation and ureteropyeloneostomy may be preferable to permanent nephrostomy drainage of a solitary kidney.

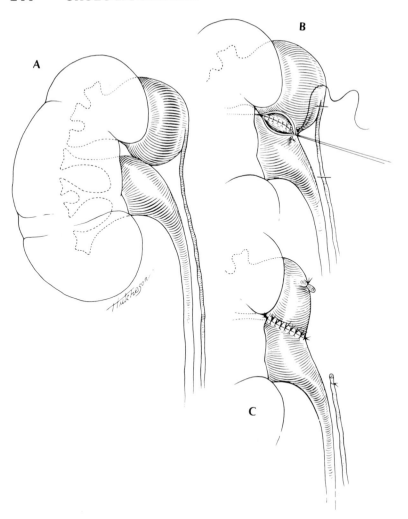

FIG. 21-17. Pyelopyelostomy. **(A)** Adjacent surfaces of the unobstructed normal lower segment of pelvis and the obstructed (abnormal) upper segment of pelvis. **(B)** A window is created between the two pelves, and the posterior margins are joined. **(C)** Anastomosis is completed. An optional resection of a portion of the upper segment of the ureter is illustrated.

ADJUVANTS TO RECONSTRUCTIVE PROCEDURES

Intubation and Drainage

The use of a ureteral stent or splint (ureteral intubation) and nephrostomy drainage (diversion) has long been considered an integral part of pelvic and ureteropelvic reconstruction operations. Currently it is perhaps more appropriate to consider the use of the stent and the diversion tube as an adjuvant to these operations. This change stems from the observations made in 1954 by Hamm and Weinberg, who advocated discontinuing the routine use of tubes.[17] Advocates of tubeless techniques believe that elimination of a route for introducing postoperative infection is the cardinal feature. Some believe that existing or preoperative infection subsides more rapidly without tubes. Parenchymal renal damage related to the placement or the presence of tubes, or to both, and ureteral injury attributable to the stent are avoided. Less tangible

benefits attributed to the tubeless technique include reduced morbidity and shorter hospital stay.

One must necessarily weigh these attractive proposed benefits against those that favor placement of stents and diversion tubes. Persistent infection is an uncommon sequel if the obstructive condition has been properly corrected. The hazards incident to postoperative pelvic distention—that is, disruption of suture lines, pyelonephritis, and the like—are avoided. Proper alignment of the ureter is maintained as the normal reparative processes fill the surgically created spaces and stabilize the ureter and ureteropelvic juncture.

The authoritative reports by Hamm and Weinberg, Smith and associates, and Webb and associates are *prima facie* evidence that certain ureteropelvioplasties can be done successfully without tubes.[18,29,32] It is equally obvious that the success of a large percentage of these operations depends on the judicious use of these adjuvants. Being a staunch advocate of the use of stents and diversion

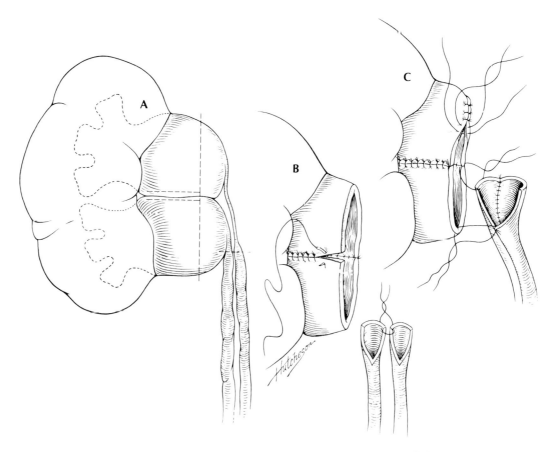

FIG. 21-18. Pyelopyelostomy and dismembered uretero-pelvioplasty. **(A)** Excision of a portion of each dilated pelvis, including a segment of adjoining surfaces and abnormal upper ureters, is shown by the *dotted lines.* **(B)** The pelvis margins are approximated to form a single pelvis, and the ureters are spatulated to form a single unit. **(C)** The joined spatulated ureters are sutured to the dependent margins of the common pelvis, and the remainder of the common pelvis is closed.

tubes, I echo the statement of my late colleague Ormond S. Culp that ". . . selection of the appropriate candidates for tubeless methods continues to be a major challenge."[5]

It is self-evident that the urologic surgeon who undertakes an operation to relieve hydronephrosis must be completely familiar with the intelligent use of stents and diversion tubes. If the circumstances are anything less than optimal, it is more judicious to use a stent and drainage tubes than not.

Personal preferences have dictated the use of various types of stents and nephrostomy tubes. Soft, pliable materials are certainly preferable to more rigid ones. Red or blue rubber catheters and those made of polyethylene are generally unsatisfactory. Silicone rubber catheters promise to be the most desirable. Silastic tubing of appropriate size can be fashioned into a stent. My colleagues and I have found that the whistle-tip catheter made of latex rubber is almost uniformly satisfactory, both for nephrostomy and for use as a stent. It provides a maximal lumen, optimal consistency, and smooth surface and tip. Two catheters are used: ordinarily a 18Fr or 20Fr catheter to serve as

a nephrostomy tube, and a smaller one of appropriate size to splint the ureter. Careful selection and fitting of the ureteral stent are mandatory.

A catheter of proper size, lubricated with water-soluble lubricant (bloody serum from the wound serves admirably), will slip easily to a point 5 cm to 8 cm below the level of repair *A catheter that fits tightly is too large.* There is no need to splint the entire ureter. Erosion and stricture at the tip of the catheter do not occur unless the catheter is too large, too rigid, or has a tip that is not smooth or tapered. Two or three small holes are made in the portion of the stent that will lie within the renal pelvis. These holes enable the urine to pass to the bladder or to the exterior if the nephrostomy tube fails to function properly.

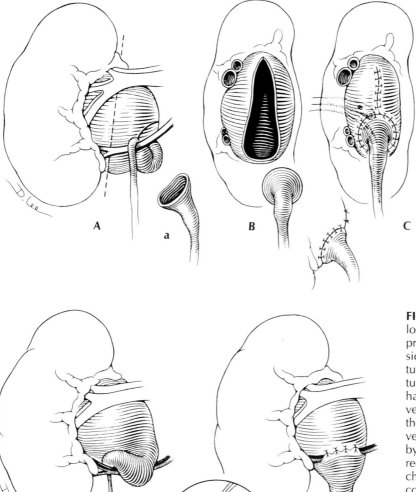

FIG. 21-19. Management of accessory vessels by dismembered pyelo-pyelostomy. Pure extrinsic obstruction of the upper ureter as it drapes over the accessory vessels, which in this instance are also aberrant in that they are posterior to the ureter, may also be managed by dismembered ureteropyeloneostomy. **(A)** A circular incision is made to leave a cuff of renal pelvis attached to the ureteropelvic juncture and the ureter **(a)**, and the excess pelvis is excised. **(B)** A medial view shows the pelvic defect. The wide margins of the superior four fifths enable closure without tension. **(C)** The ultimate relations after reapproximation are shown (see Fig. 21-24).

FIG. 21-20. Hellstrom's operation for relocation of the accessory vessels. **(A)** This procedure entails careful lysis of all adhesions between the accessory vascular structures and the pelvis, the ureteropelvic juncture, and the upper part of the ureter, which has herniated anteriorly to drape over the vessels. **(B)** The unobstructed juncture and the ureter are relocated well below the vessels, and this relationship is maintained by a sling (see cross section in *inset*) of redundant anterior pelvic wall. Several 3-0 chromic catgut sutures are placed to incorporate thickened musculoserosal layers; care must be taken to avoid mucosa.

Both tubes are brought simultaneously through a single site in the renal cortex (Fig. 21-24). This is most easily accomplished with a medium-sized, curved or right-angled hemostat, and should be done after the pelvis and ureter have been incised, partly excised, or both, and before suture reconstruction is started. An appropriate calix is selected not only to allow a gentle natural curve for the stent but also to facilitate exit through the flank wall by a stab incision rather than through the operative incision.

The tip of the hemostat is eased through the renal cortex and capsule breached by incision against the tip of the instrument. The jaws are carefully opened to permit insertion of the catheter tips, each of which is slipped over a jaw. The catheters, when drawn through the renal cortex, have a greater combined diameter than the hemostat, thus in most instances providing enough expansion effect to control hemorrage. The smaller catheter is drawn through until its apertures are well within the pelvis, and the larger catheter is positioned so that its tip lies within the pelvis. A mattress suture of 2-0 or 1-0 chromic catgut is placed to snug the renal capsule about the tubes. This suture may incorporate renal tissue, as nec-

FIG. 21-21.   Correction of the horseshoe kidney.   **(A)** The hydronephrotic left segment with a dependent ureteropelvic juncture can be corrected only by a pelvic flap operation. The projected spiral flap incisions are indicated.   **(B)** Symphysiotomy is accomplished after adequate mobilization. Two rows of vertical mattress sutures are placed, four of which serve as traction sutures. Incision against a supporting finger protects the underlying major vessels. **(b)** Fine cortical sutures control residual bleeding.   **(C)** The spiral flap reconstruction is completed. The kidney is rotated about its vertical and anteroposterior axes to accentuate dependent drainage, and it is fixed in optimal position by nephropexy.

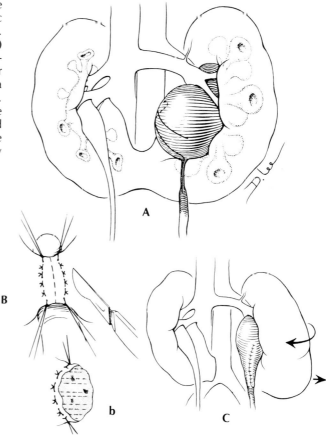

essary, for control of bleeding. The stent should be positioned in the ureter to facilitate placement of sutures, particularly those at the vertex of ureteral incisions.

The nephrostomy tube is irrigated with warm normal saline solution as soon as the pelvis has been closed. The pelvis is gently distended to demonstrate the site of any unusual leakage. Repeated lavage to wash away clots should produce clear returns by the third or fourth injection. The renal pelvis should be reopened to search for bleeding points if the return solution fails to clear satisfactorily. It is important to demonstrate the functioning capacity of the nephrostomy tube by injecting saline solution into the smaller catheter (stent). Fluid entering the pelvis through the apertures in the stent should start to flow from the nephrostomy immediately. If the return flow is delayed until the pelvis is distended, the position of the nephrostomy tube tip should be checked and perhaps adjusted. Final irrigations are done after the tubes are fixed to the skin (by sutures of heavy silk) and after the incision has been closed. The smaller catheter (stent) is then doubled over

close to the skin level and occluded with a ligature. It is inadvisable to cut away excess catheter; it is placed beneath the dressing.

Nephropexy

Nephropexy is an indicated adjuvant to surgical revision of the ureteropelvic juncture when unusual mobility is noted in the preoperative studies or at operation. Similarly, complete mobilization of the kidney should be followed by placement of sutures between its capsule and adjacent muscle and fascia, particularly when the vascular pedicle is long. A kidney with a normal or short renal pedicle and requiring only partial mobilization usually does not need stabilization sutures. Nephrostomy and splinting catheters effect a minor stabilizing influence, but use of tube techniques does not cancel the need for nephropexy in most instances. Advocates of tubeless techniques emphasize the need to position the kidney securely to prevent angulation or redundancy of the ureteropelvic juncture or upper part of the ureter.

Adequate drainage of the retroperitoneal space is imperative. One or two small-caliber (0.5-cm)

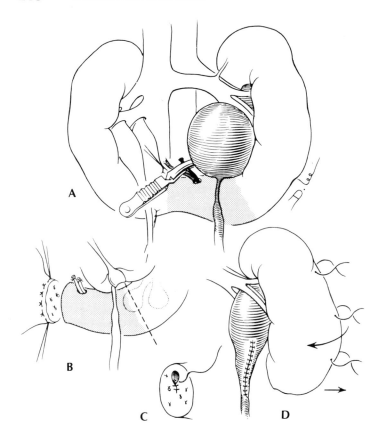

A

B

C

D

FIG. 21-22. In correction of the horseshoe kidney, anomalous vasculature must be considered the rule rather than the exception. The short arterial and venous trunks may course to the isthmus or the lower poles and interfere with the mobility necessary to achieve proper positioning in conjunction with repair. **(A)** The accessory artery is occluded with a vascular clamp to define the portion of the cortex supplied. **(B)** The vessels are ligated and divided. One row of hemostatic mattress sutures is placed, and the isthmus is divided (see Fig. 6-21). After a vascular clamp has been placed on the main renal artery, the devascularized isthmus is removed by incision. **(C)** The transected calix is closed after suture ligature of the blood vessels. **(D)** Ureteropelvic repair is effected, and the kidney is fixed in its new position.

Penrose drains with open ends placed close to, but not overlying, suture lines should exit with the nephrostomy tube and ureteral stent through a stab incision. Penrose drains, similarly placed, suffice when tubeless methods are used. It is preferable, however, to place a Hemovac drain or T tube with multiple perforations in its transverse limb in the retroperitoneal space so that blood, serum, and extravasated urine may be removed by suction devices initially and gravity drainage subsequently.

Subtotal Resection

Subtotal resection of the renal pelvis is frequently cited as an important step in surgical treatment of hydronephrosis. Occasionally the unusually large flaccid pelvis should be reduced in size by resection of redundant portions. Generally this is not necessary, however, because the muscular pelvic wall, unless severely decompensated, will contract and assume more nearly normal proportions once the obstructive features at the outlet are removed. Injudicious excision of pelvic wall may spell failure for the reconstruction procedure unless the excision is carefully planned as an integral part of the operation.

Postoperative Care

Exquisite care, including strict aseptic techniques, must be afforded the nephrostomy tube at all times. Sterile disposable plastic drainage tubes with interposed air traps to limit retrograde movement of bacteria are attached in the operating room to provide gravity drainage. Subsequent irrigation is avoided. Urine output is monitored closely. Hourly recordings provide assurance about patency of the tube.

Unusual bleeding with clot formation is occasionally a reason for further irrigation with sterile saline. Gentle syringe suction should be applied before injection of saline solution, and in any instance only a few milliliters are injected and withdrawn as one attempts to clear the tube and wash out the pelvis. Buildup of excessive pressure within the pelvis can disrupt the suture lines and destroy the pyeloplasty result. A uniformly large urine flow obviates the risk of blood clot formation unless brisk arterial bleeding has been overlooked or develops. Recently, I have requested that appropriate amounts of mannitol be given intravenously as the closure of the renal pelvis is being completed. Continued administration over a 12-hr postoperative period ordinarily causes urine pro-

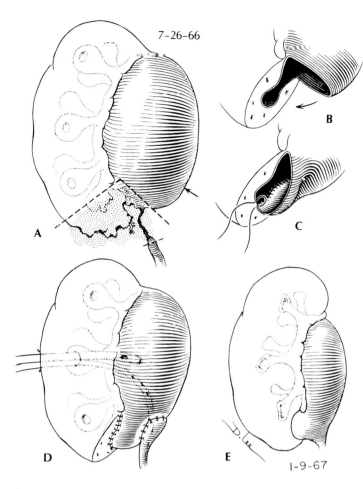

7-26-66

B

C

A

D

E

D. lee

1-9-67

FIG. 21-23. Secondary dismembered ureteropelvioplasty in an 8 year-old child. **(A)** Surgical exposure reveals an atrophic lower pole (ischemic following ligation of the polar vessels) and an obstructed ureteropelvic juncture encased in dense scar. The involved tissues are excised as indicated (*dotted lines*), because none of the flap pyeloplasties can be applied. **(B** and **C)** Mobilization of adequate extrarenal pelvis allows displacement laterally to permit suture to the margin of the calix. Residual defects in the anterior and posterior surfaces of the pelvis are closed. **(D)** The dismembered ureteropyeloneostomy provides a dependent ureteropelvic juncture. **(E)** This drawing of a urogram was made 6 months after operation.

duction at sufficient levels to keep the urine remarkably clear.

Hemovac tubes used for drainage of the retroperitoneal space are attached to a suction-collection device.

Routine use of chemotherapeutic or antibiotic agents, or both, can be the subject of considerable debate. It seems to me, however, that the beneficial effects from the routine use of these drugs far outweigh the possible hazards. It is prudent therefore to continue parenteral administration of a drug started as a therapeutic measure or a prophylactic screen before operation. Switching to a chemotherapeutic agent that can be used during the final phases of healing can be considered before dismissal from the hospital. As an enthusiastic advocate of chemotherapy, I believe it is imperative to continue administration of an effective drug in adequate doses until healing is complete (60 to 90 days).

General postoperative measures including early ambulation are used routinely and require no further discussion, except to mention that a con-

tinuously large volume of urine acts favorably to wash bits of cellular debris and fibrin from the pelvis through the nephrostomy tube, if such is present, or down the ureter when tubeless repair has been effected.

Penrose drains and Hemovac tubes should be removed about 24 hr after drainage becomes negligible. Ordinarily, removal on about the third to sixth day is indicated.

Urine leakage related to a malfunctioning or dislodged nephrostomy tube may cease after opening the stent and connecting it to straight drainage. The ureteral stent should be removed on about the tenth postoperative day, provided the postsurgical period has been uneventful. Situations that contraindicate early removal include secondary operations, infection of the kidneys, exacerbation of latent infections after operations, prolonged extravasation of urine, and intubated ureterotomy. In the last event the stent should remain in place 4 to 6 weeks; difficult problems occurring in other cases may demand similar periods.

Urographic studies may be made in each case if

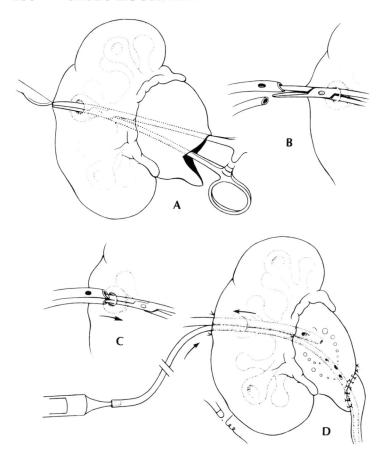

FIG. 21-24. The nephrostomy tube and stent should be positioned as indicated before suture reconstruction is commenced. **(A)** A curved or right-angled hemostat is thrust through the renal cortex, and the capsule is nicked. **(B)** The jaws of the hemostat are spread just enough to allow each tube to be slipped over a jaw. Note the position of the hemostat hinge; excursion of the jaws is minimal in the cortical tract. When difficult angles are encountered, the angled Randall calculus forceps is preferred. **(C)** The tubes should be secured to the Randall tips by ligature to ensure a successful maneuver. The tubes, firmly grasped by a curved hemostat, are drawn into the renal pelvis and positioned. **(D)** A pursestring suture of medium chromic catgut helps to secure the tubes. The pelvis is irrigated gently after reconstruction is complete.

desired, but they are actually indicated only when the operative procedure or events during the postoperative course suggest that incomplete healing or extravasation persists. After preliminary scout (plain) roentgenograms have been made, radiopaque medium is introduced under gravity. Immediate and delayed films are made, including those in oblique positions. If extravasation is demonstrated, removal of the tubes should be deferred until the defects have closed.

After the stent is removed, the nephrostomy tube may be occluded for a functional test. Impaired drainage causes leakage about the tube, pain, or both; in this event the nephrostomy tube should be opened and allowed to drain for another 48 hr. Such an occurrence need not imply failure of the operation, because residual edema or retained cellular debris or coagulum may be present. Further urograms at this point are seldom helpful; it is usually impossible to make a meaningful interpretation unless calculi or extravasation is evident. In most instances, the immediate flow of urine to the bladder constitutes a positive functional test, which carries more significance than urograms and injection of dyes and implies that the nephrostomy

tube can and should be removed. Prompt cessation of urinary drainage (within 24 hr) after removal of the nephrostomy tube is a second important confirmation of good function.

Complications that may occur early in the postoperative course include hemorrhage, infection, and accidental dislodgement of one or both tubes. Hemorrhage is ordinarily self-limited, but is has caused disruption of suture lines from obstruction by clots. Emergency measures and continuous attention must be individualized; immediate reoperation may be necessary. Infection demands vigorous use of broad-spectrum antibiotics and immediate attempts to identify the organism so that the antibiotic program may be made specific insofar as possible. If tubes are accidentally dislodged, management must be individualized. Replacement is likely to be most difficult, and attempts to do so are deferred for a time. Failure of efforts to place a ureteral catheter indicates that there is no alternative.

Late complications are those related to failure to correct the obstructive disease or to eradicate associated, often deep-seated, infection. One or more of several factors may be responsible: cicatrix and stenosis following ischemia and necrosis of tissues; unrecognized separation of suture lines with prolonged extravasation of urine; periureteral and peripelvic collections of serum, blood, and urine; and improper application of a specific operation, including attempts to preserve a kidney that should have been removed. Persistent uncontrollable infection is the rule. Hydronephrosis or loss of function is evident. Calculus formation is not uncommon.

Follow-Up Examinations

A brief inquiry into the general and specific progress achieved should be made, and routine urinalysis should be done at intervals of 2 to 3 weeks to determine whether satisfactory progress is being made and cellular and bacterial elements are being reduced or eliminated. Midstream, clean-catch specimens of urine are examined by microscopic, Gram stain, and culture methods as the postoperative chemotherapy program is completed.

Excretory urography should be repeated early when progress has been less than satisfactory. Ordinarily a urogram at the 6-month postsurgical interval demonstrates a stabilized situation of maximal improvement.

Evaluation of the result must be in terms of the individual problem originally presented. Criteria of an optimal result include, not necessarily in the order of importance, urographic evidence of significant reduction in caliceal dilatation, elimination of cellular and bacterial elements from the urine, improved renal function, and relief of symptoms. Optimal results may be unattainable in advanced and problem cases, and in these a most satisfactory result may consist only of improvement and stabilization in respect to one or more of these criteria.

Abnormalities of the renal pelvis and ureteropelvic juncture will continue to challenge the judgment, skill, and ingenuity of the urologic surgeon. Successful operative management of these fascinating conditions will continue to be a rewarding experience.

REFERENCES

1. ALBERS DD, PIRASTEHFAR K: Comparison of results of ureteroureteral anastomosis including or excluding urothelium. J Urol 96:685, 1966
2. ANSON BJ, CAULDWELL EW, PICK JW et al: Blood supply of the kidney, suprarenal gland, and associated structures. Surg Gynecol Obstet 84:313, 1947
3. BOEMINGHAUS H, GÖTZEN FJ: Partial renal infarction and hypertension resulting from ligature of aberrant renal vessels (abst). JAMA 149:1606, 1952
4. BOURNE RB: Intermittent hydronephrosis as a cause of abdominal pain. JAMA 198:1218, 1966
5. CULP OS: Treatment of tumors of the renal pelvis and ureter. Trans Am Assoc Genitourin Surg 47:101, 1955
6. CULP OS: Choice of operations for ureteropelvic obstruction: A review of 385 cases. Can J Surg 4:157, 1961
7. CULP OS, DEWEERD JH: A pelvic flap operation for certain types of ureteropelvic obstruction: Preliminary report. Proc Staff Meet Mayo Clin 26:483, 1951
8. CULP OS, WINTERRINGER JR: Surgical treatment of horseshoe kidney: Comparison of results after various types of operations. J Urol 73: 747, 1955
9. DAVIS DM: Intubated ureterotomy: A new operation for ureteral and ureteropelvic structure. Surg Gynecol Obstet 76:513, 1943
10. DAVIS DM, STRONG GH, DRAKE WM: Intubated ureterotomy: Experimental work and clinical results. J Urol 59:851, 1948
11. DORSEY JW: Pyeloplasty by modified ureteroneopyelostomy. J Urol 100:353, 1968
12. DOUVILLE E, HOLLINGSHEAD WH: The blood supply of the normal renal pelvis. J Urol 73:906, 1955
13. FOLEY FEB: New plastic operation for stricture at uretero-pelvic junction: Report of 20 operations. J Urol 38:643, 1937
14. FOOTE JW, BLENNERHASSETT JB, WIGLESWORTH FW et al: Observations on the ureteropelvic junction. J Urol 104:252, 1970
15. GIBSON, TE: The surgical treatment of hydronephrosis. West J Surg 67:193, 1959
16. GITTES RF, TALNER LB: Congenital megacalices versus obstructive hydronephrosis. J Urol 108:833, 1972
17. GLENN JF: Analysis of 51 patients with horseshoe kidney. N Engl J Med 261:684, 1959
18. HAMM FC, WEINBERG SR: Renal and ureteral surgery without intubation. Trans Am Assoc Genitourin Surg 46:109, 1954
19. HELLSTROM J, GIERTZ G, LINDBLOM K: Pathogenesis and treatment of hydronephrosis. In VIII Congreso de la Sociedad Internacional de Urología, Vol 1, p 163. Paris, Librairie Gaston Doin, 1949
20. HOLLINGSHEAD WH: Anatomy for Surgeons, Vol 2, The Thorax, Abdomen, and Pelvis. New York, Harper & Row, 1956
21. NESBIT RM: Elliptical anastomosis in urologic surgery. Ann Surg 130:796, 1949
22. NESBIT RM: Diagnosis of intermittent hydronephrosis: Importance of pyelography during episodes of pain. J Urol 75:767, 1956
23. PICK JW, ANSON BJ: The renal vascular pedicle: An anatomical study of 430 body-halves. J Urol 44:411, 1940
24. POUTASSE EF: Anterior approach to upper urinary tract surgery. J Urol 85:199, 1961
25. SCARDINO PL, PRINCE CL: Vertical flap ureteropelvioplasty: Preliminary report. South Med J 46:325, 1953

26. SCOTT RE, JR, SELZMAN HM: Complications of nephrectomy: Review of 450 patients and a description of a modification of the transperitoneal approach. J Urol 95:307, 1966

27. SHARP RF: Hydronephrosis: Development of present concept of management. J Urol 85:206, 1961

28. SMART WR: Hydronephrosis. In Campbell MF (ed): Urology, 2nd ed, Vol 3, p 2372. Philadelphia, WB Saunders, 1963

29. SMITH BA, JR, WEBB EA, PRICE WE: Ureteroplastic procedures without diversion. J Urol 83:116, 1960

30. USON AC, COX LA, LATTIMER JK: Hydronephrosis in infants and children. I. Some clinical and pathological aspects. JAMA 205:323, 1968

31. WEAVER RG: Mechanical factors in the production of hydronephrosis. J Urol 94:514, 1965

32. WEBB EA, SMITH BA, JR, PRICE WE: Plastic operations upon the ureter without intubation. J Urol 77:821, 1957

33. WEDGE JJ, GROSFELD JL, SMITH JP: Abdominal masses in the newborn: 63 cases. J Urol 106:770, 1971

Nephropexy

22

Lloyd H. Harrison

Defined as the fixation or suspension of a floating (mobile) kidney, nephropexy was performed frequently in the late 1800s and the early 1900s with approximately 170 diverse techniques described in the literature.[5] Unfortunately, poor patient selection and lack of proper understanding of the pathophysiologic structure of the ptotic kidney eventually led to the decline in popularity of this operation. A thorough search for recent data on the subject reveals little to interest or encourage today's urologic surgeon in the use of this procedure for treatment of the mobile kidney.[7] In fact, most authors have seemed determined to disassociate themselves from the original techniques described by Burford, Deming, Kelly, Lowsley, and others.[1,2,3,4,8,9]

Although renal ptosis is now considered a relatively normal condition which rarely requires surgical correction, surgeons have continued to perform fixation of the kidney, primarily in association with reconstructive renal surgery and if the clinical situation of the patient so indicates. Two basic types of nephropexy are the *superior nephropexy*, performed infrequently and always in conjunction with the mobile ptotic kidney, and the *inferior nephropexy*, the most popular operation, usually accompanying another surgical procedure that requires pexy or fixation of the kidney (*e.g.*, pyeloplasty).

The three types of surgical approaches for nephropexy that offer the highest level of success are fixation using the fatty capsule (requiring no parenchymal sutures and thus preventing parenchymal damage), fixation with foreign material, and fixation with fascial flaps or muscle bands that require some type of decapsulation. All of these operations have the same objectives:

Immobilization of the kidney by proper positioning

Uninterrupted flow of urine from the pelvis

Fixation of the kidney axis so that the lower pole of the kidney is lateral

Prevention of any tension of fixing sutures on the vascular pedicle and drainage system

Although a very large number of operative techniques for renal fixation have been described, nephropexy is employed as an isolated or rare procedure for the mobile kidney. Perhaps the simplest and most effective techniques are the Deming and Kelly operations.

Deming Operation

The Deming operation is probably the most currently accepted technique, having been modified and adapted to meet the criteria of today's urologic surgeon. It is also probably the most physiologic of any technique devised to date. The surgical procedure itself depends entirely upon the perirenal fascia and fat to hold the kidney in position. No sutures are placed in the kidney or its capsule, and the perirenal fascia and fat are sutured to the lumbar muscles below the kidney.

The kidney is stripped of all perirenal fat and delivered into the wound (along with its vessels and ureter). All adhesions must be removed from the upper and lower poles and the upper ureter should be made free. After determining the proper positioning of the kidney, it can be made to occupy practically any intrathoracic position with the lower pole lying opposite the last rib. The upper pole should be carried medially and the lower pole outward to give free drainage to the lower calix. Holding the kidney in position, a series of interrupted mattress sutures of No. 1-0 chromic catgut are placed through the perirenal fascia and peritoneum to the quadratus muscle, taking care not to include the bowel medially (Fig. 22-1*A*). The first stitch should be about 1 cm from the ureter and as high as possible on the quadratus muscle posteriorly. Extreme care should be taken not to include any nerves in these sutures. A series of five to eight sutures will close, forming a basket-type sling for the kidney and preventing it from descending. Reinforce these by bringing up all the extraperitoneal fat, suturing it with two to three mattress sutures to the quadratus muscle below the first suture line (Fig. 22-1*B*).

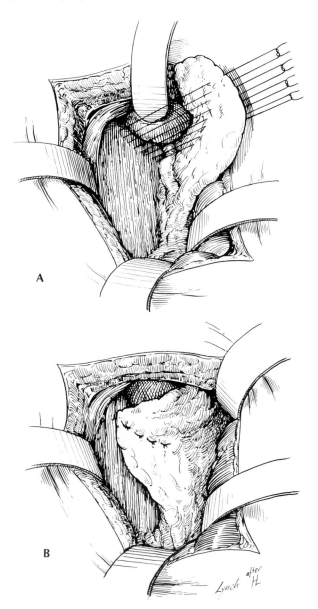

FIG. 22-1. Deming operation. **(A)** Sutures are passed through the perirenal envelope (Gerota's fascia) and through the quadratus muscle. **(B)** Four mattress sutures are placed to suture the fat and the fascia to the quadratus lumborum muscle, while the kidney is held securely in its elevated position.

Kelly Operation

In the Kelly operation, after the lower pole, the pelvis, and the upper ureter have been freed of adhesions, the kidney is retracted downward, slightly elevating the upper pole and separating all fat and adhesions from the area and from the vascular pedicle. The renal fossa is prepared by

removing all fat and fascia from the lumbar muscles well above the costal margin. Should the liver encroach upon this area, light adhesions must be broken up in order to place the kidney in a sufficiently elevated position. Kelly recommended placing three triangular sutures (Brödel) in the true capsule on the posterior surface near the external border; however, two suspending sutures will suffice (Fig. 22-2). The first suture is placed near the junction of the middle of the lower third of the kidney and carried above the 12th rib as far back as it can be placed easily. the second suture should be near the lower pole and is carried through the margin of the quadratus muscle an appropriate distance below the first suture. The upper pole of the kidney should point a little medially, thus ensuring good drainage of the lower calices. The perirenal fascia and fat are then brought across the lower pole of the kidney and sutured to the lumbar muscles immediately below the kidney, using two sutures; one in the psoas muscles immediately below the kidney and the second near the posterior margin of the quadratus lumborum, piercing the fascia about 5 cm from the first suture. Both sutures are placed beneath the lower pole of the kidney and tied, partly obliterating the kidney with the fascia and forming a sling beneath the lower pole.

FIG. 22-2. In the Kelly operation, two Brödel sutures are taken on the convex border of the kidney, including only the capsule. The upper suture, taken just below the midportion of the kidney, is carried above the 12th rib as far posteriorly as possible. The lower suture, taken at the lower pole, is sutured to the quadratus lumborum muscle at an appropriate distance below.

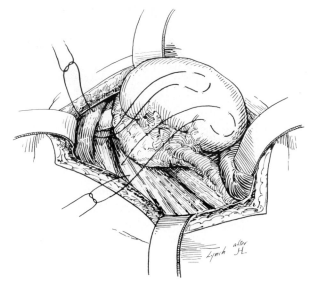

Although Kelly used silk suture material, an occasional sinus was noted. This problem led to the use of chromic catgut, which has proved to be very satisfactory.

Initially, the Deming and Kelly operations were applied to the ptotic kidney. Currently, both of these operations, with modifications, can be applied in carrying out an inferior nephropexy, which is the procedure of choice in providing tension-free anastomosis for a shortened ureter. Having survived the "test of time," it seems ironic that both the Deming and Kelly techniques have actually become surgical adjuncts, with their success depending upon another primary surgical procedure.

As stated, numerous operative methods for renal fixation have been devised, each claiming excellent results. It is common knowledge that the therapeutic value of nephropexy in the treatment of symptomatic nephroptosis is questionable due to the fact that renal ptosis is considered a relatively normal condition which does not warrant surgical correction. It is our opinion, however, that there is indeed merit in fixation of the mobilized kidney—but only as a surgical adjunct to another procedure.

REFERENCES

1. BURFORD CE: Nephroptosis with co-existing lesions. J Urol 55:220, 1946
2. DEMING CL: Nephroptosis. Causes, relation to other viscera, and correction by a new operation. JAMA 95:251, 1930
3. DODSON AI: Nephroptosis and its treatment. In Dodson AI (ed): Urological Surgery, 2nd ed, p. 227. St Louis, CV Mosby, 1950
4. GRAYHACK JT: Renal surgery. In Glenn JF, Boyce WH (eds): Urologic Surgery, 2nd ed, p. 48. Hagerstown, Harper & Row, 1975.
5. HAGMAIER U, HEBERER M, LEIBUNDGUT B et al: Long-term observations on different methods of nephropexy. Helv Chir Acta 46:351, 1979
6. LOWSLEY OS, KIRWIN TJ: Operative and non-operative treatment of the kidney. In Clinical Urology, 2nd ed., p. 1655. Baltimore, Williams & Wilkins, 1944
7. O'DEA MJ, FURLOW WL: Nephropexy: Fact or fiction? Urology 8:9, 1976
8. ROEN PR: Nephropexy. In Roen PR (ed): Atlas of Urologic Surgery. New York, Appleton–Century–Crofts, 1967
9. SMITH DR, SCHULTE JW, SMART WR: Surgery of the kidney. In Campbell MF, Harrison JH (eds). Urology 3rd ed, p. 2143. Philadelphia, W B Saunders, 1970.

Renal Ectopia and Fusion Anomalies

23

S. Lee Guice III

enal ectopia and fusion anomalies are relatively uncommon urologic findings. The fused or ectopic kidney is especially vulnerable to infection, hydronephrosis, calculus formation, and trauma because of its abnormal position, vascular supply, and pelvicaliceal drainage. These same features increase the risk of surgical intervention and necessitate modification of the usual surgical approach and procedures. The urologic surgeon must be aware of these modifications because these kidneys are also affected by all pathologic processes that can affect the normally placed and paired organ.

EMBRYOLOGY

The developmental aspects of renal ectopia and fusion anomalies seem to be centered on the metanephros.[4,6,13,22] The exact mechanism for renal ascent is not known, but it may be related to induced migration of the metanephrosis, extrusion from the true pelvis, or an apparent migration secondary to disproportionate growth of the uncurling embryonal tail and body.[17] During cephalad migration there is rotation of the embryonic kidney such that the pelvis moves from an anterior position to its final medial position (Fig. 23-1). The migration and rotation begin in the late fourth gestational week and is completed by the eighth or ninth week. If the diaphragmatic anlage has not closed or is defective, accentuated renal ascent will occur.[17]

The migrating, rotating metanephric masses approximate, and, if contact with the contralateral mass occurs, fusion may result and rotation ceases.[10] If a single mesonephric unit is met by both ureteral buds, possibly because of abnormal hindend flexion and rotation, a crossed ectopia may result.[4]

Because the migrating embryonic kidney has many temporary blood supplies, an arrest in migration will result in no loss of the temporary supply. The incomplete migration will be accompanied by renal vascularization from aberrant locations: multiple aortic levels, common internal or external iliacs, median sacral, and hypogastrics.[14] If a fusion anomaly is also present, the blood supply to the fused segment or isthmus may be from either or both common iliacs or from the aorta (Fig. 23-2).[1,12]

Horseshoe Kidney

INCIDENCE, FEATURES, AND SURGICAL INDICATIONS

Horseshoe kidney is the most commonly encountered fusion anomaly. There are two distinct renal units that lie vertically on opposite sides of the midline, with a fibrous or parenchymous isthmus being the point of fusion. The incidence of horseshoe kidney is approximately 1:400 and may be more common in males by as much as 2:1.[11,17,22] Fusion between the lower poles occurs in 95% of cases.[13]

The presence of a horseshoe kidney is often an incidental finding (34%). Even when associated with symptoms it will require surgery in only 18% to 30% of cases,[11,14] although surgical intervention is much more common (66%) in the symptomatic child. Early surgical intervention appears to decrease the morbidity of horseshoe kidney in children.[19]

The clinical presentation of a horseshoe kidney can vary widely. Most signs and symptoms are related to hydronephrosis, infection (especially in children), or calculus formation. They commonly include abdominal or flank pain, hematuria, dysuria, frequency, pyuria, and abdominal masses.[5,11,14]

Surgical intervention on the horseshoe kidney is most frequently precipitated by the presence of obstruction or calculi. Surgical intervention for Rovsing syndrome (abdominal pain, nausea, and vomiting on hyperextension of the spine) is rarely considered today because the results have been poor.[5]

DIAGNOSTIC PROCEDURES

Procedures normally employed in urologic investigations will yield the basic information about horseshoe kidney. Conventional excretory urograms will reveal pelvic rotation abnormalities and a deviation of the caliceal axis such that the upper poles point outward. Tomographic slices or radioisotope renal scanning may reveal the isthmus. Oblique projections, retrograde pyelography, and delayed films are all helpful, especially in differentiating malrotation from hydronephrosis.

In light of the frequently anomalous and occasionally bizarre vascular supply of the horseshoe kidney, it behooves the surgeon contemplating major renal surgery to obtain the best "road map" possible. Arteriography can provide an excellent guide to the complicated vascular supply and allows one to avoid either devascularizing a segment essential for renal function or causing urinary leakage.

OPERATIONS

The most common operative procedures performed on horseshoe kidneys are: pyelolithotomy, pyeloplasty, nephrectomy, and division of the isthmus with or without nephropexy. The common complications are fistula, hemorrhage, and recurrence of the primary problem (hydronephrosis, stones, and so forth). Fistula and hemorrhage are often related to the division of the isthmus and its vessels if the surgeon does not intraoperatively recognize ischema of the parenchyma, pelvis, or ureter.[18]

The indications for and principles of removal of

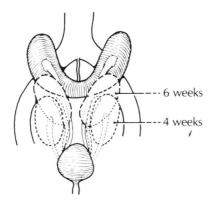

FIG. 23-1. Ascent and rotation of the kidney. Lower-pole fusion may occur at 4 to 6 weeks, resulting in horseshoe kidney.

FIG. 23-2. Three common variants of blood supply in horseshoe kidney: **(A)** single renal arteries arising from the aorta, **(B)** multiple aortic arteries, **(C)** multiple aortic and iliac arteries

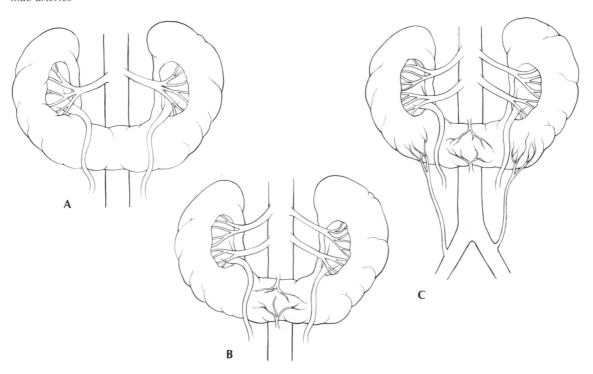

renal calculi are well discussed elsewhere (Chapter 36). The surgeon should be mindful that, because the horseshoe kidney may not drain well if left in its original state, the recurrence rate for calculi is high. The procedure for calculi is usually pyelolithotomy with pyeloplasty and possibly isthmus division. The use of isthmus division is now subject to debate, and its use is not universal, especially in children.[13,18] Whether these young patients will require reoperation for isthmus division remains to be seen.

Of the various types of pyeloplasties, only the Foley Y–V has been widely used in horseshoe kidneys.[5,18] Recently the use of dismembered pyeloplasty has been advocated.[13] Details of these procedures are in Chapter 21.

Partial nephrectomy in the patient with horseshoe kidney may be necessary because of any pathologic process that would require removal of one of the normally paired renal units. The isthmus should be handled carefully, as shown in Figure 23-3. The remainder of the nephrectomy is performed paying close attention to the anomalous vasculature. The surgical approach used will depend on each surgeon's preference. Many choose an anterior incision. The anterior transperitoneal exposure affords excellent visualization of the isthmus and both ureters. An extended subcostal can provide the same exposure. The major disadvantages of any flank approach are that the full extent of the isthmus is never appreciated and the contralateral pelvis and ureter are not well visualized. If fistula formation is to be avoided, any calix of the contralateral or remaining renal unit that is opened during isthmus division must be carefully closed, as well as a layer of parenchyma and capsule.[22]

The technique for isthmus division or resection (Fig. 23-3) is of importance in preventing the complications of fistula and hemorrhage.[22] Although some authors do not feel that nephropexy is needed, many feel that nephropexy should be accomplished if dissection of the ureter and pelvis is done (Fig. 23-4).

FIG. 23-3. Correction of a horseshoe kidney with right hydronephrosis secondary to ureteropelvic junction stenosis with high insertion. The isthmus blood supply is from the left iliac. **(A)** Incision is made around the capsule of the isthmus. **(B)** The capsule is peeled back. **(C)** The parenchyma of the isthmus is transected in a wedge fashion to facilitate closure. **(D)** Horizontal mattress sutures of absorbable 2-0 material are used to close the parenchyma for hemostasis. **(E)** The capsule is closed over the parenchyma with a continuous absorbable suture. **(F and G)** The contralateral side is handled in an identical fashion.

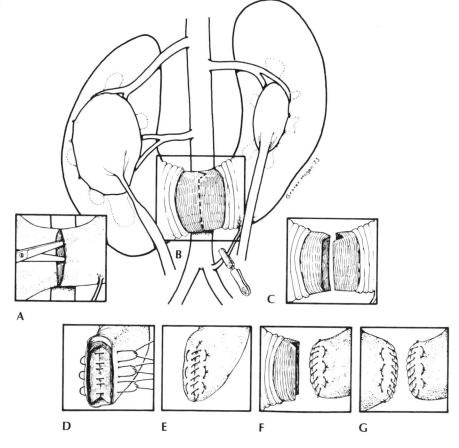

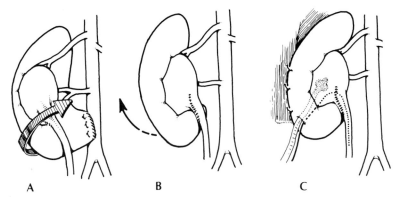

FIG. 23-4. Steps taken after those shown in Fig. 23-3 in correction of horseshoe kidney. (**A** and **B**) The pelvis is rotated medially and the lower pole is tilted laterally. (**C**) 2-0 or 3-0 absorbable mattress sutures are placed between the capsule and the lumbar musculature to secure the kidney to its new position. If pyeloplasty is performed, the ureteral stent or nephrostomy tube is in place.

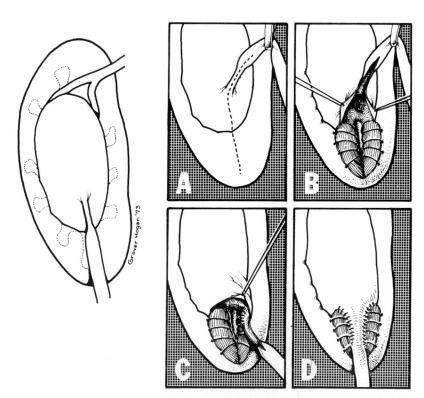

FIG. 23-5. Ureterocalicostomy for correction of ureteropelvic obstruction complicated by malrotation and a small extrarenal pelvis: (**A**) incision in the proximal ureter, through the stenotic junction to the end of the lower pole calix; (**B**) 2-0 absorbable sutures compressing the cut renal parenchyma; (**C**) the cut edges of the ureter sutured to the cut edges of the calix with 3-0 or 4-0 absorbable sutures; (**D**) completed closure. A nephrostomy tube or ureteral stent may be used.

ASSOCIATED ANOMALIES AND PROBLEMS

Patients with horseshoe kidneys appear to fall into two groups: those with serious associated anomalies and those with only non-life-threatening anomalies. Approximately one third of patients with horseshoe kidney will have an associated anomaly. The number of anomalies increase when autopsy series are reviewed. The organ systems commonly involved include the central nervous system, the cardiovascular system, the skeletal system, the gastrointestinal (especially anorectal) system, chromosomal aberrations (Turner's syndrome and trisomy 18 syndrome), and the urogenital system (ureteral duplication, vesicoureteral reflux, hypospadias, and others).[2,19,23] The multiple urogenital anomalies warrant a thorough urologic evaluation. The early use of surgical repair may decrease the morbidity of the symptomatic childhood case.[19]

Horseshoe kidney may be found in patients with abdominal aortic aneurysm. In those cases recognition and preservation of the often complicated and anomalous blood supply is of paramount importance. Division of the isthmus should be avoided, and, if technically necessary, resection of the isthmus is preferable.[3,9,20] Horseshoe kidneys have been transplanted in the divided state.[15,16]

FIG. 23-6. Reconstruction of a left pelvic kidney. **(A)** Hydroureteronephrosis and a redundant ureter are shown. **(B)** The ureter is mobilized and detached from the bladder, and the redundant length and width are excised. **(C)** The ureter has been tailored over an appropriate catheter and reimplanted into the bladder with a tunnel. **(D)** The procedure is completed with cystostomy, a ureteral stent, and nephrostomy in position.

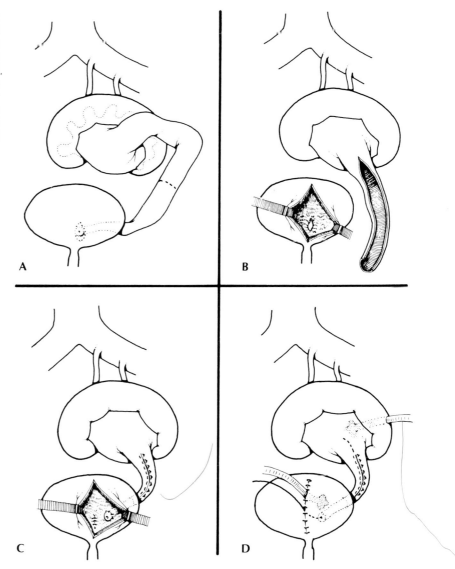

Renal Ectopia

Any mature kidney that is continually located in a position other than the renal or lumbar fossa is ectopic. Ectopia may occur as a solitary ectopic kidney or, if two renal units are present, as a unilateral or bilateral process. In crossed ectopia the ectopic renal parenchyma has its ureteral orifice on the contralateral trigone. If the parenchymas of both renal units are joined, a fused ectopia is present. Simple ectopia occurs more on the left and has an incidence of approximately 1:1000. The crossed ectopias, with and without fusion, are more rare and occur more in males, and the left renal unit is more commonly transposed.[17]

Associated anomalies are frequently seen in patients with ectopia. Genital anomalies are especially common (vaginal atresia, cryptorchidism, and hypospadias),[21] but one should also be aware of the numerous skeletal abnormalities and high incidence of imperforate anus.[17] Adult patients are usually asymptomatic or may have vague abdominal complaints which initiated evaluation.[17] Children often present with a mass, hydronephrosis, or infection.[6,13] All types of ectopia are associated with anomalous blood supply based on the principles previously discussed. Angiography is very helpful in anticipating surgery on the ectopic renal unit.

Ectopia is associated with a higher than normal incidence of hydronephrosis or calculus formation because of the abnormal pelvis or anomalous vasculature causing obstruction.[17] Thee ectopic kidney often differs radiographically from its contralateral mate because of abnormal rotation and extrarenal infundibula and calices.[7,8] Hendren and Donahoe have shown a high incidence of reflux.[13]

The diagnostic procedures described for horseshoe kidney are very helpful in evaluating the symptomatic case of ectopia. The use of voiding cystography is especially important in the child. The surgical indications are usually related to hydronephrosis (calculi or infection), reflux, or pathology which normally affects the kidney.

The most common surgical procedures in ectopic kidney include calculus removal, pyeloplasty, reflux correction, and nephrectomy.[8,13,22] The techniques for these procedures are described in Chapters 5, 14, and 21. Ureterocalicostomy instead of pyeloplasty has been used when the extrarenal pelvis is small or aberrant vasculature prevents adequate mobilization (Fig. 23-5).[22]

The solitary pelvic kidney and the discoid (lump or pancake) kidney may challenge the surgeon to preserve renal function. Extensive reconstruction of the drainage system may be required in lieu of nephrectomy (Fig. 23-6). The abnormal vasculature and absence of perinephric fat should be borne in mind.[13,22]

REFERENCES

1. BOATMAN DL, CORNELL SH, KOLIN CP: The arterial supply of horseshoe kidneys. Am J Roent 113, No. 3: 447, 1971
2. BOATMAN DL, KOLLN CP, FLOCKS RH: Congenital anomalies associated with horseshoe kidney. J Urol 107, No. 2:205, 1972
3. BROWN OW, DOSICK SM, BLAKEMORE WS: Abdominal aortic aneurysm and horseshoe kidney. Arch Surg 114:860, 1979
4. COOK WA, STEPHENS FD: Fused kidneys: Morpholgic study and theory of embryogenesis. Birth Defects XIII, No. 5:327, 1977
5. CULP OS, WINTERRINGER JR: Surgical treatment of horseshoe kidney: Comparison of results after various types of operations. J Urol 73:747, 1955
6. DONAHOE PK, HENDREN WH: Pelvic kidney in infants and children: Experience with 16 cases. J Pediatr Surg 15, No. 4:486, 1980
7. DRETLER SP, OLSON C, PFISTER RC: The anatomic radiologic and clinical charateristics of the pelvic kidney: An analysis of 86 cases. J Urol 105:623, 1971
8. DRETLER SP, PFISTER RC, HENDREN WH: Extrarenal calyces in the ectopic kidney. J Urol 103:406, 1970
9. EZZET F, DORAZIO R, HERZBERG R: Horseshoe and pelvic kidney associated with abdominal aortic aneurysms. Am J Surg 134:196, 1977
10. FRIEDLANDS GW, DEVRIES P: Renal ectopia and fusion. Urology 5:698, 1975
11. GLENN JF: Analysis of 51 patients with horseshoe kidney. N Engl J Med 261:684, 1959
12. GRAVES FT: Arterial anatomy of the congenitally abnormal kidney. Br J Surg 56:533, 1959
13. HENDREN WH, DONAHOE PK: Renal fusions and ectopia. In Ravitch MM, Welch KJ, Benson CD et al (eds): Pediatric Surgery, 3rd ed, p 1166. Chicago, Year Book Medical Publishers, 1979
14. KÖLLN CP, BOATMAN DL, SCHMIDT JD et al: Horseshoe kidney: A review of 105 patients. J Urol 107:203, 1972
15. MAJESKI JA et al: Transplantation of a horseshoe kidney. JAMA 242:1066, 1979
16. NELSON RP, PALMER JM: Use of horseshoe kidney in renal transplantation. Urology 6:357, 1975
17. PERLMUTTER AD, RETIK AB, BAUER SB: Anomalies of the upper urinary tract. In Harrison JH, Gittes RF, Perlmutter AD et al (eds): Campbell's Urology, 4th ed, p 1309. Philadelphia, W B Saunders, 1979
18. PITTS WR, MUECKE EC: Horseshoe kidneys: A 40-year experience. J Urol 113:743, 1975
19. SEGURA JW, KELALIS PP, BURKE EC: Horseshoe kidney in children. J Urol 108, No. 2:333, 1972
20. SIDELL PM, PAIROLERO PC, PAYNE WS et al: Horseshoe kidney associated with surgery of the abdominal aorta. Mayo Clin Proc 54:97, 1979
21. THOMPSON GJ, PACE JM: Ectopic kidney—A review of 97 cases. Surg Gynecol Obstet 64:935, 1937
22. WOODARD JR: Renal ectopia and fusion anomalies. In Glenn JF (ed): Urologic Surgery, 2nd ed, p 143. Hagerstown, Harper & Row, 1975
23. ZONDEK LH, ZONDEK T: Horseshoe kidney and associated congenital malformations. Urol Int 18:347, 1964

Renal Trauma

24

C. Eugene Carlton

The emergency room of the modern big-city general hospital provides a large and varied experience with all forms of trauma. In recent years, the development of sophisticated simultaneous multidisciplinary approaches to the rapid evaluation of the seriously injured patient has been responsible for a remarkable reduction in mortality and morbidity rates. This is particularly true of injury to the upper urinary tract. Properly applied, the diagnostic and therapeutic techniques described in this chapter can result in higher rates of renal salvage and restoration of functional normalcy than have heretofore been possible.

Most such injuries are caused by high-speed automobile accidents, auto–pedestrian accidents, falls, and a disturbingly common incidence of penetrating wounds due to knives, pistols, and shotguns. Many, if not most, of these injuries can be treated without surgery *provided* that in each instance a preliminary precise assessment of the nature and the extent of the injury justifies such nonsurgical management.

This chapter describes the mechanisms that produce renal injuries, the role of the diagnostic modalities useful in the delineation of the injuries, the indications for surgical and nonsurgical treatment, and the techniques of effective surgical treatment that have evolved from an extensive experience with such injuries.

Renal Vascular Injuries

PENETRATING INJURIES

Injuries of the renal artery and vein are most often the result of penetrating wounds of the abdomen. Guerriero and associates reviewed the experience in the Baylor College of Medicine affiliated hospitals with renal vascular injury; there were 43 injuries to the renal artery or vein in 33 patients.[8] The left renal vein was the most commonly injured vessel, a fact accounted for by its long length and exposed position traversing the midline. The left

renal vein crosses the aorta and is intimately associated with the superior mesenteric artery, splenic vein, and left renal artery. Multiple vascular injuries are therefore the rule rather than the exception in patients with penetrating wounds of the renal vessels.

Most patients with renal vascular injuries arrive in the emergency center in hypovolemic shock, requiring rapid and continuing efforts at resuscitation before they can be brought to the operating table. The patient's deteriorated state usually does not allow time for preoperative roentgenographic studies, but when feasible, high-dose infusion pyelography provides the assurance that there is a functioning contralateral kidney if subsequent findings dictate the need for nephrectomy.

These patients require immediate exploratory laparotomy for hemorrhage control. A midline xyphoid-to-pubis incision allows maximum speed and optimum exposure. Blood is cleared from the peritoneal cavity, and the bowel is brought out of the abdomen. The aorta is then exposed through an extended incision in the posterior parietal peritoneum, the hematoma is evacuated, and the bleeding vessels are occluded with noncrushing vascular clamps. Cross clamping the aorta and vena cava above and below the site of hemorrhage enables exact assessment of the extent and number of the vascular injuries in and about the renal pedicle.

The repair of renal pedicle injuries depends on the degree of blast effect present from the passage of the bullet (if the wound is so caused), the number of associated vascular injuries, the time allowed by the patient's condition that can be devoted to attempted salvage of a duplicated organ, and the nature of the vascular injury. Massive injury to the artery and vein with loss of most of their lengths is obviously best treated by nephrectomy. In many such cases, even if repair is immediately successful, most of the kidney has been ischemic long enough to make subsequent secondary nephrectomy almost certain.

Injuries to the left renal vein distal to the branch-

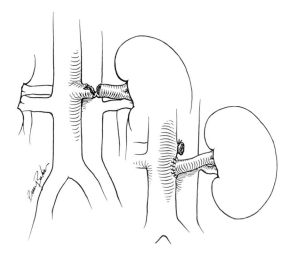

FIG. 24-1. Laceration of a renal vein treated by translocation of the vein to a new site on the vena cava

ing off of the adrenal and ovarian or testicular veins may be handled in the following manner. A clamp is placed proximal to the injured segment, and the kidney is observed. If the kidney does not swell markedly, it may be assumed that the ancillary veins will handle venous return from the kidney; thus, a simple ligation becomes the treatment of choice. If the kidney swells markedly, transposition of the left renal vein to a new site on the inferior vena cava is indicated (Fig. 24-1). Usually, enough vein length is available, especially with mobilization of the kidney, to enable this to be done without difficulty.

A simple laceration of the renal vein may be repaired using 5-0 or 6-0 arterial suture placed as a running suture. Excessive narrowing of the renal vein frequently is associated with renal vein thrombosis. In such an event, autologous vein may be used as a patch graft to increase the luminal diameter of the vessel. We prefer to use the inferior mesenteric vein or the saphenous vein for this purpose. In one of our cases, the spleen was sacrificed and the splenic vein was used to repair the injured renal vein. In our experience, injuries to the right renal vein and artery frequently result in nephrectomy. The lengths of the right renal vein and artery that are left after injury generally do not lend themselves to successful repair.

NONPENETRATING INJURIES

The renal artery may be injured by nonpenetrating trauma, usually through the contrecoup mechanism (Fig. 24-2A). This causes a marked stretching of the renal artery with a tear of the arterial intima, and a subsequent thrombosis of the renal artery (Fig. 24-2C). These renal arterial injuries are more frequent than commonly supposed; they usually occur in auto–pedestrian accidents, although they are sometimes seen with severe deceleration trauma, such as fall from heights, head-on automobile collision, and helicopter autorotation injuries.[2,4,8,9,13,14,15]

Any patient seen in an emergency center with a history of severe nonpenetrating abdominal or back trauma, auto–pedestrian injury, or severe deceleration injury should have immediate high-dose infusion urography. The failure of either one or of both kidneys to excrete the contrast medium should suggest the presence of an intimal thrombosis of the renal artery; immediate renal angiography should be performed for confirmation.

Successful reconstruction of renal artery injuries has been accomplished when the diagnosis of such arterial injury was made 9 days after injury. It should be emphasized that simple thrombectomy is inadequate in the treatment of these lesions, inasmuch as they are associated with intimal laceration and thrombus formation is a secondary phenomenon that inevitably recurs unless the injured intima is either excised or repaired. With injuries of limited extent, an arteriotomy may be done and the intima repaired. Usually, however, replacement of the injured segment with an autologous vein graft is the treatment of choice (Fig. 24-2D). In some instances, primary excision of the injured area with reanastomosis of the artery or anastomosis of the artery to a new location on the aorta is preferred (Fig. 24-2D).

Intravenous infusion of 25 g of mannitol before clamping the renal artery and flushing the kidney with cold heparinized Ringer's lactate solution before attempting repair may be of benefit in preventing subsequent small-vessel thrombosis and promoting renal survival. Autotransplantation has been performed at several institutions with fair results; it is particularly useful when it is important to remove the kidney from its original bed because of coexistent and proximate pancreatic injury or because of associated injury to the aorta or vena cava, which may compromise the repair of the renal vascular injury. It is not necessary to shorten the ureter or even modify the ureteral course in autotransplantation of this type, because ureteral dynamics remain intact if the ureter is left in its normal course.

Nonpenetrating Renal Injuries

In the immediate postinjury period, nonpenetrating renal injuries require classification regarding their location, number, and extent if they are to be placed in the proper treatment category that will yield maximum renal salvage. We are guided by the principle that primary healing of any injured tissue is more nearly ensured by early débridement, hemostasis, and primary repair before the onset of necrosis, infection, and urinary extravasation. We classify renal injuries as follows:

Contusion (Fig. 24-3*A*)

Minor cortical laceration is a laceration with or without interruption of the renal capsule and extending no deeper than the corticomedullary junction, and without urinary extravasation or the development of a large perirenal hematoma (Fig. 24-3*B*).

Major cortical laceration is a transcapsular laceration extending deeper than the corticomedullary junction and associated, in most instances, with urinary extravasation or the development of a large perirenal hematoma (Fig. 24-3*C*).

Multiple lacerations, even if minor, have a higher complication rate when treated nonsurgically than do single minor lacerations; we usually prefer to treat multiple lacerations surgically (Fig. 24-3*D* and *E*).

DIAGNOSIS

Any patient with hematuria of any degree after blunt trauma to the abdomen or flank imposes a responsibility for the exclusion of urinary tract injury. The absence of hematuria, however, should not exclude renal injury; 20% of patients with significant injury to the upper urinary tract do not have hematuria.[16]

Excretory urography using the high-dose infusion tomographic technique is indicated for any patient who has a history of blunt abdominal or flank trauma, especially if associated with any degree of hematuria or history of hematuria; any patient involved in an auto–pedestrian accident; any injured patient with unexplained ileus or abdominal pain; any patient with a penetrating abdominal wound; any patient with fractures of the lower ribs or transverse processes of the lumbar vertebrae; and any patient who has a flank mass or costovertebral angle tenderness after trauma. We agree with others that high-dose infusion nephrotomography should be the initial diagnostic study.[6,10,13,18,19] Standard excretory urography is of limited usefulness in the assessment of the traumatized kidney. Such a kidney often does not excrete contrast medium in sufficient concentration to enable the clear delineation of the extent of injury. Most often, its use results in a loss of valuable time and the need to repeat further roent-

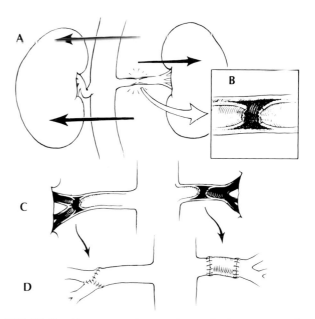

FIG. 24-2.   Nonpenetrating renal vascular injury.   **(A)** The contrecoup mechanism of marked stretching of the renal artery with laceration of the arterial intima.   **(B)** Arterial thrombus secondary to laceration of the intima.   **(C** and **D)** Common location of intimal laceration and techniques of repair.

genographic studies. In most instances, nephrotomography enables categorization of the patient into one of the preceding classifications of extent of renal injury.

Most patients with renal injuries have only a parenchymal contusion. In such injuries, nephrotomography can demonstrate sharp renal outlines without extravasation or renal laceration. Parenchymal lacerations are seen as negative defects in the brightly opacified renal parenchyma during the nephrographic phase of infusion nephrotomography. Urinary extravasation then may be seen during the excretory phase. The extent of the perirenal hematoma is that part of the retroperitoneal mass minus the dye-stained renal parenchyma.

Nephrotomography enables the proper assessment of the extent of injury in most patients. In some instances, the differentiation between major and minor injury cannot be made on the basis of nephrotomography alone; renal angiography is indicated in these cases. Selective renal arteriography is the most definitive diagnositc study available for the precise delineation of the location and extent of renal injury.[11,12] Its usefulness is such that it should be performed in any patient when there is nonvisualization of the kidney on the excretory study or when the nephrotomogram does not clearly define the extent of renal injury.

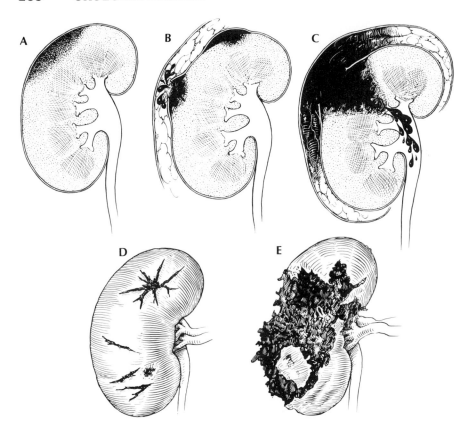

FIG. 24-3. Classification of the extent of renal injury: **(A)** contusion of the parenchyma, **(B)** minor laceration, **(C)** major laceration, **(D)** multiple laceration, **(E)** macerated kidney

Radioisotope renography in our experience has not proved to be as precise a diagnostic tool as roentgenography, but in most instances it enables the patient to be classified into the major and minor renal injury categories. It is particularly useful in patients allergic to contrast material.

Renal sonography, in many instances, demonstrates major renal lacerations quite clearly and is a useful adjunct in patients allergic to contrast material. This study, however, does not give the precise anatomic detail needed by the surgeon planning definitive repair of a major renal injury.

TREATMENT

Precise classification of the location and extent of renal injury is basic to planning treatment. Renal contusions and minor lacerations make up 85% of blunt renal injuries and can be treated conservatively with few complications. Most complications from the nonsurgical treatment of renal injury occur in the 15% of patients with major renal lacerations.

It is my opinion that renal contusion needs no treatment, and the patient may be allowed to return to normal activity as soon as recovery from associated injuries permits.

Minor cortical lacerations should be treated with bed rest, broad-spectrum antibiotics, and careful observation for secondary hemorrhage. Inasmuch as these lacerations heal secondarily, it is important that activity be limited for at least 14 to 21 days to enable the absorption of hematoma and fibroblastic proliferation across the defect in the parenchyma.

Major cortical lacerations, in our experience as well as that of others are associated with a high incidence of secondary hemorrhage, infection with abscess formation in the perirenal hematoma, pyelonephritic atrophy, and renal hypertension.[1,3,7] Early surgical repair of the injuries has, in our experience, resulted in a marked lowering of these complications and remarkably improved long-term renal salvage. The earlier in the postinjury phase this definitive surgical repair can be carried out, the easier the repair is technically and therefore the better the results are. Most of our patients with major renal injury undergo immediate surgical repair.

Technique

The peritoneal cavity is entered through a xyphoid-to-pubis midline incision, and the intraperitoneal viscera are inspected for injuries. The patient is

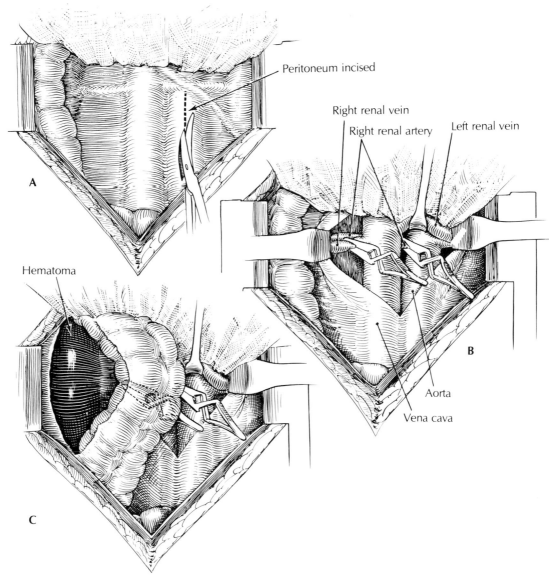

FIG. 24-4. Surgical approach to the injured kidney: **(A)** incision in the parietal peritoneum over the aorta; **(B)** exposure of the renal arteries and application of vascular clamps; **(C)** incision in the colic gutter to expose the hematoma within Gerota's fascia

then eviscerated, and an incision is made in the posterior parietal peritoneum over the aorta (Fig. 24-4*A*). This dissection is carried superiorly to expose the left renal vein, which is mobilized by sharp dissection, and retracted superiorly to expose the origins of both renal arteries from the aorta (Fig. 24-4*B*). The appropriate renal artery is mobilized by sharp dissection. A vascular tape is passed around the artery, and it is then occluded with a noncrushing vascular bulldog clamp (Fig. 24-4*C*). The appropriate renal vein is similarly occluded with a noncrushing vascular clamp. Early occlusion of the renal artery and vein is of paramount importance in the surgical repair of renal injury. It

prevents the massive hemorrhage that otherwise frequently occurs upon release of the perirenal tamponade with incision of Gerota's fascia. Attention can then be turned to the evacuation of the perirenal hematoma, the assessment of the renal injury, and the planning of its repair in a surgical field free of active renal bleeding. Certain basic principles must be kept in mind in the repair of renal injury:

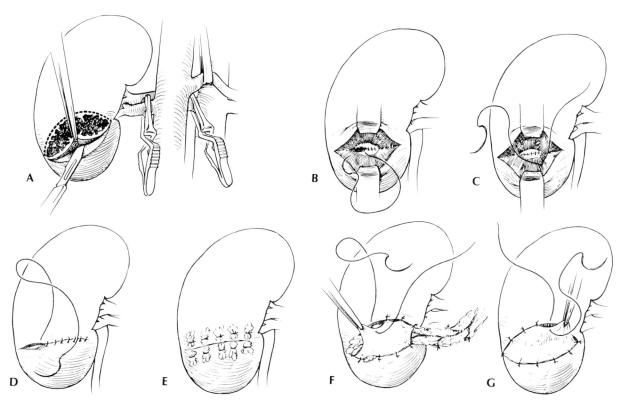

FIG. 24-5. Technique of repair of renal laceration: **(A)** débridement of the injured parenchyma; **(B)** watertight closure of the collecting system; **(C)** hemostasis with figure-of-eight sutures; **(D)** primary approximation of the superficial defect; **(E)** primary closure of the deep laceration with mattress sutures; **(F)** the large defect filled with omentum and covered with a peritoneal patch; **(G)** the denuded parenchyma covered with a patch of peritoneum

Débridement of all devitalized renal parenchyma

Meticulous hemostasis

Watertight closure of the collecting system

Primary approximation of the debrided margins or obliteration of dead space with viable tissue such as omentum or perirenal fat.

Devitalized renal parenchyma is excised by sharp-knife incision into the renal parenchyma until all torn, bruised, and ischemic renal parenchyma is excised (Fig. 24-5A). Hemostasis is achieved by individual suture ligation of the interlobar and interlobular renal arteries and veins using 4-0 chromic catgut figure-of-eight sutures (see Fig. 24-5C). After all visible vessels have been suture-ligated, venous and then arterial clamps may be released to ensure that hemostasis has been achieved. The collecting system is closed with a running suture of 4-0 or 5-0 chromic catgut to effect a watertight closure (Fig. 24-5B).

If the debrided margins of the renal parenchyma are not widely separated, primary reapproximation of the renal parenchyma may be achieved by a simple running 3-0 catgut suture in the capsule and parenchymal margins (Fig. 24-5D), or by mattress sutures of 3-0 chromic catgut tied over fat bolsters (Fig. 24-5E). The renal capsule should be resutured over the laceration, but if too much of the renal capsule has been lost, capsular integrity can be reestablished using a free graft of peritoneum (see Fig. 24-5G).

When the defect is of such magnitude as to obviate primary reapproximation, the defect should be filled with a pedicle of live fat using omentum or perirenal fat in order to obliterate dead space. Again, capsular integrity should be reestablished over the defect (Fig. 24-5F).

In instances of major lacerations of either pole of the kidney, guillotine amputation of the injured portion of the pole of the kidney is a rapid and effective means of treating renal injury. Prior to guillotine amputation of the polar portion of the kidney, the capsule is retracted for subsequent reapproximation over the amputated pole of the kidney (Fig. 24-6A). Hemostasis and collecting system closure is accomplished as previously described (Fig. 24-6B), and the capsule is reapproxi-

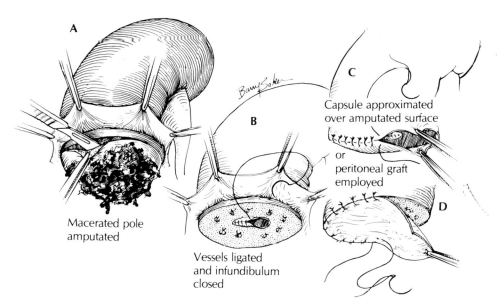

FIG. 24-6. Technique of surgical repair of a major polar injury: **(A)** reaction of capsule and débridement of the injured parenchyma; **(B)** hemostasis and closure of the collecting system; **(C)** reapproximation of the capsule; **(D)** the denuded surface covered with a peritoneal graft

mated over the denuded pole of the kidney (Fig. 24-6C). If there is not adequate capsule remaining to cover the denuded area, it may be covered with a peritoneal graft (Fig. 24-6D).

Gerota's fascia is carefully reapproximated to prevent adhesions of the kidney to the flank muscles or peritoneum, and a retroperitoneal Penrose drain is brought through a flank stab wound and left in place for 10 to 14 days. It is necessary to leave the drain in for this prolonged period because of the potential hazard of secondary hemorrhage or late urinary leak at the site of closure.

Postoperative Care

Broad-spectrum antibiotics are used in patients with penetrating wounds or in patients in whom there has been obvious contamination by intestinal leakage. It has not been our practice to use antibiotics routinely in the surgically treated noncontaminated blunt renal injuries because of the débridement of the devitalized tissue and the evacuation of hematoma, which is an integral part of this surgical treatment of renal injuries. Excretory urography approximately 4 weeks after injury documents the functional integrity of the repaired kidney. Urine cultures are obtained at weekly intervals during the first 6 weeks following repair of the injury because of the propensity of the traumatized kidney to the development of pyelonephritis. Obviously, any urinary infection should be treated vigorously and over a prolonged period.

Careful monitoring of the patient's blood pressure is mandatory during the first year after injury.[5,7] Although renal hypertension in the surgically repaired kidney has not occurred in our series of patients, it has been fairly common after nonsurgical treatment of significant renal injury.

Penetrating Renal Injuries

Review of our experience with over 3000 penetrating wounds of the abdomen reveals that 11% of gunshot wounds have significant renal injury and 6% of stab wounds are associated with injury to the kidney. Conversely, at least 80% of patients with penetrating renal injuries have associated intra-abdominal injury requiring surgical treatment.[17] For this reason, we believe that all patients with a penetrating renal injury should be subjected to exploratory laparotomy. Inasmuch as surgical exploration will be carrier out, it is of less importance in penetrating injury to delineate precisely the extent of renal injury beforehand, because this can be done on the operating table. Whenever the patient's condition permits, however, preoperative excretory urography should be used to demonstrate the functional integrity of the contralateral kidney, should subsequent findings dictate intra-operative nephrectomy.

All penetrating injuries, even minor lacerations, should be debrided and primarily closed for several reasons. First, the patient has already been subjected to surgical exploration; therefore, he should have the benefits of primary treatment of his renal injury. Second, because of the invariable penetration of the perirenal fascia, the injury may not be tamponaded as in nonpenetrating renal injury, and the incidence of secondary bleeding will be higher. Third, penetrating injuries are contaminated; and if a contaminated hematoma is left undrained or if ischemic or necrotic renal parenchyma is left *in situ*, the incidence of infection is extremely high.

The techniques of surgery are as described previously, with the exception that it may not be necessary to achieve primary control of the renal pedicle if only a small hematoma without active bleeding is found at the time of exploration.

REFERENCES

1. CASS AS, IRELAND GW: Comparison of the conservative and surgical management of the more severe degrees of renal trauma in multiple injured patients. J Urol 109:8, 1973
2. CORNELL SH, REASA DA, CULP DA: Occlusion of the renal artery secondary to acute or remote trauma. JAMA 219:1754, 1972
3. DEL VILLAR RG, IRELAND GW, CASS AS: Management of renal injury in conjunction with the immediate surgical treatment of the acute severe trauma patient. J Urol 107:208, 1972
4. EVANS A, MOGG RA: Renal artery thrombosis due to closed trauma. Trans Am Assoc Genitourin Surg 62:40, 1970
5. GLENN JF, HARVARD BM: The injured kidney. JAMA 173:1189, 1960
6. GOLDMAN HS, FREEMAN LM: Radiographic and radioisotopic methods of evaluation of the kidneys and urinary tract. Pediatr Clin North Am 18:409, 1971
7. GRAND RP, JR, GIFFORD RW, JR, PUDVAN WR et al: Renal trauma and hypertension. Am J Cardiol 27:173, 1971
8. GUERRIERO WG, CARLTON CE, JR, SCOTT R, JR et al: Renal pedicle injuries. J Trauma 11:53, 1971
9. JEVTICH MJ, MONTERO GG: Injuries to renal vessels by blunt trauma in children. J Urol 102:493, 1969
10. KRAHN HP, AXENROD H: The management of severe renal lacerations. J Urol 109:11, 1973
11. LANG EK, TRICHEL BE, TURNER RW: Arteriographic assessment of injury resulting from renal trauma. An analysis of 74 patients. J Urol 106:1, 1971
12. LANG EK, TRICHEL BE, TURNER RW et al: Renal arteriography in the assessment of renal trauma. Radiology 98:103, 1971
13. LEANDOER JL, TREMANN JA, OISHI RH et al: Bilateral renal artery thrombosis following blunt trauma: Report of two cases. J Trauma 12:166, 1972
14. PRINCE JC, PEARLMAN CK: Thrombosis of the renal artery secondary to trauma. J Urol 102:670, 1969
15. ROSS R, JR, ACKERMAN E, PIERCE JM, JR: Traumatic subintimal hemorrhage of the renal artery. J Urol 104:11, 1970
16. SCOTT R, JR, CARLTON CE, JR, ASHMORE AJ et al: Initial management of non-penetrating renal injuries: Clinical review of 111 cases. J Urol 90:535, 1963
17. SCOTT R, JR, CARLTON CE, JR, GOLDMAN M: Penetrating injuries of the kidney: An analysis of 181 patients. Trans Am Assoc Genitourin Surg 60:168, 1968
18. SMALLEY RH, BANOWSKY LH: Evaluation of renal trauma by infusion urography. J Urol 105:620, 1971
19. WATERHOUSE K, GROSS M: Trauma to the genitourinary tract: A 5-year experience with 251 cases. Trans Am Assoc Genitourin Surg 60:162, 1968

Renovascular Disorders

25

Joseph J. Kaufman

enovascular disorders to be discussed in this chapter include renal artery stenosis and renovascular hypertension, renal artery aneurysm, arteriovenous fistula, renal artery embolism, and renal vein thrombosis.

Renal Artery Stenosis and Renovascular Hypertension

Between 5% and 15% of the hypertensive population has renovascular disease.[83] This statement implies that more than 12 million persons in the United States have this condition. With improving means of establishing the diagnosis and predictability of cure by medical, surgical, or radiologic methods, there is great promise for the recognition and successful treatment of renovascular hypertension.

HISTORICAL ASPECTS

The relationship between renal disease and hypertension has been recognized for centuries. It is difficult to credit all the investigators who established a cause-and-effect relationship between renal disease and high blood pressure, but a few signal contributions deserve mention. Tigerstedt and Bergman in 1898 coined the term "renin" to describe a substance in kidney extract of rabbits that caused hypertension when injected into other rabbits.[89] Goldblatt and associates in 1934 proved experimentally that hypertension could be caused by partial clamping of the main renal artery of the dog.[31] Goldblatt, however, had no prescience that such constrictions of the renal artery occurred frequently in man as an experiment of nature. It was quickly recognized in the years following Goldblatt's remarkable discovery that hypertension in human subjects could be relieved by nephrectomy. The first documented case of hypertension cured by removal of a kidney was reported by Butler in 1937.[8] More clinical evidence of the curability of hypertension caused by renal or renovascular disease was reported in 1938 by Barker

and Walters, Boyd and Lewis, Freeman and Hartley, and Leadbetter and Burkland.[2,7,25,57]

Freeman and associates described the first case of hypertension cured by corrective renovascular surgery in 1954.[26] The operation consisted of thromboendarterectomy from above the renal arteries to the bifurcation of the common iliac arteries. On the heels of Freeman, a number of surgeons reported the surgical correction of hypertension by renovascular repair. In 1955 Ellis reimplanted the renal artery into the aorta.[17] Hurwitt in 1956 performed the first splenorenal anastomosis, and Poutasse, also in 1956, performed the first successful bilateral renal artery homograft.[42,77] One of the largest experiences in the treatment of renovascular hypertension was reported in 1960 by Morris, who popularized bypass grafts.[69]

PATHOLOGY

Two diseases, atherosclerosis and fibrous dysplasia, account for approximately 90% of all renal artery lesions. A number of less common diseases comprise the remaining 10%. Some of the lesions documented to cause human renovascular hypertension are listed in Table 25-1.

Atherosclerosis

Atherosclerosis is recognized as the most common arterial disease in human beings and the most common cause of renovascular hypertension. It has a predilection for affecting the proximal third of the main renal artery and its ostium (Fig. 25-1). Pathologically the affected segment shows eccentric or concentric intimal plaques which contain varying amounts of cholesterol, collagen, and calcium. Two thirds of renal artery lesions are caused by atherosclerosis. The left renal artery is more commonly involved than the right, and men are affected more often than women by a ratio of approximately 2:1.[21,64] Lesions are bilateral in approximately one third of patients, but one side is nearly always more severely diseased than the other.

TABLE 25-1. Etiologies of Renovascular Hypertension

Common lesions
    Atherosclerosis
    Fibromuscular diseases
        Fibromuscular dysplasia of the media
        Subadventitial fibroplasia
        Intimal fibroplasia

Uncommon lesions (intrinsic)
    Aneurysm
    Arteriovenous fistula
    Arteritis
    Embolism or thrombosis
    Arterial hypoplasia
    Neurofibromatosis
    Transplant rejection endarteritis with or without fibrosis
    Renal-splanchnic steal secondary to celiac artery stenosis
    Trauma with intimal dissection

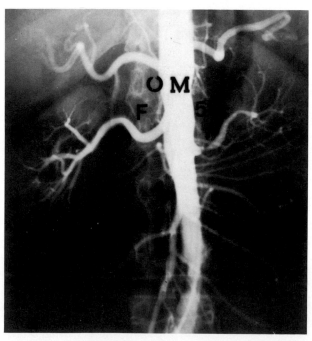

FIG. 25-1. An arteriogram shows an atherosclerotic stenosing lesion of the left renal artery in a 58-year-old woman. The stenosis involves the first portion of the renal artery. (See also Fig. 25-17.)

Complications related to atherosclerosis of the renal artery include thrombosis, aneurysm formation, and occasionally intimal dissection. Without operative intervention, progression of the disease can be expected in one third to one half of patients, but the time interval is quite variable.[67,92]

Fibrous Dysplasia

Fibrous dysplasia of the renal artery, also termed fibromuscular dysplasia, is the next common stenosing lesion of the renal arteries. This group of diseases is still poorly understood, particularly from the standpoint of their etiology. Our own view is that they probably represent the healing of variant forms of arteritis affecting the intima, subintima, media, or adventitia respectively. Medial fibroplasia is the most common variety of the disease and accounts for approximately 80% of all cases. Women, usually 20 to 50 years of age, are affected more often than men by a ratio of 4:1 or 5:1.[64,81,84] The disease is frequently bilateral, but, as a rule, the right side is more severely affected than the left. Arteriographically, the lesions are often long and multifocal with alternating stenotic and aneurysmal segments, producing the characteristic "string of beads" appearance (Fig. 25-2). Bilateral involvement of the renal arteries, although not necessarily symmetrical, occurs in approximately 35% of patients. Lesions most often involve the middle and distal thirds of the main renal artery, and branches are involved in approximately 45% of these cases (Fig. 25-3).

Histologically, the lesions show fibrous replacement of the media, disorientation of the smooth muscle fibers, and destruction and duplication of the internal elastic membrane.[60] There is conflicting information relative to the progression of this disease. It is generally believed that after the age of 35, progression is either slow or nonexistent, although we have encountered a number of patients with fibrous dysplasia of the renal arteries who subsequently developed atherosclerotic plaques in addition. The chief complication of the process is mural dissection and aneurysm formation (Fig. 25-4).[53,75]

Subadventitial fibroplasia, also termed periarterial fibroplasia, accounts for approximately 10% to 15% of lesions in this category. The disease occurs primarily in the right renal artery of young or middle-aged women and usually affects the distal half of the vessel. The stenoses tend to be tubular and affect shorter arterial segments than in the case with medial fibroplasia (Fig. 25-5). Aneurysms are rare. Histologically, dense collagen is present under the adventitia. The internal elastic membrane remains intact. The disease usually produces severe degrees of stenosis and is often rapidly progressive.[81,86]

Intimal fibroplasia is the least common of the three major forms of fibrous dysplasia and accounts for approximately 5% to 10%. The lesions appear

FIG. 25-2. Medial fibroplasia on a selective right renal arteriogram showing characteristic alternating segments of dilatation and stenosis

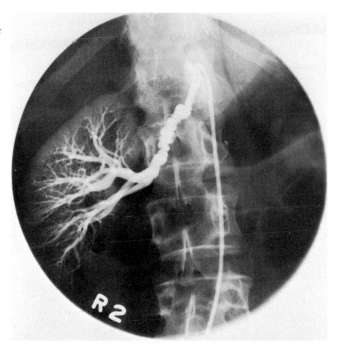

FIG. 25-3. An arteriogram shows medial fibroplasia affecting the distal half of the right renal artery and involving the primary branches.

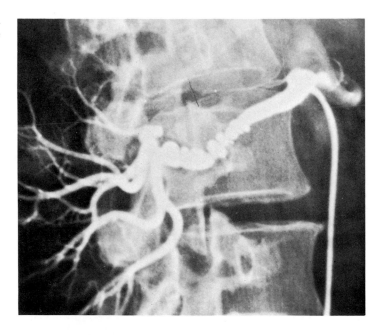

as short or long tubular stenoses arteriographically (Fig. 25-6) and affect the right and left arteries of young men and women alike. Histologically, collagenous tissue is seen inside the internal elastic membrane. Mural dissection is fairly frequent in this entity, and the disease progresses rather predictably.[81,86]

Because no clear-cut unitary etiology of fibrosing lesions of renal arteries has yet been established,

and because the lesions are not dissimilar from stenosing lesions of the main renal artery seen in kidney transplant recipients,[82] an immune pathogenesis is an attractive explanation. Positive immunofluorescence with staining for immunoglobulins IgG and IgM and C_3 nephritic factor has been found in the arteries of rejecting renal transplants.[82] Our group has also demonstrated immunochemical reactants in several resected arteries affected by

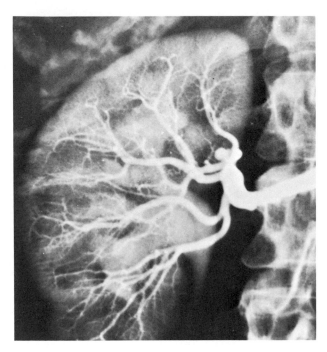

FIG. 25-4. Medial fibroplasia with stenotic changes in main renal artery and small aneurysm of one of the main branches.

FIG. 25-5. A selective right renal arteriogram shows periarterial fibrosis.

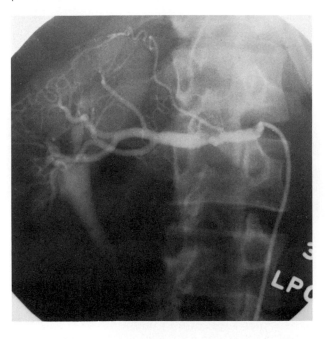

fibromuscular dysplasia.[14] The precise antigenic agent has not been identified, but the natural history of the disease suggests that viral or bacterial infections may produce an arteritis during a febrile illness. Months or years later, in the healed phase, fibrous tissue in the subintimal, medial, or subadvential layers may be responsible for stenosis.

Arteritis (Takayasu's Disease)

Takayasu's arteritis is an inflammation of undetermined etiology affecting the aorta and its primary branches. It is generally accepted to be a disease in two phases. The first phase consists of fever, arthralgia, anorexia, and, less frequently, headache, neck, or chest pain, carotid tenderness, and cardiomyopathy. Many patients have an insidious onset with no symptoms recalled. The second phase of the disease is the obstructive phase and is characterized by both stenoses and aneurysmal dilatation of the aorta or major arteries.[43,87] Although the sedimentation rate is often elevated in the early phases of the disease, it tends to return to normal later on. Nonspecific autoimmune investigation (rheumatoid factor, antinuclear antibodies, LE [lupus erythematosus] factor) has not uncovered a clear mechanism. Association between tuberculosis and Takayasu's arteritis has been suggested by several authors, and this, in fact, may be valid in those countries where tuberculosis is common.[76] However, our own series of cases of arteritis has failed to impugn tuberculosis as an etiologic agent. Rather, we submit that tuberculosis may be one of several antigenic stimuli for the development of arteritis.

Figure 25-7 demonstrates a typical case of the middle aortic syndrome with renal artery involvement, and Figure 25-8 illustrates arteritis narrowing the renal vasculature but without aortic involvement. Although Takayasu's arteritis commonly implies involvement of the aorta with or without involvement of other arteries, we believe that a spectrum of arteritides is more likely.

Neurofibromatosis

Visceral neurofibromatosis is receiving greater recognition as a cause of renal artery disease. Neurofibromatosis is a hereditary disorder of ectodermal origin, described originally by von Recklinghausen in 1882.[91] It is characterized by *café au lait* spots, cutaneous fibromas, and neurofibromas. An association of pheochromocytoma with neurofibromatosis has been clearly established.[30] In recent years, neurofibromatosis has been found to be associated with a variety of vascular lesions involving the renal arteries. In 1965 Halpern and

Currarino found reports of eight cases of renovascular hypertension in patients with neurofibromatosis and added two additional cases.[36] Our own experience now includes 12 patients varying in age from 19 months to 35 years with a variety of vascular deformities, including aneurysms and stenoses (Fig. 25-9).

The vascular lesions of neurofibromatosis can be divided into three types: an intimal form consisting of endothelial proliferation in concentric layers; an intimal and aneurysmal form which produces thickening of the intimal layer of the vessel, atrophy of the media, and disruption of the wall eventually leading to aneurysms; and a nodular form which consists of cellular nodules located in the wall of the vessel. The vessels may show long areas of stenosis, and the aorta itself is frequently involved.[32]

PATHOPHYSIOLOGY

It is now well established that renin release from the kidney is the initiating event in the biochemical chain reaction leading to hypertension. Renin is released in response either to baroreceptor stimulation, a sodium-sensing mechanism, or to neurogenic factors, but even today there is question regarding the precise sensor. There is no question that the juxtaglomerular apparatus causes renin release. Whatever the definitive stimulus for its release, renin hydrolyzes an alpha-2 globulin produced by the liver to form angiotensin I. Angiotensin I is a decapeptide with no significant vasoactive properties. It circulates through the pulmonary circulation, where it is acted upon by a converting enzyme which cleaves the decapeptide into a dipeptide and an octapeptide, angiotensin II. Angiotensin II is an extremely potent vasoconstrictor and causes hypertension as a result of this action. It also is a major stimulus for the release of aldosterone from the adrenal cortex. Aldosterone, in turn, promotes water and salt retention by the kidney(s), and this volume expansion phenomenon adds another dimension to the genesis of hypertension. This, of course, is an exquisite example of a feedback mechanism to restore homeostasis in the ischemic kidney in a futile attempt to turn off renin release. Unfortunately, the hypertension effects on the opposite kidney, the heart, and the brain are "unwittingly" misdirected.

DIAGNOSTIC METHODS

Clinical Features

No clinical features have been found to be reliable and discriminatory. It is recognized that renovas-

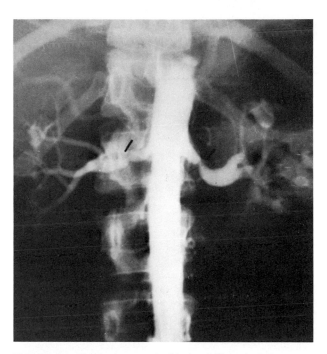

FIG. 25-6. Single stenoses (subintimal fibroplasia) are seen in the midportion of both renal arteries in this arteriogram.

cular hypertension is more likely to appear in young individuals, or in adults at a later age than is customary with essential hypertension. In the Cooperative Study of Renovascular Hypertension (CSRH), 2442 patients were evaluated, of whom 39% with atherosclerotic lesions of the renal artery had a late onset of hypertension (*i.e.*, after the age of 50), in contrast to only 17% of patients with essential hypertension whose onset of their disease occurred after middle age.[83] Patients who have a recent unexplained worsening of symptoms associated with previously benign hypertension deserve special consideration. Also, patients whose histories contain unexplained abdominal or flank pain or suggest the possibility of a renovascular accident such as renal trauma, or peripheral arterial emboli should be considered likely candidates to have renovascular hypertension.

The aforementioned criteria may be succinctly summarized as "inappropriate hypertension." A significant portion of patients with proved renal arterial hypertension fail to fulfill any of these criteria, and it is apparent that secondary hypertension may simulate essential hypertension in every respect. However, a recent publication by Davis and associates stated that malignant hypertension should alert the physician to the possibility of a renovascular cause.[12] They found a 31% incidence of renovascular hypertension in a study of

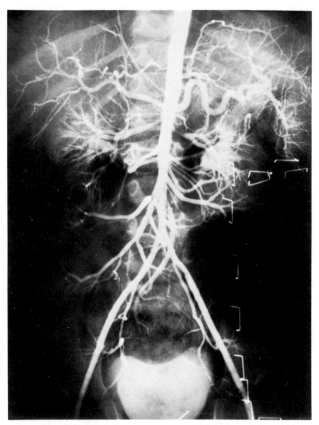

FIG. 25-7. An arteriogram shows middle aortic syndrome with narrowing of the aorta, both renal arteries, and a branch of the superior mesenteric artery.

123 patients with malignant or accelerated hypertension. On the basis of this high incidence, they propose that the hypertensive population is *not* uniform and that appropriate strategy for detecting renovascular disease should be based on a stratification of the hypertensive population according to the severity of the disease. The best diagnostic sign in their hands was Grade III or IV retinopathy.

Intravenous Urography

Despite the denigration of the intravenous urogram as a discriminatory test for renovascular hypertension, it is still one of the mainstays in the diagnosis, in our view. Rapid-sequence intravenous pyelography (IVP) is most widely used with minute sequence films for the first 5 minutes following the bolus administration of contrast material. Urographically, the major features of renal artery stenosis are decreased renal length, which reflects diminished intrarenal blood volume; delayed appearance of contrast material in the calices, which reflects a diminished glomerular filtration rate;

vascular impressions on the ureter or pelvis, suggesting collateral blood supply; atrophy of a portion of the kidney, suggesting segmental ischemia or infarct; and late hyperconcentration of contrast in the collecting system, reflecting an increased fractional reabsorption of salt and water. From CSRH, the rapid-sequence IVP was found to be positive in 83% of patients with significant unilateral renal artery stenosis and in 11% of patients with essential hypertension.[6] There were false-negative tests in 17% of patients with renovascular hypertension. In bilateral renovascular disease, the rapid-sequence IVP was positive in only 61% of patients. In light of the high incidence of false-negative tests, the IVP alone cannot reliably serve to exclude a diagnosis of renovascular hypertension.

Radioactive Renography

Analysis of the CSRH data, using a computer technique that analyzed seven variables simultaneously, indicated that 76% of patients with greater than 50% stenosis on renal arteriography had an abnormal renogram.[23,52] However, no characteristic pattern has yet been found to differentiate renovascular lesions from parenchymal disease, and it is clear that there is an even greater incidence of false-positive renograms in patients with essential hypertension than of false-negative IVPs. For this reason, the renal scan or renogram must be placed in the same category with IVPs as useful, relatively inexpensive, and safe methods of defining those patients who are most likely to benefit from more sophisticated investigational studies. Eventually, isotopic techniques may allow noninvasive determination of individual renal plasma flow and glomerular filtration rate.[20] Should this potential be realized, the value of the renal scan and renogram would be increased enormously.

Peripheral Renin Determination

Unfortunately, renin determination is not a good screening test for renovascular hypertension. In a recent review, Marks and Maxwell found that only 56% of documented cases of renovascular hypertension were associated with hyperreninemia, confirming that the incidence of false-negative tests is appreciable.[61] Moreover, at least 15% of patients with essential hypertension demonstrated elevated peripheral renin levels. Thus, hyperreninemia *per se* is neither sensitive nor specific for renovascular hypertension.

Angiotensin Blockade and Converting-Enzyme Inhibition

Recently a specific blocker of angiotensin II became available. The new compound, saralasin (1-SAR-

FIG. 25-8. An arteriogram shows an isolated left renal artery stenosis in a 6-year-old boy found following a severe upper respiratory infection. The arteritis has spared the aorta in this case.

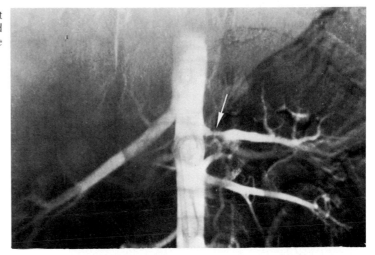

8-ALA-angiotensin II), binds to the angiotensin receptor sites and acts as a competitive inhibitor to prevent many of the usual actions of angiotensin II. Because of the specificity of the compound, a blood-pressure-lowering effect after saralasin administration indicates the presence of renin-mediated or angiotensin-dependent hypertension. The drug is administered intravenously by bolus injection or sustained infusion. If the patient has renin-mediated hypertension, the blood pressure falls often to near-normal levels within minutes after administration of the agent.[40,62,88] This must be done with the following caveats: avoidance of concomitant medication, mild rather than severe salt depletion, and a stable elevated blood pressure at the time of the test. When these conditions are present, the great majority of patients with renovascular hypertension (90%–95%) exhibit a definite vasodepressor response to saralasin. Approximately 15% of essential hypertension patients (those with high renin) also show such responses.[38]

Converting-enzyme inhibitors (CEIs) that block the formation of angiotensin II from angiotensin I hold promise of having usefulness as a diagnostic test. Parenteral teprotide (SQ 20881) and oral captopril (SQ 14225) will produce a fall in blood pressure and may have diagnostic usefulness as well.[9] Because the angiotensin-converting enzyme is identical to kininase II, captopril and teprotide may produce an increase in circulating bradykinin as well as a decrease in angiotensin II formation.

Angiography

Not all renal artery stenoses can be implicated as causing hypertension. This situation is obvious from the studies of Eyler and associates and Holley and associates.[19,39] In general, a focal stenosis is

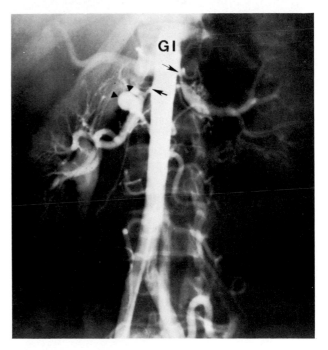

FIG. 25-9. An arteriogram shows neurofibromatosis affecting the renal arteries. An aneurysm of the right renal artery and stenosis of the left renal artery are seen. The superior mesenteric artery was also involved in this case.

most likely to cause renovascular hypertension when the lumen diameter is reduced by at least 50%. This corresponds to a cross-sectional area reduction of approximately 80%.[5] Multifocal stenoses alternating with dilatations (as in forms of fibromuscular dysplasia) may severely reduce renal blood flow, even when the stenoses appear to be relatively slight on arteriography.

"Eyeballing" the arteriogram is a poor way of

predicting the results from surgery or angioplasty. In CSRH an analysis of renal angiograms in 502 patients who underwent nephrectomy or reconstructive surgery revealed that the presence of collateral circulation was of no significant value in predicting the success or failure of surgery, nor did the presence or absence of poststenotic dilatation show a correlation with surgical results.[4]

On the horizon are computerized intravenous angiographic and angiotomographic methods (digital subtraction angiography) that appear to be promising and are less invasive than the transfemoral or transaxillary catheterization techniques currently employed.

Renal Vein Renin Determination

The concept of direct sampling of renal venous blood in hypertensive patients was established in the mid-1960s by the work of Judson and Helmer.[44] These investigators found that, in their patients with renovascular hypertension, renin levels in blood from the ischemic kidney were at least twice as high as renin levels in blood from the contralateral kidney. The concept of lateralization of renin secretion was introduced. Following this discovery, many similar investigations substantiated the finding.

In a comprehensive review of the literature, we found that, in hypertensive patients with unilateral stenosis of the main renal artery, lateralization of renin secretion to the underperfused kidney was associated with a 93% cure or improvement rate after revascularization or nephrectomy.[61] In patients with nonlateralizing renal vein renin determinations, the prognostic value is not great, because 50% of test results were false-negative. Misleading renal vein renin results may be associated with atypical renal or renovascular lesions, inaccurate renal catheter placement, inactive or declining renal secretion, or problems in the renin laboratory.[33] Our most recent experience indicates that renal vein rein ratio (ipsilateral/contralateral greater than 1.5) together with contralateral suppression (contralateral/cava less than 1.3) is predictive of cure or improvement of hypertension in approximately 95% of patients.[63] It is disconcerting that many patients lacking these criteria have also been cured or improved by operation and it is, therefore, unwise to deny a potentially beneficial operation or procedure on the basis of one set of negative renin data.

Supplemental Tests

Individual kidney function tests deserve mention even though they have not been widely practiced since the emergence of the divided renal vein renin assay. They are of great historical and physiologic interest, however. Following partial occlusion of the renal artery (50%), there is a reduction of glomerular filtration rate and a lowered filtered load of sodium, resulting in a decreased secretion of sodium and water. Increased fractional reabsorption of sodium and water leads to a higher osmolality in the final urine and to a hyperconcentration of those solutes that are poorly reabsorbed, namely, para-aminohippuric acid, inulin, and creatinine. Although divided kidney function tests are not widely employed because they are cumbersome and associated with greater morbidity than the more commonly used tests, they may be useful when other tests are equivocal. In a comparative study in which both divided kidney function tests and divided plasma renin activity determinations were done in 25 patients with arteriographically demonstrated lesions, we found 3 subjects with negative or equivocal divided kidney function tests who had positive plasma renin ratios for ischemia.[51] Furthermore, the divided kidney function tests provide the most accurate data regarding the contribution of each kidney to total renal economy.

Since **transluminal angioplasty** has been widely employed, it has been shown to have lasting therapeutic effects. Even when these effects are not achieved, dilation of the stenoisis may quickly establish a diagnosis of renal artery stenosis causing renal ischemia and renovascular hypertension. For example, if at the time of arteriography and demonstration of a stenosing lesion of the renal artery the Gruentzig balloon catheter is passed and the lesion is dilated, and if, as a result of this, the patient obtains relief of hypertension, we have a potentially definitive test available. This is not currently a routine practice because preparation is necessary prior to a planned transluminal angioplasty, and there are risks involved in the procedure. However, it is conceivable that with further refinement and firmer establishment of its indications and contraindications, the practice of diagnostic balloon dilation of a stenosis may be commonplace.

The determination of pressure/flow gradients across a stenosis was used in the past for intraoperative diagnostic purposes when preoperative studies were inconclusive. Nowadays, however, renal artery exploration is rarely undertaken unless a firm commitment to repair is made on the basis of preoperative studies. Pressure and flow determinations continue to be extremely useful in assessing the adequacy of vascular repair.

Renal biopsy is rarely done because of the relative paucity of information gained. Contrary to findings of early studies, small-vessel disease in the kidney does not rule out the possibility of surgical cure. At times, frozen-section biopsies may be useful in demonstrating interstitial fibrosis and tubular atrophy and may suggest the need for nephrectomy rather than arterial repair.[10]

TREATMENT

Treatment of renal artery stenosis and renovascular hypertension can be divided into medical treatment, transluminal dilation, and surgery.

Medical Treatment

Although effective antihypertensive drugs have become available, there are few hard data to aid in the decision as to whether operative or nonoperative therapy is preferable for a patient with renovascular hypertension. Of 214 patients with renovascular hypertension studied by Hunt and Associates in a prospective study, 100 underwent operation and 114 were treated medically.[41] In a 7- to 14-year follow-up study, 16% of surgically treated patients died, compared to 40% of those treated medically. Furthermore, more than 90% of the surgical survivors were cured or improved by the operation. Myocardial infarction, renal failure, and cerebrovascular accidents were more commonly encountered in the medical group than in the surgical cohort. Whether specific drugs such as CEIs (*e.g.*, captopril) will change this picture is undetermined at present. A number of reports indicate that hypertension can be well controlled by CEIs.[28,29] However, there are significant side-effects and occasional severe complications associated with this form of therapy. It remains to be seen whether CEIs will improve or maintain renal function in patients with renal artery stenosis.

Percutaneous Transluminal Angioplasty

Until the advent of transluminal angioplasty, the indications for surgical intervention were fairly well defined. Young individuals with severe hypertension and patients who were in satisfactory medical condition whose hypertension was correctable by reconstruction rather than nephrectomy were considered ideal candidates for operative angioplasty. With the recent development and wide use of percutaneous transluminal angioplasty (PTA), indications for open surgery are less clear. It will undoubtedly take a number of years to determine relative indications for surgical treatment as compared with PTA. Because it is now widespread practice to employ PTA prior to considering renal arterial reconstruction, this new methodology deserves brief discussion.

PTA was originally developed by Dotter and Judkins for treatment of atherosclerotic peripheral vascular disease.[15] The development of the soft, flexible, double-lumen Gruentzig balloon catheter[34] represented a definite advance over the Dotter method, which was essentially a bougie system. The initial application of the Gruentzig balloon catheter in treating peripheral vascular atherosclerosis has been expanded to include not only renal artery dilation but also coronary artery dilation.[90]

The technique of renal artery dilation is relatively simple and is currently used according to the method proposed by Katzen, Chang, and Knox.[45] Antihypertensive medications are discontinued 48 h before dilation, if possible. If blood pressure control is a problem, nitroprusside may be used. Either the femoral artery or the axillary artery may be used. The Seldinger technique is used to introduce the catheter, and the renal artery is entered with a pre-shaped catheter. A small guidewire is advanced beyond the stenosis, a catheter exchange is made, and a Gruentzig catheter with appropriate balloon diameter is placed within the stenosis over the guidewire. (Fig. 25-10 and Fig. 25-11). Heparin (5000 IU) is given through the catheter. With fluoroscopic guidance, a guidewire is passed through the stenosis and into the renal artery beyond the stenosis. The catheter is positioned under the fluoroscopic control and the balloon is inflated to between 5 atm and 8 atm of pressure (Fig. 25-12). The balloon usually must be inflated and deflated two to three times.

Blood pressure response is somewhat variable, the lowest blood pressure usually occurring between 2 hr and 6 hr following angioplasty. When dilation has been successful as proven by the angiographic appearance faollowing PTA, between 85% and 90% cure or improvement occurs for 6 months or longer in most series.[80] Although most radiologists do not distinguish between atherosclerotic stenosis and fibrous dysplastic stenoses in their results, our personal experience indicates that the technique is more difficult, more hazardous, and less predictable in treating atherosclerotic disease than in treating fibrous dysplasia.

Complications of the technique should be recognized. Massive hematoma in the inguinal or axillary regions, embolization to the toes that may require amputation, perforation of the artery with retroperitoneal hemorrhage, and dissections of the renal artery resulting in partial or complete infarction have all been reported.

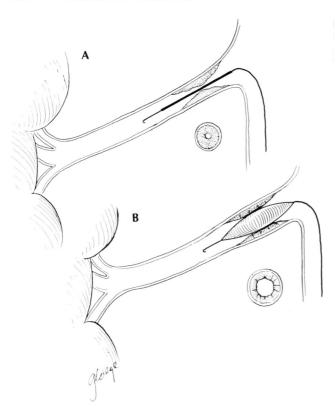

FIG. 25-10. Transluminal angioplasty using the Gruentzig balloon. **(A)** The area of stenosis is traversed with the guidewire, over which the balloon catheter is passed. **(B)** The balloon is expanded to dilate the area of stenosis.

Surgery

Should PTA prove to have long-term success and acceptable morbidity, there is little reason to believe that it will not become the treatment of choice in relatively uncomplicated cases of renal artery stenosis and hypertension. In terms of cost effectiveness and patient discomfort alone, operative correction of stenosing lesions cannot effectively compete. Surgical intervention will still maintain a secure position for the complicated cases with branch disease and for cases in which PTA has been unsuccessful in either achieving or maintaining dilatation of the renal artery. Unfortunately, these cases will be the more difficult ones, because simple stenoses that can be managed by relatively simple surgical techniques will have been managed successfully by PTA.

An intravenous infusion is begun the night before to ensure that the patient is well hydrated. It is not necessary to discontinue antihypertensive drugs before operation. Potassium is repleted preoperatively because many patients will have been on diuretic therapy and potassium depletion leads to myocardial irritability. Pulmonary wedge catheter is indicated in patients with questionable myocardial reserve. An arterial line for gas and blood pressure determinations is a helpful adjunct during the operation. A catheter is usually placed in the bladder before operation. Intraoperatively, mannitol is given intravenously. We advise 25 g of mannitol before renal artery clamping and another 25 g following restoration of blood flow. Heparin is administered systemically 5 minutes before renal artery clamping (0.5 mg/kg).

Following renovascular surgery, vital signs and urine output are closely monitored. Exacerbation of hypertension is not uncommon following operation, even with a technically adequate repair, and sometimes requires management with intravenous nitroprusside or diazoxide. We do not customarily allow ambulation until 24 h of bed rest. A renal scan is performed on the first postoperative day.

Operative procedures for renal artery stenosis and renovascular hypertension include nephrectomy and partial nephrectomy, revascularization operations, and renal autotransplantation.

NEPHRECTOMY AND PARTIAL NEPHRECTOMY. In recent years, nephrectomy has accounted for fewer than 25% of primary operations performed for renovascular hypertension. It is indicated for unilateral renal infarction with nonfunction, for extremely poor-risk patients with a relatively healthy contralateral kidney, for kidneys that have multiple branch disease not amenable to repair, for severe parenchymal disease with or without associated renal artery stenosis, and following unsuccessful previous arterial repair or partial nephrectomy. Chapter 5 presents the technical details of nephrectomy.

Partial nephrectomy (see Chap. 6) is performed when segmental renal disease makes this operation feasible, but, in our experience, fewer than 5% of patients will fall in this category. Furthermore, the cure and improvement rate following partial nephrectomy has been less than with either total nephrectomy or vascular repair; and with refined surgical techniques and magnification, it is now preferable to repair branch or segmental renal artery stenoses than to excise poorly defined ischemic renal segments.

REVASCULARIZATION OPERATIONS. Revascularization operations are most commonly done through an anterior transperitoneal approach, a chevron incision, or a vertical paramedian or midline incision. For the splenorenal bypass, we prefer a thoracoabdominal extrapleural retroperitoneal approach, excising the 11th rib or making an incision just above the 11th rib. The splenic flexure and left colon and duodenum are reflected medially and the plane between Gerota's fascia and the pancreas is developed. The pancreas and spleen are gently retracted cephalad to permit access to the splenic vessels. The splenic artery is usually palpated posterior and superior to the splenic vein.

For right-sided lesions, it is best to take down the hepatic flexure and mobilize the ascending colon and hepatic flexure along with the second portion of the duodenum to the left upper quadrant. Dividing the right gonadal vein will allow full exposure of the vena cava, and the right renal vein and renal artery. The right renal artery is best secured by placing a tape about it just to the left of the vena cava. For repair of lesions in the distal portion of the right renal artery, it may not be necessary to secure the right renal artery medial to the vena cava. For most *in situ* operations on the renal vessels, it is not necessary to mobilize the kidney.

Left-sided lesions are best handled by reflecting the small bowel upward onto the chest or into the right upper quadrant and incising along the root of the mesentery much like the approach for transperitoneal retroperitoneal lymphadenectomy. The inferior mesenteric vein should be divided below where it enters the splenic vein. The left colon and splenic flexure can usually be left intact. If inadequate exposure is obtained, however, reflection of the splenic flexure and descending colon

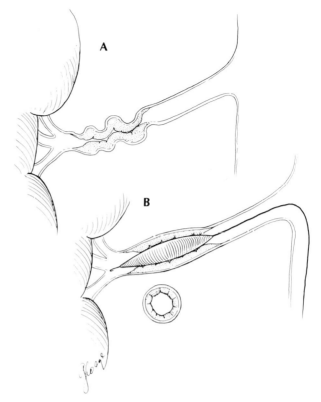

FIG. 25-11. An area of medial fibroplasia of the right renal artery (**A**) is dilated (**B**) with the balloon catheter.

to the right will permit greater access. When autotransplantation is being done, with or without *ex vivo* branch repair, we use either a transperitoneal approach or an extraperitoneal incision with the patient in the torque position, making the incision from above the 11th rib to the lateral border of the rectus above the symphysis. If it is necessary to reimplant the ureter into the bladder, we often divide the rectus muscle above the pubis.

Endarterectomy. Endarterectomy was the first reconstructive procedure performed on the renal artery. The technique is applicable when patients have localized atheromatous stenosis of the renal artery. The approach to the atheroma is by renal aortic, or aortorenal arteriotomy (Fig. 25-13). An ear curet or Cannon dissector is used to separate the plaque from the wall, after which the artery is thoroughly irrigated with heparinized saline. Care must be taken to remove the plaque as completely as possible because residual roughened portions may invite subsequent dissection or thrombosis. In addition, caution must be exercised to prevent escape of particles of atheromatous material, which may produce atheroembolism and segmental renal infarction. The arteriotomy is closed with contin-

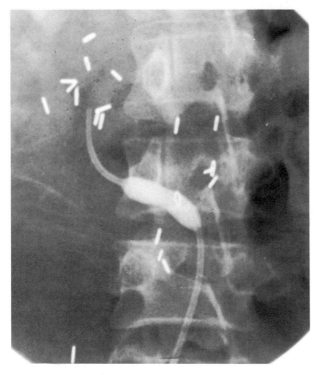

FIG. 25-12. A radiograph shows a balloon filled with contrast dilating an area of renal arterial stenosis.

uous 5-0 or 6-0 nonabsorbable sutures. If the lumen appears inadequate or if there is a tendency for the thin-walled vessel to buckle, a patch graft of vein or anterior rectus sheath is used (see Fig. 25-15). Transaortic renal endarterectomy was proposed and popularized by Wylie.[93] In this approach the aorta is cross clamped above and below the renal artery, a longitudinal aortotomy is made, and the plaques are removed from the aorta and the renal arterial ostia (Fig. 25-14). This method is particularly useful for bilateral atherosclerotic renal arterial lesions and it obviates the need to incise the renal arteries, which may require patch plasties to prevent narrowing.

The results of endarterectomy are generally acceptable, although long-term follow-up indicates that atrophy of endarterectomized vessels may occur. The advantages of endarterectomy are that it is relatively quick and simple, it involves no foreign graft material, and it permits a one-stage bilateral procedure if indicated.

Resection and end-to-end anastomosis. Resection of the diseased portion of the renal artery with reanastomosis is ideal for selected cases in which the lesion is short, well defined, and localized to the middle third of the vessel. The technique has somewhat limited application because the arteriogram often underestimates the extent of the

disease. Of the common lesions, subadventitial dysplasia is the best suited for this type of repair. Unfortunately, the disease frequently is found to be more extensive than is apparent on angiography. If the resection of the diseased portion is not complete, restenosis may occur. When applicable, we perform resection and reanastomosis with interrupted 6-0 Prolene sutures (Fig. 25-15A and 25-15B). Although we do not advocate it, an interposition graft of vein or synthetic tube can be made as illustrated in Figures 25-15C and 25-15D. However, an aortorenal bypass is preferred over interposition grafts of this type. It is best to place the first suture at the 6 o'clock position and successive sutures at the 5 and 7, 8 and 4, 9 and 3 o'clock positions, and so forth until the anastomosis is complete. Because it is difficult to ensure complete resection of diseased segments, this operation is rarely done by experienced surgeons and has, in fact, been replaced by bypass procedures for the most part.

Bypass grafts. Aortorenal bypass is currently the most popular reconstructive operation for renal artery stenosis. It is probably the simplest of repairs because dissection of the juxta-aortic portion of the renal arteries is not necessary. The saphenous vein is most widely employed because it is thick walled, the appropriate diameter, and available in long lengths. It can be adapted for anastomosis to branches of the renal artery as well as to the main trunk. Spatulated anastomoses are recommended both on the aortic and renal sides.

We usually use the aortic punch of 4.5-mm or 5-mm size to remove a plug from the full thickness of aorta and to provide a clean aortic margin (Fig. 25-16A). Figure 25-16B illustrates the placement of a free hypogastric artery graft after using the aortic punch. In the case of severe atherosclerosis of the aorta, it may be preferable to cross clamp the aorta in two places for placement of by bypass graft rather than to use a partial occlusion clamp. However, exclusion clamps are commonly used and usually a soft area of the aorta is selected for the site of origin of the bypass. An end-to-end anastomosis is generally done between the vein graft and the renal artery. On the right side the graft is brought anterior to the vena cava in preparation for the distal anastomosis. As in most arterial anastomoses, we prefer the use of interrupted sutures. Polypropylene sutures (5-0) are used for the anastomosis of the vein graft to the aorta, and 5-0 or 6-0 interrupted sutures are used for the vein-to-renal-artery union. Generally the graft is placed on the aorta first in order to limit the ischemic time for renal artery clamping. Two arterial trunks (Fig. 25-17) may be revascularized using end-to-side and

FIG. 25-13. The technique of endarterectomy of the right renal artery is shown. The arteriotomy may be closed primarily or with a patch as seen in C.

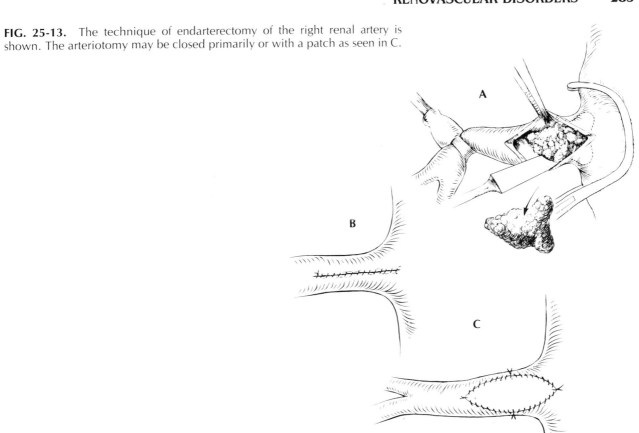

FIG. 25-14. The technique of transaortic bilateral endarterectomy is shown. Note that the aorta is cross clamped and the atheromatous plaque is removed from the aorta as well as both renal arteries.

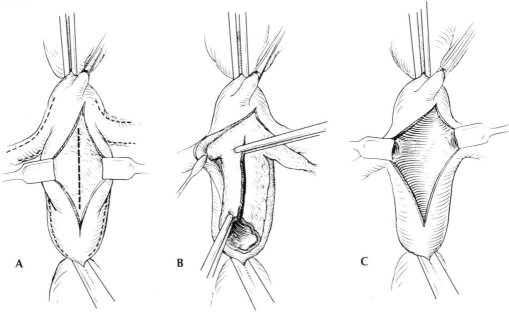

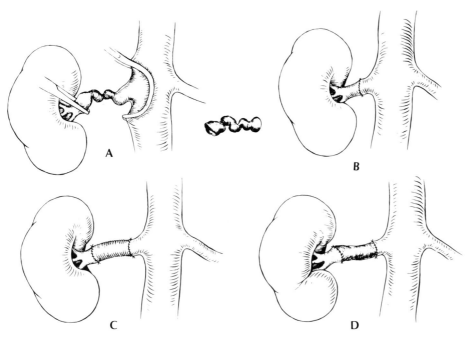

FIG. 25-15. (A and B) Resection and primary anastomosis of an area of stenosis of the right renal artery. (C) Interposition graft of Dracon. (D) Interposition graft of vein.

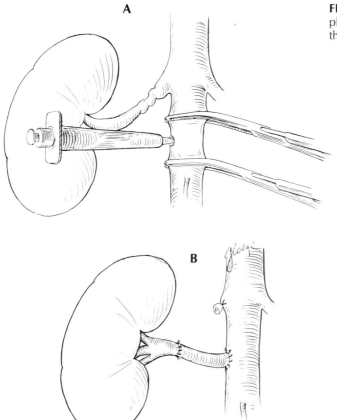

FIG. 25-16. (A) The aortic punch is used to remove a plug from the aorta for a clean area to which to anastomose the graft. (B) The hypogastric artery graft is in place.

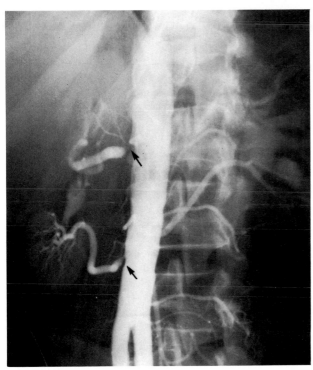

FIG. 25-17. An aortogram shows a double right renal artery with stenoses at the ostia of both trunks.

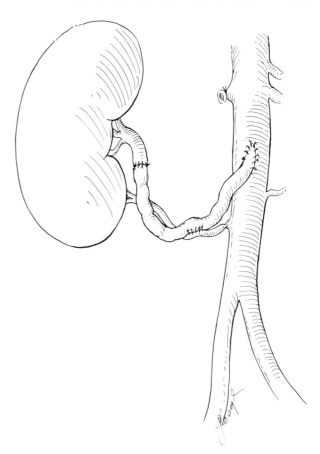

FIG. 25-18. A vein graft is used to perform a side-to-side anastomosis to the stenotic lower renal artery and then an end-to-end anastomosis with the distal stump of the divided upper renal artery.

end-to-end anastomosis as shown in Figures 25-18 and 25-19.

Long-term follow-up studies indicate that patency following vein grafts is fairly well maintained. Approximately 20% of saphenous vein grafts, however, fail during the first year because of thrombosis, stenosis, or aneurysmal dilatation.[18]

Arterial autografts have the theoretical advantage over veins of having the same general caliber and viscoelastic characteristics as the renal artery. The hypogastric artery can be sacrificed with impunity and it is not difficult to expose. On occasion, it can be taken with several branches suitable for placement into the branches of the renal artery. If more than two branches require anastomosis, we prefer *ex vivo* surgery in order to provide better cooling of the kidney and to optimize the reanastomoses of the small branches to small renal vessels. Figure 25-20 shows the use of the hypogastric artery as a free autologous graft, and Figure 25-21 shows pre-and postoperative arteriograms of a patient treated with a hypogastric artery graft. Figure 25-22 shows the hypogastric artery with two major rami as a bifurcation graft.

The disadvantages of the hypogastric artery are that it may be involved by atherosclerosis in pa-

tients over the age of 40 and that it may be too short. Our current choice for bypass grafts in young patients is the hypogastric artery autograft, which we have used in 70 reconstructions over the past 12 years with only a single long-term stenosis and two early thrombotic occlusions.

Synthetic tubes are less popular owing to the higher incidence of graft closure, particularly when runoff is poor. Newer types of synthetic grafts with external or internal velour provide a more rapid formation of a smooth-lined neo-intima.[48] The expanded polytetrafluoroethylene graft (Gore-Tex) appears to have application because the material is soft, inelastic, and easy to suture and allows for inner fibrous healing with minimal tissue reactivity. Although the material is reported to maintain patency over long periods of time, even in low-flow situations, this has yet to be established in large clinical series. The advantages of synthetics are that they are relatively easy to handle, they are

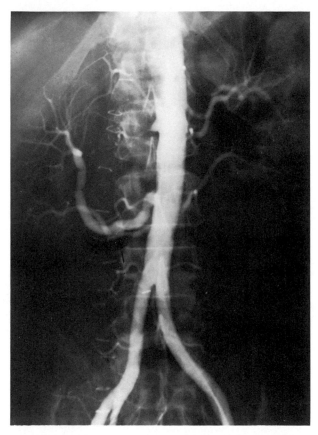

FIG. 25-19. A postoperative aortogram of the case shown in Figure 25-17, with the vein graft making a side-to-side anastomosis to the stenotic lower renal artery and an end-to-end anastomosis to the distal stump of the upper renal artery

readily available in a variety of sizes, and they entail no risk of subsequent involvement by the pathologic process (*i.e.*, fibrosis, atheroma) for which they are inserted. Figures 25-23*A* and 25-23*B* show our technique of aortorenal end-to-side Dacron bypass graft. Grafts should take origin from the anterolateral aspect of the aorta between the renal artery orifices and the inferior mesenteric artery. Long-term follow-up studies in patients undergoing Dacron aortorenal bypass grafts have recently been reported.[56] These authors found an overall patency of 78.2% on follow-up aortography in 201 patients at a mean interval of 31.5 months after operation. The patency rate was 76% (113/149) for Dacron bypass grafts, 89.7% (35/39) for saphenous vein bypass grafts, and 82% (23/28) for arteries treated by endarterectomy or patch graft angioplasty.

Splenorenal bypass. Splenoreal bypass is particularly useful for left renal revascularization when the aorta is hazardous to use because of severe atherosclerosis or previous operations. It has the advantage of employing only a single vascular anastomosis, and therefore, less operating time is required. In our early experience with transluminal angioplasty, we found that left renal artery stenosis secondary to atheromatous disease of the aorta and renal artery is frequently a situation where dilation is unsuccessful. In such cases, the splenorenal bypass is particularly applicable.

We prefer the torque position with a thoracoabdominal extraperitoneal extrapleural approach, which gives ready access to the splenic artery and

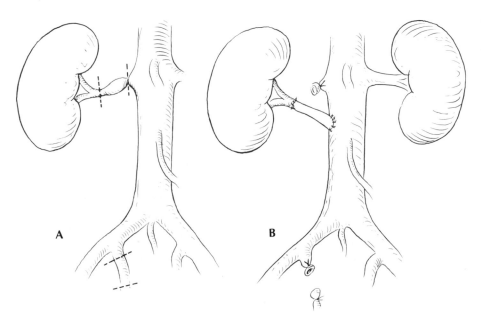

FIG. 25-20. Technique of using the hypogastric artery as a free interposition graft for right renal artery stenosis

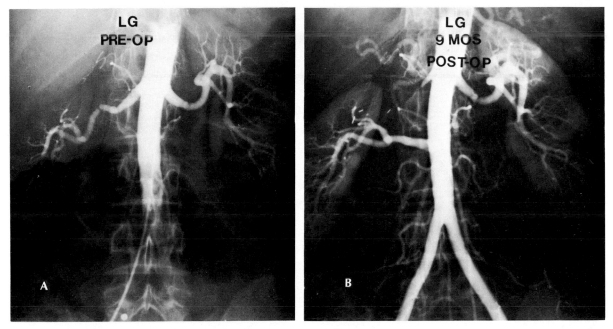

FIG. 25-21. Arteriograms show (A) pre- and (B) postoperative appearance in a patient with a right renal artery stenosis treated with an interposition hypogastric arterial graft.

FIG. 25-22. Hypogastric artery graft with two major rami anastomosed to two main renal arterial branches

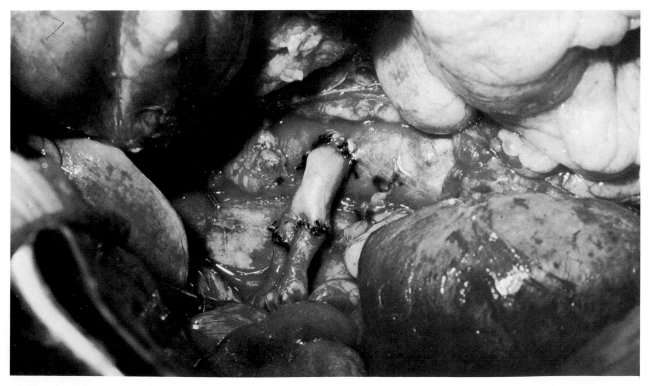

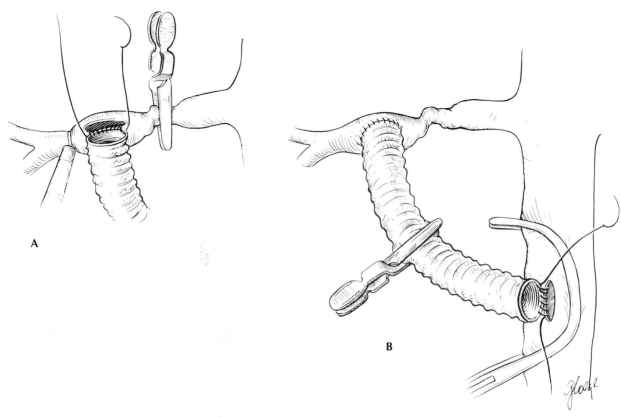

FIG. 25-23. Technique of placement of a Dacron graft side-to-side into the poststenotic main renal arterial segment. Because the anastomosis to the renal artery is the more difficult one, this is usually done first. The posterior row is placed from within.

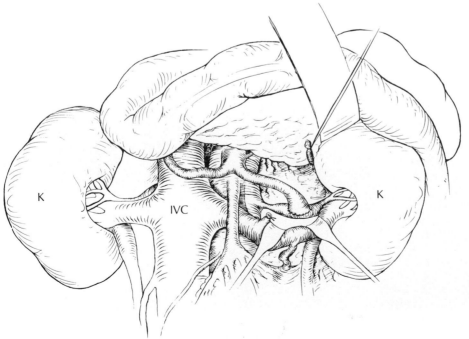

FIG. 25-24. Technique of splenorenal bypass. Note that the pancreas is lifted cephalad in order to expose the splenic artery.

the renal artery. The splenic artery must be of good size and relatively free of atherosclerosis (it should be visualized in the preoperative angiogram to ascertain its relative normalcy). After reflecting the pancreas cephalad to permit access to the splenic vessels, the splenic artery is found posterior and superior to the splenic vein. A tape is passed around the artery and the small pancreatic branches are divided between vessel clips or sutures. The splenic artery should be mobilized as close to the celiac axis as possible because the vessel is more normal and straighter proximally and gives off fewer branches than is the case more distally. A vascular clamp is then placed on the splenic artery and the artery is divided after the distal stump is doubly ligated. It is not necessary to remove the spleen, because it receives sufficient collateral circulation from the short gastric and gastroepiploic vessels. The left renal artery is then dissected free and clamped distally; it is ligated proximally and transected if an end-to-end anastomosis is planned. Otherwise end-to-side anastomosis can be done while the renal artery is temporarily occluded with vascular tapes or clamps (Figs. 25-24 and 25-25). End-to-side anastomosis is particularly applicable if there is a disparity in the size of the splenic artery and renal artery.

Results of splenorenal bypass should be 80% successful. The results are better in men than in women.[71] The major complication of splenorenal bypass is pancreatic injury or splenic injury, both of which should be possible to avoid with careful technique.

RENAL   AUTOTRANSPLANTATION.   Renal   autotransplantation of the kidney for renovascular hypertension has proven to be an acceptable surgical option in revascularizing the kidney in selected cases. We have found it particularly useful in children and in young adults. Although it would seem to be a good choice for the patient whose aorta is severely involved by atherosclerosis, such is not the case because the hypogastric artery and the iliac artery are frequently involved by atherosclerosis. On the other hand, in young patients with middle aortic disease, it may be very suitable because the iliac vessels are usually spared in this process. Although neurofibromatosis would also seem to be a reasonable instance in which to employ autotransplantation because of frequent involvement of the aorta as well as renal vessels, we have found a perplexing and disconcerting number of thromboses in a small number of patients with neurofibromatosis in whom we perform autotransplantation.

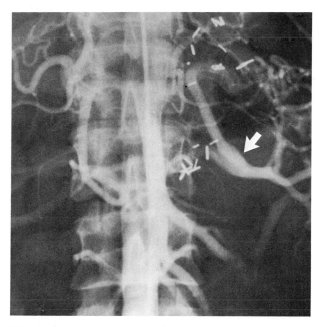

FIG. 25-25.   An aortogram shows a splenorenal end-to-side bypass.

In performing the renal transposition, the ureter is best left intact. Even though the ureter must take a redundant course to the bladder, this has presented no drainage problem in the vast majority of cases in our series in which the ureter has been left intact (Figs. 25-26 and 25-27).

A special feature of autotransplantation that is appealing is that it allows *ex vivo* surgery of branch vessels using magnification or microsurgical techniques.[54,73] With cold perfusion preparation, the kidney can be preserved for a 2 hr or 3 hr period if necessary for extracorporeal operations. Cold hyperosmolar perfusion of the kidney for 5 minutes protects the organ against ambiothermic ischemia for as long as 3 hr.[79]

For surgeons familiar with kidney transplantation who have not had ample experience with aortic surgery, autotransplantation has provided a practical and acceptable approach to the management of renal artery stenosis requiring revascularization, but *in situ* techniques should be used if at all possible. The entire operation can often be done extraperitoneally, and because extraperitoneal procedures are not generally followed postoperatively by the problems of ileus, obstruction, and so forth, this may be preferred. The kidney may also be approached transabdominally except in heavy set individuals, when the flank approach and extraperitoneal approach are preferable.

The kidney is mobilized and the renal artery is

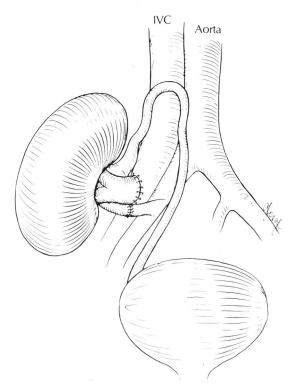

FIG. 25-26. The technique of autotransplantation is shown. The ureter is left intact.

dissected free and ligated proximally. On the right side this is usually done between the aorta and vena cava, although it is possible to divide the renal artery lateral to or under the vena cava if the disease is distal. The renal vein is easily handled, and generally a small divet of vena cava is taken if the renal vein is somewhat small. A Derra or Satinsky clamp is left on the vena cava while the kidney is moved to the iliac fossa, preferably without perfusion or cooling but with systemic mannitol and heparin administration. If simple autotransplantation is done, cooling should not be required. The autotransplantation is done as for renal allografts, first freeing the external iliac vein or common iliac vein sufficiently to encircle it with Rumel tourniquets or with an occlusion clamp. The anastomosis of the renal vein to the side of the iliac vein is done with a continuous 5-0 or 6-0 polypropylene suture in adults and with interrupted sutures in children to allow for future vessel growth. The ureter is mobilized down to the sacroiliac area and allowed to curl up in the iliac fossa and take a serpentine course to the bladder. When complicated or microsurgical anastomoses are employed, it may be necessary to divide the ureter, but we have seldom found this necessary.

The arterial anastomosis is done using interrupted 5-0 or 6-0 polypropylene sutures. Double-armed sutures prevent separation of the intima from the media when passing the needle through the vessel wall from inside out on both sides of the anastomosis. Square knots and five or six throws are mandatory when using monofilament suture material.

In dealing with stenoses involving major branches, the branched hypogastric autograft provides an excellent means of managing two renal arteries. Both branches of the hypogastric artery are isolated, dissected free, and ligated. The anastomoses of the two main rami of the hypogastric artery to the two branches of the renal artery are then made, preferably with interrupted sutures

FIG. 25-27. This intravenous urogram was taken 6 years after autotransplantation of the left kidney for renal artery stenosis. Note that, despite the redundancy of the ureter, there is no hydronephrosis.

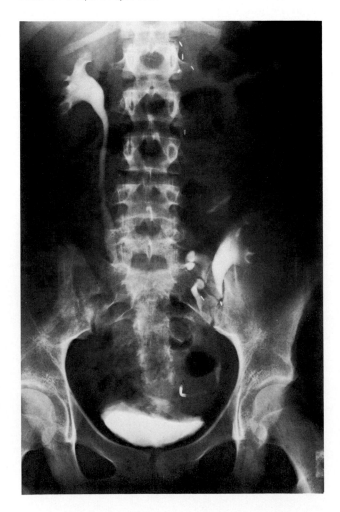

laid in first and tied later to ensure optimal visibility of the anastomotic area (Fig. 25-28). An alternative approach to handling the problems of stenoses affecting the bifurcation of the renal artery is shown in Figure 25-29. In this case, the disease involves most of the main renal artery and extends into the first portion of the bifurcation.

The kidney is flushed *ex situ* with cold hypertonic solution because the making of a pantaloon of the two branches requires additional time and dexterity. The two branches are split on their medial sides and then a double-armed suture of 6-0 polypropylene is placed through the apex. One needle is carried up one side of the two vessels to create a common wall and then the other needle is passed up the other side to complete the pantaloon. The anastomosis of the common lumen is then made either to the hypogastric artery (end to end) or to the side of the common iliac artery.

The use of segments of saphenous vein or hypogastric artery is practical for multiple vessel stenoses. The saphenous vein can be divided in three parts and segments as illustrated in Figure 25-30.[1] The segments must be oriented to maintain proper flow direction in keeping with the valves.

We have had excellent results using several branches of the hypogastric artery as a free graft, attaching these branches to branches of the renal artery distal to diseased vessels and suturing the branches end to end with 7-0 polypropylene using

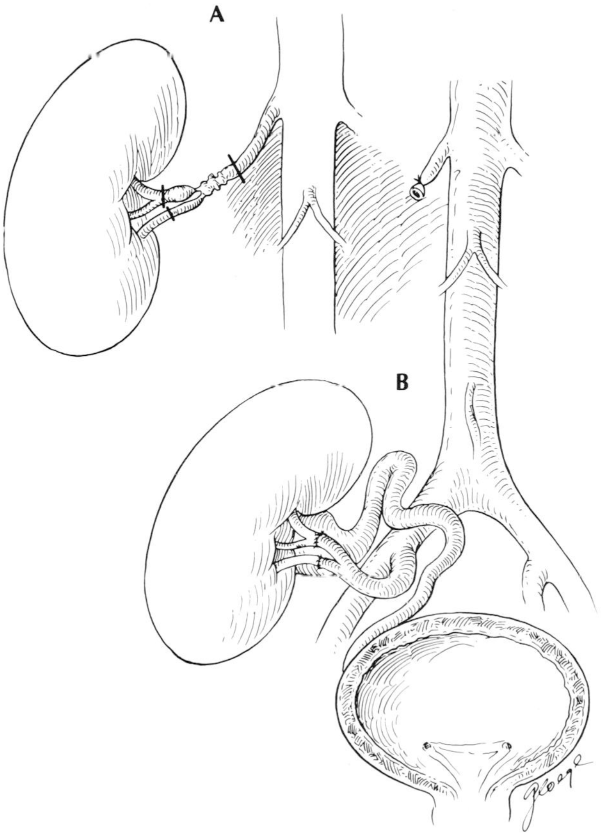

FIG. 25-28. The two primary rami of the hypogastric artery are used to anastomose the two main branches of the renal artery beyond the area of stenosis.

FIG. 25-29. Alternate method of managing disease extending into the primary branches of the renal artery. The two renal artery branches are united in a pantaloon fashion (**B**) and anastomosed end to end to the hypogastric artery (**C**) or to the side of the external iliac artery.

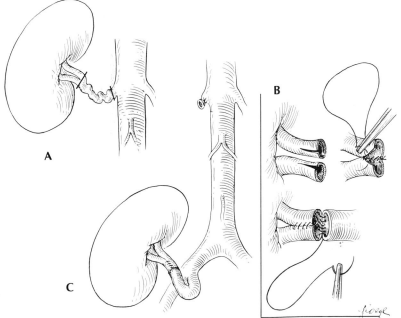

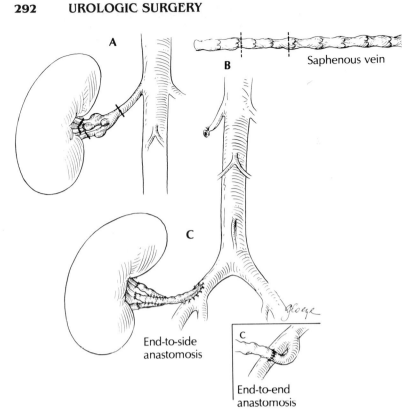

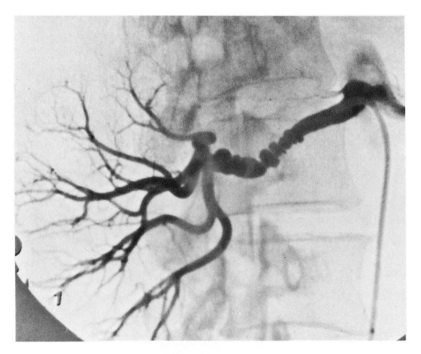

FIG. 25-30. Segments of the saphenous vein are fashioned to correct renal artery branch disease.

FIG. 25-31. An arteriogram shows complex involvement of the right renal artery by disease extending into the primary branches.

a 2-power or 3-power magnification (Figs. 25-31 and 25-32). The headlamp, in addition to magnification, makes these anastomoses much easier. Furthermore, the anastomoses can be done by threading a feeding tube or catheter through the open end of the free hypogastric artery graft and into each of the branches and then performing the anastomoses over the "stenting" catheter (Figs. 25-33 and 25-34). The base of the graft is then sewn with interrupted sutures to the end of the hypogastric artery or to the side of the external iliac artery (Fig. 25-35).

In addition to the advantages of the precise suturing for small-vessel disease, *ex vivo* radiographic techniques are more easily performed with high resolution and magnification to demonstrate intrarenal arterial disease. There are several pertinent references in the literature relation to *ex vivo* surgery.[46,49,59,66,74,79]

Complications and Mortality. Two basic patterns of surgical complications occur in renal artery disease. Myocardial infarction is the most common major complication in patients dying following simple nephrectomy. In patients undergoing complicated surgery, major causes of death are uremia or hemorrhage or both, sometimes complicated by infection. IN CSRH, more than half the surgical deaths (5.9% mortality among 102 patients) could be attributed directly to the development of postoperative uremia. In the opinion of Franklin and associates, bilaterally impaired renal function of even moderate degree is a relative contraindication for corrective surgery. However, recent papers

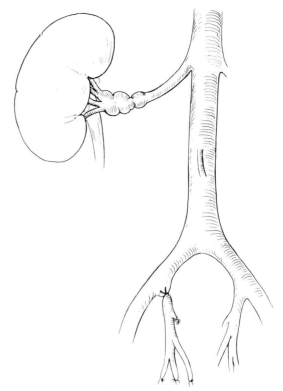

FIG. 25-32. Disease of the distal third of the right renal artery with extension into primary branches. The ipsilateral hypogastric artery and its primary branches will be used as a free interposition graft.

FIG. 25-33. Bench operation. The branches of the hypogastric artery are anastomosed to the branches of the renal artery prior to autotransplantation.

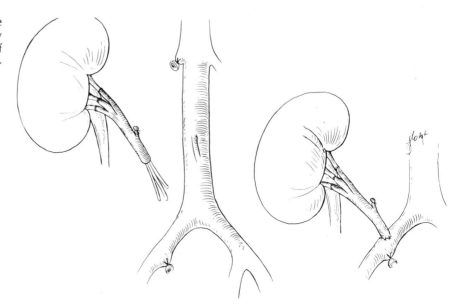

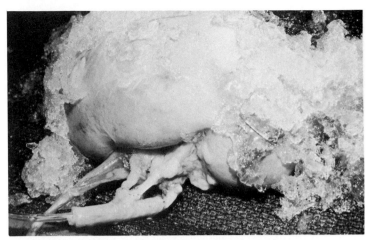

FIG. 25-34. *Ex vivo* view of kidney after anastomosing hypogastric artery and three branches to the renal arteries; the ureter is intact while the kidney is cooled by infusion and covered with slush.

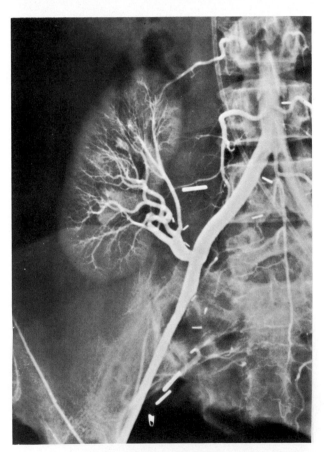

FIG. 25-35. A postoperative arteriogram of the case presented in Figures 25-31 through 25-34 shows patent anastomoses.

attest that surgery can now be undertaken in patients who are in critical condition with an acceptable mortality lower than 2%.[24,72] Naturally, when aortoiliac surgery is combined with renal arterial surgery, mortality rates will be higher. Lawrie and associates reported a mortality rate of 1.8% among 489 patients with renal artery reconstruction alone and 4.8% among 186 patients who had associated vascular procedures.[56] The crude 15-year survival in their series of 489 patients was 70%, the most common causes of death being myocardial infarction, stroke, and cancer. The conclusion of that study and others indicates that at least two thirds of patients will experience long-term relief of hypertension following reconstructive surgery and that the best long-term survival and blood pressure relief will be obtained in patients younger than 50 years of age.[21,22,55] We feel that because hypertension in women is better tolerated, perhaps younger male patients appear to have the most to gain from successful renovascular reconstruction.

Renal artery disease in children is generally caused by one of the fibrous dysplasias, usually intimal or perimedial. The lesions occurring in children are often bilateral and progressive. Although operations in children were formerly associated with a large number of technical failures, recent series suggest that surgery is suited for children with renovascular disease.[27,50,78] In general, children with renovascular disease and hypertension have severe high blood pressure, and often there is retarded growth, renal function impairment, retinopathy with visual disturbances, and other problems. Spenorenal bypasses, saphenous vein bypasses, and Dacron bypasses usually have not fared well in children. Our best results have been with the autologous hypogastric artery as a bypass. Postoperative aneurysmal dilatation of arterial autografts has not been seen, and long-tern patency has been excellent. Autotransplantation in children is done for the middle aortic syndrome and for lesions involving the branches of the renal artery. However, as mentioned earlier, the results of revascularization in children with neurofibromatosis have not been particularly encouraging.

It has been stated that if the hypertension is controllable, then growth of the child will ultimately make revascularization easier and more likely to succeed. The patient should therefore be managed medically if possible to await further maturation of renal vessels.[50] Children do not do well on the large doses of anti-hypertensive medication that are often necessary to control blood pressure, however.

The place of transluminal angioplasty in the treatment of stenosing diseases of the renal arteries in children remains undetermined. Undoubtedly, arteritis following a viral or bacterial infection accounts for transient hypertension in many children and permanent hypertension occurring when fibrosis ensues in the wake of the healing arteritis.

Renal Artery Stenosis and Renal Failure.
In clinical practice renal artery stenosis along appears to be an extremely rare cause of end-state renal disease.[47] Most patients with end-stage renal disease have instrinsic parenchymal disease, but this does not rule out the presence of renal artery stenosis, which may be a contributing factor. May and associates found eight patients with severe renal artery stenosis among a cohort with deteriorating renal function.[65] Following renal revascularization, the average creatinine of 8 mg/dl preoperative declined to approximately 4 mg/dl when reassessed up to 36 months postoperatively. Other reports have appeared indicating that patients with rapidly progressive oliguric renal failure may benefit from vascular repair. Isolated reports indicate successful revascularization after long periods of nonfunction.[13,94] The longest recorded nonfunction prior to surgical correction by atheromatous occlusion of the renal artery was 30 days.[3,35] It is logical, therefore, that renal arteriography should be considered more often in patients with renal failure, particularly when hypertension is an accompanying feature.

Renal Artery Aneurysm

Four categories of renal artery aneurysms are recognized: fusiform aneurysmal dilations associated with fibroplasia of the renal arteries (Fig. 25-36); aneurysmal dissection, either primary of indeterminate pathogenesis or following trauma (Fig. 25-37); microaneurysms usually associated with arteritis; and macroaneurysms of undetermined

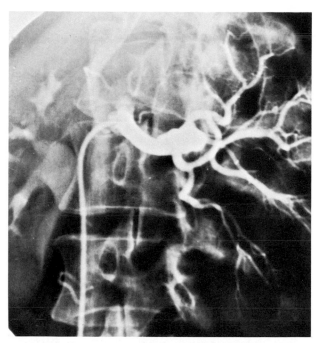

FIG. 25-36. A selective left renal arteriogram shows a fusiform aneurysm associated with fibroplasia.

FIG. 25-37. A right renal arteriogram shows an extensive dissecting aneurysm of the right renal artery causing infarction of the upper pole and segmental infarcts of the lower pole.

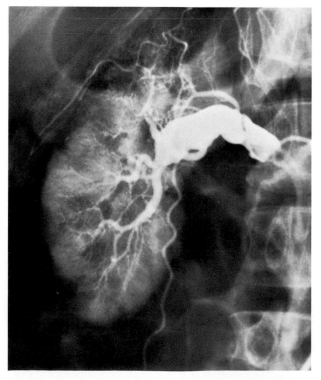

FIG. 25-38.   Four types of renal artery aneurysm

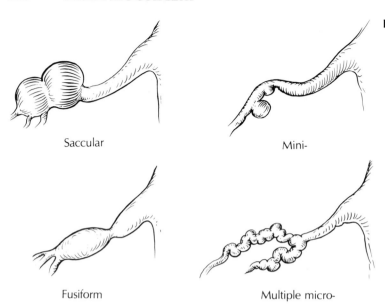

Saccular

Mini-

Fusiform

Multiple micro-

causes (Fig. 25-38). It is difficult to estimate the true incidence of renal artery aneurysms because they are rarely discovered during routine autopsies. One study in which postmortem arteriographic investigations were done disclosed saccular renal artery aneurysms in 9.7% of unselected autopsies.[85] Among patients undergoing renal arteriographic studies for hypertension, the incidence of aneurysms was found to be between 0.7% and 2.5%. In patients with renal arterial fibrous dysplasia, aneurysms occur in approximately 10% of cases. Renal artery aneurysms associated with medial fibroplasia are probably due to fragmentation and disruption of elastic tissue with loss of smooth muscle. They frequently occur at the bifurcation of vessels. Abnormalities of the media in association with neurofibromatosis also account for the development of aneurysms in this population. It is known that thinning of the media is part of the pathologic process associated with more superficial arteriosclerotic lesions.[85] Nevertheless, atherosclerosis in aneurysms appears to be a secondary rather than an inciting cause of aneurysms.

The relation of hypertension to renal artery aneurysms is well known. Arteriosclerosis has been implicated as a cause of renal artery aneurysms. Whether aneurysms *per se* cause hypertension as a result of turbulence and interruption of laminar flow is controversial. Not uncommonly, aneurysms may thrombose and such thrombosis may occlude branches of the artery. Changes in the pulsatile character of blood flow beyond an aneurysm have been proposed as causes of hypertension, but our own study has indicated that it is rare for aneu-

rysms *per se* to cause hypertension.[11] Rather, such aneurysms are generally associated with stenosing lesions, which are the cause of the hypertension. Therefore, it is important to assess renal vein renin ratios to clarify the issue as to whether an aneurysm without stenosis produces hypertension. Figure 25-39 illustrates large aneurysms in a woman without hypertension.

Large aneurysms of the renal artery may rupture, particularly during pregnancy.[85] Stanley and associates have reported an incidence of rupture of 5.6% among 72 patients with renal artery aneurysms.[85] An increased risk of rupture associated with noncalcified aneurysms larger than 1.5 cm in diameter and in hypertension patients is alleged in the literature, but size alone does not seem to be an important determinant of future rupture. Therefore, indications for operation for aneurysms are somewhat nebulous. Aneurysms associated with functionally significant renal artery stenosis should be treated operatively. In our view, PTA is hazardous in patients who have aneurysms in association with renal artery stenosis. Because of the catastrophic nature of rupture during pregnancy, prophylactic operative intervention for such lesions should be considered for women of childbearing age or who are likely to conceive in the future.

The treatment of renal artery aneurysms may be excision with primary closure, but smaller aneurysms and those associated with multiple branch disease usually require angioplastic closure of the vessel or renal artery reconstruction with autogenous vein grafts or with free autogenous hypogastric artery grafts. Macroaneurysms of the renal artery are too uncommon to make valid predictions or conclusions, and it is difficult from the sparse information available with regard to rupture of aneurysms to make categorical recommendations about their treatment. Suffice it to say that aneurysms associated with functionally significant stenosing lesions of renal arteries should be repaired by *in situ* or *ex vivo* techniques, aneurysms in women of childbearing age should be excised or repaired, and large aneurysms, even with calcification, should be repaired to prevent rupture and peripheral embolization.

Arteriovenous Fistula

Renal artery surgery for arteriovenous fistula is performed to correct hyperkinetic circulatory states and cardiac failure that may occur when there is major shunting, or to preserve renal function and cure hypertension if the kidney is ischemic beyond the area of arteriovenous diversion. Arteriovenous fistulas between the main renal artery and vein or their primary branches are usually traumatic, following penetrating injuries or mass ligation of the renal pedicle at nephrectomy. Intrarenal arteriovenous fistulas may occur congenitally in association with renal tumors or following nephrolithotomy, nephrotomy, and needle biopsy.

Intrarenal arteriovenous fistulas may be treated by ligating the artery supplying the involved segment of the kidney and resecting the resulting ischemic portion. Endaneurysmorrhaphy has been described by Ehrlich and is a suitable option. The vessels of the artery and vein are controlled with vascular clamps and the vein is opened, the fistula identified and oversewn, and the vein then closed.[16] In most cases in which there is a large communication between the renal artery and vena cava following penetrating injury, the kidney is atrophic and nephrectomy is done at the time of vascular repair of the abnormal communication.

Renal Artery Embolism

Renal artery embolism occurs most commonly as a result of underlying cardiac disease. Microembolism is not uncommon in diffuse atheromatous disease of the aorta and in association with mural thrombi within macroaneurysms of the renal artery. Typical clinical features of renal artery embolism include sudden onset of pain in the flank or upper abdomen, proteinuria, microscopic or gross hematuria, fever, leukocytosis, and elevated serum activities of SGOT (serum glutamic-oxalo-

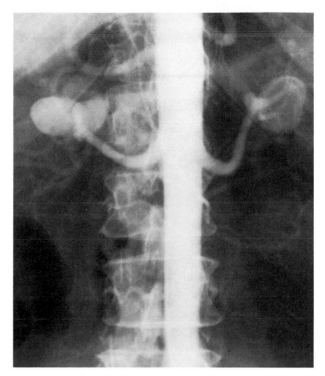

FIG. 25-39. An aortogram shows large aneurysms in a woman without hypertension.

acetic transaminase), LDH (lactate dehydrogenase), and alkaline phosphatase.[58] Usual work-up consists of intravenous and retrograde urography, renal scintiscan, and aortography, in that order. Occasionally symptoms may be vague or virtually nonexistent. Because underlying cardiac disease predisposes to embolism, the diagnosis of renal artery embolism should be considered when a patient with cardiac disease develops chest or abdominal pain in association with reduced renal function, proteinuria, or hematuria. In a recent publication we reported that underlying cardiac disease or arrythmia existed in 16 out of 17 patients. The correct diagnosis, confirmed by arteriography, was delayed beyond the second hospital day in 71%. Total renal embolization occurred in 7 and unilateral embolization occurred in 10. We found impairment of renal function in association with unilateral renal embolism in 8 out of 10 patients. In two of our cases, renal function was so compromised that dialysis was required. The cause of such a decrease in renal function was not found to be on the basis of hypotension or bilateral emboli, and the reason for diminished total renal function is not clear. Whether there was a reflex vascular spasm was not proven.

The ideal method of treating patients with renal

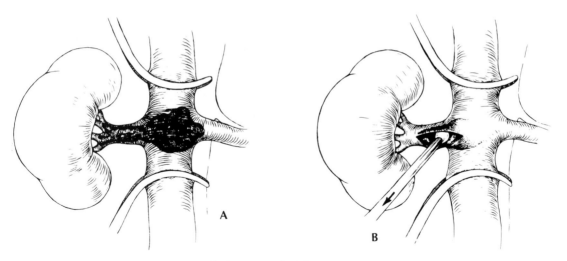

FIG. 25-40. **(A)** A phlebotomy is made for removal of the renal vein thrombus. **(B)** The primary vein is closed.

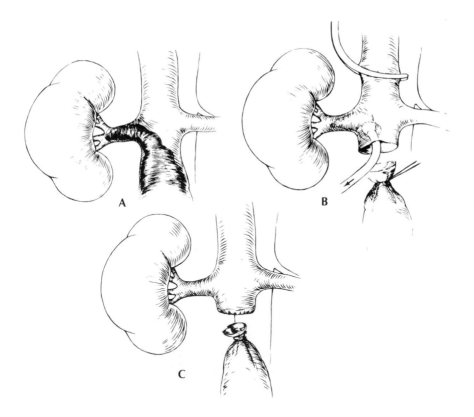

FIG. 25-41. Method of extracting the thrombus **(A)** from the inferior vena cava extending into the renal veins. **(B)** The inferior vena cava is transected caudal to the renal vein, and the thrombus is removed. The inferior end of the divided vena cava is oversewn. **(C)** The proximal end of the vena cava is ligated.

artery embolism is still undefined. An initial wave of enthusiasm for embolectomy or vascular reconstruction has been tempered by reports of successful management with expectant or medical (percutaneous catheter) treatment.[58,68,70] Moyer has stated that the mortality is greater after surgical therapy for unilateral embolic disease than follow-ing therapy with systemic anticoagulation. In our series, corrective vascular surgery was carried out in only one case. Thirteen patients received anticoagulant therapy, and only one patient died with uremic manifestations before the availability of dialysis. In patients who survived the acute illness there was a substantial return of renal function in association with treatment with anticoagulants, even in three patients with bilateral renal embolic disease. Our data suggest that surgery is not indicated in the case of unilateral embolism, particularly since the use of transcatheter infusion with anticoagulants and streptokinase.[58]

Renal Vein Thrombosis

There are several types of renal vein obstruction.[37] Thrombosis of the inferior vena cava with secondary involvement of the renal veins is commonly due to spread from pelvic or leg veins. The middle caval segment is commonly involved in the second type, obstruction of the inferior vena cava due to invasion by malignant neoplasm or external pressure. The third type is primary thrombosis of renal veins. Except during infancy primary renal vein thrombosis is rare, probably because of the brisk blood flow that normally exists. In a review of 228 patients with renal vein thrombosis, Abeshouse stated that 40% of patients were less than 2 months old.[1] The renal blood flow is relatively low in infancy and is liable to be reduced further by loss of water and salt from vomiting and diarrhea. Renal vein thrombosis, therefore, occurs especially as a complication of severe gastroenteritis. It may also be associated with acute pyelonephritis and thrombophlebitis of the renal vein. The fourth type is renal vein thrombosis secondary to primary renal disease. In adults renal vein thrombosis may occur as a result of disease causing a reduction in renal blood flow. It is found rarely in association with glomerulonephritis and pyelonephritis but is more liable to occur in renal amyloidosis.

The clinical features of renal vein thrombosis consist of sudden pain in the flank radiating around to the inguinal area or abdomen and enlargement and tenderness of the kidney. A nephrotic syndrome occurs in about 30% of patients. The diagnosis is established by vena cavagrams and selective renal venograms. If the renal artery is selectively catherized and infused with epinephrine at the time the contrast substance is injected in the renal vein, excellent filling can be obtained; whereas without reducing the renal arterial blood flow, the rapid venous washout prevents good delineation of partially obstructing thrombi. At operation the kidneys are often three to four times normal size and show diffuse hemorrhage and dilated lymphatics.

Treatment depends on the location of the thrombus. If the thrombus is located in the renal vein, the vena cava and renal veins are exposed and isolated by vascular clamps or tapes. A longitudinal phlebotomy is made (Fig. 25-40) and the clot is aspirated. Irrigation of the vein with heparinized saline is then carried out with repeated aspiration until free flow of venous blood is obtained. Following this, the phlebotomy is closed with a continous suture of 6-0 silk or synthetic material and the clamps are released from the vena cava.

If the clot is located in the vena cava and extends into one or both renal veins, the inferior vena cava is transected about 1 cm caudal to the takeoff of the renal vein and the caudal segment is suture ligated (Fig. 25-41). The thrombus is removed, the vein is aspirated and irrigated with weak heparin solution, and the inferior end of the divided inferior vena cava is oversewn with polypropylene or silk.

Nephrectomy is preferred in patients with proved unilateral thrombosis and a normal contralateral kidney, but restoration of renal venous return by removal of the thrombus may be very effective if operation is carried out promptly (within 48 hr). Systemic administration of heparin should not be used in patients with very low platelet counts subsequent to renal vein thrombosis (platelet consumption), because progression is unlikely in such patients.

REFERENCES

1. ABESHOUSE BS: Thrombosis and thrombophlebitis of the renal veins. Urol Cutan Rev 49:661, 1945
2. BARKER NW, WALTERS W. Hypertension associated with unilateral chronic atrophic pyelonephritis: Treatment by nephrectomy. Mayo Clin Proc 13:118, 1938
3. BESARAB A, BROWN RS, RUBIN NT et al: Reversible renal failure following bilateral renal artery occlusive disease: Clinical features, pathology, and the role of surgical revascularization. JAMA 235:2838, 1976
4. BLAKE WD, WEGRIA R, WARD HP et al: Effect of renal arterial constriction on excretion of sodium and water. Am J Physiol 163:422, 1950
5. BOOKSTEIN JJ, ABRAMS HL, BIGNER RE et al: Radiologic aspects of renovascular hypertension. Part III. Appraisal of arteriography. JAMA 221:368, 1972
6. BOOKSTEIN JJ, ABRAMS HL, BIGNER RE et al: Radiologic aspects of renovasular hypertension. Part II. The role of urography in unilateral renovascular disease. JAMA 220:1225, 1972
7. BOYD CH, LEWIS LC: Nephrectomy for arterial hypertension: Preliminary report. J Urol 39:627 1938
8. BUTLER AM: Chronic pyelonephritis and arterial hypertension. J Clin Invest 16:889, 1937
9. CASE TB, WALLACE JM, LARAGH JH: Comparison between saralasin and converting enzyme inhibitor in hypertensive disease. Kidney Int 15:S107, 1979
10. CROCKER DW, NEWTON RA, MAHONEY EM et al: Hypertension due to primary renal ischemia: A cor-

relation of juxtaglomerula cell counts with clinicopathological findings in twenty-five cases. N Engl J Med 267:794, 1962

11. CUMMINGS KC, LECKY JW, KAUFMAN JJ: Renal artery aneurysms and hypertension. J Urol 109:144, 1973

12. DAVIS BA, CROOK JE, VESTAL RE et al: Prevalence of renovascular hypertension in patients with Grade III or IV hypertensive retinopathy. N Engl J Med 301:1273, 1979

13. DEAN RH, LAWSON JD, HOLLIFIELD JW et al: Revascularization of the poorly functioning kidney. Surgery 85:44, 1979

14. DORNFELD L, KAUFMAN JJ: Immunologic considerations in renovascular hypertension. Urol Clin North Am 2, No. 2:285, 1975

15. DOTTER CT, JUDKINS MP: Transluminal treatment of arteriosclerotic obstruction. Circulation 30:654, 1964

16. EHRLICH RM: Renal arteriovenous fistula treated by endofistulorhaphy. Arch Surg 110:1195, 1975

17. ELLIS FH, JR, HELDEN RA, HINES EA: Aneurysm of the abdominal aorta involving the right renal artery: Report of a case with preservation of renal function after resection and grafting. Ann Surg 142:992, 1955

18. ERNST CB, STANLEY JC, MARSHALL FF et al: Autogenous saphenous vein aortorenal grafts: A ten-year experience. Arch Surg 105:855, 1972

19. EYLER WR, CLARK MD, GARMAN JE et al: Angiography of the renal areas including a comparative study of renal arterial stenoses in patients with and without hypertension. Radiology 78:879, 1962

20. FAIR WR: Renal perfusion/excretion determination renogram: A new tool in the diagnostic evaluation of renovascular hypertension. J Urol 113:595, 1975

21. FOSTER JH, DEAN RH, PINKERTON JA et al: Ten years' experience with the surgical management of renovascular hypertension. Ann Surg 177:755, 1973

22. FOSTER JH, MAXWELL MH, FRANKLIN SS et al: Renovascular occlusive disease: Results of operative treatment. JAMA 231:1043, 1975

23. FRANKLIN SS, MAXWELL MH: Clinical work up for renovascular hypertension. Urol Clin North Am 2:301, 1975

24. FRANKLIN SS, YOUNG JD, MAXWELL MH et al: Operative morbidity and mortality in renovascular disease. JAMA 231:1148, 1975

25. FREEMAN G, HARTLEY G, JR: Hypertension in a patient with solitary ischemic kidney. JAMA 111:1159, 1938

26. FREEMAN NE, LEEDS FH, ELLIOTT W.G et al: Thrombendarterectomy for hypertension due to renal artery occlusion. JAMA 156:1077, 1954

27. FRY WJ, ERNST CB, STANLEY JC et al: Renovascular hypertension in the pediatric patient. Arch Surg 107:692, 1973

28. GAVRAS H, BRUNNER HR, LARAGH JE et al: An angiotensin converting enzyme inhibitor to identify and treat vasoconstrictor and volume factors in hypertensive patients. New Engl J Med 291:817, 1974

29. GAVRAS H, BRUNNER HR, TURINI GA et al: Antihypertensive effect of the oral angiotensin converting-enzyme inhibitor SQ 14225 in man. New Engl J Med 298:991, 1978

30. GLUSHEIN AS, MANSUY MM, LITTMAN DS: Pheochromocytoma: Its relationship to the neurocutaneous syndromes. Am J Med 14:318, 1953

31. GOLDBLATT H, LYNCH, J, HANZAL RF et al: Studies on experimental hypertension: I. The production of persistent elevation of systolic blood pressure by means of renal ischemia. J Exp Med 59:347, 1934

32. GRAD E, RANCE CP: Bilateral renal artery stenosis in association with neurofibromatosis (Recklinghausen's disease): Report of two cases. J Pediatr 80:804, 1972

33. GRIM CE, KEITZER WF: Circadian rhythm of renin and aldosterone in unilateral renovascular hypertension: Pre- and postoperative studies. Ann Intern Med 80:298, 1974

34. GRUENTZIG A, KUHLMANN U, VETTER W et al: Treatment of renovascular hypertension with percutaneous transluminal dilation of a renal-artery stenosis. Lancet 1:801, 1978

35. GULBRANDSON RN, AL-BERMANI J, GASPARD DJ: Successful renal revascularization after prolonged nonfunction. JAMA 238:2522, 1977

36. HALPERN M, CURRARINO G: Vascular lesions causing hypertension and neurofibromatosis. New Eng J. Med 273:248, 1965

37. HARRISON CV, MILNE MD, STEINER RE: Clinical aspects of renal vein thrombosis. Q J Med 25:285, 1956

38. HOLLENBERG NK, WILLIAMS GH: Angiotensin as a renal adrenal and cardiovascular hormone: Responses to saralasin in normal man and in essential and secondary hypertension. Kidney Int 15:S29, 1979

39. HOLLEY KE, HUNT JC, BROWN AL, JR et al: Renal artery stenoses. A clinical–pathologic study in normotensive and hypertensive patients. Am J Med 37:14, 1964

40. HORNE ML, CONKLIN VN, KEENAN RE et al: Angiotensin II profiling with saralasin: Summary of Eton collaborative study. Kidney Int 15:S115, 1979

41. HUNT JC, SHEPS SG, HARRISON EG et al: Renal and renovascular hypertension: A reasoned approach to diagnosis and management. Arch Intern Med 133:988, 1974

42. HURWITT ES, SEIDENBERG B, HAIMOVICI H et al: Splenorenal arterial anastomoses. Circulation 4:532, 1956

43. ISHIKAWA K: Natural history and classification of occlusive thromboaortopathy (Takayasu's disease). Circulation 57:27, 1978

44. JUDSON WE, HELMER OM: Diagnostic and prognostic values of renin activity in renal venous plasma in renovascular hypertension. Hypertension 13:79, 1965

45. KATZEN BT, CHANG J, KNOX WG: Percutaneous transluminal angioplasty with the Gruentzig balloon catheter. Arch Surg 114:1389, 1979

46. KAUFMAN JJ: The middle aortic syndrome. Report of

a case treated by renal autotransplantation. Trans Am Assoc Genitourin Surg 64:39, 1972

47. KAUFMAN JJ: Renal artery stenosis and azotemia. Surg Gynec Obstet 137:949, 1973

48. KAUFMAN JJ: Dacron grafts and splenorenal bypass in the surgical treatment of stenosing lesions of the renal artery. Urol Clin North Am 2:365, 1974

49. KAUFMAN JJ, ALFEREZ C, VELA–NAVARRETTE R: Autotransplantation of a solitary functioning kidney for renovascular hypertension. J Urol 102:146, 1969

50. KAUFMAN JJ, GOODWIN WE, WAISMAN J et al: Renovascular hypertension in children: Report of seven cases treated surgically including two cases of renal autotransplantation. Am J Surg 124:149, 1972

51. KAUFMAN JJ, LUPU AN, FRANKLIN S et al: Diagnostic and predicative value of renal vein renin activity in renovascular hypertension. J Urol 103:702, 1970

52. KAUFMAN JJ, LUPU AN, MAXWELL MH: Further experiences in the diagnosis and treatment of renovascular hypertension. Part I. Clinical characteristics and diagnostic approaches. Urol Int 24:1, 1969

53. KINCAID OW, DAVIS GD, HALLERMAN FJ et al: Fibromuscular dysplasia of the renal arteries: Arteriographic features, classification, and observations on natural history of the disease. Am J Roentgenol Rad Ther Nuc Med 104:271, 1968

54. KYRIAKIDES GK, NAJARIAN JS: Renovascular hypertension in childhood: Successful treatment by renal autotransplantation. Surgery 85:611, 1979

55. LANKFORD ND, DONOHUE JP, GRIM CE et al: Results of surgical treatment of renal vascular hypertension. J Urol 122:439, 1979

56. LAWRIE GM, MORRIS GC JR, SOUSSOU ID et al: Late results of reconstructive surgery for renovascular disease. Ann Surg 191:528, 1980

57. LEADBETTER WF, BURKLAND CE: Hypertension in unilateral renal disease. J Urol 39:611, 1938

58. LESSMAN RK, JOHNSON SF, COBURN JW, KAUFMAN JJ: Renal artery embolism: Clinical features and long-term follow-up of 17 patients. Ann Intern Med 89:477, 1978

59. LIM RC, EASTMAN B, BLAISDELL FW: Renal autotransplantation: Adjunct to repair of renal vascular lesions. Arch Surg 105:847, 1972

60. MAHONEY AD, WAISMAN J: Lesions of the extrarenal segment of the renal artery and hypertension. Urol Clin North Am 2:259, 1975

61. MARKS LS, MAXWELL MH: Renal vein renin, value and limitations in the prediction of operative results. Urol Clin North Am 2:311, 1975

62. MARKS LS, MAXWELL MH, KAUFMAN JJ: Saralasin bolus test: Rapid screening procedure for renin mediated hypertension. Lancet 2:784, 1975

63. MARKS LS, MAXWELL MH, KAUFMAN JJ: Renin, sodium and vasodepressor response to saralasin in renovascular and essential hypertension. Ann Intern Med, 87:176, 1977

64. MAXWELL MH, BLEIFER KH, FRANKLIN SS et al: Cooperative study of renovascular hypertension: Demographic analysis of the study. JAMA 220:1195, 1972

65. MAY J, SHEIL AGR, HORVATH J et al: Reversal of renal failure and control of hypertension in patients with occlusion of the renal artery. Surg Gynecol Obstet 143:411, 1976

66. MCLAUGHLIN MG, WILLIAMS GM, STONESIFER GL JR: Ex vivo surgical dissection. Autotransplantation in renal disease. JAMA 235:1705, 1976

67. MEANEY TF, DUSTAN HP, MCCORMACK LJ: Natural history of renal arterial disease. Radiology 91:881, 1968

68. MILLAN VG, SHER MH, DETERLING RA, JR et al: Transcatheter thromboembolectomy of acute renal artery occlusion. Arch Surg 113:1086, 1978

69. MORRIS GC, JR, COOLEY DA, CRAWFORD ES et al: Renal revascularization for hypertension: Clinical and physiologic studies in 32 cases. Surgery 48:95, 1960

70. MOYER JH, HEIDER C, MORRIS GC JR. et al: Renal failure: I. The effect of complete renal artery occlusion for variable periods of time as compared to exposure to subfiltration arterial pressures below 30 mm Hg for similar periods. Ann Surg 145:41, 1957

71. NOVICK AC, BANOWSKY LHW, STEWART BH et al: Splenorenal bypass in the treatment of stenosis of the renal artery. Surg Gynecol Obstet 144:891, 1977

72. NOVICK AC, STRAFFON RA, STEWART BH et al: Diminished operative morbidity and mortality following revascularization for atherosclerotic renovascular disease. Presented at AUA meeting, Boston, May 1981

73. ORCUTT TW, FOSTER JH, RICHIE RE et al: Bilateral ex vivo renal artery reconstruction with autotransplantation. JAMA 228:493, 1974

74. OTA K, MORI S, AWANE Y et al: Ex-situ repair of renal artery for renovascular hypertension. Arch Surg 94:370, 1967

75. OXMAN HA, SHEPS SG, BERNATTZ PE et al: An unusual cause of renal arteriovenous fistula—fibromuscular dysplasia of the renal arteries. Mayo Clin Proc 48:207, 1973

76. PANTELL RH, GOODMAN BW, JR. Takayasu's arteritis: The relationship with tuberculosis. Pediatrics 67:84, 1981

77. POUTASSE EF: Occlusion of a renal artery as a cause of hypertension. Circulation 13:37, 1956

78. REINTGEN D, WOLFE WG, OSOFSKY S et al: Renal artery stenosis in children. J Pediatr Surg 16:26, 1981

79. SACKS SA: Renal autotransplantation and ex vivo renal surgery: Surgical treatment of renovascular hypertension. Urol Clin North Am 2:381, 1977

80. SCHWARTEN DE, YUNE HY, KLATTE EC et al: Clinical experience with percutaneous transluminal angioplasty (PTA) of stenotic renal arteries. Radiology 135:601, 1980

81. SHEPS SG, KINCAID OW, HUNT JC: Serial renal function and angiographic observations in idiopathic fi-

brous and fibromuscular stenoses of the renal arteries. Am J Cardiol 30:55, 1972

82. SIMMONS RL, TALLENT MB, KJELLSTRAND CM: Renal allograft rejection simulated by arterial stenosis. Surgery 68:800, 1970

83. SIMON N, FRANKLIN SS, BLEIFER KH et al: Clinical characteristics of renovascular hypertension. JAMA 220:1209, 1972

84. STANLEY JC, FRY WJ: Renovascular hypertension secondary to arterial fibrodysplasia in adults: Criteria for operation and results of surgical therapy. Arch Surg 110:922, 1975

85. STANLEY JC, RHODES EL, GEWERTZ BL et al: Renal artery aneurysms. Significance of macroaneurysms exclusive of dissections and fibrodysplastic mural dilations. Arch Surg 110:1327, 1975

86. STEWART BH, DUSTAN HP, KISER WS et al: Correlation of angiography and natural history in evaluation of patients with renovascular hypertension. J Urol 104:231, 1970

87. STRACHAN RW: The natural history of Takayasu's arteriopathy. Q J Med 33:57, 1964

88. STREETEN DHP, ANDERSON GH, JR: Outpatient experience with saralasin. Kidney Int [Suppl] 15:5, 1978–79

89. TIGERSTEDT R, BERGMAN PG: Niere und kreislauf. Skandinav Arch Physiol 8:223, 1898

90. TURINA M, GRUNTZIG A, KRAYENBUHL C et al: The role of the surgeon in percutaneous transluminal dilation of coronary stenosis. Ann Thorac Surg 28:103, 1979

91. VON RECKLINGHAUSEN F: Uber die Multiplen der Haut und Ihre Beziehungen zu den Multiplen Neurinomen. Berlin, Festshrift fur Rudolf Virchow, 1882

92. WOLLENWEBER J, SHEPS SG, DAVIS GD: Clinical course of atherosclerotic renovascular disease. Am J Med 21:60, 1968

93. WYLIE EJ: Endarterectomy and autogenous arterial grafts in the surgical treatment of stenosing lesions of the renal artery. Urol Clin North Am 2:351, 1975

94. ZINMAN L, LIBERTINO JA: Revascularization of the chronic totally occluded renal artery with restoration of renal function. J Urol 118:517, 1977

Lumbodorsal Surgery

26

Wolfgang Lutzeyer

The exploration of the lumbodorsal region should be done preferably by the muscle-preserving lumbodorsal incision, described by H. Lurz in 1956.[5] Despite the dorsal orientation toward the kidney and renal pelvis, this incision is not a modification of the other dorsal approaches, such as the incision of Simon; Guyon, Rosenstein, and Gil–Vernet also advocate Simon's incision.[2,3,8,10]

With only a few modifications, Lurz recommended the lumbodorsal incision for all conservative and radical operations on the kidney, adrenal glands, and upper ureter, even the removal of a calculus from a horseshoe kidney. It is, however, contradictory to both normal and pathologic anatomy to perform topographically differentiated renal surgery by a single approach.[9] A decision to use the lumbodorsal incision is based on two decisive elements:

The lumbodorsal incision, in contrast to all other approaches, demands exact anatomic definition and therefore exact anatomic surgery.

The lumbodorsal incision gives access to all dorsal renal operative targets and the upper ureter by the most direct approach and offers the surgeon a favorable horizontal working position.

Operative Technique

The lumbodorsal approach to the kidney derives its originality and clinical acceptance from its avoidance of three anatomic barriers—the quadratus lumborum muscle, the erector trunci or sacrospinal muscle, and the 12th rib. In contrast to all other lumbar and lumbodorsal incisions, the principal feature of the Lurz incision is the widening of the complete operative field by mobilization of the lower rib after cutting of the costovertebral ligament. A rib resection is never necessary.

POSITION OF PATIENT

The patient is placed on his healthy side (Fig. 26-1). The lumbar region is extended by devices of the operating table in combination with role cushions or adjustable kidney supports, increasing the distance between the costal arch and the iliac crest. The arm of the operative side is positioned upward in a right angle, without being overstretched, or it is loosely positioned to the front. The leg of the lower side is flexed at the hip and knee. A flat support is placed beneath the lower thigh. The patient is secured to the table by a strap stretched around his legs. The trunk is turned ventrally and the pelvis dorsally. The pelvis should be secured by a lateral support, and a sandbag may support the abdomen to prevent ventral rotation. Finally, the entire operating table is turned slightly ventrally. The surgeon thus has a nearly vertical view of the incision line (Fig. 26-2).

The position of the patient is most important because it brings the kidney and the adjacent organs into the appropriate position.

SKIN INCISION

Three topographic points are important for exact localization of the incision: the 12th rib, the line of the spinal processes, and the iliac crest. The skin incision begins in the costovertebral angle over the lateral part of the sacrospinal muscle just below the 12th rib, about 5 cm to 6 cm lateral from the spinal processes (Fig. 26-2). The incision extends along a slightly oblique course down to the iliac crest to a point between the anterior and middle third of a line from the spinal processes to the ventral iliac spine. If the 12th rib is long and steeply angled, the incision follows the lower edge of the rib for a certain distance.

APPROACH TO THE KIDNEY

In the superior margin of the incision, the inferior branches of the latissimus dorsi muscle and under this branches of the posterior inferior serratus muscle appear beneath the fatty tissue. Both muscle layers are incised with the scalpel (Fig. 26-3). The lateral part of the sacrospinal muscle is thus exposed, made apparent by the horizontal course of

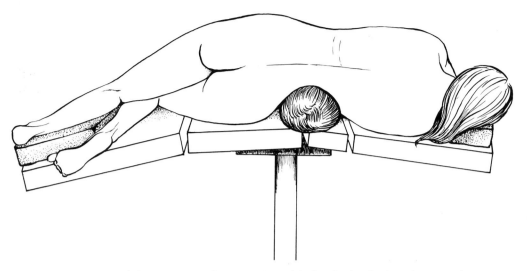

FIG. 26-1.   Position of the patient on the operating table for the lumbodorsal approach

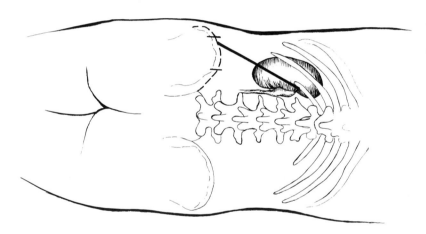

FIG. 26-2.   Lumbodorsal incision (left side). Note its relation to the 12th rib, the spine and the iliac crest, the kidney, the renal pelvis, and the upper ureter.

the muscle fibers. The previously cut musculature has a transverse course.

Along the lateral margin of the muscle, the incision comes down to the dense lumbodorsal fascia. After this fascia has been incised the quadratus lumborum muscle can be seen (Fig. 26-4). The lumbodorsal fascia is dissected 0.5 cm to 1 cm under the frontal margin of the quadratus lumborum muscle down to the iliac crest.

The very firm and tough costovertebral ligament extends from the transverse process of the first and second lumbar vertebrae to the 12th and 11th ribs. Dorsally it lies on the quadratus lumborum muscle. To expose the costovertebral ligament, the lateral margin of the sacrospinal muscle is displaced by blunt dissection and the vasa subcostalia can be seen. After complete incision of the costovertebral ligament, the transverse processes of the upper lumbar vertebrae are palpable in the depth

of the wound (Fig. 26-4). This mobilization of the 12th rib gives the same exposure as a rib resection, especially when the Finochietto rib retractor is used for generous opening of the wound.

The iliohypogastric nerve needs special attention during the exposure and later during the wound closure. In general, the nerve lies close to the inner surface of the lumbodorsal fascia (Fig. 26-4). The nerve may sometimes be found in the fatty tissue between the lumbodorsal and the retrorenal fascia, or even on this fascia. The iliohypogastric nerve is carefully mobilized at this time if it runs close to the cut edge of the fascia. Otherwise, it may be compromised during wound closure.

The retrorenal fascia (Gerota's fascia) is picked up by two forceps as far cranial as possible and incised (Fig. 26-5). The incision is extended cranially and caudally by two fingers. The iliohypogastric nerve should be located under the ventral hook

FIG. 26-3. Incision of the lumbodorsal fascia, the latissimus dorsi muscle, and the serratus posterior inferior muscle

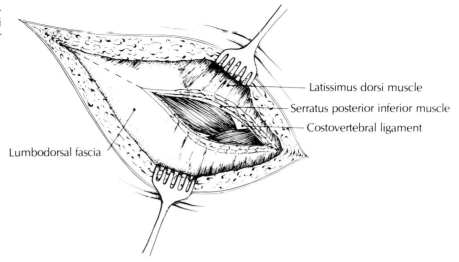

Latissimus dorsi muscle
Serratus posterior inferior muscle
Costovertebral ligament

Lumbodorsal fascia

FIG. 26-4. The costovertebral ligament is incised along the quadratus lumborum muscle up to the subcostal vessels. The pleura is not incised.

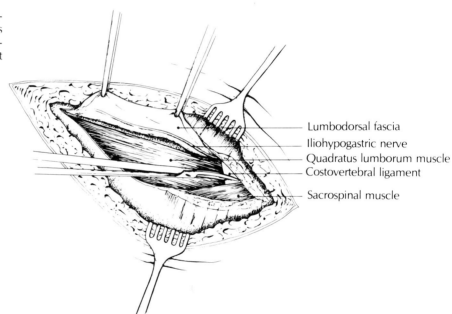

Lumbodorsal fascia
Iliohypogastric nerve
Quadratus lumborum muscle
Costovertebral ligament

Sacrospinal muscle

of the wound retractor. Spreading the wound makes the kidney visible. If necessary, the kidney may be retracted caudally by a blunt retractor of the Deaver type inserted between the adipose capsule and the renal surface (Fig. 25-6). To expose the renal hilus, it is sufficient to rotate the kidney frontally with a cotton applicator.

WOUND CLOSURE

In addition to offering rapid exposure, the lumbodorsal approach considerably simplifies wound closure. Six to eight sutures in the lumbodorsal

fascia are sufficient instead of the two- or three-layer muscle suture for closure of the standard flank incision (Fig. 26-7). It is important to take enough of the fascia with each stitch. The sutures are tied only after the kidney support has been removed and the operating table has been made horizontal. The quadratus lumborum muscle now lies like a wing beneath the fascial suture line. A surgical drain is inserted at the crossing of the sacrospinal muscle and the quadratus lumborum muscle (Fig. 26-7). In the superior wound margin, the latissimus dorsi muscle and the posterior inferior serratus muscle are reunited.

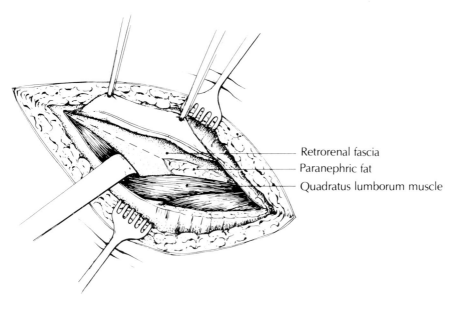

FIG. 26-5. Incision of the perinephric fascia (Gerota's) in the upper wound margin with blunt digital extension

Retrorenal fascia
Paranephric fat
Quadratus lumborum muscle

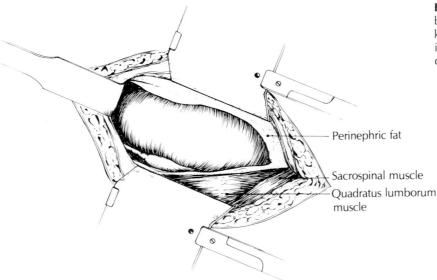

FIG. 26-6. The wound is opened by a Finochietto rib retractor. The kidney and the renal pelvis are placed into the operating position by a caudal spatula and a sponge holder.

Perinephric fat

Sacrospinal muscle
Quadratus lumborum muscle

Indications

In our experience, about two-thirds of all operations on the kidney, renal pelvis, and upper ureter may be performed using the lumbodorsal approach. It is especially recommended for secondary and repeated operations.

URETEROLITHOTOMY

The limitations for upper ureterolithotomy by the lumbodorsal incision are roentgenographically defined: a calculus *above* the iliac crest may be removed using this incision without difficulties.

PYELOLITHOTOMY (*in situ*)

The dorsal intrasinal pyelocalicolithotomy of Gil–Vernet has been found to be exceedingly valuable in the removal of staghorn or coralliform calculi, The advantages of the lumbodorsal approach, operating in a horizontal instead of a vertical position, are evident. There is no interference with the main renal vessels. Attention must be given only to the retropelvic branch of the renal artery, which crosses the renal pelvis in the upper hilar region.

The intrasinal preparation with the aid of hilar retractors in the capsular diaphragm facilitates the *in situ* procedure. Opening of the renal calices

FIG. 26-7. Suturing of the lumbodorsal fascia. A drain is placed between the wound margins. Care should be taken to avoid suturing of the iliohypogastric nerve.

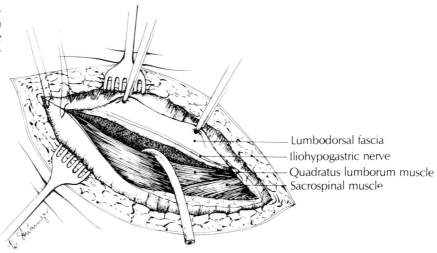

Lumbodorsal fascia
Iliohypogastric nerve
Quadratus lumborum muscle
Sacrospinal muscle

enables inspection and visual control of the intrapelvic operation, in general making intraoperative roentgenography unnecessary. If roentgenography is indicated, the kidney should be mobilized and the examination may be accomplished by cineradiography or plain film. In special cases the kidney may be mobilized and the pelvis opened, the renal calices palpated, and a nephrotomy done directly on the palpating finger.

URETEROPYELOPLASTY

Plastic corrections of the renal pelvis and the pyeloureteral segment can be easily performed using the lumbodorsal approach. Favorable drainage is obtained by the *in situ* operation, and a nephropexy is not indicated. If necessary, a nephrostomy catheter or a transrenal stenting catheter may be brought out through the middle of the incision.

PARENCHYMAL INCISIONS

The lumbodorsal approach enables partial renal resections, removal of solitary cysts, and open renal biopsies to be done. After mobilization of the kidney, even resections of the upper pole and transverse and longitudinal nephrotomies are possible with or without temporary clamping of the renal pedicle.

NEPHROPEXY

Nephropexy as a primary operation may be done with great safety using this incision. More often, nephropexy is performed after operations on the renal pelvis and ureter to give better functional and anatomic results.

NEPHRECTOMY

In contrast to Lurz's recommendations, renal tumor should not be removed using this approach. The lumbodorsal incision is only indicated for the removal of small kidneys (hypoplasia, chronic pyelonephritis). In hydronephrosis, aspiration and collapse may facilitate nephrectomy. A pyonephrotic kidney may best be removed by subcapsular nephrectomy.

NEPHROCAPSULECTOMY AND SYMPATHECTOMY

In rare cases, nephrocapsulectomy and sympathectomy of the renal pedicle may be done by the muscle-preserving lumbodorsal incision.

ADRENAL SURGERY

Only in unilateral diseases with certain diagnosis should the adrenal glands be exposed by a lumbodorsal approach. For all other cases and for bilateral exploration, other incisions are preferred (see Chap. 1).

Contraindications

KIDNEY TUMOR

Radical extirpation of a kidney tumor is not satisfactorily accomplished by the dorsal approach.

Other more extensive incisions offer improved visibility and control.

KIDNEY ANOMALIES

Generally, there is some preoperative uncertainty about the intraoperative findings in renal malformations. Because the lumbodorsal incision does not allow for the sometimes necessary widening of the incision, it should not be used in these cases. Some forms of renal duplication and hypoplastic kidney may be an exception.

COMBINED OPERATIONS

Combined operations on the kidney and the lower ureter are preferably performed using a flank incision, which can be extended to both sides, or two separate incisions. The lumbodorsal incision does not enable safe access to the lower ureter.

ADHERENT AND HIGH-PLACED KIDNEY

Relative contraindications for a lumbodorsal incision include densely adherent or an extremely high-placed kidney.

BILATERAL NEPHRECTOMY

Patients with renal insufficiency or malignant hypertension are often in poor general condition. They do not tolerate a lateral or abdominal position very well. An anterior approach may be therefore preferable for bilateral nephrectomy before or after renal transplantation.

Advantages

The advantages of the muscle-preserving lumbodorsal incision are the following:

The lumbodorsal approach is the shortest way to the dorsal aspect of the kidney.

The operative target—the renal hilus or the upper ureter—are in the center of the operating field.

The operation can be performed in a favorable natural horizontal plane instead of a frontal plane, as with a flank incision.

Except for the mentioned contraindications, nearly all operations on the renal parenchyma, the renal caliceal system, and the upper ureter can be performed without distinct dislocation of the kidney. A nephropexy as a final procedure is not necessary.

In contrast to other incisions, nearly all muscles are preserved, and the incision is anatomically exact.

Early ambulation of the patient and shortening of hospital treatment are effective prophylaxis against embolism and thrombosis.

Interventions for secondary procedures are easily done without respect to the kind of earlier incisions.

REFERENCES

1. BERGMANN EV: Über Nierenexstirpation. Berl Klin Wschr 39:46, 1885
2. GIL–VERNET J: New surgical concepts in removing renal calculi. Urol Int 20:255, 1965
3. GUYON F: Leçons Cliniques sur Les Maladies des Voies Urinaires. Paris, JB Baillière, 1881
4. ISRAEL J: Ein Fall von Nierenexstirpation. Berl Klin Wschr 37:689, 1883
5. LURZ H: Ein muskelschonender lumbalschnitt zur Freilegung der Niere. Chirurg 27:125, 1956
6. LURZ L, LURZ H: Die Eingriffe an den Harnorganen, Nebennieren und männlichen Geschlechtsorganen. In Guleke N, Zenker R (eds): Allgemeine und Spezielle Chirurgische Operationslehre, 2nd ed. Berlin, Springer–Verlag, 1961
7. LUTZEYER W, LYMBEROPOULOS S: Der lumbodorsale Zugang zur Niere (Lurz): Indikation, klinische Erfahrung, und kritische Beurteilung. Urologe [A] 9:324, 1970
8. ROSENSTEIN P: Ein funktioneller Lumbalschnitt zur Freilegung der Niere. Zeitschr Urol Chirurgie 17:119, 1925
9. SIGEL A, HELD L: Die Zugangswege der Nierenchirurgie. Urologe [A] 2:144, 1963
10. SIMON G: Exstirpation einer Niere am Menschen. Dtsch Klin 22:137, 1870

Renal Biopsy

27

Ronald P. Krueger

The indications for renal biopsy are varied, and a comprehensive discussion of these indications are beyond the scope of this chapter. It should be emphasized, however, that renal biopsy has become an important diagnostic, as well as prognostic, tool in a variety of diseases of the kidney. For this reason, the urologist should be familiar with the techniques of renal biopsy as well as the complications and contraindications of this procedure.

Although renal biopsy techniques can be used by any qualified urologist or nephrologist, biopsies should not be performed unless adequate facilities for processing the tissue are available. These facilities should include the capability for light, immunofluorescent, and electron microscopy.

Techniques

There are two basic techniques for obtaining renal tissue for diagnosis: the percutaneous needle biopsy and the open surgical biopsy. Each technique has its advantages and disadvantages, contraindications and indications, and complications. In most centers, the needle biopsy is performed by the nephrologist (or, occasionally, the radiologist) and the open biopsy is within the purview of the urologic surgeon. Nevertheless, the urologist will be called upon to treat the patient who has had a needle biopsy should serious complications occur, and for this reason, he should be familiar with needle biopsy techniques.

NEEDLE BIOPSY OF THE KIDNEY

Needle biopsy of the kidney can be done at the patient's bedside, on the ward in the treatment room, or in the operating room. The patient should go without food or drink for at least 6 hr prior to the biopsy. Premedication with promethazine and meperidine may be used, but my preference is to give intravenous diazepam just prior to the biopsy. Diazepam is particularly useful in pediatric pa-

tients, because the meperidine–promethazine combination may cause confusion and hyperactivity in some children.

The patient is placed on the operating table (or bed) in the prone position with the head turned away from the side of the biopsy, to prevent the patient from watching the operator and seeing the biopsy needle itself. This is particularly important when working with children, because the needle is a formidable-looking instrument.

Either kidney may be biopsied with the percutaneous technique, but the operator should stand on the side being biopsied rather than reach across the patient's back.

Localization of the kidney can be accomplished in a variety of ways. Ultrasound can be used to locate the kidney position as well as its depth, and the site for needle puncture can be marked on the skin. Some physicians prefer to perform the biopsy in the radiology department, using fluoroscopy at the time intravenous pyelography is being carried out. Both of these methods of localization work quite well but require coordination with other personnel, are somewhat more cumbersome, and add additional cost to the procedure. My preference is for the so-called blind technique, in which a previously obtained intravenous pyelogram or renal nephrotomogram is used to locate the kidney with relation to the 12th (or occasionally 11th) rib. The 12th rib will usually divide the kidney into the upper two thirds and lower one third. The site of needle puncture is then determined by measuring the appropriate distance medially from the tip of the 12th rib to give a needle entry point in the midportion of the lower one third of the kidney (Fig. 27-1). Care should be taken to avoid an extreme medial position so as to avoid puncturing the renal hilus.

The skin of the back is prepped with povidone and the area is draped with sterile towels. Gloves are worn by the operator, but gown and mask are not necessary. The site chosen for biopsy is infiltrated with 1% lidocaine (Xylocaine) without epinephrine and the anesthetic is infiltrated down through the skin, the subcutaneous tissues, and the lumbodorsal muscles to the perirenal fat.

Once satisfactory local anesthesia has been achieved, a 22-gauge spinal needle is used to locate the depth of the kidney. This needle is advanced in a perpendicular position through the tissues until the perirenal fat is reached. At this point, the patient is instructed to inspire deeply and hold his breath. The spinal needle is then advanced slowly until its tip enters the renal capsule. With experience, the operator can nearly always feel when the renal capsule is entered. The patient is then instructed to breathe normally. If the spinal needle is correctly placed, it will oscillate up and down as the kidney rises and falls with respiration. In addition, the needle will pulsate synchronously

with the patient's pulse. These two movements confirm proper placement of the spinal needle (Fig. 27-2). The patient is again instructed to inspire deeply and hold his breath, and the spinal needle is removed. The operator places his thumb and forefinger on the needle at the skin level so that after removal the distance from the operator's fingers to the needle tip will equal the depth of the kidney capsule. It is imperative that the operator not hold or restrict the motion of either the spinal needle or the biopsy needle unless the patient is holding his breath. To do so when the patient is breathing may result in a renal laceration.

The renal biopsy needle with obturator is then inserted into the same site as the spinal needle and advanced to the previously measured depth. The Franklin modification of the Vim–Silverman biopsy needle is suitable for adult patients, but the Metcoff biopsy needle, because of its lighter hub, is preferable for use in children. Before advancing the biopsy needle the last centimeter, the patient is instructed to inspire deeply again and hold his breath. The final centimeter of needle is then advanced, and the tip of the biopsy needle should be through the renal capsule. Entry into the capsule can be felt by the experienced operator. at this point, the patient is asked to breathe normally and the needle location is confirmed by the oscillation and pulsation of the biopsy needle.

The patient again is asked to hold his breath and the obturator is removed and replaced by the cutting element. The cutting element is advanced into the needle sheath slowly until resistance is encountered. This occurs when the cutting element tip has reached the same depth as the tip of the sheath. At this point, the patient is again asked to breath so that reconfirmation of the needle position can be made.

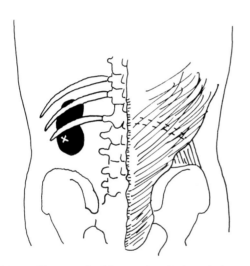

FIG. 27-1. The needle biopsy site (x) in relation to the anatomic structures

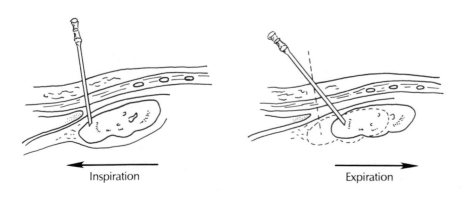

Inspiration

Expiration

A

B

FIG. 27-2. (A) The needle is placed during inspiration. **(B)** The position of the needle is confirmed by oscillation of the needle with expiration.

The patient then inspires and holds his breath, and the kidney is biopsied. This is done by sharply advancing the cutting element into the renal substance. The cutting element is then grasped by the operator and stabilized while the sheath is advanced and rotated 360 degrees around the cutting element. Both the sheath and cutting element are then removed as a unit and the patient is allowed to breathe normally. The core of tissue is removed from the cutting element and placed on a gauze moistened with normal saline. The procedure can be terminated at this point, or a second core of renal tissue can be obtained in the same fashion.

Following completion of the biopsy, the patient should be kept in the prone position for 1 hr and then allowed to turn over. Absolute bed rest should be maintained for 24 hr. The patient should be warned that he may have some gross hematuria for the next several voidings and reassured that this is not unexpected. In fact, transient gross hematuria occurs following needle biopsy in between 5% and 22% of patients but usually subsides within 24 hr.[2] If it does not subside within 24 hr, the patient should be kept in bed until it does.

The hematocrit should be measured at 6 hr at and 24 hr after after biopsy and should not change significantly from the prebiopsy level. Pulse and blood pressure should be measured frequently during the first few postbiopsy hours. My routine is to measure them every 15 minutes for the first hour, every 30 minutes for the next 4 hr, then hourly for the next 4 hr, then every 4 hr during the next 24 hr. If pulse, blood pressure, and hematocrit are stable and the patient has no or decreasing hematuria, then he may be out of bed after 24 hr and discharged (if appropriate) after 48 hr. If significant postbiopsy bleeding occurs then, of course, appropriate observation and management should be carried out.

OPEN RENAL BIOPSY

Access to the kidney for open biopsy can be gained either by placing the patient in the standard flank position and making an incision off the tip of the 12th rib or by using the posterior approach with the patient placed prone on the operating table. The supine position with an anterior subcostal incision can also be used, but it is the least preferable approach.

Although the standard flank incision is probably the most widely used, the posterior approach with a vertical paraspinal incision affords easy access to the lower pole of the kidney and is associated with a considerable reduction in postoperative pain and discomfort as compared to the standard flank incision. In addition, the cosmetic advantage of a paraspinal scar over that following a flank incision is worth considering.

In either case, after division of the anterior oblique or lumbodorsal muscles, the retroperitoneal space is entered and Gerota's fascia is incised. The perirenal fat is mobilized from the lower pole of the kidney. A Deaver retractor can be used to retract the kidney caudally several centimeters for better exposure if necessary (Fig. 27-3).

The biopsy is taken by making a deep elliptic incision into the cortex. The surgeon should lift the specimen out with sharp scissors rather than damage it by picking it up with forceps. The specimen should be placed on a gauze sponge moistened with saline.

Closure of the renal capsule over the incision site is best accomplished using 3-0 chromic catgut on a ⅝-inch (16-mm) circle taper needle. The needle must be carefully rotated through the renal parenchyma below the depth of the biopsy incision. After the suture is placed, it is tied using a surgeon's knot. As the first knot is tied, equal tension should be applied on both ends of the suture, and both forefingers should be placed on the knot as it is tightened. Several similar stitches may be required to close the biopsy incision to achieve hemostasis.

Following the open biopsy, a needle biopsy under direct vision should be obtained also. The reason for this is that some glomerular diseases

FIG. 27-3. A Deaver retractor in the perinephric space displaces the kidney caudally.

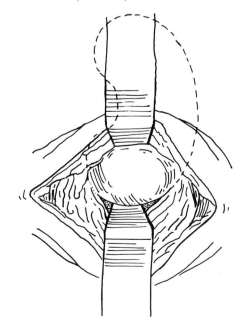

involve the deep cortical or juxtamedullary nephrons preferentially and a needle biopsy will provide a deep core of tissue for analysis, whereas the elliptic biopsy may not always be adequate for this purpose. This tissue should also be placed on a saline-moistened gauze. Bleeding is usually minimal and self-limited following the needle biopsy, but if significant bleeding occurs, it can be stopped with a single figure-of-eight stitch of 3-0 chromic catgut.

Following completion of the biopsies, the would is irrigated and carefully inspected for hemostasis. No drains are left. Gerota's fascia is closed with a continuous 3-0 chromic catgut suture. The muscles are closed in layers with interrupted 2-0 or 1-0 chromic catgut. Subcutaneous closure is effected with 3-0 chromic suture. For skin closure in adults, 4-0 nylon interrupted sutures or metal clips are satisfactory, but in children a continuous 4-0 Dexon subcuticular closure is preferable.

In most circumstances, the skin sutures or clips can be removed at several days, but in edematous or immunosuppressed patients, 10 to 12 days is probably safer.

The Biopsy Specimen

Regardless of the method of biopsy, the specimen should be immediately placed on a saline-moistened sponge (never in formalin).[6] Disposition of the specimen varies from hospital to hospital and according to the preference of the pathologist.

At present, in most institutions, the tissue is divided into three parts. One portion is placed in 10% formalin for routine light microscopy preparation. The second portion is placed in 2% Glutaraldehyde for electron-microscopic processing. The third portion should be quick frozen in an acetone–dry ice mixture or liquid nitrogen for immunofluorescent staining.

Whether the tissue is divided by the operating surgeon or pathologist varies by institution, but the tissue should be divided and fixed within minutes after it is obtained. Allowing the tissue to stay on the saline-soaked gauze for any period of time will render it unsatisfactory for interpretation, particularly by electron microscope or immunofluorescent techniques.

As a general rule, the biopsy specimen should yield adequate tissue for interpretation.[6] For most renal lesions, at least five glomeruli must be available for evaluation. Using the surgical biopsy technique, low tissue yield should not be a problem, but with the closed needle technique, occasionally no renal tissue or renal tissue with fewer than five glomeruli will be obtained. However, in experienced hands, the yield of satisfactory tissue following needle biopsy should be between 90% and 95%. If, following closed needle biopsy, insufficient tissue is obtained, then needle biopsy may be repeated or the patient may undergo open surgical biopsy.

Contraindications to Renal Biopsy

There are several absolute contraindications to renal biopsy either by the percutaneous needle technique or the open technique. These contraindications include severe uncontrolled hypertension, renal malignancy or perinephritis, coagulation disorders, renal tuberculosis, patient unwillingness, and unlikelihood of obtaining information beneficial to the patient.[1,4,5]

There are also specific contraindications to performing renal biopsy by the percutaneous needle technique. These are presence of a solitary kidney; atypical position of the kidney; small, contracted kidneys; an uncooperative patient or who is unable to lie still during the biopsy procedure; a glomerular filtration rate of less than 20 ml/min; and marked obesity. In any of these situations, however, an open renal biopsy may usually be performed successfully and with safety to the patient.

I believe that needle biopsy should not be performed in infants and small children (usually under age 4), because patient cooperation is essential. Some authors advocate general anesthesia in these patients to allow needle biopsy to be performed, but if one is going to invest the time and personnel necessary for general anesthesia, then it would seem more sensible to proceed with open surgical biopsy. In this way, one can be assured of obtaining an adequate tissue specimen as well as absolute control of hemostasis.

Complications of Renal Biopsy

Although a variety of complications have been reported following both closed (needle) biopsy and open renal biopsy, the constant improvement in biopsy techniques over the past 20 years has resulted in a continuing decline in the number of complications.[2,3,5] The principal complication associated with renal biopsy, either open or closed, is postoperative bleeding. This occurs more commonly in hypertensive patients and those with minor coagulation disorders or renal insufficiency. One of the principal advantages of the open biopsy technique is the ability of the surgeon to identify and control any bleeding points following the removal of renal tissue. However, even under ideal circumstances using the open biopsy technique, postoperative bleeding occasionally occurs.

Gross hematuria may occur following needle biopsy, but this ordinarily will resolve within the first 24 hr while the patient is still at bed rest. Prolonged bleeding rarely is a problem but has been reported and, on occasion, has required nephrectomy for control of bleeding. Retroperitoneal hematoma also occurs. Severe bleeding leading to circulatory collapse is rare.

In addition to acute postbiopsy bleeding, there is some risk of late hemorrhage in patients undergoing needle biopsy of the kidney. This most often occurs between the 7th and 10th day postbiopsy. For this reason, patients undergoing needle biopsy of the kidney should be cautioned to restrict physical activities, including sports, heavy exercise, and bicycle or motorcycle riding, for at least 2 weeks after needle biopsy.

Another reported complication of needle biopsy of the kidney is that of arteriovenous aneurysm. This appears to be the result of needle puncture of either the main artery or a large intrarenal vessel.

An infrequent complication of closed needle biopsy is that of needle puncture of some organ other than the kidney. Presumed needle biopsy specimens of the kidney have yielded such tissues as gastric or colonic mucosa, spleen, liver, pancreas, adrenal gland, and diaphragm. Fortunately, there usually are no associated complications when these unintended organs are biopsied.

The complications of open biopsy include untoward reactions to anesthesia, wound infection, and, of course, bleeding. Although patient death has been reported as a complication of both needle and open renal biopsy, fortunately this is a rare occurrence.

In summary, renal biopsy, whether percutaneous or surgical, is a relatively safe diagnostic procedure associated with minimal morbidity or mortality when performed by experienced physicians.

REFERENCES

1. BURKE SC: Urinalysis, the investigation of hematuria and renal biopsy. In Kelalis PP, King LR (eds): Clinical Pediatric Urology, pp 139–143. Philadelphia, WB Saunders, 1976
2. KARAFIN L, KENDALL AR, FLEISHER DS: Urologic complications in percutaneous renal biopsy in children. J Urol 103:332, 1970
3. KARK RM: Renal biopsy. JAMA 105:220, 1968
4. PRIMACK WA, EDELMANN CM, JR: Technique of renal biopsy. In Edelmann CM, Jr (ed): Pediatric Kidney Disease, pp 262–269. Boston, Little, Brown & Co, 1978
5. SCHREINER GE: Renal biopsy. In Strauss MB, Welt LG (eds): Diseases of the Kidney, 2nd ed, pp 197–209. Boston, Little, Brown & Co, 1971
6. ZOLLINGER HU, MIHATSCH MJ: Renal Pathology in Biopsy, pp 1–7. Berlin, Springer-Verlag, 1978

Dialysis Access Surgery

28

John M. Barry

The purpose of this chapter is to provide the practicing urologist and the urologist-in-training with the common surgical techniques of access as practiced by the Division of Urology at the University of Oregon School of Medicine. These techniques are based on 21 years of experience with the surgery of end-stage renal disease and an annual average of 61 vascular access and 36 chronic peritoneal dialysis access procedures during the past 5 years.

Vascular Access

ARM ARTERIOVENOUS SHUNT

Surgical Anatomy

The radial artery lies just under the antebrachial fascia in the lower part of the forearm (Fig. 28-1) and is the artery of choice for forearm arteriovenous shunting and fistula formation. Proximally it lies between the brachioradialis and flexor carpi radialis muscles. The superficial radial nerve is lateral to it and must be avoided when the shunt is tied in place to prevent chronic pain. The venae comitantes which accompany the radial artery are too small for cannulation. The ulnar artery is the forearm artery of second choice for arteriovenous shunting. In the distal forearm it lies on the radial side of the ulnar nerve and is covered by the flexor carpi ulnaris muscle.

The distal cephalic vein, which receives the dorsal veins of the thumb, ascends at the radial border of the wrist, and runs parallel to the anterior border of the brachioradialis muscle, is the vein of choice for forearm arteriovenous shunting (Fig. 28-2). Alternate veins for shunting procedures are the accessory cephalic vein, which arises on the dorsum of the forearm and ascends diagonally, where it usually joins the cephalic vein; the proximal cephalic vein in the lateral bicipital groove; and the basilic vein, which ascends along the ulnar border of the forearm and turns into the antecubital fossa, where it receives the median cubital vein

and continues in the medial bicipital groove. The median cubital vein is usually unsatisfactory for cannulation because flexion of the elbow results in vessel tip pressure against the posterior wall of the vein, with obstruction and eventual perforation.

Preoperative Preparation

Whenever possible the nondominant arm is used for arteriovenous shunts of fistulas, but one should not hesitate to use the dominant arm when the blood vessels in the nondominant arm are of questionable quality. Collateral circulation to the hand is determined by occluding both the radial and ulnar arteries at the wrist, having the patient form several fists in rapid succession, and then releasing the ulnar artery. Rapid filling of the finger capillaries indicates that adequate collateral circulation will be present when the radial artery is used for the shunt. The same test can be used to determine the adequacy of radial artery filling of the hand when the ulnar artery is to be sacrificed in the creation of a shunt.

The venous anatomy for the individual patient can be determined preoperatively by placing a warm moist pack on the arm for an hour, then applying a proximal tourniquet and examining the veins. The patient has a shower and shampoo the night before surgery, including preparation of the hand and fingernails with a surgical scrub brush and nail cleaner. Included in the patient's preoperative medications are a narcotic, a tranquilizer, and a prophylactic antibiotic of the surgeon's choice.

Surgical Technique

The winged-in-line Ramirez shunts are preferred because they are easily declotted.[7] In addition to the items in a simple cut-down tray and rolling stools for the surgeon and assistant, two winged-in-line shunt tubes, two small vessel tips, two medium vessel tips, two large vessel tips, one straight connector, 100 ml of a 1% solution of neomycin–polymyxin B irrigation, 100 ml of heparinized saline, a 10-ml syringe without a Luer lock for shunt irrigation with heparinized saline, and

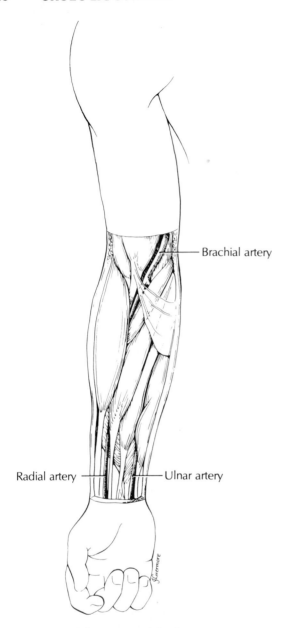

FIG. 28-1. Arterial anatomy of the forearm

1% lidocaine (Xylocaine) for local anesthesia are all the materials that are required.

After surgical preparation and draping of the arm from midhumerus to fingertips, a tourniquet is applied and a sterile marking pencil is used to outline the courses of the forearm veins and the radial artery. For the occasional vascular access surgeon, this helps preserve blood vessel orientation after local anesthetic infiltration. If the distal cephalic vein and radial artery are chosen and lie close to one another, a transverse incision is planned

3 finger-widths above the wrist to prevent vessel tip erosion of the vessels with wrist flexion (Fig. 28-3). The skin and subcutaneous tissue are infiltrated with 1% Xylocaine, and the incision is deepened through the skin. Electrocautery with a needle electrode is extremely helpful for the small bleeders in the skin and subcutaneous tissue. The cephalic vein is isolated with hemostat dissection for a distance of 1.5 cm to 2 cm, and two 2-0 silk ligatures are passed around the isolated venous segment. The subcutaneous tissue over the antebrachial fascia is cleared, and the underlying radial artery is palpated. Perforation of the antebrachial fascia in its transverse plane and then longitudinal incision of the fascia for 1.5 cm to 2 cm exposes the radial artery and its venae comitantes. Small muscular arterial branches are ligated with 4-0 silk, and two 2-0 silk ligatures are passed around the isolated segment of radial artery.

An estimate of the needed vessel tips is made and each is inserted into the end of its trimmed, winged-in-line shunt until the scored area is within the tubing (Fig. 28-4). A 2-0 silk ligature is triply tied around the shunt tubing to anchor the vessel tip. One limb of this ligature is cut. The remaining limb will be used to anchor the shunt assembly. The shunt tubing and vessel tip assembly are filled with heparinized saline, and the end of the tubing opposite the vessel tip is clamped. The distal ligature on the vein is tied and left long. A No. 11 blade is passed halfway through the vein with the cutting edge upward to form a slight visor incision. This is grasped with atraumatic forceps, the opening is gently dilated with a small, closed hemostat, and the vessel tip is gently introduced into the vein (Fig. 28-5). The proximal 2-0 silk ligature is now tied around the vein, and one limb of this ligature is cut. This ligature is now tied to the one anchoring the vessel tip within the tubing (Fig. 28-6). The ends of the distal venous ligature are passed around the shunt tubing and tied to complete the anchoring of the shunt assembly within the vessel. A subcutaneous tunnel is created distally to allow the wings of the shunt to further stabilize the assembly. The vein is now irrigated through the shunt tubing with heparinized saline to be certain there is no obstruction, and the shunt tubing is reclamped.

Attention is now directed to the radial artery. The distal ligature is tied and left long and the proximal ligature is elevated to prevent bleeding while the radial artery is incised in a manner similar to that used for the vein. The radial artery is gently dilated with a small, closed hemostat, and the previously assembled shunt tubing and vessel tip

FIG. 28-2. Arm venous anatomy. **(A)** The distal cephalic vein is the vessel of choice for venous return. **(B)** The venous "M" of the antecubital fossa must be remembered when the veins are not visible or palpable because of obesity.

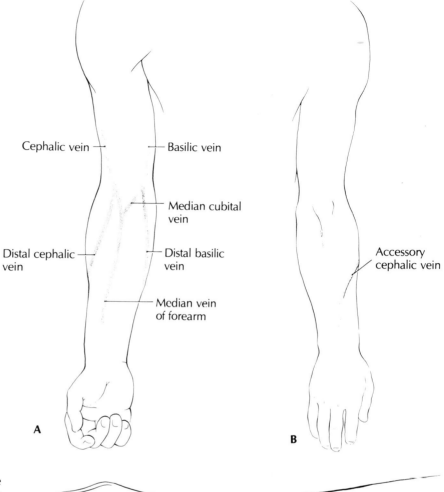

FIG. 28-3. The skin incision for the arteriovenous shunt must be well above the wrist to allow joint mobility without shunt obstruction.

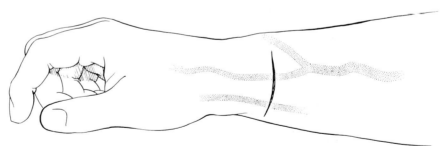

are placed into the radial artery and anchored in the same fashion as described for venous cannulation. After the shunt tubing is brought through its stab wound in the skin, the air is removed by allowing the radial artery blood to fill the shunt tubing. A shunt connector is used to join the two limbs, and the shunt is completed (Fig. 28-7). Shunt tape is used to secure the tubing ends over the connector. The subcutaneous tissue is closed with interrupted 4-0 polyglycolic acid suture, and the skin is closed with either a running, subcuticular

4-0 polyglycolic acid suture on a cutting needle, or a running suture of 4-0 monofilament nylon.

The same principles can be applied to any of the alternate veins previously mentioned, and to the ulnar artery. If it is necessary to cannulate the proximal cephalic vein in the bicipital groove, it is extremely helpful to create a long subcutaneous tunnel across the elbow joint and to bring the shunt tubing out the proximal forearm. This removes the necessity of a dressing going across the elbow joint.

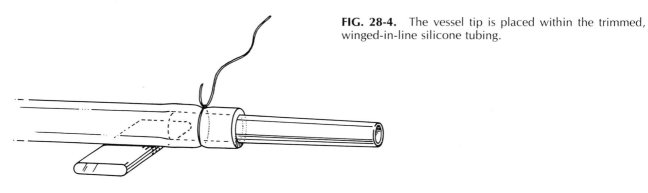

FIG. 28-4. The vessel tip is placed within the trimmed, winged-in-line silicone tubing.

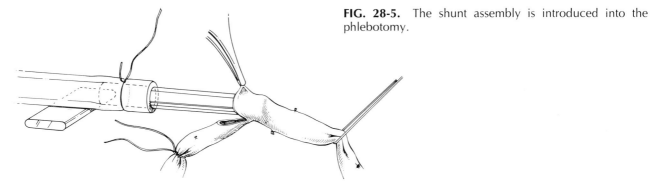

FIG. 28-5. The shunt assembly is introduced into the phlebotomy.

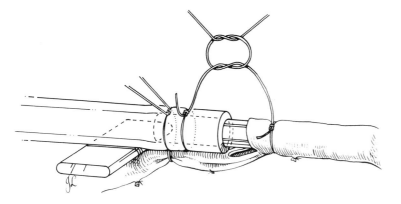

FIG. 28-6. The shunt tubing and the vessel tip are anchored to the vein.

FIG. 28-7. Completed arteriovenous shunt demonstrating distal stab wounds

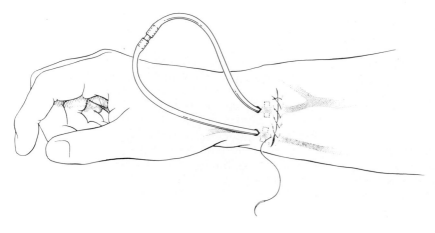

A dry sterile dressing is applied, and the shunt is ready for immediate use. Daily shunt care is necessary to prevent ascending infection, and consists of washing the tubing exit sites with soap and water and applying an antibiotic ointment prior to redressing. Nonabsorbable skin sutures are removed 10 to 14 days after surgery.

Common Problems

Clotting of a winged-in-line shunt is managed by prepping and draping the forearm shunt, and then performing the following procedure in an aseptic field. The shunt tubing is separated at its connector, and a No. 3 Fogarty embolectomy catheter is passed up the venous limb. The balloon is partially inflated and very gently withdrawn through the venous limb of the cannula, which is then gently irrigated with 5 ml to 10 ml of heparinized normal saline with a plastic syringe that has no Luer lock, allowing it to readily fit into the shunt tubing without a blunt needle. After the venous limb is declotted, it is clamped and attention is turned to the arterial limb. The declotting procedure is repeated on the arterial limb and the shunt is reconnected. If the problem recurs, a cannulogram will often demonstrate a ball thrombus or damage to the blood vessels. The latter requires moving the shunt proximally on the same vessel or to a secondary vessel in that extremity. Recurrent arteriovenous shunt thrombosis can be prevented with sulfinpyrazone, 200 mg, three times daily or warfarin (Coumadin) with a goal of prothrombin time maintenance at 1.5 times the normal control.[3]

ARM ARTERIOVENOUS FISTULA

Preoperative Preparation

The preoperative preparation is the same as that described for an arteriovenous shunt.

Surgical Technique

The smooth venous loop arteriovenous fistula is preferred over the pioneering Brescia–Cimino side-to-side fistula because of the better flow mechanics of the former.[1,4] In addition to the simple instrument set used for the shunt procedure, the following materials are necessary: one straight Castroviejo needle holder, one pair of Westcott scissors, two fine serrated forceps, two double-armed 7-0 polypropylene sutures, two white sewing towels, two vessel loops, one Heifitz clip, and one No. 3 Fogarty embolectomy catheter. A 2.5-power binocular loop is helpful for the smaller vessel anastomoses. All irrigation solutions should be warmed to body temperature to prevent vasospasm.

The previously described horizontal incision for shunt placement is usually extended cephalad in a hockey stick fashion to allow further mobility of the radial artery. Care is taken to preserve as many branches of the radial nerve as possible. A triangular flap of skin and subcutaneous tissue is raised to allow extensive mobilization of the cephalic vein so that the cut end will form a gentle curve after its anastomosis to the side of the radial artery (Fig. 28-8). The radial artery is mobilized as previously described except that its small branches are doubly ligated with 4-0 silk and divided between ligatures

FIG. 28-8.   A triangular flap of skin and subcutaneous tissue is elevated to allow formation of a smooth loop arteriovenous fistula.

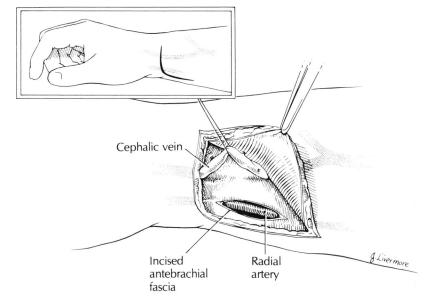

Cephalic vein

Incised antebrachial fascia

Radial artery

J. Livermore

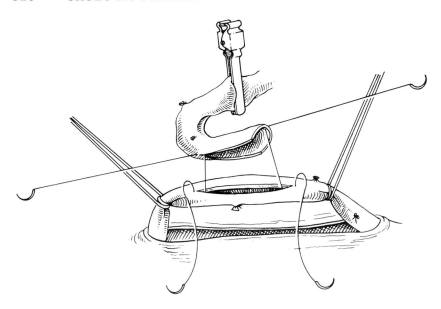

FIG. 28-9. Isolation of a radial artery segment with vessel loops and control of the cephalic vein with a Heifitz clip. Polypropylene cardiovascular sutures (7-0) are placed at either end of the proposed anastomosis.

to allow complete mobilization for 2 cm to 4 cm for a tension-free anastomosis. The cephalic vein is transected distally as far as possible, the distal end is ligated with 2-0 silk, and the outer margin is incised with Westcott scissors for 5 mm. Dilute heparinized saline is injected into the cut end of the cephalic vein, and a Heifitz clip is used to temporarily occlude the vessel after passage and withdrawal of a partially inflated No. 3 Fogarty embolectomy catheter to gently dilate, but not overstretch, the vein. Vessel loops are doubly passed around the radial artery and clipped to the drapes, isolating 1.5 cm to 3 cm of this vessel and eliminating the need for vascular clamps (Fig. 28-9). Retracting the vessel tapes and attaching them to the drapes on the radial side of the forearm will bring the radial artery closer to the spatulated cephalic vein and ensure complete visualization of the radial side of the anastomosis from the outside. Sewing the back wall of this small anastomosis from the inside results in an internal ridge which can result in clotting.

After incising the radial artery for 5 mm to 10 mm to match the opening in the spatulated cephalic vein, a double-armed 7-0 polypropylene cardiovascular suture is passed through the midportion of the distal end of the cephalic vein and then from inside out of the proximal end of the radial artery incision. The apex of the spatulated cephalic vein is similarly managed and tagged distally, thus setting up the anastomosis. The heel stay suture is left untied to allow complete visualization when coming around the corner, and it is unnecessary to tie the other suture because it will be held in place as soon as the suture line is continued beyond

three stitches. The radial side of the anastomosis is completed first, beginning proximally and extending to the heel of the spatulated vein. Having the first assistant follow the suture with gentle outward traction prevents inclusion of the ulnar wall with this suture line and eliminates the need for triangulating sutures. Without tying the suture, it is handed to the first assistant who comes around the heel of the anastomosis for two to three stitches, then tags it, picks up the proximal suture, and completes the suture line along the ulnar surface of the radial artery (Fig. 28-10). The distal stay suture is then tied, the Heifitz clip is removed, the arterial vessel loops are loosened, and a dry sponge is gently placed on the anastomosis for 5 minutes to aid suture line hemostasis. The wound is irrigated with warm antibiotic solution, and the subcutaneous tissue is loosely approximated with interrupted 4-0 polyglycolic acid sutures, beginning at the apex of the hockey stick incision. If the thrill over the arterialized cephalic vein decreases after completion of the subcutaneous stitches, they are removed and the skin is approximated with either a running, subcuticular 4-0 polyglycolic acid suture or a simple running suture of 4-0 monofilament nylon.

For the alternate antecubital fossa arteriovenous fistula, the arm is surgically prepped from the axilla to the fingertips after preoperative preparation as previously described. A tourniquet is applied to the mid-upper arm to demonstrate the antecubital veins. A sterile marking pencil is used to outline the visible or palpable "M" pattern, and the skin and subcutaneous tissue are infiltrated transversely across the antecubital fossa. A 5-cm transverse

FIG. 28-10. Partially completed end cephalic vein to side radial artery suture line

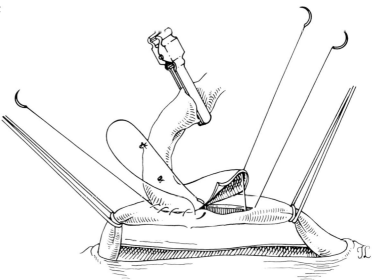

incision is made across the antecubital fossa, beginning midway between the medial epicondyle and the palpable brachial artery, which is medial to the tendon of the biceps muscle, and crossed by the bicipital aponeurosis (Fig. 28-11). Deepening the incision through the superficial fascia exposes the antecubital veins.

After the median cubital vein is dissected in its entirety, the perforating vein and distal median vein are ligated. The dissection is then continued laterally to expose the junction of the distal cephalic vein with the median cubital vein, and the distal cephalic vein is ligated with 2-0 silk just distal to this junction. The deep fascia is incised over the brachial artery, and additional Xylocaine is injected because this tissue plane has not been anesthetized by the previous Xylocaine infiltration. The medial portion of the bicipital aponeurosis is incised, exposing the brachial artery with its venae comitantes and the median nerve, which lies medial to it (Fig. 28-12). With sharp and blunt dissection, the venae comitantes can usually be rolled medially or laterally and not require ligation and division. The brachial artery is isolated for 2 cm to 4 cm, doubly ligating and dividing the muscular branches which are most common on the medial side. The median vein is then ligated with 2-0 silk where it joins the basilic vein, occluded with a Heifitz clip to prevent back bleeding, and spalutated on its medial surface.

Vessel loops are doubly passed proximally and distally to elevate and isolate the brachial artery segment. Clipping the ends of the vessel loops to the drapes on the lateral side of the arm provides room for a tension-free anastomosis with the spat-

FIG. 28-11. A transverse antecubital fossa incision exposes the venous "M" and the brachial artery. The incision may be extended as a "Z" to prevent contracture across the joint.

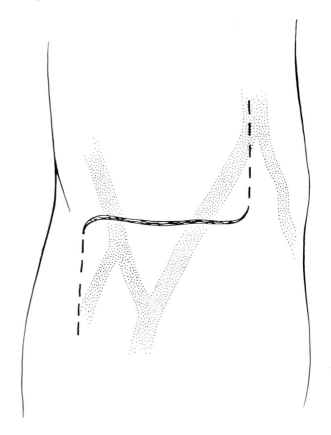

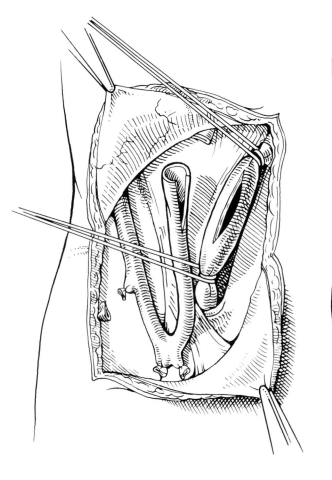

FIG. 28-12. Median cubital vein to brachial artery anastomosis fistula with ligation of unnecessary venous tributaries

ulated median cubital vein. A longitudinal arteriotomy is made on the anterior surface of the isolated brachial artery with a No. 11 blade. The same suture technique as described for the cephalic-vein-to-radial-artery fistula is then used to anastomose the median cubital vein to the side of the brachial artery. After release of the Heifitz clip, arterial vessel loops, and control of suture line bleeding with 5 minutes of gentle sponge pressure, the subcutaneous tissue and skin are closed as previously described.

When the valvular venous anatomy prevents use of this technique, the cephalic vein can often be mobilized sufficiently to make an end-cephalic-vein-to-side-brachial-artery fistula (Fig. 28-13).

Postoperative care for both fistula techniques includes leaving a warm pack on the arm overnight to promote vasodilatation. If nonabsorbable skin sutures have been used, they are removed 10 to 14 days after surgery. It usually requires 3 to 6

weeks for maturation of the arterialized vein before hemodialysis is instituted.

Common Problems

Early clotting of a native arteriovenous fistula usually requires exploration with revision of the subcutaneous closure, repeating the anastomosis, or creation of another fistula. Clotting of the fistula after a hemodialysis run is managed by prepping and draping the extremity and then, after local anesthesia, making a transverse incision over the proximal arterialized vein, incising the vein and gently passing a Fogarty embolectomy catheter first up the venous return limb, then towards the arterial anastomosis. After bright red forward bleeding and venous back bleeding or ease of venous irrigation have been demonstrated, thumb pressure by the first assistant on either side of the arterialized phlebotomy allows rapid closure with a running 7-0 polypropylene suture. The skin and

FIG. 28-13. Distal cephalic vein to side brachial artery fistula

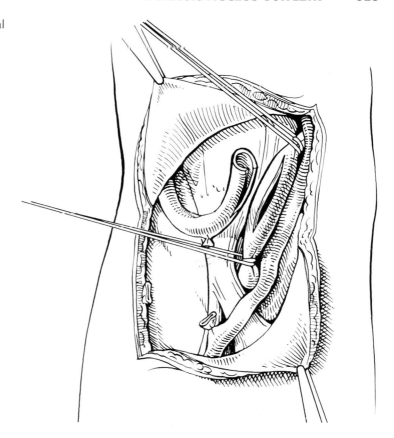

subcutaneous tissue are then closed as previously described.

LOOP FOREARM GRAFTS

When there is insufficient time for maturing a native arteriovenous fistula, when the vessels are inadequate for native fistula formation, or when the patient is obese with deep veins, a loop arteriovenous fistula can be created in the forearm and used within hours of surgery.[5] Although saphenous vein interposition is rarely used in our program, we have extensive experience with both bovine and expanded polytetrafluoroethylene vascular grafts. Bovine carotid arteries which have been subjected to enzymatic digestion with ficin and tanned with dialdehyde starch are available in diameters of 6 mm to 10 mm and lengths of 20 cm to 45 cm. The usual diameters and lengths used at the University of Oregon are 8 mm and 35 cm, respectively.

Preoperative Preparation

The preoperative preparation is the same as that described for arm shunts and native vessel fistulas.

Surgical Technique

In addition to the standard arteriovenous fistula materials, the following are necessary: two more 7-0 polypropylene sutures; 2 liters of normal saline; a splash basin; a glass bulb syringe; 16Fr, 20Fr, 24 Fr, and 30Fr van Buren sounds; and a catheter stylet with the distal end bent into a 3-mm-diameter loop.

Two transverse incisions are made in the arm, one in the antecubital fossa and one in the midportion of the forearm (Fig. 28-14). The largest vein in the antecubital fossa is chosen for the venous limb of the anastomosis, and is isolated between vessel loops as previously described. Occasionally it will be necessary to use one of the venae comitantes for the venous return limb. The brachial artery is also isolated between vessel loops. One percent Xylocaine is infiltrated into the proposed tunnels between the two transverse incisions, and a 16Fr Van Buren sound is passed from the distal forearm incision into the incision in the antecubital fossa. The sound is withdrawn into the tunnel for 2 cm, then rotated so that its tip points upward, then further withdrawn through the tunnel to widely dissect the subcutaneous tissue. The pro-

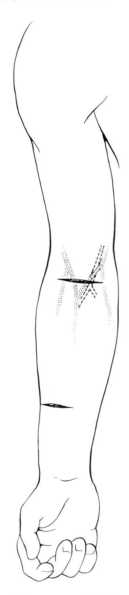

FIG. 28-14. Parallel transverse incisions for a loop forearm graft fistula. Subcutaneous tunnels are created with Van Buren sounds.

cedure is repeated with 20Fr, 24Fr, and finally 30Fr sounds. The same procedure is then used for the other limb of the tunnel.

The bovine graft is removed from its container and irrigated at least ten times with a bulb syringe containing normal saline. The outside is then thoroughly rinsed to prevent carry-over of preserving fluid. The larger end of the graft is used for the venous anastomosis. The vessel loops isolating the segments of artery and vein are clamped to the drapes, and longitudinal incisions are made in the artery and vein that correspond to the tangential

cuts in the graft (Fig. 28-15). The most difficult anastomosis is completed prior to passing the graft through the tunnel. A double-armed 7-0 polypropylene suture on a Castroviejo needle holder is used to suture the bovine graft in the manner previously described for the cubital-vein-to-brachial-artery fistula. The heavy wire urethral catheter stylet with a 3-mm loop is passed from the distal horizontal forearm incision through one of the tunnels into the antecubital fossa. The open bovine graft is passed over the end of the catheter guide and gently tied in place with a 2-0 silk. The graft is then withdrawn through the tunnel, and the holding 2-0 silk ligature is cut. The catheter guide is then passed from the antecubital fossa into the distal forearm incision through the other tunnel, and the procedure is repeated to draw the open end of the graft into the antecubital fossa for the second anastomosis. The graft is then gently distended with heparinized normal saline to be certain there are no kinks, and the remaining graft-to-native-vessel anastomosis is completed with a running 7-0 polypropylene suture. The venous vessel loops are removed, the arterial vessel loops are removed, and the suture lines are covered with a dry sponge for 5 minutes. The final position of the graft is checked in the tunnels, and the subcutaneous tissue and skin are closed as previously described (Fig. 28-16).

The procedure is the same for the expanded polytetrafluoroethylene vascular grafts, except that their rigidity usually requires a slightly heavier needle, such as that found on a 5-0 or 6-0 polypropylene suture. These grafts should not be preclotted or wetted prior to establishing blood flow because the latter action interferes with the hydrophobic properties of the graft and may allow persistent plasma leakage.

Although we have successfully used these grafts within 2 hr of implantation, 10 to 30 days are usually required for the surrounding edema to resolve, and for fibrosis around the graft to prevent extensive subcutaneous hematomas after needle puncture.

Common Problems

Clotting of a vascular graft is managed in a fashion similar to that described for the native arteriovenous fistula. Unless the clotting is directly related to a pressure bandage following a hemodialysis run, the usual problem is plaque buildup in the patient's vein at the venous anastomosis. This is manifested by increasing back pressure on serial hemodialysis runs. We have satisfactorily managed this problem with Gruentzig transluminal dilata-

FIG. 28-15. Anastomosis technique for graft loop arteriovenous fistula. Polypropylene sutures (5-0 or 6-0) are usually necessary with synthetic grafts because they are more rigid than the bovine grafts.

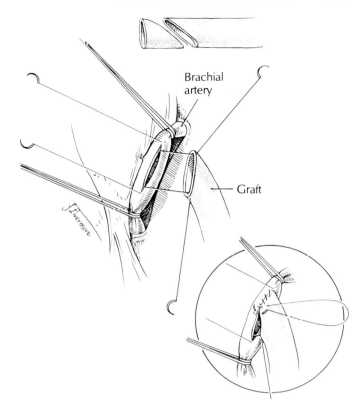

tion as previously described for coronary and renal arteries.[2] When this fails, surgical revision with a patch angioplasty is necessary.[5]

CHRONIC PERITONEAL DIALYSIS ACCESS

We have adopted the Toronto Western Hospital catheter and procedures, and found them extremely satisfactory for chronic peritoneal dialysis catheter placement.[6] The two flat Silastic discs in the distal part of the abdominal portion of the catheter prevent dislodgement in the pelvis and catheter obstruction by the omentum and intestines (Fig. 28-17).

Preoperative Preparation

The patient has a preoperative shower and shampoo with a surgical soap, with special attention directed to the abdomen. Tobramycin (1.5 mg/kg) and a cephalosporin are given intravenously within 1 hr of skin incision and continued for 24 hr.

Surgical Procedure

After shaving the lower abdomen and a surgical scrub, the skin, subcutaneous tissue, fascia, and peritoneum are infiltrated in the infraumbilical midline for 5 cm to 10 cm (Fig. 28-18). Following the skin incision, electrocautery is used to deepen the incision into the fascia, using suction to keep the field free of edema fluid and local anesthetic. The incision is deepened through the fascia and into the peritoneal cavity. The distal disc is guided into the pelvis with forceps. A pursestring suture of 3-0 polyglycolic acid is placed in the peritoneum and tied around the catheter. A single stitch is then taken in the cuff closest to the discs to anchor the disc between the peritoneum and fascia. The fascia is closed with interrupted 2-0 polyglycolic acid sutures. One percent Xylocaine is infiltrated into the subcutaneous tissue and skin to develop a tunnel for the catheter. This tunnel is developed with a hemostat so that the second cuff will be 1 cm to 2 cm away from the exit stab wound. Passing a uterine sound through the stab wound and threading the catheter onto the sound for 2 cm to 3 cm will allow the catheter to be drawn through the subcutaneous tunnel and out the exit wound.

Peritoneal dialysis should be started immediately in the operating room during closure. This dialysis should be continued for 24 hr to 48 hr. At the end of the first dialysis, 500 ml of dialysate is left inside the peritoneal cavity and 3 ml of heparin

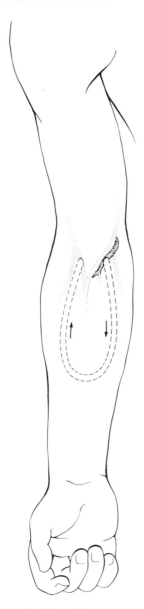

FIG. 28-16. Completed graft loop arteriovenous fistula

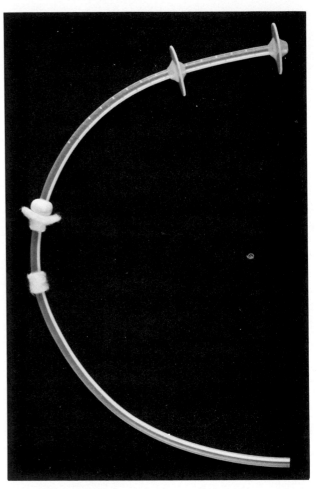

FIG. 28-17. The Toronto Western Hospital chronic peritoneal dialysis access catheter has cuffs to provide ingrowth of fibrous tissue and to prevent bacterial invasion along the subcutaneous tunnel.

(1000 units/ml) is left inside the catheter. This heparin solution is instilled at the end of every dialysis run. Heparin, 500 units/liter of dialysate, is recommended for the first 2 months to prevent fibrin clot formation.

Common Problems

Patients who form fibrin clots in the dialysate will require heparinized dialysate indefinitely.

Peritonitis is managed by the addition of appropriate antibiotics to the dialysate, and the catheter is not removed.

Catheter obstruction is usually manifested by progressive difficulty in the drainage cycle. A plain film of the abdomen will demonstrate whether or not the radiopaque catheter has been dislodged from the pelvis. If so, occasionally it can be replaced under aseptic conditions by passing a wire obturator into the catheter lumen and redirecting it into the pelvis. If this gentle manipulation is unsuccessful, catheter replacement is usually required.

In children, a patent processus vaginalis can result in scrotal or labial filling with dialysate. This requires herniorrhaphy, and can be prevented if a peritoneogram is performed in infants and children prior to or at the time of chronic dialysis catheter placement.

FIG. 28-18. Placement of the Toronto Western Hospital chronic peritoneal dialysis access catheter

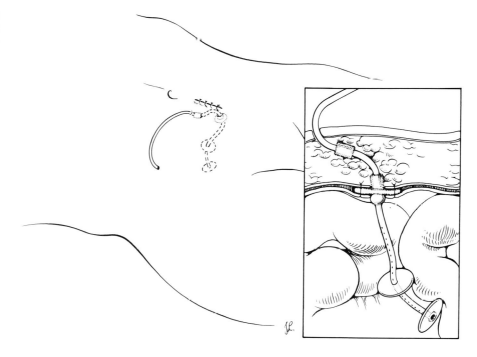

REFERENCES

1. BRESCIA MJ, CIMINO JE, APPEL K et al: Chronic hemodialysis using venipuncture and a surgically created arteriovenous fistula. N Engl J Med 275:1089, 1966
2. GRUENTZIG A, KUHLMANN U, VETTER W et al: Treatment of renovascular hypertension with percutaneous transluminal dilatation of a renal artery stenosis. Lancet 1:801, 1978
3. KAEGI A, PINEO GF, SHIMIZU A et al: Arteriovenous shunt thrombosis: Prevention by sulfinpyrazone. N Engl J Med 290:304, 1974
4. KARMODY AM, LEMPERT N: "Smooth loop" arteriovenous fistulas for hemodialysis. Surgery 75:238, 1974
5. LEFRANK EA, NOON GP: Surgical technique for creation of an arteriovenous fistula using a looped bovine graft. Ann Surg 182:782, 1975
6. OREOPOULOS DG, IZATT S, ZELLERMAN G et al: A prospective study of the effectiveness of three permanent peritoneal catheters. Proceedings Dialysis Transplant Forum 6:96, 1976
7. RAMIREZ O, SWARTZ C, ONESTI G et al: The winged in line shunt. Trans Am Soc Artif Intern Organs 12:220, 1966

Cadaver-Donor Nephrectomy

29

Michael G. Phillips

Only 25% to 30% of patients with end-stage renal disease, desiring a kidney transplant, will be able to receive a graft from a living related donor.[10,13,20] The remaining 70% to 75% must rely on cadaveric donor kidneys. Because of ethical, social, legal, and medical considerations confronted when using a living related donor, some transplant centers are reluctant to transplant kidneys from these donors and rely solely on cadaveric kidneys.[21] The kidney waiting list at transplant centers around the world is increasing each year, and the availability of cadaveric kidneys is considered to be the limiting factor determining the number of kidney transplants performed.[5,10,18,20]

Because transplant centers alone are unable to supply an adequate number of cadaveric kidneys for transplantation, nontransplant hospitals are rapidly becoming a major source of cadaveric donor kidneys.[2,5,10] Developing community-hospital, cadaveric-kidney procurement programs is a major step in meeting the demands for these kidneys. It is important that the same medical and legal protocol—based on standard guidelines for brain death, donor evaluation and management, and donor nephrectomy—be practiced in all hospitals within any procurement program. Permission from hospital professional and administrative staffs and from medical examiners, and consent from the donor prior to death or from the immediate family at the time of death, must be made certain before donation procedures begin.[4,10,20]

Donor Criteria

Generally, cadaveric kidney donors are between 5 and 55 years of age; however, neonates and patients well into their 60s have been successfully used as cadaveric kidney donors.[11,16,20]

The primary sources of suitable cadaveric kidneys are patients suffering total and irreversible brain destruction from traumatic accidents, strokes, drug overdose, primary brain tumors, cardiac ar-

rest, and drowning in which heart–lung resuscitation was successful within 10 to 20 minutes.[10,18,20]

The past history and present hospital records of potential donors must be carefully reviewed. Patients with prolonged hypotension, oliguria, hypoxia, unexplained hyperthermia, bacterial sepsis, diabetes mellitus, hypertension, renal disease, renal stone history, and neoplasia outside the central nervous system are usually disqualified as suitable kidney donors. Patients with prerenal azotemia or with transient shock are sometimes suitable; however, caution and clinical judgment must be exercised when considering such patients as kidney donors.[18,19] Laboratory studies should include arterial blood gases, plasma creatinine, blood urea nitrogen (BUN), urinalysis, blood typing, hematocrit, VDRL (Venereal Disease Research Laboratories) antigen, hepatitis-associated antigen, white blood cell count, and, when feasible, a creatinine clearance. A thorough review of all laboratory results, as well as a review of the donor's fluid and electrolyte status, is essential in the management of cadavers whose kidneys are to be harvested. Serial evaluation of laboratory findings such as plasma creatinine, BUN and urinalysis may be needed to evaluate the resuscitative measures. Blood and urine cultures are an added safeguard, but not mandatory in the routine donor work-up.

Donor Management

Most transplant centers and procurement agencies employ an organ recovery team, which is under the direction of an experienced physician. The team is usually comprised of specially trained, nonphysician personnel such as physician's assistants, nurses, and technicians. Team members are on emergency call 24 hr day, because potential donor availability is unpredictable.

Once notified, it is the responsbility of the recovery team personnel to assist the potential donor's attending physician in following the donor's or his immediate family's wishes for kidney

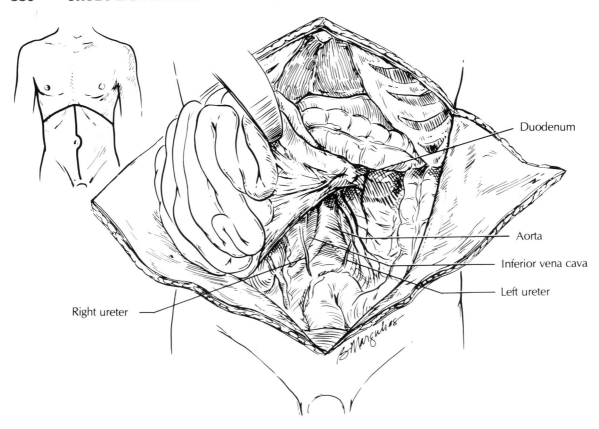

FIG. 29-1. Opening incision and general abdomi

donation. The attending physician must establish brain death as state laws and hospital policies dictate. The medical–legal guidelines for each institution, permission from the medical examiner, and donation permission must all be well documented and confirmed for each kidney donor.[15]

Following the pronouncement of brain death the recovery team personnel may become directly responsible for donor care. Usually, the recovery team is capable of assisting the surgeon during the donor nephrectomy; their knowledge of specialized procedures and protocols for donor nephrectomy and postnephrectomy kidney management is a valuable component of optimal kidney harvesting.

When possible, tissue typing should begin immediately after family consent is obtained. Often donor typing and selective recipient crossmatching can be completed before the donor nephrectomy. Immunologic pretreatment of the donor, usually 1 g of methylprednisolone intravenously (IV) over a 10-minute period, should be administered *after* 10 ml of coagulated and 20 ml of heparinized blood are drawn for tissue typing. Some investigators suggest larger doses of methylprednisolone and

cyclophosphamide for immunologic pretreatment.[8,9,22]

The success of a kidney transplant begins early in the donor care, because all too often there is irreversible injury of the kidneys during preharvest and harvest. Because the kidneys are very sensitive to hypoxia and hypotension and because urine output is a reasonable initial indicator of renal function, the "Minimum Hundreds Criteria" may be used as a guideline for adult donors. These criteria are systolic blood pressure > 100 torr, po_2 > 100 torr, and hourly urine output > 100 ml.

The selection of appropriate medication for the donor during the preharvest and harvest periods requires a thorough understanding of the individual patient's condition as well as the effects of brain death on renal physiology. A minimum of two intravenous lines should be established to allow rapid replacement of fluids from either iatrogenic or endogenous diuresis. A central venous catheter for fluid replacement and volume monitoring is ideal but not mandatory. Once donor maintenance has begun, rapid fluid replacement may be necessary: isotonic, crystalloid, and colloid

FIG. 29-2. The kidneys, the ureters, and the great vessels are exposed after the abdominal contents have been removed.

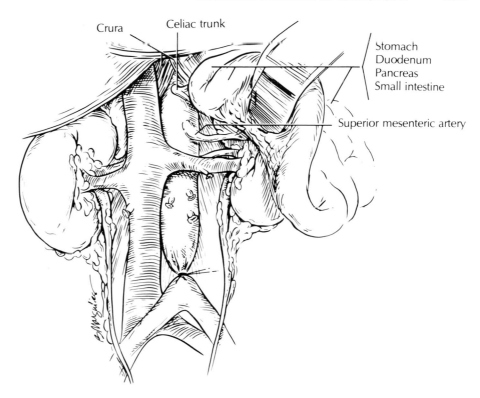

Crura — Celiac trunk — Stomach — Duodenum — Pancreas — Small intestine — Superior mesenteric artery

solutions may all be used to maintain intravascular volume and urine production. The use of whole blood products should be avoided, if possible, so as not to compromise tissue typing.

In addition to fluid replacement, diuretics such as mannitol and furosemide are frequently required to protect the kidneys and to sustain diuresis during the donor maintenance phase. Prolonged or extreme diuresis secondary to diabetes insipidus can cause renal cellular swelling and even capsular rupture of the kidneys. Severe diabetes insipidus in kidney donors can be well controlled by titration of aqueous vasopressin (Pitressin)—20 units/liter D_5W ¼ N.S.—initiated at 2 ml/min for 30 minutes. Generally after a period of 60 minutes, the urine output can be stabilized at an optimum level of 100 ml/hr to 150 ml/hr. It should be noted that Pitressin can have an additive effect with other vasopressors such as dopamine, the sympathomimetic drug of choice in maintaining blood pressure and adequate renal perfusion.[3,7,17,19] The Pitressin should be discontinued approximately 1 hr prior to nephrectomy.

Surgical Approach

Heart-beating, cadaveric (brain-dead) donors usually allow for a scheduled procedure referred to as a cadaver-donor nephrectomy. Occasionally this procedure must be done on an emergency basis. In addition to a standard major laparotomy instrument set, with additional vascular instruments, a second sterile area is required for the kidney flush basin and vascular instruments necessary to prepare the organs for preservation. An intravenous stand is placed at the second sterile table to allow the flush solution to be raised approximately 36 inches above the flush table. The donor is brought to the operating room with respiratory maintenance provided and a gastric drainage tube in place. The donor is prepared with iodophor from the nippleline to the symphisis pubis using standard sterile techniques. The donor's blood pressure and urine output are recorded continuously and, when appropriate, fluids and medication changes are initiated during the procedure.

EN BLOC RESECTION

A wide range of surgical techniques have been employed for cadaveric donors that would be unsuitable in living related donors.[1,6,12,14] The *en bloc* nephrectomy is one such technique, by which both kidneys and segments of aorta and vena cava are included as a single specimen.[1,12] One incision is made obliquely from the xiphoid process to the

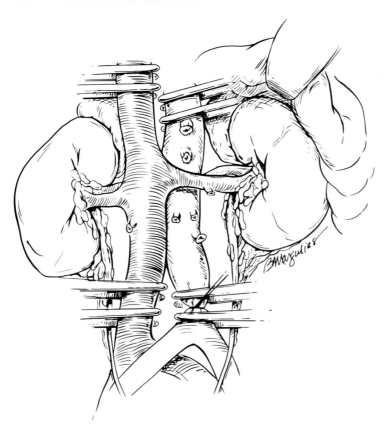

anterior axillary line bilaterally at the level of the 8th, 9th, and 10th ribs, and a second incision is made from the xiphoid process to the symphysis pubis (Fig. 29-1). This type of high incision will allow for access to the superior mesenteric trunk, the proximal abdominal aorta, and the vena cava. The abdominal wall flaps are then pulled away from the midline and secured laterally with towel clips. The entire abdomen is now exposed (Fig. 29-1). A general exploration must be performed and abnormal findings documented, with a copy to the medical examiner when pertinent. Mannitol (12.5 g to 25 g IV) are given early to increase diuresis and to minimize renal cellular edema.[19]

Beginning in the right lower quadrant, the mesocolon is freed along the line of Toldt from the cecum to the diaphragm and medially to the midline. The posterior peritoneum is then cut from the cecum along the mesentery to the aortic bifurcation. Dissection is continued from the aortic bifurcation along the descending mesocolon ending deep within the pelvis. Care must be taken to avoid injury to the ureters during this part of the procedure. Next, the posterior peritoneum over the aorta is incised to the level of the inferior mesenteric artery, which is ligated and divided.

The dissection is continued along the posterior peritoneum in a cephalad direction along the mesenteric base of the descending colon, ligating and transecting the inferior mesenteric vein. The ligament of Treitz is divided and the duodenum and other retroperitoneal structures are dissected free of the left renal vein using blunt and sharp dissection. The abdominal contents are rotated to the left upper quadrant and eviscerated out of the abdominal cavity. The abdominal aorta is isolated and ligated securely above the bifurcation (Fig. 29-2). (If the donor's blood pressure is unstable, this part of the operation can be done sooner to aid in increasing the blood pressure during the remainder of the procedure.) The distal vena cava is now isolated. Both ureters are freed from deep within the pelvis to the lower pole of each respective kidney. Special care must be taken to leave extra adventitia around the ureter's entire length, because this adventitia contains the blood supply for the transplanted ureter.

Frequently, before freeing the kidneys, 100 mg IV of furosemide is given to attempt to increase the renal vascular blood flow and to maximize diuresis. Also, a slow infusion of an α-adrenergic blocking drug such as Regitine may be started

FIG. 29-4. The flush table is checked for readiness.

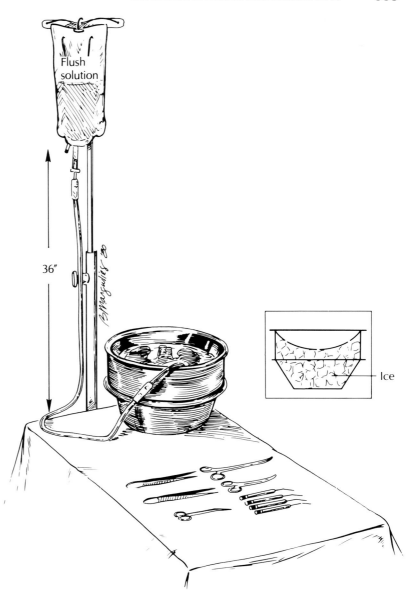

before kidney manipulation is initiated. Constant monitoring of the blood pressure is required during the infusion of the α-blocker because of the vasodilating effect.

Using blunt and sharp dissection, isolation of the kidneys is now begun. They may or may not remain within Gerota's fascia, according to the surgeon's preference. Dissection of the lower pole should be minimal to protect the blood supply of the ureter in this region. No dissection in the renal hilus should be necessary in freeing the kidneys. The gonadal veins are ligated, and the distal ureters are divided deep within the pelvis and placed out of the abdomen so that urine production may be

observed. The superior mesenteric artery and frequently the celiac artery are isolated, ligated, and cut. Dissection here may be difficult, because autonomic nerve fibers and ganglia as well as muscle fibers of the crura of the diaphragm are adjacent to the aorta in this area. The proximal aorta and the proximal vena cava are isolated. Large vascular clamps are placed around the great vessels in an open position (Fig. 29-3). The distal vena cava and aorta are double clamped just proximal to their bifurcation, and both distal great vessels are cut. The vascular clamps holding the great vessels are lifted and retracted toward the chest. The lumbar arteries and veins are hemoclipped up to and above

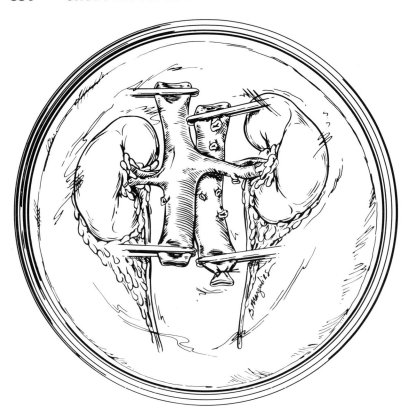

FIG. 29-5. The removed *en bloc* specimen is placed in the cooling basin.

the renal arteries and veins, when possible. Copious urine production should be maintained at this time. If not, adjustment of fluids and diuretics may be required before the administration of 15,000 units to 20,000 units of heparin. The second sterile table should now be rechecked for instruments and solutions. The flush solution of choice, usually Sacks or Collins solution, should be hung on the intravenous stand and made ready for use (Fig. 29-4).

Approximately 5 minutes after the addition of the heparin, the vascular clamps around the proximal aorta and vena cava are gently pushed forward toward the diaphragm and clamped. The aorta is clamped first and the time recorded. The level of cutting of the proximal aorta is very important because there is frequently less than 1 cm between the superior mesenteric artery and the left renal artery. A mistake in the placement of the vascular clamp too inferiorly results in cutting the great vessels through the origin of the renal arteries and can compromise the specimen, especially if multiple arteries are present. Lifting the distal vessel clamps as well as both ureters and both kidneys cephalad, the remaining dissection is completed.

The entire *en bloc* specimen is now removed and immersed in the cooled (5° C–7° C) normal saline

solution (Fig. 29-5). Not all transplant surgeons agree with immediate immersion, because they believe this causes vasospasm. Prompt flushing of the *en bloc* specimen, while immersed in the cooled bath, is begun through either the aorta or each individual renal artery or both, until the effluent from the renal veins is clear. (For descriptions of specially constructed cooling units, see text and art, Chap. 32). Usually 400 ml to 500 ml of flush solution is required for each kidney. Inspection of each kidney for complete blanching is mandatory, to rule out undetected aberrant vessels.

Before closing the abdominal cavity numerous lymph nodes from the small bowel mesentery or periaortic region as well as the entire spleen should be removed and preserved according to established protocols for tissue typing and crossmatching. Also, the great vessels should be tied securely to assist with postmortem preparation of the cadaver. Following a secure abdominal closure, the cadaver is prepared in the usual manner and transported to the appropriate holding area.

Using the surgical technique of *en bloc* nephrectomy for cadaveric kidney donors at all network hospitals allows for uniformity of kidneys for transplantation. This relatively simple and quick surgical technique can be successfully performed by a local surgeon and a nonphysician member of the affiliated transplant procurement team. Because this surgical technique requires minimal dissection in and around the renal hilus and very little kidney manipulation, vasospasm and surgical injury to the kidneys during nephrectomy are minimized. *En bloc* nephrectomy is clearly the surgical technique of choice when removing cadaveric kidneys for transplantation.

REFERENCES

1. ACKERMANN JR, SNELL ME: Cadaveric renal transplantation: A technique for donor kidney removal. Br J Urol 44:515, 1968

2. BELZER FO, SALVATIERRA O, JR: The organization of an effective cadaver renal transplantation program. Transplant Proc 6:93, 1974

3. BROWN JAY HJ: Anesthesia for renal transplantation. A Review. Anesthesiology Review 11:22, 1976

4. DAVIS JH, WRIGHT RK: Influence of the medical examiner on cadaver organ procurement. J Forensic Sci 22:834, 1977

5. ETHEREDGE EE, MAESER MN, SICARD GA et al: A natural resource. Prevalence of cadaver organs for transplantation and research. Special communication JAMA 241:2287, 1979

6. FREED SZ, VEITH FJ, TELLIS V et al: Improved cadaveric nephrectomy for kidney transplantation. Surg Gynecol Obstet 137:101, 1973

7. GOLDBERG LI: Dopamine-clinical uses of an endogenous catecholamine. Engl J Med 291:707, 1974

8. GUTTMANN RD: Manipulation of allograft immunogenicity by pretreatment of cadaver donors. Urol Clin North Am 3:475, 1976

9. GUTTMANN RD, MOREHOUSE DD, MEAKINS JL et al: Donor pretreatment in an unselected series of cadaver renal allografts. Kidney Int (Suppl) 8:S-99, 1978

10. KAUFMAN HH, HUCHTON JD, MCBRIDE MM et al: Kidney donation: Needs and possibilities. Neurosurg 5:237, 1979

11. KOOTSTRA G, WEST JC, DRYBURGH P et al: Pediatric cadaver kidneys for transplantation. Surgery 83:333, 1978

12. LINKE CA, LINKE CL, DAVIS RS et al: Cadaver donor nephrectomy. Urology 51:133, 1975

13. MARY JL: Improving the success of kidney transplants. Science 209:673, 1980

14. MERKEL FK, JONASSON O, BERGAN JJ: Procurement of cadaver donor organs: Evisceration technique. Transplant Proc 4:585, 1972

15. MILNE JF, CHIR B: Psychosocial aspects of renal transplantation. Suppl Urol 9:82, 1977

16. MORLING N, LADEFOGED J, LANGE P et al: Kidney transplantation and donor age. Tissue Antigens 6:163, 1975

17. RAFTERY AT, JOHNSON RWG: Dopamine pretreatment in unstable kidney donors. Br Med J 1:522, 1979

18. ROSENBERG JC, KROME RL, MCDONALD FD et al: Identifying and managing the potential transplant donor in the emergency department. JACEP 4:328, 1975.

19. SALVATIERRA O, JR, OLCOTT C IV, COCHRUM KC et al: Procurement of cadaver kidneys. Urol Clin North Am 3:457, 1976

20. SOLHEIM BG, THORSBY F, OSBAKK TA et al: Letter to the editor. Tissue Antigens 7:251, 1976

21. WEINERTH JL: Renal preservation. In Glenn JF ed: Urologic Surgery, 2nd ed, pp 966–972. New York, Harper & Row, March 1975

22. ZINCKE H, WOODS JE, KHAN AU et al: Immunological donor pretransplant in combination with pulsatile preservation in cadaveric renal transplantation. Transplantation 26:207, 1978

Special thanks to John L. Weinerth, M.D., for his guidance in preparing this chapter.

Live-Donor Nephrectomy

30

Russell K. Lawson

Live-related-donor kidney transplantation offers an improved graft functional survival of 30% to 45% when compared to cadaver-donor transplantation.[5] This improved graft survival is reflected in improved patient survival and improved quality of life posttransplant.[8] Approximately one third to one half of patients with renal failure who are considered transplant candidates have potentially usable familial donors. Unfortunately, there has been a gradual decrease in the use of live donors as compared to cadaver donors over the past 10 years. When suitable familial donors are found who have the correct blood type and who are either identical or half-identical at the HLA (human leukocyte antigen) gene complex, every effort should be extended to use that donor source.[1]

The use of live donors may increase if the recent improved results seen with donor-specific transfusions are substantiated in larger series of patients.[3] The surgeon who undertakes live-donor nephrectomy must exercise particular care and caution in preoperative selection, conduct of the operative procedure, and postoperative management. The live donor is making a major sacrifice to help a relative with renal failure. Donors deserve the utmost in consideration and care to help them through this experience.

Selection

Donors should be 18 years of age or older so that they may give consent for the operation. Children have been used in the past as donors, particularly in identical-twin transplants; court permission has been obtained in such cases.[2] Use of children as donors raises serious ethical questions and should not be considered in today's practice of transplant surgery.

The older patient is more problematic. Generally, individuals over the age of 60 have not been considered candidates for live-donor nephrectomy. However, there are many exceptions to this guideline that have resulted in an excellent outcome for the recipient and no problems for the donor. The most important factor in selecting older people for the procedure is to exclude those individuals who have even minor health problems.

Live related donors must have a compatible blood group with the recipient and should share one or both HLA haplotypes. Totally mismatched siblings at the HLA locus should not be transplanted. Siblings or parents who have a history of upper urinary tract infection, diabetes, hypertension, renal calculi, cancer, or familial renal disease should be excluded from donation. Because live-donor nephrectomy requires that a healthy individual undergo an operative procedure with its attendant mortality and morbidity for no physical benefit to himself, it is important to adhere rigidly to very strict criteria for selection of live donors.

Work-up and Preparation

The work-up should include a complete history and physical examination and laboratory and radiographic studies to determine if prospective donor has two normal kidneys and no other major organ system diseases. Evaluation of the kidneys should include a urinalysis, serum electrolytes, blood urea nitrogen (BUN), creatinine clearance, and intravenous pyelography. Renal angiography should be carried out at the end of the evaluation if all other studies indicate that the patient will be a suitable donor.[7] The angiograms should include selective renal arteriograms of the kidney that will be used for transplant. Small polar vessels are best seen by examining both an aortic flush and a selective renal artery injection.

Special studies may be considered in donors with the potential for inherited kidney disease. Donors with a family history of diabetes should have a glucose tolerance test and in some cases a steroid stress glucose tolerance test with plasma insulin levels. Young patients with a family history of polycystic kidney disease should have abdominal computed tomography scanning to look for small renal cysts. Occasionally, highly motivated

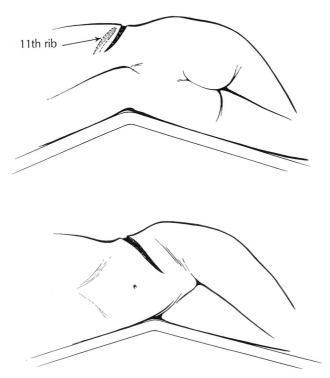

FIG. 30-1. Anteriorly, the incision for live-donor nephrectomy is extended downward to permit extended exposure of the ureter. The 12th rib may be resected, or the incision may be between the 11th and 12th ribs.

potential donors from families with familial nephritis may require renal biopsy before being accepted for kidney donation.

A number of steps can be taken in the preoperative preparation of donors that will minimize the risk to the donor and improve immediate graft function in the recipient. In our transplant program, donors are told that they are required to ambulate the evening following surgery. Considerable time is spent discussing the importance of early ambulation with the donor, which usually results in better cooperation in the postoperative period. The skin is prepared for 24 hr in advance of surgery by use of antibacterial soap showers, shampoos, and flank skin scrubs. An intravenous flow is started the evening before surgery, and the patient is given 1500 ml to 2000 ml of half-normal saline through the night so that he arrives in the operating room well hydrated. Prophylactic antibiotics are used in the form of a cephalosporin, which is given with the premedication and is continued for 3 days postoperatively. After the donor is anesthetized, a Foley catheter is placed in the bladder and left indwelling.

Nephrectomy

The left kidney is preferred for transplantation because of the longer length of the renal vein. However, the right kidney may be used if there are multiple arteries on the left side. A 12th-rib incision should be used unless there is some specific reason to use another approach, such as a high-lying kidney. The incision is slightly modified from the standard flank approach as shown in Fig. 30-1. The incision is curved downward into the left or right lower quadrant after passing the tip of the rib in order to allow better exposure for dissection of the distal ureter. I prefer to resect the 12th rib, but intercostal incisions with the 12th or 11th rib hinged down are equally as good. Details of this incision, other than placement, are not described because the anatomy is shown in Chapters 5 and 7.

Several reports have appeared in the literature stating that transabdominal and even thoracoabdominal incisions are preferred for donor nephrectomy. We have found that the standard flank incision is best for live-donor nephrectomy. Patients ambulate better, eat sooner, and generally recover faster from flank incisions as compared to abdominal incisions. There is also some increased risk to the donor of developing a bowel obstruction from postoperative adhesions when the abdominal approach is used.

A very important technical aspect in donor nephrectomy is gentle handling of the kidney during dissection of the vessel. Rough handling of the kidney or traction on the renal vessels may result in severe vasospasm, acute tubular necrosis, and poor initial function in the recipient. Particular care should be taken not to dissect in the renal hilus inferior to the renal artery and lateral to the ureter because of risk of injury to the ureteral blood supply (Fig. 30-2). The only blood supply available to the ureter following nephrectomy usually arises from the renal artery or from its first posterior branch near the renal pelvis. It may also arise from an inferior polar artery or directly from a large renal pelvis artery. Injury may also occur to the distal ureteral artery as the ureter is freed from the retroperitoneum. The ureter should be handled with care and a margin of periureteral fibrous and areolar tissue removed with it to ensure preservation of its blood supply.

Multiple renal arteries are often encountered and require special consideration. Small second renal veins can be ligated and cut without difficulty. If there are two renal veins of equal size, three alternatives are available: (1) one of the veins may be ligated with some increased risk of venous

FIG. 30-2. The ureteral blood supply is preserved by limiting dissection in the renal hilus and inferiorly.

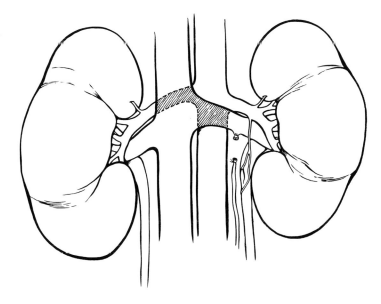

hypertension in the graft, (2) the veins can be spatulated and sewn together to form a common lumen, or (3) two separate venous anastomoses can be carried out at the time of transplantation. I prefer the third method when there is a question of possible venous congestion if the second vein is ligated.

A great deal has been written about management of multiple renal arteries.[9] The techniques that have been described for cadaver donors are generally not applicable to live donors because of the need to remove segments of aorta and vena cava with the renal vessels. The preoperative arteriogram provides a "road map" of the renal arterial blood supply, including the number and location of the accessory arteries. With this road map the accessory arteries can be carefully dissected free without injury. Upper pole vessels that supply only a small segment of kidney can be ligated and cut without difficulty. Before cutting an upper pole vessel, a small bulldog clamp should be placed on the vessel and the amount of renal tissue that will infarct can be readily seen. Small patches of parenchyma less than 2 cm in diameter in adult kidneys do not cause problems when infarcted. Larger areas of infarction can be dangerous because they may lead to necrosis and blowout of an upper pole calix. Accessory vessels to the midportion of the kidney and the lower pole must be preserved because they may supply blood to the renal pelvis and ureter.[4]

Dissection of the vessels on the left side should be carried out down to the left lateral border of the aorta. It is not necessary to free the left renal vein all the way to the vena cava. Adequate vein length is obtained by transecting it over the center of the aorta. On the left side, small branches from the renal artery to the adrenal gland are often encountered and should be ligated and cut. The left renal vein usually has two or three branches: the gonadal vein inferiorly, one or more adrenal veins superiorly, and often a very large vertebral vein which is found lying under the renal vein that passes posteriorly toward the spine. This vertebral vein can be particularly troublesome to control if torn during dissection of the left renal vein.

After completing dissection of the vessels down to the level of the aorta, the ureter should be transected at a point below the common iliac artery. This can be best accomplished by placing a Deaver retractor in the retroperitoneum to provide exposure of the distal ureter. A long-handled, right-angled clamp is placed around the ureter at a point below the vessels, and the ureter is cut proximal to the clamp. The distal ureteral stump is ligated with a 2-0 silk ligature. The transected ureter is dissected from its bed, taking care not to injure its blood supply. The kidney is then inspected and all remaining attachments, other than the renal vessels, are severed. Approximately 10 minutes prior to clamping of the renal vessels, the donor is given 100 units/kg of heparin and 20 mg of furosemide (Lasix) intravenously. The vessels are clamped and the kidney removed when a brisk diuresis is noted from the severed end of the ureter. The vessels are doubly clamped with right-angle vascular clamps and transected. The kidney is passed off of the table for perfusion and cooling and any vascular reconstruction that may be re-

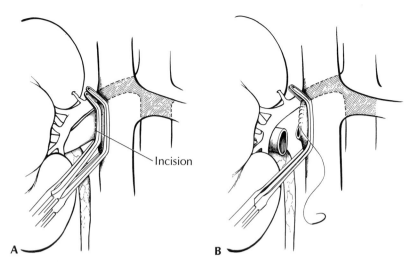

Incision

A   B

FIG. 30-3.   Management of the right renal vein.   **(A)** Two Satinsky clamps of different size are applied to the vena cava at the insertion of the renal vein.   **(B)** After transecting the vein, the outer clamp is removed and the vena cava is closed with a running suture.

quired for multiple vessels. The renal vein is doubly ligated with 1-0 silk. A 1-0 silk ligature is placed on the renal artery, followed by a 2-0 suture ligature through the wall of the vessel as a second distal ligature. The heparin is then reversed by giving 1 mg/kg of protamine by slow intravenous drip. Heparin gives an extra margin of safety for the donor kidney in case unforeseen problems develop at the final stages of kidney removal that delay perfusion and cooling.

Management of the vessels on the right side is different than on the left side. The renal artery passes under the vena cava, and it is often necessary to ligate and cut several vertebral veins on the right side. Mobilization of the right border of the vena cava allows an easier and safer dissection of the right renal artery in order to gain adequate arterial length. A second problem encountered on the right side is the short right renal vein. Occasionally the vein is less that 2 cm long and it is important for the recipient operation to obtain the entire length of the vein. This can be safely accomplished by using two Satinski clamps of dissimilar size as shown in Figure 30-3. After cutting the renal vein flush with the vena cava the outer clamp can be removed, which provides an edge for closure of the vena cava with a running 4-0 Prolene suture. This suture is run twice as a "baseball stitch." The right renal artery is doubly ligated as previously described.

Following nephrectomy the wound is irrigated with 500 ml of antibiotic solution (50,000 units/500 ml of bacitracin and 1 g/500 ml of kanamycin). The 11th and 12th intercostal nerves are infiltrated near their exit from the foramina with 20 ml of 0.75% bupivacaine (Marcaine)—10 ml/nerve. The wound is closed in layers using interrupted 1-0 Tevdek

sutures in the fascia and muscle layers, taking care not to trap the intercostal nerve in the sutures.

If the pleural space has been entered during the procedure, I prefer to place a small chest tube (20Fr Argyle) between the 9th and 10th or 10th and 11th interspace. The chest tube is placed for water-seal drainage and removed the first postoperative day if no air leak is present. The lung can be expanded at the operating table with a small catheter, but often there is a moderate pneumothorax postoperatively. I feel that it is important that the lung be fully expanded in the live kidney donor, and a small chest tube is a simple and certain way of avoiding any postoperative problems with a pneumothorax.

No drains are placed in the wound, except on the rare occasion when there is generalized oozing from the renal bed. If a Penrose drain is placed in the wound, it is removed as soon as the drainage stops—usually in less than 24 hr. Young female donors are often concerned about appearance of the scar, and closure of the skin in these individuals can be carried out with a subcuticular nylon pull-out suture.

Flushing and Cooling of the Kidney

Some transplant surgeons prefer not to flush or cool the donor kidney prior to transplantation. The kidney contains approximately 50 ml of donor blood, and it has recently been suggested that recipient transfusion with donor blood at the time of surgery may have a beneficial effect on the immunologic response of the recipient to the donor kidney. If the kidney is not flushed following donor nephrectomy, then it is imperative that the donor be heparinized prior to clamping of the renal vessel. When there are no unusual vessel problems that

FIG. 30-4. Perfusion of the transplant kidney

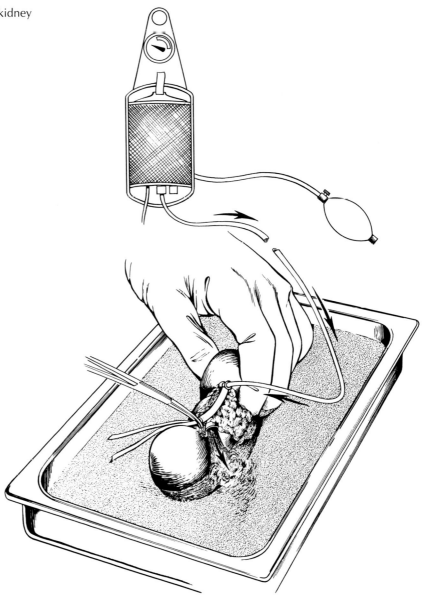

might slow the transplant operation and if the recipient surgeon can revascularize the kidney in 15 to 20 minutes, I believe it is preferable not to perfuse or cool the kidney. Reconstruction of polar vessels, adult to child transplants, and other technical problems that may prolong the revascularization time are all reasons requiring that the kidney be perfused and cooled.

A large number of perfusion solutions have been devised and all seem to work equally effectively for the short-term preservation required in live-donor transplantation. I prefer to perfuse with cold (4°C) Ringer's lactate solution that has had

the pH adjusted to 7.2 by the addition of sodium bicarbonate. This solution is readily available and provides excellent preservation for up to 4 hr— more than an adequate time to accomplish any vascular reconstruction and transplant the kidney.

The perfusion setup is shown in Figure 30-4. The bag of chilled Ringer's solution is placed in a blood pump with a manometer attached. Cannulas for the main renal artery are constructed from straight 8Fr, 10Fr, and 12Fr rubber catheters by cutting off and beveling the tip. These rubber catheters are soft and are not likely to injure the intima of the renal artery. The cannulas are held

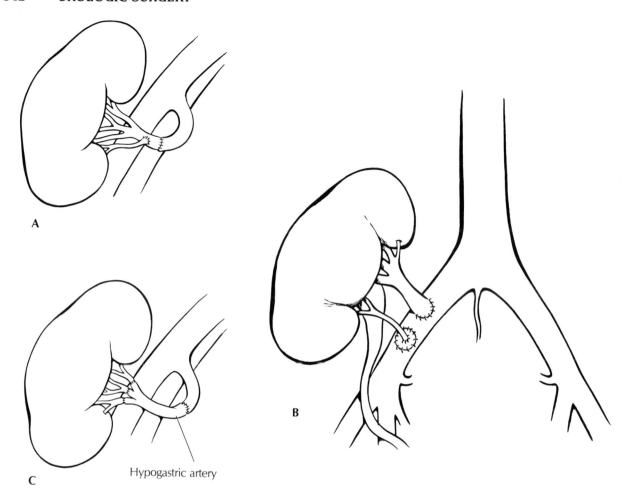

FIG. 30-5.   Techniques of managing multiple arteries.   **(A)** Small polar vessels are anastomosed with interrupted sutures.   **(B)** A venous patch may be used to facilitate an anastomosis
of a small, thin-walled vessel to a larger, thicker-walled vessel.   **(C)** The hypogastric artery
with its branches may be employed.

in place during perfusion with rubber vessel loop
nooses. Perfusion should be carried out at a pressure of 60 torr to 80 torr. Smaller polar vessels are
best perfused with small plastic cannulas that are
used for venous and arterial fluid administration,
such as 14- or 16-gauge Angiocaths. If the polar
vessel is small, it is sometimes advantageous to
gently perfuse it by hand, using a 50-ml syringe.
During flushing, the kidney should be placed in a
basin with chilled saline solution and saline slush
to begin surface cooling. The adult kidney is usually
flushed free of blood and cooled sufficiently by
perfusion with 500 ml of perfusate. Adequacy of
flushing can be judged by a uniform pale appearance of the kidney when the blood is removed and
by observing clear efflux of perfusate from the
renal vein.

Multiple Vessels

Potential live donors should not be excluded because of multiple renal arteries. Current methods
of extracorporeal renal artery surgery allow reconstruction of almost all multiple vessel problems so
that the kidney can be used for transplantation.
Numerous techniques have been described for the
management of these problems. Some of the solutions are shown in Figure 30-5.

Certain principles should be followed when
dealing with small arterial anastomoses. When
small polar vessels are sutured to the side of the
main renal artery, interrupted sutures of 7-0 or
8-0 Prolene should be used to avoid any bunching
and narrowing of the main artery (Fig. 30-5A).
There is often a problem in maintaining patency
when suturing a thin-walled vessel to a thick-

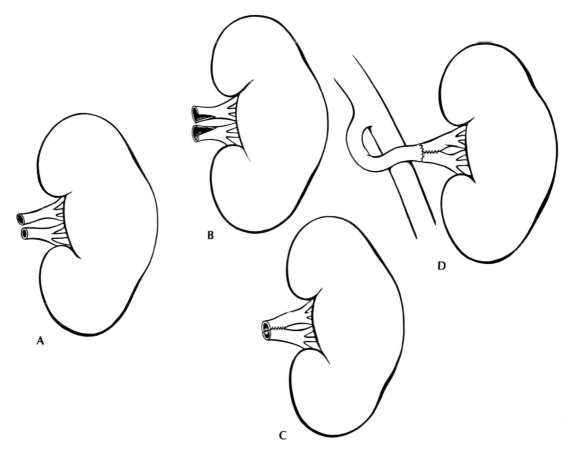

FIG. 30-6. Management of dual arteries. **(A)** Renal arteries of approximately equal size and in good proximity may be joined. **(B)** Each artery is spatulated. **(C)** The two vessels are joined with running or interrupted sutures. **(D)** The hypogastric artery is anastomosed end to end to the common lumen.

walled vessel. The use of a small venous patch to serve as a site for anastomosis on the common or external iliac is an excellent solution to this problem (Fig. 30-5B). If multiple small renal arteries are present, it is usually technically easier to remove the hypogastric artery and its branches from the recipient and to perform the anastomoses of the renal arteries to the hypogastric artery branches as an extracorporeal procedure (Fig. 30-5C). The hypogastric artery serves as an excellent graft, and this technique will allow more precise anastomoses while the kidney is preserved in the ice bath. These fine anastomoses are best accomplished using optical aids, microvascular instruments, and 7-0 or 8-0 suture material. The distal stump of the hypogastric artery can then be sutured end to side to the common or external iliac artery in the recipient. Two renal arteries of equal size that are long enough or close enough together can be spatulated and sewn to form a common lumen (Fig. 30-6). The

common vessel can then be sutured end to end or end to side to the recipient's hypogastric or iliac artery.

Postoperative Management

The two most common serious problems that may develop in the live donor during the postoperative period are wound infection and deep vein thrombosis. The donors are given antibiotics preoperatively and for 3 days postoperatively. Additional measures to help prevent wound infections are preoperative skin preparation with antibacterial soap and wound irrigation with antibiotic solution during surgery. Early ambulation is helpful in preventing deep vein thrombosis, and the donor is asked to walk about the room and in the hall the evening of the surgery. Injection of the intercostal nerves with local anesthetic prior to closure of the wound helps the patient with deep breathing and coughing during the first postoperative day.

Often a brisk diuresis occurs postoperatively from the preoperative fluid load and the intraoperative administration of Lasix. The urine output is replaced with 0.45% saline at a volume of 80% of the previous hour's urine output. The diuresis usually subsides within 6 hr to 8 hr following surgery. A chest tube is used in all patients in whom the pleura was entered during surgery. The chest tube is attached to water-seal drainage on low suction. A chest radiograph is taken in the recovery room to ensure that the lung is fully inflated. The tube is usually removed on the first postoperative day, and a second chest radiograph is taken after removal of the chest tube to again ensure that the lung is fully inflated.

The Foley catheter is removed the morning following surgery, and the patient is encouraged to begin oral fluid intake. A majority of the donors will be able to eat solid food by the second postoperative day. The donors remain in the hospital for 1 week and skin sutures are removed at 1 week. Donors are cautioned not to strain or engage in vigorous physical activity for 1 month following surgery. A urinalysis, urine culture and sensitivity, BUN, creatinine clearance, serum electrolytes, and complete blood count are performed when the patient returns for follow-up after discharge from the hospital.

REFERENCES

1. FARRELL RM, STUBENBORD WT, RIGGIO RR et al: Living renal donor nephrectomy: Evaluation of 135 cases. J Urol 110:639, 1973
2. HARRISON JH, BENNETT AH: The familial living donor in renal transplantation. J Urol 118:166, 1977
3. LEARY FJ, DEWEERD JH: Living donor nephrectomy. J Urol 109:947, 1973
4. MERKEL FK, STRAUS AK, ANDERSEN O et al: Microvascular techniques for polar artery reconstruction in kidney transplants. Surgery 79:253, 1976
5. PENN I, HALGRIMSON CG, OGDEN D et al: Use of living donors in kidney transplantation in man. Arch Surg 101:226, 1970
6. RUIZ R, NOVICK AC, BRAUN WE et al: Transperitoneal live donor nephrectomy. J Urol 123:819, 1980
7. SHERWOOD T, RUUTU M, CHILSHOLM GD: Renal angiography problems in live kidney donors. Br J Radiol 51:99, 1978
8. SMITH RB, WALTON KN, LEWIS EL et al: Operative morbidity among 40 living kidney donors. J Surg Res 12:199, 1972
9. SPANOS PK, SIMMONS RL, BUSELMEIER TJ et al: Kidney transplantation from living related donors with multiple vessels. Am J Surg 125:554, 1973

Recipient Nephrectomy

31

Donald C. Martin

Nephrectomy of the end-stage kidneys in transplant recipients was once widely practiced in many major transplant centers;[11] today this procedure is performed only in carefully selected patients. Pretransplant nephrectomy is not without risk.[15] These patients are chronically ill and must undergo repeated dialysis with its attendant heparinization associated with a risk of postoperative hemorrhage.[13]

Indications

The indications for bilateral nephrectomy in the past included elimination of infection, removal of refluxing systems (vesicoureteral reflux), control of hypertension, elimination of the diseased kidneys as a possible source for extension of glomerulonephritis to the newly transplanted kidney, and ease of patient management because volume and constituents in the urine all come from the graft.[4,6]

URINARY TRACT INFECTION

The need to eliminate infection from the urinary tract of the recipient is the most important and enduring indication for nephrectomy.[8]

Urinary infection in the immunosuppressed recipient is a great risk during transplantation and can lead to wound infection, vascular infection, hemorrhage, and death. The recipient must have bacteriologically sterile urine prior to transplantation. Even if the new kidney is not being connected to the recipient urinary system but is being drained to the skin through the ureter or an ileal conduit, an infected urinary tract is still a hazard in the presence of immunosuppression.

Nephrectomy to eliminate urinary infection must be done prior to renal transplantation. If the infection is associated with vesicoureteral reflux, both ureters and kidneys are removed. This is best accomplished by a transperitoneal midline incision. Separate flank incisions for the kidneys and a lower midline incision for the terminal ureters remains an option.

We favor bilateral nephroureterectomy through a long midline transperitoneal incision when both ureters are also to be removed. The right kidney is exposed by an incision in the posterior parietal peritoneum lateral to the duodenum, right colon, and cecum. The duodenum must be reflected medially to expose the right renal pedicle. The end-stage kidney will have an attenuated arterial system, thus one may ligate the artery and vein together with 1-0 silk just lateral to the vena cava, or, if desired, the artery and vein may be individually ligated. With the renal pedicle divided the ureter is readily dissected from the retroperitoneum. The ureter is mobilized down behind the bladder and secured with a suture ligature of 3-0 chromic catgut.

The left kidney is exposed by incising the posterior parietal peritoneum lateral to the left colon. The colon is reflected medially over the kidney. The renal pedicle is isolated and ligated after complete mobilization of the kidney. The ureter is dissected out by medial reflection of the colon. The distal one third of the left ureter is exposed by elevating the sigmoid colon anterior to trace the ureter behind the colon and bladder. The distal ureter is suture ligated behind the bladder.

Occasionally urinary tract infections will occur after transplantation with involvement of the upper urinary tract. We have localized such infections on clinical grounds and by the use of selective catheterization of the ureters to obtain bacteriological specimens from right, left, and transplanted kidneys. In these patients, we have removed only those old end-stage kidneys which have been proven to be the site of chronic infection. A standard extraperitoneal flank incision is the usual approach in these cases.

In the patient with a large polycystic kidney with infection, a transperitoneal approach provides better access to the pedicle and is a safer approach. Removal of an infected adult polycystic kidney is a very large and hazardous operation which must be approached with this knowledge in mind. The patient's fluid and electrolyte balance and other

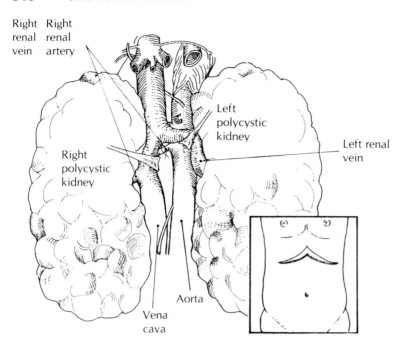

Right renal vein

Right renal artery

Left polycystic kidney

Left renal vein

Right polycystic kidney

Aorta

Vena cava

FIG. 31-1. Nephrectomy of the right polycystic kidney. The right renal artery is ligated initially with exposure at its origin from the aorta. The exposure is made by dissection on the left side of the vena cava.

factors such as arterial blood gases must be in optimum status prior to surgery. Judicious use of fluid management, dialysis, cardiac drugs, and antibiotics must all precede surgery. The patient should have a central venous catheter and arterial line placed in surgery.

We prefer the chevron, bilateral subcostal incision for the polycystic patient. The right kidney is approached by reflecting the right colon medially. The right renal artery is not easily found lateral to the vena cava because of the size of the kidney. We recommend initial exposure and ligation of the right renal artery by dissection on the medial side of the vena cava to expose the renal artery at its origin from the aorta. This is a very inaccessible part of human anatomy. One must find the junction of the left renal vein with the vena cava and reflect the left renal vein superiorly and the vena cava to the right. The right renal artery is thus exposed and ligated in continuity with 1-0 silk (Fig. 31-1). With the right renal artery ligated, one can then ligate the right renal vein adjacent to the vena cava. Dissection of the right polycystic kidney will involve exposure up to the diaphragm.[10]

The left polycystic kidney is approached by reflecting the left colon medially. Great care must be taken not to injure the spleen. We have had the spleen come off its retroperitoneal bed and require removal in the process of left nephrectomy for polycystic disease. The left renal pedicle is a little easier to visualize than the right. The left renal artery is ligated at its origin from the aorta.

The left renal vein is ligated at a similar level. The dissection of the left polycystic kidney is hazardous because of the proximity of the tail of the pancreas and the spleen. Great care must be exercised not to injure the pancreas. There have been fatalities associated with pancreatic injury during nephrectomy.

STERILE REFLUX

On occasion we have transplanted kidneys into recipients with vesicoureteral reflux without infections. These patients have done well and have not required ureterectomy. At the present time we do not consider vesicoureteral reflux without infection and absolute indication for nephroureterectomy. The antecedent history of the patient is an important consideration. In the patients we have not nephrectomized, there was no history of infection at any time. In the past, many transplant surgeons have considered vesicoureteral reflux an absolute indication for nephroureterectomy.

HYPERTENSION

Many patients with end-stage renal disease have hypertension, which can be controlled by dietary and medical therapy. This is also true of the patient after a successful transplant. Most of our patients with a successful graft receive one or more medications for hypertension. The development of newer drugs and increased skill of physicians in the management of these agents reduces greatly the number of patients to be considered for nephrectomy either before or after transplantation. Pretransplant nephrectomy for hypertension has become an infrequent procedure.[9]

Nephrectomy of the old kidneys must be considered for recipients who have severe hypertension after successful transplantation. We have obtained renal vein renins from all three kidneys in an attempt to localize the source of excess renin production. While this sounds logical and desirable, in practice, we have not convincingly demonstrated the old kidneys to be the source of excess renin production. Despite a failure of precise localization, bilateral nephrectomy may be carried out.[3] In these patients several surgical approaches are open to the surgeon. We prefer either a midline upper abdominal transperitoneal or a bilateral extraperitoneal exposure with the patient in the prone position.[1,2] This latter approach is very satisfactory for the patient and the surgeon because there is minimal trauma and direct access to the kidneys is achieved. The only additional hazard relates to the anesthesiologist's limited access to the airway in the prone position. These patients in the prone position must be carefully intubated and a good airway must be maintained.

The small contracted end-stage kidneys of glomerulonephritis or pyelonephritis are readily mobilized and removed through two incisions made with resection of the 12th rib or with lumbar lumbotomy.[14] The patient is postured on bolsters to support the chest and abdomen. Slight flexion at the hips is desirable. In the prone position, it is easy to resect the 12th ribs bilaterally and thus gain access to the retroperitoneum. The small end-stage kidney is completely mobilized and pulled up out of the wound. The pedicle is attenuated and the artery and vein may be ligated together in continuity. Separate ligation of the renal artery and vein may be readily accomplished if desired.

The alternative incisions for the patient operated upon in the prone position are the lumbotomy incisions described by Young in 1936. These incisions are made from the 12th rib to the iliac crest just medial to the lateral margins of the erector spinal muscle group. The lowermost fibers of the latissimus dorsi are incised at the cephalad aspect of the incision. The lumbodorsal fascia is exposed by slight retraction of the lateral margins of the erector spinal muscles. The lumbodorsal fascia is incised to expose the transversalis fascia, which is incised in the line of the incision to enter the retroperitoneum. The self-retaining Balfour retractor may be placed superiorly to inferiorly rather than left to right. The pleura is occasionally apparent at the upper extremity of the incision (Fig. 31-2). Gerota's fascia is entered sharply and the small end-stage kidney is completely mobilized. The pedicle is ligated with 1-0 silk, and the ureter is ligated and transected at the level of the lower pole of the kidney.

The posterior approach allows for simultaneous bilateral nephrectomy by two surgical teams and

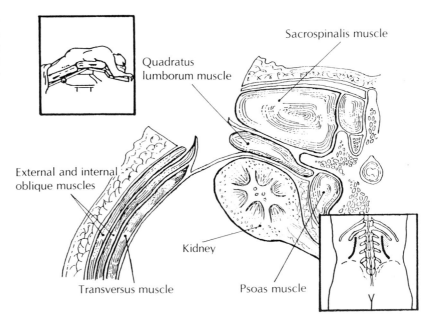

FIG. 31-2. Bilateral synchronous nephrectomy through lumbotomy incisions. The patient is positioned prone on bolsters. The exposure requires incision of the lumbar fascia, but no major muscles must be incised.

Sacrospinalis muscle

Quadratus lumborum muscle

External and internal oblique muscles

Kidney

Transversus muscle

Psoas muscle

is associated with less postoperative pain and less ileus.[5,7]

DISEASED KIDNEYS AS A SOURCE OF EXTENSION OF GLOMERULONEPHRITIS TO THE NEW KIDNEY

The elimination of the old, diseased kidneys as a source of extension of glomerulonephritis to the new kidney is a theoretical indication for pretransplant nephrectomy that has not stood the test of time. It was applied to identical-twin recipients, 25% of whom experience recurrent glomerulonephritis in the new kidney. Preliminary nephrectomy does not protect against this event.

PATIENT MANAGEMENT

As surgeons and physicians have gained experience in the management of patients with transplanted kidneys, the presence of a small amount of residual function in the old kidneys has rarely presented a major clinical problem. The source of urine volume is rarely a concern. The source of protein, red blood cells, and casts may occasionally present a clinical problem.

Bilateral nephrectomy at the same time as renal transplantation is rarely performed today. It is only done in conjunction with a live-donor transplant. The technique is by the transperitoneal approach already described. Bilateral nephrectomy has been recommended and performed in patients with the nephrotic syndrome who lose large amounts of protein in the urine despite advanced renal insufficiency. Thiebot and associates have described extensive embolization of the kidneys as an alternative to surgical removal.[12] Severe protein losses in the urine were controlled by this method of renal destruction. Hypertension was not adequately relieved by this method of renal destruction, because islands of renal tissue remained viable owing to the presence of collateral circulation.

Contraindications

The major contraindication to recipient nephrectomy is the loss of this source of erythropoietin. This, of course, is only of concern while the patient is on dialysis. Because many renal transplants have a limited functional life, many patients return to dialysis after transplantation.

The anephric patient on dialysis has a significantly compromised life. There is usually a much more profound anemia with the need for blood transfusions each month. This can ultimately lead to hemosiderosis and hepatic insufficiency. The anemia on dialysis is one major reason for not performing recipient nephrectomy without a precise indication.

Postoperative Care

The most critical patients are those in whom the bilateral nephrectomy is done prior to transplantation. These patients are rendered anephric. Fluid balance must be monitored carefully in the postoperative period. Anuric patients require only 300 ml/day to 400 ml/day of fluid for insensible losses. The serum potassium must be checked every 4 hr in the initial 24 hr after surgery. Hyperkalemia is the greatest immediate risk to the patient. A serum potassium in excess of 5.5 mEq/liter must be lowered with sodium polystyrene sulfonate (Kayexalate) enema. Kayexalate (50 g in 200 ml of 20% sorbitol) is used every 4 hr as necessary.

Dialysis is not performed on the day of nephrectomy nor on the following day if possble to reduce the risk of postoperative hemorrhage.

Nephrectomy in renal transplantation recipients is now performed only with a precise, individualized indication. Most recipients of renal grafts are able to retain their old kidneys without untoward effects on the outcome of the graft.

REFERENCES

1. BANOWSKY LH: The role of adjuvant operations in renal transplantation. Urol Clin North Am 3:527, 1976
2. BREDAEL JJ, CARSON CC III, WEINERTH JL: Bilateral nephrectomy by the posterior approach. Eur Urol 6:251, 1980
3. CURTIS JJ, LUCAS BA, KOTCHEN TA et al: Surgical therapy for persistent hypertension after renal transplantation. Transplantation 31:125, 1981
4. DAGHER FJ, RAMOS E, ERSLEV A et al: Erythrocytosis after renal allotransplantation: Treatment by removal of the native kidneys. South Med J 73:940, 1980
5. FREED SZ: Bilateral nephrectomy in transplant recipients. Urology (Suppl) 10:16, 1977
6. KONNAK JW, HYNDMAN CW, CERNY JC: Bilateral nephrectomy prior to renal transplantation. J Urol 107:9, 1972
7. LEE C, NEFF MS, SLIFKIN RF et al: Bilateral nephrectomy for hypertension in patients with chronic renal failure on a dialysis program. J Urol 119:20, 1978
8. MENDEZ R, MENDEZ RG, PAYNE JE et al: Renal transplantation. Urology 5:26, 1975
9. MROCZEK WJ: Malignant hypertension: Kidneys too good to be extirpated. Ann Intern Med 80:754, 1974

10. SALVATIERRA O, JR, KOUNTZ SL, BELZER FO: Polycystic renal disease treated by renal transplantation. Surg Gynecol Obstet 137:431, 1973

11. STARZL TE: Experience in renal transplantation. Philadelphia, WB Saunders, 1964

12. THIEBOT J, MERLAND JJ, DUBOUST A et al: Nephrectomie bilaterale par embolisation des arteres renales. Sem Hop Paris 56:670, 1980

13. VINER NA, RAWL JC, BRAREN V et al: Bilateral nephrectomy: An analysis of 100 consecutive cases. J Urol 113:291, 1975

14. WARD JP, SMART CJ, O'DONOGHUE EPN et al: Synchronous bilateral lumbotomy. Eur Urol 2:102, 1976

15. YARIMIZU SN, STEWART BH, SUSAN LP et al: Mortality and morbidity in pretransplant bilateral nephrectomy. Urology 12:55, 1978

Renal Preservation

32

John L. Weinerth

Each year 62,000 patients develop renal disease of such magnitude that chronic hemodialysis or renal transplantation must be considered to preserve their lives. The majority of patients who are candidates for transplantation do not have relatives of sufficiently similar antigenicity to provide a living-donor graft and must rely on cadaver-renal grafts. The time required for immunologic testing and recipient preparation, the uncertainty of graft availability and transportation arrangements, and the logistics of transplant team assembly make extended graft preservation a highly desired adjunct to renal transplantation. In recent years increased emphasis has been applied to extending both the quality and the length of renal preservation to use fully cooperative cadaver-graft sharing programs (local, state, and national) as well as to allowing sufficient time for exhaustive immunologic testing and preoperative recipient preparation. In addition, the principles and methods of current renal preservation have been applied to *ex vivo* bench surgery of the kidney in difficult clinical situations (see Chap. 11).[13,29]

The origins of modern renal preservation reside in the early work of the Nobel-prize winner Alexis Carrel and the engineer–aviator Charles Lindbergh. In 1938 while logically extending Carrel's tissue culture techniques, they developed an "organ culture" and in the process proved that kidneys could be kept viable outside of the body using a very complicated blood-perfusing apparatus. The short period of viability produced by these methods discouraged further attempts at long-term preservation until renal transplantation became a reality in the 1950s. Hypothermia was then discovered to significantly prolong the period of viability,[6,30] and simple surface cooling of the kidneys was employed extensively. Subsequent studies led to the employment of intravascular gravity perfusion of various cold electrolyte solutions to speed the cooling process, preserve additional viable renal tissue, and increase the effective preservation.

Preservation studies then returned to the donor, and the importance of adequate donor preparation prior to nephrectomy and preservation was clarified. Various manipulations of the donor were emphasized, particularly the importance of induced diuresis using mannitol and furosemide, the use of antispasmotics, and the support of the donor's vascular compartment.[1,15,37]

Interest then shifted back to Carrel's work and the possibility of hypothermic perfusion. Foremost of the advances were the experiments of Belzer and associates and Humphries.[3,4,16,17] Belzer succeeded in 1968 in applying a very successful system of pulsatile perfusion with hypothermia and membrane oxygenation to the preservation of human kidneys. This method extended the time of effective preservation from several hours to as long as 50 hr.[4,37]

Most recently preservation studies have been in the following areas: elucidation of the limiting factors in perfusion preservation; combining simple flush-out techniques to facilitate harvesting and transportation over long distances; development of more efficient and more compact technology; and determination of the suitability of various perfusates and of the importance of various additives.[1,15,24,38]

In the span of one generation, renal preservation for transplantation has advanced from an armchair possibility to an efficient methodology, with acceptable time limits, accompanied by an increase in physiologic information regarding the effects of various technologic maneuvers, drug therapy, hypothermia, and altered physiology on the kidney. A new approach to temporary preservation in renal surgery has been proposed by Wickham and associates using intra-arterial administration of inosine (a purine nucleoside) followed by normothermic ischemia.[40] Initial results seem promising. The obvious next step in organ preservation is organ banking by means of freezing. This is as yet unobtainable on the organ level, but information is rapidly accumulating, as indicated by several excellent reviews.[5,38]

Principles

TISSUE OXYGENATION

The oxygen supply of the kidney is vitally important in renal graft survival, because the kidneys are among the most sensitive organs of the body to normothermic hypoxia. The avoidance of hypoxia of potential renal grafts starts long before *in vitro* renal preservation. The concern for renal preservation must begin in the donor, because the effects of vasoconstriction, decreased blood flow, and cardiac failure can lead to deterioration and loss of the renal graft. The transition from a normal kidney to acute tubular necrosis to permanent damage from cortical necrosis is markedly short and deserves important consideration.

These precautions are particularly pertinent in the cadaveric donor as opposed to the living-related donor in whom the metabolic environment is reasonably normal. It is estimated that the adenosine triphosphate (ATP) of the renal cortex is exhausted within minutes, leaving the kidney to depend on anaerobic metabolism with the accumulation of waste products and pH changes which are responsible for intrarenal blood coagulation and enzymatic dysfunction.[8] It has been clearly shown that hypoxia changes renal vascular flow, decreasing renal cortical supply and compounding the hypoxemia and resultant damage.[27] In several clinical studies a large majority of renal grafts were not successful after transplantation when exposed to normothermic hypoxia for 15 minutes following cardiovascular collapse in a cadaver donor. This was true even when one of the best available techniques of renal perfusion was employed.[12]

It is imperative for effective renal preservation to attend closely to the donor with the maintenance of satisfactory blood pressure, blood volume, and renal blood flow and the avoidance of arterial hypoxemia. Once the renal graft is removed from the donor, other maneuvers—such as hypothermia or metabolic inhibition, or both—must be employed because the delivery of normal blood flow (3 ml/g/min–5 ml/g/min)[1] to the kidney is not possible in an *in vitro* environment (see Chap. 29).

METABOLIC REQUIREMENTS AND WASTE REMOVAL

The metabolic requirements of the human kidney undergoing preservation are altered, and the extent and significance of these alterations are still not fully understood. Glucose requirements of the kidney are low at 5° C, but not absent. Because the renal cortex preferentially uses fatty acid metabolism, it is suggested that the success of plasma or albumin solutions is secondary to the binding of fatty acids.[14] The electrolyte content of perfusates is important to maintain membrane and lysosomal integrity, especially the concentrations of calcium and magnesium.[1,37] Potassium is necessary for enzymatic activity, but the actual concentration needed in perfusates during preservation is still in dispute.[7,28,36] Obviously the total requirements of the kidney are still poorly understood, and many necessary factors have not yet been elucidated. The necessity for energy stores at low temperature is not clear, but continuous perfusion has resulted in higher ATP and total adenine nucleotides in the renal cortex with suggested improved function after preservation.[8]

Perfusates have ranged from simple electrolyte solutions to modified plasma in attempts to elucidate or to supply blindly all metabolic needs. This very complex area is well reviewed.[1,15,37]

As important as the delivery of metabolites to the preserved kidney is the removal of waste products. Despite low temperatures, anaerobic metabolism persists with the accumulation of metabolic waste products, decreasing the pH and increasing the accumulation of ammonia in the distal tubules.[41] The inference can be drawn that even with nonoxygenated solutions, low flow with the removal of waste products is better than no perfusion at all.[8]

HYPOTHERMIA

The main effect of hypothermia is to decrease the metabolic rate and the need for oxygen. Levy has demonstrated that oxygen consumption is reduced from 100% at 37° C to approximately 5% at 10° C.[21] Hypothermia also protects against oxygen toxicity.[34] Although hypothermia causes hemoglobin to bind oxygen to a greater degree at low temperatures, decreasing its availability to the cells, hemoglobin-free solutions are adequate for the metabolic needs of the kidney at low temperatures.[1] The general inhibitory effect of hypothermia is not uniform, as exemplified by decreased glucose metabolism but normal amino acid transport.[22] Hypothermia decreases enzymatic activity with the inability of cellular membranes to maintain the sodium pump mechanism. This disadvantage results in intracellular potassium loss, but neither the degree of loss nor its significance has been clearly stated. This loss of potassium is the rationale for the use of electrolyte concentrations in perfusion solutions which approximate intracellular concentrations.[36]

Because tissues respond differently to hypothermia, Downes and associates suggest that the inability to preserve livers with the same system that adequately preserves kidneys is due to the specific high degree of inhibition of the sodium–potassium pump (at 10° C) exceeding the limits of reversibility in liver perfusion.[11] In kidneys, however, there is a residual amount of sodium–potassium pump activity remaining at 10° C, which may explain this particular organ's success in low-temperature preservation.

PERFUSION HEMODYNAMICS

The kidney has an autoregulatory mechanism in the preglomerular arterioles that maintains the glomular pressure at 60 torr to 90 torr. Although preservation perfusion has been carried out at pressures greater than 90 torr in the arterial system, the best results have been obtained with those systems that keep the pressure below 60 torr to 90 torr.[1,37] Our preference is systolic pressure lower than 60 torr. Pressures greater than 90 torr lead to edema with obstruction from interstitial swelling and increased resistance.

Arterial Pressure

Flow is felt to be the most important parameter in organ perfusion as long as arterial pressure is kept lower than 60 torr, but recent studies indicate that constant pressure regulation is more desirable, providing that initial flow rates are adequate.[31] The regulation of pressure is undoubtedly important at low temperatures because there is paralysis of the vasomotor system, and pressures greater than 90 torr would not be regulated by the kidney, exposing the arterioles to pressures higher than normal.[35] The lower level of pressure is dictated by the closing pressure of the precapillary sphincters (10 torr).

Clinically the lower limits of adequate renal flow in man is 100 ml/min;[19] it is calculated that with oxygen tensions of 200 torr to 300 torr, 0.25 ml to 0.5 ml per gram of kidney per minute can supply renal oxygen requirements at 5° C to 10° C.[1]

Venous Pressure

Several investigators maintain that a venous pressure is essential, especially because it contributes to total vascular flow as described by Poiseuille's law.[1] DeFalco and associates suggested that flow in transplanted kidneys is affected by intratransplantation vascular collapse and inadequate venous pressure during storage.[10] Estimates of optimal venous pressure during isolated perfusion have ranged from 4 cm to 20 cm of water;[1] however, current isolated perfusion systems do not use a venous pressure gradient. Although both bile and urine flow are influenced by venous outflow gradients,[37] the ultimate need for this particular parameter is unclear and is not generally considered in renal preservation.

Pulse Pressure

The use of pulsatile flow has been accepted by most active preservation methods. Certainly in the normothermic preparation, pulsatile perfusion has been clearly shown to preserve optimal function.[25,43] Increased edema and vascular resistance are the consequence of nonpulsatile flow.

This particular problem has recently been restudied, with the decision that lymphatic flow and vascular integrity appear to be significantly influenced by an adequate pulse pressure.[19,39] Until this problem is clearly resolved, it is felt that the maintenance of pulse pressure of 20 torr to 30 torr is justifiable.

PERFUSATE COMPOSITION

No area of organ preservation is the subject of greater controversy than the suggested composition of perfusates. The controversies entail the precise composition of the electrolyte solutions, the use of modified plasma *versus* synthetic solutions, and the need for additives such as steroids, glucose, insulin, and diuretics. The actual composition of the solutions has ranged from simple extracellular electrolytes to intracellular salt solutions to tissue culture media, dextran solutions, albumin solutions, and plasma in many forms. These solutions are discussed in detail in several excellent reviews.[1,15,37]

The general criteria for simple flush hypothermic technique solutions are normal or slightly elevated osmolarity and ready availability. Both modified Ringer's solutions and Collins C-3 solution[9] meet these requirements and are used in many institutions for short-term preservation. Concerning solutions for continuous pulsatile perfusion, oncotic pressure becomes an important addition to the criteria. Our incomplete knowledge of the renal metabolic requirements under hypothermic conditions prompted the use of a modification of Belzer's cryoprecipitated plasma. Belzer and associates have shown that low-density lipoproteins form emboli during perfusion, leading to increased vascular resistance and decreased or spotty perfusion of the kidney.[4] The difficulty was eliminated by freezing the plasma and precipitating out the low-density lipoproteins. Recent studies show that hyperosmolarity may prevent edema with longer preservation.[36] Presently, a survey of 54 transplant centers indicates that only 2% are using cryoprecipitated plasma. Sixty-five percent are using commercial plasma protein fraction, and 25% are using an albumin solution.

Pharmacologic additives to the perfusion solutions are diverse and are employed to buffer the kidney against the nonphysiologic conditions imposed by hypothermic perfusion or simple hypothermic storage. Membrane stabilizers, such as phenothiazines and corticosteroids, have been shown to increase membrane resistance to hypoxia and to stabilize lysosomal membranes, preventing cellular destruction from released enzymes.[24] Several metabolic inhibitors, such as furosemide and magnesium ions, allegedly work in concert with hypothermia to obtain a more complete metabolic depression. Agents such as papaverine, procaine, and phenoxybenzamine decrease pre- and post-harvest vasoconstriction and promote maximal flow. Mannitol is added to increase osmolarity and to prevent edema in the perfused organ.

Several buffers, such as bicarbonate or trisaminomethane, are added to counteract acid metabolites. Antibiotics are added to suppress bacterial proliferation in the longer perfusions. Insulin and glucose cover the minimal glucose needs of the hypothermic organ. A more complete discussion of the myriad of possible additives is dealt with in the literature,[1,15,37] but the general trend is to use as few additives as possible.

Methods of Preservation

The two most common methods of renal preservation are simple flush hypothermic storage and continuous pulsatile hypothermic perfusion. Both methods provide adequate renal preservation over short periods (up to 12 hr), and the continuous pulsatile hypothermic perfusion has produced consistent results for as long as 50 hr.[4] The actual choice depends on the local need of the renal transplantation team.

For the simple flush technique there is a choice of three general solutions. An extracellular solution (Table 32-1) used at many centers for short-term renal preservation is used both in flushing and cooling of living-related-donor grafts and for the initial preparation of cadaver grafts destined for continuous pulsatile perfusion. Table 32-2 shows the composition of two intracellular solutions proposed by Collins and Sacks respectively, the main difference being that the Sacks solution is hyper-

TABLE 32-1. **Extracellular Electrolyte Solution**

Modified Ringer's Solution	
COMPONENT	CONCENTRATION PER LITER
NaHCO$_3$	20 mEq
NaCl	102 mEq
KCl	4 mEq
CaCl$_2$	3.0 mEq
Heparin	5000 U
Albumin	25 g

TABLE 32-2. **Intracellular Electrolyte Solutions***

Collins C-3		Sacks	
KH$_2$PO$_4$	2.05	KH$_2$PO$_4$	2.05
K$_2$HPO$_4$ · 3H$_2$O	9.7	K$_2$HPO$_4$ · 3H$_2$O	9.70
KCl	1.12	KCl	1.12
NaHCO$_3$	0.84	NaHCO$_3$	0.84
Procaine HCl	0.10	Mannitol	25
Heparin	5000 U/ liter		
Glucose	25		
MgSO$_4$ · 7H$_2$O	7.38		
330 mosmoles/ liter		410 mosmoles/ liter	

* Concentration is in grams per liter unless otherwise indicated.

osmolar.[9,36] Reports state that these solutions can preserve kidneys from 12 hr to 24.

Regardless of the solution selected, the methodology of simple flush hypothermic storage is the same. Immediately after the kidney is removed from the donor (either living or cadaveric), the renal artery is gently dilated. A soft Silastic cannula is introduced and secured with a tourniquet tie. The kidney is perfused with the solution of choice at approximately 5° C. After the effluent has remained clear for several minutes, the kidney is placed into two sterile plastic bags and then immersed in ice water. Using polystyrene plastic containers, the kidneys can be kept at 5° C to 10° C until ready for transplantation. It is important that a full description of renal vascular anomalies and the status of the donor accompany the kidneys, because it is difficult to reinspect the kidneys under these circumstances.

When continuous pulsatile hypothermic perfusion is chosen, the perfusate composition is the preference of the preservation center and may include cryoprecipitated plasma, plasma protein fraction (PPF), or albumin solutions. Various solution compositions are available from the Southeastern Organ Procurement Foundation, Richmond, Virginia. The solutions appear to give comparable results, and the main differences are ease of preparation (PPF and albumin) and absence of possible deleterious globulins (albumin).

In practice, after the kidneys are removed from the donor and flushed with a cold electrolyte solution of choice, they are immediately put on the perfusion apparatus with the arterial pressure set at 40 torr to 60 torr. Gas flows are adjusted to provide a pO_2 at approximately 150 torr to 200 torr, and the CO_2 flow is adjusted to keep the pH within normal limits. Temperature control is set automatically at 5° C to 7° C. Periodic flow measurements are determined, because a flow rate less than 100 ml/min is associated with poor posttransplant function.[19] Some experimental evidence also suggests that there is immediate improvement in renal function during the first few hours of perfusion.[38] The exact reason for this improvement is not clear but may be related to the relaxation of precapillary sphincters and the washout of accumulated metabolic wastes.

Recent experiences show that human kidneys are preserved adequately by a combination of techniques.[18] This flexibility in the application of storage techniques diminishes many of the logistic problems in cadaver-graft procurement and transportation.

A useful adjunct to preparing and repairing renal grafts is a sterile controlled temperature organ bath (Fig. 32-1), used for the initial dissection, flushing, holding during living-related transplants, and repair of grafts, such as arterial lesions during cadaver procedures. The "double-boiler" apparatus (made in the hospital instrument shop) allows for complete sterility and avoidance of the profound hypothermia (< 0° C) occasionally associated with ice-slush preparations. Connected to standard preservation pumps, the bath solution can be held at 3° C to 7° C with ease.[42]

Clinical Results

Results of preservation vary according to method and preservation time, but both flush and perfusion methods provide excellent results up to 12 hr to 18 hr storage, with some groups claiming no difference at 24 hr.[2,5] Others report immediate function rates of 66% with flush methods and 65%

FIG. 32-1. The double-boiler apparatus is used for continuous maintenance of sterile hypothermic (3°C–7°C) fluid for renal preservation and storage.

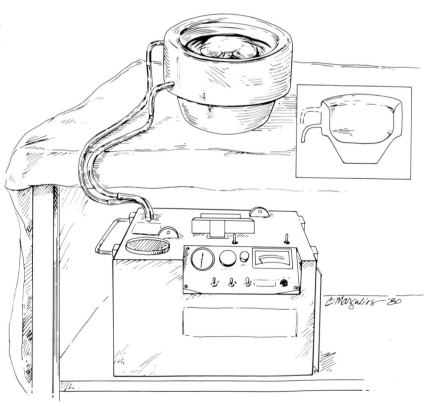

to 80% immediate function using pulsatile perfusion. However, average storage time for the flush method was 5.8 hr, as opposed to 21.5 hr for the perfusion method.[7,28]

Our results over an 8-year period involving 253 kidneys transplanted and using cryoprecipitated plasma initially, followed by silica gel fraction cryoprecipitated plasma, PPF, and finally albumin solutions with pulsatile perfusion have been encouraging considering the average storage time was 24 hr. Sixty-nine percent of the transplanted kidneys had immediate function; 3% had delayed function but did not necessitate dialysis; 16% had delayed function which required dialysis but subsequently regained satisfactory function; 10% were lost due to rejection, vascular problems, or patient death before function could be assessed; and 2% never functioned.[32] By evaluating the kidneys while they are on the perfusion apparatus and discarding those organs with low flow rates or high diastolic pressures, we believe that the percent of immediate functioning kidneys in our series approximates the more favorable results of other investigators.[28]

Our evaluation also included the injection of phenolsulfonphthalein (PSP) directly into the arterial line as a bolus at 60 torr to ensure uniform perfusion. At the same time, by watching the ureter with 2.5-power ocular loupes of the 100 lost cadaver kidneys, ureteral vascular integrity could be demonstrated by visualization of the dye in the small ureteral vessels. The two kidneys that failed this test proved to have had their ureteral blood supply interrupted by hilar dissection at time of harvest.[33] The use of PSP also avoids the theoretical adverse effects of methylene blue injections.[26]

The main types of renal preservation (simple flush hypothermic storage and continuous pulsatile perfusion) will adequately preserve the kidney for short-term storage (up to 18 hr). For periods longer than 18 hr the continuous perfusion method is both reliable and the method of choice in many centers. The additional storage time of the continuous pulsatile perfusion provides a greater flexibility in recipient preparation, tissue matching, assessment of the functional capacity of the organ, and time for long-distance transportation. The advantages of simplicity and less expense of the simple flush hypothermic storage procedures make necessary a continuous assessment of the current literature for documented improvements in this method of renal preservation.

REFERENCES

1. ABBOTT WM, WEINERTH JL: The perfusion of isolated whole organs. Cryobiology 8:113, 1971

2. BARRY JM, METCALFE JB, FARNSWORTH MA et al: Comparison of intracellular flushing and cold storage to machine perfusion for human kidney preservation. J Urol 123:14, 1980

3. BELZER FO, ASHBY BS, DUNPHY JE: Twenty-four and seventy-two hour preservation of canine kidneys. Lancet 2:536, 1967

4. BELZER FO, ASHBY BS, HUANG JS et al: Etiology of rising perfusion pressure in isolated organ perfusion. Ann Surg 168:382, 1968

5. BELZER FO, SOUTHARD JH: The future of kidney preservation. Transplant 30:161, 1980

6. BOGARDUS GM, SCHLOSSER RJ: Influence of temperature upon ischemic renal damage. Surgery 39:960, 1956

7. CLARK EA, MICKEY MR, ODELL G et al: Evaluation of Belzer and Collins Kidney—Preservation methods. Lancet 2:361, 1973

8. COLLESTE H: Preservation of kidneys for transplantation. Acta Chir Scand (Suppl) 425:5, 1972

9. COLLINS GM, BRAVO–SHUGARMAN M, TERASAKI PI: Kidney preservation for transportation. Lancet 2:1219, 1969

10. DEFALCO AJ, MUNDTH ED, JACOBSON YG et al: A possible explanation for transplantation anuria. Surg Gynecol Obstet 120:748, 1965

11. DOWNES OL, MARTIN DR, SCOTT DF et al: Cold sensitivity of active cation transport—A major problem in liver and heart preservation. Surg Forum 22:256, 1971

12. FROST AB, ACKERMAN J, FINCH WT et al: Kidney preservation for transportation. Lancet 6:620, 1970

13. GUERRIERO WG, SCOTT R, JOYCE L: Development of extracorporeal renal perfusion as an adjunct for bench renal surgery. J Urol 107:4, 1972

14. HORSBURGH T: Possible role of free fatty acids in kidney preservation media. Nature (London) 242:122, 1973

15. HUMPHRIES AL: Organ preservation: A review. Transplantation 5:1138, 1967

16. HUMPHRIES AL, HEIMBURGER RA, MORETZ WH: Homotransplantation of canine kidneys after 24 hour storage. Invest Urol 4:531, 1967

17. HUMPHRIES AL, RUSSELL R, STODDARD LD et al: Successful five-day kidney preservation. Invest Urol 5:609, 1968

18. KAUFMAN HM, RODGERS RE, GROSS WS et al: Human kidney preservation and shipping. Transplantation 15:465, 1973

19. LANTON RL, ROGERS J, KEMMER SR et al: Perfusion characteristics of nonfunctional and functional canine kidneys. Transplantation 16:67, 1973

20. LARGIADIER F, MANAX WF, LYONS GW: Prolonged in vitro hypothermic perfusion of the canine lung. Trans Am Soc Artif Intern Organs 11:197, 1965

21. LEVY MN: Oxygen consumption and blood flow in the hypothermic perfused kidney. Am J Physiol 197:1111, 1959

22. LOWENSTEIN LM, HUMMELER K, SMITH I: The effect of storage of 4° C on amino acid transport by rat kidney cortex slices. Biochim Biophys Acta 150:415, 1968

23. MARBERGER M, EISENBERGER F: Regional hypothermia of the kidney: Surface or transarterial perfusion cooling? A functional study. J Urol 124:179, 1980

24. MCCABE RE, LATTES LG, LORRIED DR et al: The protective effect of methylprednisolone on the machine-preserved kidney. Am Surg 46:335, 1980

25. MCLAUGHLIN ED, AUSTEN WG: Perfusion of the isolated canine liver in vivo and in vitro. Trans Am Soc Artif Intern Organs 12:259, 1966

26. MEREDITH JE, WALLEY BD, TODO SK et al: Effect of methylene blue on hypothermically preserved canine kidneys. Transplant 26:366, 1978

27. MILLER HC, ALEXANDER JW, NATHAN P: Effect of warm ischemic damage on intrarenal distribution of flow in preserved kidneys. Surgery 72:193, 1972

28. MILLER HC, ALEXANDER JW, SMITH EJ: Evaluation of kidney preservation methods. Lancet 2:880, 1973

29. NOVICK AC, STEWART BH, STRAFFON RA: Extracorporeal renal surgery and autotransplantation; Indications, techniques, and results. J Urol 123:806, 1980

30. PEGG DE, CALNE RY, PRYSE–DAVIES J et al: Canine renal preservation using surface and perfusion cooling techniques. Ann NY Acad Sci 120:506, 1964

31. PEGG DE, GREEN CJ: Renal preservation by hypothermic perfusion: 1. The importance of pressure control. Cryobiology 10:56, 1973

32. PETERSON CJ, WEINERTH JL, PHILLIPS MG: Accumulated results of perfusion preservation techniques (in press)

33. PHILLIPS MG, WEINERTH JL, PETERSON CJ: Use of PSP dye to evaluate ureteral blood supply in cadaver kidneys (in press)

34. POPVIC V, GERSCHMAN R, GILBERT DL: Effect of high oxygen pressure on ground squirrels in hypothermia and hibernation. Am J Physiol 206:49, 1964

35. RUDOLF LE, JONES RE, RAMSBURGH SR: The vasculature in isolated perfusion. In Malinin TL, Zeppa R, Gollan F et al (eds): Reversibility of Cellular Injury due to Inadequate Perfusion, pp 466–468. Springfield, Charles C Thomas, 1972

36. SACKS SA, PETRITSCH PH, KAUFMAN JJ: Canine kidney preservation using a new perfusate. Lancet 2:1024, 1973

37. SELL KW: Tissue and organ preservation. In Najarian JS, Simmons RL (eds): Transplantation, pp 404–417. Philadelphia, Lea & Febiger, 1972

38. SELL KW, BENJAMIN JL, GARTIVER S et al: Improvement in renal function during hypothermic in vitro perfusion. In Malinin TL, Zeppa R, Gollan F, et al (eds): Reversibility of Cellular Injury due to Inadequate Perfusion, pp 481–490. Springfield, Charles C Thomas, 1972

39. TOLEDO–PEREYRA LH, NAJARIAN JS: Pulsatile flow and viability of isolated perfusion kidneys. Transplantation 16:63, 1973

40. WICKHAM JE, FERNANDO AR, HENDREY WF et al: Inosine: Clinical results of ischaemic renal surgery. Br J Urol 50:465, 1978

41. WICKHAM JE, SHARMA JP: Endogenous ammonia formation in experimental renal ischemia. Lancet 2:195, 1965

42. WEINERTH JL, PHILLIPS MG, PETERSON CJ: Surgical cooling bath for kidneys. (in press)

43. WILKENS H, REGELSON W, HOFFMEISTER FS: The physiologic importance of pulsatile blood flow. N Engl J Med 267:443, 1962

Renal Transplantation

33

Oscar Salvatierra, Jr.

The consequences of vascular, urologic, or infectious wound complications in renal transplantation, with their associated morbidity, mortality, and graft loss, are well documented. Complications in our series of more than 1800 renal transplants have been minimal, which can be attributed to strict adherence to techniques and principles outlined in this chapter.

Transplantation of the kidney graft in a renal-failure patient demands precision and careful surgical technique, because there is no other operation that is routinely performed under the same high-risk constraints attendant with uremia and immunosuppression. These conditions give no latitude for surgical error that risks graft loss. Currently the goal of transplantation surgery is to ensure that immunologic rejection is the primary, if not the only, reason for graft loss.[4] A high graft-loss rate from surgical complications, in addition to immunologic rejection, would make the risks of renal transplantation unacceptable.

PREPARATION OF THE PATIENT

The prospective transplant recipient should be in metabolic and electrolyte balance so as to avoid perioperative hyperkalemia and difficult operative hemostasis associated with inadequate dialysis. When dialysis can be scheduled in advance, as with living-related transplantation, it should be performed on the day prior to surgery.

We prefer to shave the patient after the induction of anesthesia so that careful skin prepping without skin injury or contamination can be achieved. An indwelling Foley catheter is also best inserted after the patient is anesthetized. Any urine present in the bladder is evacuated and submitted for culture, after which the bladder is distended to approximately 80 ml or 100 ml with a saline solution containing Neosporin G.U. Irrigant. This greatly facilitates an accurate anterior cystotomy later in the procedure and, in addition, protects against possible wound contamination when the bladder is opened. After instillation of the antibiotic solution, the catheter is clamped. The clamp is removed prior to the cystotomy closure.

Incision and Iliac Fossa Dissection

A lower quadrant incision is made in a gentle curvilinear fashion extending from near the symphysis pubis to 1.5 cm to 2 cm medial to the anterior superior iliac spine and up to approximately 2 cm below the lower thoracic cage (Fig. 33-1A). The upper four fifths of the incision is extended through the external oblique, internal oblique, and transversus abdominis muscles, and in the lower one fifth of the incision the rectus fascia is incised. The rectus muscle can thus be dissected inferiorly to its tendinous insertion to the symphysis pubis, where it is divided. The inferior epigastric vessels are identified and skeletonized as they pass across the incision, and then divided and ligated. There is an anterior extraperitoneal thin fascial layer that, on division in the direction of the incision, permits entry into the extraperitoneal space and easy development of an essentially avascular plane immediately adjacent to the peritoneum.

With medial retraction of the peritoneum, the spermatic cord in the male patient or round ligament in the female patient is easily identified. In the male patient, some of the connective tissue around the cord is freed to permit easier retraction of the cord when the self-retaining retractor is inserted later. Cord ligation should be avoided to prevent posttransplantation testicular atrophy or hydrocele formation. In the female patient, the round ligament is divided and ligated. Further development of the extraperitoneal space over the iliac fossa can now be accomplished, with exposure of the distal common and external iliac artery. The insertion of a self-retaining retractor at this point ensures adequate exposure for the subsequent iliac vessel dissection and vascular anastomoses.

The dissection and skeletonization of the iliac vessels must be performed in a manner that allows secure ligature of the divided lymphatics passing

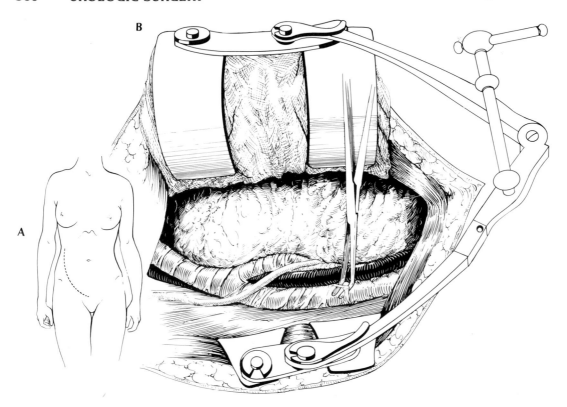

FIG. 33-1. **(A)** The incision is depicted for the right abdomen, and subsequent illustrations will represent graft implantation in the right iliac fossa. The renal transplant, however, can be performed on either the right or left side. **(B)** The iliac vessels are best exposed with a self-retaining retractor. Segmental separation, ligature, and division of perivascular tissue containing lymphatics are essential and must precede skeletonization of the iliac vessels.

over these vessels. This is best accomplished by the use of a Gemini–Mixter forceps to develop the plane of Leriche over the external and distal common iliac arteries (Fig. 33-1B). The tissue overlying the arteries and containing the lymphatics sequentially is segmentally separated, doubly ligated with 4-0 suture, and divided, a maneuver that has greatly reduced the incidence of lymphocele. This tissue should be doubly ligated before it is incised, in contrast to double clamping and division of the tissue. With the latter procedure, some of the contained lymphatics may be lost, which could predispose to lymphocele formation. The anterior separation of tissue over the iliac artery is more easily performed in an inferior to superior direction. Following this procedure, the iliac artery can be skeletonized and freed up from adjacent tissue by sharp scissor dissection.

At this point, palpation of the common iliac bifurcation and internal iliac artery will determine whether the internal iliac artery should also be skeletonized in preparation for an end-to-end an-

astomosis with the renal artery. If there is moderate atherosclerosis extending into the bifurcation, an end-to-side anastomosis with the iliac artery is preferred. However, if an endarterectomy can be safely performed, or if there is no evidence of atheroma in the internal iliac vessel, then skeletonization of this vessel can also be accomplished. Before skeletonization is begun, the traversing longitudinal lymphatics on the medial aspect of the iliac bifurcation should be doubly ligated and divided. If the internal iliac artery is to be used, it may be clamped proximally with the Wylie hypogastric artery clamp and distally divided with appropriate ligation of the distal stump. The freed internal iliac artery should be irrigated with a heparinized saline solution.

The iliac vein can now be skeletonized with the same segmental ligature and division of anterior lymphatic-containing tissue as was done with the iliac artery. Posterior venous tributaries are often encountered and must be divided to permit maximum anterior mobility of the iliac vein. It is preferable to doubly ligate these posterior tributaries with 2-0 or 3-0 suture prior to division, because the double clamping maneuver may sometimes result in injury or avulsion of the distal stump during ligature. Hemostasis can then only be achieved with difficulty and with risk of obturator nerve injury.

Graft Implantation and Vascular Anastomoses

The iliac vein is prepared for the end-to-side renal vein anastomosis by placement of clamps proximal and distal to the proposed venotomy for the anastomosis. We customarily use a bent-handle DeBakey curved aortic clamp for proximal occlusion and an angle DeBakey clamp for distal occlusion. A venotomy is fashioned to accommodate the caliber of the renal vein and can best be accomplished with a curved DeBakey endarterectomy scissors that permits removal of a smooth ellipse of vein. The isolated segment of the iliac vein can now be irrigated with heparinized saline. Following this, four 5-0 or 6-0 cardiovascular sutures are placed at the superior and inferior apexes of the venotomy and at the midpoints of the medial and lateral margins of the venotomy. These sutures will later be passed through corresponding points on the renal vein for a four-quadrant end-to-side attachment of the renal vein to the iliac vein. brings the renal vein into juxtaposition with the

If a cadaver kidney is being used, the graft is at this time removed from storage (cold storage or perfusion preservation). With living-related transplantation, the graft is obtained from the live donor in an adjacent operating room and is placed in a container with cold Ringer's lactate. The renal artery is additionally flushed with Ringer's lactate plus additives at 5° C. The formula for this solution is

> 1000 ml Ringer's lactate
> 15 ml NaHCO$_3$
> 10 ml 1:1000 heparin
> 10 ml 1% procaine

The kidney is secured in a sling and held in position for the vascular anastomosis by the assistant. A clamp is used to secure the sling to prevent the assistant from holding the kidney in position with his hands, which might accelerate warming of the kidney during the period of the vascular anastomoses.

The previously placed four sutures through the iliac vein are now passed through the corresponding points of the renal vein and secured, which brings the renal vein into juxtaposition with the

iliac vein venotomy (Fig. 33-2A). The medial and lateral sutures are retracted with mosquito clamps, which separate the venotomy opening to facilitate rapid anastomosis without inadvertent suture of the back wall. The superior suture is used as a running suture down one side of the renal vein, and the inferior suture is used as a running suture up the other side of the renal vein. The vascular clamps on the iliac vein may be left in place until after completion of the arterial anastomosis, although I prefer to use a bulldog clamp across the renal vein at this time and to remove the iliac vein clamps. This allows for earlier establishment of venous return from the lower extremity.

If the internal iliac artery is to be used for the arterial anastomosis, an end-to-end anastomosis is then performed with the renal artery (Fig. 33-2B). The two vessels are positioned so as to allow a gentle upward curve from the iliac bifurcation to the kidney by fixating the superior and inferior arterial apexes with interrupted 5-0 or 6-0 cardiovascular suture. The anastomosis is completed with interrupted sutures. With the kidney resting in the iliac fossa, the initial interrupted suture is placed midway between the apical sutures on the anterior vessel walls facing the operator, thus allowing better approximation of the opposing arterial margins, particularly when a discrepancy in the size of the vessels exists. Subsequently, the remaining interrupted sutures are placed to approximate each anterior quadrant. Following this, the previously placed apical sutures are used to rotate the arteries so that the posterior vessel walls will be in the anterior position for subsequent suture placement. Just as before, a suture is placed midway between the apical sutures, which again divides the rotated posterior vessel walls into quadrants for subsequent interrupted suture placement. The preference for interrupted sutures instead of a running suture to effect this end-to-end anastomosis relates to the ability to absolutely avoid any pursestring effect as might occur from a running suture and the allowance of better accommodation of the two vessels to each other when a size discrepancy exists. Using this technique, our experience has revealed a less than 1% incidence of subsequent renal artery stenosis.

If extensive arteriosclerotic plaques extend into the bifurcation of the common iliac artery, then an end-to-side anastomosis of the renal artery to the external or common iliac artery is preferred. Usually this anastomosis is performed superior to the level of the venous anastomosis. A bent-handle DeBakey curved aortic clamp is placed superiorly and an angle DeBakey clamp is placed inferiorly

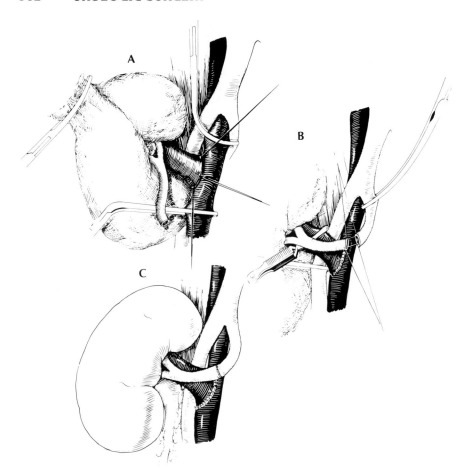

FIG. 33-2. **(A)** The renal vein is brought into exact juxtaposition with the iliac vein phlebotomy by previously placed four-quadrant sutures. A running suture anastomosis will follow. **(B)** The renal artery is positioned to the end of the internal iliac artery by superior and inferior apical sutures. Subsequent placement of interrupted sutures will complete the anastomosis. Note the occluding bulldog clamp on the renal vein. **(C)** The completed venous and arterial anastomoses are demonstrated.

on the iliac vessel isolating the segment for anastomosis. The location of clamp placement must be carefully selected so as not to injure or disrupt existing arteriosclerotic plaques. A longitudinal incision is then made on the anterior or anterolateral portion of the iliac segment with a No. 11 blade knife. Following incision, regional heparinization of the lower extremity is accomplished by instilling approximately 80 ml of heparinized saline (1000 units/100 ml) into the distal iliac limb. Systemic heparinization is not necessary during the procedure. Following regional heparinization, ellipses of arterial wall are removed on each side with a curved DeBakey endarterectomy scissors that allows a smooth, oval arteriotomy to accommodate the end of the renal artery. This anastomosis is also performed with interrupted sutures after initial fixation of the ends of the renal artery to the apexes of the arteriotomy with superior and inferior sutures. The intervening interrupted sutures may then be placed according to the operator's preference.

The previously placed sling around the kidney is now removed. It is extremely important to have obtained preoperative assessment of the recipient for existing cold agglutinins, because moderate to high titers of these agglutinins will require warming the kidney before the circulation is reestablished.[1] The vascular clamps can then be released, with the venous clamps removed before the arterial clamps.

Multiple Renal Vessels

A cadaver kidney with multiple renal arteries perfused through the aorta is best transplanted with an end-to-side anastomosis of a Carrel patch encompassing the multiple arteries (Fig. 33-3). If the vessels are in close proximity to each other, a single Carrel patch will suffice.[3] If the vessels are some distance apart, two Carrel patches are preferable. The Carrel patch of donor aorta is fashioned to accommodate the multiple vessels, and its anastomosis to the common or external iliac artery is performed after an arteriotomy that accommodates the width and length of the Carrel patch. This anastomosis is best performed by fixing the patch at the superior and inferior apexes of the arteriotomy with 5-0 cardiovascular suture. The superior suture is then used as a running suture down one side of the arterial anastomosis, and the inferior suture is used as a running suture up the opposite side of the arterial anastomosis.

The presence of multiple arteries in related transplantation is known in advance because all live related donors have preoperative arteriograms. Most donors have at least a single artery to one of their kidneys, but, at times, a donor kidney with double arteries or triple arteries must be used. However, these arteries cannot be taken with a Carrel patch because of the risk to the live donor. In these instances the following arterial anastomoses are possible: double end-to-side renal artery to iliac artery, end-to-end superior renal artery to internal iliac artery with end-to-side inferior renal artery to external iliac artery, and implantation of an accessory artery end to side into the larger main stem renal artery, with the larger renal artery anastomosed to the internal, external, or common iliac artery. An accessory artery to main renal artery anastomosis should be performed with *ex vivo* technique before the renal vein anastomosis.

Pediatric Cadaver Kidneys

We have previously shown that it is not necessary to transplant both kidneys from young children *en bloc*, but that each kidney can be used for a different recipient as is the case with adult-cadaver donors.[5] All pediatric kidneys at our center have been transplanted as single units, with the arterial anastomosis formed by using a Carrel patch of donor aorta and, whenever possible, a Carrel patch of vena cava for the venous anastomosis (Fig. 33-4). A Carrel patch is mandatory because direct implantation of a small vessel into a much larger vessel may result in actual thrombosis or produce functional stenosis concomitant with graft hypertrophy. If a Carrel patch of vena cava cannot be used, the venous anastomosis should be performed with interrupted sutures. The arterial and venous anastomoses are usually carried out on the iliac vessels, with the aorta and vena cava used only in small pediatric recipients. In our experience, pediatric kidneys have proved to be excellent donor grafts in both adults and children, with considerable early hypertrophy occurring in the immediate posttransplant period. At our center, pediatric-cadaver kidneys transplanted as single units have provided good renal function to more than 80 recipients whose ages range from 18 months to 53

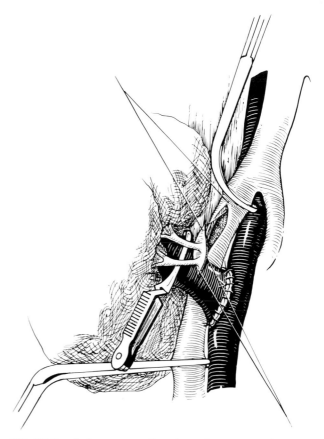

FIG. 33-3. A donor aorta Carrel patch encompassing two renal arteries is positioned by apical sutures to an iliac arteriotomy fashioned to accommodate the length and width of the patch.

years. At 6 months posttransplantation, these recipients have graft survival and serum creatinine levels equivalent to those obtained following adult-cadaver kidney transplantation.

Ureteroneocystostomy

A modification of the Politano–Leadbetter submucosal tunnel technique is used for ureteral implantation and is performed through a counter-anterior cystotomy incision.[7] Previous filling of the bladder facilitates a longitudinal anterior cystotomy with minimal handling of the bladder wall. A submucosal tunnel is fashioned near the bladder floor where angulation of the ureter upon vesical distention is prevented. The tunnel is constructed between two transverse mucosal incisions about 2 cm to 2.5 cm apart, with the distal aspect of the tunnel in close proximity to the trigone.

A small No. 8Fr Robinson catheter is then passed through the tunnel in retrograde fashion. Follow-

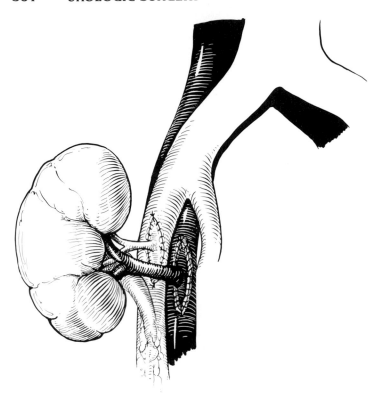

FIG. 33-4. Small pediatric-cadaver renal vessels are anastomosed to larger recipient iliac vessels using Carrel patches of donor aorta and vena cava.

ing this, a muscular ureteral hiatus is created with a right-angle forceps adjacent to the superior aspect of the submucosal tunnel through which the previously placed Robinson catheter is brought. This catheter now lies in the contemplated position of the ureter to be implanted (Fig. 33-5A). The end of the catheter is then secured extravesically to the end of the ureter with a 2-0 suture, and the ureter is pulled down and brought into position in the bladder by gentle interior traction on the catheter. This maneuver avoids any handling of the ureter, which is important because the ureter of the transplanted kidney receives its blood supply exclusively from the renal vessel branches that course in its adventitia.[6] In the male patient, it is important to pass the ureter below the spermatic cord. Intravesically, the ureter is divided transversely approximately 1 cm distal to its exit from the submucosal tunnel. The remaining distal intravesical portion of the ureter is spatulated anteriorly and then secured to the adjacent mucosa and muscularis of bladder with three interrupted sutures of 5-0 plain catgut that incorporate the corners of the spatulation and the distal midportion of the ureter (Fig. 33-5B). An additional 5-0 plain catgut suture approximates the proximal apex of the spatulation to the distal margin of the submucosal tunnel. The superior mucosal opening is then approximated with two or three interrupted sutures of 5-0 plain catgut. The ureter is not stented postoperatively.

Certain principles are important in successful transplant ureteroneocystostomy:

1. A "no touch" technique is essential so as not to produce vascular insufficiency (and subseqeuent ureteral necrosis and urinary extravasation) from injury to the adventitial anastomotic network of the ureter.

2. The submucosal tunnel and muscle hiatus must comfortably accommodate the ureter to avoid postoperative obstruction from edema, particularly because no stent is used.

3. An oblique upward course of the muscular hiatus must be ensured so that the course of the ureter is straight and unobstructed from the kidney to the superior aspect of the tunnel. Care must be taken to avoid making the muscle hiatus directly beneath, and at a right angle to, the superior end of the tunnel, because angulation of the ureter may result. This consideration is important because the ureter of a transplanted kidney takes a more direct upward course than the native ureter and crosses the iliac vessels in a much more caudal position because of the location of the transplanted kidney in the iliac fossa.

FIG. 33-5. Utereroneocystostomy. **(A)** A small Robinson catheter lies in the submucosal tunnel and bladder wall hiatus and is secured extravesically to the transplant ureter, which will be brought into proper position by gentle inferior traction on the catheter. **(B)** The completed transplant ureteroneocystostomy is demonstrated. Four interrupted sutures secure the spatulated ureteral orifice.

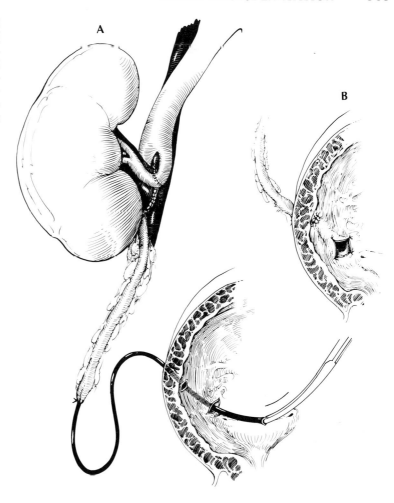

4. A little redundancy of the ureter is established above the bladder to ensure that the ureteroneocystostomy is done without tension.

5. Four sutures are usually sufficient to secure the ureter to the bladder and to avoid ischemia and subsequent necrosis of the distal ureter.

6. Patency of the ureteroneocystostomy is confirmed by gently passing a No. 8 soft Robinson catheter toward the renal pelvis.

Kidneys with a double ureter can also be successfully transplanted with strict adherence to these principles.[6,7] However, the double ureters cannot be used unless they have been dissected *en bloc* with their common adventitial sheath and periureteral fat so that the ureteral blood supply is protected. The technique of ureteroneocystostomy is essentially the same as with a single ureter, except that the ureters are brought through together side by side in a generous submucosal tunnel. The distal end of each ureter is spatulated, and the

adjacent margins are approximated with 5-0 plain catgut.

To ensure a watertight closure, the cystotomy incision is closed in three layers.[7] The first layer is with continuous 4-0 plain catgut for the mucosa, the second is with continuous 4-0 Vicryl or Dexon for the muscularis, and the third is with interrupted 4-0 Vicryl or Dexon that includes the adventitia and muscularis with minimal inversion. If the bladder wall is thick, 3-0 Vicryl or Dexon can be used. The second and third layers should overlap the immediately underlying layer about 0.5 cm at each end of the cystotomy closure to avoid urinary extravasation at these two points.

Wound Closure

The ureter of the transplanted kidney is not stented, and the Retzius space and iliac fossa are not drained. If good hemostasis has been obtained, and if the principles of implantation as outlined in

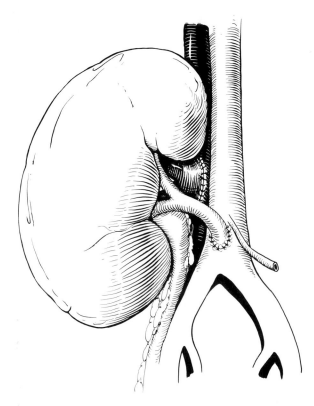

FIG. 33-6. Anatomic relationships of an adult-donor kidney in a small child are shown with renal vessel anastomoses to the inferior vena cava and aorta.

this chapter have been followed, there will be no need whatsoever for postoperative drainage other than a urethral catheter. The length of Foley catheter drainage is debatable. In our series, bladder decompression has been maintained for approximately 1 week, and this practice appears to account in part for our low incidence of urinary vesical extravasation, even in insulin-dependent juvenile diabetics with "sensory-loss" bladders.

Prior to wound closure, the wound is thoroughly irrigated with an antibiotic solution composed of 50,000 units of bacitracin and 1 g of neomycin in 150-ml saline, which is aspirated before the actual closure.[2] The wound is then closed using a No. 1 Vicryl or Dexon running suture to approximate transversus abdominis and internal oblique muscles in a single-layer closure; the adjacent fascia is included inferiorly at the tendinous insertion of the rectus muscle. Secure approximation of these muscle layers is important to prevent postoperative bleeding should hemodialysis with heparinization become necessary. Following this, the rectus fascia anteriorly and the fascia of the external oblique are approximated with interrupted 2-0 or 1-0 braided nylon suture (Surgilon or Nurolon). In obese patients, internal retention sutures through all muscle layers have also been used.

The subcutaneous tissue is thoroughly irrigated with a more concentrated antibiotic solution containing 50,000 units of bacitracin and 1 g of neomycin in 50-ml saline and is then approximated with interrupted satures of 4-0 Vicryl or Dexon. These sutures are placed approximately 2 cm apart and include both Scarpa's fascia and the underlying fascia superficially. In this manner, one can obliterate dead space in the subcutaneous area in which a seroma in an immunosuppressed patient might become secondarily infected. The skin is approximated with interrupted fine nylone sutures.

Pediatric Transplantation

In small children, the iliac fossa is not large enough to accommodate a kidney from an adult donor, which is the case with living-related transplantation and frequently the case with cadaver transplantation. In addition, the pelvic vessels in a small child are so small that the disparity in size between the donor renal vessels and the recipient vessels negates the technique described for adults. In these small children, graft implantation must use the recipient aorta and vena cava, which is best accomplished through a midline abdominal incision that provides ready access to the great vessels as well as the urinary bladder. After the lateral posterior parietal peritoneum is incised, the right colon is reflected medially and the right kidney is usually removed. The vena cava is then freed from the level of the right renal vein inferiorly to its bifurcation. Posterior lumbar veins are doubly ligated with 5-0 silk and divided. Mobilization of the vena cava is important to facilitate the end-to-side anastomosis of the renal vein, which is performed with running 6-0 cardiovascular suture, as described for the adult (Fig. 33-6). Performing the venous anastomosis superiorly allows room for an end-to-side anastomosis of the renal artery to the inferior abdominal aorta, which is facilitated by the previous superior mobilization of the vena cava. Aortic mobilization should be limited to its distal portion, from the level of the inferior mesenteric artery inferiorly and including both common iliac arteries. The segment of the aorta to be used for the end-to-side renal artery anastomosis can be isolated by a superior pediatric vascular clamp and by two inferior clamps on the common iliac arteries. The end-to-side anastomosis is performed with interrupted 6-0 cardiovascular sutures.

Important to the revascularization of an adult kidney in these small children is the realization that vascular clamp release will result in immediate renal consumption of several hundred milliliters of their effective blood volume. We prefer to initiate blood transfusion prior to beginning the vascular anastomoses so as to avoid hypotension after release of the vascular clamps. When the vascular anastomoses are completed, the superior aortic clamp must be kept loosely in place until it is ensured that hypotension is not a problem. Immediately after establishing circulation in the graft, the anesthesiologist must obtain blood pressures at 30-second or 1-minute intervals until stabilization is ensured.

The ureteral implantation is carried out as previously described except that the ureter must be passed retroperiotoneally behind the intact inferior peritoneum. Following ureteral implantation, the graft and superior ureter are reperitonealized by developing and freeing up the lateral peritoneal margin. The lateral peritoneal margin is then approximated to the medial peritoneal margin adjacent to the mobilized colon with a running suture, thus ensuring a retroperitoneal position for the kidney and ureter. The midline abdominal incision can be closed according to the operator's preference.

REFERENCES

1. BELZER FO, KOUNTZ SL, PERKINS HA: Red cell cold autoagglutinins as a cause of failure of renal allotransplantation. Transplantation 11:422, 1971
2. BELZER FO, SALVATIERRA O, SCHWEIZER RT et al: Prevention of wound infections by topical antibiotics in high risk patients. Am J Surg 126:180, 1973
3. BELZER FO, SCHWEIZER RT, KOUNTZ SL: Management of multiple vessels in renal transplantation. Transplant Proc 4:639, 1972
4. SALVATIERRA O, AMEND W, VINCENTI F et al: 1500 renal transplants at one center: The evolution of a strategy for optimum success. Am J Surg 142:14, 1981
5. SALVATIERRA O, BELZER FO: Pediatric cadaver kidneys: Their use in renal transplantation. Arch Surg 110:181, 1975
6. SALVATIERRA O, KOUNTZ SL, BELZER FO: Prevention of ureteral fistula after renal transplantation. J Urol 112:445, 1974
7. SALVATIERRA O, OLCOTT C, AMEND WJ et al: Urological complications of renal transplantation can be prevented or controlled. J Urol 117:421, 1977

Transplantation Biology

34

Hilliard F. Siegler

For centuries people have been inspired by the possibility of transplanting tissues and organs of the body from one person to another. Legends of these feats have been expounded in Chinese, Indian, Greek, and Roman documents. Most of the early accounts involved reconstruction of the nose or ears that had been removed in combat or as punishment. Hindu surgeons described their techniques in the Susruta Sanhita, written in approximately 700 B.C.[7] In the 16th century, Tagliacozzi reported his technique of nasal reconstruction using a forearm flap.[3] Also in the 16th century, Pare reported on the transplantation of teeth,[11] and 200 years later attempts at this practice were reported by Hunter.[4] In 1804, Baronio first reported successful free skin graft transplantation. Sixty years later Bert documented that skin exchange from one individual to another was not successful, but that skin transplanted from one part of the body to another on the same individual was successful. His most significant observations went almost completely unnoticed until the middle of the 20th century.

Modern transplantation immunology requires an understanding of certain basic terminology. There are four possible genetic relationships between the donor of the graft and the recipient: *autograft*, which is transplantation between different areas of the same individual; *isograft*, which is transplantation between a donor and a recipient of the same species that are genetically identical (transplantation between monozygotic twins); *allograft*, which is transplantation between a donor and a recipient of the same species that are genetically dissimilar; and *xenograft*, which is transplantation between a donor and a recipient of different species. The immunologic reaction against a transplant is directed against a multiplicity of protein and glycoprotein molecules of varying structure and function that are present on the cell membrane. These molecules are accepted as cells by the lymphoid system of the original host, but many of them function as highly potent antigens when transferred or transplanted to another individual. Cell surface molecules that are recognized in this way are defined as transplantation or histocompatibility antigens. They present the major barrier to the successful transplantation of tissue and organs.

Early reports by Jensen and Little indicated the influence of genetic factors of the host when foreign tissues were transplanted.[3,11] The importance of blood group antigens in tissue transplantation was discussed in numerous treatises by Lansteiner during the first half of this century. Accelerated rejection in a previously sensitized host was early recognized and reported by Jensen.[3] Medawar's classic description in the mid-1940s concerning skin graft rejection is known to all students in transplantation biology and has served as a cornerstone for the mechanisms of graft rejection as we understand it today.

Major Histocompatibility Complex

Gorer, Lyman, and Snell described the H-2 locus in the mouse in 1948.[11] Analogous to H-2, the major histocompatibility complex (MHC) in the mouse, are the less familiar and considerably more complex antigens of the MHC in humans, which has been termed *HLA*. Numerous similarities between the mouse H-2 system and the human HLA system are evident. Each system occupies a considerable segment of chromosome (a haplotype), and each includes a number of genetic loci of varying functions, all of which appear to have some relevance to the functioning of the immune system. The HLA system is now known to include five histocompatibility loci—HLA-A, HLA-B, HLA-C, HLA-D and HLA-Dr—and there are at least 100 separate antigens controlled by those loci. Other components known to be within the HLA region or closely linked to it include genes for complement proteins, genes determining disease susceptibility, structural genes for red cell enzymes and antigens, regulatory genes, and genes for various types of receptor or binding protein. Antigens determined by the MHC in humans are implicated in both thymus and bone marrow cell-specific differentiation, as are linked genes that govern our ability to mount a humoral or cell-mediated immune response against bacteria, viruses, or transplanted allogeneic tissues.

HLA has been localized to the sixth chromosome using hybridization techniques and family studies. There are now 20 recognized antigens at the HLA-A locus, 33 at HLA-B, 6 at HLA-C, 11 at HLA-D, and 7 at HLA-Dr. If the two C6 chromosomes of the father are designated as AB and the two of the mother CD, there are four possible combinations in the offspring—AC, AD, BC, and BD—because each child inherits one paternal and one maternal chromosome. The HLA chromosomal complex, including HLA-A, HLA-B, HLA-C, HLA-D, and HLA-Dr antigens, is termed a *haplotype*. Recombination, the crossing over between homologous chromosomes during mioses, occurs among all HLA loci. HLA recombination occurs with a frequency of just less than 1%. The HLA-A and HLA-B antigens are glycoproteins expressed on the plasma membrane of most nucleated cells. HLA-C antigens have been less well studied but are now thought to be very similar to the A and B molecules.

HLA antibodies usually require prior sensitization of the host by mechanisms including skin grafting, blood transfusion, experimental immunization, organ transplantation, and most frequently pregnancy. The sera used for HLA typing are most commonly from highly selected multiparous women, transplant recipients, or experimentally immunized subjects. These antibodies also are responsbile for the necessity of doing crossmatches prior to performing tissue transplants between human subjects.

When lymphocytes from two HLA-distinct individuals are cultured together, a number of mononuclear cells are stimulated to undergo blast transformation and proliferation. This proliferation is quantitated by incorporation of tritiated thymidine. The genes responsible for this cellular stimulation comprise the HLA-D locus. The HLA-D locus has been mapped on the chromosome close to HLA-B. At present there are 11 detectable HLA-D antigens definable only by a mixed lymphocyte reaction. Until recently HLA-D typing could be accomplished only in families, because mixtures of cells from unrelated individuals almost invariably gave strong stimulation. This observation gave strength to the theory that a large number of alleles for HLA-D were present and codominantly expressed. Therefore, no definition of individual alleles in a heterogeneous population was possible. More recently, however, it has been noted that some

individuals in a more homogeneous population fail to stimulate in a mixed lymphocyte reaction, especially if they are phenotypically identical for the HLA-A and HLA-B alleles. This observation led to the realization that lymphocytes from HLA-D homozygotes could provide reference standards that have been termed *HLA-D homozygous typing cells*. Such homozygotes have provided cells for typing other family members, members of different families, and even unrelated panels. Most of the homozygous typing cells are selected by screening the mixed lymphocyte reaction capacity of individuals homozygous for HLA-B.

The HLA-D antigens are, by definition, expressed on cells which will stimulate in a mixed lymphocyte culture. These include B lymphocytes, epidermal cells, monocytes and macrophages, endothelial cells, and spermatozoa. Very similar antigens present on the B lymphocyte have been classed as D-related or Dr. These antigens have a distribution distinct from but similar to HLA-D. A basic cytotoxicity assay is used for Dr typing. Because B cells represent only 10% to 20% of the total peripheral blood mononuclear cells, the remaining monocytes and T cells are separated in order to allow B-cell typing. B-cell-specific antisera have been raised both through planned immunizations and using hybridoma technology. The Dr molecules are expressed on B lymphocytes, macrophages, epidermal cells, endothelial cells, and sperm. The correspondence between Dr and D is close, so in the great majority of individuals, D and Dr alleles coincide. To date, seven Dr antigens have been defined.

The results of consanguineous organ transplants have clearly shown that HLA is a major factor to be taken into account in such transplants.[9] HLA is a polymorphic system and two unrelated individuals are rarely exactly alike. However, the situation is simplified within a family group. As was previously stated, the entire HLA complex is inherited as a gametic unit. If the paternal haplotypes are represented by the symbols A and B and the maternal haplotypes by C and D, then the children must inherit either A or B from the father and either C or D from the mother. The only possible HLA genotypes of the children are AC, AD, BC, or BD. If there are five children, two of them must inherit the same pair of haplotypes, for example, AC. This sibling pair is referred to as HLA identical. If one haplotype is shared and one is distinct, such family pairs are referred as *HLA haploidentical*. These sib–sib pairs and parent–sib pairs experience more severe graft rejection than HLA-identical sibling pairs but foster a more favorable course than unrelated subjects. Some sib pairs differ at both haplotypes and are referred to as *HLA-non-identical* combinations. A representative family pedigree is shown in Figure 34-1.

Experimental and clinical evidence suggests that HLA-A, HLA-B, and HLA-C antigens probably can serve as targets for host cell-mediated immunity. The molecules coded for by the HMC do not, however, serve as simple antigens in the way that A and B blood group antigens do, but consist as antigenic mosaics on the cell surface which are recognized as foreign or as self by complementary molecular groupings on other cells. No single component of the HMC has been shown to be solely responsible for the rejection phenomenon. There is no simple relationship between MHC responses and response to a transplant, nor has any single HLA antigen been shown to be uniquely associated with accelerated rejection of kidney transplants.

Cellular Immune Functions

Human thymic-dependent lymphocytes have been divided into separate subpopulations by the presence of cells bearing Fc receptors for the immunoglobulin classes, IgG, IgM, IgA, and IgE. Using monoclonal antibodies, cell surface determinants have been characterized for human T cells in the peripheral blood population. Between 50% and 75% of humoral peripheral blood mononuclear cells are identifiable thymic-dependent cells. Between 5% and 15% of human T cells bear Fc receptors for IgG and are referred to as T_γ cells. Functional analysis of this T-cell subpopulation has demonstrated that this subset is able to suppress poke-weed mitogen-induced B-cell differentiation and immunoglobulin synthesis. In addition to immunoregulation of B-cell differentiation, this subpopulation of T cells appears to mediate certain natural-killer cell functions and antibody-dependent cellular cytotoxicity. Natural killing activity is

a well-recognized phenomenon in which lymphoid cells have cytotoxic activity in the absence of apparent antigenic stimulation. The significance of such natural killing as a mechanism for immunosurveillance has promoted considerable interest.

T-cell subpopulations bearing Fc receptors for IgM are referred to as T_μ cells and have been shown to function as helper cells for promoting cell-mediated cytotoxic reactions. The production of humoral antibodies is carried out by bone-marrow-dependent lymphocytes referred to as B cells. Undoubtedly, hybridoma technology permitting production of a vast array of monoclonal antibodies will lead to the discovery of an ever-growing number of lymphocyte cell surface markers. An increasing discrimination of subsets of lymphocytes will result from these investigations. A correlation of these cell surface markers with cellular activity will undoubtedly lead to an increasingly complex picture.

An important and as yet unresolved question involves the nature of the cell surface structures that enables T cells to recognize antigens. B lymphocytes have been shown to bind antigen by means of cell surface immunoglobulins, and the interaction of cell surface immunoglobulin and antigen may lead to their activation and to clonal expansion. The continuing lack of definition of the T-cell receptor is of central importance not only for transplantation biologists but also for immunologists in general. The fact that many of the immune response genes are linked to the genes that determine major histocompatibility antigens provides evidence that the discrimination of "self" from "non-self" may depend on the presence of histocompatibility antigens. Cell-mediated cytotoxic responses, either to cells infected with viruses or to cells modified with chemical reagents, are directed toward both the foreign and the self-antigens; this finding indicates that thymic-dependent lymphocytes react preferentially with foreign antigens that are presented in association with self-antigens. The

FIG. 34-1. Representative family pedigree

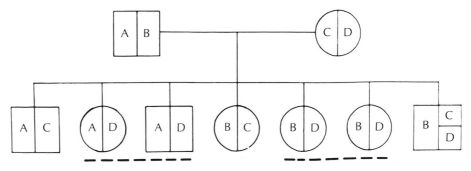

real biologic foundation of the major histocompatibility antigens, therefore, may not be their role as a barrier for tissue transplantation. The major histocompatibility antigens may have evolved as a mechanism for ensuring that the T-cell system will be triggered into response only by modified self-antigens.

Suppression of the Immune Response

Clinical organ transplantation in the past 25 years has stimulated most of the important discoveries in immunosuppression that have benefited other subspecialties of immunopathology. The first clinical application of irradiation was carried out in the late 1950s in renal transplantation when the first kidney transplants were performed in Boston.[6] Almost simultaneously the immunosuppressive effect of 6-mercaptopurine on the production of antibodies against bovine serum albumin was described.[8] The knowledge of the effect of this pharmacologic agent on renal allograft survival was quickly demonstrated by clinical application. At the present time the immunosuppressive regimen received by renal transplant recipients includes azathioprine, steroids, antilymphocyte globulin, and external irradiation.

Azathioprine is a purine analog and as such most probably interferes with nucleic acid synthesis. It is felt that this agent has a T-cell preference and acts by interfering with antigen recognition by T cells. Steroids continue to be the most efficient therapy for acute rejection crises. Steroids interfere with protein and thus with antibody synthesis. They have a definite interfering effect on macrophages and T-cell subsets. The exact mode of action of antilymphocyte globulin continues to escape definition. Recent randomized clinical trials have, however, documented that antilymphocyte serum can indeed, for the most part, abate the early acute rejection phenomenon. Additional data suggest that antilymphocyte globulin might also reverse late rejection that has been unresponsive to azathioprine and steroid therapy.

There is a continuing observation that blood transfusion prior to renal transplantation is associated with an improved allograft survival rate. The exact mechanisms of this observation remain to be explained. In experimental animal model systems, recipients that received donor-specific blood transfusions were observed to have a specific state of unresponsiveness. Thymocytes, spleen cells, peripheral blood lymphocytes, and lymph node cells from blood-conditioned recipients were

adoptively transferred to irradiated hosts, and it was found that suppressor cells were present in the spleen and thymus of unresponsive recipients but not in the peripheral blood or lymph nodes. Adoptive transfer of such spleen cells led to permanent survival of allografts in approximately 50% of the cases, whereas transfer of a similar number of thymocytes always resulted in permanent graft survival. Fractionation of suppressor spleen cells into T and B enriched populations and macrophages revealed that the suppressor was mediated by T cells. Renal allograft survival rates in first cadaveric renal transplants in humans are improved if recipients are prospectively transfused prior to transplantation.[5] There does not seem to be a statistically significant difference between graft survival rates in patients who receive more than 6 units of blood and those receiving less than 6 units. Graft survival in the preoperative transfused patients seems to be intermediate between the never-transfused and the prior-transfused patients. Patients receiving a living-related transplant also seem to experience improved survival with pretransplant blood transfusion. Such observations seem to be confined to the HLA-haplotype-disparate renal recipients, and no such effect has been observed on the survival of HLA-identical transplants.

Chronic thoracic duct drainage has also been reported to improve renal engraftment. Patients treated by at least 1 month of thoracic duct drainage before cadaveric renal transplant are reported to require only half the dosage of steroids and suffer only half the instance of acute rejection as do patients not receiving chronic thoracic duct drainage. Graft survival in the thoracic duct drainage patients is reported to be double that of the non-thoracic duct drainage patients at all time intervals.

The use of irradiation as an immunosuppressive regimen was of questionable efficiency until recent investigations into total lymphoid irradiation or total body irradiation and autologous marrow recovery. Lethal total body irradiation and organ transplantation, followed 2 days later by hematopoietic reconstitution of the host with autologous cryopreserved marrow, have resulted in permanent engraftment of 70% of the animals studied.[1] The same regimen, with methotrexate added on posttransplant days 1, 3, and 6 and with no further immunosuppression, has also been associated with marked prolongation of allograft survival when nonidentical dogs were treated. Fractionated total lymphoid irradiation and allogeneic bone marrow injection have been reported to produce stable chimerism without graft-*versus*-host disease in both rodents and mongrel dogs. In these experimental models, transplantation tolerance for skin, heart, and renal allografts has been reported.[10] Early results in humans have been encouraging, and this particular immunosuppressive regimen will continue to undergo intensive study.

Cyclosporin A is a new antilymphocytic drug with potent immunosuppressive properties. This drug was developed as part of an investigation of fungal products with antifungal activity. Cyclosporin A has been reported to be effective in inhibiting cell-mediated cytolysis using spleen cells sensitized with allogeneic tumor cells. Borel has shown that cyclosporin A prolongs survival of skin grafts between different strains of mice and has extended these studies in multiple species with various experimental models demonstrating successful engraftment across major histocompatibility barriers.[2]

The biologic activity of cyclosporin A is to a degree selective against lymphocytes. Hematopoietic cells in animals treated *in vivo* remain relatively normal in animals receiving this immunosuppressive agent. The mode of action appears to be mainly on T-lymphocytes. The ability of the drug to inhibit antibody formation seems to be confined to T-dependent antigens. Experiments performed *in vitro* with both human and nonhuman primate peripheral blood lymphocytes have been conducted in an effort to study the effect of cyclosporin A on suppressor cell activity. The agent did not affect the generation or function of concanavilin A-induced suppressor lymphocytes as measured by their ability to suppress thymidine uptake of lymphocytes in secondary cultures. No evidence of suppressor-cell induction was noted by incubation of lymphocytes with only cyclosporin A. These data suggest that cyclosporin A does not generate or induce suppressor-cell lymphocytes, nor does it spare them. The immunosuppressive mechanism of this unique compound may result from inhibition or killing of T-helper subpopulations and some sparing of T-suppressor-cell fractions, resulting in an imbalance of immunoregulation that culminates in profound suppression.

In an *in vivo* rodent renal allograft model, large doses of cyclosporin A administered from day 4 after transplantation did not prolong graft survival, suggesting that this agent has no effect on an established rejection response. Histologic study of allograft biopsies in animals receiving cyclosporin A prior to and following renal transplantation demonstrated very little rejection activity even when this agent was used as the sole immunosuppressive regimen. Early clinical trials have revealed rather significant side-effects of cyclosporin A that seem to be dose related, including a high incidence of infection and lymphoma occurrence. At this point in time one would have to say that cyclosporin A is a powerful immunosuppressive agent that has the attractive feature of being steroid sparing. It is also relatively nontoxic to the bone marrow. Most patients have been grateful for the lack of steroid side-effects. Cyclosporin A is a move in the direction of selective activity against subpopulations of lymphocytes. Serious side-effects of the agent, however, make continued investigation necessary.

Transplantation and Malignancy

The tumor immunologist has been the beneficiary of important concepts and observations resulting from organ transplantation. Tumor transplantation in animals has been an important area of cancer research. Early observations indicated that most tumor transplants failed because of histocompatibility differences between the tumor donor and the recipient. In order to transplant tumors across histocompatibility barriers, it became obvious that impairment of the immune response using immunosuppressive agents was necessary. Tumors will survive, grow, and spread provided the animal is kept sufficiently immunosuppressed; if the immunosuppressive therapy is discontinued, the immune system may recover and destroy the tumor. Immunologically impaired animals such as the athymic nude mouse will grow human tumor xenografts without difficulty. Transplantation of malignancies into immunologically normal humans is extremely rare. In organ transplantation, immunosuppressive therapy may, however, permit the survival of cancer cells inadvertently transplanted with a renal allograft procured from a donor with a malignancy. These cells may remain locally invasive or may disseminate widely. Approximately 40% of renal allograft recipients that received kidneys from donors with documented noncentral nervous system malignancies subsequently developed tumors compatible with donor origin. Most of the renal allograft recipients died secondary to the neoplasia; however, with cessation of immunosuppressive therapy and removal of the transplant there have been cases in which the immune system has recovered and rejected the tumor transplants.

The overall incidence of spontaneous malignancy in the chronically immunosuppressed renal allograft recipients is approximately 6%. The types of malignancy commonly seen in the general population show very little, if any, increase. Certain types of neoplasms are seen with increased frequency in organ transplant recipients. Non-Hodgkin's lymphomas are increased 50- to 100-fold over the incidence seen in the general population. Skin cancer is increased fourfold to sevenfold in areas of low sun exposure, but is increased almost 20-fold in areas of high sun exposure. *In situ* carcinoma of the cervix or the uterus is increased 14-fold.

It is not yet clear to what the cause of the malignancies seen in the transplant recipient is secondary. It has been proposed that it results from the depression of immunity, but other investigators would point out that there is a known oncogenic effect of the immunosuppressive agents used to prevent rejection. Other explanations include activation of oncogenic viruses, genetic predisposition or resistence to malignancy, and stimulation of cellular proliferation. The investigative paths of the tumor immunologists and the transplant immunologists are thus densely interwoven. Understanding the etiology of malignancy, the nature of the host's defense against the neoplasia, and the tumor–host relationship, and finding the immunologic means of prevention or treatment of malignancy represent the common scientific goals of the transplantation and tumor immunobiologists.

REFERENCES

1. BLUMENSTOCK DA, CANNON FD, HALES CA et al: Pulmonary function of DLA-nonidentical lung allografts in dogs treated with lethal total-body irradiation, autologous bone marrow transplantation and methotrexate. Transplantation 28:223, 1979

2. BOREL JF: Comparative study of in vitro and in vivo drug effects on cell-mediated cytotoxicity. Immunology 31:631, 1976

3. CALNE RY: Renal Transplantation. London, Edward Arnold & Co, 1967

4. CONVERSE JM, CASSON PR: The historical background of transplantation. In Rappaport FT Dausset J (eds): Human Transplantation, pp 3–11. New York, Grune & Straton, 1968

5. CORREY RJ, WEST JL, HUNSICKER BA et al: Effect of timing of administration and quality of blood transfusion on cadaver renal transplant survival. Transplantation 30:425, 1980

6. MERRILL JP, MURRAY JE, HARRISON JH et al: Successful homotransplantation of the kidney between nonidentical twins. N Engl Med 262:1251, 1960

7. PEER LA: Transplantation of Tissues. Baltimore, Williams & Wilkins, 1955

8. SCHWARTZ RS, DAMESHEK W: Drug-induced immunological tolerance. Nature (London) 183:1682, 1959

9. SEIGLER HF, GUNNELLS JC, ROBINSON RR et al: Renal transplantation between HLA identical donor-recipient pairs. J Clin Invest 51:3200, 1972

10. SLAVIN S, GOTTLIEB M, STROBER: Transplantation of bone marrow in outbred dogs without graft versus host disease using total lymphoid irradiation. Transplantation 27:139, 1979

11. WOODRUFF MFA: Transplantation of Tissues and Organs. Springfield, Charles C Thomas, 1960

Surgical Complications of Renal Transplantation

35

Lynn H.W. Banowsky

During the first decade of clinical renal transplantation, surgical complications were a significant contributor to postoperative morbidity and mortality. Surgical complications were common (25%) and the associated mortality (33%) was high.[11] The most frequent and devastating problems were urinary fistulas and wound infections. It has been estimated that 10% of renal allografts were lost as a direct result of technical errors. Although the early transplant surgeons were skilled and resourceful, it soon became apparent that transplantation surgery was different. The renal transplant recipient represented an especially fragile operative candidate in that the surgeon's oldest and most formidable ally, the patient's immune system, had been altered both by the disease process itself and by postoperative immunosuppression. Wounds healed grudgingly and the patient was extremely vulnerable to local and systemic infections.

At the present time, serious postoperative complications are uncommon in the renal transplant recipient.[5] Patient mortality or allograft loss directly related to a technical error are even more uncommon. In the last 151 consecutive renal transplants at the University of Texas Health Science Center (UTHSC) at San Antonio, only one patient has lost an allograft as the direct result of a surgical error (0.06%).

The most effective management of any surgical complication is prevention. Preventing surgical complications in renal transplant recipients depends on both a technically sound recipient operation and an appreciation of the importance of the donor nephrectomy. Regardless of the care exercised during the recipient operation, surgical errors during the donor nephrectomy may preordain the development of vascular, ureteral, or infectious complications. Although the recipient operation is not technically difficult, the surgeon must have sufficient mental discipline to avoid shortcuts and to recognize that all parts of the operation—the preparation of the allograft bed, vascular and ureteral anastomosis, and wound closure—are of equal importance. The operation must be constructed to withstand the rigors of postoperative immunosuppression. Even minor technical imperfections allowed by the surgeon may result in a serious penalty to the patient.

Postoperative Anuria or Oliguria

Anuria and oliguria are common problems in the immediate posttransplant period. The differential diagnosis is a lengthy one and includes problems that may be trivial (e.g., blockage of the urethral catheter) or catastrophic (e.g., hyperacute rejection). Technical causes include obstruction of the urethral catheter, ureteral obstruction, urinary fistula, hemorrhage, and arterial thrombosis. Nontechnical causes include hyperacute rejection, hypovolemia, and acute renal failure (ARF) secondary to ischemic injury. Attention here will be focused on a general plan of evaluation (Fig. 35-1) and on the nontechnical problems of hyperacute rejection, hypovolemia, and acute renal failure.

HYPERACUTE REJECTION

Hyperacute rejection occurs in 4% to 6% of renal transplant recipients who have preformed cytotoxic antibodies specific for the donor's HLA histocompatibility antigens.[16] Sensitization of the recipient is accomplished by blood transfusion,[46] pregnancy, or previous transplantation.[45] The most prominent pathologic finding is extensive renal intravascular coagulation. The incidence has probably decreased as crossmatching techniques have become more sensitive and more centers are using the antiglobulin crossmatch.

The phenomenon of hyperacute rejection is classically noted as a kidney with poor turgor and a darkly mottled surface. The renal vein is poorly filled and urinary output is absent. Initially the allograft may produce small amounts of bloody urine prior to the onset of complete anuria. A febrile response is common and hyperkalemia is frequently present. Evaluation of coagulation stud-

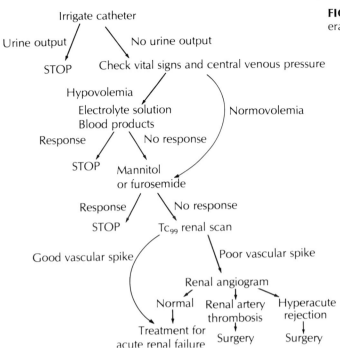

FIG. 35-1. Evaluation and management of early postoperative anuria or oliguria

ies may reveal a drop in the patient's platelet count and an elevation in fibrin split products.

Hyperacute rejection should be considered whenever the renal transplant recipient is anuric in the immediate postoperative period. A presumptive diagnosis can be made with a ^{99}Tc renal flow scan. The renal scan will show no or very poor perfusion. A renal angiogram will distinguish hyperacute rejection from renal artery thrombosis. In hyperacute rejection, the renal angiogram characteristically shows prolonged clearance time of the contrast media, absent filling of cortical vessels, and thrombi in small and medium arterial branches (Fig. 35-2). If the diagnosis of hyperacute rejection is suspected during the operation, the renal allograft should be biopsied before closure of the wound, and, if confirmed, transplant nephrectomy is the only effective treatment. Failure to immediately remove the renal allograft merely prolongs the patient's exposure to immunosuppressive drugs.

HYPOVOLEMIA

The diagnosis of hypovolemia is the same in all surgical patients; the transplant recipient does not represent an exception. Measurements of central venous pressure, blood pressure, pulse rate, and urine output are correlated with the patient's clinical condition to establish the diagnosis. Careful records of blood loss and fluid replacement should

be included in the written operative note for future reference.

Postoperative hypovolemia should be promptly treated with adequate amounts of colloids or electrolyte solutions. The exact amount and type of fluid will vary with the cause of hypovolemia and the condition of the patient. It is preferable to replace the deficit rapidly with a bolus of fluid over 30 to 45 minutes. The object should be to return the patient to a normovolemic state using central venous pressure, blood pressure, pulse, and urine output to indicate the desired end point. In patients who have significant cardiac disease, consideration should be given to the preoperative placement of a Swan–Ganz catheter so that pulmonary wedge pressure can be measured during the intra- and postoperative period. If the patient is carefully watched, rapid fluid replacement rarely causes fluid overload.

When the blood volume has been restored and the patient remains anuric or oliguric, diuretics should be given in adequate doses. Uncomplicated hypovolemia will respond with a brisk diuresis.

ACUTE RENAL FAILURE

ARF is caused by ischemic injury to the allograft. The injury may occur during the donor's agonal period, donor nephrectomy, organ preservation, or recipient operation. Far from being an all-or-none phenomenon, ARF represents a spectrum of ischemic injury. Acute renal failure occurs clinically in two forms, oliguric and nonoliguric.[37] In many instances oliguric ARF can be converted to nonoliguric ARF by the prompt replacement of any fluid deficit and the aggressive use of diuretics. Conversion of oliguric to nonoliguric ARF significantly decreases the need for postoperative hemodialysis and the frequency of complications commonly associated with ARF. In addition, the presence of urinary output facilitates the postoperative diagnosis of rejection.

The diagnosis of ARF can be made safely only after the exclusion of all other possibilities. A renal flow scan with ^{99}Tc is usually sufficient to exclude serious problems such as renal artery thrombosis or hyperacute rejection. Should the clinical picture suggest the possibility of a technical problem with the urinary tract (urinary fistula or ureteral obstruction), the integrity of the ureter and bladder must be promptly determined by ultrasonography, cystography, retrograde pyelography and other studies.

When diuresis is not forthcoming after revascularization of the allograft, treatment of possible ARF should begin in the operating room. The emphasis in treatment should be directed at converting oliguric ARF to nonoliguric ARF. Hypovolemia should be corrected. When this alone is inadequate to promote diuresis, 12.5 g of mannitol and 40 mg of furosemide are given intravenously. If the patient is still oliguric, furosemide is repeated, doubling the previous dose, until a dose of 160 mg to 320 mg has been reached. A maximum of 15 mg/kg of furosemide can be given, but one must be aware of the side effects of ototoxicity and gastrointestinal ulceration. Furosemide not only is a safe, potent diuretic, but also seems capable of shortening the period of severe oliguria.

Vascular Complications

Hemorrhage

Postoperative hemorrhage is most often due to inadequate hemostasis by the surgeon and only occasionally by the faulty coagulation mechanisms in the recipient. Hemorrhage may occur from the vascular anastomosis, the retroperitoneal space, or the renal allograft. Coagulation defects are most often due to poor-quality platelets (uremia),[37] inadequate numbers of platelets (azathioprine or antilymphocyte globulin), or disseminated intravascular coagulation (rejection or sepsis).[42] The

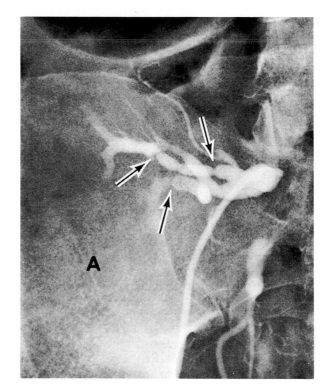

FIG. 35-2. Renal angiogram in a patient with hyperacute rejection shows thrombi in small and medium arteries *(arrows)* and absent filling of cortical vessels **(A).**

presence of these coagulation defects can be determined by preoperatively determining the patient's platelet count, prothrombin time, and partial thromboplastin time.

Although postoperative hemorrhage is usually not life threatening, it does represent a serious postoperative complication. Episodes of hypotension associated with the bleeding may contribute to postoperative ARF. The most serious sequelae of postoperative hemorrhage, however, is wound infection. Early series, reported wound infections being associated with 25% of patients who had postoperative hemorrhage.[4]

The qualitative platelet defect associated with uremia can be corrected by frequent hemodialysis. All end-stage renal disease patients should be hemodialyzed for 2 consecutive days before any elective surgery.

In order to prevent postoperative hemorrhage from inadequate hemostasis, the surgeon must be meticulous in the preparation of the allograft bed and carefully inspect all areas of the wound prior to closure. Regardless of size all bleeding points must be controlled with either electrocautery or ligatures. Bleeding at the vascular suture lines should be stopped by carefully placed interrupted sutures of 6-0 vascular silk or polyethylene. The temptation to assume that troublesome oozing will stop with time should be resisted.

To avoid serious bleeding from the donor organ, its integrity should be determined before and after revascularization. When cadaveric organs are used, defects can be identified during the period of organ preservation. The most common injury to the donor organ is a laceration of the main renal vein or its branches.[15] Venous injuries can be recognized by temporarily occluding the vein during pulsatile perfusion or flushing. Any injury can be repaired easily at this time.

Once the patient has been stabilized and a coagulopathy has been excluded, the patient's wound should be explored immediately. At the time of reoperation the allograft bed, the vascular suture lines, and the allograft itself are carefully inspected for bleeding points. Frequently the bleeding will have stopped spontaneously and the origin of the bleeding cannot be determined. Regardless of the etiology of the bleeding, evacuation of the hematoma to avoid subsequent wound infection is mandatory. The operative site should be copiously irrigated with 2 liters to 3 liters of normal saline and an antibiotic solution. Several reports have shown a significant reduction in wound infections when the wound is closed without drainage.[4,5] If hemostasis has been adequate, drains are superfluous and only provide a portal of entry for bacteria.

ARTERIAL INFECTION

The arterial system has a formidable resistance to infection. Although this resistance is somewhat diminished by the administration of corticosteroids and azathioprine, arterial infection only occurs in the presence of gross bacterial contamination that is present for an extended period of time. The response to the infection may be leakage, arterial wall dissolution, or the formation of a mycotic aneurysm. Although this problem occurs infrequently (1.6%), it does represent a common cause of major postoperative hemorrhage from the transplant wound.[29,32]

Arterial infection occurs primarily in postoperative patients who have a deep bacterial wound infection that has been diagnosed late or inadequately drained. Owens and associates reported that a period of 2 to 5 weeks was usually necessary before the infection became clinically apparent.[29] The most common clinical presentation is a small amount of bleeding from the wound followed in several days by major hemorrhage. This clinical picture represents dissolution of the arterial wall from infection. Less commonly a mycotic aneurysm may be formed. Arterial infection can be prevented by the early diagnosis and prompt treatment of deep wound infections. Surgical drainage should be extensive, and the entire wound should be left open to heal by secondary intention. At the time of incision and drainage, any sign of arterial or venous infection is sufficient indication for transplant nephrectomy.

Once arterial wall infection is established, vascular repair is not feasible. Attempts at repair may actually lead to massive secondary hemorrhage and the demise of the patient. The involved vascular wall will be extremely friable, and ligation of the vessel is usually the only safe surgical option. In order to create the greatest margin of safety, one should ligate the involved vessel a sufficient distance from the site of infection so that the ligature is around normal arterial wall. The stump of the vessel should be oversewn with a double layer of 5-0 vascular suture.

Patients tolerate ligation of the major pelvic arteries surprisingly well. Ligation of the hypogastric artery creates no disability. Ligation of the common or external iliac artery also creates few clinical problems. The vast majority of patients will have no significant ischemic signs or symptoms of the involved extremity. Low-dose heparin may be helpful postoperatively. Should any signs of ipsilateral lower extremity ischemia develop, this can be corrected surgically by a femorofemoral or axillofemoral bypass graft. All patients should be treated for 6 weeks with the appropriate parenteral antibiotic.

RENAL ARTERY THROMBOSIS

The vascular complications of thrombosis or stenosis are only rarely related to an immunologic phenomenon, immunosuppressive drugs, or recurrence of the patient's primary renal disease. When these complications occur, it should be assumed that they are due to an ill-conceived or poorly performed operation.

Thrombosis or stenosis of the renal vessels are both due to the same types of surgical errors and differ only in a matter of degree. The worst mistakes result in thrombosis, while more minor imperfections result in late postoperative stenosis. Breaches in technique that are most commonly made are poor alignment of the intima, intimal injury, disparity in vessel size, and excessive of deficient length of the two vessels being joined. Less commonly, thrombosis or stenosis may occur from perfusion or cannulation injury to the renal artery, excessive periadventitial stripping, intravenous administration of antilymphocyte globulin, and severe rejection reactions.[5]

Failure to accurately realign the vascular endothelium causes both a rough surface at the suture line and uncovered areas of subendothelial collagen.[2] Laminar flow is converted to turbulent flow by the rough surfaces, and platelets and fibrin adhere to the denuded areas of collagen. It is my opinion that arterial vascular endothelium can be best aligned by an interrupted anastomosis with double-armed needles. This type of anastomosis is not only less constricting, but also offers the advantages of starting all sutures from within the vessel's lumen and placing all sutures under direct vision.[3]

When constructing an end-to-end arterial anastomosis, the vessels are frequently of unequal size. A disparity in size of up to 50% can usually be compensated for without difficulty. A discrepancy of greater than 50% causes the smaller vessel to be crimped and creates a very uneven endothelial surface. This irregular surface predisposes to leakage, stenosis, or thrombosis. When faced with this clinical situation, rather than force an end-to-end anastomosis, other surgical options, such as an end-to-side anastomosis, should be exercised.

Excessive or deficient vessel length can cause torsion, kinking, or tension at the suture line. The more common error is to leave the vessels too long. This overcompensation to avoid tension can result in either stenosis or thrombosis. Vessels should be trimmed so that the length is adequate but not excessive. Tension at the suture line frequently results in stenosis. When vessels are too short to be handled safely, a segment of autogenous saphenous vein should be used to bridge the defect.

Renal artery thrombosis, rarely seen after the second postoperative day, is fortunately a rare complication occuring in up to 2% of postoperative renal transplant patients.[11] The diagnosis should be suspected in any patient who suddenly becomes anuric in the immediate postoperative period. Some transplant surgeons advocate immediate surgical exploration of patients who become anuric, but it has been our policy to perform a ^{99}Tc renal flow scan or renal angiogram. Surgical exploration is reserved for those patients who lack renal blood flow on either study. This policy seems reasonable when one considers that renal artery thrombosis is a much less likely possibility than ARF; none of the last 151 consecutive renal transplant recipients at our instutition have had renal artery thrombosis.

Because of excessive delay in establishing the diagnosis, all too often the only possible treatment for renal artery thrombosis is transplant nephrectomy. When the diagnosis has been made promptly, the patient should be explored, the previous anastomosis taken down, and the thrombus extracted. Fogarty catheters should be passed into the segmental renal arteries and any distal clots extracted. Dilute heparin solution should be flushed through the kidney to try and establish backbleeding. It can be assumed that the previous arterial anastomosis was improperly constructed and a new anastomosis should be done. Treatment with low-dose heparin may be helpful in the postoperative period.

RENAL ARTERY STENOSIS

Significant diastolic hypertension has been reported to occur in 24% to 60% of renal transplant recipients. Posttransplantation hypertension can originate from the administration of corticosteroids, acute or chronic rejection, retained native kidneys, recurrence of the primary renal disease, and renal artery stenosis.[10]

Inadequate arterial flow to the renal allograft can be the result of occlusive lesions originating primarily in either the donor or recipient vessels. These lesions occur with a frequency that has varied from 1% to 12%. Four basic types of stenotic lesions can be identified: stenosis of the recipient's common or internal iliac artery or arteries, suture line stenosis; a smooth, tubular stenosis of the donor artery distal to the suture line; and multiple stenotic areas distal to the suture line involving both the main renal artery and its branches (Fig. 35-3).[30]

Occlusive arterial lesions of the recipient's vessels proximal to the suture line are the result of arteriosclerosis obliterans (ASO) or a vascular injury during the transplant operation. The hypogastric artery is commonly involved with ASO. When an arteriosclerotic plaque is found during revascularization, an endarterectomy should be done. If the hypogastric artery is too extensively diseased for local endarterectomy to be feasible, the renal artery should be anastomosed end to side to the external iliac artery. Control of the hypogastric artery during revascularization of the allograft should be achieved with an atraumatic vascular clamp. The clamp should be closed only enough to interrupt the arterial flow. An inappropriately selected or applied clamp will damage the vascular endothelium and can result in stenosis at a later date.

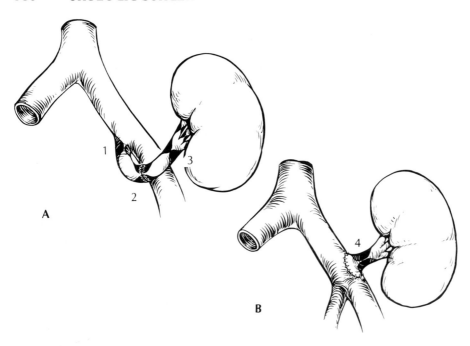

FIG. 35-3. **(A)** Schematic representation of three types of renal artery stenosis involving **(1)** the recipient artery, **(2)** suture line, and **(3)** donor artery. **(B)** The smooth, tubular type of stenosis **(4)** usually seen only in an end-to-side arterial anastomosis.

Stenosis at the suture line appears on angiography as a short segment of irregular narrowing (Fig. 35-4). The stenosis is virtually always secondary to one or more of the technical errors previously described. Intimal injury from the cannula used for pulsatile perfusion of cadaveric organs can also cause late renal artery stenosis. The segment of renal artery in contact with the cannula should always be trimmed off before doing the arterial anastomosis.

A relative suture line stenosis can occur when a pediatric kidney is used in an adult recipient. There is usually sufficient discrepancy in size between a pediatric renal artery and an adult hypogastric artery to preclude an end-to-end anastomosis. An end-to-side anastomosis between the renal artery and external iliac artery is usually necessary. If this anastomosis is not done with a Carrel aortic cuff, late renal artery stenosis is common. This may be due to the inherent stenosis caused by joining a thin-walled vessel to a thick-walled vessel.[5] The stenosis can also be related to a discrepancy in growth of the main renal artery and kidney as compared to the limited possible enlargement of the renal arterial ostium. It has been our policy not to use pediatric kidneys in adult recipients unless an aortic cuff is available.

Stenotic lesions that primarily involve the donor artery distal to the anastomosis can either be a smooth, tubular type of stenosis or multiple areas of stenosis affecting the main renal artery or its branches. The smooth, tubular type of stenosis is usually seen only with an end-to-side anastomosis. This type of stenosis may be due to the altered hemodynamics associated with an end-to-side anastomosis or to excessive stripping of the vasa vasorum.[30] Multiple focal areas of stenosis of the main renal artery and its branches may be seen in patients who have had severe or recurrent rejection reactions. Histologically these lesions represent intimal proliferation and are thought to represent response of the renal arteries to immunologic injury.[14]

Renal artery stenosis should be considered as a serious diagnostic possibility whenever the patient has severe or uncontrollable hypertension or hypertension associated with a decline in renal function.[40] The presence or absence of an arterial bruit over the renal allograft has not been helpful in predicting which patients have renal artery stenosis. Many normotensive transplant patients have a soft, systolic bruit adjacent to the renal allograft.[6] Should there be a change in the character of the bruit, especially if it becomes harsh and develops a diastolic component, renal artery stenosis should be suspected.

There is no valid screening test to select patients who should have renal angiography. The usual screening tests (minute sequence intravenous pyelography, renal scan, renography, and so forth) depend on comparing one kidney with the other and are, therefore, not helpful in the renal transplant recipient. Selective biplanar renal angiography is the only method of accurately evaluating

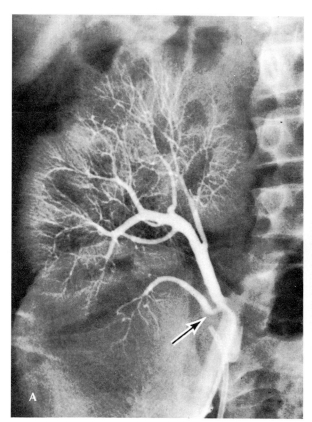

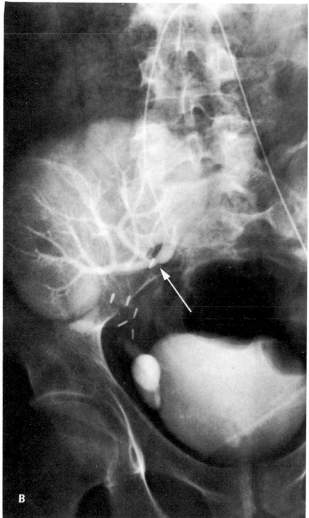

FIG. 35-4. **(A)** Donor kidney with two arteries, with stenosis occurring in the smaller vessel. **(B)** Renal artery stenosis at the suture line *(arrow).*

the integrity of the renal arterial tree.[40] Significant stenosis will be missed unless the artery can be viewed in several projections. A flush film of the common iliac and hypogastric arteries should be done initially to exclude any occlusion of those vessels secondary to ASO or operative trauma. In order to minimize any renal impairment from the contrast media, the patient should be well hydrated and undergoing a brisk diuresis.

The detection of a renal arterial lesion does not imply that the anatomic abnormality is the cause of either the hypertension or any existing functional impairment. It is necessary to attempt to define the interrelationship between the native kidneys (if they are present) or any coexisting parenchymal disease of the renal allograft, that is, chronic rejec-tion or recurrence of the patient's primary renal disease.[10,25]

Renal transplant patients who have retained their native kidneys present a perplexing diagnostic problem. Peripheral or selective plasma renin levels have not been sufficiently reliable in predicting either the source of the hypertension (native kidneys or renal allograft) or the patient's response to surgery (nephrectomy or arterial reconstruction) to be used with confidence. Patients with "three kidneys" will commonly have an elevated peripheral plasma renin, but elevated values may not localize to either the native kidneys or the renal allograft. It is uncommon for one-kidney patients (renal allograft) to have an elevated peripheral plasma renin activity.

There is evidence that removal of the patient's native kidneys may be the most effective initial surgical treatment for severe posttransplant hypertension. Curtis and associates studied ten posttransplant patients with severe or uncontrollable hypertension.[10] All ten patients had normal renal function and were on maintenance doses of alternate-day corticosteroids. Four of the patients had renal artery stenosis and all ten patients had elevated peripheral renin activity, although selective renins did not necessarily implicate the native kidneys as the cause of the hypertension. Bilateral nephrectomy was done in all ten patients in an attempt to surgically control the hypertension. Nine out of ten patients were either cured or improved. The only failure occurred in a patient who had significant parenchymal disease (chronic rejection) documented by renal transplant biopsy. All four of the patients who had coexisting arterial stenosis of the transplanted kidney had their hypertension either cured or improved by bilateral nephrectomy alone.

Based on current information it is possible to outline a reasonable plan of management for the post-renal transplant patient with severe or uncontrollable hypertension. Patients who have severe hypertension and normal renal function are treated medically. The dosage of corticosteroids is reduced at a somewhat faster rate than normal in the hope that the hypertension will be less severe once the patient is on a daily maintenance dose. As long as the hypertension can be controlled and renal function does not deteriorate, no evaluation is done. If the hypertension is poorly controlled or renal function changes, biplanar renal angiography and renin levels are obtained. Patients who have a significant renal artery stenosis, no significant parenchymal disease on transplant biopsy, and already had their native kidneys removed are felt to be candidates for either transluminal angioplasty or surgical repair. This decision is made regardless of the results of peripheral or selective renin activity.

The three-kidney patient is a more difficult therapeutic problem. In deciding on the initial surgical therapy (revascularization of the renal allograft *vs* bilateral nephrectomy), one must clearly identify whether intervention is necessary primary to control hypertension or because of the concern that the lesion is so severe that renal arterial thrombosis is a real concern. If control of hypertension is the primary goal and renal function is normal or nearly so, removal of the native kidneys would be our initial therapy. Renal revascularization would be reserved for those patients in whom

the primary consideration was preservation of renal allograft function.

Currently renal arterial stenosis may be corrected by either conventional means (*e.g.* bypass grafts) or by transluminal angioplasty.[13,18,21,26,27,30] Although there is not yet sufficient experience with transluminal angioplasty to accurately define its benefits or limitations, it does appear to be a reasonable first option for some patients, especially those with suture line stenosis.

Although the type of revascularization will depend on the nature and extent of the renal arterial lesion(s), saphenous vein bypass has been our most commonly employed technique. Resection of the stenotic segment followed by end-to-end anastomosis is usually not practical if the new suture line is to be free of tension. Patients who have the tubular form of stenosis are also treated primarily with a bypass graft. Simple freeing of the artery from its surrounding investment of scar tissue is usually inadequate.

Revascularization of the renal allograft is possible through a midline incision, but our preference is to go through the previous transplant incision. Dissection of the vessels is facilitated by early opening of the peritoneal cavity so that the iliac or hypogastric artery(s) can be identified outside of the dense scar tissue surrounding them in the retroperitoneal space. The various specific techniques of revascularization are described in detail in Chapter 25.

RENAL VEIN THROMBOSIS

Thrombosis of the renal vein is a rare surgical complication having a reported incidence of up to 3.6%.[5,12] Although the thrombus usually involves the main renal vein, segmental renal vein occlusion can also occur.

Primary renal vein thrombosis can originate from a variety of causes. Because of the large diameter of the renal vein and relatively rapid flow rates, technical problems with the anastomosis are uncommon. The most frequent surgical errors are excessive length of the renal vein resulting in tension or the inadvertent incorporation of the anterior and posterior venous walls during the anastomosis. Primary renal vein thrombosis can also result from the steroid-resistant nephrotic syndrome, membranoproliferative glomerulonephritis, hyperacute rejection, or cortical necrosis. Compression of the iliac or renal veins by a lymphocele, abscess, or edematous renal allograft can also cause renal vein thrombosis. Propagation of an ipsilateral iliofemoral thrombosis can secondarily involve and occlude the renal vein.

Patients with renal vein thrombosis present with oliguria, hematuria, proteinuria greater than 2 g/day, a swollen allograft, and deterioration of renal function. This clinical picture can be confused with more commonly occurring rejection reactions. If during surgery there were technical problems with the renal vein or if any of the predisposing problems (e.g., recurrent nephrotic syndrome or ipsilateral lower-extremity venous thrombosis) are present, renal vein thrombosis should be a serious diagnostic consideration.[41]

Unless there is good reason to suspect a technical problem, the treatment of renal vein thrombosis is anticoagulation with heparin. If there is a technical problem, it should be surgically corrected and the patient should be anticoagulated with heparin. The indications for vena caval ligation or insertion of a caval umbrella do not differ in renal transplant recipients.

Urologic Complications

URINARY FISTULA

During the first decade of renal transplantation urinary fistulas occurred at an alarming rate (3%–10%).[1,15,31] This surgical complication was especially distressing not only because of its frequency, but also because it was associated with high rates of allograft loss and patient mortality (25%).[15] Ureteral fistulas were usually secondary to devascularized ureteral segments, and bladder fistulas were the result of inadequate closure of the cystotomy. Diagnosis of the urinary fistula was frequently late. Late diagnosis decreased the likelihood of a successful repair and increased the possibility of wound infection.

An appreciation of why urinary fistulas occurred and the importance of prompt diagnosis and treatment allowed transplant surgeons to take appropriate steps to reduce the frequency, morbidity, and mortality previously associated with this surgical complication. Current data place the frequency of urinary fistulas at 0.5%–3.5%.[34,35] Salvatierra and associates reported 29 urinary fistulas; none died, and 25 out of 29 retained their renal allografts. Urinary fistulas should no longer be a common problem and should be managed successfully.

Urinary fistulas originating from the ureter may be the result of ureteral devascularization, tension in the anastomosis, or rejection. The most common cause by far is ureteral devascularization. Injury to the ureteral blood supply during the donor nephrectomy represents an error that cannot be compensated for during the recipient operation, regardless of the high quality of subsequent urinary tract reconstruction.[19] In order to prevent a ureteral fistula from ischemic injury, a practical knowledge of the ureteral blood supply is necessary. Although the arterial supply of the ureter is multiple, the primary ureteral artery arises from the renal artery. Excessive dissection in the renal hilus during the donor nephrectomy will damage this tiny artery and ureteral sloughing is inevitable. Of equal importance is the interlocking arterial system located in the ureteral adventitia. These arteries are not end arteries, and they communicate freely with one another. This arterial system gives off muscular penetrating branches that nurture the ureteral wall. Stripping of the ureteral adventitia will cause devascularization of that segment of the ureter and eventual ureteral necrosis. When the main renal arterial supply is multiple, the primary ureteral branch most commonly arises from the lower pole vessel.[5]

Although this is less common than ureteral ischemia, some fistulas are the result of technically inadequate urinary tract reconstruction. Selection of the best operation for reestablishing urinary tract activity is the initial step in minimizing ureteral fistulas due to poor surgical technique. Ureteroneocystostomy, ureteroureterostomy, and ureteropyeloneostomy are all surgical options for establishing urinary drainage for the renal allografts.[9] Although it should be well known, it bears repeating that in virtually any clinical situation ureteroneocystostomy is superior to ureteroureterostomy. The experience at many institutions indicates that ureteroneocytostomy has an extremely low complication rate. When compared with ureteroureterostomy or ureteropyeloneostomy, it has a significantly lower rate of urinary fistulas.[15,20,42,43] Ureteroureterostomy and ureteropyeloneostomy should be reserved for secondary operations in the treatment of urinary fistulas. They should be used as a primary means of urinary tract reconstruction only when the length of the donor ureter precludes ureteroneocystostomy.

Many acceptable techniques are available for reimplanting the donor ureter into the recipient's bladder. Regardless of the technique used, some basic principles should be followed to avoid ureteral complications. The hole in the bladder and the submucosal tunnel should be sufficiently large to easily accommodate the ureter without causing compression. Some excessive ureteral length should be left outside the bladder to avoid tension on the suture line, and an excessive number of sutures should not be used or the ureter tip will become devascularized.[35]

Bladder fistulas are always the result of poor technique. The bladder should be closed in three layers. Each layer after the first should overlap its predecessor to ensure watertight closure of the corners of the suture line. The bladder should be kept at rest during the postoperative period by drainage with an appropriately sized indwelling catheter for 5 to 7 days. If the patient has insulin-dependent diabetes mellitus or has had previous bladder surgery, the urethral catheter is left for 10 to 14 days. Earlier removal of the catheter offers little advantage. Colonization of the bladder with bacteria should be feared less than overdistention of the bladder and excessive stress on the suture line.

Urinary fistulas should be considered in patients with a floating urinary output, oliguria, anuria, declining renal function, unusual wound pain, unexplained ileus or fever, a mass in transplant wound, or fluid leaking from the transplant incision. The diagnosis of urinary extravasation is made with the standard urologic tools of cystography, intervenous pyelography,[131]I hippurate renal scan, and the intravenous injection of Indigo Carmine. A normal cystogram alone is not sufficient to exclude urinary leakage. It is essential to obtain postvoid films on both the intravenous pyelogram (IVP) or ^{131}I hippurate renal scan to demonstrate small amounts of urinary leakage from the distal ureter. Of paramount importance in reducing the morbidity and mortality associated with urinary fistulas is the correct differentiation of urinary fistulas from a rejection reaction.

The treatment of urinary fistulas is predicated on the following factors: the presence of infection, the condition of the ureter and bladder, and the condition of the patient. Under virtually all circumstances urinary extravasation should be considered a urologic emergency, and immediate operation is indicated. Several surgical methods are available for dealing with urinary fistulas.[36,42] Unless specifically mentioned, drains, stents, or nephrostomy tubes are not used.

Repeat ureteroneocystostomy is the secondary procedure of choice only if the ureter is unquestionably viable. The distal ureteral segment should be trimmed away until an area with obviously good blood supply is reached. To avoid tension on the ureteral anastomosis to the bladder wall, it is frequently necessary to hitch the bladder wall to the psoas muscle.

Ureteroureterostomy or ureteropyeloneostomy is applicable to almost any situation and is fre-quently the secondary procedure of choice. Care should be exercised in mobilization of the recipient's ureter as well as in selecting a segment of donor ureter or pelvis that is unquestionably viable. Every effort should be made to effect a watertight anastomosis with fine running or interrupted sutures of 5-0 or 6-0 chromic catgut. In placing the sutures, one should take disproportionately larger bites of seromuscular tissue while including minimal bites of ureteral or pelvic mucosa. This technique minimizes both stricture formation and leakage of urine from the suture line. If the patient's native kidneys are in place, the ipsilateral ureter can be safely used without removal of that kidney.

Even under ideal circumstances both of these anastomoses have a tendency to leak. This represents one of the few instances in transplant surgery in which drainage of a noninfected wound is advocated. Hemovac drainage is preferred because it is felt that the opportunity for bacterial entrance into the wound is decreased, and aseptic wound care can be more easily given. Drains, regardless of type, should be removed as soon as the wound is dry.

Patients with recurrent fistulas or in whom infections or sepsis have occurred require deviation from the surgical treatment just described. To close persistent fistulas, proximal diversion with nephrostomy tube drainage may be necessary.[28] Patients with persistent fistulas and wound infections require not only nephrostomy drainage but also complete incision and drainage of the entire wound. The wound is allowed to heal by granulation and when clean is suitable for application of split-thickness skin grafts. Use of this technique allows allografts to be saved that otherwise would be lost. If the patient's condition is poor or questionable, transplant nephrectomy should be performed without hesitation.

To avoid significant morbidity and mortality from a urinary fistula, not only must the patient have the fistula diagnosed early and have prompt surgical repair, but also the immunosuppressive regimen must be modified. Even with early diagnosis and prompt therapy some reduction in the level of immunosuppressive therapy is temporarily necessary. If the patient is septic, the corticosteroid dose should be rapidly reduced to maintenance levels and the azathioprine should be discontinued.

URETERAL OBSTRUCTION

Ureteral obstruction has been reported to occur with a frequency that varies from 1.1% to 10.7%.[11,42] Most recently reported series have indicated that currently this is a rare complication and should not occur in more than 2.5% of patients (obstruction from lymphoceles being excluded).[35] In the last 151 consecutive renal transplants at the UTHSC at San Antonio, only one patient has had ureteral obstruction (0.06%). A variety of causes for ureteral obstruction have been postulated, including ureteral ischemia, torsion, blood clots, impingement of the spermatic cord and periureteral fibrosis, anastomotic stricture, and rejection of the ureter.[17]

Significant early ureteral obstruction always represents a technical error. Most commonly this problem is created by an inadequate opening in the bladder wall, a constricting suture at the ureterovesical anastomosis, or torsion of the ureter. These technical errors can only be corrected surgically. Transient or intermittent early ureteral obstruction can be caused by ureteral edema or the passage of blood clots. These problems are self-limiting and if necessary can be treated by short-term drainage of the kidney with a ureteral stent.

Although it is not a common problem, late ureteral obstruction is a more common and significant problem than early ureteral obstruction. Late ureteral obstruction is most frequently due to ureteral ischemia, compression by the spermatic cord, periureteral fibrosis, and anastomotic stricture. Although chronic rejection has been implicated as a cause of ureteral and caliceal ectasia, it is rarely responsible for clinically significant hydronephrosis. Devascularization during the donor nephrectomy is the most likely cause of late ureteral obstruction. Ureteral ischemia is a continuum of complications ranging from early ureteral slough and fistula formation to late ureteral obstruction.

The diagnosis of ureteral obstruction is made using standard diagnostic techniques (intravenous pyelography, retrograde pyelography, and so forth.) Surgical correction of ureteral obstruction should be carefully considered. An abnormal urogram alone without the complications of infection or deteriorating renal function does not represent an indication for reoperation.

Relief of the ureteral obstruction is usually best accomplished by using the recipient's own ureter and performing a urethroplasty.[42] This obviates the problem of mobilizing the donor ureter from the ever-present bed of scar tissue and also ensures that the anastomosis will be done in an area with the best possible blood supply (the renal pelvis of the allograft). The results with late reconstruction of the urinary tract in renal transplant recipients are surprisingly good. Once the patient is on maintenance doses of immunosuppressive drugs,

the complication rate is basically not different from that observed in nonimmunosuppressed patients.

URETHRAL STRICTURES

Loening and associates reported an incidence of postoperative urethral strictutres of 6.1% of 211 consecutive men undergoing renal transplantation.[23] All of the patients presented with obstructive voiding symptoms. The cause of the strictures was believed to be the postoperative use of an indwelling urethral catheter. Use of a large catheter (24 Fr) seemed to especially predispose to stricture formation. These patients were primarily managed by periodic urethral dilation. No patients or allografts were lost as a result of the urethral strictures or the treatment of these strictures.

Routine use of a smaller urethral catheter in men (16Fr–18Fr) should decrease the incidence of posttransplant urethral strictures. In the last 91 consecutive men transplanted at the UTHSC at San Antonio, no postoperative urethral strictures have been identified. It is still prudent, however, to reevaluate the lower urinary tract of men who have had a first renal transplant fail before proceeding with a second transplant. Treatment of strictures, if they occur, should be consistent with the current urologic management of this disease, that is, visual urethrotomy, skin graft urethroplasty, and so forth.

HYDROCELE

An ipsilateral hydrocele may occur in approximately 70% of male renal transplant recipients.[42] The formation of the hydrocele may be related to division of the vas deferens and the gonadal vessels. It is usually asymptomatic and rarely requires surgical treatment.

Deep Wound Infections

Subfascial infection of the transplant wound can be a potentially lethal complication resulting in loss of the renal allograft, major arterial hemorrhage, or wound sepsis.[29,32] The operative wound of a renal transplant recipient is unusually vulnerable to infection. Patients are frequently anemic and hypoalbuminemic. Host defenses have been severely compromised by chronic renal failure and are further impaired during the postoperative period by the administration of immunosuppressive drugs. Dietary restrictions imposed by chronic hemodialysis may lead to poor nutritional status of the patient. In spite of these handicaps, the successful prevention and treatment of deep wound infections is a crucial part of decreasing the surgical morbidity and mortality of renal transplant recipients.[4]

Even with the conditions favoring asepsis found in modern operating rooms, some bacterial contamination of the surgical wound is inevitable. For a wound infection to occur, the bacteria must have sufficient resources to make the transition from contamination to colonization. This usually implies a relatively large or continued inoculum or local conditions in the wound that especially favor the replication of bacteria. Thus, primary efforts at avoiding wound infections should be directed at minimizing the size of the inoculum (good sterile technique) and creating an unfavorable environment in the wound for bacterial multiplication (good surgical technique).

The most effective surgical tactic for preventing bacterial colonization is to have a dry, well-closed wound that is free of devitalized tissue. Most body fluids can sustain and promote bacterial multiplication, therefore the complications of bleeding, urinary fistula, or lymphocele encourage bacterial contamination of the wound. If these local wound problems do not occur, the infection rate in uncomplicated transplant wounds should not exceed 3%.[5] In addition to good surgical technique, the use of local or systemic antibiotics has been reported to decrease the incidence of wound infections.

Wound contamination can occur during the postoperative period as well. Although the skin may be sealed in 24 hr to 28 hr, the incision is not impervious to bacterial invasion until granulation tissue has formed. For this reason it has been our policy to keep all wounds covered, to change dressings under sterile conditions, and to apply an antibiotic ointment to the skin surface.

Just as clean wounds should not be drained, wounds that have become infected must be opened widely to avoid sepsis or recurrence of the closed-space infection. Drainage of pus through counterincisions with Penrose drains or sumps is frequently ineffective. The most conservative treatment is to leave all layers of the wound open (including the fascial layers) over the area of infection. If the renal allograft is still in place, any sign of infection at either vascular anastomosis warrants the immediate removal of the kidney and ligation of the involved vessels.

Healing of the open wound is by secondary intention. Although the healing process is lengthy, the added margin of safety should be adequate compensation. Skin grafting the defect is rarely necessary. Using the regimen described here to manage deep transplant wound infections, there have been no fatalities from wound sepsis in our last 151 renal transplant recipients.

Lymphatic Complications

Lymphatic complications have been reported to occur in 8% to 10% of postoperative renal transplant patients.[24,44] Lymphatic leakage can occur from the renal allograft or from lymphatic channels around the iliac vessels.[33] Because the renal allograft is in a retroperitoneal position, extravasated lymph is inadequately absorbed. This extravastated lymphatic fluid can either find its way to the outside (lymph fistula) or become encysted (lymphocele).

Lymphatic channels that have been severed during the donor or recipient operations do not heal for 21 days. During the hearling period they may be called upon to handle an increased amount of lymphatic fluids. Many medications commonly used in the posttransplant period stimulate pelvic or renal lymphatic flow. Prominent among these medications are corticosteroids, diuretics, and anticoagulants.[7] Rejection reactions also stimulate renal lymphtic flow. Lymphatic complications should be viewed as a technical mistake and can only be minimized by meticulous ligation of the renal and pelvic lymphatics.

LYMPHOCELE

Lymphoceles are clinically significant because they are capable of depressing renal function and mimicking the more serious complications of rejections and urinary extravasation. Renal function can be adversely effected by the lymphocele mechanically compressing the renal parenchyma, the renal vessels, or the ureter.[39]

Lymphoceles can be present with a variety of symptoms or signs and mimic either immunologic or technical problems seen in post-renal transplant patients. When a lymphocele is suspected, the diagnosis can be made safely and simply by ultrasonography (Fig. 35-5). Lymphoceles also produce distinctive findings on cystography or intravenous pyelography (Fig. 35-6). The findings on the IVP consist of hydronephrosis with lateral and superior displacement of the bladder. Lymphangiography is usually unnecessary.

LYMPH FISTULA

In evaluating lymphatic fistulas the main problem is in differentiating a lymphatic fistula from a

FIG. 35-5. Sonogram reveals a normal renal allograft *(left arrow)* and a moderately large lymphocele *(right arrow).*

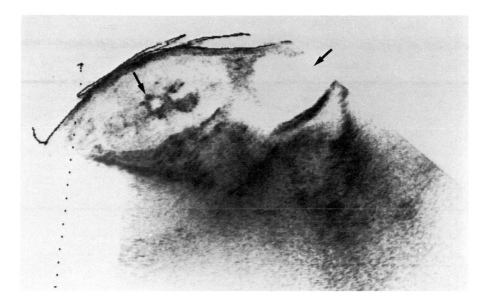

urinary fistual. This differential can be made by intravenous pyelography, renal scan, or a chemical analysis comparing the composition of the wound drainage with serum and urine.

Sonography has been such a safe, easy, and accurate diagnostic tool to detect perinephric collections of fluid that the treatment of lymphoceles has become more complicated.[8,22] Previously lymphoceles were detected by virtue of their size or by their adverse effect on renal function, and patients who had large, symptomatic lymphoceles or who had hydronephrosis were obviously candidates for surgical drainage. Routine sonography of postoperative renal transplant patients will not uncommonly reveal small, asymptomatic collections of fluid. In our experience these do not require routine drainage and if followed will frequently disappear without intervention. Drainage of a lymphocele is still reserved for those patients who have a symptomatic lymphocele, a lymphocele in conjunction with altered renal function, or a lymphocele associated with infection.

Lymphoceles may be aspirated, drained internally into the peritoneal cavity, or marsupialized externally.[7,38] Aspiration of a lymphocele is ineffective and potentially hazardous. It is the rule rather than the exception that lymphoceles treated in this manner will recur. In addition, the introduction of the needle may infect an otherwise sterile collection of fluid. Williams and Howard have advocated the injection of 5mc of [198]Au into the lymphocele or lymph fistula.[44] This technique has been used successfully in treating malignant pleural effusions and was successful in all six of his patients treated with this technique.

Schweizer has advocated draining the lymphocele internally into the peritoneal cavity.[38] Through a transperitoneal incision the retroperitoneal lymphocele is identified. A peritoneal window is fashioned to allow free drainage of the lymph into the peritoneal cavity, where it is readily absorbed. This internal drainage procedure is safe and effective.

Lymphoceles may also be drained externally by marsupializing the lymphocele to the skin. This procedure, can be done under local anesthesia, avoids the possible complications of a laparotomy, and has a low recurrence rate. The potential infectious problems associated with an open wound have never materialized.

Before the incision is made, the patient's bladder should be drained to avoid inadvertent injury. A 22-gauge spinal needle is used to confirm the presence and location of the lymphocele. The old incision is usually opened in its medial aspect. A window is made in the fascia over the lymphocele, which is incised and drained. The wall of the lymphocele is sutured to the previously created fascial window. A Penrose drain and gauze pack impregnated with neosporin solution are placed in the cavity. The wound is left open and covered with a sterile dressing.

If contamination is to be avoided, meticulous wound care must be given post-operatively. The wound should be repacked daily under sterile conditions. Dressings should not be allowed to soak through and should be changed as often as

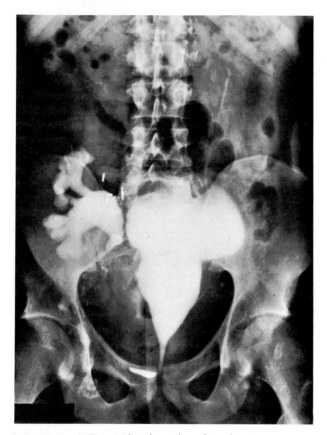

FIG. 35-6. IVP reveals a large lymphocele.

necessary to avoid this source of external contamination. The gauze pack serves three useful functions: it prevents premature closure of the cavity with subsequent loculation, it facilitates scarring of the lymphocele walls, and it serves as a sponge for the Neosporin solution that is used daily. The wound is allowed to heal by granulation.

The bulk of the drainage ceases in 48 hr to 72 hr, at which time the Penrose drain is pulled. The wound should be healed in 3 to 4 weeks. Patients can be trained to dress their own wounds, and hospitalization is usually unnecessary after 5 to 7 days.

REFERENCES

1. ANDERSON EE, GLENN JF, SIEGLER HF et al: Ureteral implantation in renal transplantation. Surg Gynecol Obstet 134:494, 1972
2. BANOWSKY LH: Basic Prinicples and Techniques of Vascular Surgery. In Novick AC, Stroffon RA (eds): Vascular Problems in Urologic Surgery. Philadelphia, W B Saunders, (in press)
3. BANOWSKY LH: Optical Magnification in Urological Surgery. In Silber SJ (ed): Microsurgery, pp 443–465. Baltimore, William & Wilkins, 1979
4. BANOWSKY LH, MONTIE JE, BRAUN WE et al: Prevention of wound infections in recipients of renal transplants. Urology 4:656, 1974
5. BELZER FO: Technical Complications after Renal Transplantation. In Morris PJ (ed): Kidney Transplantation, Principles and Practice. London, Academic Press; New York, Grune & Stratton, 1979
6. BRAUN WE: The renal-allograft bruit as an indicator of good function. N Engl J Med 286:1350, 1972
7. BRAUN WE, BANOWSKY LH, NAKAMOTO S et al: Lymphoceles associated with renal transplantation. Am J Med 57:714, 1974
8. CAHILL PJ, SACHIKO C, SAMPLE WF: Conventional radiographic and ultrasonic imaging in renal transplantation. Urology 10, No. 1, 1977
9. CORRIERE JN, JR, PERLOFF LJ, BARKER CF et al: The ureteropyelostomy in human renal transplantation, J Urol 110:24, 1973
10. CURTIS JJ, LUCAS BA, KOTCHEN TA et al: Surgical therapy for persistent hypertension after renal transplantation. Transplantation 31: February 1981
11. EHRLICH RM, SMITH RB: Surgical complications of renal transplantation. Urology 10, No. 1, 1977
12. FIGUEROA JE, CORTEZ LM, DECAMP PT et al: Renal vein thrombosis after transplantation. Br Med J 1:288, 1971
13. KAUFFMAN HM, SAMPSON D, FOX PS et al: Prevention of transplant renal artery stenosis. Surgery 81:161, 1977
14. KAUFMAN JJ, EHRLICH RM, DORNFELD L: Immunologic considerations in renovascular hypertension. Trans Am Assoc Genitourin Surg 67:40, 1975
15. KISER WS, HEWITT CB, MONTIE JE: The surgical complications of renal transplantation. Surg Clin North Am 51:1133, 1971
16. KISSMEYER–NIELSEN F, OLSEN S, PETERSON VP et al: Hyperacute rejection of kidney allografts associated with pre-existing humoral antibodies against donor cells. Lancet 2:662, 1966
17. KRANE RJ, CHO SI, OLSSON CA: Renal tranplant ureteral obstruction simulating retroperitoneal fibrosis. JAMA 225:607, 1973
18. LEE HM, LINEHAN D, PIERCE J et al: Renal artery stenosis and gastrointestinal hemorrhage in human renal transplantation. Transplant Proc 4:681, 1972
19. LEE HM, SULKIN M, HUME D: A standard technique for procurement of cadaveric donor organs. Transplant Proc 4:583, 1972
20. LEITER E, KIM KH, GLABMAN S et al: Urinary reconstruction by pyeloureteral anastomosis in human renal transplants. J Urol 109:28, 1973
21. LINDFORS O, LAASONEN L, FRYHRQUIST F et al: Renal artery stenosis in hypertensive renal tranplant recipients. J Urol 118:240, 1977
22. LIPSHULTZ LI, WEIN AJ, ARGER PH et al: Post-transplantation lymphocyst. Use of ultrasound as adjunct in diagnosis. Urology 8:624, 1976

23. LOENING SA, BANOWSKY LH, BRAUN WE et al: Bladder neck contracture and urethral stricture as complications of renal transplantation. J Urol 114:688, 1975

24. MADURA JA, DUNBAR JD, CERILLI GJ: Perirenal lymphocele as a complication of renal hemotransplantation. Surgery 68:310, 1970

25. MARKS LS, MAXWELL MH, SMITH RB et al: Detection of renovascular hypertension: Saralasin test versus renin determination. J Urol 116:406, 1976

26. MORRIS PJ, YADOV RVS, KINCAID-SMITH P et al: Renal artery stenosis in renal transplantation, Med J Aus 1:1255, 1971

27. NERSTROM B, LADENFOGED J, LUND FL: Vascular complications in 155 consecutive kidney transplantations. Scand J Urol Nephrol (Suppl) 15:65, 1972

28. OLSSON CA, MANNICK JA, SCHMITT GW et al: Nephrostomy in renal transplantation. Am J Surg 121:467, 1971

29. OWENS ML, WILSON SE, MAXWELL JG et al: Transplantation 27:285, 1979

30. PALLESCHI J, NOVICK AC, BRAUN WE et al: Vascular complications of renal transplantation. Urology 16:61, 1980

31. PALMER JM, KOUNTZ SK, SWENSON RS et al: Urinary tract morbidity in renal transplantation. Arch Surg 98:352, 1969

32. PAYNE JE, STOREY BG, ROGERS JH et al: Serious arterial complications following removal of failed renal allografts. Med J Aust 1:274, 1971

33. PONTES JE, MCDONALD FD, MIGDAL SD et al: Lymphatic complications in renal allografts—A new look. Urology 17:26, 1981

34. SALVATIERRA O, JR, KOUNTZ SL, BELZER FO: Prevention of ureteral fistula after renal transplantation. J Urol 112:445, 1974

35. SALVATIERRA O, JR, OLCOTT C IV, AMEND WJ, JR et al: Urological complications of renal transplantation can be prevented or controlled. J Urol 117:421, 1977

36. SCHIFF M, JR, MCGUIRE EJ, WEISS RM et al: Management of urinary fistulas after renal transplantation. J Urol 115:251, 1976

37. SCHRIER RW: Acute renal failure: Pathogenesis, diagnosis, and management. Hosp Prac 16:93, 1981

38. SCHWEIZER RT, CHO SI, KOUNTZ SL et al: Lymphoceles following renal transplantation. Arch Surg 104:43, 1972

39. SMELLIE WAB, VINICK M, HUME DM: Angiographic investigation of hypertension complicating human renal transplantation. Surg Gynecol Obstet 128:963, 1969

40. SMITH RB, COSIMI AB, LORDON R et al: Diagnosis and management of arterial stenosis causing hypertension after successful renal transplantation. J Urol 115:639, 1976

41. STARZL TE, BOEHMIG HJ, ANEMIJA H et al: Clotting changes including disseminated intravascular coagulation during rapid renal-hemograft rejection. N Engl J Med 283:383, 1970

42. STARZL TE, GROTH CG, PUTNAM CW et al: Urologic complications in 216 human recipients of renal transplants. Ann Surg 172:1, 1970

43. WEIL R, SIMMONS RL, TALLENT MD et al: Prevention of urological complications after kidney transplantation. Ann Surg 174:154, 1971

44. WILLIAMS G, HOWARD N: Management of lymphatic leakage after renal transplantation. Transplantation 31:134, 1981

45. WILLIAMS GM, DEPLANQUE B, LOWES R et al: Antibodies and human transplant rejection. Ann Surg 170:603, 1969

46. WILLIAMS GM, STERWIFF S, BIAS W: Hyperacute and acute fulminating rejection of human renal allografts. Transplant Proc 4:665, 1972

Retroperitoneal Fibrosis, Tumors, and Cysts

36

Joseph K. Wheatley

For many years, the problems associated with delineating the retroperitoneal space (excluding the urinary tract) meant that many lesions in this area were diagnosed only in advanced stages or at autopsy. Retroperitoneal tumors belong in the differential diagnosis of any abdominal mass, and the emergence of high-quality, rapid-sequence computed tomography (CT) scanners has changed this to one of the best-delineated regions. The urologist, general and vascular surgeon, and gynecologist all have an interest in this area, but it is the urologist who is usually most experienced with inflammatory and neoplastic processes found here.

Sweetser was among the first to discuss primary retroperitoneal masses.[48] In this chapter we will attempt to deal with the management of primary benign and malignant lesions of the retroperitoneum, excluding the adrenals, kidneys, ureters, or gastrointestinal tract.

RETROPERITONEAL SPACE

The retroperitoneal space is bounded superiorly by the thoracic diaphragm and inferiorly by the pelvic diaphragm. The posterior aspect is bounded by the psoas, quadratus lumborum, and transversalis muscles. The anterior aspect consists of the posterior layer of the parietal peritoneum and nonperitonealized aspects of the duodenum, colon, rectum, and liver. The lateral boundaries are the tips of the 12th ribs and iliac crests.

The contents of the retroperitoneal space are multiple and varied (Table 36-1). The compliance of the peritoneal cavity anteriorly allows unrestricted growth of some masses to large proportions before producing symptoms. Even embryonic remnants of the urogenital ridge may give rise to both benign and malignant tumors in this area.

The lymphatics are an important component of the retroperitoneum. The parietal lymphatic aggregates consist of iliac channels that coalesce at the level of the upper sacrum and continue as the periaortocaval plexus. Visceral channels course with the mesenteric vessels. The cisterna chyli is the dilated ampullar origin of the thoracic duct and is formed by the coalescence of the parietal and visceral channels. It lies dorsal and slightly medial to the aorta at the level of the L1 and L2 vertebral bodies. As many as 50% of individuals do not have a discrete cisterna chyli.[18] However, there is always a coalescence of lymphatics at this area to form a thoracic duct. This is at the level of the renal pedicles and is often encountered in a node dissection. It must be carefully and completely ligated to prevent chylous ascites from subsequent leakage.

DIAGNOSTIC IMAGING

The intravenous pyelogram (IVP) remains the most available, cost-effective, and useful screening tool to evaluate the retroperitoneal space. It permits the estimation of renal size, position, function, and internal anatomy. Displacement of the kidney or ureters or bladder deformities are clues to retroperitoneal pathology. Tomographic cuts enhance these details and often demonstrate the adrenal glands.

Although the IVP is valuable as an initial or screening procedure, its limitations are obvious. The normal position of the ureters is so variable that small retroperitoneal lesions may be unsuspected. Displacement of the kidney or bladder deformities are more sensitive, but remain considerably less sensitive than the CT scan.

CT is highly effective for evaluation of the retroperitoneum because the abundance of fat that is usually present in this area permits exquisite, direct demonstration of both normal and abnormal structures (Fig. 36-1). CT is increasingly the next logical step when an abnormality is suspected on an IVP. It is an excellent way to plan and monitor therapy for retroperitoneal abnormalities and may one day become the primary screening tool for suspected nonurinary disorders such as adrenal or lymphatic lesions.

Retrograde pyelography has a role when the use of contrast is not indicated, when decreased renal function results in poor demonstration of the urinary tract, or to demonstrate the ureter distal to an obstruction. Ultrasound is less expensive than CT and is more available but requires skilled personnel for its performance and lacks the clarity of CT. Arteriography helps define the origin of retroperitoneal masses and aids in planning a surgical approach. Vena cava studies are also useful in planning surgical therapy for larger masses which may occlude or invade this structure. Gastrointestinal studies are helpful in selected patients. Lymphangiography has value with tumor spread to normal or slightly enlarged nodes but is less effective than the CT scan with bulky nodal disease. Retroperitoneal pneumography has essentially been replaced by the diagnostic techniques discussed here.

Retroperitoneal Fibrosis

Retroperitoneal fibrosis was first described by Albarran in 1905.[2] In 1948, Ormond described two more cases and defined this as a clinical entity.[36] The topic was reviewed by Koep and Zuidema and more recently by Lepor and Walsh.[22,23]

Retroperitoneal fibrosis is a hard, grayish white fibrous plaque that is often centered about the sacral promontory and may envelop the ureters, aorta, vena cava, and nerves. Involvement of almost every retroperitoneal and mediastinal structure has been reported. The fibrosis consists of a deposition of collagen with areas of cellular inflam-

TABLE 36-1. Retroperitoneal Contents

Vascular
    Aorta and vena cava with their branches, portal vein
Gastrointestinal
    Pancreas, portions of duodenum and colon
Urinary
    Kidneys and ureters
Adrenal glands
Embryonic remnants
    Urogenital ridge, wolffian, mullerian
Neural tissue
    Celiac, superior and inferior hypogastric and sacral plexus
    Ilioinguinal, iliohypogastric, lateral cutaneous, genitofemoral, femoral, obturator, sciatic, and pudendal nerves; sympathetic trunks
Lymphatic tissue
    Parietal and visceral chains, cisterna chyli, thoracic duct

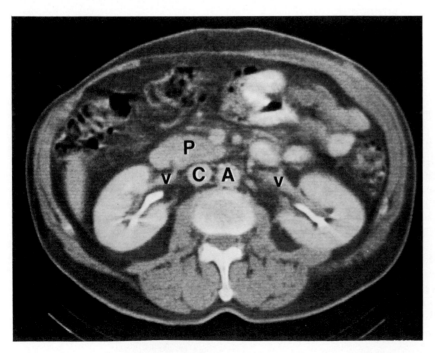

FIG. 36-1. A CT scan using intravenous and gastrointestinal contrast demonstrates normal retroperitoneal anatomy. *P* = head of the pancreas, *C* = vena cava, *A* = aorta, *V* = renal vein

mation, representing the maturation of nonspecific, nonsuppurative inflammation.[15,25,37,52] The cellular elements consist primarily of lymphocytes, plasma cells, eosinophils, and polymorphonuclear leukocytes.

As described by Lepor and Walsh, the process may be secondary or idiopathic.[23] Causes of secondary retroperitoneal fibrosis include malignancy, injury (trauma, surgery, inflammation, urinoma, aneurysm), infection, drugs (methysergide, amphetamines, phenacetin, methyldopa, LSD [lysergic acid diethylamide]), and an autoimmune process such as vasculitis. When these are excluded it may be considered idiopathic.

DIAGNOSIS

Idiopathic retroperitoneal fibrosis has a male predominance (2.9:1). The average age is 49 years, although some cases have been reported in children.[7] Pain the most common presenting complaint, is most often referred to the abdomen or back, but may also be testicular or in the loin, thigh, or pelvis. It is noncolicky and dull in character. Other complaints include weight loss, gastrointestinal complaints, fever, and occasionally anuria.[20] The most common physical finding is an abdominal or rectal mass. Other findings include pedal or scrotal edema or jaundice. Abnormal laboratory findings include an elevated sedimentation rate, elevated blood urea nitrogen, and anemia.

The "classic" finding on IVP is bilateral narrowing of the ureters at the level of L5 with medial deviation and proximal dilatation. Sometimes the ureteral involvement is unilateral and rarely it is displaced laterally.[43] Even the most severely narrowed ureter usually admits a ureteral catheter. CT generally demonstrates a mass effect with a density in the range of muscle or solid organs. Aortography, vena cava studies, and lymphangiography have value in clinically selected cases. The diagnosis is ultimately established by surgical exploration with multiple deep tissue biopsies.

MANAGEMENT

Surgical exploration may be deferred if there is a clear-cut etiology (e.g., methysergide use) or if the patient is debilitated and a poor surgical risk. Methysergide withdrawal in the former case and steroid therapy in the latter case may give a good response. As with all inflammatory processes, steroids have little effect on advanced, acellular

fibrotic lesions. The use of ureteral catheters or percutaneous nephrostomy has a role with azotemic patients or those who are poor operative risks. Unless a tissue diagnosis is obtained, errors in diagnosis may result in improper or delayed treatment.[35]

A generous midline incision permits exposure from the level of the renal pedicles to the bladder. The abdominal viscera are palpated to exclude malignancies. Multiple deep biopsies are taken. Because most patients have bilateral disease, conservative treatment is indicated. On each involved side, the parietal peritoneum is incised lateral to the colon from the level of the iliac vessels to the hepatic or splenic flexure, respectively. The colon with its mesentery is reflected medially, exposing the fibrotic process (Fig. 36-2). The ureter is identified at the level of the iliac artery and isolated. Ureterolysis is performed from the level of the ureteropelvic junction to an area near the bladder. The fibrotic process can usually be unwrapped or stripped from the ureter like a peel, although some sharp dissection may be required. If this dissection is especially difficult, the surgeon should suspect neoplasm. Except for the biopsies, no attempt is made to excise the fibrotic process.

Ureterolysis alone is inadequate treatment unless something else is done to keep the ureter separated from the fibrotic process. This is accomplished by either intraperitoneal or lateral displacement of the ureter. With the former, the parietal peritoneum incision is closed posterior to the ureter with 2-0 chromic catgut suture. If possible, the entire ureter from the renal pelvis to the peritoneal reflection is placed intraperitoneally (Fig. 36-3). The entrance and exit windows must be loose enough to avoid stenosis and subsequent obstruction.[16]

When the fibrosis is especially extensive or there is intraperitoneal involvement, lateral displacement and fixation offer the best results. Ureterolysis is followed by displacement of the ureter laterally away from the fibrotic process. Three to five interrupted mattress sutures of 2-0 chromic catgut between the parietal peritoneum and the psoas or quadratus lumborum muscles are placed medial to the ureter, fixing it laterally (Fig. 36-4). The peritoneal defect is closed. Tressider and Blandy improved their results with intraperitoneal ureter placement by wrapping the ureter in an omental sleeve.[51]

These procedures usually result in the prompt resolution of symptoms and the normalization of laboratory data. On occasion, tight or dense involvement of a short ureteral segment will require

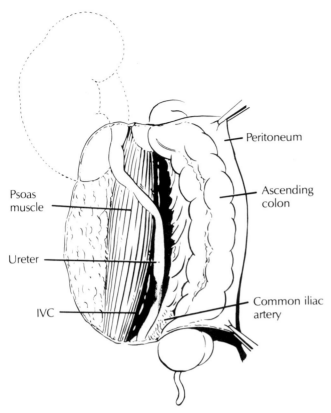

FIG. 36-2. Incision of the parietal peritoneum in the right colic gutter with mobilization of the ascending colon

primary excision and reanastomosis. Longer defects may need a bladder flap, ileal segment interposition, or even autotransplantation. Nephrectomy has a limited role because of the propensity for bilateral disease.

Corticosteroids have value in the management of recurrent obstruction following ureterolysis and as an adjunct to ureterolysis.[19,44] Long-term follow-up is mandatory to detect progressive disease.[42]

Retroperitoneal Tumors and Cysts

CLASSIFICATION

Primary retroperitoneal tumors are rare, representing as few as 0.2% of tumors in some series. Different series report lymphoma or sarcoma as the most common histopathologic type.[5,13,29,38] The many tissue types in the retroperitoneum, both mature and embryologic, may give rise to a broad spectrum of neoplasms or cystic lesions.[1] Eighty-five percent of primary retroperitoneal tumors are malignant, with lymphomatous tumors being the most common. Others include leiomyosarcoma, liposarcoma, rhabdomyosarcoma, and fibrosarcoma.[5,38,40] Most lesions are unresectable at initial exploration,[4,53] and the mortality after attempted resection is substantial.[12]

Lymphomatous tumors include lymphosarcoma, reticulum cell sarcoma, and Hodgkin's disease. CT (Fig. 36-5) and lymphangiography are valuable in delineating the extent of these tumors. Diagnosis can often be made through biopsy of a peripheral node. Treatment consists primarily of chemotherapy for systemic disease and irradiation for local control. The lesions are usually unresectable, but exploration is sometimes necessary for diagnostic purposes.

Leiomyosarcomas arise from blood vessels, the spermatic cord, and embryonic or wolffian elements. They grow rapidly and have a lobulated appearance with a pseudocapsule, cystic degeneration, hemorrhages, or calcifications. Benign leiomyomas are very rare. Treatment is surgical excision, although adjunctive irradiation has value.

Liposarcomas are among the most common retroperitoneal sarcomas. They have variable histologic features and can be divided into three types, with significant differences among them: lipomyxosarcoma, which has a high incidence of local recurrence but low metastatic propensity; differentiated liposarcoma, which is very difficult to distinguish from a lipoma (Fig. 36-6), has minimal metastatic potential, and is curable but only if totally excised; and pleomorphic liposarcoma, which is highly malignant and bears a resemblance to fibrosarcoma or rhabdomyosarcoma. Pre- and postoperative irradiation has value because these lesions are generally radiosensitive.

The majority of **rhabdomyosarcomas** are found in children less than 5 years of age and arise in undifferentiated mesenchyma. Treatment consists of combination chemotherapy and attempted surgical extirpation.

Retroperitoneal fibrosarcomas are rare, and benign fibromas are even more so. Surgery with wide excision is the treatment of choice. They are relatively radioresistant, but the likelihood of surgical removal of large fibrosarcomas and other nonlymphomatous retroperitoneal sarcomas is enhanced by preoperative chemotherapy or irradiation. Intra-arterial chemotherapy administration is favored if a specific major tumor vessel can be identified and cannulated. Cyclophosphamide, actinomycin D, doxorubicin (Adriamycin), and vincristine are among the agents shown to have value.

Most benign lesions are lipomas, abscesses, hematomas, or cysts. Thirty-five percent of **retroperitoneal lipomas** arise from perirenal fat. They are slow growing but have a tendency to recur, and some may in fact have elements of well-differentiated liposarcoma in them. They are treated by wide and complete excision because of this.

Retroperitoneal abscesses are more common in males. In children, they are usually caused by a gram-positive coccus metastatic from the tonsils, skin, or middle ear. In adults, the organism is commonly a gram-negative rod or anaerobe and arises from direct extension of inflammatory bowel disease or follows instrumentation of an infected lower urinary tract.[45] Common symptoms are fever, back pain, and often pain on leg extension (psoas sign). Treatment consists of extraperitoneal incision and drainage with appropriate antibiotic therapy.

Retroperitoneal hematomas are most commonly the result of blunt or penetrating trauma, anticoagulant therapy, or an iatrogenic cause. Flank ecchymosis, occasionally a mass effect, or hypotension are some clinical findings. Those hematomas due to anticoagulants and most iatrogenic causes can be managed conservatively as long as the clinical status is stable. Penetrating injuries are usually explored. Expanding hematomas due to blunt trauma require exploration.

Retroperitoneal cysts are rare and are classified according to the tissue of origin. Urogenital cysts arise from persistent remnants of the primitive urogenital system.[38] They are more common in females, perhaps arising from persistent wolffian elements. Cysts of mesocolic origin develop as a result of defective fusion of the peritoneal layers. Teratomatous and dermoid cysts are composed of multiple tissue types in varying degrees of histologic differentiation. Lymphatic or chylous cysts result from mechanical obstruction or defective development of these structures. Enterogenous cysts are of intestinal origin, including from a Meckel's diverticulum. Surgical excision is curative.

DIAGNOSIS

Most patients present late in their disease course with large, extensive tumors. Many have had symptoms for 6 months or more prior to seeking medical care. Pain is the most common complaint and is referred to the abdomen, back, or flank. Other symptoms include abdominal swelling, weight loss, weakness, nausea, constipation, edema, anorexia, adenopathy, anuria, fever, or painful varicocele. An abdominal mass or tenderness is the

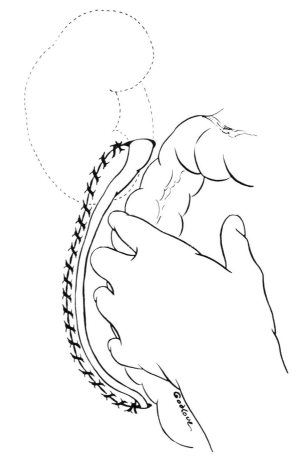

FIG. 36-3. Intraperitoneal displacement of the right ureter from the renal pelvis to the peritoneal reflection

most common physical finding. The differential diagnosis includes abnormalities of the kidney, liver, pancreas, gastrointestinal tract, spleen, ovary, or omentum, or abdominal aortic aneurysm.

The evaluation of retroperitoneal masses (excluding metastases from a known testicular primary) includes an IVP, CT scan, applicable gastrointestinal studies, and a lymphangiogram (for Hodgkin's disease or lymphoma). VMA (vanillylmandelic acid) studies and serum catecholamines are done for possible neuroblastoma, ganglioneuroma, or pheochromocytoma. Serum α-fetoprotein or serum β-subunit human chorionic gonadotropin may be elevated in primary retroperitoneal germ cell tumors.[46] With large masses, arteriography and venacavography provide a surgical road map to the mass, may demonstrate vena cava thrombosis and collateral formation, and provide a parameter to monitor therapy. Here again the CT scan plays a prominent diagnostic role. Before CT scans were used, the incidence of correct preoperative diag-

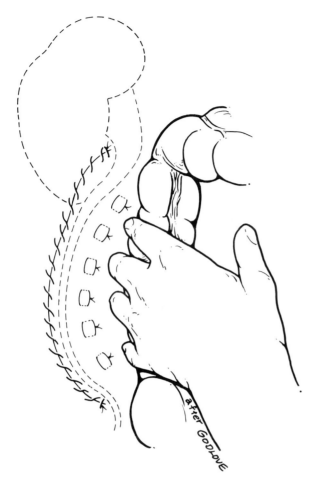

FIG. 36-4. Lateral displacement of the right ureter, with chromic catgut mattress sutures placed medially

nosis ranged from 37% to 64%.[3,34] The addition of this diagnostic tool should improve these statistics.

Pretreatment with chemotherapy or irradiation will render many lesions surgically resectable. A definite tissue diagnosis is necessary to establish a treatment plan, and in some patients a diagnostic laparotomy is needed. In others, more accessible lesions provide the diagnosis.

SURGICAL MANAGEMENT

Modern surgical management of retroperitoneal tumors uses the combined efforts of surgery, radiation therapy, and chemotherapy. Curative resection as a single mode of therapy is often futile because of the extensive disease at presentation. Recurrences are common and changes in histopathologic types can occur.[29] The high recurrence rate relates to the lack of encapsulation of these tumors and their easy spread along fascial planes and nerve trunks. Except for lymphomas, survival of patients with a malignant retroperitoneal mass correlates with its complete surgical resection.[21]

Incisions

Midline Transabdominal Incision. Roberts performed the first reported retroperitoneal node dissection in 1902.[41] This was performed transperitoneally and unfortunately the patient subsequently died of peritonitis. Because of this, the transabdominal approach fell into disfavor until the 1950s. Mallis and Patton stressed the relative safety of the midline transperitoneal incision for retroperitoneal surgery as the result of modern anesthesia, antibiotics, and surgical techniques.[27] Tobenkin, Binkley, and Smith described the combined mobilization of the right colon and the small intestine, so important in obtaining good exposure in retroperitoneal surgery.[50] This approach is now favored by many surgeons. The patient is supine and the incision is made in the midline from xiphoid to pubis, circumventing the umbilicus (Fig. 36-7A). Young recommends elevation of the kidney rest or the placement of rolled sheets under the lumbar spine to correct the relative concavity of this area when supine.[54] When there is extensive neoplastic thrombus in the vena cava, a midline abdominal incision can be extended with a median sternotomy to permit cardiopulmonary bypass. Chest tubes are advised in this circumstance.

Extraperitoneal Incision. Chevassu described an extraperitoneal node dissection in 1910.[6] Hinman proposed an extraperitoneal incision (Fig. 36-7B) extending from the tip of the 12th rib anteriorly to the lateral border of the rectus muscle and then inferiorly to the superior border of the pubis.[17] Lewis and associates described an incision (Fig. 36-7C) beginning at the posterior axillary line between the 10th and 11th ribs that was continued anteriorly and inferiorly the same as Hinman's.[24] If the pleural cavity was entered inadvertently, it was immediately closed without the routine use of a thoracotomy tube. Nagamatsu combined his dorsolumbar flap incision with a Cherney incision that extended across the lower abdomen (Fig. 36-7D).[32,33] This extensive incision provides a considerable exposure of the retroperitoneum, but staying out of the pleural cavity can be difficult. Exposure adequate for most procedures can be obtained with a transabdominal or thoracoabdominal approach that requires less time and dissection.

Thoracoabdominal Incision. Advantages of the thoracoabdominal incision for high retroperitoneal masses were described in the 1940s.[8,28,31,47]

FIG. 36-5. A CT scan demonstrates massive retroperitoneal lymph node enlargement (N) due to lymphoma; C = vena cava; A = aorta with calcifications in its wall

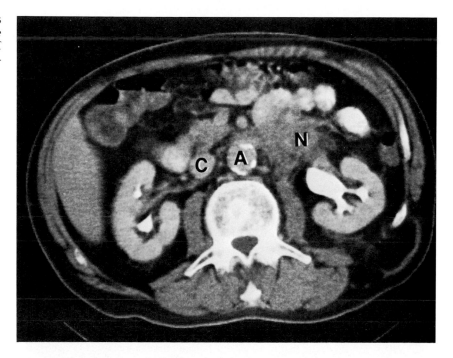

FIG. 36-6. A CT scan demonstrates a massive retroperitoneal liposarcoma. The peritoneal contents are displaced far anteriorly. C = vena cava, A = aorta

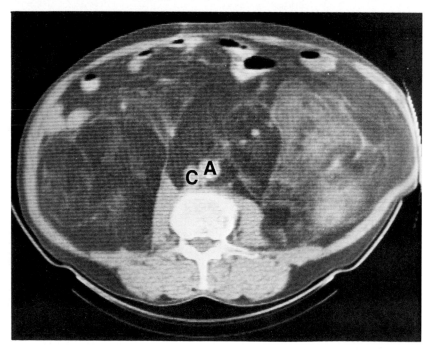

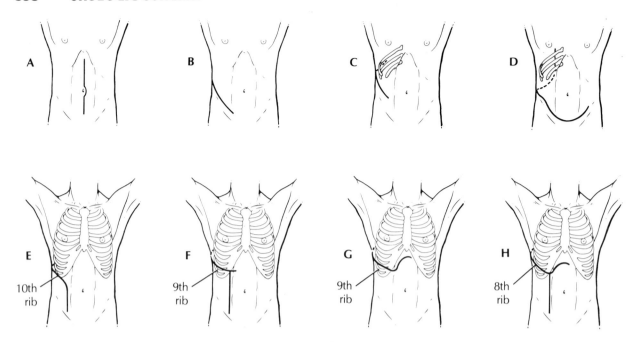

FIG. 36-7. Incisions for exposure of the retroperitoneal space: **(A)** classical midline, **(B)** Hinman, **(C)** thoracoabdominal approach (Lewis), **(D)** extrapleural extraperitoneal (Nagamatsu), **(E)** Cooper and associates, **(F)** Fraley and associates, **(G)** Cole and associates, **(H)** Merrill

Cooper and associates advocated its use for lymphadenectomy with testes tumors (Fig. 36-7E).[10] They used an incision through the bed of the 10th rib. Fraley and associates raised the thoracic incision to the 9th rib bed. It was extended to the midline and a paramedial vertical incision dropped from the appropriate position (Fig. 36-7F).[14] This increased the access to the contralateral retroperitoneum. Cole and associates described a thoracosubcostal incision arising in the 9th rib bed and continuing to the contralateral border of the rectus muscle (Fig. 36-7G), permitting wider exposure of the contralateral upper retroperitoneum.[9] Merrill combined the efforts of Cole and Fraley and raised the thoracic incision to the 8th rib bed (Fig. 36-7H).[30] This combines the wide upper retroperitoneal and caudal exposures necessary in some patients, although a less extensive incision will usually suffice.

The pelvis is rotated slightly by the placement of a small rolled sheet or sandbag under its ipsilateral aspect. The upper torso is rotated until the shoulders form an angle of 50 to 60 degrees with the table. The arm on the ipsilateral side is supported on an armrest on the opposite side of the table. Rolled sheets help to maintain this position. The table is flexed, increasing the distance between

the rib margin and the anterior superior iliac crest. Adhesive tape placed from the operating table over the ipsilateral shoulder to the armrest and a similar tape over the bony prominence of the hip help support the position. An axillary roll should be used in this surgical position to protect the brachial plexus (Fig. 36-8).

The incision is carried down from the midaxillary line over a rib at the level appropriate for the position and size of the mass. It is continued medially to a point determined by the type of incision chosen. The inferior arm of the incision continues as an ipsilateral paramedian or occasionally a midline incision to a point sufficient for the dissection.

Pitts and Marshall reviewed their experience with 210 radical retroperitoneal excisions using transabdominal or thoracoabdominal incisions.[39] They found that the flank thoracoabdominal approach was superior for access to the ipsilateral renal hilus, the suprarenal area, and the ipsilateral chest and mediastinum.

Operative Techniques

The surgeon should be prepared for any eventuality, including resection of the vena cava, aortic replacement, and bowel or partial pancreatic re-

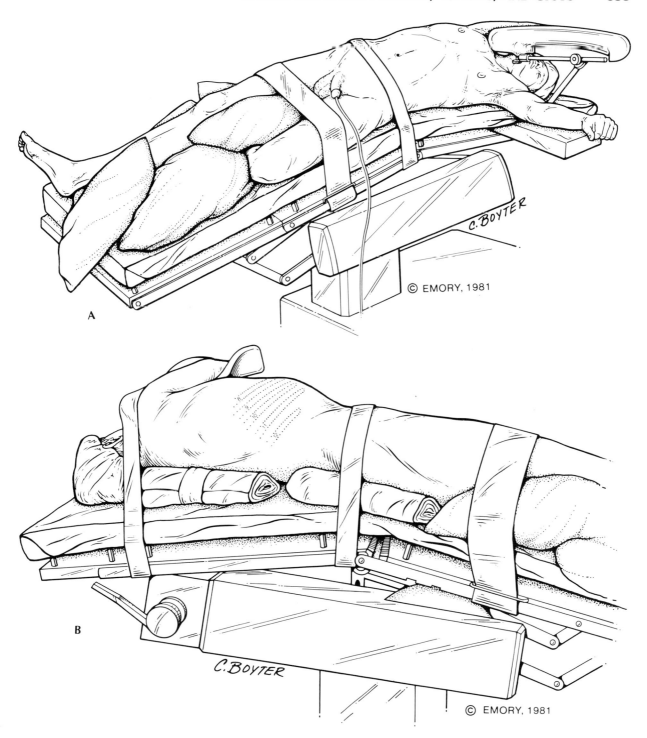

FIG. 36-8. Patient position for a thoracoabdominal incision

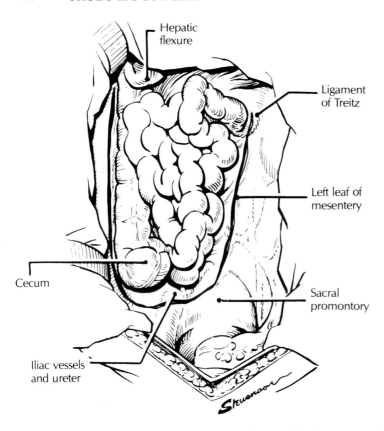

Hepatic flexure

Ligament of Treitz

Left leaf of mesentery

Cecum

Sacral promontory

Iliac vessels and ureter

FIG. 36-9. Mobilization of the small intestines and ascending colon

section, or have ready access to specialists skilled in these procedures. A bowel prep is a wise precaution with extensive lesions.

Upon entering the abdominal cavity, the liver, kidneys, pancreas, spleen, and retroperitoneal nodes are palpated to gauge the extent of disease. The small bowel is reflected to the right and the retroperitoneum is entered by incising the parietal peritoneum from below the cecum to the ligament of Treitz, which is then divided. This incision is extended up the right lateral gutter to the hepatic flexure (Fig. 36-9). The small bowel, ascending and transverse colon, pancreas, duodenum, and spleen, if necessary, are completely mobilized on a superior mesenteric artery pedicle and reflected out of the abdomen into an intestinal bag. This pedicle must be protected carefully because the superior mesenteric artery is not expendable (Fig. 36-10). The inferior mesenteric artery is ligated, if necessary, to provide increased exposure of the lesion. Incision of the left lateral gutter is usually not necessary. In younger patients, the inferior mesenteric artery may be ligated with impunity if the marginal artery is intact. However, in some older patients bowel ischemia may occur with postoperative diarrhea or mild mesenteric angina. This maneuver permits mobilization of the mesentery of the de-

scending colon and completes the exposure of the retroperitoneum. If a segment of the descending colon does not appear viable, this segment is resected with a primary reanastomosis and diverting colostomy.[46]

As part of a tumor or node resection, lumbar vessels may be ligated below the level of the renal vessels with little risk of spinal cord ischemia, because a significant proportion of its blood supply originates above the renal vessels.[11,46,49] In older patients or those with clinical atherosclerosis or diabetes, alternate contralateral lumber arteries may be preserved without excessive loss of exposure.[30] Lumbar vessels should be ligated and not clipped if possible. In selected cases, aortic resection with bypass graft or vena cava resection is required because of tumor invasion. Many cases of vena cava resection require *en bloc* removal of the right kidney. McCullough and Gittes and Skinner stress the importance in these situations of maintaining a connection between the left renal vein and the remaining vena cava.[26,46] Postoperative morbidity is substantial when this is not accomplished.

As mentioned earlier, the cisterna chyli lies dorsal and slightly medial to the aorta at the level of the L1 and L2 vertebral bodies. Careful ligation

FIG. 36-10. Exposure of the retroperitoneal space. The inferior mesenteric and marginal arteries are intact.

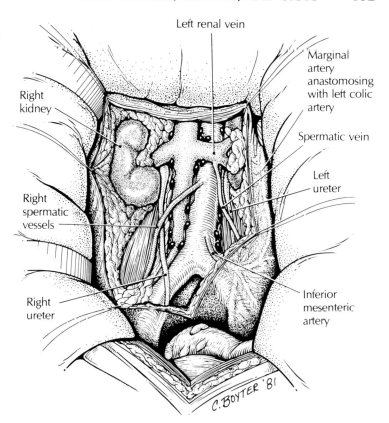

Left renal vein

Right kidney

Marginal artery anastomosing with left colic artery

Spermatic vein

Left ureter

Right spermatic vessels

Inferior mesenteric artery

Right ureter

C. BOYTER '81

of all lymphatic channels in this area is important to prevent a leak with subsequent chylous ascites. Cauterization of the cisterna chyli or major lymphatics is not adequate, and clips may dislodge. If dissection around the renal vessels is anticipated, mannitol should be administered prior to this dissection to induce a diuresis. The topical application of 1% lidocaine to the renal vessels at intervals during the dissection also helps prevent the spasm and subsequent oliguria sometimes seen in this setting. The ureters must be identified and their location ascertained throughout the procedure. The ureter's adventitial sheath must be widely preserved.

At the completion of the resection, the kidneys are inspected to be certain that the perfusion appears adequate. The abdominal viscera are replaced, and the parietal peritoneum is reconstructed with interrupted 3-0 silk sutures placed 2 cm to 3 cm apart. This is reapproximated along both the right colic gutter and the base of the small bowel mesentery. The spacing of the sutures permits free flow of lymphatic fluid and exudate into the peritoneal cavity, where absorption can occur because no retroperitoneal drains are used. If the procedure is performed through a completely retroperitoneal approach, then drains are advisable.

With thoracoabdominal incisions, a chest tube is inserted through an interspace above the incision in the midaxillary line, positioned along the posterior chest under direct vision, and sutured securely to the skin. This is attached to underwater seal for 2 to 3 days after surgery. The pleura is closed with a continuous 3-0 polyglycolic suture. The proper position of the nasogastric tube in the stomach is confirmed, and the operating table is unflexed to facilitate wound closure. The diaphragm is closed with interrupted, figure-of-eight 0 silk sutures. The thoracic part of an incision is closed with a continuous 0 Prolene suture, interrupted at every fourth or fifth stitch and tied. The abdomen is closed with a No. 1 Prolene suture using the same technique, taking good bites of the fascia. Nasogastric drainage is usually required for 3 to 4 days.

Complications

Complications are similar to the complications seen after any major abdominal procedure and include atelectasis, prolonged ileus, small bowel obstruction, wound infection, and phlebitis. Two complications deserve special mention: lymphocele formation and ejaculatory disturbances. Lymphoceles are uncommon following upper retroperitoneal surgery, especially with transperitoneal approaches. When they do occur, a transabdominal approach with marsupialization of the collection into the peritoneal cavity generally solves the problem. Ejaculatory disturbances are not uncommon following extensive retroperitoneal surgery and are related to the extent of injury of the lumbar sympathetic chains. This is discussed in greater detail in Chapter 37.

REFERENCES

1. ACKERMAN LV: Tumors of the retroperitoneum, mesentery and peritoneum. In Atlas of Tumor Pathology, sect. 6, fascs 23 and 24, p 136. Washington, DC, Armed Forces Institute of Pathology, 1954

2. ALBARRAN J: L'Rétention rénale par petriuréterite; Liberation externe de l'uretére. Ass Fr Urol 9:511, 1905

3. ARMSTRONG JR, COHN I, JR: Primary malignant retroperitoneal tumors. Am J Surg 110:937, 1965

4. BEK V: Primary retroperitoneal tumours. Neoplasma 17:253, 1970

5. BRAASCH JW, MON AB: Primary retroperitoneal tumors. Surg Clin North Am 47:663, 1967

6. CHEVASSU M: Deux cas d'epithéliome du testicule traités par la castration et l'ablation des ganglions lomboaortique. Bull Mem Soc Chir Paris 36:236, 1910

7. CHAN SL, JOHNSON HW, MCLOUGHLIN MG: Idiopathic retroperitoneal fibrosis in children. J Urol. 122:103, 1979

8. CHUTE R, SOUTTER L, KERR WS, JR: Value of thoracoabdominal incision in removal of kidney tumors. N Engl J Med 241:951,1949

9. COLE AT, FRIED FA, BISSADA NK: The supine subcostal modification of the thoracoabdominal incision. J Urol 112:168, 1974

10. COOPER JF, LEADBETTER WF, CHUTE R: The thoracoabdominal approach for retroperitoneal gland dissection: Its application to testis tumors. Surg Gynecol Obstet, 90:486, 1950

11. COUPLAND GA, REEVE TS: Paraplegia: A complication of excision of abdominal aortic aneurysm. Surgery 64:878, 1968

12. DEWEERD JH, DOCKERTY MB: Lipomatous retroperitoneal tumors. Am J Surg 84:397, 1952

13. DONNELLY BA: Primary retroperitoneal tumors; A report of 95 cases and a review of the literature. Surg Gynecol Obstet 83:705, 1946

14. FRALEY EE, MARKLAND C, KEDIA K: Treatment of testicular tumors. Minn Med 56:593, 1973

15. HACHE L, UTZ DC, WOOLNER LB: Idiopathic fibrous retroperitonitis. Surg Gynecol Obstet 115:737, 1962

16. HEWITT CB, NITZ GL, KISER WS et al: Surgical treatment of retroperitoneal fibrosis. Ann Surg 169:610, 1969

17. HINMAN F: The Principles and Practice of Urology. Philadelphia, W B Saunders, 1935

18. IKARD RW: Iatrogenic chylous ascites. Am Surg 38:436, 1972

19. KEARNEY GP, MAHONEY EM, SCIAMMAS FD et al: Venacavography, corticosteroids and surgery in the management of idiopathic retroperitoneal fibrosis. J Urol 115:32, 1976

20. KERR WS, JR, SUBY HI, VICKERY A et al: Idiopathic retroperitoneal fibrosis: Clinical experience with 15 cases, 1956–1967. J Urol 99:575, 1968

21. KINNE DW, CHU FC, HUVOS AG et al: Treatment of primary and recurrent retroperitoneal liposarcoma. Twenty-five year experience at Memorial Hospital. Cancer 31:53, 1973

22. KOEP L, ZUIDEMA GD: The clinical significance of retroperitoneal fibrosis. Surgery 81:250, 1977

23. LEPOR H, WALSH PC: Idiopathic retroperitoneal fibrosis. J Urol 122:1, 1979

24. LEWIS EL, JOHNSTON RE, ROWE RB et al: Retroperitoneal lymph node resection: The intercostoinguinal approach. J. Urol 67:338, 1952

25. LONGMIRE WP, JR, GOODWIN WE, BUCKBERG GD: Management of sclerosing fibrosis of the mediastinal and retroperitoneal areas. Ann Surg 165:1013, 1967

26. MCCULLOUGH DL, GITTES RF: Ligation of the renal vein in the solitary kidney: Effects on renal function. J Urol 113:295, 1975

27. MALLIS N, PATTON JF: Transperitoneal bilateral lymphadenectomy in testis tumor. J Urol 80:501, 1958

28. MARSHALL DF: Urogenital wounds in an evacuation hospital. J Urol 55:119, 1946

29. MELLICOW MM: Primary tumors of the retroperitoneum: A clinicopathologic analysis of 162 cases; Review of the literature and tables of classification. J Int Coll Surg 19:401, 1953

30. MERRILL DC: Modified thoraco-abdominal approach to the kidney and retroperitoneal tissue. J Urol 117:15, 1977

31. MORTENSEN H: Transthoracic nephrectomy. J Urol 60:855, 1948

32. NAGAMATSU G: A new extraperitoneal approach for bilateral retroperitoneal lymph node dissection in testis tumor. J Urol 90:588, 1963

33. NAGAMATSU GR, LERMAN PH, BERMAN MH: The dorsolumbar flap incision in urologic surgery. J Urol 67:787, 1952

34. NEWMAN HR, PINCK BD: Primary retroperitoneal tumors; A summation of 33 cases. Arch Surg 60:879, 1950

35. NITZ GL, HEWITT CB, STRAFFON RA et al: Retroperitoneal malignancy masquerading as benign retroperitoneal fibrosis. J Urol 103:46, 1970

36. ORMOND JK: Bilateral ureteral obstruction due to envelopment and compression by an inflammatory retroperitoneal process. J Urol 59:1072, 1948

37. OSCHNER MG, BRANNAN W, POND HS et al: Medical therapy in idiopathic retroperitoneal fibrosis. J Urol 114:700, 1975

38. PACK GT, TABAK EJ: Collective review; Primary retroperitoneal tumors; A study of 120 cases. Surg Gynecol Obstet 99:209, 1954

39. PITTS WR, JR, MARSHALL VF: Radical retroperitoneal surgery: A 25 year experience. J Urol 119:37, 1978
40. RHAMY RK: Retroperitoneal Tumors. In Glenn JF, Boyce WH (eds): Urologic Surgery, 2nd ed, p 859. New York, Harper & Row, 1975
41. ROBERTS JB: Excision of the lumbar lymphatic nodes and spermatic vein in malignant disease of the testicle. Ann Surg 36:539, 1902
42. SANDERS RC, DUFFY T, MCLOUGHLIN MG et al: Sonography in the diagnosis of retroperitoneal fibrosis. J Urol 118:944, 1977
43. SAXTON HM, KILPATRICK FR, KINDER CH et al: Retroperitoneal fibrosis. A radiological and follow-up study of fourteen cases. Q J Med 38:159, 1969
44. SHAKEEN DJ, JOHNSTON A: Bilateral ureteral obstruction due to envelopment and compression by an inflammatory retroperitoneal process: Report of two cases. J Urol 82:51, 1959
45. SIROKY MB, MOYLAN R, AUSTEN G, JR et al: Metastatic infection secondary to genitourinary tract sepsis. Am J Med 61:351, 1976
46. SKINNER DG: Considerations for management of large retroperitoneal tumors: Use of the modified thoracoabdominal approach. J Urol 117:605, 1977
47. SWEET RH: Carcinoma of the esophagus and cardiac end of the stomach: Immediate and late results of treatment by resection and primary esophagogastric anastomosis. JAMA 135:485, 1947
48. SWEETSER TH: Retroperitoneal tumors influencing the kidneys and ureters. J Urol 47:619, 1942
49. TAVEL FR, OSIUS TG, PARKER JW et al: Retroperitoneal lymph node dissection. J Urol 89:241, 1963
50. TOBENKIN MI, BINKLEY FM, SMITH DR: Exposure of the retroperitoneum for radical dissection of lymph nodes. J Urol 86:596, 1961
51. TRESSIDDER GC, BLANDY JP, SINGH M: Omental sleeve to prevent recurrent retroperitoneal fibrosis around the ureter. Urol Int 27:144, 1972
52. WEBB AJ: Cytological studies in retroperitoneal fibrosis. Br J Surg 54:375, 1967
53. WILEY AL, WIRTANEN GW, JOO P et al: Clinical and theoretical aspects of the treatment of surgically unresectable retroperitoneal malignancy with combined intra-arterial actinomycin D and radiotherapy. Cancer 36:107, 1975
54. YOUNG JD, JR: Retroperitoneal Surgery. In Glenn JF, Boyce WH (eds): Urologic Surgery, 2nd ed, p 854. New York, Harper & Row, 1975

Retroperitoneal Lymphadenectomy

37

John P. Donohue

Retroperitoneal lymphadenectomy is currently undergoing careful scrutiny, and rightly so. Improvements in noninvasive surgical staging such as computed tomography (CT) scans combined with lymphangiogram and serologic markers are refining the accuracy of clinical noninvasive staging. Our own experience reveals a 30% false-negative clinical-staging rate, but the technology of our CT scanning was a relatively early state of the art and was not combined with lymphangiography. Several important clinical studies here and abroad are comparing clinical staging and careful follow-up (with chemotherapy at relapse) to retroperitoneal lymphadenectomy for pathologic staging (with chemotherapy at relapse). Although the studies are in the early phases, preliminary evidence suggests that the role for retroperitoneal lymphadenectomy for staging alone may sharply diminish and even disappear; however, such data are not yet available in large enough numbers nor long enough follow-up. Therefore, there remains a role for retroperitoneal lymphadenectomy in the accurate pathologic staging of testicular cancer and the assignment of appropriate possible adjuvant chemotherapy in those with resected nodal disease. Clearly, those with positive nodes have had a therapeutic procedure as well as a pathologic staging procedure. Yet even those with "negative nodes" enjoy a survival advantage and a reduced subsequent relapse rate (only 7% in our experience). However, clinical Stage A patients bypassing node dissection entirely have subsequent relapse rates from 20% to 40%. Micrometastatic disease resected but not sampled by the pathologist may explain this enhancement of disease-free state after node dissection in patients with negative nodes.

Special Preoperative Preparation and Medical Notes

Patients who are to undergo a retroperitoneal lymphadenectomy are prepared, as a donor for renal transplantation would be, with overnight intravenous hydration. We use no antibiotics preoperatively or postoperatively.

The bladder is catheterized at the time of draping in surgery. The catheter is usually removed on the second postoperative day. The patient is in the supine position, with the right arm suspended from an ether screen or with both arms extended. Topical 1% lidocaine (Xylocaine) is used on the renal vessels during the dissection. Otherwise, falsely high, misleading hematocrit values may follow. An increased need for crystalloid also is apparent, because the losses from the intravascular space into the large, raw third space created in the retroperitoneum can produce significant contraction of effective blood volume. Transfusions of whole blood are often unnecessary in uncomplicated cases if enough colloid replacement is given.

Preoperative emphasis is put on pulmonary physiotherapy to assist the patient postoperatively in this regard. Again, no prophylactic antibiotics are used. If fever develops, appropriate cultures and investigations are made and then the drug is selected, but this is rarely necessary.

Surgical Approach

The surgical approach to the retroperitoneum can be either anterior (transabdominal midline) or anterolateral (thoracoabdominal). Each has its advantages.

The rationale and technique of the anterior approach for retroperitoneal lymphadenectomy for the purpose of staging nonseminomatous germinal cell tumors of the testis have been well described by Patton and Mallis, Staubitz and associates, Van Buskirk and Young, Whitmore.[13,20,21,23] Also, Young described this approach in the second edition of this text, Urologic Surgery.[25]

An alternative approach to the retroperitoneum for staging testicular tumors by lymphadenectomy was championed by Leadbetter and colleagues.[1,19] He preferred the thoracoabdominal approach, which affords exposure above the renal hili. This approach has been followed, with some modifications, by Fraley and associates and Skinner.[11,18]

Fifteen years ago, we asked ourselves, "Can the midline approach also be developed to allow ex-

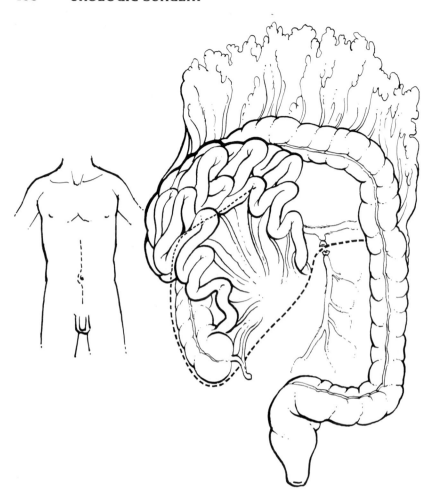

FIG. 37-1. The basic mesenteric divisions are made: the right mesocolon into the foramen of Winslow, the root of the small bowel to the ligament of Treitz, division of the inferior mesenteric vein and the right colic mesentery to the renal upper pole. The bowel is then separated from Gerota's fascia below it and placed in a plastic bowel bag on the patient's chest.

cellent exposure of the suprarenal-hilar zones for the purpose of lymphadenectomy?'' Postmortem dissections of the retroperitoneum were done through a midline incision from xiphoid to pubis to determine whether this approach could equal the high exposure afforded by the thoracoabdominal approach. As of this writing, more than 300 patients with nonseminomatous germinal tumors of the testis have been staged by high retroperitoneal lymphadenectomy through the anterior approach, using the techniques described herein to afford optimum exposure and nodal clearance.

Surgical Technique

EXPOSURE

The incision is midline, xiphoid to pubis. Drapes are sewn in place and an 11-inch (28-cm) circular plastic wound protector is used; then two Balfour abdominal retractors are placed. The abdomen is explored carefully by palpation, and the basic mesenteric divisions are made in order to mobilize the entire small bowel and right colon so that they can be placed on the patient's chest in a plastic bowel bag (Fig. 37-1). First the hepatic flexure is taken down and then the mesocolon is incised from the foramen of Winslow to the cecum. It is important to extend this posterior peritoneal incision through the base of the foramen of Winslow, which covers the anterior surface of the vena cava, because later dissection must extend above this area.

After the right mesocolon is divided, the incision is turned around and the root of the small bowel is incised cephalad to the ligament of Treitz. This incision is carried along the root of the bowel until the inferior mesenteric vein is encountered. This vein must be divided to carry the incision in an oblique manner further cephalad, still further into the left upper quadrant, paralleling the inferior border of the pancreas. If the inferior mesenteric vein is not divided, it will restrict the exposure in this area. When the inferior mesenteric vein is divided, the pancreas can be mobilized fully and retracted off the anterior surface of Gerota's fascia. The anterior surface of Gerota's fascia is then separated bluntly and sharply from the undersurface of the bowel and the pancreatic head and body, as well as the duodenum and cecum. All of this is now completely mobilized and the bowel is placed on the chest in a bowel bag. We no longer recommend a routine appendectomy (the appendiceal stump leaked in one of our cases, producing massive peritonitis and abscess formation). The retroperitoneum is a rich culture medium postoperatively; all potential sources of contamination should be avoided.

INFRARENAL DISSECTION (AORTOCAVAL DISSECTION)

In infrarenal dissection, or aortocaval dissection, the nodal package is split anteriorly down over the inferior vena cava and aorta. The specimen is then rotated off the vessels. It is useful to divide every lumbar vessel, both aortic and caval, so as to get complete mobilization and central vascular control. Another important maneuver is the squaring out of the upper corners of the nodal package at each renal hilus and taking it down off the posterior body wall at the foramen of L2-L3 (Figs. 37-2 and 37-3). The lateral borders of the dissection are the ureters; the psoas fascia is tripped down parallel to this. The gonadal vein is divided on the left from the renal vein or on the right from the inferior vena cava. The involved gonadal vein is then followed down to its origin in the groin and dissected out separately and submitted to the pathologist separately.

Care is taken to obtain the divided stump of the spermatic cord with its original ligtures, if at all possible. The vas deferens is clipped and divided so that the distal portion can be submitted with the spermatic vein and cord stump. On the left side this is then tunneled under the left colic mesenteric artery. The aortic dissection is continued distally by dividing the inferior mesenteric artery. The left colic mesentery is then further mobilized off Gerota's fascia, and the sphlanchnic nervous and venous connections are clipped where necessary to mobilize this thoroughly and hence expose the iliac areas from the medial approach without having to divide the left mesocolon. The left ureter is then easily seen over the pelvic brim. As noted earlier, the nodal packages are rotated

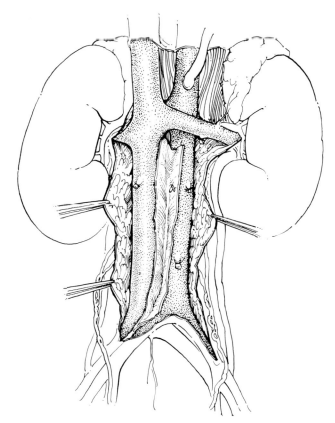

FIG. 37-2. The infrahilar aortocaval dissection involves the anterior longitudinal splitting of the nodal and vascular adventitia over the vena cava and the aorta, its lateral rotation, and the squaring out of the posterolateral nodal tissue.

off the anterior surfaces of both vessels, the dissection being advanced in the subadventitial planes. This allows easy exposure of each lumbar artery and vein and their division between 2-0 silk ligatures. Now the great vessels are completely mobilized (Figs. 37-4 and 37-5). The only thing holding the unfurled nodal package is its posterior and lateral attachments.

Each lumbar artery and venous penetration into the posterior body wall is divided between clips or ligatures. Bleeding venous tributaries are often controlled by Bovie coagulation or additional suture ligature (see Fig. 37-4). Once the posterior attachments are divided at the foramina, the nodal package can be wiped off the anterior spinous ligaments with a gauze sponge and drawn under the vessels either medially or laterally. It is convenient for the nodal analysis to submit the aortocaval package of nodes separately and then later to submit the two iliac dissections separately. Formerly, the entire specimen was obtained *en bloc*

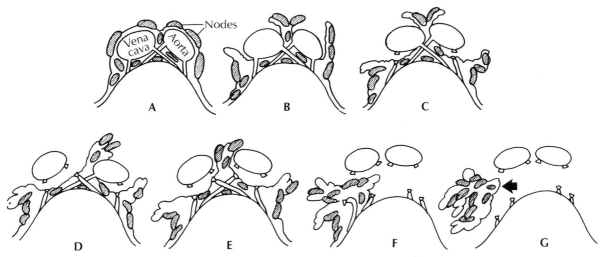

FIG. 37-3.   An axial view showing the anterior split of the nodal package in the subadventitial plane **(B)** and its rotation off the vena cava and aorta after the division of each lumbar vessel **(C, D,** and **E).** The specimen is removed from the posterior body wall by ligating and sharply dividing all the lumbar vessels and ganglia as they emerge from the foramina. After these posterior attachments are divided, the specimen is easily rotated under the mobilized great vessels.

FIG. 37-4.   At the conclusion of the dissection, the anterior spinous ligaments and the medial psoas muscle are seen stripped bare. The lumbar vessels are tied off on the body wall as well as on the great vessels. Each foramen is clear of nodal tissue. Fully mobilized great vessels allow thorough inspection.

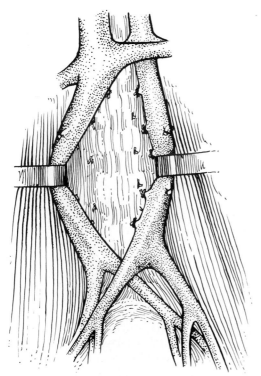

and laid out on a predrawn template for the pathologist. There were some errors in nodal location once the tissue was placed in formalin, because occasionally the tissue would float off the paper template.

The iliac dissections extend several centimeters beyond the bifurcation of the hypogastric artery on either side. The same principal of nodal rotation beneath the vessels is employed. The anterior division of the arteries and veins is carried out and the tissue is rotated below these after the division of any lumbar attachments. It is important to mobilize the psoas muscle in retractors because the nodal chain in the paravertebral area here is often large but not clearly visible without mobilization of the psoas. Again, the right iliac and left iliac nodal packages are submitted separately.

The wound is then thoroughly inspected and irrigated. When tumor invasion of the nodes is grossly evident, we irrigate with distilled water, which might lyse any tumor cells that might have been spilled in the wound during dissection. Then we close the mesenteric attachment with running 1-0 chromic catgut beginning at the left posterior colonic mesentery in the left upper quadrant and proceeding below the pancreas to the ligament of Treitz. Closure is then carried down, closing the root of the small bowel to the cecum up to the foramen of Winslow. We believe that this helps to prevent postoperative bowel complications and that it limits the escape of bloody lymphatic fluid into the peritoneal cavity. The omentum is drawn down over the bowel. The position of the Levin tube is checked. The midline incision is closed with interrupted No. 1 Ethibond sutures placed in the manner of Tom Jones. Buried knots are tied below the fascia to avoid uncomfortable nodules in the subcutaneous tissue in thin patients.

SUPRARENAL HILAR DISSECTION

Suprarenal hilar dissection refers to nodes above the level of the renal artery extending for several centimeters both above and below the crura of the diaphragm (Figs. 37-6 and 37-7). The lymphatic drainage of the retroperitoneum above the renal vessels is largely retrocrural as it moves into the cisterna chyli just above this level. The cisterna is between the aorta and cava on the anterior spinous ligaments at the L1, T12 levels. Most of the major lymphatic drainage from the retroperitoneum moves cephalad through this posterior route. There are also smaller nodes and lymphatics on the surface of the crura and medial to each adrenal gland, intermingled with nerves and ganglia. Whereas the major nodes below the level of the renal veins lie mostly anterior and lateral to the great vessels, these smaller nodes and lymphatics assume a posterior lateral relationship to the aorta above the renal vessels. CT scans confirm this as the locus of most bulky suprahilar metastases; they can be seen lying below the crura of the diaphragm on axial views extending to the posterior mediastinum in the chest.

Earlier communications have demonstrated the impracticality of dissecting the suprarenal hilar zones in patients with no gross disease.[5] Our experience has been largely negative in analysis of nodal tissue taken from this zone in patients with Stage B_1 disease. No patient with right-sided primary tumor and a grossly unimpressive retroperitoneum had positive suprahilar nodes. In like manner, only three patients with left-sided primaries and Stage B_1 disease had suprahilar nodes; two of these three had their nodes lying just above the renal artery in what could be called the renal hilus. There was only one patient with a discrete node 1 cm or 2 cm above the renal artery medial to the left adrenal who had negative nodes below the hilum. Therefore, on a "net yield" basis, such an extended dissection in patients without gross disease is unnecessary and unwarranted.

On the other hand, patients with gross disease in the retroperitoneum, particularly those with multiple grossly enlarged nodes (larger than 3 cm in diameter), had positive suprahilar nodes in about

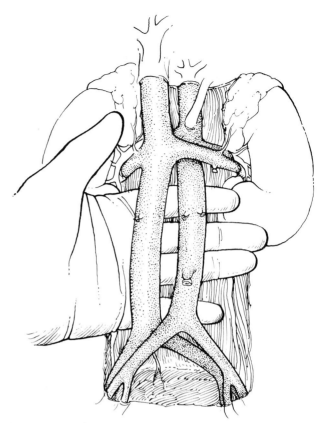

FIG. 37-5. The aorta and the inferior vena cava can be manipulated easily during and after the dissection when all the lumbar vessels and the inferior mesenteric artery have been divided. Hemostasis is easily secured with this exposure and vascular mobility. Complete clearance of nodes and removal of bulky tumor deposits are achieved better with this central vascular control.

one out of four cases. Also, those patients with massive (B_3) disease had positive involvement in this area by direct extension of their nodal tumor, which was centralized below the hilus but extended above it. In early-stage disease (B_1) suprahilar involvement and contralateral involvement are rare. Therefore, in grossly negative retroperitoneal dissections, the modified bilateral dissection as proposed by Ray, Hajdu, and Whitmore should suffice.[15] In cases where there is gross disease, a suprahilar dissection can be developed.

In recent times we have found it convenient to save the suprahilar dissection until the infrahilar (main aortocaval) dissection is done. The major suprahilar nodes are posterior at the foramina and medial to the crura of the diaphragm. Their exposure and removal is facilitated by prior complete aortic and caval mobilization, renal vascular dissection, and removal of infrahilar nodal tissue from

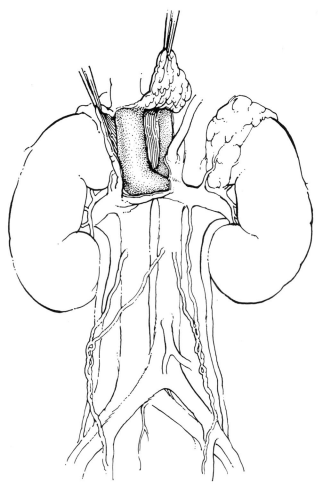

FIG. 37-6. The right suprahilar dissection (unnecessary in the absence of gross disease) extends up the aorta from the superior mesenteric artery, onto the crus of the diaphragm, over to the medial aspect of the right adrenal gland 4 cm to 6 cm above the right renal artery, then down the medial border of the right adrenal gland to the right renal artery and along the renal artery back to the aorta. The major nodes are retrocrural.

the posterior body wall. The extension of nodal tissue from infrahilar to suprahilar zones is then readily appreciated by elevating the renal vessels in vein retractors. Also, the crural muscle fibers can be seen to cover these nodes. The crural muscle can be retracted or split to gain access to the occasional large node here. Usually they can be grasped in broad Russian or Shingley forceps and extracted from this space, with care taken to secure approximate lymphatic channels in vascular clips.

The dissection on the surface of the crura begins at the base of the superior mesenteric artery. With the head and body of the pancreas padded and elevated by two deep Harrington retractors, both

the right and left crus can be dissected clean. The basic technique involves clipping along the base of the superior mesenteric artery and celiac artery, then across along the dorsum of each respective renal artery, and finally laterally along the border of the adrenal. This small wedge of tissue contains fat lymphatics, ganglia, and lymph nodal tissue, but these are not the major nodes draining the testis. As noted earlier, the major nodal tissue is below the surface of the crus and posterolateral to the aorta.

Cytoreductive Surgery Following Chemotherapy

There are several special considerations of a technical nature when approaching the patient pretreated with combination chemotherapy for cytoreduction of masses or disseminated disease. Preoperative considerations are assessment of the bulk and location of the tumor by CT scan. This will direct the choice of incision. The very large persistent lesion in the hilar or suprahilar region is best approached by thoracoabdominal incision on the ipsilateral or involved side. If the disease is very extensive and equally bulky across the midline, the incision can be carried transabdominally as well. Also, preoperative pulmonary function studies and pO_2 values on room air are very useful in assessing the patient's postoperative blood gases. Many patients tolerate relatively low pO_2 postoperatively because it represents their preoperative status quo. It is important to get them off the ventilator as soon as possible and to avoid excessive hydration with crystalloid.[7,12]

At surgery, the bowel is reflected in the usual manner and set aside in a bowel bag for optimal exposure of the retroperitoneal mass lesion (Fig. 37-8). We have demonstrated in an earlier report the immense variety of histologic subtypes in these tumor masses.[6] A mere biopsy will be insufficient in providing accurate tissue diagnosis. Therefore, a full retroperitoneal lymph node dissection (RPLND) should be done for ideal clearance of potential tumor and complete histopathology sampling.

In order to do a complete RPLND in a retroperitoneum occupied by bulky disease, it is often necessary to dissect either below or on the adventitia of the great vessels and reflect the tumor off in this manner (Fig. 37-9). Usually sharp dissection with scissors or scalpel blade will effectively roll off a tumor, provided it is gently retracted with right-angle clamps or attached to the adventitia and tumor capsule (Fig. 37-10). The inferior mesenteric artery and the lumbar arteries are best divided prospectively after ligature and clipping to give the vessels mobility and allow resection from the posterior body wall more safely. The tumor mass can usually be separated from the ureter and the kidney. At times, however, these structures are inseparably bound within the tumor mass and are best removed *en bloc* with the tumor, provided the contralateral renal unit is established as functional and is not also involved with tumor.

Our experience suggests that a plane of cleavage can often be established in the subadventitial plane, especially when dealing with the vena cava (Fig. 37-11). However, the aorta in certain cases is so diseased by virtue of tumor involvement of the wall and by postchemotherapy changes that it is quite cheesy and does not suture well. Therefore, it is best to leave an additional layer on the aortic side of the dissection so that fibrous tissue can support sutures placed in the aorta. Pre- and para-aortic dissection should be in the extra-adventitial plane to provide this extra support to hold suture ligatures when needed. Should the situation prove technically impossible, or should the aorta give evidence of weakness or rupture, it should be replaced with a Dacron interposition tube graft or branched graft if the iliac vessels are also involved; we have done this on three occasions. The venous side is less of a problem. As long as the renal veins can be spared, the cava can be resected with impunity below this level, and we often do if it is quite involved with tumor. In such cases, we try to spare iliac lumbar contributions whenever possible.

Results and Discussion

At the time of this writing some 300 patients have been staged with retroperitoneal lymphadenectomy as described in this chapter. Crude 2-year survival rates are available for 194 patients.[2,8,24] These patients can be divided roughly into two groups.

The first group can be assigned to the pre-PVB era (before Platinol, Velban, bleomycin). There were 30 patients with Stage A disease, 3 of whom subsequently developed Stage C disease with pulmonary metastases. All three were salvaged by the use of single-agent chemotherapy (actinomycin D), pulmonary lobectomy, and, in one instance, chest local radiotherapy. These 30 patients continue well and disease-free. Another 28 patients were proven to be Stage B with nodal involvement in the retroperitoneum. Of these 28, 24 (86%) survive, all clinically tumor-free. Their management in those days consisted of monthly chest radiographs and

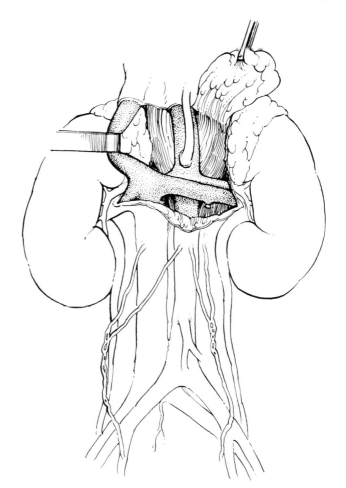

FIG. 37-7. The left suprahilar dissection (unnecessary in the absence of gross disease) extends from the superior mesenteric artery up the left side of the aorta, onto the crus and up 4 cm to 6 cm above the left renal artery. The left renal vein and artery are mobilized caudad, the adrenal vein is divided, and the adrenal gland is rotated cephalad after all its medial attachments are divided between clips. The tissue is taken off the crus and foramina by sharp dissection between clips. The crus is elevated and the nodes below are removed. Large nodes may require crural splitting for removal.

actinomycin D, 1 mg/day intravenously for 4 consecutive days at monthly intervals for the first year postoperative. Therefore, 54 of the 58 patients with Stage A or B disease still survive, all clinically tumor-free, for a cumulative survival rate of 93% in this group of patients.[2]

The second group represents the post-PVB era (after the introduction of Platinol-Velban-bleomycin for treatment of clinical relapse; *i.e.*, Stage C disease). This group of 136 patients have also been reported.[24] These patients are divided into two

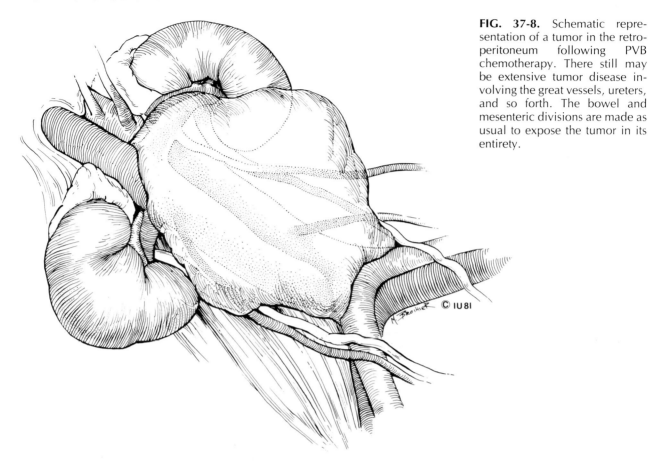

FIG. 37-8. Schematic representation of a tumor in the retroperitoneum following PVB chemotherapy. There still may be extensive tumor disease involving the great vessels, ureters, and so forth. The bowel and mesenteric divisions are made as usual to expose the tumor in its entirety.

major groups: histologic Stage I and histologic Stage II.

All Stage I patients continue alive and well. None received adjuvant chemotherapy after retroperitoneal lymphadenectomy. Of the 57 Stage I patients, there were four relapses at 3, 4, 10, and 22 months postoperatively. Each was salvaged with PVB chemotherapy at the time pulmonary metastases became evident. Presently all 57 patients are in complete remission with no evidence of disease.

The Stage II patients were treated in three different ways. One group was treated with surgery alone and followed expectantly; the second group was treated with single-drug adjuvant actinomycin D, monthly for 1 year; and the third group was treated with adjuvant PVB as a pilot study. The dosages of PVB have been reported elsewhere.[4] Of the 24 Stage II patients who were treated with surgery alone, there were seven relapses (30.4%), all of whom were treated with PVB at time of discovery. Twenty-three enjoy NED (no evidence of disease) status. One died of unrelated causes and at postmortem was tumor-free. Of the 31

patients treated with adjuvant actinomycin D, there were 15 relapses (48.4%), although the incidence of advanced disease seemed no higher in this group than in the surgery-alone group. Thirty patients enjoy NED status (96.8%), and one died of progressive metastatic disease after initial partial remission. In the third Stage II subset, the small pilot group given adjuvant PVB, seven patients have been followed for a minimum of 24 months, and the status of all remains continuously NED. We have reported these in more detail (Table 37-1).[4] In summary, our post-PVB era survival in Stage I remains 100% and in Stage II is 96.7% (Table 37-2). Currently we are participating in a group study whereby our Stage II patients either receive adjuvant chemotherapy (PVB in the dosages noted elsewhere[4] for two courses) or are merely observed, with crossover to PVB treatment only in the event of clinical relapse (see Fig. 37-12). In such a case, their PVB treatment would be a four-course program.[9]

It is our feeling that thorough retroperitoneal lymphadenectomy provides accurate pathologic

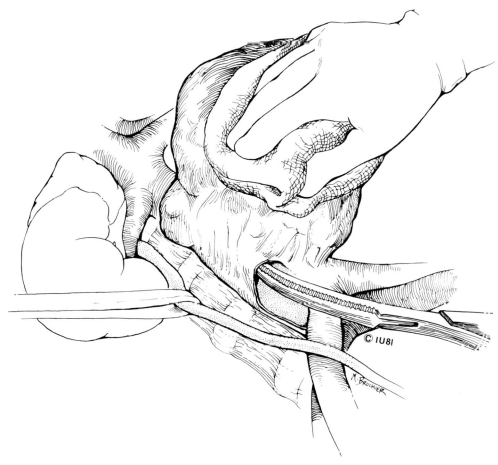

FIG. 37-9. The tumor can be dissected off of the vena cava usually in the subadventitial plane below the fibrous capsule of the tumor. When it is extremely dense, subadventitial dissection can assist caval extraction from the tumor. If the tumor grows through the wall of the cava, the cava itself can be resected provided it is below the level of the renal veins.

TABLE 37-1.   1973–1978 Stage I and II NSGTT, Indiana

Stage	No. of Patients	Ŗ p̄ RPLND	Relapse	Cure with PVB	Survival
I	57	None	4	4	57/57 (100%)
II	55	Actinomycin D (31)	14	13	53/55 (96%)
II		None (24)	7	7	
II	7	PVB (7)	0		60/62 (96.7%)

* One dead, unrelated cause, mental institution

staging. It therefore offers true information on the disease status and possibly will assist in optimal assignment of therapy. For example, our current adjuvant study is based on accurate histologic information as opposed to merely clinical noninvasive data which, in our experience, are significantly falsely negative.[16] Although the future of retroperitoneal lymphadenectomy is still unclear and improvements in noninvasive staging will doubtless continue, it would seem unlikely that completely accurate staging can be obtained without surgical dissection and histologic nodal examination.

Our position is that the more thorough the

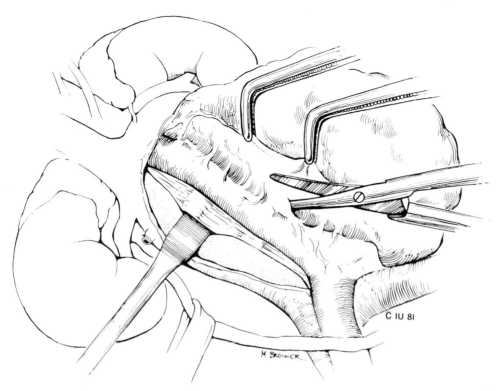

FIG. 37-10. The tumor is now dissected free of the cava and the aorta is being dissected free of the tumor. It is important to preserve the adventitia of the aorta if possible. Subadventitial dissection may leave a very weakened wall, which can rupture spontaneously and also is difficult to repair. An effort to leave adventitia on the aorta is shown in this diagram.

TABLE 37-2. Indiana RPLND Results

Era	Survival	
	STAGE A	STAGE B
Pre-PVB 1965–1974	30/30 (100%)	24/28 (86%)
Post-PVB 1974–1978	57/57 (100%)	60/62 (97%)

lymphadenectomy, the more accurate the staging. The merits of a bilateral dissection versus a unilateral dissection remain debatable. The report by Ray, Hajdu, and Whitmore of their standard infrahilar dissections indicates that contralateral spread is rare in the face of tumor-free ipsilateral nodes.[15] Our own experience confirms this.[5] Perhaps one purpose of the unilateral dissection was to preserve ejaculation, but it appears that the majority of patients are still unable to ejaculate even after this form of dissection. Also, the fact that contralateral spread sometimes occurs, particularly in the face of multiple ipsilateral nodal involvement with tumor, suggests the possible merit of a thorough bilateral dissection in such cases.

The merits of a suprahilar dissection in combination with the standard hilar and infrahilar approach are still less well known. Admittedly, it is rare that a patient would have disease in the suprahilar nodes in the face of tumor-free infrahilar nodes (it happened in only 2 of our 104 Stage B patients). But it is not rare to have the suprahilar nodes involved when the infrahilar nodes contain gross tumor; in our series, one of every four patients with gross tumor in infrahilar nodes also had tumor in the suprahilar nodes. It seems reasonable then, in such cases, to clear out the nodal drainage pathways of the testis completely if we are to stage and treat with surgery as thoroughly as possible. The frequency of suprahilar nodal involvement is directly proportional to the number of nodes involved below the hilus. Stage B_1 disease has from none (right side) to 7% to 14% (left side) positive suprahilar nodes. Stage B_2 has from 13% to 33% (right) and 16% to 42% (left) positive

FIG. 37-11. The ureter is dissected out from the tumor after the appropriate lumbar arterial divisions are made. This allows dissection of the tumor off the posterior body wall and the foramina. Note that right-angle clamps holding this tumor fibrous capsule or vessel adventitia help in providing traction on the tumor specimen.

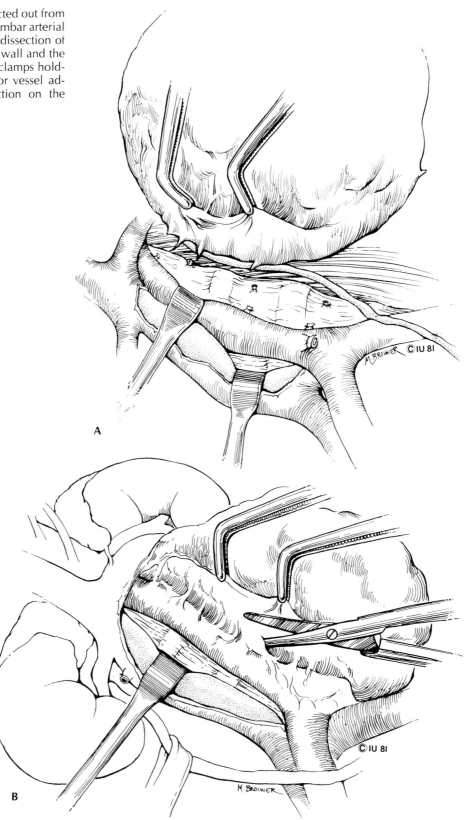

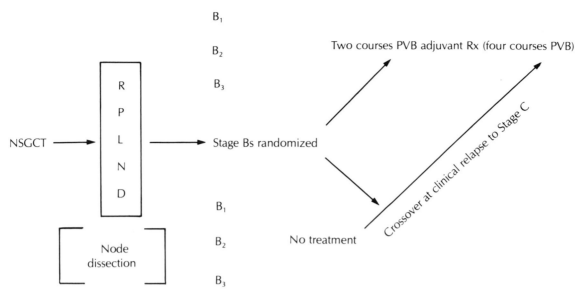

FIG. 37-12. Scheme of managing non-seminomatous germinal cell tumors (NSGCT) by retroperitoneal lymph node dissection (RPLND) and combination chemotherapy employing platinum, vinblastine, bleomycin (PVB).

suprahilar nodes. Hence, the value of routine bilateral suprahilar dissection in a grossly normal retroperitoneum is doubtful. On the other hand, it seems useful in Stage B_2 and B_3 disease.

Questions are often asked about the value of total vascular mobilization by dividing all the lumbar vessels. In our series there have been no spinal cord complications from this procedure. Ferguson, Bergan, and Conn, in a literature review, reported 28 cases of paraparesis following total infrarenal aortic replacement for aneurysm in older males.[10] This study, however, relates to an older group of patients who had lost their primary anterior descending spinal blood supply because of atherosclerotic cardiovascular disease in the thoracic aorta and its branches and who had been depending on their lumbar arteries for collateral circulation. In our younger patients this is not a problem. We believe that vascular mobilization is necessary because lateral views and dissection studies have shown that there are as many nodes and lymphatics behind the great vessels and posterolateral to them as there are above them, particularly high in the retroperitoneum. Also, the lymphatics occupy each lumbar foramen, and there are many tumor-containing nodes found in these foramina in patients with Stage B disease.

It is a fact that the best results in the last decade in the management of patients with testicular tumors are to be found in those medical centers in which the surgical staff is committed to a thorough retroperitoneal lymphadenectomy.[4,11,18,20] Those authors espousing a partial and less aggressive lymphadenectomy do not have the data to support their contention that this is a superior method of staging and treatment.

Still another area of controversy that should be mentioned concerns the role of radiotherapy in the management of these patients. In brief, it can be said that the need for radiotherapy as treatment for nonseminomatous testis cancer is diminishing sharply in the face of great advances in chemotherapy. In our earlier experience, radiotherapy was a negative factor if the patients developed Stage C disease, as all Stage B patients are at risk of doing. The impact of prior radiotherapy on the bone marrow is lasting. More persistent and profound leukopenia in patients treated earlier with radiotherapy (especially if the chest is included) limits the chemotherapist in his ability to deliver effective doses of chemotherapy. Still, it must be said that radiotherapy is an effective alternative to RPLND in controlling low-stage disease in areas where RPLND is not employed or available.[14]

Conclusions

Several conclusions can be drawn from our experience. Chemotherapy is opening new avenues in the management of these patients. It allows us to leave patients with proven Stage A disease untreated with close follow-up. Should Stage C disease develop, the patient can be salvaged with appropriate and aggressive combination chemotherapy, as our cases were. Patients with Stage A disease should have a 100% survival rate if the retroperitoneum is dissected appropriately and the patient is followed closely postoperatively. Several options exist for the postoperative management of patients with Stage B disease. Two courses are under cooperative study: (a) no treatment after lymphadenectomy, as in Stage A; (b) combination chemotherapy after lymphadenectomy (Table 37-2). Those patients in the no-treatment group who develop Stage C disease cross/over to combined chemotherapy with PVB. Since 1974, all but two of our patients with Stage B disease who progressed to Stage C have achieved complete remission with this three-drug combination. Another new horizon is the potential for chemical cytoreduction of disseminated Stage C disease; persistent abdominal disease can be resected. It is my opinion that chemotherapy provides a safer, more extensive initial cytoreduction than the contrary approach of primary surgical cytoreduction and postoperative chemotherapy.[3,17,22]

Serotesting for the β-subunit of human chorionic gonadotropin and for α-fetoprotein has been a helpful means of following patients with Stage B disease and for detecting tumor before it can be seen by any of the conventional radiologic methods.

Although the future of retroperitoneal lymphadenectomy is still unclear and improvements in noninvasive staging will doubtless continue (serotesting for tumor-associated antigens, ultrasound, CT, and lymphangiography), it would seem unlikely that completely accurate staging can be obtained without surgical dissection and histologic nodal examination. We have had recent experience with several patients in whom all these preoperative tests for metastases (including serotesting) were negative, yet they had evidence of multiple tumorous nodes on microscopic examination.[16] This suggests that the role of surgical staging with histologic nodal study will remain central to the accurate definition of the disease status and direction of therapy. Furthermore, in this disease, retroperitoneal surgery completely done seems to have positive influence on patient survival.

REFERENCES

1. COOPER JF, LEADBETTER WF, CHUTE R: The thoracoabdominal approach for retroperitoneal gland dissection: Its application to testis tumors. Surg Gynecol Obstet 90:486, 1950

2. DONOHUE JP: Retroperitoneal Lymphadenectomy, Urol Clin North Am 4:517, 1977

3. DONOHUE JP, EINHORN LH, WILLIAMS SD: Cytoreductive surgery for metastatic testis cancer: Considerations of timing and extent. J Urol 123:876, 1980

4. DONOHUE JP, EINHORN LH, WILLIAMS SD: Is adjuvant chemotherapy necessary following retroperitoneal lymphadenectomy for non-seminomatous testis cancer? Urol Clin North Am 7:747, 1980

5. DONOHUE JP, PEREZ JM, EINHORN LH: Improved management of non-seminomatous testis tumors. J Urol 121:425, 1979

6. DONOHUE JP, ROTH LM, ZACHARY JM et al: Cytoreductive surgery for metastatic testis cancer: Tissue analysis of retroperitoneal tumor masses after chemotherapy. Accepted for publication in J Urol 127:1111, 1982

7. DONOHUE JP, ROWLAND RG: Complications of retroperitoneal lymph node dissection. J Urol 125:338, 1981

8. EINHORN LH, DONOHUE JP: Improved chemotherapy for germinal testis tumors. Cancer 42:293, 1978

9. EINHORN LH, DONOHUE JP: Improved chemotherapy in disseminated testicular cancer. J Urol 117:65, 1977

10. FERGUSON LRJ, BERGAN JJ, CONN J, JR et al: Spinal ischemia following abdominal aortic surgery. Ann Surg 181:267, 1975

11. FRALEY EE, KEDIA K, MARKLAND C: The role of radical operation in the management of nonseminomatous germinal tumors of the testicle in the adult. In Varco RL, Delaney JP (eds): Controversy in Surgery, p 497. Philadelphia, W B Saunders, 1976

12. GOLDINGER PL, SCHWEIZER O: The hazards of anesthesia and surgery in bleomycin treated patients. Semin Oncol 6:121, 1979

13. PATTON JF, MALLIS N: Tumors of the testis. J Urol 81:457, 1959

14. PECKHAM MJ: Combined management of malignant teratoma of the testis. Lancet 2:267, 1979

15. RAY B, HAJDU SI, WHITMORE WF, JR: Distribution of retroperitoneal lymph node metastases in testicular germinal tumors. Cancer 33:340, 1974

16. ROWLAND RG, WEISMAN D, WILLIAMS SD et al: Accuracy of preoperative staging in stage A and B nonseminomatous germ cell testis tumor. J Urol (in press)

17. SCARDINO PT: Adjuvant chemotherapy is of value following retroperitoneal lymph node dissection for non-seminomatous testicular tumors. Urol Clin North Am 7:735, 1980

18. SKINNER DG: Non-seminomatous testis tumors: A plan of management based on 96 patients to improve survival in all stages by combined therapeutic modalities. J Urol 115:65, 1976

19. SKINNER DG, LEADBETTER WF: The surgical management of testis tumors. J Urol 106:84, 1971

20. STAUBITZ WJ, EARLY KS, MAGOSS IV et al: Surgical treatment of nonseminomatous germinal testis tumors. Cancer 32:1206, 1973

21. VAN BUSKIRK KE, YOUNG JG: The evolution of the bilateral antegrade retroperitoneal lymph node dissection in the treatment of testicular tumors. Milit Med 133:575, 1968

22. VURGRIN D, CVITKOVIC E, WHITMORE WF, JR et al: Adjuvant chemotherapy in resected non-seminomatous germ cell tumors of testis: Stages I and II. Semin Oncol 6:94, 1979

23. WHITMORE WF, JR: Treating germinal tumors of the adult testes. Cont Surg 6:17, 1975

24. WILLIAMS SD, EINHORN LH, DONOHUE JP: High cure rate of stage I or II testicular cancer with or without adjuvant chemotherapy. Proc Am Soc Clin Surg 21:421, 1980

25. YOUNG JD, JR: Retroperitoneal Surgery. In Glenn JF, Boyce WH (eds): Urologic Surgery, 2nd ed, p 848. New York, Harper & Row, 1975

Ureterolithotomy

38

Jack Hughes

Ureteral calculi originate in the kidney. Most of these calculi that have a diameter of 5 mm or less will pass into the bladder spontaneously, and those that do not but reach the lower ureter usually can be removed cystoscopically. Ureteral calculi that do not pass and are not suitable for cystoscopic extraction are removed by open operation.

Surgical Anatomy

The ureter is divided into upper, middle, and lower portions. The upper ureter extends from the ureteropelvic junction to the level of the upper margin of the sacrum, where there is a physiologic narrowing of the ureter as it crosses over the iliac vessels. The middle portion courses posteriorly and lies in front of and near the lateral margin of the sacrum. The lower or pelvic portion extends from the inferior margin of the sacrum to the ureteral meatus. The lower ureter is divided into extramural and intramural parts, the latter being the narrowest of the entire ureter.

The upper ureter lies on the posterior abdominal wall lateral to the transverse processes of the lower three or four lumbar vetebrae. In the midlumbar area it is separated from the psoas muscle by the posterior layer of Gerota's fascia, and it is in front of and very close to this thin fascial layer. The close anatomic relation of the ureter, the posterior layer of Gerota's fascia, and the psoas muscle is used to advantage in approaching the midlumbar ureter. On the right the duodenum is near the proximal 1 cm or 2 cm of the ureter, but only in the most complicated situations is the relationship apt to be important. Also on the right the vena cava is sometimes bared unexpectedly and is an obvious signal to move slightly lateralward. The gonadal vessels may be encountered on either side and if necessary may be divided without consequence.

The lower ureter is attached loosely to the peritoneum and at operation is found on the posterior surface of the medially reflected peritoneum. Transperitoneally, the relationship is seen readily. Near the bladder the ureter courses under the vas deferens in the man and the fallopian tube in the woman.

Preoperative Procedures

The diagnosis of ureteral calculus having been made previously by intravenous or retrograde pyelograms, a kidney, ureter, and bladder radiograph is made on the way to the operating room to determine the exact location of the calculus at the moment and the appropriate operative approach. Inserting a catheter up to or by the ureteral calculus preoperatively makes location of the ureter less difficult, and the catheter can be left indwelling for 2 or 3 days to reduce urinary drainage through the incision. However, there is always the risk that preoperative placement of a catheter will displace the calculus upward, particularly when the location is the upper ureter and when there is considerable hydroureter above the calculus. In a debilitated patient with obstruction and sepsis, retrograde or percutaneous passage of a catheter can be lifesaving. By establishing drainage the infection can be managed better, and the operation postponed until a less unfavorable time.

Appropriate antibacterial drugs should be given prophylactically starting 1 hr to 2 hr before the incision is made and continued for 3 days. Longer courses of treatment are given when indicated.

Operative Approach

To remove ureteral calculi, we approach the ureter through the flank, varying levels of the lower abdominal quadrant, or the suprapubic area. Transvaginal ureterolithotomy (Fig. 38-1) has been advocated for calculi near the ureterovesical junction in the woman. However, not since our early experiences have we encountered a situation in which the transvaginal operation was thought to be the procedure of choice. We use a transperitoneal approach when a calculus is located close to a

419

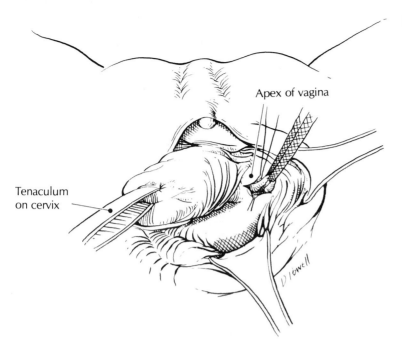

FIG. 38-1. Vaginal approach

Apex of vagina

Tenaculum
on cervix

ureteroileal or ureterosigmoid anastomosis, when the ureter cannot be mobilized extraperitoneally, and sometimes when the peritoneal cavity is already open for another purpose.

Approximately 65% of ureterolithotomies are done for calculi in the upper ureter, 15% in the middle ureter, and 20% in the lower ureter.

UPPER URETER

Calculi in the upper ureter are removed through the conventional flank incision parallel to and 1 cm below the 12th rib (Fig. 38-2). The skin, subcutaneous tissues, and muscles are divided sharply, and the retroperitoneal space is entered. The posterior layer of Gerota's fascia is gently stripped from the muscles on which it lies to the level of the transverse processes. Deaver retractors can be used effectively to pull the fascia away from the muscles. When the calculus is in the upper 2 cm of the ureter, the posterior layer of Gerota's fascia is opened longitudinally at the level of the lower pole of the kidney, the periureteral fat is pushed aside with ring forceps, and the ureter is identified. Often a bulging is seen at the site of the calculus, and there may be dilatation of the ureter proximally. If the ureter is not located readily, the area is explored gently with the thumb and index finger.

As soon as possible after locating the calculus, a Babcock or Coppridge ureteral clamp is placed around the ureter above the calculus before mobilization is carried out because of the possibility

of dislodging the calculus. Mobilization of the ureter is limited to the degree necessary to identify the calculus and to permit a ureterotomy directly over it using a knife with a hawk-bill blade. The calculus is teased out of the ureter using the tip of the knife blade or is extracted with a small forceps or clamp. To ensure patency of the distal ureter, an 8Fr urethral catheter or a smaller ureteral catheter is passed gently to the bladder and withdrawn. A Babcock clamp is placed around the ureter below the ureterotomy and the one above is removed. Urine flows out of the ureteral opening while the operator watches carefully for additional calculi or fragments. A culture of the urine may be done at this point. When indicated, a small rubber catheter or malleable cannula is passed up to the renal pelvis and irrigations are carried out. The ureterotomy is closed with one or two sutures of 4-0 chromic gut, and the ureter is returned to its original position. The incision is closed in layers around a 5/8-inch (16-mm) Penrose drain brought out through a stab wound or through the posterior angle of the incision.

Calculi located between the transverse processes of the third and fourth lumbar vertebrae often can be removed through a Foley muscle-splitting incision (Fig. 38-3). This approach offers to the patient the considerable advantages of reduced morbidity, hospital stay, and disability. A flank incision is made at the approximate level of the calculus. The external and internal oblique muscles and the latissimus dorsi muscles are freely mobilized but

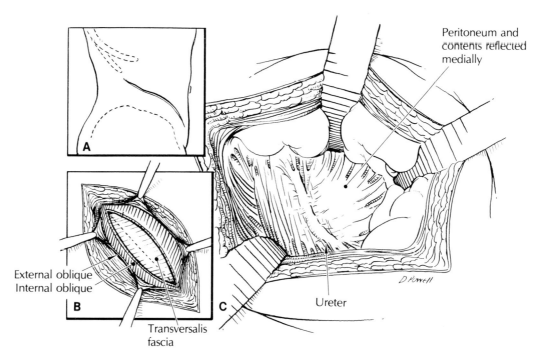

FIG. 38-2. Approach to the upper ureter: **(A)** Incision is made for exposure of the upper third of the ureter. **(B)** The peritoneum is exposed through the transversalis muscle and fascia. **(C)** Retraction of the peritoneum exposes the ureter on the psoas muscle.

FIG. 38-3. Foley muscle-splitting incision for uncomplicated upper ureteral calculi: **(A)** line of incision; **(B)** the external and internal oblique muscles are retracted from the edges of the latissimus dorsi to expose the lumbodorsal fascia; **(C)** the ureter is exposed retroperitoneally.

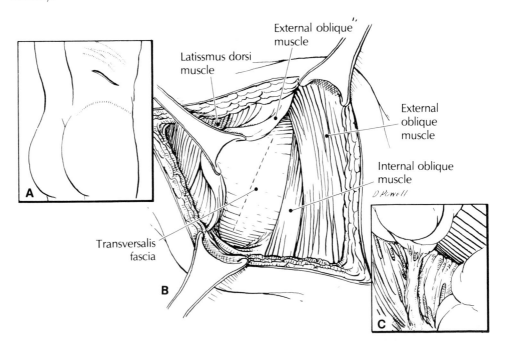

not cut. The oblique muscles are pulled forward and the latissimus dorsi backward, exposing the lumbar fascia. The fascia is opened parallel to the line of its fibers, the edges are retracted, and the retroperitoneal space is entered. With the help of two narrow Deaver retractors, the posterior layer of Gerota's fascia is separated from the posterior abdominal wall to the level of the transverse processes medially and the ureter is located. Periureteral edema is often seen before the ureter is identified and indicates that the ureter is close by. In all but the most obese patients the ureter can be seen lying very close to and in front of the posterior layer of Gerota's fascia. The fascia is opened vertically directly over the calculus, and a Babcock or Coppridge clamp is placed around the ureter above the calculus. The location of the calculus is confirmed by palpating the ureter with the tips of the DeBakey forceps, and the calculus is removed as previously described. The Foley operation must be performed with the hands outside the lumbar fascia because of the small opening. However, with a good assistant to handle the Deaver retractors, the operation can be performed satisfactorily in most patients except the obese and those with very thick muscles. If the calculus cannot be identified readily or if local complications occur, the Foley incision can be enlarged easily by cutting the muscles anteriorly or posteriorly.

MIDDLE URETER

Ureteral calculi at L5 and in the middle ureter can be removed through a muscle-splitting incision at the appropriate level, termed the high Gibson incision (Fig. 38-4). The patient is placed on the operating table in the dorsal recumbent position with a sandbag under the hip. The skin and subcutaneous tissue are divided in the line of cleavage at the approximate level of the calculus. The fascia and muscles are separated bluntly parallel to the line of their fibers for a distance of 4 cm to 6 cm. The underlying peritoneum is mobilized and reflected medially. The fat is pushed aside with ring forceps, and the ureter is located. In the area of the iliac vessels, obviously the ureter must be approached carefully because of the close relationship. When for any reason the ureter is difficult to locate, the incision can be enlarged medially by incising parallel to the line of fibers the fused aponeuroses of the internal and external oblique muscles. When the calculus-bearing ureter is located, a clamp is placed around it above the calculus and a ureterotomy is done, using a hawk bill knife. The ureteral incision is closed with one

or two sutures of 4-0 chromic gut, and the incision is closed around a ⅝-inch (16-mm) Penrose drain. The muscle and fascial layers are closed separately using two or three sutures of 1-0 or No. 1 chromic gut, and the subcutaneous tissue and skin are reapproximated.

LOWER URETER

A calculus in the lower ureter can be removed usually through a muscle-splitting incision (Fig. 38-5) in the lower quadrant (modified Gibson incision) similar to but placed slightly lower than the high Gibson (Fig. 38-6). The incision is made at the approximate level of the calculus, and the retroperitoneal space is entered. The peritoneum is mobilized and retracted medially. The ureter is found attached loosely to the posterior surface of the peritoneum and is traced to the calculus. A clamp is placed around the ureter above the calculus, and the operation is completed as described previously. When it is difficult to locate the lower ureter, the peritoneum can be mobilized superiorly and the ureter can be found as it crosses the iliac vessels. When necessary this lower quadrant incision can be extended medially even across the midline.

MANAGEMENT OF SPECIAL PROBLEMS

When calculi are impacted in or very near the intramural ureter or when the operation is expected to be difficult for any reason, the preferred approach to the lower ureter is through a vertical or transverse midline hypogastric incision (Fig. 38-7). Adequate exposure is obtained by making the incision as large as desired. When necessary, the bladder can be opened and the calculus palpated between a thumb and index finger placed on either side of the bladder wall. If indicated, the ureter can be opened transvesically. When a meatotomy is done or a ureterocele is incised to facilitate removal of a calculus from the intramural ureter, the cut edges should not be sutured. Only very rarely will a secondary ureteroneocystostomy be necessary because of reflux or stricture.

Calculi are sometimes dislodged upward and rarely downward during the process of identifying and mobilizing the ureter and thus cannot be located readily. Before enlarging the incision or calling for the radiology technician, it is sometimes most productive to open the ureter and explore it up and down using a Dormia basket. Even a calculus dislodged into the renal pelvis can sometimes be removed using a plain tip basket. When

FIG. 38-4. Approach to the middle ureter: **(A)** incision; **(B)** exposure

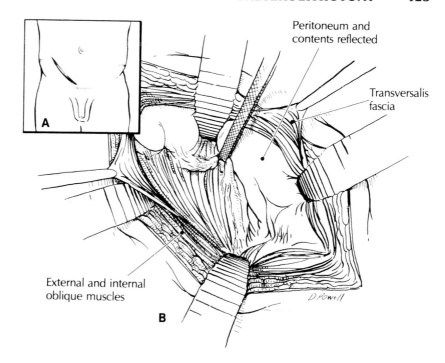

Peritoneum and contents reflected

Transversalis fascia

External and internal oblique muscles

B

D. Powell

FIG. 38-5. Approach to the lower ureter through a modified Gibson incision, including hockey stick extension: **(A)** incision; **(B)** exposure

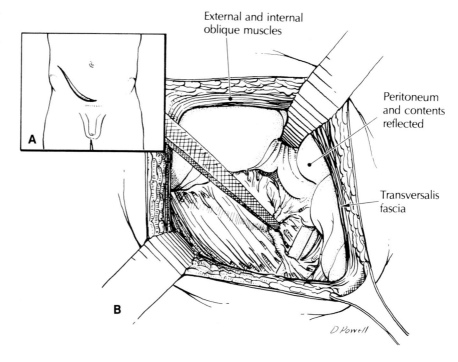

External and internal oblique muscles

Peritoneum and contents reflected

Transversalis fascia

B

D. Powell

calculi are located at two or more levels of the ureter, often it is possible to remove the remaining ones with a basket passed through the ureterotomy, or when close enough by "milking" into the ureterotomy.

A ureterolithotomy for a small stone performed 24 hr to 72 hr after one or more unsuccessful cystoscopic manipulations can be very difficult and has a high rate of complications. If relief of obstruction is imperative and a catheter cannot be passed cystoscopically, percutaneous nephrostomy or open pyelostomy may be the procedure of choice.

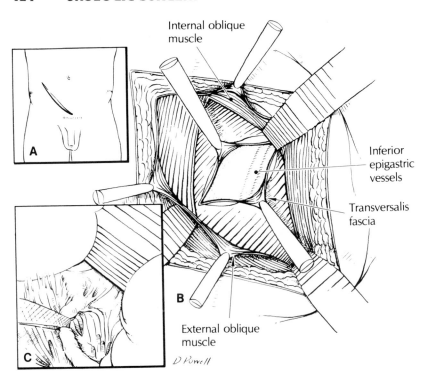

Internal oblique muscle

Inferior epigastric vessels

Transversalis fascia

External oblique muscle

B

C

A

D Powell

FIG. 38-6. Approach to the lower ureter through a high Gibson incision: **(A)** incision; **(B)** exposure; **(C)** exposure of ureter

FIG. 38-7. Low transverse incision

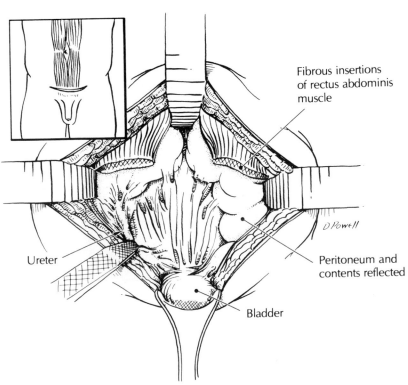

Fibrous insertions of rectus abdominis muscle

Peritoneum and contents reflected

Ureter

Bladder

D Powell

Postoperative Complications

Temperature elevations of 1° C for 24 hr to 48 hr postureterolithotomy are not unusual, particularly when general anesthesia is used. Postoperative sepsis occurs rarely, even when urinary infection is present preoperatively, and failure to respond promptly to the appropriate antibacterial drugs suggests obstruction of the ureter or an infected urinoma.

Urinary drainage from the operative site for 48 hr postoperatively occurs in about 50% of patients. Drainage beyond 4 days is an indication for an indwelling ureteral catheter for 24 hr to 48 hr. Rarely will the catheter have to be reinserted. Prolonged drainage requiring that the patient be discharged from the hospital with a ureteral stent curled up in the bladder occurs about once in 200 ureterolithotomies. The stent is removed in 2 to 3 weeks. Penrose drains can be removed 24 hr after cessation of urinary drainage provided the drain has been shortened at least 24 hr earlier. Occasionally, prolonged urinary drainage decreases dramatically or ceases shortly after the drain has been shortened, suggesting that the drain may have been lying on the ureterotomy and preventing closure.

The incidence of ureteral stricture is unknown, but it has to be extremely rare following uncomplicated ureterolithotomy. Some of the apparent ureteral strictures are actually ureters compressed by extramural fibrosis. Urinomas are also rare and are caused most often by the Penrose drain coming out prematurely, particularly if a muscle-splitting incision (Foley or Gibson) has been used.

Retroperitoneal herniation of the bowel can occur if a rent in the peritoneum is not closed. The pelvic peritoneum is opened unintentionally most often and is the usual site of herniation.

REFERENCES

1. FOLEY FEB: Management of ureteral stone. JAMA 104:1314, 1935
2. FROHBOSE WJ: Vaginal approach to calculus disease in the lower urinary tract. J Urol. 88:480, 1962
3. GIBSON CL: The technique of operations on the lower portion of the ureter. Am J Med Sci 139:65, 1910

Ureteroureterostomy and Transureteroureterostomy

John D. Young, Jr.

39

Ureteroureterostomy

Ureteroureterostomy is defined as surgical anastomosis of any segments of the ureter to each other, or anastomosis of ipsilateral ureters to each other.

The indications for ureteroureterostomy include disruption of the ureter by blunt, penetrating, or surgical trauma; resection of short fibrotic strictures resulting from surgical clamping or ligation; periureteral inflammation; radiation damage to short segments; reflux or obstruction in a duplicated or ectopic ureter, which might be anastomosed to a nonrefluxing uninjured mate or to a refluxing mate to facilitate reimplantation into the bladder; congenital stricture; and occasionally, vascular obstructions such as retrocaval ureter and resection of a segment of ureter for neoplasm.

Contraindications to ureteroureterostomy include inadequate length to permit a completely tension-free anastomosis; sepsis or urinema for more than 1 or 2 days, involving a significant portion of the ureter to be anastomosed; previous dissection or mobilization of the ureter; a ureter extricated from retroperitoneal fibrosis from any cause or from a site of previous injury; previous injury; previous exposure of the ureter to therapeutic doses of radiation; and ureteral involvement in the field of dissection for a previous aortic or iliac graft or by-pass.

SURGICAL TECHNIQUE

If disruption of the ureter is recognized immediately, or within hours, surgical anastomosis is to be considered. Exposure of the ureter might be through the incision at hand in the case of an intraoperative injury, or through an extraperitoneal approach. I prefer a lower midline incision for approaching the lower third of the ureter, for although the ureters are perceived as "right" and "left," they really are closer to the midline in the pelvic region. After the rectus muscles are separated, the retropubic space is entered and blunt finger dissection is continued around the antero-

lateral surface of the bladder on the side of interest. The processus vaginalis is encountered on entering the internal inguinal ring and is divided. The round ligament is divided and ligated in the female. The spermatic cord strictures are separated from the reflected peritoneum and preserved in the male.

The umbilical artery is identified, ligated, and divided as the only remaining structure preventing medial retraction of the lateral bladder wall. The ureter lies medial to the umbilical artery near its junction with the hypogastric artery. Excellent exposure of the lower third of the ureter to a point well above the pelvic brim is thus obtained. Whereas injuries to the lower end of the ureter might best be treated by ureteroneocystostomy, ureteroureterostomy is usually indicated if the ureter is injured more than 5 cm from the bladder.

For the middle third of the ureter, a muscle-splitting, "large McBurney" incision is appropriate. The midportion of this incision should be 2 cm to 5 cm medial to the anterior superior iliac spine on a line between this structure and the umbilicus.

The upper third of the ureter is best approached through a conventional flank or 12th rib incision, the same as that used for exposing the kidney. If a ureteral injury is discovered during an intra-abdominal or retroperitoneal procedure, it is usually managed through the exposure at hand. If the right or left colon has been mobilized from its respective lateral gutter, the ureter usually is readily available for exploration and repair. However, if there is a suspected or an apparent transperitoneal injury to the ureter during an intraperitoneal operation, either ureter is best exposed by incising the left peritoneal leaf of the small bowel mesentery (Fig. 39-1). This can be extended to include the ligament of Treitz and the peritoneum over the promontory and body of the sacrum. The only structure anterior to either ureter through this approach is the inferior mesenteric artery crossing the left ureter; this artery can safely be sacrificed if the remainder of the left colon–sigmoid blood supply is intact. Because the lower left and sigmoid

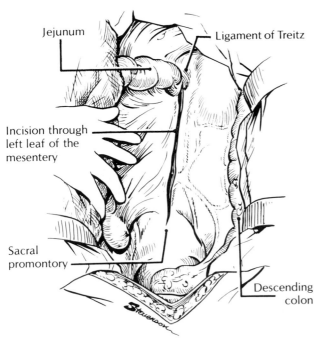

FIG. 39-1. Exposure of retroperitoneal space. Abdominal viscera are displaced to permit vertical incision of left leaf of mesentery for exposure of retroperitoneal space.

colon is the easiest and safest portion of the large bowel to reflect medially, it is an alternative route of exposure for the lower half of the left ureter.

After exposure and identification of the ureteral segment in question, the following questions must be addressed:

1. Is there a missing or nonviable segment and if so, how long is it?

2. Were the periureteral area and ureter previously nonirradiated, uninjured, surgically nonmobilized, and uninvolved in acute or chronic inflammation?

3. Is there more than one ureter on the side in question?

4. Does the ureter show evidence of acute or chronic obstruction?

5. Do the freshly cut ends of the ureter show evidence of an adequate vascular supply?

When it has been determined that ureteroureterostomy is an appropriate solution for the problem at hand, the ends of the ureter to be connected must be mobilized sufficiently to provide anastomosis without tension. The dissection to free the ends of the ureteral segments must include all tissue, from the peritoneum anteriorly to psoas muscle posteriorly and the vena cava or the aorta medially (Fig. 39-2). The gonadal vessels should be included with the periureteral tissue, which serves as a sort of mesentery not always readily apparent to the surgeon. The dissection is adequate when the ends of the ureter remain in opposition when lying without attached suture or instruments. Additional mobility of the upper end of the ureter might be obtained in selected cases by mobilizing the kidney downward as far as its pedicle will permit.[10]

With fulfillment of the above criteria, the method of anastomosis, the type of suture material, and the use of a stent are of relatively secondary importance. If the ureter is 1 cm in diameter or less, I prefer to spatulate the end by an incision parallel to the long axis, perpendicular to the cut end of the ureter, and about one half the diameter of the ureter in length.

If a stent is to be used, it should be placed before the anastomosis is begun. In a larger, well-vascularized ureter, a stent is less essential. If there is a question of tension on the anastomosis or any question of viability, a properly used stent may increase significantly the chances for a successful ureteroureterostomy. The stent should be the largest caliber of medical grade silicone that will fit loosely in the ureter. Standard ureteral catheters and rubber catheters have been used successfully and are acceptable if silicone tubing or feeding tubes are not available. Although earlier models of the self-retaining ureteral stents ("double-J," etc.) are not easily tailored to the precise needs of a stent inserted at open operation, more recent modifications show promise of meeting the requirements for flexibility, length, size, and softer consistency. This would be a major contribution to ureteral anastomoses. While some have condemned the T-tube as a ureteral stent, I have found the 6Fr to 10Fr silicone T-tube very useful and dependable. This tube has limbs long enough to reach from renal pelvis to bladder.

It is important that the proximal end of any ureteral stent be in the renal pelvis. It is desirable, but less important, that the distal end be in the bladder. The distance between the anastomosis site and the renal pelvis is determined by passing a calibrated ureteral catheter (4Fr–7Fr) and locating the pelvis by aspiration and irrigation. The distance to the bladder is measured in the same manner. Extra holes are cut in the pelvic and bladder ends of the T-tube or other stent, and holes smaller than the internal diameter of the stent are cut 2 cm apart in the entire length. If a T-tube is used, it is necessary to remove a V-segment opposite the junction of the vertical limb to facilitate its removal at a later date. The vertical limb junction of the T-tube should be tested by manual stretching after excision of the V to make sure the remaining junction of the limbs will not break at the time of withdrawal.

The advantages of the T-tube are ready access for urographic studies and drainage; less need for nephrostomy, suprapubic and urethral catheters; and removal without cystoscopy. The disadvantages are that a T-tube does not provide adequate nephrostomy drainage when that is indicated and that angulation of the ureter may occur at the time of removal, particularly if it is removed during the first 2 weeks. When possible, the T-tube stent should be inserted into the ureter distal to the site of the ureteroureterostomy, so that urine transport through the anastomosis will be encouraged after its removal. However, I have also seen good results when the T-tube has been inserted into the ureter above the ureteral anastomosis, so this is not a major consideration. A generous incision 1 cm to 1.5 cm in length, exactly parallel to the long axis on the anterolateral surface of the ureter, is required for insertion of the T-tube.

About equally often, I use an indwelling straight 5Fr to 10Fr clear silicone tubing or a feeding tube stent. I measure length and place holes as described above for the T-tube. The straight stent tends to migrate downward on occasion. This can be prevented by placing a 5-0 or 6-0 plain or chromic gut suture through the ureter and the side of the stent and tying it loosely on the external surface of the ureter. If the anticipated duration of the stenting is 10 to 14 days, plain gut is used; if more than 10 days, chromic gut is preferred. These sutures break fairly easily, thus permitting removal of the stent by cystoscopy forceps at the desired time. Internal straight ureteral stents can be held in place also by a removable, nonabsorbable suture such as a 2-0 silk or Tevdek suture through ureter and stent, bringing the ends to the skin surface to be tied over a button.[7] When the suture is cut free from the button, both stent and suture can be withdrawn through the bladder. I have placed a 2-0 or 3-0 monofilament synthetic nonabsorbable suture through the ureter with a tangential bite through the wall of the stent, and have brought both ends through the flank about an inch apart and tied them loosely on the surface. This suture has been left in place for as long as several months; then one end was cut and the suture was pulled out, leaving the stent in place for several more months in a patient who had an extraordinary number of recurrent urinary calculi. If the upper end of the ureter is exposed and the kidney is available, a

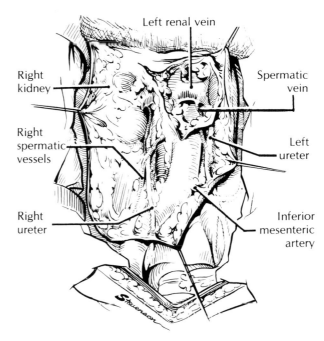

FIG. 39-2. Exposure of the entire midline and right retroperitoneal space may be gained with reflexion of the intestines upward and onto the abdominal wall and lower chest.

straight indwelling stent can be brought through the renal cortex into a calix, through the renal pelvis, and down the ureter in the manner described above. The proximal end of this stent can be brought to the exterior from the kidney surface where it will be available for injection of contrast material, for drainage if needed, and for easy removal at the desired time. This latter maneuver is particularly useful in children.

After the preferred stent has been placed, the fixation of choice accomplished, and the ureteral ends spatulated as described above, the ureteroureteral anastomosis is begun by placing one right angle of each cut end into the angle of the spatulating incision on the opposing cut end of the ureter and suturing it in place with 5-0 chromic gut (Fig. 39-3). The anastomosis is then completed with interrupted sutures of 5-0 chromic gut placed 2 mm apart. As mentioned above, the spatulating incisions are made only if the ureteral ends are 1 cm or less in diameter. This method best increases the diameter of the ureter at the site of anastomosis. Less ischemia of the suture line results from interrupted sutures, and follow-up studies suggest that this suture line does not leak if bites 2 mm thick are taken 2 mm apart. However, good results have been obtained with the running lock stitch (Fig. 39-4). Reports indicate satisfaction with straight

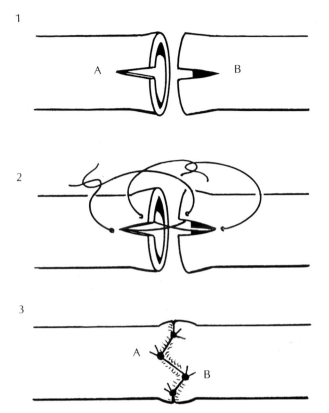

FIG. 39-3. Spatulation of the ends of the ureter prevents narrowing of the ureter at the site of anastomosis.

FIG. 39-4. Technique of primary repair of ureteral laceration: **(A)** Spatulation of ureteral margins and placement of running sutures. **(B)** Running locked sutures are completed.

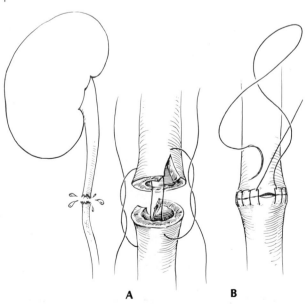

transverse, Z-plasty, oblique, and fishmouth anastomoses (Fig. 39-5). The goal should be a watertight suture line that produces a minimum of ischemia for the healing edges and does not decrease the diameter of the ureteral lumen. It seems likely that anastomosis under tension, devitalized or poorly perfused ureter, improper or no stenting, and inadequate postoperative periureteral drainage have led to more ureteroureterostomy complications than have the type of suture and the method of anastomosis.

Provision for drainage of collections of urine, serum, blood, pus, or other exudate from the ureteroureterostomy site is mandatory. A Penrose drain or some of the prefabricated suction-drainage systems cannot be trusted for this purpose. The author uses a 14Fr to 18Fr clear silicone or rubber tube with two or three side holes cut within 5 cm of the internal end. The end of this drain is sutured to tissue, usually psoas muscle, with 5-0 chromic gut 1 cm to 2 cm from the ureteroureterostomy suture line after the ureter has been carefully returned to its normal position.

This precise fixation also prevents the peritoneal reflection from falling back into place, excluding the drain, and permitting an accumulation of urine or other fluid in the periureteral space. (A drain outside the peritoneal reflection was the cause of a huge urinoma following a ureteropyeloplasty in one of the author's patients.) The tube drain is irrigated with 5 ml to 10 ml of normal saline during daily rounds to ascertain its patency. It is left in place for at least 1 week but is not removed until after it has been essentially dry for 5 days. If the drainage is sufficient to cause a continued wet dressing, the drain is connected to straight drainage with IV tubing. Suction is not needed because the normal intra-abdominal pressure tends to obliterate extraperitoneal spaces as long as there is a patent outlet for any fluid collection. On several occasions, after prolonged drainage through a Penrose drain, eventual removal, and replacement with a 14Fr rubber or silicone tube, I observed a gush of fluid from the space and rather prompt cessation of drainage.

Following completion of the ureteroureterostomy with or without a stent and after careful placement of the drain, the tube drain may be brought out through the incision or (if the course seems more direct) through a stab wound, when it is sutured to the skin. If a T-tube has been used, the vertical limb is brought to the surface with minimal tortuosity and no kinking—usually through a separate stab wound—and is sutured to the skin with a 2-0 silk suture. If there is any question about

FIG. 39-5. Ureteroureterostomy: techniques of anastomosis: **(A)** oblique; **(B)** Z-plasty; **(C)** fishmouth

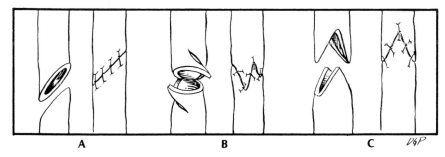

its patency, the vertical limb can be irrigated and connected to straight drainage. It is usually clamped by folding over the end and wrapping it with a small rubber band. Hoffman clamps and other devices are cumbersome and tend to get caught in the dressing. The vertical limb of the T-tube can be opened at any time to check residual urine in the renal pelvis, to obtain urine for culture, or to provide access for injection of contrast medium for pyeloureterograms. Unless there is some special indication (fever, renal pain, hematuria), the T-tube injection pyeloureterogram is done 5 to 7 days after ureteroureterostomy,. If there is no evidence of extravasation of the contrast medium at the site of anastomosis, the retroperitoneal extraureteral tube drain can be removed after 1 week *and* after it has been dry for 5 days.

If a straight ureteral stent has been used, an intravenous urogram is performed 1 week postoperatively. The same criteria are used for removing the tube drain.

Appropriate antibiotics are administered if infection is known to be present, but routine use of broad spectrum antimicrobials should be avoided until specific indications arise.

If a stent has been used and is functioning properly, it is left in place for a minimum of 4 weeks. A T-tube usually is not removed for 6 weeks. This allows time for more complete healing and for the ureter to become fixed in its bed, from which it has been partially removed during disruption and repair. I have not seen angulation of the ureter at the site of T-tube insertion if the tube is removed after 4 weeks. The T-tube is pulled through the skin opening by gradual traction until the junction of the vertical and horizontal limbs appears. The horizontal limbs are then grasped with a Kelly clamp to aid in the gradual withdrawal. (The length of the horizontal limbs can be determined from the radiographs or from measurements recorded in the operative note.) One of the two limbs of the T-tube is left as a drain down to the ureterotomy site from which it has been withdrawn. If a segment of the tube is to be left as a drain, one must be certain that this internal end has been withdrawn from the ureter so that the ureterotomy will heal. There usually is no drainage, but the segment is left in place as a preventive measure and is removed in 1 week.

The Lowsley grasping forceps has been used most frequently for transvesical removal of the straight ureteral stent, but any of several cystoscopic biopsy forceps or flexible rongeurs can be used for this purpose.

If there is any question of viability of the ureter, stricture at the site of anastomosis, or extravasation on the urographic studies, the ureteral stent should be left in place.[6] In the absence of infection, urinary precipitate will rarely obstruct silicone stents. I have seen silicone stent obstruction from urinary precipitate encrustation after 2 and 4 weeks respectively in two patients, both of whom had urea-splitting urinary infections. More ureteral stents have been removed too soon than too late. Seldom is there urgency to remove a silicone stent unless it is obstructed or symptomatic.

Patients with indwelling stents should have an intravenous urogram 1 month after removal and thereafter as indicated. If there is any evidence of stricture at the site of repair, more frequent follow-up examinations, periodic ureteral dilatations, and replacement of a stent such as the double-J retention ureteral catheter, all are to be considered. It should be added that although ureteral dilatations are not effective for congenital ureteral narrowing, such as most ureteropelvic obstructions, postoperative strictures seen after ureterolithotomy and ureteroureterostomy do respond to progressive dilatation by ureteral catheterization through a cystoscope. Additional benefit may be obtained by leaving the ureteral catheter in place for 24 hours. Although there appears to be an increasing tendency to perform ureteral dilatations through the kidney with fluoroscopic or ultrasonic guidance, in most cases it can be done more quickly, more economically, and with no more discomfort through a cystoscope. However, the percutaneous approach to the kidney and ureter is a welcome and useful addition to our armamentarium.

Anastomosis between ureters on the same side has become more popular as a method of managing reflux, ectopia, and other problems in one ureter when the ipsilateral mate is normal.[2,5,9,14] The procedure has been recommended also for reflux into both ipsilateral duplicated ureters as an alternative to reimplanting the ends of two large ureters into the bladder. Some have expressed concern about retrograde flow into one or both ureters, the "yo-yo" effect, proximal to the ureteroureterostomy, but this would appear to be an infrequent occurrence.[1]

In anastomosing the end of a ureter to the side of its ipsilateral mate, the surgeon must be particularly cautious on two counts. First, the end of a larger ureter is often being connected to the side of a smaller one, creating the hazard of damaging the recipient ureter. Second, great care must be used in clearing a site on the surface of the recipient ureter by using only careful blunt dissection with a small hemostat and without dissecting any segment of recipient ureter from its bed.

The incision in the recipient ureter must be exactly parallel to its long axis, and the incision must be long enough to receive the obliquely cut end of the donor ureter. If both ureters are relatively large and healthy, stenting is not necessary. If the donor ureter is large and the recipient ureter is normal or small in size, I would use a stent. The stent could be as small as a 5Fr feeding tube or plain silicone tube, with holes cut 1 cm apart along the side of the tube. The distal end of the stent is fed down the recipient ureter to the bladder; the proximal end is directed up the donor ureter to the renal pelvis. If the size of the recipient ureter permits, a second 5Fr silicone tube with holes cut 1 cm apart can be passed down to the bladder and the proximal end can be directed upward to the renal pelvis of the recipient ureter.

As mentioned above, stents should be as large as they can be while still fitting loosely in the ureter. In smaller children, the distal ends of the stents can be brought out through the bladder along with a suprapubic cystostomy tube to facilitate eventual removal. If the kidney is available in the surgical field, the stents can be brought into the renal pelvis through a calix in the manner of a nephrostomy.

A metal malleable 12Fr or 14Fr bougie à boule is useful in pulling a tube into a small kidney. This instrument is easily shaped into any size hook and inserted through a small opening in the renal pelvis. The end is blunt and can be manipulated through the renal cortex to the surface. One end of a 2-0 silk suture is tied proximal to the bulb on the bougie; the other is sutured to the end of the stent to be pulled into the kidney. The stent can then be fed down the ureter into the bladder where, with holes cut along the side of its indwelling portion, it can serve for nephrostomy drainage if needed and it can be easily removed at the desired time. If it is working properly it can be tied off externally and left in place for several weeks or longer. The end-to-side anastomosis of the donor ureter to its ipsilateral recipient mate is performed with interrupted sutures of 5-0 chromic gut placed 2 mm apart. Only 1-mm bites—through the entire wall including the urothelium—can be taken in the recipient ureter if it is normal size. Larger bites can be taken if the ureter is dilated and thickened. Bites 2 mm thick can be taken in the edges of the obliquely cut end of the donor ureter, and the thicker bites are an aid in making the anastomosis water tight. When the anastomosis is completed, and the ureters are replaced in the normal location, an extraureteral drain should be placed in the same manner as described above for ureteroureterostomy.

Transureteroureterostomy

When all or part of the lower half of one ureter is damaged, diseased, obstructed, or involved in a pathologic process and the contralateral ureter is functionally normal, a transureteroureterostomy provides a means of conserving the kidney with the damaged ureter. For the operation to succeed, at least the proximal (upper) half of the ureter *must* have sufficient length to cross the midline for anastomosis to its mate on the opposite side.[3] Contraindications to transureteroureterostomy include those listed under ureteroureterostomy plus stones in either or both kidneys. Transureteroureterostomy has been useful in urinary diversion from both kidneys through a single ureterostomy stoma, in undiversion procedures to avoid reimplantation of two large ureters into the bladder, and, more rarely, in making use of a normal ureter after nephrectomy when the ureter to the remaining kidney is diseased or injured.[15,18] Although earlier reports of transureteroureterostomy have been most encouraging,[4,11,12,17] later communications spelling out some of its complications and pitfalls should be reviewed before undertaking the operation.[8,16] Of particular interest is the observation that the risk to the recipient ureter might be greater than was originally thought, but the risk is not prohibitive if all precautions are taken.

Transureteroureterostomy is best performed

through an anterior midline abdominal incision. We again remind the reader that the ureters are closer to the midline than to the right and left extremes of the retroperitoneal space. As mentioned above, the exposure of both ureters is best accomplished by incising the peritoneum that forms the left leaf of the small bowel mesentery just anterior and parallel to the abdominal aorta (Figs. 39-1 and 39-2).

The inferior mesenteric artery is the only real anatomic obstacle to complete exposure of the lower left ureter though this approach, and the left ureter usually can be mobilized without sacrificing it. As the small bowel mesentery is mobilized carefully and reflected to the right, there is literally no anatomic barrier to mobilization of the right ureter. Whether it be left or right, the donor ureter should be brought across the midline above the inferior mesenteric artery, even for anastomosis at the level of the pelvic brim. The inferior mesenteric artery may be divided if the remainder of the left colon vascular supply is intact, but this usually is unnecessary.

The donor ureter should be transsected as low as possible. All periureteral tissue, including the gonadal artery and vein, should be mobilized with the ureter, leaving a clean anterior surface of psoas muscle. The dissection should begin just lateral to the gonadal vessels and continue medially toward the ureter. The fibroareolar tissue on the lateral surface of the vena cava on the right and of the aorta on the left is dissected off those vessels and carried laterally toward the respective ureter. No portion of the ureter should be isolated and retracted with a tape or a vascular loop. The end of the donor ureter is brought across the midline as the dissection progresses. When this end reaches the contralateral recipient ureter while lying free with no traction and following a gentle course with no acute angulation, the donor ureter has been mobilized adequately.

Attention is then directed to a site for its anastomosis on the recipient ureter. The recipient ureter should not be mobilized at all. An opening is made in its fibroareolar sheath with the end of a hemostat. An adequate area should be cleared to receive the obliquely cut end of the donor ureter at the appropriate level on the anteromedial surface of the recipient ureter. An incision as long as the corner-to-corner oblique end of the donor ureter is made exactly parallel to the long axis into the lumen of the recipient ureter with a No. 12 scalpel blade. Again, a stent is optional, but the rule is, "When in doubt, stent, but stent properly." Stenting is less needed in well-vascularized ureters of larger diameter (more than 1 cm).

If the recipient ureter is normal in caliber, a 5Fr or 6Fr silicone tube or feeding tube is used, with holes smaller than the internal diameter cut in the side of the tube at 1-cm intervals. The distances to the bladder and to the renal pelvis are measured with a calibrated 5Fr ureteral catheter. These distances are carefully measured on the stent and marked with a temporary ligature that is removed after the stent is secured in place.

One end of the stent is fed upward into the donor renal pelvis and the other end is fed down the recipient ureter into the bladder. If the distal recipient ureter is large enough, a second stent is fed down into the bladder with the proximal end inserted upward into the recipient renal pelvis. It is important that the distal ends of stents are in the bladder for the purpose of future removal. The holes 1 cm apart in the stent are most essential at each end and in the 5-cm segment proximal and distal to the anastomosis. In the younger child, the proximal end of the stent might be brought out through the kidney to provide access for possible drainage, diagnostic studies, and eventual removal.

Once the stent is positioned, it should be fixed in place with 6-0 or 5-0 chromic gut suture through the recipient ureter and the wall of the stent and be tied loosely on the external surface of the ureter. The marking ligature should be removed from the stent before beginning the anastomosis. The oblique end of the donor ureter is sutured to the opening in the recipient ureter with interrupted 5-0 chromic gut sutures, 2 mm apart. If the recipient ureter is normal in caliber, suture bites should be only 1 mm thick. If the recipient ureter is larger than normal, 2-mm bites are taken. Another option is to make the posterior anastomotic suture line continuous (Fig. 39-6).[13] *Note* that the length of the incision in the recipient normal-sized ureter can be made long enough to receive the oblique end of the donor ureter without undue risk to the recipient ureter as long as the recipient ureter is not freed from its bed, the incision is exactly parallel to the long axis of the ureter, and small suture bites are taken. The site of the anastomosis is drained in the manner described above for ureteroureterostomy. The 14Fr tube surfaces in the ipsilateral flank through a stab wound made over the end of a Kelly clamp, which is passed posterior to the colon on the side of the anastomosis.

After the drain has been placed precisely, the left leaf of the small bowel mesentery is reapproximated with sutures of 3-0 chromic gut every 2 cm to 3 cm. The incision is closed according to the surgeon's preference. A 5-ml balloon Foley catheter is left in the bladder for 24 hours unless there is

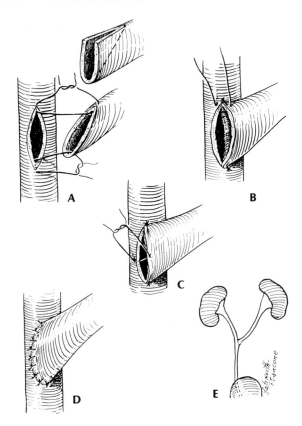

FIG. 39-6. Transureteroureterostomy. The ureteroureteral anastomosis is done end to side using a running layer of 4-0 chromic catgut suture for posterior layer. The anterior layer is approximated with interrupted sutures of the same material.

reason to leave it longer. A nasogastric tube is used as long as needed. The patency of the retroperitoneal drain should be checked daily with 5 ml to 10 ml of normal saline.

An intravenous urogram is performed 7 to 10 days postoperatively. If there is no extravasation and no significant drainage *and* the retroperitoneal drain has been dry at least 5 days, the drain may be removed any time after 7 days. When a stent cannot be removed from a child by cystoscopy without general anesthesia and it has been brought to the surface through a suprapubic cystotomy or a nephrostomy, there is some urgency to remove the stent as soon as possible after 10 days. When the end of the stent has not been brought through the skin surface, and it is functioning well, its removal is less urgent and can be deferred until maximum benefit has been obtained. Unless otherwise indicated, a second postoperative intravenous urogram is made in 4 to 6 weeks and thereafter as dictated by the findings.

Transureteroureterostomy is a rewarding oper-

ation if the surgeon adheres to the criteria spelled out for its success and avoids the conditions leading to its failure.

REFERENCES

1. BARRETT DM, MALEK RS, KELALIS PP: Problems and solutions in surgical treatment of 100 consecutive ureteral duplications in children. J Urol 114:126, 1975
2. BELMAN AB, FILMER RB, KING LR: Surgical management of duplication of the collecting system. J Urol 112:316, 1974
3. BOYARSKY S: Ureteral surgery. In Glenn JF (ed): Urologic Surgery, 2nd ed, pp 197–232. Hagerstown, Harper & Row, 1975
4. BRANNAN W: Useful applications of transureteroureterostomy in adults and children. J Urol 113:460, 1975
5. BUCHTEL HA: Ureteroureterostomy. J Urol 93:153, 1965
6. CARLTON CE, JR: Upper urinary tract trauma. In Glenn JF (ed): Urologic Surgery, 2nd ed, pp 154–168. Hagerstown, Harper & Row, 1975
7. DORR RP, RATLIFF RK, HYNDMAN CW: Technique of ureteral repair using an indwelling ureteral stent. J Urol 111:481, 1974
8. EHRLICH RM, SKINNER DG: Complications of transureteroureterostomy. J Urol 113:467, 1975
9. FOLEY FEB: Ureteroureterostomy as applied to obstruction of the duplicated upper urinary tract. J Urol 20:109, 1928
10. HARADA N, MORIHIKO T, KAZUHIRO F et al: Surgical management of a long ureteral defect: Advancement of the ureter by descent of the kidney. J Urol 92:192, 1964
11. HIGGINS CC: Transureteroureteral anastomosis: Report of a clinical case. J Urol 34:349, 1935
12. HODGES CV, MOORE RJ, LEHMAN TN et al: Clinical experiences with transureteroureterostomy. J Urol 90:552, 1963
13. LAWSON RK: Ureteral substitution. In Glenn JF (ed): Urologic Surgery, 2nd ed, pp 259–260. Hagerstown, Harper & Row, 1975
14. LYTTON B, WEISS RM, BERNEIKE RR: Ipsilateral ureteroureterostomy in the management of vesicoureteral reflux in duplication of the upper urinary tract. J Urol 105:507, 1971
15. OBRANT KO: Cutaneous ureterostomy with skin tube and plastic cup appliance, together with transureteroureteral anastomosis. Br J Urol 29:135, 1957
16. SANDOZ IL, POULL DP, MACFARLANE CA: Complications with transureteroureterostomy. J Urol 117:39, 1977
17. UDALL DA, HODGES CV, PEARSE HM et al: Transureteroureterostomy: A neglected procedure. J Urol 109:817, 1973
18. YOUNG JD, ALEDIA FT: Further observations on flank ureterostomy and cutaneous transureteroureterostomy. J Urol 95:327, 1966

Ureterocalicostomy

40

Bruce A. Lucas

U reterocalicostomy is a very useful technique which has not been sufficiently appreciated by many practicing urologists. Every urologic surgeon who performs renal stone surgery or reconstructive surgery should be familiar with ureterocalicostomy as an option in dealing with difficult cases of ureteropelvic junction (UPJ) obstruction or injury. Usually some type of UPJ repair of pyeloplasty can be performed, but occasionally an intrarenal pelvis will be inaccessible for a suitable ureteral anastomosis.

The urologist's expertise in reconstructing the UPJ has evolved steadily since Foley's[4] introduction of the Y–V plasty in 1937. Scardino and Prince[9] and Culp and DeWeerd[2] in the early 1950s devised flaps that gained popularity among those surgeons who were reluctant to interrupt UPJ continuity. Anderson and Hynes,[1] however, in 1949 broke with the Foley tradition and demonstrated that ureteral peristalsis would return within several weeks after a dismembered pyeloplasty. With this conceptual advance, nearly all UPJ repairs now involve total transection of the ureter and ureteropyeloneostomy. Ureterocalicostomy, as first reported by Jameson, McKinney, and Rushton[6] in 1957, follows naturally, involving ureteral anastomosis to the lower pole calix rather than the renal pelvis. Ureteropyelocalicostomy, a variant of the procedure described in this chapter, can be applied to the kidney with a large extrarenal pelvis requiring a lowerpole partial nephrectomy and UPJ repair.

Indications and Contraindications

The urologist is most likely to choose ureterocalicostomy over the other available options when the renal pelvis is entirely intrarenal, the lower pole calix is dilated, the overlying renal parenchyma is very thin or scarred, and the patient has had previous surgery for renal calculi or UPJ reconstruction. Common causes of postoperative stenosis or obliteration of the UPJ include extension of a pyelotomy or ureterotomy through the UPJ, stent trauma to a narrow upper ureter, loss of UPJ blood supply, and kinking.

When the renal pelvis is even partially extrarenal, traditional pyeloplasty techniques (see Chap. 21) are almost always preferred for relief of chronic UPJ obstruction requiring repair. If the strictured segment is long, Davis intubated ureteropyelotomy,[3] mobilization of the kidney caudad, autotransplantation, or bowel interposition may be applicable.

When the renal pelvis is inaccessible or not dependent, ureterocalicostomy may be the surgeon's best choice. Reported examples of suitable cases, other than an intrarenal pelvis undergoing repeated surgery, include traumatic UPJ transection and horseshoe kidney.[8] Recently, based on their experience with 15 cases, Levitt and associates advocated ureterocalicostomy as a primary procedure in some children with congenital UPJ obstruction.[7]

A stenotic lower pole infundilbulum would prevent optimal drainage of urine from the upper pole through the ureterocalicostomy. Advanced age, diffuse renal atrophy or scarring with minimal function, and ureteral abnormalities below the UPJ or a normal contralateral kidney may render nephrectomy preferable to ureterocalicostomy if no other options are feasible. Thick cortex in the lower pole may necessitate the sacrifice of much functioning parenchyma, but does not absolutely contraindicate ureterocalicostomy.

Patient Selection and Preparation

The first determination to be made is the need for reconstructive surgery for UPJ obstruction or disruption. If surgical repair is deemed necessary, all other options should be considered as previously noted and ruled out.

Standard evaluation usually includes excretory urography (IVP), voiding cystoureterogram (VCUG), and retrograde ureteropyelograms. Most patients should have cystoscopic passage of a ureteral catheter preoperatively even if it will not traverse

435

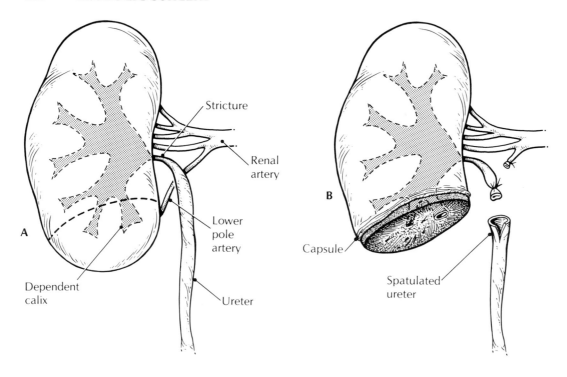

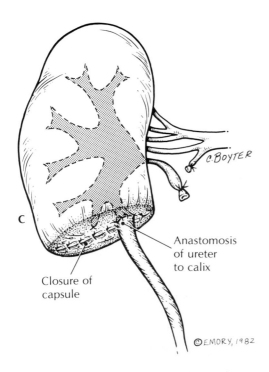

FIG. 40-1. Kidney with a thick parenchyma. **(A)** The lower-pole artery is ligated with demarcation of the infarcted lower pole. **(B)** The lower pole is resected. The calix and the spatulated ureter are prepared for anastomosis. **(C)** The ureterocalicostomy is completed.

the UPJ. The presence of the catheter may aid indentification and mobilization of the upper ureter at surgery and facilitate passage of a double-J stent down to the bladder intraoperatively if desired.

Because many ureterocalicostomy candidates have had previous renal surgery or have high-grade impassable UPJ stenosis, a traditional nephrostomy or percutaneous nephrostomy may be in place during the preoperative evaluation period. This urinary diversion catheter facilitates precise assessment of anatomic and physiologic abnormalities of the obstructed kidney. Differential creatinine clearances can be done. Antegrade pyelograms supplement retrograde ureterograms to optimally define the morphology and drainage characteristics of the upper collecting system. Hippuran radionuclide scan and renogram of the diverted, unobstructed kidney may be helpful, as may a Whitaker test.

Surgical Technique

A flank approach is usually preferable. Thorough mobilization of the kidney is desirable. The stenotic or obliterated UPJ may be resected or left *in situ*. The upper ureter is transected, mobilized as little as possible, and spatulated.

If the renal pelvis can be entered, the most

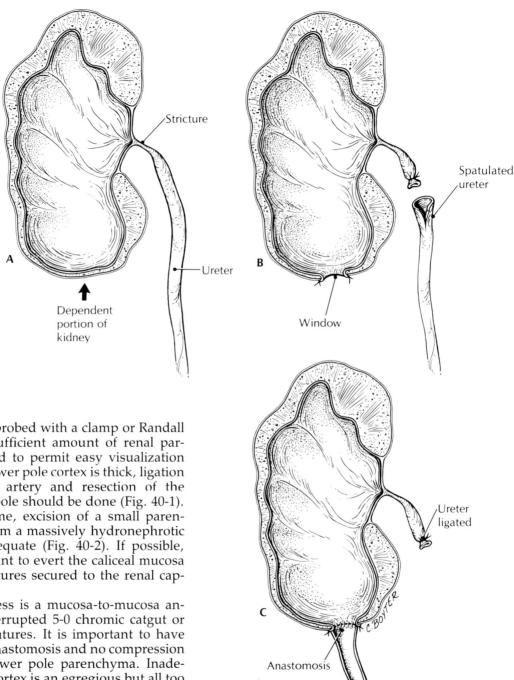

dependent calix is probed with a clamp or Randall stone forceps. A sufficient amount of renal parenchyma is resected to permit easy visualization of the calix. If the lower pole cortex is thick, ligation of the lower pole artery and resection of the demarcated lower pole should be done (Fig. 40-1). At the other extreme, excision of a small parenchymal window from a massively hydronephrotic system may be adequate (Fig. 40-2). If possible, the surgeon will want to evert the caliceal mucosa with absorbable sutures secured to the renal capsule.

The key to success is a mucosa-to-mucosa anastomosis with interrupted 5-0 chromic catgut or polyglycolic acid sutures. It is important to have no tension on the anastomosis and no compression of the ureter by lower pole parenchyma. Inadequate resection of cortex is an egregious but all too frequent error.

The ureterocaliceal anastomosis should always he stented. I prefer a Silastic double-J catheter which can be extracted from the bladder endoscopically 6 weeks later. A No. 5 or No. 8 polyethylene pediatric feeding tube stent alongside a nephrostomy tube is also acceptable. Penrose drains or Jackson–Pratt flat suction drains should be brought to the skin from below the kidney.

FIG. 40-2. Massively hydronephrotic kidney. **(A)** The most dependent calix is selected. **(B)** A parenchymal window is created with eversion of the caliceal mucosa. The ureter is spalutated. **(C)** The ureterocalicostomy is completed.

Results and Complications

Insufficient numbers of cases have been reported to assess the success rate of ureterocalicostomy. No one has a very large series, but the approximately 100 cases in the literature represent a small proportion of those actually done. Excellent long-term results are likely to be reported as worldwide experience with this neglected procedure increases.

Expected complications are the same as for other surgery involving the renal collecting system. Recurrent obstruction can be prevented by attention to the technical points described in this chapter. Errors in judgment concerning drains, stents, and nephrostomy should be on the side of leaving them in place too long, avoiding persistent extravasation and sepsis. The nephrostomy tube, if present, should be clamped when the stent is removed in order to prevent cicatrization of a "dry anastomosis."

REFERENCES

1. ANDERSON JC, HYNES W: Retrocaval ureter: Case diagnosed preoperatively and treated successfully by plastic operation. Br J Urol 21:209, 1949
2. CULP OS, DEWEERD JH: Pelvic Flap operation for certain types of ureteropelvic obstruction: Observations after 2 years' experience. J Urol 71:523, 1954
3. DAVIS DM: Intubated ureterotomy: New operation for ureteral and ureteropelvic strictures. Surg Gynecol Obstet 76:513, 1943
4. FOLEY FEB: New plastic operation for stricture at uretero-pelvic junction; report of 20 operations. J Urol 38:643, 1937
5. HAWTHORNE NJ, ZINCKE H, KELALIS PP: Ureterocalicostomy: An alternative to nephrectomy. J Urol 115:583, 1976
6. JAMESON SG, MCKINNEY JS, RUSHTON JF: Ureterocalycostomy: A new surgical procedure for correction of ureteropelvic stricture associated with an intrarenal pelvis. J Urol 77:135, 1957
7. LEVITT SB, NABIZADEH K, MUHAMMAD J et al: Primary calycoureterostomy for pelviouretal junction obstruction: Indications and results. J Urol 126:382, 1981
8. MOLONEY GE: Avulsion of the renal pelvis treated by ureterocalycostomy. Br J Urol 42:519, 1970
9. SCARDINO PL, PRINCE CL: Vertical flap ureteropelvioplasty: Preliminary report. South Med J 46:325, 1953
10. SINGER J: Ureterocalycostomy: A case report and discussion. Br J Urol 34:178, 1962
11. WESOLOWSKI S: Uretero-calicostomy. Eur Urol 1:18, 1975

Ureteroplasty and Ureteral Replacement

41

Victor A. Politano

Ureteral Substitution

On occasion, the urologic surgeon is faced with the dilemma of replacing all or part of both ureters. Many substitutes have been tried, which run the gamut from vessels, skin, glass, and fallopian tubes to synthetic materials.[3,4,9,12,13,16] For a variety of reasons, including stone formation, infections, stricture formation, and hydronephrosis, these substitutes have not been successful.[1] Of the possible synthetic substitutes, hydrogels seem to hold the best promise at this moment.[5]

Davis demonstrated the remarkable capacity of the ureter to regenerate if continuity can be maintained.[8] However, most lesions encountered do not fall into this category, but require substitution of all or part of the ureter. The most satisfactory method for substitution of a lower ureter that is not amenable to direct implantation is use of a tubularized bladder flap.[6] Autotransplantation is another option. Substitution of the entire ureter is best accomplished with small or large intestine.

Bladder Flap Methods

Ockerblad popularized the Boari bladder flap technique in this country.[18] The ureter may be reimplanted submucosally in the tubularized bladder flap to prevent reflux. This method is excellent for replacing as much as 15 cm of ureter when the bladder is normal. Flocks described constructing such a tube all the way to the renal pelvis.*

Operative Procedure

The bladder flap is constructed by making two parallel incisions across the anterior bladder wall with the base of the flap posteriorly. The width of the flap must be sufficient to accept the ureter. A distal end of approximately 3 cm is the width necessary for a normal or only slightly dilated ureter. The base of the flap should be 1 cm or 2 cm wider to ensure good blood supply to the distal end of the tube. A submucosal tunnel is

---

* Flocks R: Personal communication

made in the distal end of the flap for 2 cm to 3 cm to prevent reflux. The ureter is pulled through the tunnel and sutured with several interrupted sutures of 4-0 chromic catgut to the mucosa. An appropriate-size ureteral stent is passed up the ureter and the flap is closed as a tube. I prefer to use a running suture of 5-0 chromic catgut in the mucosa as a hemostatic suture followed by a running suture of 4-0 chromic catgut in the muscularis. The bladder is closed similarly. A few interrupted sutures of the same material may be used to reinforce the suture line; they are placed in the serosa of the bladder and the tube flap (Fig. 41-1). The area must be drained adequately with a Penrose drain. Care is taken to keep the drain away from the suture line. Bilateral bladder flaps may be developed if replacement of both lower ureteral segments is necessary and if the bladder size and mobility are adequate. Additional length for bridging large defects can be gained by incorporating a psoas hitch.

Ileal Substitution

Injuries, retroperitoneal disease, or intrinsic lesions of the ureter may necessitate partial or total replacement. Occasionally, bilateral replacement may be necessary. The experience gained with use of the ileum as a cutaneous urinary conduit has encouraged ureteral substitution with isolated intestinal segments.[2,7,10,11,17,20,21] The ileum has been used most commonly, but large intestine may be used with equal success. Obviously, disease of the intestinal tract, such as Crohn's disease, regional ileitis, or diverticulitis, is a contraindication to use of the intestinal segment as substitution for the ureter.

Increasing experience with the use of intestine as a ureteral substitute has broadened the indications for its use. We have used intestine for such diverse conditions as large, adynamic, or aperistaltic ureters; severe retroperitoneal fibrosis and pelvic lipomatosis (leading the intestine intraperitoneally rather than placing it in a retroperitoneal position); carcinoma of the ureter in a solitary

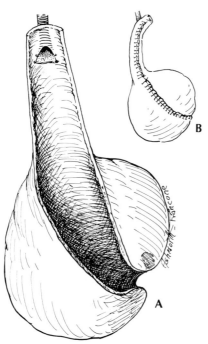

FIG. 41-1.   Boari–Ockerblad bladder flap for replacement of lower ureteral segment. This modification of the original procedure shows the ureter passing through a submucosal tunnel to prevent reflux. The spatulated ureter is sutured to the bladder mucosa using 4-0 chromic catgut. The bladder and the flap are closed with a 4-0 chromic catgut sutures.

kidney; severe or multiple ureteral strictures; and undiversion of cutaneous conduits.

Certain criteria should be met before substitution is undertaken. The bladder must be usable or a bladder substitute such as the cecum must be provided. Renal function must be sufficient to handle adequately the absorption of electrolytes that may occur during transport of the urine through the intestine. The creatinine clearance should be at least 20 ml to 25 ml per minute. The bladder outlet must be adequate to allow passage of the mucus without difficulty.

If small intestine is to be used, the patient is placed on clear liquids for at least 2 days prior to surgery. Antibiotics are used when the urinary tract is infected. If large intestine is used, laxatives and enemas are given to clean the intestine. In addition, neomycin sulfate, 1 g, q.i.d., is given 12 to 24 hours prior to surgery.

Operative Procedure

A generous midline, paramedian, or flank (twist-position) incision is made to allow access both to the renal pelvis or upper ureter and to the bladder.

When small intestine is to be used, a segment long enough to bridge the defect is isolated, usually 20 cm to 25 cm in an adult. It is important to select a segment that has a mobile mesentery. The isolated segment of intestine may be left as an intraperitoneal structure, or it may be passed through the mesocolon of the ascending or descending colon into the retroperitoneal space, after first taking down the colon and reflecting it medially. The continuity of the intestine is reestablished by the surgeon's choice of a single-layer closure, two-layer closure, or staples. It is important to close the intestine carefully, to close the mesentery, and to suture the mesocolon around the root of the mesentery to the isolated ileal segment to prevent herniation of the intestine through any of these potential spaces. The intestine should be placed in an isoperistaltic manner. When the right ureter is being substituted, the root of the mesentery may have to have a half twist or be folded over on itself to make it isoperistaltic. Care must be taken to ensure an adequate blood supply to the isolated ileal segment.

The upper end of the ileum may be anastomosed directly to the renal pelvis or to a dilated ureter as an end-to-end anastomosis. When the ureter is not dilated, it is preferable to close the end of the ileum and do a side-to-side anastomosis of the ureter to the ileal segment. The ureter is spatulated and the anastomosis is performed with interrupted 4-0 chromic full-thickness sutures, through ureter and intestine. The anastomosis may be reinforced with additional sutures, serosa to serosa (Fig. 41-2).

When the problem is related to obstruction of the ureteropelvic junction, ileocaliceal anastomosis may be performed using the same principles as apply to any ureterocaliceal anastomosis. It is necessary to resect the renal parenchyma surrounding the calix or infundibulum to be used.

The bladder is opened and the distal end of the ileum is brought into the bladder, preferably along the posterior wall or near the base. My preference is to pull several centimeters of ileum into the bladder and turn it back on itself as a cuff. The ileum is fixed to the serosal surface of the bladder with several interrupted sutures of 3-0 chromic. The turned-back cuff of ureter is sutured to the bladder mucosa with several interrupted sutures of 4-0 chromic. The cuff acts as a flutter valve and may eliminate or reduce reflux into the ileal segment (Fig. 41-3). The ileum can enter the bladder at any point, but when brought in at the dome, any redundancy must be eliminated to prevent the ileum from kinking or angulating as the bladder fills.

FIG. 41-2. Ileal ureter. The descending colon is retracted to show the retroperitoneal position of the ileal segment. The entire ileal segment is passed through a window in the mesocolon.

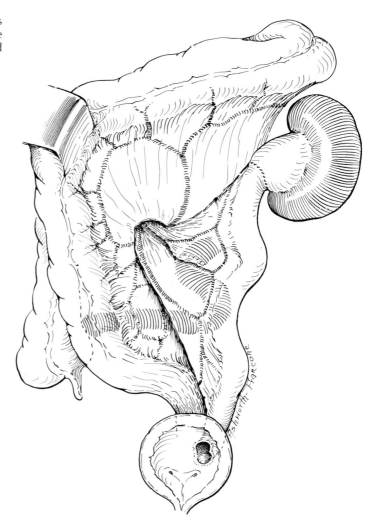

Bilateral replacement can be performed using the same ileal segment, running the proximal end from one pelvis to the other and down into the bladder. When the upper ureters are available, they are brought through the posterior peritoneum toward the midline and anastomosed to the ileal segment in the same fashion as an ileal conduit; thus, the entire ileal substitute lies intraperitoneally.

In the presence of retroperitoneal disease, the proximal ileum is passed through the mesocolon at the renal level, the anastomosis is performed, and the ileal segment remains intraperitoneal. The edges of the mesentery of the isolated segment are sutured to the posterior peritoneum to prevent the small bowel from becoming caught behind the mesentery. Because of the large amount of mucus that is given off by the intestine, it is advisable to use a large catheter suprapubically as well as a urethral catheter. The bladder is closed in the usual two- or three-layer closure and is adequately drained. Large intestine may be used in exactly the same manner as ileum, and there appears to be little or no difference in the final results.

ILEAL SLEEVE

When an adynamic or aperistaltic ureter is encountered, an alternative to total replacement is the use of the ileal sleeve.[14,15,19] This is especially useful when renal function is marginal and the added workload on the kidney from absorption through the mucosa may be hazardous. The ileal segment for the sleeve is isolated in the same manner. The pedicle of the mesentery is clamped with a rubber-shod clamp, and the ileum is opened along the antimesentery border (Fig. 41-4). The mucosa is stripped away, using the back of a knife

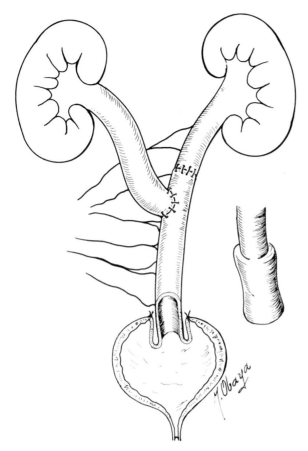

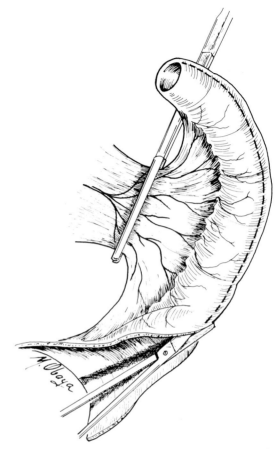

FIG. 41-3. The distal ileal segment is turned back on itself for 5 cm or 6 cm. The cuff acts as a flutter valve to eliminate or reduce reflux.

FIG. 41-4. Ileal sleeve. A segment of ileum is isolated. The mesentery is clamped with a rubber-shod clamp and is opened along the antimesentery border in preparation for stripping of the mucosa.

blade or an open clamp. Once the plane has been established, the mucosa strips easily. The open intestine is placed over the surgeon's finger for countertraction as the mucosa is stripped away. It is important that all of the mucosa be removed in order to prevent formation of a mucocele, which could be obstructive.

The ileum, once isolated, is passed behind the ascending or descending colon. The upper end of the mucosa-free segment is sutured to the hilus of the kidney, incorporating all of the renal pelvis if possible (Fig. 41-5). The ureter from the renal pelvis down to the bladder is encompassed by the ileum; the edges of the now-denuded ileal segment are sutured together with a continuous interlocking suture of 3-0 chromic (Fig. 41-6). The sutures through the ileum are placed so that about every third suture picks up the serosal covering of the ureter. The ureter is mobilized, kinks are removed, and excess or redundant ureter is resected. A

reduction ureteroplasty can be made, if necessary. The distal end of the ureter is reimplanted into the bladder through a submucosal tunnel and the distal end of the mucosa-free ileal segment is sutured to the serosa of the bladder at the entry point of the ureter into the muscularis of the bladder. The ileum is sutured to the bladder with interrupted 3-0 chromic catgut sutures (Fig. 41-7). The surgical areas should be drained adequately.

The ileal sleeve has certain advantages over complete ileal replacement. It may be used when renal function is very marginal, because the ureter remains intact and there is no absorption of electrolytes from its surface. It restores or improves absent or sluggish peristaltic action. Because urine is transported through the ureter, there is no absorption, nor is there mucus to eliminate. The ileal sleeve has been used when external diversion would have been the only other choice.

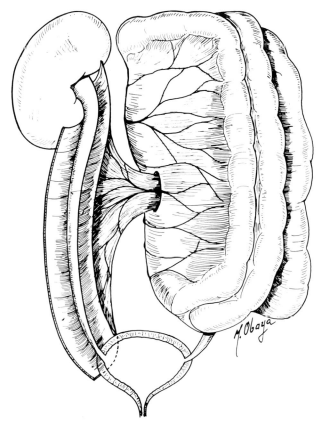

FIG. 41-5.   The ileum, free of mucosa, is passed through a window of the mesocolon of the ascending or descending colon to encompass the ureter.

Reduction Ureteroplasty

When ureters have become dilated and tortuous from obstruction or reflux, longitudinal reduction ureteroplasties may be necessary prior to ureteral reimplantation. Dilated, tortuous ureters are best approached extravesically, mobilizing the ureters, detaching the distal end from the bladder, removing the kinks, and straightening the ureter. The ureter is opened and inspected for valves or mucosal folds that may be obstructive. A longitudinal strip of ureter is removed and the ureter is closed over a 14Fr or 16Fr catheter (Fig. 41-8). Excessive length of ureter is amputated. Care is taken to leave the adventitia of the ureter intact during the mobilization and not to reduce the diameter of the ureter excessively. The ureter may be mobilized totally, completely, and without jeopardy from the renal pelvis to the bladder, providing the adventitia, which carries the blood vessels, has not been stripped. The ureter is closed in two layers over the stenting catheter with a continuous suture of 4-0 chromic. The suture line is reinforced with

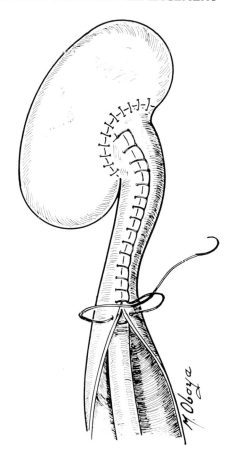

FIG. 41-6.   The upper end of the sleeve encompasses the renal pelvis and is sutured to the hilus of the kidney. An interlocking suture is used to approximate the edges of the ileum. About every third stitch catches the adventitia of the ureter.

interrupted sutures of the same material. The distal end of the ureter is reimplanted into the bladder by a submucosal tunnel technique in the manner preferred by the surgeon. It is advisable to leave a 10Fr or 12Fr catheter in the ureter for a week or 10 days, bringing it out through the bladder suprapubically. It is important to leave adequate drains along the course of the ureters. These drains should be left in place until the stents have been removed.

Reduction ureteroplasties may be performed transvesically. The ureter is mobilized as for a reimplantation, the excess ureter is removed, and a longitudinal strip is excised from the last 6 cm or 8 cm of ureter. The ureter is closed and reimplanted submucosally. It is my personal preference to do the reduction ureteroplasty extravesically and to begin the ureteroplasty much higher on the ureter, at or near the renal pelvis, or certainly well

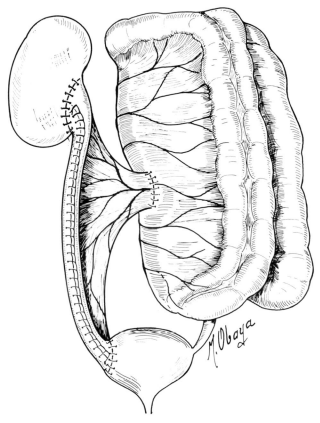

FIG. 41-7. The completed ileal sleeve. The lower end is sutured directly to the bladder at the point of ureteral entry.

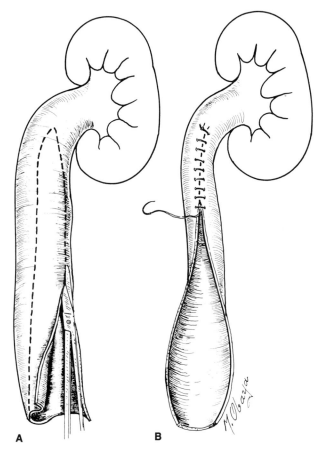

A   **B**

FIG. 41-8. **(A)** Reduction ureteroplasty is accomplished by excising a longitudinal strip of ureter. **(B)** The ureter is closed in two layers using 4-0 chromic. The distal end is reimplanted into the bladder using a submucosal tunnel.

above the iliac vessels. Most important for a successful ureteroplasty are preservation of the blood supply to the lower ureter, careful closure, and adequate drainage.

NONEXCISIONAL REDUCTION URETEROPLASTY

An alternative to the excision of a longitudinal strip of ureter for reduction of the diameter is simply to mobilize the ureter, straighten it, and remove the kinks and adhesions. Cut off the excess length of ureter, then do an imbrication of the ureter beginning well above the pelvic brim. The ureter is imbricated with 4-0 Dexon or catgut, with interrupted sutures. When the sutures are taken as illustrated in Figure 41-9, the ureteral circumference can be reduced by as much as or more than half. The distal end is reimplanted submucosally.

The advantages of this technique are that it is more rapid and that there is no drainage, because the ureter has not been opened. It is especially

useful in cases that have had previous ureteral surgery, in whom the blood supply may be tenuous to start with. Since the ureter remains intact and no longitudinal strip is removed, there is less chance for devascularization. A ureteral catheter may be left in the ureter for several days, until edema at the reimplantation site has subsided.

REFERENCES

1. BAUM N, MOBLEY DF, CARLTON CE: Ureteral replacements. Urology 5:165, 1975
2. BAUM WC: The clinical use of terminal ileum as a substitute ureter. J Urol 72:16, 1954
3. BETTMAN AG: Anastomosis between the ureter and urinary bladder by means of a subcutaneous skin tube. Plast Reconstr Surg 2:80, 1947
4. BLASUCCI E: Substitution of segments of ureters with arterial hemografts. Minerva Chir 12:1590, 1957
5. BLOCK NL, STOVER B, POLITANO VA: A prosthetic ureter

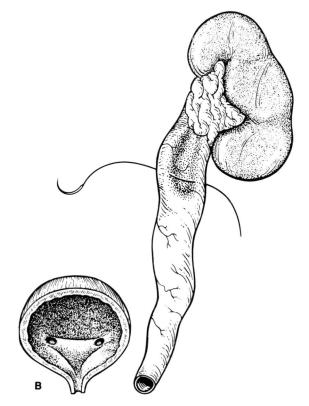

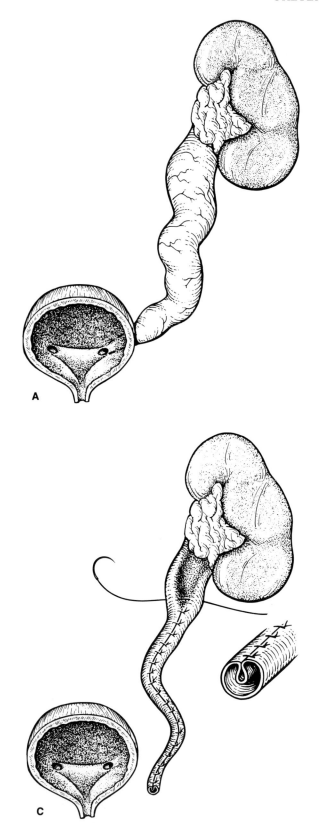

FIG. 41-9. **(A)** The dilated ureter is mobilized completely and straightened out. **(B)** After dissection from the bladder, imbrication to reduce the caliber is started well up on the ureter and continued to the distal end. 4-0 Dexon is used for the imbrication. **(C)** The completed imbrication. The distal end is reimplanted in a submucosal tunnel.

in the dog. Am Assoc Artif Internal Organs, April, 1977

6. BOARI A: Chiurgia dell' uretere con prefazione del dott. I. Albarran, 1900. Contributo sperimentale alla plastica delle ureter. Quoted by Spies JW, Johnson CW, Wilson CS: Reconstruction of the ureter by a bladder flap. Proc Soc Exp Biol Med 30:425, 1932

7. BOXER RJ, FRITZSCHE P, SKINNER DG et al: Replacement of the ureter by small intestine: Clinical application and results of the ileal ureter in 89 patients. J Urol 121:728, 1979

8. DAVIS DM: Intubated ureterotomy: A new operation for ureteral and ureteropelvic structure. Surg Gynecol Obstet 76:514, 1943

9. FANTINO M, RANGONI AG: Arterial and venous autoplastic grafts in reparative surgery of the ureter: Experimental research. Arch Sci Med (Torino) 107:640, 1959

10. FRITZSCHE P, SKINNER DG, CRAVEN JD et al: Long-term radiographic changes of the kidney following the ileal ureter operation. J Urol 114:843, 1975

11. GOODWIN WE, WINTER CC, TURNER RD: Replacement of the ureter by small intestine: Clinical application and results of the "ileal ureter." J Urol 81:406, 1959

12. HARDIN CA: Experimental repair of ureters by polyethylene tubing and ureteral and vessel grafts. Arch Surg 68:56, 1957

13. HARVARD BM, CAMILLERI JA, NADIG PW et al: Experimental transplantation of freeze-dried homologous and autologous ureteral segments. J Urol 86:385, 1961

14. HIRSCHHORN RC: The ileal sleeve. I. First case report with clinical evaluation. J Urol 92:206, 1964

15. HIRSCHHORN RC: The ileal sleeve. II. Surgical technique in clinical application. J Urol 92:120, 1964

16. HORTON CE, POLITANO VA: Ureteral reconstruction with split skin grafts: An experimental study. Plast Reconstr Surg 15:261, 1955

17. MOORE VE, WEBER R, EDWARD WR et al: Isolated ileal loops for ureteral repair. Surg Gynecol Obstet 102:87, 1956

18. OCKERBLAD NF: Reimplantation of the ureter into the bladder by a flap method. J Urol 57:845, 1947

19. POLITANO VA, LYNNE CM, SMALL MP: The ileal sleeve for the dilated ureter. J Urol 107:31, 1972

20. PROUT GR, JR, STUART WT, WITTUS WS: Utilization of ileal segments to substitute for extensive ureteral loss. J Urol 90:541, 1963

21. SKINNER DG, GOODWIN WE: Indications for the use of intestinal segments in management of nephrocalcinosis. J Urol 113:436, 1975

Ureteral Stricture, Fistula, And Trauma

42

Saul Boyarsky

The purpose of this chapter is to describe how to repair and restore ureteral morphology and function after stricture, fistula, or other trauma. The chapter emphasizes the surgical technique and decisions and only summarizes or alludes to surgical rationale and pathophysiology. It emphasizes techniques and questions that should be kept in mind by the surgeon and does not attempt to provide complete answers. Many of the answers are still controversial.

ANATOMICAL AND PHYSIOLOGICAL ASPECTS

Anatomically, for a repair of the ureter to be successful, the mucosa must be constituted of normal urinary epithelium without abnormal folds, pockets, or diverticula. The lumen must be patent and distensible enough to offer low resistance to the flow of urine from the pelvis and the nephron. The muscularis must show a normal number and direction of smooth muscle bundles with interspersed blood vessels and sparse innervation. The adventitia should be free of inflammatory infiltrate and periureteral adhesions so that the entire ureter can be free to glide in its sheath longitudinally and to expand transversely to receive a peristaltic bolus. No periureteral adhesions should trap the ureter so as to kink or compress it.

Physiologically, the ureter must be actively peristaltic so as to empty itself completely without residual urine or infection and to allow it to meet its functional demands of rhythm and bolus conduction. Urinary absorption and extravasation should not occur, nor should calculus formation.[1–3]

The normally constituted ureter is free of stricture, ulceration, diverticula, calcification, stones, and extravasation.

REGENERATION OF THE URETER

The processes of ureteral healing, regeneration, and reconstitution have been studied in animal models in a series of papers from 1950 to 1970 to which the interested reader is referred.[1,9,12,15–17] Current physiologic theory has been developed from this research to describe a process of rapid uroepithelial outgrowth over a ureteral defect, in a matter of 4 to 7 days, followed by a slower bridging of a ureteral defect by the ingrowth of muscular tissue into the exudate and granulation tissue covering the defect. In the absence of urine, inflammation, foreign body, and tissue detritus, rather large gaps in ureteral continuity are bridged successfully. Otherwise, the process is incomplete and normal ureteral architecture is disturbed in three dimensions, not two, leading to diverticula and false passages as well as stricture formation. In the absence of normal smooth muscle, scar replacement and even calcification can result, leading to aberrations of shape and caliber.

Small gaps in muscular continuity, such as those due to fine scars, offer little delay or blockage to the passage of a peristaltic impulse; the same is not true for larger defects. For a large defect it may take 6 to 8 weeks to bridge the gap by a combination of smooth muscle and fibrous tissue. Research has shown that in the absence of urinary extravasation the regenerative process overcomes many difficulties, but it produces strictures, bone, and diverticula in the presence of extravasation.[5,9,10,13] Lapides and others have shown the importance of the periureteral fatty sheath in preventing adherence to surrounding muscle or tendon to prevent fixation, angulation, traction, and dense, fibrous encapsulation.[12] The Davis intubated ureterotomy (Fig. 42-1) is still successfully employed.[4]

Indications and Timing

It is beyond the scope of this chapter to discuss in great detail diagnosis, except to stress the importance of differential diagnosis—the discovery of those conditions that would alter the operative plan. It is especially important to rule out a vesi-

Acknowledgment is gratefully made to Dr. Robert Royce for a critical reading of and several additions to the manuscript.

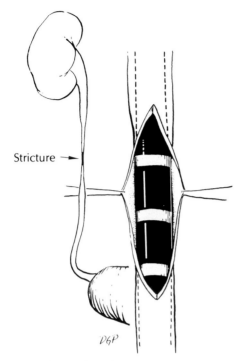

FIG. 42-1. In the intubated ureterotomy, the defect in the ureter is left to close spontaneously around the catheter.

covaginal fistula when operating for a ureterovaginal fistula and to differentiate between periureteral fibrosis and retroperitoneal malignancy as a cause of ureteral obstruction. During surgery, it is most important to distinguish normal or nearly normal ureteral wall from scarred, aperistaltic, or necrotic wall.

Surgery is indicated to meet the following needs:

To preserve renal function

To restore ureteral continuity

To remove ureteral obstruction

To prevent repetition of a clinical insult such as urinary tract infection or calculus due to ureteral stricture or scar

Occasionally, to excise a ureteral scar because of intermittent hydronephrosis with or without associated renal colic.

The timing of surgery deserves consideration. First, the lesion must be shown to have damaged or threatened to damage renal function or integrity. The mere presence of ureteral pathology is often not enough to indicate surgery unless a progression of renal damage is demonstrated or infection is actually localized to the renal and ureteral unit involved, not to the urinary tract as a whole. Second, the patient and the local lesion must be placed in the best possible condition for the surgery. This requires that infection be controlled as best possible, by antibiotic therapy and that any urine soaked tissues recover from chemical insult by preliminary urinary diversion, particularly in the case of the ureterovaginal fistula. Third, proper evaluation and judgment must be used for any past, present, or future vascular insult, including radiation injuries, bullet injuries, crushing clamps, and constricting ligatures that produce vascular damage at varying time frames to produce ischemia.

Preoperative Preparation

The preoperative preparation requires that infection be properly identified bacteriologically and treated to the utmost possible; that preexisting damages of irradiation, scarring, adhesions, and the like be recognized; that any urinary extravasation be treated by prior diversion when feasible; and that the patient be in the best possible condition for surgery. Bowel extravasation or contamination requires antibiotic therapy and possible fecal diversion. It is recognized that for the trauma patient, especially in the presence of multiple injuries, or the patient with malignancy, the procedure may need to be performed before the patient can be ideally readied for surgery.

Operative Approach and Technique

Ureteral repairs must be performed through a wide variety of operative incisions. Specific incisions are not discussed here because the discussion would repeat the approaches used for malignancies, stones, abdominal crises, and elective procedures.

The surgeon must be ready to enlarge the original incision or to close it and make another, depending upon the need of the moment and the condition of the patient. He may need to expose the kidney, the bladder, or the opposite ureter, and he may need to enter the peritoneal cavity. The original dissection may have been performed by a gynecologist, a general surgeon, or a vascular surgeon, and the urologist may need to complete the exposure or to expose more of the urinary tract. The patient's condition may compel him to perform a temporary urinary diversion, or even a nephrectomy, rather than to attempt repair of the ureteral injury.

The immediate or long-term threat of urinary infection, the response to diversion by the periureteral tissues, the extent of devascularization or postirradiation ischemia, and the distribution of the healthy residual tissue are factors that enter into the choice of techniques of ureteral repair, especially in regard to the use of stents and drainage tubes.

LOCATION AND DISSECTION OF THE URETER

Tricks in locating the ureter include being aware that the ureter follows the peritoneum during the operative approach and crosses the bifurcation of the iliac artery. The surgeon should aspirate the urine with a fine needle and should not hesitate to enter the peritoneal cavity. The ureter can be found immediately underneath the obliterated umbilical ligament when that structure can be identified. When tweaked gently with thumb forceps, the ureter usually manifests rather active peristalsis that can very readily be appreciated.

The ureterolysis is limited to that necessary for efficient surgery in order to preserve the periureteral blood supply as much as possible. The ureter receives multiple fine arterioles throughout its course. Needless dissection should be avoided. However, for a successful repair of a damaged ureter, it will be necessary to appose good tissue to good tissue. Hence, the ureter should be freed enough to demonstrate the entire scar and the normal tissue on either side, all other factors being equal.

Ureterolysis may be the definitive procedure and all that is necessary when the ureter is trapped either in fibrous tissue owing to retroperitoneal fibrosis or by a traction adhesion secondary to overlying bowel inflammation or previous ureteral surgery. An indwelling ureteral catheter placed preoperatively by cystoscopy may help identify the encased ureter. Dissecting the ureter from its surrounding bed is difficult, particularly when the ureteral wall is fibrosed and thickened so as to be indistinguishable from the surrounding fibrous tissue. Here, care must be taken to preserve the integrity of the ureteral wall by careful, gentle, and sharp dissection. The ureter may be manipulated by traction suture, tape (rubber, plastic, or umbilical), or finger, or by gently grasping the adventitia, but it must never be grasped with an instrument that can crush it and produce local necrosis. A seriously damaged ureter must be considered for wrapping with omentum, transplantation to the peritoneum, or even replacement. If the decision is made to preserve it, then urinary diversion by nephrostomy catheter or ureterostomy proximal to the injury during the postoperative period may be helpful. The surgeon should not optimistically jump to conclusions on the assumption of normal multiple ureteral blood supply when he is dealing with a reoperated or scarred urinary tract in which the normal anastomotic pathways may have been altered or completely destroyed.

DÉBRIDEMENT

After the ureter is freed completely enough to allow planning of the repair and reanastomosis, the edges of the damaged, destroyed, or scarred area are excised and the edges are freshened and prepared for reanastomosis. In the preliminary incision, if it is a linear one, the incision must be carried from normal ureteral wall through the scar to normal wall on the other side. The color, pinkness, and thickness of the tissue, and its prior peristaltic motility, are the standard guides to normality. The edges should be smooth according to the requirement of the type of anastomosis chosen. The lumen should be patent as demonstrated by ureteral catheters or probes.

Even though the ureteral wall appears to be normal, if the patient has suffered a high-velocity bullet injury, the extent of vascular damage may be greater than is first apparent. If there is bacterial contamination, then the healing will be impaired. If the patient has undergone irradiation or the ureter has been crushed by a clamp, the pinkness or apparent normalcy may be misleading. Of course, if there is a cancer nearby, then micrometastases may be present even though the ureteral wall appears to be normal.

REANASTOMOSIS

The technique of reanastomosis (Fig. 42-2) is rarely end to end or side to side but is usually a spatulated, diagonal, or elliptic reanastomosis which combines the advantages of both end-to-end and side-to-side closure: not producing a kink or pocket in the channel and not producing a short circular scar that can constrict and cause a stricture. The fishmouth, the Z-plasty, or the U-flap may be used to lengthen the suture line when the ureteral wall is dilated. Whichever technique the surgeon selects to facilitate reanastomosis, the two ends of ureter must be appropriately prepared. It helps to place a small 4-0 chromic or similar guide suture to identify opposite points so that the final anastomosis is more accurately performed.[14,15,16]

Some surgeons prefer to dilate the ureter prior to making the anastomosis in order to facilitate the surgery. This should be done gradually and gently and within physiologic limits up to 8Fr, rather than

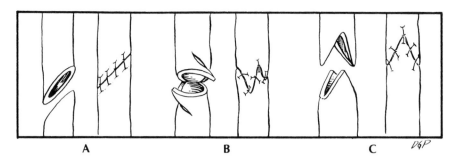

FIG. 42-2. The techniques of reanastomosis include **(A)** oblique, **(B)** Z-plasty, and **(C)** fishmouth.

traumatically (beyond 10Fr–12Fr suddenly and forcibly). It is more helpful to intubate the two ends of the ureter with a catheter or stent during the anastomosis to hold the opposite wall away from the area of suturing and to distribute the lengths of the edges more evenly around the circumference. Such an indwelling catheter may be removed after the anastomosis has been completed or may be left indwelling postoperatively as a stent for 10 to 14 days.

What should one do when the ureter does not fall into place easily with adequate length? Be sure that the recommended techniques have been followed:

The previously described methods of preparing the edge by spatulation, fishmouthing, Z-plasty, and the like gain length to bridge the surgical defect.

Gentle dissection and tension on the ureter suffice to gain 1 cm or 2 cm to close a gap. However, if the gap is much larger or if the ureter is adherent, compromised, or otherwise immobilized, then the use of tension to lengthen the ureter would be counterproductive and possibly disastrous.

Attention must be given to dissecting large lengths of ureter or to performing a downward nephropexy or even autotransplantation of the kidney.[7]

From below, a bladder flap can be raised or, more commonly, a psoas hitch can be used to elevate the bladder toward the ureter on the ipsilateral side.

A long defect in which it is necessary to gain width of ureteral wall is better handled by the intubated ureterotomy technique. Essentially, this technique involves performing a linear ureterotomy through the desired area and splinting the ureter with an indwelling catheter or a stent until the ureteral wall has closed and reconstituted itself. A period of 2 to 6 weeks will be required, depending upon the health and integrity of the wall, the size of the gap, and the absence of interfering extra-

vasation, infection, and other deleterious influences.[4]

To bridge a larger ureteral gap than can be healed by conventional surgery requires the use of an inert plastic splint, a split-thickness skin graft, a renal capsular flap, and possibly a biological material such as umbilical vein and procedures that are experimental or infrequently used. A segment of ileum has been used to good advantage to bridge long ureteral defects and is no longer considered experimental.[6]

A ureteral diversion may be necessary by ureteroneocystostomy, if the defect is in the lower portion of the ureter. The diversion is facilitated by a bladder flap or a psoas hitch. Transureteroureterostomy has been performed to great advantage in many instances.[8,11] It may be necessary to perform a cutaneous ureterostomy or an ileal segment type of urinary diversion. Even a nephrectomy may be necessary in some cases if the opposite side is normal or adequately functional. Renal autotransplantation has been performed in several instances.

APPOSITION AND SUTURE TECHNIQUE

Before the actual suturing is performed, it is useful to appose the edges of the ureter to be sure that the edges fall into place at the desired level. In this way, any tendency for postoperative disruption or undue tension can be discovered and corrected.

Fine absorbable sutures are used, whether 4-0 chromic, 5-0 chromic catgut, Dexon, or other suture. Silk or other nonabsorbable suture is not used conventionally because of the possibility of erosion into the lumen or incrustation, with stone formation. If used, care must be taken to avoid engaging the ureteral mucosa with this suture material.

The ureter must be handled gently, with fine instruments. It should be grasped, if at all, only very superficially by its surrounding corrective tissue. It should not be stretched, pulled, or tugged. It should not be handled any more than is necessary, but rather allowed to lie in place as if it were brain tissue or delicate conjunctiva.

Interrupted sutures produce the least constricting effect upon the ureteral edges, but continuous or locking sutures provide the most watertight closures, granting the same accuracy of apposition.

GEROTA'S FASCIA AND OMENTAL WRAP

The ureter may be replaced into the retroperitoneum where it will receive some new blood supply. Usually, the ureter should be separated from the psoas muscle, a large artery, or an arterial graft by interposing retroperitoneal fat, fascia, or omentum. This is done to prevent periureteral adhesions, which limit longitudinal contractions of the ureter that are necessary for effective ureteral peristalsis.

MECHANICAL AIDS TO SURGERY

The binocular loupe is helpful to those who are familiar with its use. It enables one to detect irregularities or pouting of the suture line and inversions or eversions of the delicate ureteral wall from a strict mucosa-to-mucosa and muscularis-to-muscularis apposition. The operating microscope has not found great favor in ureteral surgery, although it has been used to great advantage in the experimental laboratory in vas deferens surgery.

Tissue adhesives may eventually prove to be the ultimate method in the closure of visceral incisions and wounds. The stapler has also been used experimentally on the ureter as well as in the bowel, but not clinically. A headlamp is useful.

STENT

A ureteral stent or indwelling catheter provides a scaffolding for the actual repair and healing processes. The stent need not fill the entire ureter to be effective. In fact, if it does, it may produce pressure ischemia by displacing blood from capillaries in its stretching of the ureter. The other price to be paid for using the stent is the presence of a foreign body, which encourages the perpetuation of infection. However, stents, if properly placed, can prevent the formation of secondary kinks in the course of the ureter as well as facilitate reconstitution of the ureteral wall over large defects that might not otherwise close primarily.

The stenting catheter should be properly fashioned and placed so as to be a diverting catheter as well as a scaffold. The stent may be placed cystoscopically, preoperatively, or postoperatively,

and it may be a semipermanent diversion like the Gibbon or Cook catheter.

DIVERSION

In this section we discuss temporary urinary diversion to facilitate repair, not permanent diversions such as transureteroureterostomy, ureteroneocystostomy, psoas hitch or bladder flap or ureteroileostomy.

Diversion can be effected through an indwelling catheter stent, a percutaneous nephrostomy, a permanent stent such as a Gibbon or Cook catheter, or a conventional nephrostomy (Fig. 42-3). A nephrostomy can be a U-tube nephrostomy, a straight-catheter, a Foley-catheter, or a combination mushroom-type or balloon-type catheter nephrostomy, with its own extension as a stent. Other forms of diversion are ureterotomy, pyelostomy, and ureterostomy (Fig. 42-3) above the anastomosis, or a slash-venting pyelostomy or ureterostomy with a Penrose drain down to the level of the vent.

The patient's diagnosis and condition and the type of injuries found determine the choice of diversion as much as the surgeon's preference and habit. The surgeon must have an open mind to do what is best called for by the immediate situation. No single recipe can be given for the many types of diversion that may be required.

A more important issue is whether to divert or not. The controversies of the past decade have subsided in intensity, but they have not disappeared. In general, the guideline is to divert unless one is sure that it is unnecessary or that a patient's condition can withstand the possible consequences of failure to divert. Hence, a poor risk, a serious infection, a widely contaminated abdomen, impaired renal function, or similar serious factors will press for diversion. On the other hand, the easily performed well-taken anastomosis which is watertight in virgin tissues may tempt one to rely on internal stenting or on no diversion. The extravasation of urine will disrupt normal healing processes, even in this antibiotic age when most infections can be suppressed or eradicated.

DRAINAGE

A Penrose drain should be left indwelling, down to the side of any potential extravasation of urine or hemorrhage. It should be left as long as there is a possibility of leakage of urine from the urinary tract, and then should be removed in steps over several days. Once the drain is loosened from its anchoring suture, it falls out easily with a change

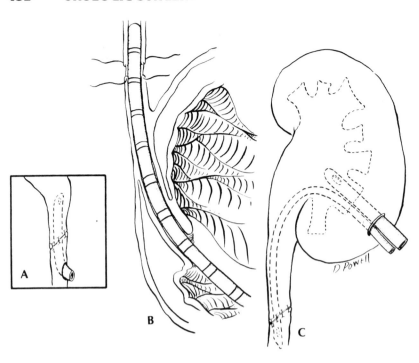

FIG. 42-3. The techniques of splinting and diversion include (**A**) ureterostomy, (**B**) indwelling catheter, and (**C**) nephrostomy with stent.

Follow-Up

The patient should be followed clinically insofar as symptoms, abdominal findings, fever, urinalysis, and urine culture are concerned. Subsequently, intravenous urograms or retrograde pyelograms will delineate the success of restoration of ureteral continuity and peristalsis and drainage.

The postoperative ureter will remain aperistaltic for 1 or more weeks, depending upon its initial state and on the degree of operative handling and trauma. The ureteral edema may not subside for several months, so that any impairment of lumen may be due to edema rather than permanent stricture. Certainly, the preoperatively overly distended system cannot be expected to resume a normal configuration postoperatively until an adequate amount of time has been allowed for resumption of ureteral muscular tone.

Removal drains and stents are individualized considering each patient's clinical course and anticipated ureteral regenerative processes.

The urologist should not hesitate to perform cystoscopy and ureteral catheterization postoperatively if there is any question of the integrity of the anastomosis. This may be necessary to minimize urinary extravasation in the immediate postoperative period.

It may be helpful to dilate a soft ureteral stricture in the course of healing if one should be demonstrated. Such a maneuver should not be done unless necessary, because the tissues are soft and the catheter can penetrate the kidney or the ureteral wall to extravasate or disrupt the suture line. Hence, ureteral catheterization is a minor surgical procedure in its own right and is associated with a certain amount of risk.

Long term follow-up should include urinalyses, cultures, and intravenous urograms at appropriate intervals, and possibly renal function studies.

REFERENCES

1. BOYARSKY S, DUQUE O: Ureteral regeneration in dogs. An experimental study bearing on the Davis intubated ureterotomy. J Urol 73:53, 1955
2. BOYARSKY S, GOTTSCHALK CW, TANAGHO EA et al: Urodynamics. New York; London, Academic Press, 1971
3. BOYARSKY S, LABAY P: Ureteral Dynamics. Baltimore, Williams & Wilkins, 1971
4. DAVIS RM: Intubated ureterotomy. J Urol 66:77, 1951
5. ESTES R, BOYARSKY S, GLENN JF: The use of microsurgery for experimental ureteral re-anastomosis. J Urol 96:443, 1966
6. GOODWIN WE, WINTER CC, TURNER RD: Replacement of the ureter by small intestine: Clinical application and results of the ileal ureter. J Urol 81:406, 1959

of dressing, position, or hospital personnel. The drain should be sutured to the skin, but care should be taken not to suture the drain accidentally when closing the deeper layers of the wound.

7. HARADA N, TANIMURA M, FUKUYAMA K et al: Surgical management of a long ureteral defect: Advancement of the ureter by descent of the kidney, J Urol 92:192, 1964

8. HIGGINS CC: Transuretero-ureteral anastomosis: Report of a clinical case. Trans Am Assoc Genitourin Surg 27:279, 1934

9. HINMAN F, JR: Ureteral repair and the splint. J Urol 78:376, 1957

10. HINMAN F, JR, OPPENHEIMER R: Ureteral regeneration. IV. Fascial covering compared with fatty connective tissues. J Urol 76:729, 1956

11. HODGES CV, MOORE RJ, LEHAMN TH et al: Clinical experience with transureteroureterostomy. J Urol 90:552, 1963

12. LAPIDES J, CAFFREY EL: Observation on the healing of ureteral muscle: Relationship to intubated ureterotomy. J Urol 73:47, 1955

13. NARATH PA: Renal Pelvis and Ureter. New York, Grune & Stratton, 1951

14. ORKIN LA: Trauma to the Ureter. Philadelphia, FA Davis, 1964

15. PERSKY L, CARLTON CE, JR: Urinary diversion in ureteral repair. In Scott R (ed): Current Controversies In Urologic Management, pp 169–173. Philadelphia, WB Saunders, 1972

16. WEINBERG SR: Injuries of the ureter. In Bergman H (ed): The Ureter, p 355. New York, Harper & Row, 1967

17. WEINBERG SR, HARMON FC, BERMAN B: The management and repair of lesions of the ureter and fistula. Surg Gynecol Obstet 110:575, 1960

Carcinoma of the Ureter

43

Abraham T. K. Cockett

The rapid passage of urine by peristalsis from the renal pelvis to the ureter and finally to the bladder, where it is stored, accounts for the higher incidence of bladder carcinoma because of this reservoirlike function. Ureteral tumors arising from carcinogens in the urine are relatively uncommon. It should be emphasized that patients with a history of bladder carcinoma have a higher incidence of tumors in the lower ureter.[5] The incidence of ureteral tumors seen in autopsies is probably 1 in 1000. There is a predominance of men to women (2.5:1). The incidences of renal pelvic tumor and ureteral tumor are equal, but the incidence of primary tumor involving lower ureter is five times higher than that of carcinoma in the upper ureter.

From a historical perspective, inhabitants of certain Balkan countries represent a high-risk group for ureteral tumors regardless of sex.[10] The natural course in these select group of patients is slow but progressive. There may be multiple foci in the upper urinary tract. The exact etiology is obscure, but careful epidemiologic studies in the future may uncover specific environmental factors.

Chronic analgesic ingestion with a consequent nephropathy is well known in selected patients.[2] The relationship of chronic renal damage in such patients and subsequent pelvic transitional cell carcinoma is obscure. There appears to be a higher incidence in women who provide a history of analgesic ingestion. It should be emphasized that infection or inflammation are important local factors that can promote growth of the tumor. Ureteral tumors arise after chronic irritation. Squamous ureteral carcinomas, which are rare, arise because of metaplastic degeneration. In some patients squamous cell carcinoma of the lower ureter can arise from schistosomal infestation.

Squamous cell carcinoma of the pelvis is associated with a calculus in 50% of cases. Usually chronic infection is also present. Sarcomas have been reported but are rare.

Pathologic Classification

A useful pathologic classification consists of four stages. Stage A carcinoma is characterized by submucosal involvement. Muscular invasion without extension through the outer muscular coat of ureter defines Stage B. In Stage C there is invasion into the periureteral fat or the renal parenchyma adjacent to pelvis. In Stage D extension is now outside the ureter into retroperitoneal tissues.

The histologic spectrum of ureteral tumors is the same as for bladder tumors and consists of benign papilloma, transitional cell carcinoma (four histologic grades), and papillary or broad-based (sessile) growths. Squamous cell carcinoma and adenocarcinoma are extremely rare.

Clinical Evaluation

The urologist faces the dilemma of a poorly functioning or nonfunctioning kidney on the side of the ureteral tumor. If urine is traversing the tumor surface, gross hematuria is an important clue. At times the urologist cannot be certain whether he is looking at a nonopaque calculus, a blood clot, or a primary ureteral tumor. Fortunately, the advent of the computed tomographic (CT) scan has been quite useful in focusing on a ureteral tumor. If this modality is available, then a CT scan of the involved area may be quite illuminating and can reveal neoplastic tissue densities. The CT scan is also effective in ruling out the presence of a poorly opaque calculus.[12]

The urologist as a first step will perform intravenous urography. If the kidney is nonfunctioning, then this study may not be diagnostic, except to denote the presence of a contralateral normal kidney. A radiolucent defect on the papillary surface may be helpful.

Retrograde urography with passage of a special brush-tip catheter permits collection of cell washings for cytology. Brush biopsy is helpful if the special catheter can reach the tumor area.

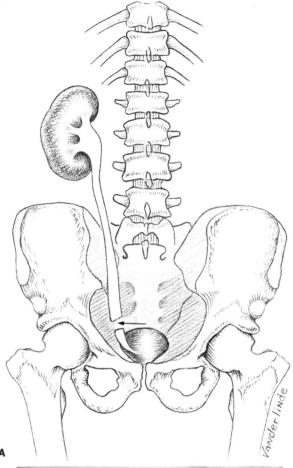

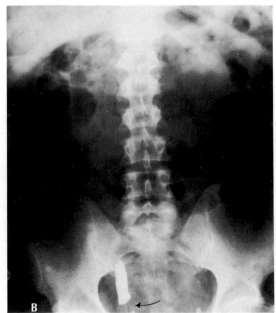

FIG. 43-1. Napkinlike deformity (*arrow*) of right lower ureter

Antegrade urography, which was popularized by Goodwin in 1955,[8] is exceedingly useful and diagnostic because approximately 35% of the ureteral tumors may progress to a nonfunctioning kidney. In the case of a poorly functioning kidney, the placement of an antegrade nephropyelocutaneous catheter may restore function. The intrinsic, irregular, small-napkin-ring appearance is suggestive of a ureteral carcinoma (Fig. 43-1). A nonopaque calculus or blood clot can be moved about, particularly in the renal pelvis.

Hematuria may be present in the patient; therefore, cystoscopy is mandatory to rule out the presence of a bladder lesion. Observation of the ureteral orifice may reveal a bloody efflux. A low ureteral tumor with a long stalk may also protrude at the orifice (Fig. 43-2). When one encounters a low-lying tumor, gross hematuria will be continuous. If the ureteral tumor is in the upper half of the ureter, then the finding of blood may coincide only with ureteral peristalsis; therefore, hematuria is intermittent.

Angiography is not useful except in the renal pelvic tumor which has extended into the parenchyma. Abnormal vascularity may be present in these few, select cases.

Because metastases tend to spread to the lung, the liver, and bone, routine chest radiographs and bone and liver scans are helpful.

Surgical Treatment

The classic two-incision technique of nephroureterectomy including a cuff of bladder was developed approximately four decades ago. The cuff of bladder was added because of ipsilateral tumor recurrence in 84% of cases.[4] The previous concept was that tumor arose in the renal pelvis and by distal implants involved the lower ureter. Dodson suggested that ureteral tumor arose from "carcinogenic irritation" and represented a "multiplicity of origin."[7] Deming and Harvard underscored the spread of tumor from the ureter to the adjacent bladder.[6]

We prefer a two-incision technique for the high-grade lower ureteral tumor invading the ureteral wall muscle (Fig. 43-3).[3] The kidney and attached ureter are explored through an anterior lateral approach. The kidney is removed as demonstrated in Fig. 43-4, and the renal artery and vein are ligated separately and in that order. For the vascular structures we prefer 1-0 silk ligatures. The inferior retroperitoneal cleavage plane is prepared for passage of the kidney and the intact ureter inferiorly. The second incision is now made. The

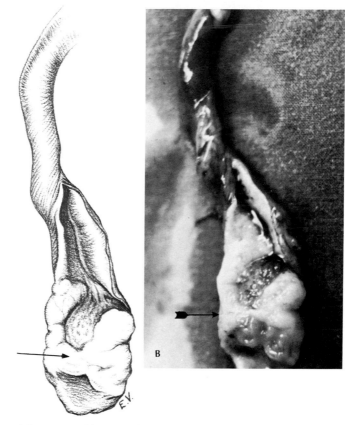

FIG. 43-2.   Tumor of lower right ureter with protrusion (*arrow*)

extraperitoneal ureter is isolated, still attached to the kidney and the upper ureter. A cuff of bladder is removed, and the entire specimen is removed through the inferior incision (Figs. 43-5 and 43-6). The bladder opening is closed in two layers using interrupted 2-0 and 3-0 catgut sutures. A small Penrose drain is used inferiorly for 2 to 3 days.

The increased accuracy of preoperative diagnosis coupled with careful cytology using brush biopsies has led to an improved understanding of the pathogenesis of a ureteral tumor. Low-stage, Grade I or II ureteral tumors without muscular invasion can be best handled by segmental resection of the tumor and adjacent ureter. Scott and McDonald reviewed 300 cases and treated 20% by excision of the ureteral tumor.[11] Perhaps 30% to 40% of cases today can undergo this kidney-preserving procedure. If a 5-cm to 7-cm segment of ureter is excised from the lower ureter, a bladder flap can be raised to reach the shortened ureter. The two best methods to reanastomose the ureter are demonstrated in Figures 43-7 and 43-8. Each technique involves a widening of lumen at the anastomotic sites. We use 4-0 chromic catgut and

FIG. 43-3.   Two-incision technique for right nephroureterectomy (Cockett ATK, Koshiba, K: Manual of Urologic Surgery. In Egdahl RH (ed): Comprehensive Manuals of Surgical Specialties, Vol. 5. New York, Springer-Verlag, 1979)

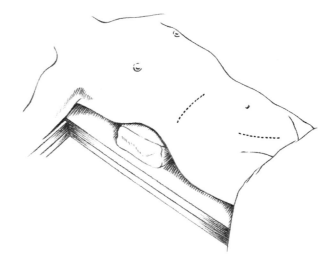

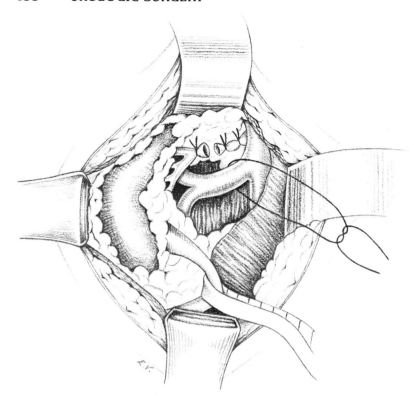

FIG. 43-4. The right renal artery has been doubly ligated proximally and divided. A ligature is around the right renal vein. A Penrose drain is around the ureter. (Cockett ATK, Koshiba K: Manual of Urologic Surgery. In Egdahl RH (ed): Comprehensive Manuals of Surgical Specialties. Vol. 5. New York, Springer-Verlag, 1979)

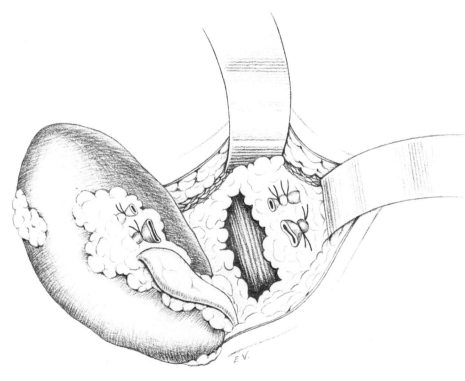

FIG. 43-5. The ischemic kidney is free in the upper wound except for the ureteral attachment. (Cockett ATK, Koshiba K: Manual of Urologic Surgery. In Egdahl RH (ed): Comprehensive Specialties, Vol. 5. New York, Springer-Verlag, 1979)

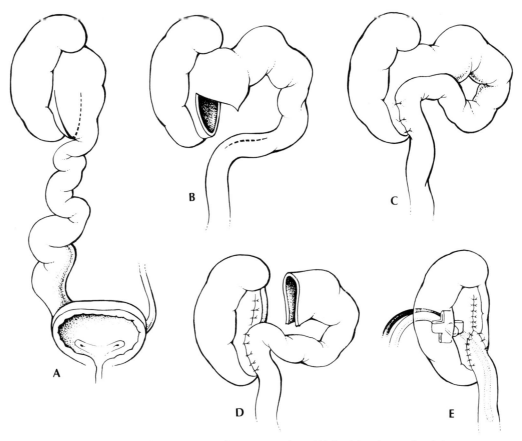

FIG. 44-1. Renal and upper ureteral reconstruction: **(A)** incision in renal pelvis preparatory to ureteral mobilization; **(B)** V-shaped pyelotomy with ureter mobilized for incision; **(C)** preliminary anastomosis of ureter to renal pelvis; **(D)** ureteropelvic junction dismembered and pelvis closed; **(E)** nephrostomy with Malecot catheter and stenting ureteral catheter with renal pelvis closed

quate, the lower ureter is straightened, reduced in caliber, and reimplanted into the bladder (Fig. 44-2). The ureter is mobilized from above the iliac vessels down to the posterior aspect of the bladder and is transected. The bladder is opened in the midline from the urachus to the bladder outlet, or from the urachus in the direction of the involved ureter. If the latter method is used, one must be sure to terminate the incision 3 cm to 4 cm proximal to the old ureteral orifice to allow room for an adequate submucosal tunnel. The bladder is inspected, and a ureteral catheter is passed up the opposite ureter to identify it. If the involved ureter is tortuous, it is mobilized in the retroperitoneal space, avoiding the medial aspect, if possible, so as not to jeopardize the blood supply. The ureter is opened in a cephalad direction, and the opening is carried up above the iliac vessels. The adventitia, which contains the blood vessels, is then dissected off the ureter, beginning in the most cephalad

portion of the incision in the ureter. Careful dissection guarantees the viability of the ureter. The dissection is carried out with sharp iris scissors, on both sides, from the apex of the opened ureter caudally to its terminus. At the uppermost part of the opened ureter, the adventitia is mobilized for only a millimeter or more, and as one progresses distally, more and more adventitia is mobilized from each side.

A small catheter (8Fr–12Fr) is placed in the ureter, and the muscular portion is excised, beginning at the top, taking only a millimeter from each side and increasing the amount taken from each side until the ureter fits snugly about the splinting catheter. The ureter is approximated with mattress sutures of 4-0 atraumatic chromic catgut. When this is accomplished, the ureter is gradually tapered with all the adventitia intact; the ureter, of necessity, is quite bulky. A submucosal tunnel is then developed with its termination on the trigone. The

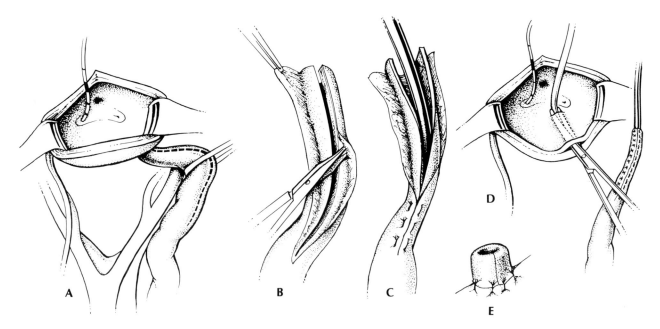

FIG. 44-2. Lower ureteral reconstruction and reimplantation. **(A)** The ureter is mobilized with the incision marked; the contralateral ureter has been catheterized for identification. **(B)** The ureteral adventitia containing the blood supply is carefully dissected and mobilized from the ureteral muscular wall. **(C)** The ureter and adventitia are closed over the indwelling catheter. **(D)** The submucosal tunnel is developed. **(E)** A Paquin cuff is used for ureterovesical anastomosis.

tunnel must be more spacious than a routine ureteral reimplantation in order to accept the large ureter. The long-pointed dissecting scissors can be used to create the submucosal tunnel. A whistle-tip catheter is grasped and pulled through the tunnel. The ureter is sutured to the catheter and pulled through the submucosal tunnel. The distal ureter is excised, and the ureter is anastomosed to the bladder with interrupted 4-0 atraumatic chromic catgut sutures. Each suture takes a bite of the bladder wall and of the lateral wall of the ureter, and the terminus of the ureter is turned back upon itself as a French cuff.[11] If the ureteral orifice is gaping, the edges of the French cuff can be approximated to narrow the orifice. It is important to make sure the ureter is not rotated in the tunnel or outside the bladder in a manner that might produce obstruction.

A small splinting catheter is left in place as a splint (8Fr–12Fr) or pediatric gastric feeding tube, and the bladder is closed in a routine manner. The splinting catheter and cystostomy tube (Malecot catheter) are brought out in the midline and sutured to the skin. The operative area is always drained with Penrose drains.

The ureteral splint is removed 7 to 10 days postoperatively. Approximately 10 to 14 days after

surgery, pyelograms are obtained using the nephrostomy tube. Manometric studies are also performed. If there is no extravasation and no obstruction, the nephrostomy tube is attached to a buret.[17] It is hoped that the intrapelvic pressure will be 15 cm of water or less. If pressures are less than 20 cm of water, the nephrostomy tube is clamped for 24 hrs, and it is opened if the patient has flank pain or fever. If there are no complications due to clamping the nephrostomy tube and the residual urine is less than 30 ml, the tube is removed. When there is no obstruction, the sinus heals promptly. Frequently, there is evidence of extravasation at the site of the wedge resection, obstruction at the site of the anastomosis, or both. In such cases, the patient is discharged with the nephrostomy tube in place and is readmitted in 4 to 8 weeks for retesting.

Although approximately 90% of the involved units have a good result, some have required a second operative procedure because of persistent reflux or obstruction at the site of anastomosis.

Case Management and Results

Severe hydronephrosis or hydroureter, other than the isolated ureterovesical junction obstruction, can result from many causes, including ectopic ureter, ureterocele, vesical outlet obstruction with or without vesicoureteral reflux, prostatic urethral valves, urethral valves, urethral diverticulum, and urethral meatal obstruction. The treatment varies according to the etiology, the stage of the disease, the age of the patient at the time of diagnosis, and whether the disease is unilateral or bilateral.[7,18] When surgical therapy is indicated, the procedure we use is as previously described. In addition, the source of the obstruction (e.g., ureterocele and valves) is removed at the time of reimplantation. If the bladder has a thick wall, a Y–V revision of the anterior bladder neck is performed.

In 21 years of experience with ureteral reimplantation in 701 children with 1050 ureters, we have been successful in eliminating the reflux without causing obstruction in 93% of the patients (96% of the girls and 84% of the boys).[4] In this group there were 136 patients with 186 ureters that were sufficiently dilated to require preliminary nephrostomy. In 24 of the patients and 34 of the ureters, a pyeloplasty was required in addition to the nephrostomy. However, only 60 patients with 73 ureters required distal wedge resection to reduce the ureteral caliber; stated differently, 18% of the ureters were dilated to the extent that preliminary nephrostomy was performed, but only 7% of these ureters required wedge resection to reduce the caliber. The preliminary nephrostomy apparently decompressed the ureter sufficiently in 93% of the cases to eliminate the need of decreasing the caliber before reimplantation.

REFERENCES

1. ALLEN TD: Congenital ureteral strictures. J Urol 104:196, 1970
2. BISCHOFF P: Observations on the genesis of megaureter. Urol Int 2:257, 1961
3. CAULK JR: Megaloureter: The importance of the ureterovesical valve. J Urol 9:315, 1923
4. COLEMAN JW, MCGOVERN JH: A 20 year experience with pediatric ureteral reimplantation. Surgical results in 701 children. In Hodson JR (ed): Reflux Nephropathy, Chap 30. New York, Masson, 1979
5. CREEVY CD: The atonic distal ureteral segment (ureteral achalasia). J Urol 97:457, 1967
6. HENDREN WH: Operative repair of megaureter in children. J Urol 101:491, 1969
7. JOHNSTON JH: Reconstructive surgery of megaureter in children. Br J Urol 39:17, 1967
8. KING LR: Guest Editorial: Megaloureter: Definition, diagnosis and management. J Urol 123:222, 1980
9. MACKINNON KJ, FOOTE JW, WIGLESWORTH FW et al: The pathology of the adynamic distal ureteral segment. J Urol 103:134, 1970
10. MONIE IW, NELSON MM, EVANS HM: Abnormalities of the urinary system of rat embryos resulting from transitory deficiency of pteroylglutamic acid during gestation. Anat Rec 127:711, 1957
11. PAQUIN AJ, JR: Ureterovesical anastomosis: The description and evaluation of a technique. J Urol 82:573, 1959
12. PITTS WP, MUECKE EC: Congenital megaloureter: A review of 80 patients. J Urol 3:468, 1974
13. ROUX C, DUPUIS R: Urohydronephroses par carence pantothenic. Arch Pediatr 18:1337, 1961
14. SWENSON O, MCMAHON HE, JAQUES WE, et al: A new concept of the etiology of megaloureters. N Engl J Med 246:41, 1952
15. TANAGHO EA, SMITH DR, GUTHRIE TH: Pathophysiology of functional ureteral obstruction. J Urol 104:73, 1970
16. VERMOOTEN V: A new etiology for certain types of the dilated ureters in children. J Urol 41:455, 1939
17. WALZAK MP, JR, PAQUIN AJ, JR: Renal pelvic pressure levels in management of nephrostomy. J Urol 85:697, 1961
18. WILLIAMS DI: Megaureter in children. In Riches E (ed): Modern Trends in Urology, 2nd ser, p 147. New York, Paul B Hoeber, 1960

Prune-Belly Syndrome

45

Panayotis P. Kelalis

The congenital anomaly complex in which urinary tract abnormalities are associated with absence of abdominal muscles and abdominal testes is well known; it occurs almost exclusively in males. Less well known, however, are incomplete forms of the syndrome which also clearly exist.[4,6,7,10]

The multiplicity of the disorders and their varying severity have important implications for the therapeutic approach. For this reason, a "standard" approach to treatment is not possible; and even though a few generalities can be made, treatment should be individualized. When urinary stasis with intractable infection and diminution of renal function becomes a continuous problem, procedures to improve urinary drainage—temporary or permanent, extensive or limited—are clearly necessary.[15,16] However, in the majority of cases no treatment is required or limited surgical interference suffices.

Pathologic Spectrum

Prune-belly syndrome occurs in a spectrum of forms and severity, and treatment varies accordingly.[2] In the most severe form of the disorder, the neonate has complete urethral obstruction, patent urachus, renal dysplasia, and severe pulmonary difficulties that are beyond treatment, and therefore support of life is not justified. In the least severe form, although uropathy is present, the renal parenchyma is of good quality and no surgical interference is required in the absence of stasis and urinary tract infection. Between these two extremes are the majority of patients in whom the full-blown syndrome is present. Some, because of increasing uremia and urinary infection, may require surgical intervention early in life. Anesthetic hazards are significant, and in general because of the delicate nature of the problem, these patients should be transferred to an expert pediatric urologic unit. On the other hand, despite the alarming urographic appearance of the kidneys, the ureters, and the bladder, most patients do surprisingly well, grow into adulthood, and maintain stable renal function and exhibit improved radiologic findings. In this group, deterioration is likely to result later in life from progressive inability to empty the bladder and recurring urinary infection.

Investigation and Management

Prompt evaluation is imperative upon recognition of the syndrome, which is likely to take place at birth or soon thereafter. Any cardiac and pulmonary problems must be evaluated on an urgent basis, because they have a bearing on subsequent treatment. In particular, pulmonary hypoplasia, pneumothorax, or pneumomediastinum are likely to be severe when associated with urethral obstruction and therefore may be incompatible with life.[1]

Excretory urography, renal function studies, and urine examination for bacteriuria generally suffice. The need for voiding cystourethrography should be weighed in relation to the danger of introducing infection in this very vulnerable urinary tract. Such an infection may be extremely difficult to eradicate and may eventually necessitate surgical drainage. If the basic studies are satisfactory, urethral instrumentation for purposes of voiding cystourethrography is best deferred until surgical intervention is contemplated if such becomes necessary. Otherwise, such an examination should be carried out under the most aseptic precautions and with antibiotic coverage.

Treatment

NONSURGICAL OR MINIMAL SURGICAL INTERFERENCE

In the majority of cases, the urinary tract remains stable and free of infection, and careful monitoring of renal function and control of infection with suppressive chemotherapeutic agents when indicated will suffice. The urinary tract may deteriorate later in life because of inability to empty the

467

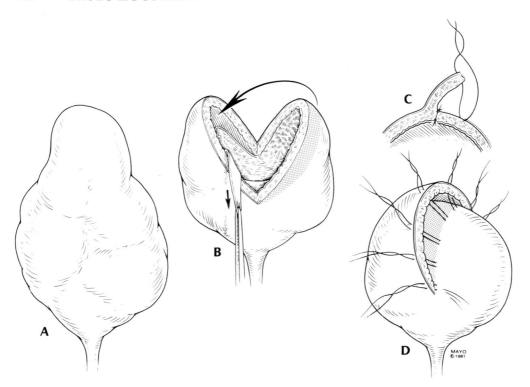

FIG. 45-1. Technique of reductive cystoplasty used on (**A**) anomalous bladder includes (**B**) excision of dome of bladder and removal of mucosa on one side and (**C** and **D**) modified closure of new dome to increase detrusor thickness and efficiency

bladder, and as a result progressive ureterectasis and difficulty in controlling infection may arise. In such instances, procedures to improve bladder emptying are necessary and generally prove satisfactory.[19]

The prostatic urethra is generally dilated, but it comes to a narrow point in the membranous region.[5] Even though no clear-cut point of obstruction can be found, some obstructive element is likely to be present on the basis of this narrowing.[14] The flow rate is improved and bladder-emptying enhanced by urethrotomy to 24Fr to 36Fr in the membranous region by means of the cold knife or the Bugbee electrode (3Fr) and cutting current, or by means of transurethral resection of the membranous zone. The cut is made anteriorly or anterolaterally, and it should be followed by 1 or 2 days of catheter drainage. This procedure should precede any formal upper urinary tract reconstruction, but in cases of severe abnormalities of the dome of the bladder, I prefer to combine or follow this approach with reductive cystoplasty.

Encouraging results have followed the use of reductive cystoplasty, even though it is too soon to state that this improvement will be permanent.[3,11] The entire dome of the bladder should be excised because it is the most anomalous portion (Fig. 45-1A); a modified closure results in a spherical detrusor muscle that theoretically improves bladder emptying. The mucosa is removed on one side (Fig. 45-1B). The overlapping (vest-over-pants) three-layer closure, producing a double-thickness bladder muscle in the new dome, is preferable to simple closure and appears clinically to improve bladder emptying (Figs. 45-1C and D and 45-2).

TEMPORARY DIVERSION

When renal function is impaired, urinary infection is present, and ureteral dilatation is considerable, early surgery may be necessary.[6,9] Very severely ill children who are obviously unsuitable for major reconstruction require prompt management, and a simple diversionary procedure such as tubeless cutaneous vesicostomy will probably drain the urinary tract satisfactorily in the majority of cases, despite the dilatation and tortuosity of the ureters. Because of its simplicity, ease of execution, and

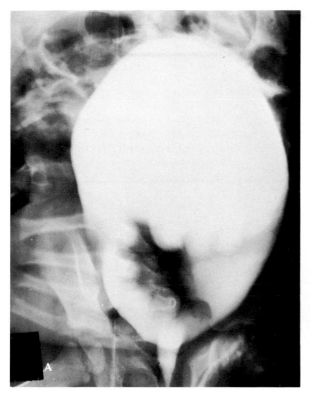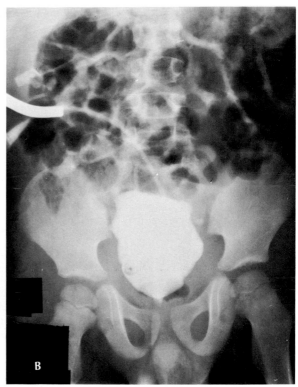

FIG. 45-2.   Cystograms taken before **(A)** and after **(B)** reductive cystoplasty

prompt reversibility, it is the procedure of choice.

Rarely, if good drainage is not achieved, proximal diversion becomes necessary. Loop ureterostomy is a simple and expedient technique which offers good proximal drainage; at the same time, it allows biopsy of the kidney. Its disadvantages are that it interferes with the proximal ureter, which is essential in subsequent reconstruction, and it is relatively difficult to reverse. Cutaneous pyelostomy is an attractive alternative in that the upper good ureter is left undisturbed for subsequent use, but it does have a tendency to retract unless the pelvis is greatly dilated. If upper tract drainage is necessary, nephrostomy over a short period is probably a good compromise approach because it offers good drainage and can be removed without formal operation after surgical reconstruction of the ureters and bladder.

EARLY TOTAL RECONSTRUCTION

Extensive surgical reconstruction early in life has its appeal because the static and grossly dilated urinary system is unlikely to be protected indefinitely from infection.[12,18] Such a procedure involves

excision of the distal ureters—the most abnormal portion histologically—and reimplantation into the bladder, often in combination with reductive ureteroplasty and also reductive cystoplasty (Fig. 45-2). Furthermore, anatomic considerations at this time of life make conventional orchiopexy quite possible, and this is another attractive feature of the procedure. Its disadvantage lies in the technical difficulty inherent in such a procedure and the likelihood that failure will lead to urinary diversion.

Even though such procedures are best carried out early in life before long-standing infection has led to fibrosis of the ureter, the decision must be weighed in the light of the possibility that such surgery may be unnecessary, because of the tendency of the urinary tract to improve spontaneously, or that limited surgical interference can achieve the desired result in the majority of cases.

NEPHROURETERECTOMY

Asymmetric upper tract damage is sometimes present. When massive unilateral reflux is demonstrated, it is likely to be associated with a functionless, dysplastic system. Efficient function can be restored to the urinary tract in such instances by nephroureterectomy.

ORCHIOPEXY

In the cryptorchidism associated with this syndrome, the limiting factor for a successful orchiopexy is insufficient length of the spermatic vessels. However, the well-developed artery to the vas deferens provides an adequate blood supply to the testis, and if it is carefully preserved, it permits one to divide the spermatic vessel.[8,17] It should be performed by age 2 (Chap. 102).

URETHROPLASTY

In some cases a flabby penis with upward curvature is associated with a greatly enlarged urethra in its pendulum portion. In such patients, a reductive urethroplasty that reduces the caliber to normal levels appears also to improve the cosmetic appearance of the organ. A distal circumferential incision is made. The skin is dissected proximally from the shaft of the penis to the penoscrotal angle, and the urethra is opened. The redundant portion is then excised and reconstructed over a catheter of appropriate size in a two-layer closure.

ABDOMINAL WALL MANAGEMENT

A characteristic finding is absence of the muscles of the medial and lower abdominal wall but development of the upper rectus and outer oblique muscles. This defect causes little disability. Plication of the abdominal wall by excision of the redundant skin in the deficient area and plication of the fibrous underlying layer have been said to improve respiratory, urinary, and bowel function, but in general the indication for surgery is mostly cosmetic.

Recently, an even more extensive approach—incision beginning at the 12th rib and extending to the central suprapubic area in full thickness—has produced further cosmetic improvement because tightening of the area is enhanced.[13] However, in most instances, an elastic corset will disguise the abdominal defect and produce an aesthetically satisfactory physique in these patients.

REFERENCES

1. ALFORD BA, PEOPLES WM, RESNICK JS, et al: Pulmonary complications associated with the prune-belly syndrome. Radiology 129:401, 1978

2. BERDON WE, BAKER DH, WIGGER HJ, et al: The radiologic and pathologic spectrum of the prune-belly syndrome: The importance of urethral obstruction in prognosis. Radiol Clin North Am 15:83, 1977

3. BINARD JEC, ZOEDLER D: Treatment of the hypotonic, decompensated urinary bladder. Int Surg 50:502, 1968

4. BURKE EC, SHIN MH, KELALIS PP: Prune-belly syndrome: Clinical findings and survival. Am J Dis Child 117:668, 1969

5. DEKLERK DP, SCOTT WW: Prostatic maldevelopment in the prune-belly syndrome: A defect in prostatic stromal–epithelial interaction. J Urol 120:341, 1978

6. DUCKETT JW, JR: The prune-belly syndrome. In Kelalis PP, King LR, Belman AB (eds): Clinical Pediatric Urology, vol 2, p 615. Philadelphia, W B Saunders, 1976

7. DUCKETT JW, JR: The prune-belly syndrome. In Holder TM, Ashcraft KW (eds): The Surgery of Infants and Children, p 802. Philadelphia, W B Saunders, 1980

8. GIBBONS MD, CROMIE WJ, DUCKETT JW, JR: Management of the abdominal undescended testicle. J Urol 122:76, 1979

9. GOULDING FJ, GARRETT RA: Twenty-five-year experience with prune-belly syndrome. Urology 12:329, 1978

10. NUNN IN, STEPHENS FD: The triad syndrome: A composite anomaly of the abdominal wall, urinary system and testes. J Urol 86:782, 1961

11. PERLMUTTER AD: Reduction cystoplasty in prune-belly syndrome. J Urol 116:356, 1976

12. RABINOWITZ R, BARKIN M, SCHILLINGER JF, et al: Urinary tract reconstruction in prune-belly syndrome. Urology 12:333, 1978

13. RANDOLPH JG: Total surgical reconstruction for patients with abdominal muscular deficiency ("prune-belly") syndrome. J Pediatr Surg 12:1033, 1977

14. SNYDER HM, HARRISON NW, WHITFIELD HN, et al: Urodynamics in the prune-belly syndrome. Br J Urol 48:663, 1976

15. WILLIAMS DI, BURKHOLDER GV: The prune-belly syndrome. J Urol 98:244, 1967

16. WILLIAMS DI, PARKER RM: The role of surgery in the prune-belly syndrome. In Johnston JH, Goodwin WE (eds): Reviews in Paediatric Urology, p 315. Amsterdam, Excerpta Medica, 1974

17. WOODARD JR, PARROTT TS: Orchiopexy in the prune-belly syndrome. Br J Urol 50:348, 1978

18. WOODARD JR, PARROTT TS: Reconstruction of the urinary tract in prune-belly uropathy. J Urol 119:824, 1978

19. WOODHOUSE CRJ, KELLETT MJ, WILLIAMS DI: Minimal surgical interference in the prune-belly syndrome. Br J Urol 51:475, 1979

Vesicoureteral Reflux

46

Edmond T. Gonzales, Jr.

As long ago as 1898, Young postulated that vesicoureteral reflux might endanger the kidneys by allowing bladder infections to spread to the upper urinary tract.[64] He conducted simple experiments in cadavers and demonstrated that reflux did not occur normally in the adult. Following a description of a clinical case of vesicoureteral reflux and ascending pyelonephritis by Sampson in 1903,[45] several authors explored the relationship of reflux and pyelonephritis in the laboratory.[16,17,57] But the clinical significance of vesicoureteral reflux remained unrecognized until the pioneering work of John Hutch, who noted a high incidence of vesicoureteral reflux in association with renal damage in paraplegics.[21] He suggested that reflux resulted from weakening of the bladder wall (often manifest by a paraureteral diverticulum) and thereby loss of the normal support of the intramural segment of ureter, and he suggested an operative procedure for its correction. Shortly after his publication, several articles demonstrated a relationship between urinary infection and reflux in children.[23,60] Since that time, an extensive literature on vesicoureteral reflux has developed and defined more clearly indications for operative and nonoperative management of this common disorder.

Reflux and Urinary Tract Infection

There is little doubt today regarding the relationship of vesicoureteral reflux and acute pyelonephritis in children, and the association between urinary infection, vesicoureteral reflux, and renal scarring is striking.[49] Nearly one third of children evaluated urologically because of urinary tract infection will be found to have reflux, and one third of these will already have scars at the time of diagnosis.[9,47] In the presence of reflux and continued infection, fresh scars or the progression of established scars can occur.[12,29]

However, implicating vesicoureteral reflux as a cause of urinary infection during childhood is not so easy. Fair and Govan have shown that the incidence of recurrent bacilluria is the same in girls with infection who never had reflux, in girls who had reflux corrected, and in girls with continuing reflux.[11] The difference was that in the first two groups, the infections were limited to episodes of cystitis, but in the last one they experienced recurrent pyelonephritis. Thus, it would appear that mild to moderate degrees of reflux act not to increase the incidence of urinary infection, but rather to allow pyelonephritis rather than cystitis to occur and thus markedly change the risk of bacilluria. Not all authors, however, have reported such a high post-reimplantation infection rate, suggesting that antireflux surgery reduces the incidence of symptomatic bacilluria.[61] More severe degrees of reflux, which result in large, false, postvoid residuals, would be expected to increase the incidence of infection.

Although the relationship of renal scars and the presence of vesicoureteral reflux is well established, the pathophysiologic mechanism whereby renal parenchymal atrophy occurs remains controversial. Hodson and associates have demonstrated in a pig model the focal nature of pyelonephritic atrophy in relationship to the nephrons draining into a particular papilla, have defined different types of scarring, and have suggested that the presence of intrarenal reflux (IRR) significantly increases the risk of focal atrophy in the affected renal lobule.[20] In the presence of infravesical obstruction and reflux, atrophy was seen to occur in the absence of infection. Ransley and Risdon studied the anatomy of the papilla of the pig and demonstrated that compound papilla were more likely to demonstrate IRR, and thus presumably be more likely to sustain parenchymal atrophy.[43] Rolleston and associates followed a series of infants with massive reflux and IRR and demonstrated the progression of established scars or the appearance of new scars in the absence of infection.[44] They postulated that the presence of IRR initiated an interstitial nephritis which resulted in atrophy, and that correction of reflux associated with IRR was essential. IRR was seen only in massive degrees of reflux and only in very young infants.

This concept of sterile reflux causing renal atrophy remains controversial, but it is apparent clinically that most children with reflux and renal scarring present initially with about as much atrophy as they ultimately will develop. Because most children present for evaluation after an infection, Ransley has proposed that those segments of the kidney with papillae that allow IRR will be affected severely and simultaneously with the first urinary infection, and thus the most susceptible portions of the kidney will all undergo atrophy after the first or second urinary infection.[42]

It is not entirely clear, however, that all small kidneys associated with vesicoureteral reflux are a result of postinfectious atrophy. Whereas Ambrose and associates have suggested that the great majority of these small kidneys are a result of postinflammatory atrophy, Mackie and Stephens have argued convincingly that some of these renal units are primarily dysplastic.[2,34] They have proposed that the quality of the renal parenchyma induced by the ureter depends on the site of budding of the ureteral orifice and that, in cases of severe reflux, the ureter buds abnormally close to the orifice of the mesonephric duct into the urogenital sinus. Duckett has shown that the combination of reflux and infravesical obstruction is particularly detrimental to renal embryogenesis, demonstrating a high incidence of nonfunctioning kidneys in association with massive vesicoureteral reflux and posterior urethral valves.*

A less well discussed problem related to reflux and parenchymal atrophy is the development of renin-dependent hypertension in later years.[26,46,48,51,52,58] Increasingly, articles are emphasizing the relationship, although prospective studies, needed to define the exact incidence of this problem, are only now beginning.

Of most concern to physicians who manage children with reflux is the possibility of progressive renal failure despite correction of reflux and prevention of recurring urinary infection.[26] Although the condition is rare, Torres and associates have defined those children who are at risk of developing progressive renal failure, predominantly by the finding of significant proteinuria.[55] Reimplantation will not halt the relentless progression of renal failure in this entity.

In summary, the challenge to the urologic sur-

geon managing a child with reflux is to reduce morbidity and to prevent renal atrophy and possibly renal failure. There is overwhelming evidence now that antireflux surgery can accomplish the former goal, although continuous chemoprophylaxis in most instances is just as effective. The role of surgery in preventing parenchymal atrophy, hypertension, and renal failure is less clear. Unfortunately, most children with severe parenchymal disease are already affected at the time of presentation. It is possible that some of these are primarily dysplastic kidneys, but the evidence suggests that evaluating children after their first urinary infection may already be too late.

Anatomy of the Ureterovesical Junction

As early as 1812, Bell recognized that the muscles of the terminal ureter continued on as the superficial muscles of the trigone, and Wesson subsequently demonstrated that they continued into the urethra to the verumontanum, effectively fixing the terminal ureter to the bladder neck.[5,59] Gruber, in the late 1920s, studied the anatomy of the terminal ureter and trigone in a number of animals and concluded that the absence of reflux was solely dependent on the length of the intravesical segment of ureter and the degree of muscular support.[18] With the current interest in vesicoureteral reflux, several studies were reported regarding muscularization and fibrosis of the distal ureter, and controversies developed over whether the antireflux mechanism was active or passive.[19,53,54] Clinically, however, Gruber's hypothesis has been upheld by several carefully done studies which support the concept that the presence and persistence of vesicoureteral reflux is directly related to the length of intravesical ureter and the degree of muscular backing to this segment.[7,27,32]

Several studies are available which demonstrate that reflux is not normally present, even in premature infants, and it is tempting to assume that all reflux in children is congenital[24,39]—that delays in recognition of its presence are dependent on the development and diagnosis of urinary infection. But it is well known that the incidence of reflux increases in the presence of severe urinary outflow obstruction (as with posterior urethral valves) and can develop in previously nonrefluxing units (as in acquired neurogenic bladders). Based on these observations, both Allen and Koff and associates have suggested that some cases of reflux in older childhood may be acquired secondary to dysfunctional voiding.[1,28]

* Duckett JW: Personal communication, 1980

Management of Vesicoureteral Reflux

It was recognized early that reflux was much more common in children than in adults. At first this was misinterpreted to mean that many children with reflux developed renal failure and died, but it soon became evident that many children simply ceased refluxing as they got older. Around this observation has developed a controversy which continues unabated: the operative versus the non-operative management of reflux.[30] There is now overwhelming evidence that in the absence of infection, children with reflux will not show progressive atrophy and can be followed safely for many years. Although this is a surgical text, one cannot discuss the surgical management of reflux without maintaining a proper perspective of the nonoperative approach.

Numerous clinical studies have shown that a significant number of children with reflux will cease refluxing as they grow older.[9,26] Perhaps the two best known are those by Edwards and associates and King and associates.[10,27] In the latter series, the length of the submucosal tunnel, measured endoscopically, was the most reliable factor in predicting whether reflux would cease or not. Spontaneous cessation was extremely unlikely when the tunnel measured 2 mm or less and was the rule with intravesical segments of 9 mm or greater. Other authors have shown that lesser degrees of reflux (Grades 1–2 of the International Classification) are more likely to cease than more severe degrees,[9] but, in general, 50% to 75% of children will stop refluxing on nonoperative management. Thus, in planning a program of management for a child with vesicoureteral reflux, one must take into account several factors: the age of the child, degree of renal parenchymal damage (if any), degree of reflux (Grades 1–5 of the International Classification), ability to control recurrent urinary infection, compliance in maintaining continual chemoprophylaxis, presence or absence of true bladder outlet obstruction, and the appearance of the orifices endoscopically. Of these, only the inability to prevent recurring urinary infection can be considered an absolute indication for surgical management. The rest are relative indications and must be assessed *in toto* in order to plan appropriate management.

Of the factors to be considered in planning a program of management, the appearance of the ureteral orifice and the length of the intravesical ureter have stimulated the most interest. The more severe the anomaly, the more likely it is that surgery will be necessary.[27,32] But even significant orifice anomalies, such as duplication anomalies or paraureteral diverticula, cannot be considered primary indications for surgery, because reflux has been reported to cease on long-term follow-up even in the presence of these defects.

Approaches vary from surgeon to surgeon, but it is my preference to offer the majority of children with primary reflux a nonoperative approach (on continual chemoprophylaxis) until 3 to 5 years of age so long as infection or drug allergy is not a problem. I have found it difficult to make an assessment of the degree of ureterovesical orifice distortion in the neonate and young infant. In addition, rather marked degrees of ureteral dilatation in association with reflux in the neonate will often improve as the child gets older, and what may have required ureteral tailoring during infancy in order to accomplish a successful ureteral reimplantation can be handled later by a simple reimplantation. At a predetermined time, a complete reassessment is undertaken and a decision made regarding surgery or continued medical management, based primarily on the degree of anomaly of the ureterovesical junction.

OPERATIVE MANAGEMENT

The **surgical management** of vesicoureteral reflux occupies a prominent role in the history of the development of pediatric urology. Many techniques, such as those by Hutch (Fig. 46-1), Bischoff (Fig. 46-2), and Paquin (Fig. 46-3), can now be described as of historical interest and will not be discussed in this chapter.[6,21,37] The interested reader is referred to the chapter on vesicoureteral reflux by Politano in the second edition of *Urologic Surgery* and to a paper by Paquin in 1962 for a more complete description of these techniques.[38,40] The Lich procedure (Fig. 46-4) has never been embraced with much enthusiasm in the United States, but in some centers it is used frequently and with good success.[31,33,35] Reimplantation requiring ureteral tailoring will be discussed elsewhere in this edition. Whether the reimplantation is for obstructive megaloureter or massive reflux, the technical considerations in handling the ureter are the same.

In my opinion, there is little reason today to routinely accomplish ureteroneocystostomy by means of extravesical approach. The techniques to be described in this chapter employ a transvesical approach entirely and allow for an adequate submucosal tunnel to ureteral caliber ratio. Even dilated ureters can be tailored and reimplanted transvesically. The extravesical approach requires more dissection of the perivesical space than is necessary and carries the theoretic risk of partially denervating the bladder. This approach is necessary only when a psoas hitch or Boari flap is felt to be indicated. Even when planning an extravesical approach, dissection is initiated intravesically if at all possible. However, this commitment to a transvesical approach is not to discourage an extravesical look at the ureter if the surgeon is concerned that he may have damaged the peritoneum or if the ureter appears to have kinked as it enters the bladder.

Pre-reimplantation cystoscopy is always performed prior to any open procedure in order to evaluate the anatomy of the orifice and the length of the submucosal tunnel. In older children, this is often done in conjunction with a planned ureteral reimplantation under the same anesthetic. If the orifices appear such that I feel that there is a reasonable chance for reflux to cease, the open procedure is canceled.

When only unilateral reflux has been identified, endoscopic assessment of the contralateral orifice is important. Even if contralateral reflux has never been evident, I would choose a bilateral reimplantation if the orifice were laterally positioned and had a shortened tunnel.

TRANSVESICAL APPROACHES

The bladder is exposed through a small Pfannensteil incision and opened anteriorly in a longitudinal fashion. It is then fixed in position with silk sutures on the Dennis–Browne ring retractor, which has been found eminently satisfactory for this procedure. The ureter is then secured to a small feeding tube (usually 5Fr) by placing a suture through the mucosa around the orifice. With gentle traction, the distal ureter can now be inverted into the bladder.

The mucosa surrounding the orifice is incised sharply, either with fine, pointed scissors or a knife, exposing the muscles of the superficial trigone. With the ureter on gentle traction, these muscles are most obvious medially and inferiorly as they sweep toward the bladder neck. The dissection of the ureter is usually begun at this point,

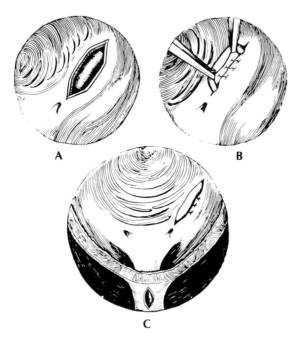

FIG. 46-1. The Hutch procedure as originally described, emphasizing the importance of a good muscular backing to the intravesical ureter (Hutch JA: Vesicoureteral reflux in the paraplegic: Cause and correction. J Urol 68:457, 1952)

FIG. 46-2. Bischoff's technique of lengthening the intravesical mucosal segment without mobilization of the ureter

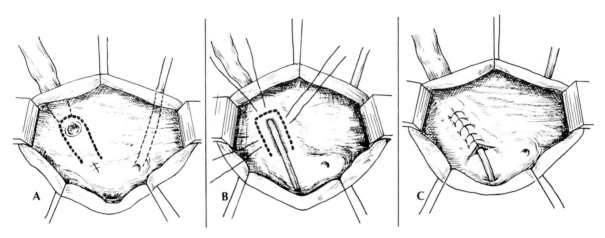

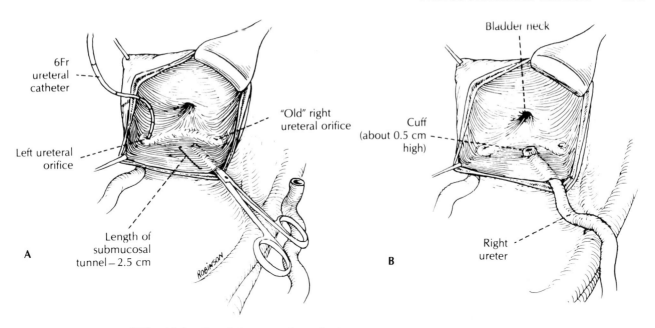

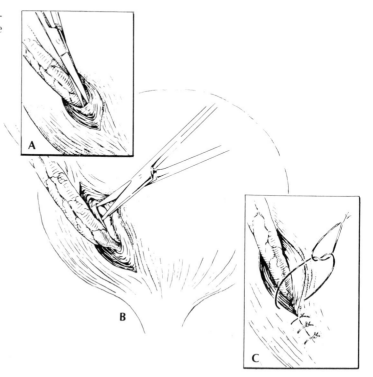

FIG. 46-3. Paquin's original method of ureteroneocystostomy, combining extravesical and intravesical approaches, required an extensive dissection of the superior, lateral, and posterior bladder wall and encouraged a long submucosal tunnel. (Paquin AJ, Jr: Ureterovesical anastomosis: The description and evaluation of a technique. J Urol 82:573, 1959)

FIG. 46-4. A completely extravesical approach ·described by Lich to lengthen the segment of intravesical, submucosal ureter

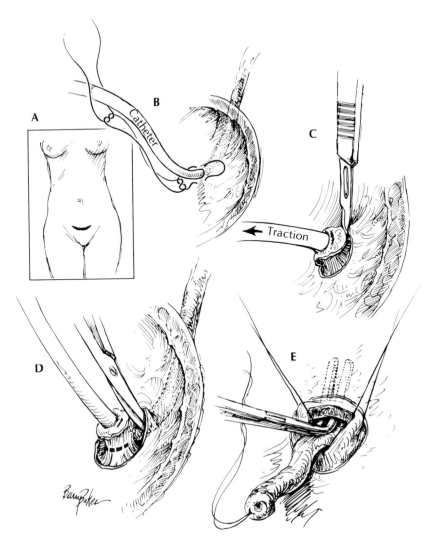

FIG. 46-5. Initial dissection of the ureter transvesically. The prominent muscle band of the superficial trigone is emphasized in **D**. Control of the superior margin of the muscular hiatus (**E**) with traction sutures allows more complete dissection of the ureter and for mobilization of the peritoneum off of the posterior bladder wall.

detaching this muscle band from the ureter. The surgeon wants to stay as close to the ureteral adventitia as possible, and with experience the proper plane can be entered with the first muscular cut.

The ureter is then freed of all detrusor attachments by blunt and sharp dissection, with care being taken not to damage the adventitial blood supply. At the completion of the ureteral dissection, two silk traction sutures are placed in the detrusor muscle medially and laterally in the superior edge of the ureteral hiatus to allow for control of the posterior wall of the bladder. With these sutures on gentle traction the superior margin of the hiatus can be elevated and a blunt dissector, right-angled clamp, or Kittner dissector can be used under vision to be sure that all peritoneal attachments to the ureter and bladder wall have

been disrupted (Fig. 46-5). The choice of a particular technique for reimplantation from this point on depends largely on the experience and preference of the surgeon. Three variations are recognized: the Politano–Leadbetter technique, the Glenn–Anderson advancement technique, and the Cohen transtrigonal advancement.

Politano–Leadbetter Technique

In the Politano–Leadbetter technique,[41] the ureter is passed extravesically and brought back into the bladder superior to the original hiatus (Fig. 46-6). One must be careful not to place the new muscular hiatus more lateral than the original one; rather it is preferable to have the ureter swing slightly medially in order to prevent placing the hiatus in the more distensible, lateral bladder wall where obstruction may result from kinking or "J-hooking"

FIG. 46-6. The Politano–Leadbetter technique. A somewhat longer tunnel can be achieved by combining this maneuver with a short distal tunnel (see also Fig. 46-7).

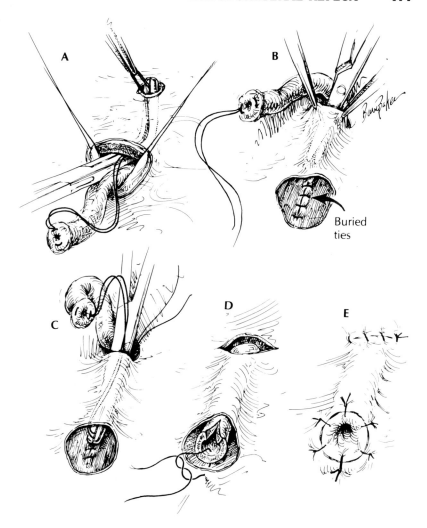

Buried ties

during bladder filling. To achieve this, a pocket must be carefully dissected around the ureter toward the midline of the bladder. A submucosal tunnel is then fashioned toward the previous hiatus, which has been closed with interrupted 4-0 chromic catgut.

One of the criticisms of this technique is that it is entirely "blind," and in order to achieve a satisfactory tunnel of about 2 cm, one must go well up onto the posterior bladder wall. Indeed, perforations of the peritoneum, the bowel, and the vagina have all been reported.[3] But with traction sutures and careful dissection of the posterior bladder wall, the ureter can actually be passed under direct vision. I have found the technique more risky in relation to perforation of the peritoneum in infants, in whom the bladder is small and the reflection of the peritoneum comes down closer to the bladder neck.

Glenn–Anderson Advancement Procedure

Although Hutch and Williams and associates described advancement techniques, Glenn and Anderson improved and popularized this approach.[13,22,60] In its simplest form, a submucosal tunnel is fashioned inferiorly and medially toward the bladder neck from the site of the original hiatus (Fig. 46-7). The ureter is never passed extravesically, and the risk of obstruction to the ureter or perforation of the peritoneum and its contents is minimized. However, this technique is applicable only when the trigone is very large. At times, the new ureterovesical anatomosis is so near the bladder neck that the mucosal anastomosis is technically more demanding than in other procedures.

Glenn and Anderson have recently suggested incising the muscular hiatus superiorly and medially and then closing the detrusor inferior to the

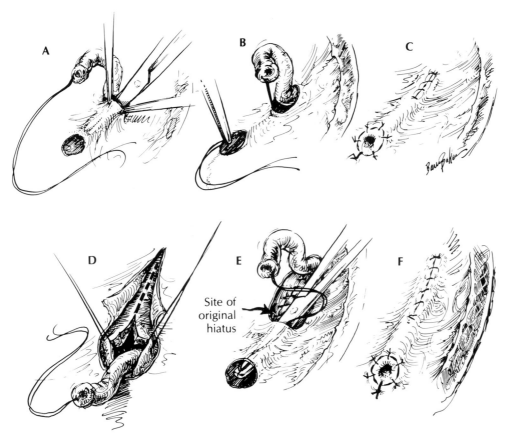

FIG. 46-7.   The advancement technique as described by Glenn and Anderson.   (**A** to **C**) The ureteral orifice is advanced from its original location to a more distal one.   (**D** to **F**) If the trigone is not large enough to provide an adequate distal tunnel, the ureter can be placed more cephalad by incising the muscle above the ureteral hiatus and closing the muscle below the ureter.

ureter.[14] This allows for a more limited distal tunnel but a long submucosal segment. I have found this approach universally applicable and use it extensively. In addition, as the posterior bladder wall is reconstructed, the detrusor muscle can be closed in a stepwise fashion, allowing for a more gentle entrance of the ureter into the bladder. Kelalis has suggested another modification of this approach: using a short Politano–Leadbetter suprahiatal placement and a short distal tunnel.[25]

Cohen Technique

Cohen's technique is a modification of the transtrigonal advancement approach transversely rather than inferiorly (Fig. 46-8).[8] It is technically easy and allows for a long submucosal tunnel and an accessible ureterovesical anastomosis. The only criticism of this technique regards the theoretic difficulty of catheterizing the ureter should retrograde studies be advisable in the future, but the

development of antegrade pyelography and percutaneous nephrostomy should lessen this concern. The Cohen technique is rapidly being accepted as the preferred approach for routine reimplantation in children.

REIMPLANTATION WITH PSOAS HITCH

Occasionally for a primary reimplantation with a slightly dilated ureter or for a secondary reimplantation one cannot achieve a sufficiently long tunnel with one of the intravesical techniques, and an extravesical approach will be chosen. If the ureter is placed high in the posterior bladder wall, it may enter a more mobile portion and likely obstruct from kinking. The use of a psoas hitch provides for fixation of this otherwise mobile portion and allows for a long tunnel without angulation. Middleton has suggested that fixation of the bladder should be routine,[36] although this seems unnecessary for routine reimplantation of the undilated

FIG. 46-8. Cohen's technique of transtrigonal advancement

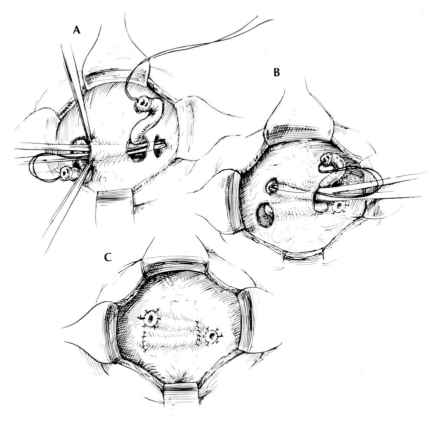

ureter. I prefer to fix the bladder with heavy Dexon just over the iliac vessels, establishing a ureteral hiatus medial to the fixation stitches (Fig. 46-9).

POSTOPERATIVE MANAGEMENT

Indwelling ureteral catheters are not used routinely, and the vesical catheter is generally removed on the first postoperative morning. Maintenance chemotherapy with nitrofurantoin or trimethoprim–sulfamethoxazole is continued for 1 month.

If bilateral ureteroneocystostomy was accomplished, a limited intravenous urogram is obtained at 1 month. A standard urogram and a voiding cystourethrogram are done at 4 months postoperatively. If only a unilateral reimplantation was chosen, the 1-month postoperative intravenous pyelogram is not usually done.

RESULTS OF URETERAL REIMPLANTATIONS

Any of the techniques described in this chapter should provide a success rate of 95% or greater (as judged by correction of reflux and prevention of obstruction) for reimplantation of the normal or minimally dilated ureter into a normal bladder.[15,40,63] Abnormal bladders secondary to obstruction or neurogenic disease, markedly dilated ureters that require tapering, and reimplantations for the second or third time are factors that lessen the chance for success.

As mentioned earlier, it does not appear that the correction of reflux reduces the incidence of bacilluria; rather it only reduces the incidence of ascending pyelonephritis and prevents the development or progression of atrophic renal scars. But other potential benefits may result from antireflux surgery. Atwell and Vejay and Willscher and associates have reported a significant increase in ipsilateral renal growth,[4,62] and Uehling and Wear have observed an increase in concentrating ability following successful antireflux surgery.[56] The significance of these findings remains unclear, especially when compared to the results of nonoperative management of reflux, and they deserve further study.

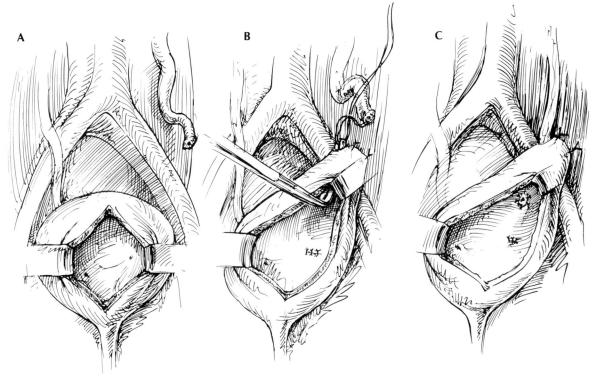

FIG. 46-9. The psoas hitch fixes the otherwise mobile posterolateral portion of the bladder and allows higher placement of a shortened ureter.

REFERENCES

1. ALLEN TD: Vesicoureteral reflux as a manifestation of dysfunctional voiding. In Hodson J, Kincaid-Smith P (eds): Reflux Nephropathy, p 171. New York, Masson, 1979

2. AMBROSE SS, PARROTT TS, WOODARD JR et al: Observations on the small kidney associated with vesicoureteral reflux. J Urol 123:349, 1980

3. ANDERSON EE: Complications of ureteral reimplantation. In Glenn JF (ed): Urologic Surgery, p 294. Hagerstown, Harper & Row, 1975

4. ATWELL JD, VEJAY MR: Renal growth following reimplantation of the ureters for reflux. Br J Urol 50:367, 1978

5. BELL C: Account of the muscles of the ureters and their effects in the irritable state of the bladder. Med Chir Trans Land 3:171, 1812

6. BISCHOFF PF: Megaureter. Br J Urol 29:416, 1957

7. CLARK P, HOSMANE RU: Reimplantation of the ureter. Br J Urol 48:31, 1976

8. COHEN SJ: The Cohen reimplantation technique. Birth defects 13:391, 1977

9. DWOSKIN JY, PERLMUTTER AD: Vesicoureteral reflux in children: A computerized review. J Urol 109:888, 1973

10. EDWARDS D, NORMAND ICS, PRESCOD N et al: Disappearance of vesicoureteric reflux during long-term prophylaxis of urinary tract infection in children. Br Med J 2:285, 1977

11. FAIR WR, GOVAN DE: Influence of vesico-ureteral reflux on the response to treatment of urinary tract infections in female children. Br J Urol 48:111, 1976

12. FILLEY RF, FRIEDLAND GW, GOVAN D et al: Development and progression of clubbing and scarring in children with recurrent urinary tract infection. Radiology 113:145, 1974

13. GLENN JF, ANDERSON EE: Distal tunnel ureteral reimplantation. J Urol 97:623, 1967

14. GLENN JF, ANDERSON EE: Technical considerations in distal tunnel ureteral reimplantation. J Urol 119:194, 1978

15. GONZALES ET, GLENN JF, ANDERSON EE: Results of distal tunnel ureteral reimplantation. J Urol 107:572, 1972

16. GRAVES RC, DAVIDOFF LM: Studies on the ureter and bladder with special reference to regurgitation of the vesical contents. J Urol 10:185, 1923

17. GRAVES RC, DAVIDOFF LM: Studies on the ureter and bladder with special reference to regurgitation of the vesical contents. J Urol 18:321, 1927

18. GRUBER CM: A comparative study of the intravesical ureters (ureterovesical valves) in man and in experimental animals. J Urol 21:567, 1929

19. HAMMAR E, HELIN I: Microanatomy of the intravesical ureter in children with and without reflux. J Urol 117:353, 1977

20. HODSON CJ, MALING TMJ, MCMANAMON PJ et al: The pathogenesis of reflux nephropathy (chronic

atrophic pyelonephritis). Br J Radiol (Suppl) 13, 1975

21. HUTCH JA: Vesicoureteral reflux in the paraplegic: Cause and correction. J Urol 68:457, 1952

22. HUTCH JA: Ureteric advancement operation: Anatomy, technique, and early results. J Urol 89:180, 1963

23. HUTCH JA, BUNGE RG, FLOCKS RH: Vesicoureteral reflux in children. J Urol 74:607, 1955

24. JONES BW, HEADSTREAM JW: Vesicoureteral reflux in children. J Urol 80:114, 1958

25. KELALIS PP: The present status of surgery for vesicoureteral reflux. Urol Clin North Am 1:457, 1974

26. KINCAID–SMITH P, BECKER G: Reflux nephropathy and chronic atrophic pyelonephritis: A review. J Infect Dis 138:774, 1978

27. KING LR, KAZMI SO, BELMAN AB: Natural history of vesicoureteral reflux: Outcome of a trial of nonoperative therapy Urol Clin North Am 1:441, 1974

28. KOFF SA, LAPIDES J, PIAZZA DH: Association of urinary tract infection and reflux with uninhibited bladder contractions and voluntary sphincteric obstruction. J Urol 122:373, 1979

29. LENAGHAN JD, WHITAKER G, JENSEN F et al: The natural history of reflux and long-term effects of reflux on the kidney. J Urol 115:728, 1976

30. LEVITT SB: Medical versus surgical treatment of primary vesicoureteral reflux: Report of the International Reflux Study Committee, Pediatrics 67:392, 1981

31. LICH R, HOWERTON LW, DAVIS LA: Recurrent urosepsis in children. J Urol 86:554, 1961

32. LYON RP, MARSHALL S, TANAGO EA: The ureteral orifice: Its configuration and competency. J Urol 102:504, 1969

33. MCDUFFIE RW, LITIN RB, BLUNDON KE: Ureteral reimplantation: Lich method. Urology 10:19, 1977

34. MACKIE GG, STEPHENS FD: Duplex kidneys: A correlation of renal dysplasia with position of the ureteral orifice. J Urol 114:274, 1975

35. MARBERGER M, ALTWEIN JE, STRAUB E et al: The Lich–Gregoir antireflux plasty: Experiences with 371 children. J Urol 120:216, 1978

36. MIDDLETON RG: Routine use of psoas hitch in ureteral reimplantation. J Urol 123:352, 1980

37. PAQUIN AJ, JR: Ureterovesical anastomosis: The description and evaluation of a technique. J Urol 82:573, 1959

38. PAQUIN AJ, JR: Ureterovesical anastomosis. A comparison of 2 principles. J Urol 87:818, 1962

39. PETERS PC, JOHNSON DE, JACKSON JH: The incidence of vesicoureteral reflux in the premature child. J Urol 97:259, 1967

40. POLITANO VA: Vesicoureteral reflux. In Glenn JF (ed): Urologic Surgery, p 272. Hagerstown, Harper & Row, 1975

41. POLITANO VA, LEADBETTER WF: An operative technique for correction of vesicoureteral reflux. J Urol 79:932, 1958

42. RANSLEY PG: Vesicoureteral reflux: Continuing surgical dilemma. Urology 12:246, 1978

43. RANSLEY PG, RISDON RA: Renal papillae and intrarenal reflux in the pig. Lancet 2:1114, 1974

44. ROLLESTON GL, MALING TMJ, HODSON CJ: Intrarenal reflux and the scarred kidney. Arch Dis Child 49:531, 1974

45. SAMPSON JA: Ascending renal infection with special reference to the reflux of urine from the bladder into the ureters. Johns Hopkins Hosp Bull 14:334, 1903

46. SAVAGE JM, SHAH V, DILLON MJ et al: Renin and blood pressure in children with renal scarring and vesicoureteric reflux. Lancet 1:441, 1978

47. SCOTT JES, STANSFELD JM: Ureteric reflux and kidney scarring in children. Arch Dis Child 43:468, 1968

48. SIEGLER RL: Renin-dependent hypertension in children with reflux nephropathy. Urology 7:474, 1976

49. SMELLIE JM, EDWARDS D, HUNTER N, et al: Vesicoureteric reflux and renal scarring. Kidney Int 4:565, 1975

50. SMELLIE JM, NORMAND ICS: The clinical features and significance of urinary tract infection in childhood. Proc R Soc Med 59:415, 1966

51. SMELLIE JM, NORMAND ICS: Reflux nephropathy in childhood. In Hodson J Kincaid–Smith P (eds): Reflux Nephropathy, p 14. New York, Masson, 1979

52. STECKER JF, READ BP, POUTASSE EF: Pediatric hypertension as a delayed sequela of reflux-induced chronic pyelonephritis. J Urol 118:644, 1977

53. TANAGHO EA, GUTHRIE TH, LYON RP: The intravesical ureter in primary reflux. J Urol 101:824, 1969

54. TANAGHO EA, HUTCH JA, MEYERS FA et al: Primary vesicoureteral reflux: Experimental studies of its etiology. J Urol 93:165, 1965

55. TORRES, VE, VELOSA JA, HOLLEY KE et al: The progression of vesicoureteral reflux nephropathy. Ann Intern Med 92:776, 1980

56. UEHLING DT, WEAR JB: Concentrating ability after antireflux operation. J Urol 116:83, 1976

57. VERMOOTEN V, SPIES JW, NEUSWONGER C: Transplantation of the lower end of the dog's ureter: An experimental study. J Urol 32:261, 1934

58. WALLACE DMA, ROTHWELL DL, WILLIAMS DI: The long-term follow-up of surgically treated vesicoureteric reflux. Br J Urol 50:479, 1978

59. WESSON MB: Anatomical, embryological, and physiological studies of the trigone and neck of the bladder. J Urol 4:279, 1920

60. WILLIAMS DI, SCOTT J, TURNER–WARWICK RT: Reflux and recurrent infection. Br J Urol 33:435, 1961

61. WILLSCHER MK, BAUER SB, ZAMMUTO PJ et al: Infection of the urinary tract after anti-reflux surgery. J Pediatr 89:743, 1976

62. WILLSCHER MK, BAUER SB, ZAMMUTO PJ et al: Renal growth and urinary infection following antireflux surgery in infants and children. J Urol 115:722, 1976

63. WOODARD JR, KEATS G: Ureteral reimplantation: Paquin's procedure after 12 years. J Urol 108:891, 1973

64. YOUNG HH: Hydraulic pressure in genitourinary practice especially in contracture of the bladder. Johns Hopkins Hosp Bull 9:100, 1898

Ureterocele

47

Claude C. Schulman

Ureterocele is a congenital cystiform dilatation of the terminal ureter within the bladder that may extend into the urethra. On the basis of location of the orifice, ureteroceles are usually divided into simple and ectopic types. In the simple or orthotopic form, the intravesical dilatation arises from a normally located ureteral orifice. In the ectopic type, the ureterocele arises from a ureter opening in the bladder neck or urethra, some portion of the ballooning extending extravesically down into the urethra.[4,7,8,12]

Simple Ureterocele

Simple ureteroceles are more common in adults than in children and are relatively small, causing only mild or no obstruction and hydronephrosis (adult-type). They are usually associated with a single ureter or, rarely, with the upper pole ureter of a duplicated collecting system with minimal dilatation and good renal function. These small, entirely intravesical ureteroceles are seldom seen in children, which suggests that they are acquired rather than congenital, but most authors consider that ureteroceles result from the persistence of the Chwalla membrane. The etiology of ureterocele is debatable, and an extensive discussion is beyond the scope of this chapter.

Simple ureteroceles may be symptomless until complicated by stasis, infection, and stone formation. The diagnosis is usually made on intravenous urography; the classic finding of a "cobra head" or "spring onion" deformity is pathognomonic. Reflux is uncommon with this type of ureterocele, and voiding cystourethrography or other diagnostic modalities are not usually thought to be necessary for accurate diagnosis.

In most instances of simple ureterocele, the upper urinary tract changes are not as severe as those associated with an ectopic ureterocele and kidney function is preserved; thus treatment should focus on the ureterocele only. In some small, uncomplicated cases, no treatment is needed. Transurethral resection of ureteroceles was widespread in the past, but today most surgeons agree that it is seldom indicated because it invariably results in reflux. There remains, however, a place for minimal endoscopic incision of a small adult ureterocele complicated by a stone or infection and minimal dilatation (Fig. 47-1). That approach is not applicable to cases seen in children or to larger ureteroceles in adults in which treatment should be operative. The recommended operation is excision of the ureterocele with ureteral reimplantation, using one of the advancement techniques or the Politano–Leadbetter procedure.[5] When the involved ureter is dilated, lower tapering should be considered.

In the uncommon situation of a simple intravesical ureterocele associated with a duplication, the renal parenchyma related to the ureterocele keeps a satisfactory functional value and the ureter is minimally or not at all dilated, the condition being very similar to simple ureterocele with a single

FIG. 47-1. Simple ureterocele in the adult, if complicated by stasis, infection, or stone formation, may be treated by endoscopic incision. A small knife electrode is introduced in the ureteral orifice, cutting toward the base of the ureterocele or horizontally, which leads to less reflux, then unroofing with a conventional loop electrode.

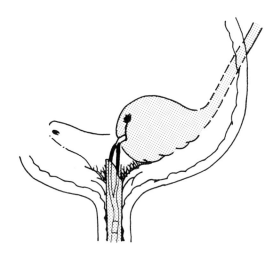

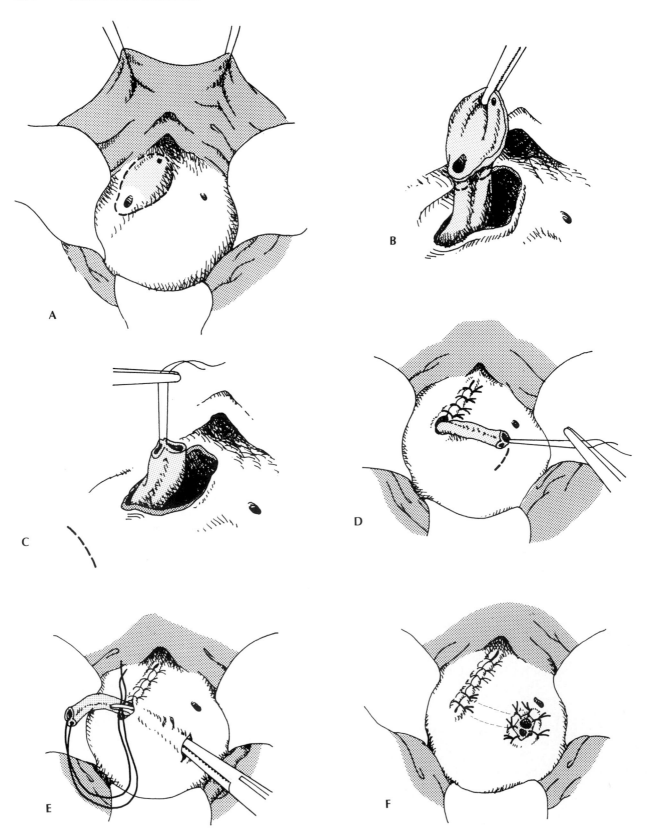

◄ **FIG. 47-2.** Simple intravesical ureterocele associated with duplication. **(A)** Ureteral dilatation is usually moderate, and the treatment is similar to simple ureterocele with a single ureter, consisting in excision of the ureterocele with common sheath ureter reimplantation. **(B)** The bladder is opened, and a circumferential incision is made at the base of the ureterocele. Previous injection of saline into the ureterocele is helpful for its dissection from the trigone. **(C and D)** After excision of the ureterocele, the hiatus may be quite large and is closed with 2-0 chromic catgut. The two ureters are treated as a single unit. **(E and F)** The ureters are reimplanted, using one of the advancement techniques or the Politano–Leadbetter procedure. A transverse submucosal tunnel, as is used in the Cohen reimplantation procedure, is illustrated here. Ureteral catheters are usually left for a few days with bladder drainage.

ureter. Reflux may be present in the lower pole ureter. Treatment is similar to that used when there is a single ureter, removing the ureterocele with common sheet reimplantation of both ureters using an antireflux procedure (Fig. 47-2).

Ectopic Ureterocele

Ectopic ureteroceles are a common and severe anomaly in pediatric urology. There is a marked predominance in girls. The anomaly is bilateral in about 10% of the cases.[6,7] These large ureteroceles, which frequently extend extravesically into the urethra, are related to the upper pole of a duplex system. Rarely, ectopic ureteroceles occur without duplication, usually in boys. There is a wide variety of anatomic forms and Stephens has attempted to classify ectopic ureteroceles as stenotic, sphincteric, or cecoureteroceles,[10] but the classification is not of great clinical importance, as stressed by several authors.[5,12] Of more importance to the surgeon is the eventual extravesical extension of the ureterocele, which causes bladder outlet obstruction, and the strength or weakness of the underlying detrusor muscle backing, which might appear as an extensive defect after excision of the ureterocele.[11]

The patient often presents during early childhood with symptoms of urinary infection or failure to thrive. The ureterocele may sometimes appear as a genital deformity in the female child, when it is prolapsed in the vulva. A flank mass may be palpated during physical examination. Mostly, the diagnosis is made on well-performed excretory urography. Typical urographic findings include a duplicated collecting system with poor opacification or nonopacification of the upper pole on the side of the ureterocele. This is associated with downward and lateral displacement of the lower pole collecting system (drooping lily sign) and a large filling defect in the bladder base. A micturating cystogram should be performed to demonstrate the frequently associated reflux in the ipsilateral and contralateral ureter.[11]

The renal parenchyma drained by the ectopic ureterocele is characteristically small and dysplastic, whereas the ureter is grossly dilated. The lower pole ureter is very often refluxing, and the associated parenchyma presents with pyelonephritis. In other cases, the ureter is dilated from obstruction by the ureterocele, which may also affect the contralateral ureter. The diagnosis can be confirmed by endoscopy.

The **surgical management** of a large, infant-type ureterocele depends on several factors, including the child's age, his clinical condition, the presence of renal failure or sepsis, the presence of associated lesions of the lower pole and contralateral kidney or bilateral ureteroceles, and the surgeon's expertise. There is no general agreement on the optimum treatment method for ectopic ureteroceles (Fig. 47-3), but there is definitely no place for simple endoscopic unroofing as the only treatment for this anomaly. With a few exceptions, there is no justification to use a conservative approach, because there is gross damage or dysplastic lesions of the upper pole parenchyma associated with the ureterocele. Procedures such as ureteropyeloneostomy would only be considered in solitary kidney or when both kidneys are damaged. Thus, in most cases, heminephrectomy is the procedure of choice. It is easily accomplished through a retroperitoneal, flank incision with resection of the proximal portion of the involved ureter (Fig. 47-4). The controversial question is whether or not ureterocele excision is necessary after the upper pole nephrectomy.[9] Several pediatric urologists suggest its excision with extensive reconstruction of the bladder floor and reimplantation of the ipsilateral and sometimes also contralateral ureter as the standard procedure.[5,6,12]

The removal of the ureterocele may be done in various ways. Simple unroofing through a transvesical incision may suffice in the unusual case when the ureterocele is small and the detrusor backing is strong. Even in these cases, the unroofing should usually be combined with an anti-

A   B   C   D   E

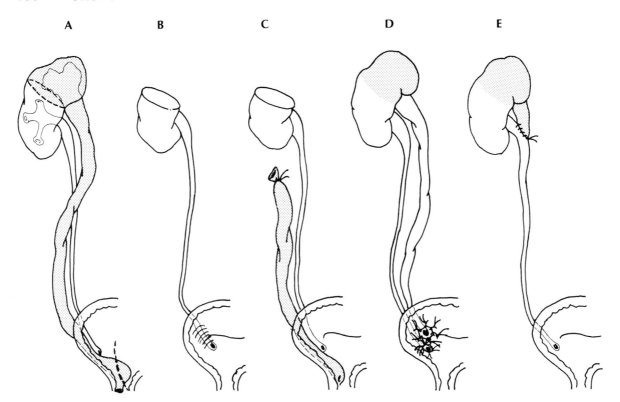

FIG. 47-3. Different surgical procedures for a large ureterocele associated with ureteral duplication and eventual extravesical ectopic extension: (**A**) endoscopic unroofing to provide temporary relief of obstruction followed by reconstruction (especially in a septic neonate); (**B**) complete correction with upper pole nephroureterectomy and ureterocele excision with usual lower pole ureter reimplantation; (**C**) upper pole nephrectomy with partial ureterectomy, leaving the ureterocele to collapse; (**D**) ureterocele excision with reimplantation of a small ureterocele with minimal dilatation and good renal function (rare); (**E**) ureteropyeloneostomy with or without removal of the small ureterocele

reflux reimplantation of the lower pole ureter, because both ureters are closely bound together in their terminal portion and the excision of the ureterocele often makes it essential to remove also the terminal lower pole ureter, where there is often reflux. When unroofing the ureterocele, it is important to remove the entire wall of the ballooning, in particular near the bladder neck and in the posterior urethra to avoid having a retained lip of incised ureterocele act as a valvular fold, causing obstructive problems.[5,9]

In most cases, however when the ureterocele is large, a complete excision is preferable, particularly if the detrusor backing is weak, if there is ipsilateral and even contralateral reflux, and if the ureterocele extends down into the urethra. Complete dissection of the ureterocele may be very difficult, especially at the lower end, where it may adhere closely to the bladder neck and urethra. In these cases, a combination of intravesical and extravesical

approaches is useful for complete downward dissection of the ureterocele with entire mobilization of the bladder. During the dissection of the ureterocele, one should be careful not to injure the external sphincter area. After complete excision of the ureterocele, the urethra and the trigone should be reconstructed with reimplantation of the lower pole ureter and even the contralateral one, following a standard antireflux (Politano–Leadbetter) or advancement procedure (Fig. 47-5).

In the last decade, an increasing number of authors have advocated a more conservative approach, consisting of heminephrectomy with removal of the upper pole ureter to the level of the iliac vessels, if excision of the ureterocele is not considered mandatory. Complete decompression of the ureterocele as well as disappearance of mild to moderate reflux in the ipsilateral lower pole ureter can be anticipated.[1,2,3] This approach avoids the risk and potential complications of extensive

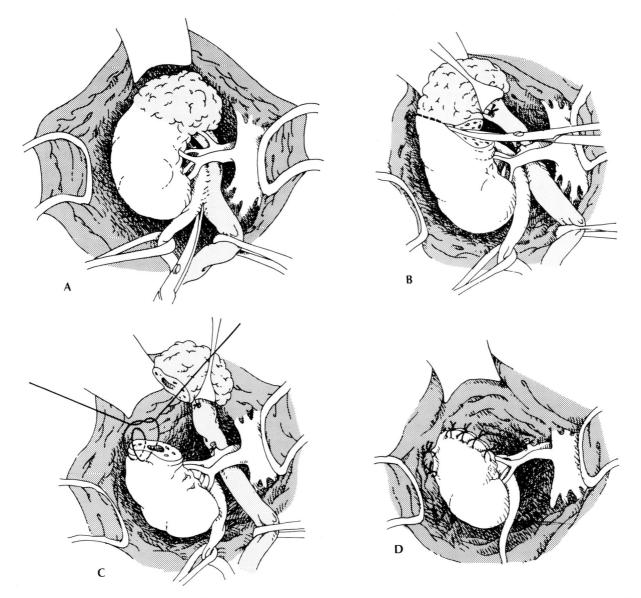

FIG. 47-4.   Upper pole nephrectomy.   **(A)** In the classic lumbotomy both ureters are carefully dissected, preserving the blood supply of the lower pole ureter.   **(B)** Dissection of the various branches of the renal pedicle and ligation of the upper pole vascular supply. A clear demarcation is often visible between the destroyed upper pole and the normal lower pole. The renal capsule is incised to cover the later suture of the renal parenchyma.   **(C)** After removal of the upper pole, deep catgut sutures complete the hemostasis of the parenchymal section.   **(D)** Suture of the parenchyma is completed with capsular covering. Fixation of the remaining lower pole to the posterior muscles prevents rotation on a pedicle that is often stretched.

surgical reconstruction at the bladder level because the bladder is never entered, the procedure being completed entirely through a single retroperitoneal flank incision. The ureteral stump is left open and drained so that urine remaining in the ureterocele and distal ureter will empty in a retrograde fashion when the child voids and intravesical pressure rises. If reflux was noted in the obstructed system or if the ureterocele was willfully or inadvertently incised causing reflux, then the distal stump is ligated.

This more conservative approach gives satisfac-

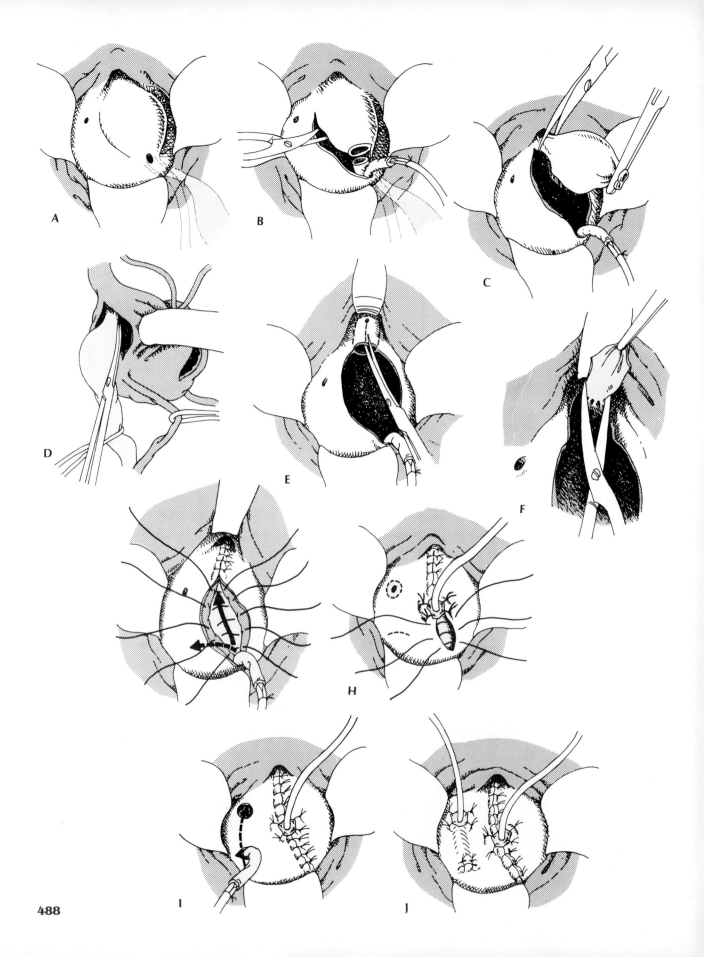

◀ **FIG. 47-5.** Complete excision of an ectopic ureterocele with reimplantation of the lower pole ureter and sometimes of the contralateral ureter also. Upper pole nephroureterectomy has been done first during the same operative session through a retroperitoneal flank incision. Cautious extravesical dissection will separate both ureters; great care must be taken to preserve the periureteral adventitia of the lower pole ureter with its blood supply. **(A)** The bladder is opened through a long median incision or, even better, by a T-shaped incision, so as to expose the entire bladder and bladder neck. **(B)** The ureterocele is dissected from the trigone by incision of the vesical mucosa, which includes the lower pole ureteral orifice. **(C)** The entire intravesical part of the ureterocele is removed down to the bladder neck. **(D)** Extravesical mobilization and dissection of the ureterocele facilitate its removal. Previous complete mobilization of the bladder is necessary to allow easy access. **(E)** Extravesical extension of the ureterocele is difficult to remove where it is fixed to the bladder neck and urethra. This excision is facilitated by opening the upper wall of the ureterocele extension in the bladder neck and urethra. **(F)** The lateral and posterior walls of the ureterocele extension are carefully dissected from the bladder neck and urethra and removed. **(G)** The urethra, trigone, and posterior bladder wall are reconstructed by a series of 2-0 chromic catgut sutures to ensure a strong backing to the bladder. Reimplantation of the lower pole ureter is done by advancement (*solid arrow*) or by a transverse submucous tunnel following Cohen's procedure (*broken arrow*). **(H)** The advancement procedure is illustrated. The lower pole ureter is covered by the vesical mucosa. **(I and J)** The contralateral ureter, which may be refluxing, obstructed, or sectioned during the dissection of the ureterocele, will be reimplanted by a standard antireflux procedure.

tory results in about two thirds of the cases. However, if the ureterocele fails to collapse and remain obstructive, or if reflux persists in the lower pole ureter, it is likely to result in recurrent infections, bladder outlet obstruction, or bladder diverticulum or reflux, which will necessitate an additional operation through a suprapubic incision in a second stage some months later in one third of the cases.[1,2,3] This expectant approach allows also total reconstruction at separate times, and sometimes in easier and safer conditions, in "naturally" selected cases which really need it.

Another option may be considered in the severely ill and septic neonate, when preliminary drainage is dictated by the poor clinical situation and endoscopic incision of the ureterocele provides temporary internal drainage of the obstructed bladder and upper pole. After the condition has improved, single- or two-stage repair is undertaken with upper pole nephroureterectomy and complete removal of the unroofed ureterocele with reimplantation of the associated lower pole ureter.[9]

It is clear that there is no unanimity on how to manage surgically complex infant-type ureterocele cases and that all the points of view have certain advantages and drawbacks. For the surgeon who is not familiar with the condition and rarely operates on infants, upper pole nephrectomy alone is the safest initial procedure. In the newborn with sepsis and poor general condition, preliminary drainage may be necessary, and simple unroofing

of the ureterocele by endoscopy or a transvesical incision is advisable because these neonates are poor candidates for a major procedure. For older children in good general condition, the experienced surgeon will consider a total, single-stage complete reconstruction. In some rare cases, total nephroureterectomy is indicated when the lower pole is also destroyed by obstruction or reflux.

REFERENCES

1. BARRETT DM, MALEK RS, KELALIS PP: Problems and solutions in surgical treatment of 100 consecutive ureteral duplications in children. J Urol 114:126, 1975
2. BELMAN AB, FILMER RB, KING LR: Surgical management of duplication of the collecting system. J Urol 112:316, 1974
3. CENDRON J, MELIN Y, VALAYER J: Simplified treatment of ureterocele with pyelo-ureteric duplication. Eur Urol 7:321, 1981
4. ERICSSON NO: Ectopic ureterocele in infants and children: A clinical study. Acta Chir Scand (Suppl) 197:1, 1954
5. HENDREN WH, MITCHELL ME: Surgical correction of ureteroceles. J Urol 121:590, 1979
6. JOHNSTON JH, JOHNSON LM: Experiences with ectopic ureteroceles. Br J Urol 41:61, 1971
7. MALEK RS, KELALIS PP, BURKE EC: et al: Simple and ectopic ureterocele in infancy and childhood. Surg Gynecol Obstet 134:611, 1972

8. SCHULMAN CC: Ureteroceles. Acta Urol Belg 40:687, 1972

9. SCHULMAN CC, GREGOIR W: Ureteric duplication. In Eckstein HB, Hohenfellner R, Williams DI (eds): Surgical Pediatric Urology, p 244. Stuttgart: Philadelphia, Georg Thieme Verlag, 1977

10. STEPHENS FD: Caecoureterocele and concepts on the embryology and aetiology of ureteroceles. Aust NZ J Surg 40:239, 1971

11. WILLIAMS DI, FAY R, LILLIE JG: The functional radiology of ectopic ureterocele. Br J Urol 44:417, 1972

12. WILLIAMS DI, WOODARD JR: Problems in the management of ectopic ureteroceles. J Urol 92:635, 1964

Ureteral Diversion

48

Herbert B. Eckstein

Ureteral diversion, or cutaneous ureterostomy, is a useful method of providing effective drainage of the upper urinary tract in patients with vesical dysfunction when this is associated with marked ureteral dilatation. The procedure is especially applicable in infancy and childhood. Ureteral diversion has advantages over intubated nephrostomy, pyelostomy, or ureterostomy on the one hand and intestinal conduits on the other. Its use is limited by the size of the ureter, and there are various methods of temporary and permanent ureteral diversion. Ureteral diversion may be indicated as a temporary measure in patients with such conditions as urethral valves, severe bladder outflow obstruction, megacystis syndrome, dysplasia of the abdominal wall muscles (prune-belly syndrome), and severe refluxing megaloureters. Permanent ureteral diversion is indicated in some patients with noncorrectable bladder outflow obstruction or neuropathic disease of the bladder, especially in relation to myelomeningocele, and in patients with bladder tumors and associated ureteral dilatation.[1,2]

Temporary Cutaneous Ureterostomy

The indications for temporary cutaneous ureterostomy have already been mentioned; they by and large are confined to infancy. In most patients with conditions such as urethral valves, definitive corrective surgery is usually feasible, but reimplantation of the ureter into the bladder to prevent reflux or to remove an obstruction at the ureterovesical junction may be necessary. It is therefore important that the distal portion of the ureter remain undisturbed during the original diversion procedure so that there is no interference with the subsequent distal ureteral surgery.[5,11]

LOOP URETEROSTOMY

Loop ureterostomy is the simplest method of cutaneous ureteral diversion that affords adequate drainage of the kidneys while leaving the distal ureter undisturbed (Fig. 48-1). With the patient supine, bilateral V-shaped skin incisions are made (Fig. 48-1A). The size of the incision depends on the age of the patient and the thickness of the abdominal wall, but in infancy, a flap some 5 cm in length suffices. The base of the skin flap should be lateral so that there is no interference with the blood supply of the flap. A full-thickness skin flap is raised, and the muscle layers are divided (Fig. 48-1B). Dissection is carried down to the peritoneal level, and great care must be maintained not to open the peritoneum accidentally.

The dilated ureter is mobilized, with care taken not to interfere with its blood supply, and the ureter is retracted from the wound (Fig. 48-1C). The skin flap is then pulled underneath the loop of ureter to prevent its retraction, and its apex is sutured back into position (Fig. 48-1D). A longitudinal incision is made into the ureter (shown by the dotted line in Fig. 48-1E), and this is everted and sutured to the skin and skin edges with interrupted 3-0 catgut or 4-0 Dexon sutures. The final appearance is shown in Figure 48-1F. The ureterostomy usually drains spontaneously. If free urine drainage is not established within 12 hr, a catheter can be inserted into the upper limb of the ureterostomy to overcome any possible postoperative edema.

Once bladder outflow obstruction (e.g., urethral valves) has been dealt with, the ureters have, if necessary, been reimplanted, and renal function has recovered satisfactorily, the ureterostomy is closed by full mobilization of the exteriorized loop, which is then resected, and an oblique end-to-end anastomosis of the ureter is performed. The anastomosis should be sufficiently oblique to provide a lumen of 1 cm in diameter, because some contraction of the anastomosis inevitably occurs. The anastomosis is again performed with absorbable sutures. The ureter need not be intubated, but an extraureteral drain should be inserted and brought out through the incision.

The loop ureterostomy provides a total diversion that results in complete nonfilling of the bladder.

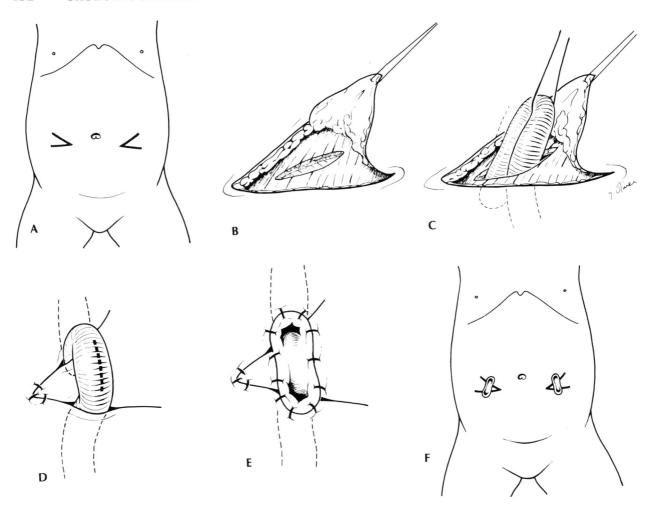

FIG. 48-1. Technique of cutaneous loop ureterostomy

This may be disadvantageous in some patients in whom reconstructive surgery is contemplated after a period of several months.

RING URETEROSTOMY

Ring ureterostomy, described by Williams and Cromie,[10], has the advantage that some urine will pass through the ureteral anastomosis into the bladder while the kidneys are effectively drained and decompressed. The various steps of the operation are shown in Figure 48-2 and are similar (except for the anastomosis) to the loop ureterostomy. However, for this procedure a simple longitudinal incision is preferred to the skin flap previously described. The other great advantage of the ring ureterostomy is the ease with which it can be closed once the need for decompression has been eliminated (Fig. 48-2D).

Y-URETEROSTOMY

In the Y-ureterostomy, bilateral anterolateral incisions are made to expose the renal pelvis and the upper ureter extraperitoneally. If the ureter is grossly tortuous, it should be mobilized and a part resected (Fig. 48-3A). The divided end of the ureter is then brought out through a circular skin incision at a convenient point, and a lateral incision is made in the ureter (Fig. 48-3B). The renal pelvis is then anastomosed to the side incision in the ureter (Fig. 48-3C). The end of the divided ureter is fashioned into a nipple and sutured to the skin (Fig. 48-3D). This procedure provides free drainage from the kidney; at the same time, some urine will pass into the bladder so that the vesical function is maintained. Once definitive surgery has been performed, the cutaneous ureterostomy is mobilized, the ureter is dissected down to the level of the

FIG. 48-2. Technique of ring ureterostomy

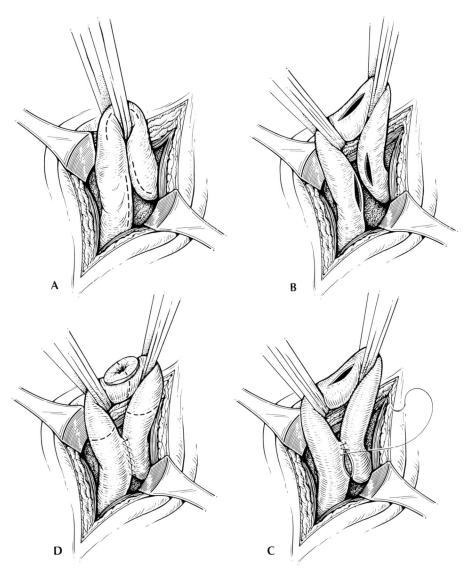

A

B

D

C

pyeloureteral anastomosis, and the excess portion of the ureter is resected.

END URETEROSTOMY

End ureterostomy (see Fig. 48-4A) is not recommended for temporary ureteral diversion because subsequent reconstruction procedures, such as reimplantation of the ureter into the bladder, are extremely difficult. The surgical technique in end ureterostomy is essentially the same as that in permanent ureteral diversion.

The indications for temporary ureteral diversion must be assessed in relation to pyelostomy, nephrostomy, and intubated ureterostomy. If upper urinary tract drainage is likely to be required for only 3 weeks or less, nephrostomy or pyelostomy is undoubtedly preferable. If prolonged drainage is likely, cutaneous ureteral diversion is preferable. Intubated ureterostomy has, in our hands, been singularly unsuccessful because the displaced catheter cannot be reintroduced without a major operation. The advantages of cutaneous ureterostomy are that the patient can be discharged quickly and infection due to a foreign body inserted in the urinary tract is avoided. Although adhesive bags can easily be applied around the ureterostomy to collect urine for the purpose of fluid balance and electrolyte studies, the temporary cutaneous ureterostomy in the infant can be well managed by placing a diaper around the infant's abdomen and changing this as necessary. The routine use of

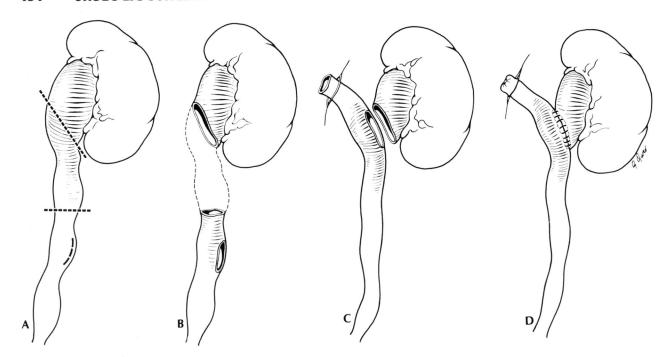

FIG. 48-3. Cutaneous Y-ureterostomy

appliances for temporary ureterostomy is not recommended.

Permanent Ureteral Diversion

The most frequent indication for permanent ureteral diversion is a neuropathic bladder associated with gross dilatation of the ureters.[4,6] Some patients with megacystis syndrome, grossly dilated refluxing megaloureters, or bladder tumors obstructing outflow also fall into this category. The advantage of ureteral diversion is that it avoids the necessity for intestinal surgery required to produce an ileal or colonic conduit and the necessary intraperitoneal procedures. The possible reabsorption and mucus production caused by such an intestinal conduit are also avoided.

On the other hand, only patients with at least one grossly dilated ureter are suitable for a permanent ureteral diversion. In my experience, most surgical disasters after cutaneous ureterostomy have resulted from the wrong selection of patients—those whose ureters have really not been wide enough or tortuous enough to enable ureteral diversion to be performed satisfactorily. The acutely dilated thin-walled ureter is quite unsuitable.

The four options of ureteral diversion are indicated in Figure 48-4. Figure 48-4*A* shows a bilateral cutaneous ureterostomy, which is simple to perform but should be used only in emergency situations. This procedure, resulting in two stomas that require the fitting of two separate appliances, is not generally recommended. In the double-barreled ureterostomy (Fig. 48-4*B*), the site of the stoma should usually be placed on the side of the less dilated of the two ureters. However, if stomal complications develop later, a right-sided cutaneous ureterostomy can only be converted into an ileal conduit, whereas a left-sided cutaneous ureterostomy must be converted into a colonic conduit. In addition, the site of the stoma must bear a relation to the patient's other physical disabilities, especially kyphoscoliosis. Whenever possible, the stoma should be situated on the side of the abdomen that has the greater length; that is, on the convex side of the scoliosis.

Figure 48-4*D* shows the use of a unilateral cutaneous ureterostomy in a patient who has a grossly dilated ureter on one side but an essentially normal upper urinary tract on the other. The grossly dilated ureter can be exteriorized as shown, and subsequently (depending on the basic pathologic condition) the exteriorized ureter may be reimplanted into the bladder or alternately the nonexteriorized ureter can be anastomosed end to side to the dilated ureter to convert this situation to the ureteroureterostomy shown in Figure 48-4*C*.

FIG. 48-4. Various modules of cutaneous ureterostomy: **(A)** bilateral cutaneous ureterostomy, **(B)** double-barreled ureterostomy, **(C)** ureteroureterostomy, **(D)** unilateral cutaneous ureterostomy

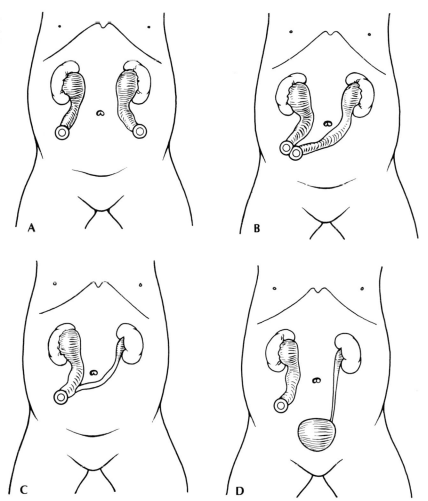

DOUBLE-BARRELED CUTANEOUS URETEROSTOMY

The double-barreled cutaneous ureterostomy (Fig. 48-5) is the most usual type of permanent ureteral diversion. The site of the stoma depends on the relative length of the two ureters, but the exact site should be determined by the appliance fitter or the stomatologist to make subsequent appliance fitting less troublesome.

The abdomen is opened through a paramedian incision, which should be on the side opposite to the intended site of the stoma. Dissection is carried out extraperitoneally, and both ureters are mobilized down to the bladder and divided. One ureter is brought extraperitoneally across to the opposite side, and both ureters are incised by approximately 2 cm (Fig. 48-5B). The incised edges of the ureters are anastomosed to each other with interrupted absorbable sutures. A stoma is fashioned at a predetermined site through a circular skin incision, which is then deepened using an adequate cruciate incision into the rectus sheath or the external oblique muscle, and the stoma is everted and sutured to the skin so that it projects approximately 1 cm (Fig. 48-5C).

URETEROURETEROSTOMY

When one ureter is grossly dilated and the other ureter is either normal or only moderately dilated, a satisfactory ureteral diversion can be performed using the grossly dilated ureter as the stoma and anastomosing the less dilated ureter obliquely end to side (see Fig. 48-4C).[7,8] A paramedian incision should be made on the side opposite to the proposed stoma, and a V-shaped skin incision 1 cm to 2 cm in length should be made at the stoma site (Fig. 48-6A).

A transperitoneal approach is preferred, and

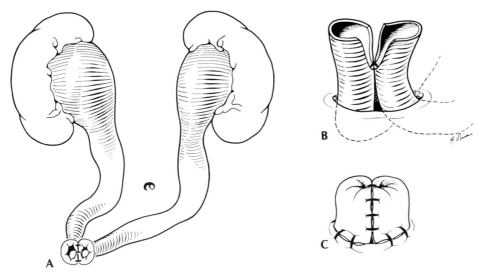

FIG. 48-5. Double-barreled cutaneous ureterostomy

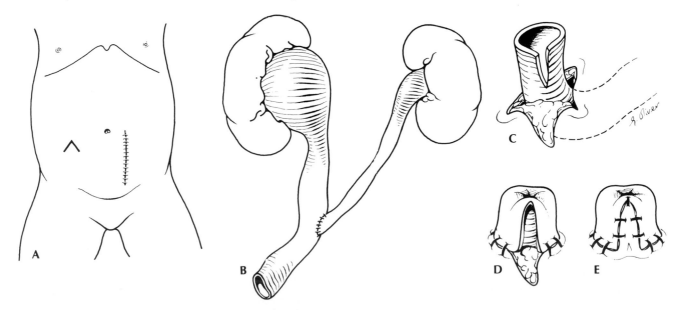

FIG. 48-6. Cutaneous ureterostomy with ureteroureterostomy

suitable incisions are made through the posterior peritoneum to mobilize both ureters. The less dilated ureter is brought retroperitoneally across to the opposite side and is anastomosed obliquely end to side to the more dilated ureter (Fig. 48-6B). The anastomosis should be no less than 1 cm in length to allow for subsequent contraction. The dilated ureter is then brought out retroperitoneally through the stomal incision and is incised for 1 cm to 2 cm longitudinally (Fig. 48-6C). The V-shaped skin flap at the stomal incision is carefully sutured into the defect produced by the ureteral incision (Fig. 48-6D and E). The introduction of such a skin

flap prevents subsequent scarring and contracture of the ureterostomy stoma.

The ureteroureteral anastomosis must be drained with a corrugated or similar drain brought out extraperitoneally through a separate stab incision well away from the stoma. The improvement in renal function and renal anatomy that can be produced by a ureteral diversion is shown on the excretory pyelographic films of one patient (Fig. 48-7). The ureteral stoma is eminently satisfactory initially and tends to epithelialize gradually by the apparent migration of skin cells (Fig. 48-8).

FIG. 48-7. Excretory urograms demonstrate improvement in renal function after cutaneous ureterostomy; **B** was taken 3 years after **A**.

COMPLICATIONS AND RESULTS OF PERMANENT URETEROSTOMY

Both early and late complications follow cutaneous ureterostomy. The most serious early complication is necrosis of the ureterostomy stoma. This may result from excessive mobilization or rough handling, which can interfere with the blood supply of the ureter; from too tight an opening in the abdominal wall muscle or skin; or from eversion of the ureter to form a stoma. Such a stomal necrosis can usually be avoided by meticulous surgical technique, by ensuring an adequate incision through the abdominal wall and, most important, by introducing the V-shaped skin flap into the ureterostomy stoma in the case of single ureters (see Fig. 48-6D and E).

Because there is usually insufficient ureter to resect the necrotic section and to produce an adequate stoma, the cutaneous ureterostomy usually must be converted into an ileal or colonic conduit, depending on the side on which the ureterostomy has been made. Ureteral dysfunction may prevent the drainage of urine in the early postoperative period, either because of operative trauma or because of excessive distention of the ureter before surgical relief had been undertaken. This can usually be overcome by the insertion of a catheter through the stoma. In the case of the double-barreled ureterostomy, separate catheters must be inserted into the two ureters; in the case of the Y-ureterostomy, the catheter should only be inserted for a few centimeters and should on no account reach as high as the interureteral anastomosis, because the catheter may well damage it.

Late complications of the cutaneous ureterostomy include stomal stenosis and stomal retraction. Stomal stenosis was common in the past, but its incidence has considerably decreased since we have used the method of interpositioning the skin flap into the stoma. Once the obstructed ureter has been decompressed, it will shrink both in diameter and in length; thus, a straightforward revision of the ureterostomy stoma is not only very difficult but also very unsatisfactory. For these reasons, stenosis of the ureterostomy or retraction of the stoma should be treated by the interposition of an intestinal conduit using either ileum or colon.

Although the early results of cutaneous ureterostomy are quite satisfactory, the late results are disappointing. In our experience, well over half

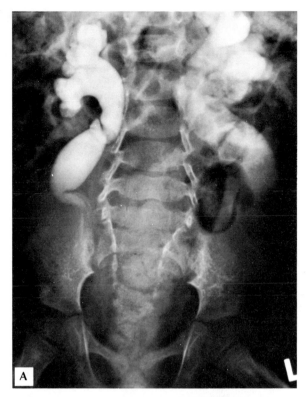

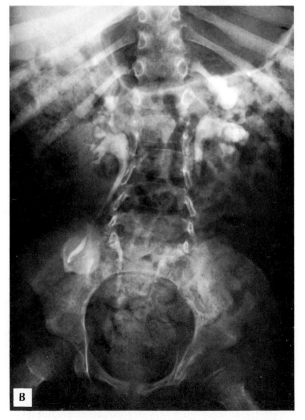

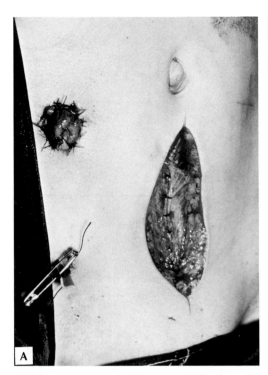
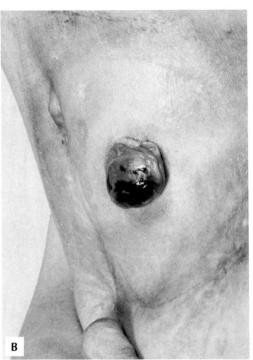

FIG. 48-8.   **(A)** Ureteral stoma exhibits everted mucosal surface.   **(B)** A few years later, epithelialization will be noted.

FIG. 48-9.   **(A)** Disposable urinary diversion appliance manufactured by Downs Surgical Ltd., Mitcham, Surrey, England. Note the transparency of the appliance and the nonreturn valve in the bag.   **(B)** Appliance fitted on the patient

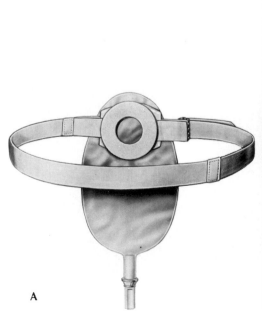
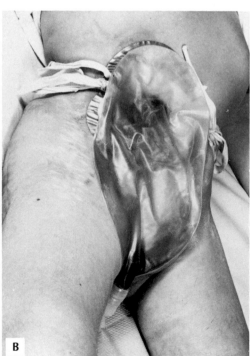

the patients with permanent cutaneous ureterostomies have required the conversion of these ureterostomies to intestinal conduits within 7 years of the original diversion because of stomal complications. In other patients, the cutaneous ureterostomy has given no reason for concern for as long as 10 years, and the stoma has remained satisfactory. Despite the high late stomal complication rate and the need for conversion to an intestinal conduit, cutaneous ureterostomy remains an operation of choice in patients with grossly dilated ureters who usually have some degree of renal insufficiency.[3,9]

URETEROSTOMY APPLIANCES

The choice of appliances in relation to ureteral diversion is of paramount importance. Rubber or latex bags are condemned because they are impossible to clean satisfactorily or to sterilize. Urinary diversion appliances should be made of plastic materials and should be disposable. Various makes of appliances are available; one that I favor is shown in Figure 48-9. The appliance must be translucent so that the stoma can be observed and must contain a nonreturn valve so that accidental detachment does not result in a calamity.

REFERENCES

1. ECKSTEIN HB: Cutaneous ureterostomy. Proc Soc Med 56:749, 1963
2. ECKSTEIN HB, KAPILA L: Cutaneous ureterostomy. Br J Urol: 306, 1970
3. ECKSTEIN HB, SHAH K: Ileal conduit urinary diversion, a review of 126 patients. Actuelle Urologie 5:1, 1974
4. GRAF RA, FLOCKS RH, SMITH JH et al: Urinary tract changes associated with spina bifida and myelomeningocele. Am J Roentgenol 92:255, 1964
5. HOHENFELLNER R, WULFF HD: Zur Harnableitung mittels ausgeschalteter Dickdarmsegmente. Actuelle Urologie 1:18, 1970
6. LISTER J, COOK RCM, ZACHARY RB: Operative management of neurogenic bladder dysfunction in children; Ureterostomy. Arch Dis Child 43:672, 1968
7. MADDEN JL, TAN PY, MCCANN WJ: An experimental and clinical study of cross uretero-ureterostomy. Surg Gynecol Obstet 124:483, 1967
8. SHAFIK A: Cutaneous uretero-ureterostomy. Br J Urol 40:568, 1968
9. SMITH ED: Ileo-cutaneous ureterostomy in children. Aust NZ J Surg 33:169, 1964
10. WILLIAMS DI, CROMIE WJ: Ring ureterostomy. Br J Urol 47:789, 1976
11. WILLIAMS DI, RABINOVITCH HH: Cutaneous ureterostomy for the grossly dilated ureter of childhood. Br J Urol 40:696, 1968

Ileal and Jejunal Urinary Diversion

49

Clarence V. Hodges

Urinary diversion is necessary when the urinary conduit system is incompatible with the maintenance of renal function, the prevention or eradication of urinary tract infection, the prevention or eradication of secondary skin lesions, or social acceptability. Diversion is always a reluctant compromise, because there is no satisfactory substitute for the normally functioning urinary system. Yet temporary procedures are too often employed when the available evidence points to the need for permanent urinary diversion.[9]

The need for adequate methods of urinary diversion has long been recognized, and the development of successful techniques has coincided with progress in medical knowledge and improvement in technical skills. The first attempt to divert urine to the bowel was made by Simon in the mid-19th century. Nesbit described mucosa-to-mucosa anastomosis of ureter to bowel to prevent strictures, and Bricker, in 1950, revived the concept of ileal conduit urinary diversion as originally proposed by Tizzoni and Foggi in 1888.[3,14,15] Modifications of the ureteroileal conduit by placing the conjoined ureters onto the butt of the ileal segment have been popularized by Albert and Persky and by Wallace.[1,17]

Urinary diversion by bowel segment may be indicated for ureteral or bladder incompetence, after cystectomy, or to bypass infravesical obstruction. The type of diversion is determined by the location of the lesion, the pathologic process, the age and condition of the patient, and the ability and inclination of the urologist.

ANATOMIC AND PHYSIOLOGIC CONSIDERATIONS

The small bowel lumen diminishes in caliber from above downward. There is an increase in the mesenteric fat toward the ileum and a change in the distribution of the mesenteric blood vessels. The jejunum is characterized by rather long vasa recta with very large lunettes, or clear spaces, free of mesenteric vessels. The ileum has secondary arcades with shorter straight vessels and smaller lunettes, and preservation of the distal arcade with vertical incision of the ileal mesentery will allow an ileal conduit to span an obese abdominal wall without vascular compromise of the stoma (Fig. 49-1).

The bowel, when interrupted and anastomosed, seals by adherence of the very highly reactive and poorly differentiated serosal tissues; an enteric anastomosis is functionally sealed within hours. The major strength of the bowel is contained in the submucosa, and all suture techniques make use of this strength by including the submucosa in the anastomoses.

If an ileal segment is to be the conduit, it must be isoperistaltic, and the stoma is usually on the right side of the abdomen. Concern over the absorption of urinary solutes from the ileal segment has prompted extensive investigations.[7,16] The bowel mucosa absorbs large quantities of water and solutes in proportion of their concentrations, ion gradients, and duration of contact with the mucosal surface. Therefore, minimum length and rapid passage are desirable to keep absorption to a minimum and to prevent symptomatic hyperchloremic metabolic acidosis. Lack of the manifestations of absorption will depend on the kidneys' ability to compensate for this internal shunt.

Preoperative Care

A thorough evaluation of the patient is essential. If urinary diversion is an elective procedure, any physiologic abnormalities should be corrected prior to surgery. The nutritional status and fluid and electrolyte balance should be as good as possible.

Previous administration of digitalis, antihypertensive agents, cortisone, insulin, or other potent drugs requires a presurgical treatment plan. Prophylactic antibiotic therapy is not necessary unless the patient harbors pathogenic organisms which cannot be eradicated before surgery. In the presence of a persistent urinary or other infection, the most suitable antibiotic based on sensitivity studies

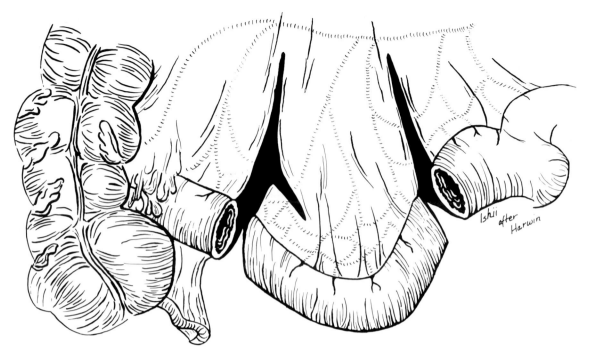

FIG. 49-1. Isolation of ileal segment. Note the additional incision parallel to the ileum and proximal to the vascular arcade. This will provide additional length to the mesentery, allowing it to span an obese abdominal wall.

and renal function is given before, during, and after surgical management.

Because of the long duration of some surgical procedures, especially if they are combined in one stage with cystectomy, every possible measure to avoid pulmonary complications should be taken. Wrapping the legs with elastic bandages and early ambulation are of value in the prevention of deep vein thrombosis, the most common source of pulmonary emboli. Patients with cardiopulmonary symptoms or decreased pulmonary or cardiac reserve may require special evaluation and preoperative preparation, such as training in the use of the respirator.

Before deciding to use segments of bowel, the surgeon needs pertinent information on the structural and functional integrity of the gastrointestinal tract. A history of regional ileitis, diverticulitis, polyps, malignancy, or functional disturbances must be evaluated. The prospective stoma site must be carefully selected with the patient in sitting, supine, and erect positions. Care should be taken to find a site free of scars, ridges, or deep infoldings of the panniculus. The intended appliance should be selected and worn preoperatively. Many appliances are available, and we prefer clear ileostomy bags. A number of adhesives are avail-

able, and several brands can be applied preoperatively to diagnose contact dermatitis. The development of a dermatitis at the site of the urinary stoma can cause considerable postoperative morbidity.

The intestinal tract may be prepared mechanically or mechanically in combination with antibiotics. We prefer to prepare the patient over a 3-day period immediately prior to surgery. A low-residue diet is instituted on the patient's admission to the hospital. Laxatives are employed only on the first day and enemas are kept to a minimum. No antibiotic preparation is necessary in newborn infants. For other patients, neomycin can be given orally the 3 days prior to surgery and oral administration of nystatin is added for children. Erythromycin base is added as indicated in Table 49-1. This preparation results in a relatively sterile bowel.[5] If more rapid bowel sterilization is necessary, neomycin can be given orally for 24 hr in the dosages prescribed in Table 49-2.

Ureteroileal Urinary Conduit

Ureteroileal urinary conduit, currently the most popular method for supravesical diversion, does not furnish a bladder substitute. The ileal segment

TABLE 49-1.   Bowel Preparation for Ileal Conduit Urinary Diversion

Day	Diet	Mechanical Preparation	Antibiotic*
1	Low residue	Castor oil, 0.5 ml/kg	Neomycin by mouth; nystatin†
2	Low residue	Saline enemas in evening	Neomycin by mouth; nystatin†
3	Liquid; intravenous fluids	Saline enemas in evening	Neomycin by mouth; nystatin†
4 (Surgery			Erythromycin base 1.0 g q 4 hr × 3

*See Table 49-2.
†Nystatin is optional.
Adapted from Cotlar AM, Cohn, I, Jr: Antimicrobial therapy for surgical gastrointestinal disease. In Kagan BM (ed): Antimicrobial Therapy, p 331. Philadelphia, WB Saunders, 1970

functions as a conduit to bridge the gap from ureter to skin. If cutaneous ureterostomy were always successful, there would be little need for the ileal conduit. The latter can be regarded as a distal ureteral substitute, useful because of its efficient blood supply, favorable location, maneuverability, and expendability. The previously selected stoma site should be marked prior to the abdominal incision, and a nasogastric tube is passed by the anesthesiologist.

If the urinary diversion is part of an exenteration, the ureters can be transected and left ligated throughout the excisional surgery, the surgeon completing the ureteroileostomy as the final step in the operation. While the ureters are ligated, they tend to dilate and become easier to handle. The construction of the ureteroileostomy at the onset of the procedure handicaps the excisional portion of the operation. If the patient's condition deteriorates during the exenteration, rapid ureterocutaneous or ureterosigmoid diversion can be performed.

After the excision is completed, the ureters are mobilized proximally, care being taken not to remove the adventitia which carries the blood supply from above. A devascularized ureter will result in leakage and disruption of the ureteroileal anastomosis or future stricture. An appendectomy is performed.

The terminal ileum is inspected and its mesentery examined by transillumination. The ileocolic artery is identified and avoided because ligation of this vessel may result in ischemia of the cecum and right colon. A site for distal transection of the ileum is selected approximately 10 cm proximal to

TABLE 49-2.   Antibiotic Bowel Preparation by Age

Age	Drug	Dose*
Neonate	Neomycin; nystatin	None; none
1 yr	Neomycin; nystatin	250 mg; 50,000 μ
1–3 yr	Neomycin; nystatin	333 mg; 100,000 μ
3–6 yr	Neomycin; nystatin	500 mg; 100,000 μ
6–15 yr	Neomycin; nystatin	1 g; 500,000 μ
Adult	Neomycin	1 g

*1 dose every 4 hr for 4 doses, then 1 dose every 6 hr until NPO for surgery.
Adapted from Cotlar AM, Cohn I, Jr: Antimicrobial therapy for surgical gastrointestinal disease. In Kagan BM (ed): Antimicrobial Therapy, p 331. Philadelphia, WB Saunders, 1970

the ileocecal junction (Fig. 49-1). The length of the ileal segment is determined by a rough measurement of the direct distance from the projected stomal site on the abdominal surface to the left side of the sacral promontory plus 3 cm to allow for variation in the route of the segment. If the segment is too long, it can be shortened at the close of the procedure. The segment, when finally constructed, should be neither under tension nor markedly redundant. The latter consideration is especially important in children, because the ileal conduit will grow with the child and provide a large absorptive surface and reservoir of infection.

The area of section is identified, the mesenteric surfaces are cleared of fat, and the blood vessels are ligated and divided over an area of 4 cm. The bowel is divided in the midportion of this area between clamps or occluding ligatures. The mes-

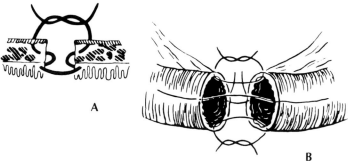

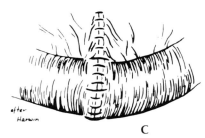

FIG. 49-2.   Technique for one-layer bowel anastomosis

FIG. 49-3.   Two methods of conjoined ureteral anastomosis. Any number of ureters can be sutured together prior to suturing their common lumen onto the butt of the ileal segment.

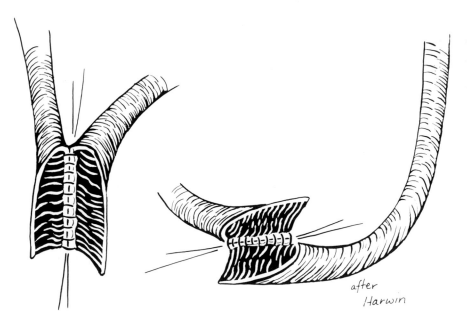

entery is incised at right angles to the bowel for a distance of 10 cm to 15 cm distally to allow the distal end of the segment to be brought through the abdominal wall and for 5 cm proximally to allow room to close the ileum or to suture the conjoined ureters onto the butt of the conduit. The mesenteric vessels are ligated with fine nonabsorbable sutures. Bowel continuity is reestablished with a one- or two-layer closure superior to the isolated conduit.

Open Anastomosis

The one-layer open anastomosis described by Gambee and modified by Hodges and associates is simple, rapid, and remarkably free of complications.[8,12] The ends of the ileum are apposed with vertical mattress sutures of 3-0 silk (Fig. 49-2). These sutures are placed in the four quadrants and engage 3 mm of the serosa and muscularis of either

segment and a thin portion of mucosa. The sutures are tied on the serosal side under sufficient tension to just bring the bowel ends into close approximation. The anastomosis is completed by placing interrupted sutures of the same material between each of the four quadrant sutures.

In the two-layer closure, the posterior bowel wall is approximated with interrupted seromuscular sutures of 3-0 silk. Full-thickness continuous sutures of 3-0 chromic catgut invert the mucosa on the posterior wall and are continued with a Connell stitch for the anterior wall and corners. Interrupted seromuscular silk sutures are then taken anteriorly to complete the second layer. The anastomotic lumen is checked at this point and should admit a single finger. The ileal mesentery is approximated with 3-0 chromic catgut sutures, making the ileoileal anastomosis superior to the isolated conduit.

Stapling devices for bowel anastomosis have become popular in recent years. In the hands of

FIG. 49-4. Technique of ureteroileal anastomosis and optional retroperitonealization of ureteroileal anastomosis. Note the smooth, left-to-right retroperitoneal course of the left ureter.

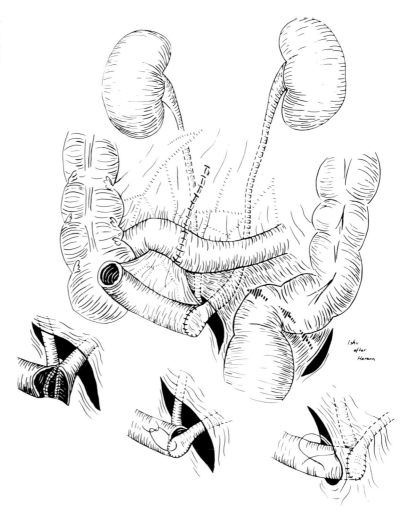

experienced surgeons, a reproducible, technically satisfactory procedure is accomplished smoothly and with significant reduction in operating time. The details are beyond the scope of this chapter but are well described by Bredael, Kramer, and Anderson.[2]

Attention is then redirected to the ureters. The left ureter is brought medially through a 6-cm incision in the mesosigmoid after being bluntly freed proximally to make its left-to-right course in a long smooth arc without kinking. The blood supply of the ureter at this point is from its medial surface, and dissection laterally will not devascularize it.

The ureters are laid side by side and are spatulated and joined on their posterior edges or by the "soixante neuf" technique (Fig. 49-3). The anastomosis is made with interrupted or running sutures of 4-0 chromic catgut or polygalactic or polyglycolic acid. Some surgeons employ a sec-

ond, external layer of interrupted sutures to reinforce the running suture line. The conjoined ureters are anastomosed to the butt of the ileal segment beginning with the posterior wall and using the same suture technique and material (Fig. 49-4). The proximal end of the conduit is retroperitonealized with catgut or synthetic absorbable seromuscular sutures.

The previously selected stoma site is identified. Care should be taken that the vertical opening through the skin, the fascia, the muscles, and the peritoneum is in a straight line; otherwise the abdominal layers which move independently may turn an initially clear passage into a shuttered defect, thus obstructing the conduit. It has been suggested that the ileal stoma be constructed through all thicknesses of the abdominal wall prior to making the initial skin incision. We prefer to put tension with Kocher clamps upon the edges of the fascia and peritoneum to approximate the midline

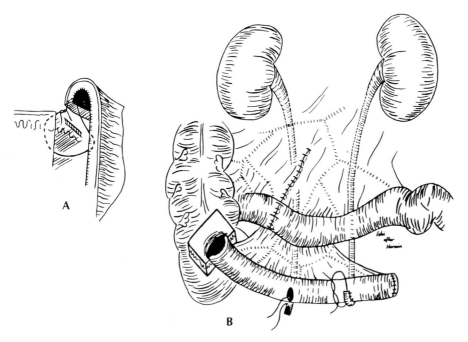

FIG. 49-5. Ileal conduit construction. **(A)** The 5-mm nipple at the ileal stoma employs buried absorbable sutures in its construction to prevent peristomal scars. **(B)** Modification of the ureteroileal conduit when prior pelvic irradiation has been used. The ureters are transected as high as possible and the conduit is brought to the ureters.

and then make a full-thickness defect 3.5 cm in diameter through the skin, the fascia, and the peritoneum, with all layers under tension.

On wound closure the layers will maintain their nonobstructing relationship. The ileum is brought up through this defect; its course should be quite straight from the sacral promontory through the hiatus in the anterior abdominal wall. Bringing the conduit through a two-finger split in the rectus muscle, rather than incising the muscle, will prevent peristomal herniation. Fine chromic sutures are placed between the ileum and surrounding peritoneum and posterior fascia. The distal end of the conduit is brought out and sutured to the cutis, producing a 5-mm nipple with buried, absorbable sutures (Fig. 49-5A). This provides an easy target for the appliance, has a lower incidence of stenosis than the flush stoma, and eliminates peristomal radical scars. It is not necessary to close the large opening between the right border of the conduit mesentery and the abdominal wall, because it is too large to cause a bowel obstruction.

The previous technique is modified if the patient has received prior curative radiotherapy. The ureters are mobilized as little and as high as possible to use minimally irradiated ureters with the best possible blood supply.[11] The intestinal conduit butt is closed with an inverted running 3-0 chromic catgut suture reinforced with seromuscular stitches (Fig. 49-5B). The ureters are spatulated on their anterior surfaces for 2 cm, and the intestinal conduit is then brought to the spatulated ureters, which are sutured to the antimesenteric side of the conduit with interrupted 4-0 absorbable sutures, placing the apical suture first. The remainder of the procedure is the same as that described for the conjoined ureterointestinal conduit except abdominal wall retention sutures are routinely used.

A temporary collecting device is applied in the operating room. No catheter is inserted into the ileum, and no ureteral stents are necessary. Nasogastric suction is applied.

Ureterojejunal Urinary Conduit

The jejunum may be substituted for the ileum as a conduit if the ileum has been heavily irradiated or if postdiversion radiation is planned. The operative technique is essentially similar to that described for using the ileum. However, the description by Golimbu and Morales in 1975 of a syndrome characterized by hypochloremic acidosis, hyperkalemia, hyponatremia, and uremia when jejunal segments were used has resulted in diminished interest.[10] Reduced renal function, a long conduit, or salt depletion increases the problem; salt dietary supplements are indicated for patients who undergo jejunal diversion.

Postoperative Care

The extent of bowel trauma determines the duration of postoperative ileus. The use of nasogastric tube and avoiding early oral feedings will usually

TABLE 49-3. Ileal Conduit Follow-Up

Date	Stoma check	Urine pH	Urine C & S	BUN	Electrolytes	IVP	Loopogram
1 wk	X	X	X	X	X		
1 mo	X	X	X	X	X		
3 mo	X	X	X	X	X	X	prn
6 mo	X	X	X	X	X	X	prn
9 mo	X	X	X	X	X		prn
1 yr	X	X	X	X	X	X	prn
Annually	X	X	X	X	X	X	prn

BUN = blood urea nitrogen; IVP = intravenous pyelogram; prn = according to need

prevent significant distention. If the bowel is kept at rest, peristalsis and function will resume in 3 to 5 days. If bowel function does not return within 1 week, an underlying cause of irritation such as hematoma, infection, or urinary or fecal leakage must be suspected. A fecal fistula usually closes spontaneously if the patient's nutritional needs can be met. Hyperalimentation may be necessary.[13] Urinary anostomotic leakage usually seals within 8 days; persistent leakage beyond 2 weeks requires excretory urography and retrograde "loopograms" to determine the site of urinary drainage, followed by surgical repair. Fluid and electrolyte disorders are not encountered if accurate balance and replacement are observed.

An important aspect of the operation is the proper care and management of the stoma and the urinary collection device.[4] Often the stoma will shrink, requiring new disks at 1, 3, and 12 months. A leaking device and excoriated skin make for a miserable patient. Stenosis of the stoma may require dilatation or surgical revision.[6]

Renal function and structure must be checked regularly throughout the life of the patient (Table 49-3). Some mild hydronephrosis is expected during the first year.

REFERENCES

1. ALBERT DJ, PERSKY L: Conjoined end-to-side uretero-intestinal anastomosis. J Urol 105:201, 1971
2. BREDAEL JJ, KRAMER SA, ANDERSON EE: Ileal loop urinary diversion by the auto suture stapling technique. Brochure, US Surgical Corp, 1980
3. BRICKER EM: Bladder substitution after pelvic evisceration. Surg Clin North Am 30:1511, 1950
4. BROOKE BN: The management of an ileostomy including its complications. Lancet 2:102, 1952
5. COTLAR AM, COHN I, JR: Antimicrobial therapy for surgical gastrointestinal disease. In: Kagan BM (ed), Antimicrobial Therapy, p 331. Philadelphia, W B Saunders, 1970
6. DERRICK WA, JR, HODGES CV: Ileal conduit stasis: Recognition, treatment and prevention. J Urol 107:747, 1972
7. EISEMAN B, BRICKER EM: Electrolyte absorption following bilateral ureteroenterostomy into an isolated intestinal segment. Ann Surg 136:761, 1952
8. GAMBEE LP: A single-layer open intestinal anastomosis applicable to the small as well as the large intestine. Western Journal Surgery, Obstetrics and Gynecology 59:1, 1951
9. GIESY JD, LEHMAN TH, MOORE, RJ et al: Urinary diversion for bladder dysfunction in children. J Urol 93:46, 1965
10. GOLIMBU M, MORALES P: Jejunal conduits: Technique and complications. J Urol 113:787, 1975
11. HECKER GN, HODGES CV, MOORE RJ et al: Radical cystectomy after supervoltage radiotherapy. J Urol 91:256, 1964
12. HODGES CV, LEHMAN TH, MOORE RJ et al: Use of ileal segments in urology. J Urol 85:573, 1961
13. MACFADYEN BV, JR, DUDRICK SJ, RUBERT RL: Management of gastrointestinal fistulas with parenteral hyperalimentation. Surgery 74:100, 1973
14. NESBIT RM: Ureterosigmoid anastomosis by direct elliptical connection: A preliminary report. J Urol 61:728, 1949
15. TIZZONI A, FOGGI P: Die Wiederherstellung der Harnblase; Experimentelle Untersuchungen. Zentralbl Chir 15:921, 1888
16. VISSCHER MB, VARCO RL, CARR CW et al: Sodium ion movement between the intestinal lumen and the blood. Am J Physiol 141:488, 1944
17. WALLACE DM: Ureteric diversion using a conduit: A simplified technique. Br J Urol 38:522, 1966

Sigmoid Conduit

50

Earl Haltiwanger

Although the practice of diversion of urine into the intestinal tract is well accepted, there is no standard procedure. The type of operation chosen can be influenced by the location and nature of the underlying abnormality, the availability of suitable segments of intestinal tract, the general condition of the patient, and the life expectancy. Currently, the use of bowel as a conduit is more popular than diversion into the intact functioning bowel.

A major advantage in choosing the colon over the small bowel is that this permits an antireflux ureterointestinal anastomosis.[1,3,5] As experience with long-term follow-up of patients with ileal conduits has accumulated, there has been observed a disturbing trend toward upper tract deterioration, particularly in the presence of infected urine. There is evidence implicating reflux in the etiology of this undesirable change.[10,11] Another advantage of the larger stoma of the colon conduit is the fewer postoperative complications than with the stoma of the ileum.[4,8,9] The decreased incidence of stricture of the ureterointestinal anastomosis reported in the early experience of colon conduits has not been borne out by longer-term observations. Like the ileal loop, the colon conduit is not usually associated with the electrolyte abnormalities sometimes found with ureterosigmoidostomy in the intact colon.

A sigmoid conduit should not be created in a patient with a history of diverticulitis or ulcerative colitis. This operation is also not advised in the face of radical cystectomy and irradiation for carcinoma of the bladder, because of the risk of poor healing secondary to altered blood supply to the rectum and the sigmoid colon. The presence of hydroureter precludes the nonrefluxing anastomosis unless ureteral tapering is done. This tapering increases the risk of complication, particularly in the adult.

Preoperative preparation of the colon is done, as for any open large bowel surgery, with low-residue diet and oral administration of antibiotics such as neomycin and erythromycin base. A stoma site is selected and marked prior to operation and is usually placed in the upper section of the left lower quadrant. Care should be taken to ensure the presence of an area of smooth skin to which a collection appliance may be sealed.

The patient is placed in the supine position and a midline incision is made from the umbilicus to the symphysis pubis. An appendectomy is performed at this time. A 15-cm to 20-cm portion of the sigmoid colon is selected to be the conduit and should have its blood supply based on the inferior mesenteric artery. An effort should be made to select a segment that may be positioned in an isoperistaltic position (Fig. 50-1), although this is not essential. The sigmoid colon is mobilized from its lateral and posterior attachments as required. It may be necessary to free the sigmoid medially to the sacral promontory and cephalad to the inferior mesenteric artery. The splenic flexure may be released if needed for additional mobility. With adequate freeing of the sigmoid mesentery it is possible to rotate this segment a full 180 degrees if desired. After the loop has been selected and marked, it is isolated by division of the bowel and incision of the mesentery. In incising the lower border of the mesentery leaf, the superior hemorrhoidal branch of the inferior mesenteric artery is often divided. This will give increased mobility to the distal end of the loop and can be done safely because of the rich blood supply to the rectum and the lower sigmoid. The colon is restored medial to the new conduit with a standard two-layer closure. The proximal end of the sigmoid segment is closed with two layers of absorbable suture.

The ureters are now mobilized and detached from the bladder. The right ureter usually can be seen through the retroperitoneum as it crosses the iliac artery. The retroperitoneum is incised over the ureter to allow mobilization to the bladder. The ureter is detached as close to the bladder as possible to allow adequate room to pass it beneath the newly anastomosed colon and into the conduit. Any excess ureter is resected at the time of implantation. In the case of children in whom undiv-

509

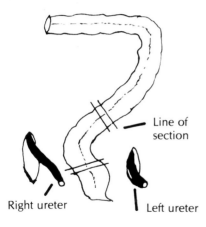

Line of section

Right ureter   Left ureter

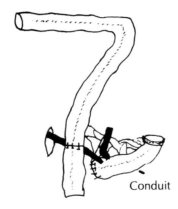

Conduit

FIG. 50-1. Technique of sigmoid conduit. The redundant portion of the sigmoid is selected and placed in an isoperistaltic position with the ureters anastomosed near the closed end.

ersion is a later consideration, this technique must be modified so that no ureter is discarded. The left ureter frequently can be seen during the mobilization of the sigmoid mesentery. It is mobilized and divided in the same manner as the right side.

Tunnels are created with two staggered 4-cm linear incisions in the taenia near the proximal end of the conduit. The areas of the incisions first are infiltrated with 1:200,000 epinephrine to facilitate dissection and to suppress oozing. The incision for the right ureter is made near the right side of the taenia and near the closed end of the conduit. It is made down completely through the muscle but with care being taken not to puncture the mucosa. With the aid of the previously mentioned infiltration, the mucosa can be freed from the muscularis of the bowel with ease.[6] This dissection is made lateral from the taenia and is extensive enough to allow the ureter to lie freely in the tunnel without undue compression. The ureter and the loop are measured in their final positions before the excess ureter is resected. The end of the ureter may be beveled or splayed to present a larger orifice for the anastomosis. The ureter is laid in the tunnel in the technique of Leadbetter[7] and anastomosed to a small mucosal incision in the distal end of the tunnel with 4-0 absorbable sutures. The tunnel is closed over the ureter with interrupted black silk. Optional stents may be used for 10 days but are not necessary. The other ureter is sewn into the conduit in the same fashion through the left side of the taenia in a more distal position.

The proximal end of the conduit is anchored to the posterior body wall, usually the psoas muscle. One may place retroperitoneal flaps over this if desired. A retroperitoneal drain is optional.[2] The distal end of the conduit is brought through the abdominal wall in the preselected ostomy site with excision of a circle of fascia. The everted stoma is created in the usual fashion. The abdomen is closed, and a collection bag is attached to the stoma.

REFERENCES

1. ALTHAUSEN AF, HAGEN–COOK K, HENDREN WH, III: Non-refluxing colon conduit; Experience with 70 cases. J Urol 120:35, 1978
2. BAGLEY DH, GLAZIER W, OSIAS M et al: Retroperitoneal drainage of uretero-intestinal conduits. J Urol 121:271, 1979
3. DAGEN JE, SANFORD EJ, ROHNER TJ, JR: Complications of the non-refluxing colon conduit. J Urol 123:585, 1980
4. ELDER DD, MOISEY CU, REES RW: A long-term follow-up of the colonic conduit operation in children. Brit J Urol 51:462, 1979
5. HENDREN WH: Nonrefluxing colon conduit for temporary or permanent urinary diversion in children. J Pediatr Surg 10:381, 1975
6. JACOBS JA, YOUNG JD, JR: The Strickler technique of ureterosigmoidostomy. J Urol 124:451, 1980
7. LEADBETTER WF, CLARKE BG: Five years' experience with uretero-enterostomy by the 'combined' technique. J Urol 73:67, 1954
8. MOGG RA: The result of urinary diversion using the colonic conduit. Br J Urol 97:684, 1967
9. MOGG RA, SYME RRA: The result of urinary diversion using the colonic conduit. Br J Urol 41:434, 1969
10. PAGANO F: Ureterocolic anastomosis: description of a technique. J Urol 123:355, 1980
11. RICHIE JP: Nonrefluxing sigmoid conduit for urinary diversion. Urol Clin North Am 6:469, 1979

Ureterosigmoidostomy

51

Sam S. Ambrose

When functioning normally, the urinary transit system is an unappreciated mechanism that affords optimal protection for the kidneys and simultaneously frees man for sustained social encounters unencumbered by urinary odor and moisture. A satisfactory substitute for this transit system has not been devised. A decision to divert the urinary output to an alternative system must be supported by compelling circumstances. Those circumstances include surgical removal of the bladder, irreparable congenital malformations of the bladder and urethra, and irreparable bladder or bladder outlet dysfunction that jeopardizes kidney function or the general health or social activity of the patient.

If permanent urinary diversion becomes necessary, the wide variety of alternative methods must be fully understood and considered by the responsible urologic surgeon. The advantages, the disadvantages, and the capability to provide a successful procedure must be objectively considered by the surgeon before recommending a particular form of diversion to a patient or guardian. The patient and family should be fully informed and understand the necessity of the diversion. They must understand the advantages and disadvantages of alternative procedures, and their expectations for their future course must be realistic.

When a decision for diversion is final, every effort must be made to have the patient in optimal condition for a successful procedure. The surgical application must be well planned and meticulously executed; few surgical disasters exceed those resulting from poorly conceived or executed urinary diversions.

The purpose of this chapter is not to outline and discuss the relative merits of all the various methods of urinary diversions but to present ureterosigmoidostomy as one of the alternatives.

History

Reports for the past 130 years by surgeons of their efforts to provide a satisfactory urinary diversion are remarkable testimony to their ingenuity, craftsmanship, and tenacity. Techniques tried include formation of a fistulous tract between the ureter and the colon, direct anastomosis of the ureter to the bowel, use of the muscularizing principle, transplantation of the trigone or ureteral orifice, ureteral anastomosis to an excluded portion of the bowel, use of the submucosal tunnel and the combined technique, and use of intracolonic nipple (Fig. 51-1).

The principle of a delayed ureterocolonic fistula was used in the hope of avoiding peritonitis, local infection and leakage at the anastomosis, and acute pyelonephritis—the most frequent complications during the preantibiotic era. The earliest planned ureterocolonic anastomosis used this principle and was performed by Simon in 1851.[44] Subsequent efforts to use and improve this technique were reported by Lloyd (1851), Kirwin (1930), Coffey (1930), Hinman (1936), and Jewett (1940).[7,20,23,49] Frequent obstruction at the anastomosis has prevented general acceptance.

Hope of reducing the incidence and degree of postoperative obstruction at the ureterocolonic junction prompted attempts at direct ureterocolonic anastomosis. The major contributions to this technique include those of Smith (1878), Chaput (1892), Peterson (1900), Nesbit (1949), and Cordonnier (1950).[9,20,23,36,49] Persistent coloureteral reflux, infection, and anastomotic leakage were the deterrents to general use.

The muscularizing principle was initially used to reduce the chance of urinary leakage at the ureterocolonic anastomosis. Later it was recognized that the potential for reflux had been reduced. Those who contributed to this development were Bardenheuer (1886), Martin (1899), Stiles (1907), and Thompson (1973).[20,23,49] Ureteral obstruction in the long tunnel was the principal complication.

Exstrophy of the bladder provided the ideal model for the technically simple extraperitoneal approach of transplantation of the trigone or the ureteral orifice. Maydl[33] first used this principle in

1894 and was followed by Bergenhem[3] in 1895. The technique is appealing but reflux is a common complication.

Ascending urinary sepsis was recognized early as a major complication of ureterocolonic anasto-

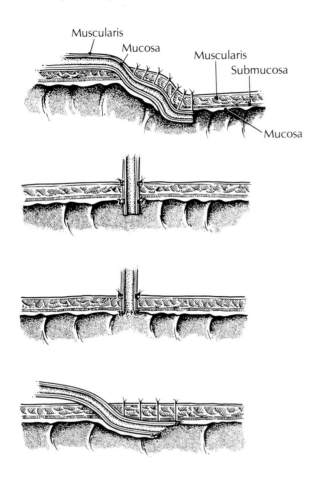

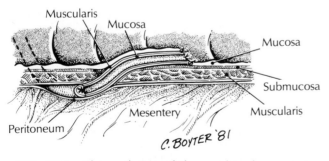

FIG. 51-1. The evolution of the combined mucosa-to-mucosa anastomosis with a submucosal tunnel is illustrated sequentially and demonstrates that the transcolonic procedure incorporates the combined principle. The procedures shown are **(A)** Coffey No. 1, **(B)** direct, **(C)** Cordonnier, **(D)** combined, and **(E)** transcolonic.

mosis and was attributed to the fecal stream. Efforts to remove the ureter from the fecal stream resulted in many innovative surgical procedures. Mauclaire (1894), Gersuny (1898), Kronig (1906), Verhoogen (1908), Heitz–Boyer (1912), Hovelacque (1912), and Lemoine (1913) were the first to use excluded bowel segments for urinary diversion.[16,20,22,23,32,49] Recent trials of the Gersuny and Heitz–Boyer techniques met some success but fecal or urinary incontinence has been the chief deterrent to wide application of the procedures.

Quite early in the development of ureterosigmoidostomy, the passage of the ureter through a colonic submucosal tunnel was perceived as possibly the most effective way to simultaneously reduce anastomotic leakage and also prevent ureteral reflux. The submucosal tunnel is now the basic principle of the most frequently used techniques of ureterocolonic anastomosis. Those surgeons who contributed most to the general adoption of this technique were Kryrnski (1896), Coffey (1910), Mayo (1912), Leadbetter (1955), Weyrauch (1952), Gallo (1951), Goodwin (1953), and Strickler (1965).[7,15,19,20,23,27,49,50] The unique contribution of Gallo and Goodwin was the demonstration that a transcolonic approach to the ureterocolonic anastomosis was feasible. The addition of the spatulated, direct mucosa-to-mucosa anastomosis to the submucosal tunnel (the combined technique) has resulted in our current lower incidence of postoperative obstruction, leakage, reflux, and infection.

Mathieson[31] in 1953 described the formation of an intracolonic nipple that provided good protection against reflux. Clinical trials have produced results comparable to the combined technique.

Contraindications

Contraindications to ureterosigmoidostomy relate to life expectancy, general physical condition of the patient, renal function and the presence of calculi or pyelonephritis, liver function, ureteral dilation, primary colon disease, anal sphincter ability, radiation therapy, and psychologic stability.

Those patients with a poor prognosis for survival should be considered for a simpler form of temporary urinary diversion. Debilitating disease of such severity that wound healing and resistance to infection are significantly impaired is also a relative contraindication to ureterosigmoidostomy. Neurologic impairment that demands excessive nursing attention for frequent bowel elimination may justify consideration of another form of diversion. Fecal incontinence is an absolute contraindication to ureterosigmoidostomy.

Patients with moderate to severe impairment of renal function are not satisfactory candidates, because postoperative obstruction or infection may rapidly compromise their remaining renal reserve. Additionally, they are more susceptible to hyperchloremic acidosis. The presence of renal calculi or active pyelonephritis is, unless corrected, also a contraindication to ureterosigmoidostomy.

Encephalopathy due to hyperammonemia has been reported in patients with cirrhosis of the liver and ureterosigmoid diversions. Recent studies in rats with ureterocolostomies revealed chronic hyperammonemia in the absence of liver damage. This condition was attributed to hepatic overloading by an increased portal ammonia supply caused by intestinal absorption of urinary ammonia and increased intestinal ammoniagenesis induced by hydrolysis of urinary and circulating urea.

Anastomosis of a severely dilated ureter to the colon increases the risk of reflux and pyelonephritis and should be avoided. Urinary diversion to the colon in patients with colon carcinoma, diverticulosis, or colitis should also be avoided. Preoperative evaluation should include barium enema and proctosigmoidoscopy.

Patients with incontinence of liquid feces are not candidates for ureterosigmoidostomy. Particular care must be taken in evaluating the anal sphincter of patients with any neurologic deficit, history of anal surgery, and exstrophy of the bladder with colon prolapse. All should be tested for their ability to retain 300 ml to 400 ml of normal saline.

Radiation therapy doses in excess of 5000 rads to the pelvis are associated with a higher incidence of complications.

Some patients are psychologically unable to cope with a state of mild, chronic diarrhea, occasional nocturnal soiling, and inability to release flatus except at stool. Their attitudes need to be assessed in time to avoid what may become an intolerable burden.

Preoperative Patient Preparation

The nutritional, pulmonary, renal, urinary, electrolyte, and hemodynamic status should be brought to the best possible level preoperatively. When bacteriuria is present, reliable bacterial identification and sensitivity to antibacterials must be determined preoperatively so that precise and adequate antibacterial coverage can be started 24 hr prior to surgery and maintained intra- and postoperatively.

Adequate bowel preparation can be achieved in 24 hr with mechanical cleansing (enemas) and neomycin sulfate given orally 1 g/hr for four doses and then 1 g/4 hr for a total of 7 g, accompanied by 80 mg of gentamicin intramuscularly 2 hr prior to surgery. When time allows, a more optimal program, which I prefer, includes 72 hr of a clear-liquid or low-residue diet, a laxative on the first day, and a cleansing enema each of the 3 nights prior to surgery. This not only provides a mechanically clean bowel for surgery but also reduces the fecal load during the early postoperative period.

To reduce the incidence of postoperative venous thrombosis and embolus, full-length stockings should be used during surgery and through the entire postoperative stay.

Procedure

The combined procedure includes a submucosal ureteral segment, direct anastomosis of the spatulated ureter to the bowel mucosa, and extraperitonealization of the anastomotic site, which isolates the anastomosis from the peritoneal cavity and affords anatomic fixation and stability for the anastomotic site. A large (28Fr–30Fr) rectal tube with multiple drainage holes is inserted to the rectal ampulla immediately before surgery and secured in position by suture or tape to the perianal skin. The tube provides drainage of urine, flatus, and liquid feces. It usually effectively decompresses the colon during surgery and the critical, early phase of healing of the ureterocolonic anastomosis and provides continuous monitoring of urinary flow. The catheter may be safely removed when normal peristalsis returns and there is no evidence of an anastomotic leak.

With the patient supine and in a slight Trendelenburg position, adequate exposure is obtained through a midline, suprapubic incision carried a few centimeters above the umbilicus. The peritoneal cavity and contents are explored, any restricting adhesions are taken down, both ureters are identified at the pelvic brim, and the sigmoid colon is carefully examined. Ideally, the ureteral anastomosis should be low in the sigmoid colon approaching the rectosigmoid junction. It must be achieved without tension on the ureter and the sigmoid must be positioned against the posterior pelvic wall so that its course and the ureteral course are unobstructed and as natural as possible. The mobility of the sigmoid should be determined prior to incising the peritoneum over the ureters, because

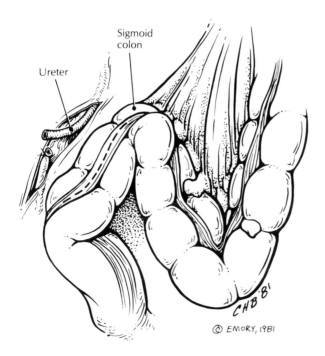

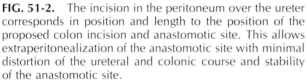

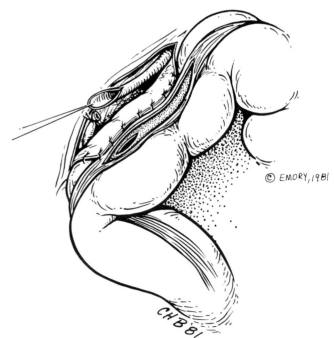

FIG. 51-2. The incision in the peritoneum over the ureter corresponds in position and length to the position of the proposed colon incision and anastomotic site. This allows extraperitonealization of the anastomotic site with minimal distortion of the ureteral and colonic course and stability of the anastomotic site.

FIG. 51-3. The ureter is trimmed to the appropriate length and spatulated. The longitudinal colon incision is carried down to the submucosa, and a small plug of mucosa is removed at the distal extremity of the colon incision. The colon mucosa should be elevated from the muscularis sufficiently to provide room for the ureter in its ultimate submucosal position. Note that the medial peritoneal reflection has been sutured to the adjacent colon wall parallel to the colon incision.

the edges of the incised peritoneum will be sewn to the colon. The medial edge of the incised peritoneum will be approximated to the posterolateral wall of the colon prior to the ureteral anastomosis. The lateral peritoneal edge will be approximated to the anteromedial colonic wall after completion of the ureteral anastomosis. This extraperitonealizes the anastomotic site and provides essential stability for the anastomosis without restricting colonic or ureteral function.

If the full length of ureter is available bilaterally, the left anastomosis is performed quite low by rotating the anterior bowel wall posterolaterally. The right ureteral anastomosis is done at a slightly higher level by rotating the anterior colon wall to the right posterolateral peritoneal incision.

If the ureteral length is limited to the pelvic brim or slightly below, bowel positioning usually dictates that the right anastomosis be at the lowest level.

When the final position of the anastomosis has been determined, the peritoneum is incised longitudinally over each ureter (Fig. 51-2), and the ureters are freed proximally with care to protect the adventitia and the longitudinal blood supply.

The vessels supplying these longitudinal ureteral vessels are lateral to the ureter below the pelvic brim and medial above the pelvic brim, and if necessary for ureteral mobility they are divided and ligated or clipped. The ureters are divided as near the bladder as possible and the distal stumps are either tied off with 1-0 chromic catgut or clipped. I prefer large clips on both cut ends with the proxmal clip left in place until the time of actual anastomosis, when the ureter is trimmed to appropriate length and spatulated. Leaving the ureter obstructed until the anastomosis prevents the constant flow of urine into the operative site and results in ureteral diltation, which facilitates the anastomosis.

The most appropriate site in the bowel wall is selected for each anastomosis, and the medial peritoneal reflection is sutured with interrupted 3-0 absorbable sutures to the posterolateral surface of the bowel posterior to the site of the ureterocolonic anastomosis. A longitudinal 5-cm incision is made in the bowel wall through the tenia or

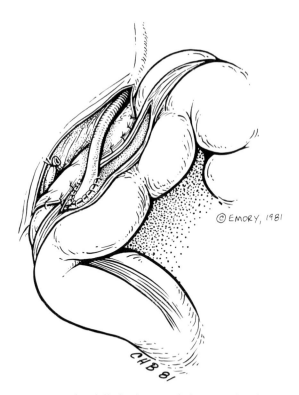

FIG. 51-4. The full thickness of the spatulated ureteral wall is sutured to the full thickness of the colon mucosa and submucosa. I prefer a running lockstitch of 5-0 absorbable material interrupted at each extremity of the spatulated orifice.

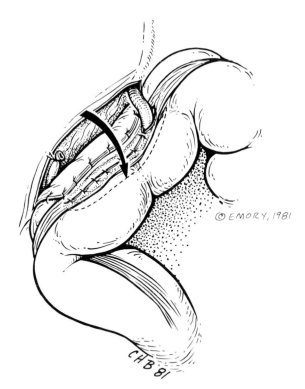

FIG. 51-5. The colon muscularis and visceral peritoneum are approximated over the distal ureter with interrupted 3-0 absorbable sutures. The ureteral hiatus should be at least twice the diameter of the ureter. Note that the lateral posterior parietal peritoneum is sutured to the colon wall to the left of the colotomy, effectively rotating the anastomotic site to the normal course of the ureter, extraperitonealizing the anastomotic site, and providing stability for the site.

immediately lateral to the tenia and is carried down to the submucosa, which is freed for 0.5 cm on each side from the overlying muscularis. The ureter is trimmed to appropriate length and spatulated, and a small (0.5 cm) plug of colon submucosa and mucosa is sharply removed at the distal extremity of the colon incision (Fig. 5l-3). The full thickness of spatulated ureteral wall is approximated to the colon submucosa and mucosa with two running, interlocking absorbable 5-0 sutures (Fig. 51-4). This should produce a watertight, unobstructed ureterocolonic junction. The distal ureter is covered by approximating the colon muscularis with interrupted 3-0 absorbable sutures, allowing the ureter to emerge from the colon wall at the superior angle of the colon incision (Fig. 51-5). A 3-cm to 5-cm submucosal ureteral segment is formed by this colon closure and should be sufficient to prevent reflux. If obstruction of the ureter is to be avoided where the ureter emerges from the bowel wall at the superior angle of the incision, the hiatus should be approximately twice the diameter of the ureter. The lateral edge of the peritoneum is pulled over the ureterocolonic anastomosis and is approxi-

mated to the colon wall with interrupted 3-0 absorbable sutures (Fig. 51-6). The anastomosis is extraperitoneal in position and the bowel wall is fixed in position, providing needed stability for the anastomosis during the critical early phase of healing.

The same procedure is performed on the opposite side.

The small bowel and omentum are returned to their normal position and the abdominal wall is closed without drains (Fig. 51-7).

Postoperative Complications

The early complications of ureterosigmoidostomy include infection, urinary leakage at the anastomosis, ureteral obstruction, and ileus. Infection that does not respond to appropriate and intensive antibacterial therapy is often secondary to urinary leakage or obstruction and will require local drain-

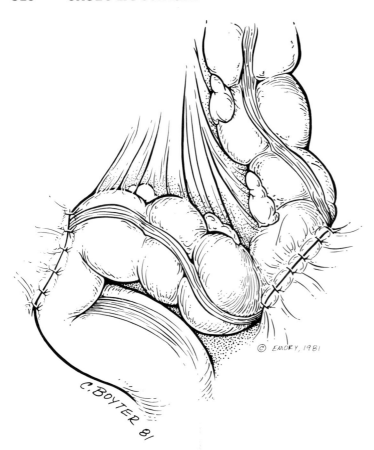

FIG. 51-6. The completed bilateral anastomosis is shown and demonstrates the anastomotic positions when ureteral length dictates a high anastomosis. Note that the course of the rectosigmoid is relatively normal.

age, correction of the leakage or obstruction, or proximal temporary diversion. If the infection can be controlled with antibacterials, patience may be rewarded with spontaneous closure of the leak or resolution of temporary obstruction at the anastomosis. Renal isotope scanning is reliable in evaluating obstruction and may reveal leakage if present in significant volume. If leakage or obstruction persists without infection, surgical correction will be necessary. Simple revision of the anastomosis may be feasible, but reanastomosis, ureteroureterostomy, conversion to ileal conduit, or nephrostomy may be indicated.

Late complications attributable to ureterosigmoidostomy include hyperchloremic acidosis, potassium and magnesium deficit, ammonia encephalopathy, ureteral obstruction, pyelonephritis, urinary calculi, and colonic tumors at the anastomosis.

Acidosis secondary to hyperchloremia produced by selective reabsorption of chloride will occur in the majority of cases and is caused or aggravated by excessive exposure of urine to the colonic mucosa. This may be controlled when mild by

more frequent bowel evacuation or by a rectal tube during sleep. Oral sodium bicarbonate or citrate is effective in controlling hyperchloremia and acidosis and may be required if more frequent bowel evacuation does not resolve the acidosis.

Potassium and magnesium deficiency may reach severe, symptomatic levels in patients with diarrhea or persistent acidosis. A high index of suspicion and determination of blood levels are necessary for their detection; and when found, the treatment is appropriate replacement by parenteral or oral means.

Encephalopathy due to hyperammonemia has been reported in patients with cirrhosis of the liver and ureterosigmoidostomies and in rare individuals without cirrhosis. The hyperammonemia is attributed to hepatic overloading by high ammonia levels in the portal return from the colon caused by absorption of urinary ammonia and ammonia produced by intracolonic bacterial hydrolysis of urea. If hyperammonemia is encountered, it is best controlled by reducing urinary pooling time in the colon.

Late ureteral obstruction (usually at the anas-

FIG. 51-7. The transcolonic procedure is accomplished through an anterior longitudinal colotomy with minimal disturbance of the normal course of the ureters or bowel. This procedure facilitates a very low anastomosis in the rectal ampulla or lower sigmoid, the most desirable level for ureterocolonic diversion. The entire completed anastomosis is extraperitoneal, with a combined spatulated mucosa-to-mucosa anastomosis and a submucosal segment of adequate length. The lower sigmoid and ampulla are relatively fixed in position, providing stability for the anastomotic site.

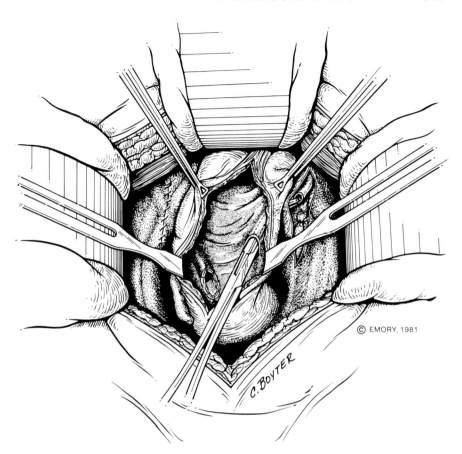

© EMORY, 1981

C. BOYTER

tomosis) occurs in 10% to 30% of cases, and if severe, may require reoperation with reanastomosis, transureteroureterostomy, or an alternate form of diversion.

Acute pyelonephritis is usually related to an underlying complication such as obstruction, reflux, or stones. Episodes will usually respond to antibacterial therapy but do rarely require temporary external diversion. Suppressive antibacterial therapy can be used, but if pyelonephritis persists, the cause must be corrected. If pyelonephritis cannot be controlled, reoperation with an alternative form of diversion is advisable.

Renal calculi are reported in 8% to 18% of cases with long-term follow-up. They are probably secondary to chronic infection, stasis, reflux of colonic material that may act as a nidus, or hypercalciuria in patients whose bones are demineralizing from immobility or persistent acidosis.

Intracolonic tumors at the anastomosis are now a well-recognized late complication of ureterosigmoidostomy and have been reported to occur from 5 to 50 years after surgery. The true incidence is unknown, but it has been estimated to be from 100 to 500 times that of normal contemporaries. The median age at detection of reported cases is 33 years. The type of neoplasm encountered in the majority of cases has been colonic adenocarcinoma, with benign colon neoplasms and transitional cell carcinomas occurring less frequently. The cause of these neoplasms is unknown, but the intriguing studies of Gittes suggest that the presence of combined urine and feces is essential for the carcinogenic effect of ureterosigmoidostomy.

It is now clear that careful regular follow-up of these patients is essential and should include annual sigmoidoscopy or barium enema. Any blood in their stools should alert the patient to return for earlier evaluation.

Conclusions

In view of the significant complications that may occur following ureterosigmoidostomy, are we justified in the continued use of this form of diversion as an alternative to the more frequently used ileal conduit? Are the complications of ureterosigmoidostomy of sufficient magnitude to preclude an

TABLE 51-1. Comparison of Ureterosigmoidostomy and Ileal Conduit Results

	Uretersigmoidostomy		Ileal Conduit		
	Series 1	Series 2	Series 3	Series 4	
		Total—Group B 1954–1963			
Number of patients	37	94	34	90	96
Follow-up (yr)	6.5–52	5–35	5–18	10–16	2–16
Median	28 > 10	18		11	8
Mortality (%)					
Operative	0	2.1	0	4.4	3.1
Total	11	13	3	16	10
Complications requiring secondary surgery (%)	32	66	24	87	76
Satisfactory pyelograms during follow-up (%)	50	47	74	71	67
Free of clinically apparent pyelonephritis (%)	54		82	83	93
Urinary calculi (%)	18	19	3	16	13
Required other forms of diversion (%)	8	13	5	9	0
Undiversion (%)				11	

Data from Series 1—Spence HM, Hoffman WW: Exstrophy of the Urinary bladder treated by ureterosigmoidostomy: Long-term follow-up in a series of 37 cases. Birth Defects: Original Article Series 13, No. 5:185–192, 1977; Series 2—Bennett AH: Exstrophy of bladder treated by ureterosigmoidostomies. Long-term evaluation. Urology 2, No. 2:165–168, 1973; Series 3—Shapiro SR, Lebowitz R, Colodny AH: Fate of 90 children with ileal conduit urinary diversion a decade later: Analysis of complications, pyelography, renal function and bacteriology. J Urol 114:289, 1975; Series 4—Schwarz GR, Jeffs RD: Ileal conduit urinary diversion in children: Computer analysis of follow-up from 2 to 16 years. J Urol 114:285, 1975

effort to provide patients with the obvious advantages of the procedure—no abdominal stoma, reduced operative time and trauma, urinary continence, and a relatively undisturbed small bowel? These questions are currently best evaluated in the light of available data on long-term results in similar patient patient groups with nonmalignant disease. The questions could be answered with more confidence if long-term data were available on a series of ileal conduits performed on patients with nonmalignant disease and essentially normal urinary tracts at the time of diversion.

Table 51-1 records the results of ileal conduit and ureterosigmoidostomy in four groups of patients of similar age whose primary disease was nonmalignant. The results are remarkably similar for both forms of diversion and again emphasize the fact that a totally satisfactory form of diversion is not available. No clear advantage as to complications is apparent for either procedure. Certainly, there is no compelling evidence that patients who are suitable candidates for ureterosigmoidostomy should arbitrarily be denied an opportunity for life with urinary continence and freedom from an abdominal appliance. Ureterosigmoidostomy, meticulously provided to an appropriate patient and carefully monitored for life, should remain a desirable alternative to other forms of urinary diversion.

REFERENCES AND SUGGESTED READING

1. AMBROSE SS, PUPPEL AD: Use of anal sphincter to sustain fecal and urinary control in neovesical formation (abstract). Surgery 30:274, 1951
2. BENNETT AH: Exstrophy of bladder treated by ureterosigmoidostomies. Long-term evaluation. Urology. 2:165, 1973
3. BERGENHEM B: Ectopia vesicae et adenoma destruens vesicae: exstirpation af blasan; implantation of ureterena i rectum. Eira 19:268, 1895
4. BOYCE WH: The absorption of certain constitutents of

urine from large bowel of the experimental animal (dog). J Urol 65:241, 1951

5. BRICKER EM: Current status of urinary diversion. Cancer 45:2986, 1980

6. COFFEY RC: Physiologic implantation of the severed ureter or common bile-duct into the intestine. JAMA 56:397, 1911

7. COFFEY RC: Production of aseptic ureteroenterostomy. JAMA 94:1748, 1930

8. CORBETT CRR, LLOYD–DAVIES RW: Long-term survival after urinary diversion: A reappraisal of ureterosigmoidostomy. Eur Urol 2:221, 1976

9. CORDONNIER JJ: Ureterosigmoid anastomosis. J Urol 63:276, 1950

10. CORDONNIER JJ: Urinary diversion. Arch Surg 71:818, 1955

11. CRISSEY MM, STEELE GD, GITTES RF: Rat model for carcinogenesis in ureterosigmoidostomy. Science 207:1079, 1980

12. CULP DA, FLOCKS RH: The diversion of urine by Heitz–Boyer procedure. J Urol 95:334, 1966

13. DRETLER SP: The pathogenesis of urinary tract calculi occurring after ileal conduit diversion: I. Clinical study. II. Conduit study. III. Prevention. J Urol 109:204, 1973

14. ENSOR RD, ATWILL WH, SECREST AJ et al: The modified Gersuny procedure for urinary diversion. J Urol 104:93, 1970

15. GALLO D, DUPONT CHACON JL: Tecnica transcolica de utera colostomia. Ginec. Obstet. Mex 6:14, 1951

16. GERSUNY, R: Cited by Foges: Officielles protokll der K. K. Gesellschaft der Aerzte in Wien. Wien Klin Wochenschr. 11:989, 1898

17. GIESY JD, HODGES CV: Flaccid paralysis associated with hyperchloremic acidosis and hypokalemia following ileal loop urinary diversion. J Urol 94:243, 1965

18. GOODWIN WE: Complications of ureterosigmoidostomy. In Smith RB, Skinner DG (eds): Complications of Urologic Surgery, Prevention and Management, p 229. Philadelphia, WB Saunders, 1976

19. GOODWIN WE, HARRIS AP, KAUFMAN JJ et al: Open, transcolonic ureterointestinal anastomosis; a new approach. Surg Gynecol Obstet 97:295, 1953

20. GOODWIN WE, SCARDINO PT: Ureterosigmoidostomy. J Urol 118:169, 1977

21. HARVARD BM, THOMPSON GJ: Congenital exstrophy of the urinary bladder: Late results of treatment by the Coffey–Mayo method of uretero-intestinal anastomosis. J Urol 65:223, 1951

22. HEITZ–BOYER M, HOVELACQUE A: Creation d'une nouvelle vessie et d'un nouvel uretre. J Urol Nephrol 1:237, 1912

23. HINMAN F, WEYRAUCH HM, JR: A critical study of the different principles of surgery which have been used in uretero-intestinal implantation. Int Abstr Surg, p 313, April 1937

24. HINMAN F, JR: The technique of the Gersuny operation (ureterosigmoidostomy with perineal colostomy) in vesical exstrophy. J Urol 81:126, 1959

25. IMLER M, SCHLIENGER JL, BATZENSCHLAGER A: Hyperammonemia following ureterocolostomy in the rat. Surg Gynecol Obstet 149:183, 1979

26. JOHNSON TH: Further experiences with a new operation for urinary diversion. J Urol 76:380, 1956

27. LEADBETTER WF, CLARKE BG: Five years' experience with ureteroenterostomy by combined technique. J Urol 73:67, 1955

28. LOWSLEY OS, JOHNSON TH: A new operation for creation of an artificial bladder with voluntary control of urine and feces. J Urol 73:83, 1955

29. MCCONNELL JB, MURISON J, STEWART WK: The role of the colon in the pathogenesis of hyperchloraemic acidosis in ureterosigmoid anastomosis. Clin Sci 57:305, 1979

30. MADSEN PO: The etiology of hyperchloremic acidosis following urointestinal anastomosis: An experimental study. J Urol 92:448, 1964

31. MATHISEN W: New method for ureterointestinal anastomosis: Preliminary report. Surg Gynecol Obstet 96:255, 1953

32. MAUCLAIRE. De quelques essais de chirurgie experimentale applicables au traitement (a) de l'exstrophie de la vessie; (b) des abouchements anormaux du rectum; (c) des anus contre nature complexes. Congres Francais de Chirurgie, p 546, 1895

33. MAYDL K: Uber die Radikaltherapie der Ectopia vesicae urinariae. Wien Med Wochenschr 44:1113, 1894

34. MOGG RA: Neoplasms at the site of ureterocolic anastomosis. Br J Surg 64:758, 1977

35. MOUNGER EJ, BRANSON AD: Ammonia encephalopathy secondary to ureterosigmoidostomy: A case report. J Urol 108:411, 1972

36. NESBIT RM: Ureterosigmoid anastomosis by direct elliptical connection: A preliminary report. J Urol 61:728, 1949

37. NESBIT RM: Another hopeful look at ureterosigmoid anastomosis. J Urol 84:691, 1960

38. O'DEA MJ, BARRETT DM, SEGURA JW: Ureterosigmoidostomy after pelvic irradiation. J Urol 118:386, 1977

39. PARSONS CD, THOMAS MH, GARRETT RA: Colonic adenocarcinoma: A delayed complication of ureterosigmoidostomy. J Urol 118:31, 1977

40. PIERCE EH, JR, ZICKERMAN P, LEADBETTER GW, JR: Ureterosigmoidostomy and carcinoma of the colon. Trans Am Assoc Genitourin Surg 70:92, 1979

41. SCHWARTZ GR, JEFFS RD: Ileal conduit urinary diversion in children: Computer analysis of followup from 2 to 16 years. J Urol 114:285, 1975

42. SHAPIRO SR, LEBOWITZ R, COLODNY AH: Fate of 90 children with ileal conduit urinary diversion a decade later: Analysis of complications, pyelography, renal function and bacteriology. J Urol 114:289, 1975

43. SIKLOS P, DAVIE M, JUNG RT et al: Osteomalacia in ureterosigmoidostomy: Healing by correction of the acidosis. Br J Urol 52:61, 1980

44. SIMON J: Ectopia vesicae (absence of the anterior walls of the bladder and pubic abdominal parietes); operation for directing the orifices of ureters into the rectum: Temporary success: Subsequent death: Autopsy. Lancet 2:568, 1852

45. SPECHT EE: Rickets following ureterosigmoidostomy and chronic hyperchloremia. J Bone Joint Surg 49-A:1422, 1967

46. SPENCE HM, HOFFMAN WW: Exstrophy of the urinary bladder treated by ureterosigmoidostomy: Long-term follow-up in a series of 37 cases. Birth Defects 13:185, 1977

47. SPENCE HM, HOFFMAN WW, FOSMIRE GP: Tumour of the colon as a late complication of ureterosigmoidostomy for exstrophy of the bladder. Br J Urol 51:466, 1979

48. STAMEY TA: Pathogenesis and implications of electrolyte imbalance in ureterosigmoidostomy. Surg Gynecol Obstet 103:736, 1956

49. WEYRAUCH HM: Landmarks and development of uretero-intestinal anastomosis. Ann R Coll Surg Engl 18:343, 1956

50. WEYRAUCH HM, JR, YOUNG BW: Evaluation of common methods of uretero-intestinal anastomosis: An experimental study. J Urol 67:880, 1952

51. WILLIAMS RE, DAVENPORT TJ, BURKINSHAW L et al: Changes in whole body potassium associated with uretero-intestinal anastomoses. Br J Urol 39:676, 1967

52. WILSON KS, DOIG A, FOWLER JW: Renography in the assessment of patients with uretero-sigmoid diversion. Br J Urol 49:195, 1977

Rectal Bladder Diversion

52

Geraldo de Campos Freire, Jr.

The complete separation of feces and urine is one of the most important goals to be achieved when diverting urine to the intestine. It can be achieved by using isolated intestinal segments in which stomas are opened on the anterior abdominal wall. If the ureters are implanted in the excluded rectal segment, a continent rectal bladder can be constructed, once the anal sphincter is intact. These are the principles upon which the rectal bladder diversion was based.

In 1895 Mauclaire presented the rectal bladder experimentally, but with left iliac terminal colostomy.[21] Gersuny in 1898 was the first to describe the use of a perineal sigmoidostomy anterior to the rectum, in an experimental work. In 1912 Heitz–Boyer and Hovelacque described a clinical case of bladder exstrophy operated upon by Marion, who performed a rectal bladder procedure with perineal sigmoidostomy but posteriorly to the rectum. In 1957 Duhamel presented five children with bladder exstrophy in whom he accomplished a rectal bladder operation with a slight modification of the Heitz–Boyer procedure.[10]

The operation has been indicated in cases in which the bladder is malformed or irreparable or must be removed. It also has been used in untreatable urethral lesions. The basic prerequisite for the operation is the anatomic and functional integrity of the anal sphincter.

Extensive experience with rectal bladder diversion has been described by Bracci and associates, Campos Freire, Constantini and associates, Menezes de Góes, and Hanley.[2,4,6,14,15]

Techniques

GERSUNY'S OPERATION

The bowel is prepared for Gersuny's operation by restricting the patient to a low-residue diet for 4 days. The patient receives preoperatively a solution of 10% mannitol given orally, 250 ml every 15 minutes for a total of 1.5 liters in 24 hr before the surgery. Usually this is associated with oral kanamycin, 2 g/day for 3 days.

The patient is placed in the Rose–Weyrauch position, which affords adequate simultaneous exposure of both abdominal and perineal operative fields. A left paramedian incision from the pubis to a point 5 cm or 6 cm above the umbilicus affords excellent abdominal exposure with the patient in the Trendelenburg position (Fig. 52-1). The bladder and pelvic cavity are thoroughly examined after the abdomen is opened to determine the extent of the disease process, particularly in malignancies. Both ureters are dissected in their lower portions as far as the bladder. Total radical cystectomy may be performed at this stage. In bladder exstrophy, the repair or the removal of bladder is done at a later stage. In female patients, anterior pelvic exenteration (cystectomy plus radical hysterectomy) may also be carried out.

The perineal approach is performed usually as described by Belt and associates in 1939 for perineal prostatectomy (Fig. 52-2).[1] Because of the observation of some cases of stenosis of perineal sigmoidostomy, a modification of the perineal skin incision has been tried to prevent this complication. A cruciate incision is performed to provide four triangular skin flaps, which are sutured to the intestinal mucosa when the resection of the rectal stump is performed (usually 8–10 days postoperatively). The circular and the longitudinal fibers of the anal sphincter are separated by blunt dissection. The rectum is depressed posteriorly and in so doing the free space between these fibers is entered. Thus a tunnel is created with is completed from inside by making a circular opening in the pelvic peritoneum. The tunnel is then ready for the passage of the intestine.

The major sigmoid vessels are secured, taking care to preserve the marginal arcade (Fig. 52-3). The rectosigmoid is transected between intestinal clamps at the level of the promontory (Fig. 52-4), and the proximal stump is closed with a continuous

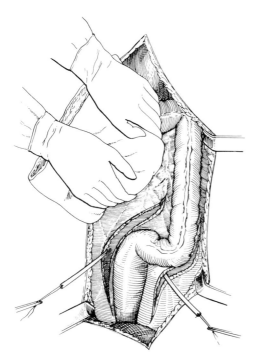

FIG. 52-1. In the Gersuny procedure, a left paramedian incision is made and the posterior peritoneum is opened vertically to the left and the right of the sigmoid colon, giving access to the ureters which are mobilized and transected. (Campos Freire JG, Góes GM: Annals XII Congress Soc Int Urologie, 1961)

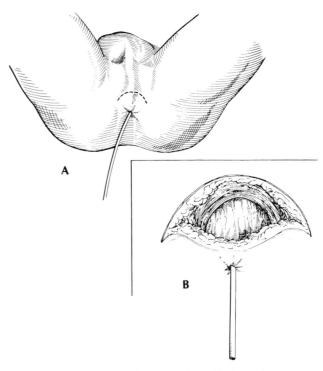

FIG. 52-2. The perineal approach. **(A)** A curving transverse perineal incision, about 2 cm anterior to the anus, may be employed. **(B)** The superficial and deep external sphincters are dissected bluntly from the anterior wall of the rectum. A urinary catheter is maintained in the rectum. (Campos Friere JC, Góes GM: Annals XII Congress Soc Int Urologie, 1961)

row of 1 chromic atraumatic catgut sutures of 2-0 cotton. The distal stump is closed as usual and sutured to the posterior parietal peritoneum.

The ureters are implanted into the rectum according to Cordonnier's technique after closure of the distal stump (Fig. 52-5).[7] Goodwin's technique may also be employed.

At this point it is necessary to elongate and liberate the proximal stump of the sigmoid colon. The sigmoid attachments are freed after ligation of either the main trunk of the inferior mesenteric artery or its branches (the superior hemorrhoidal and sigmoid arteries). The marginal arcade is always preserved. The peritoneum lying to the left side of the sigmoid colon is transected to gain complete mobilization. It is necessary to preserve an efficient blood supply to this mobilized portion of sigmoid colon.

The sigmoid stump is drawn downward to the perineum and pulled beyond the skin level for at least 8 cm to 10 cm (Fig. 52-6). It is fixed to the skin with interrupted 2-0 cotton sutures. The alternative perineal incision (Fig. 52-7) previously mentioned may be used.

The redundant perineal stump is left closed for 24 hr to 48 hr. The bowel is opened at the end of that time, but the perineal stump is allowed to project for an additional 6 to 8 days.

Penrose drains are left in the abdominal and perineal wounds. The perineal drain is brought out through a stab wound in order to prevent contamination from the sigmoid colon. The abdominal wound is closed in routine fashion with three layers of sutures: continuous 1-0 chromic catgut for the peritoneum and the fascia, and interrupted skin sutures of 2-0 cotton.

By the 8th or 10th postoperative day the perineal stump of colon has become well fixed, and the redundant portion is divided a short distance beyond the perineal skin. This delay in cutting the perineal stump is necessary to prevent retraction, which can be a serious complication. Opening of the perineal colostomy may be done in plastic fashion to prevent stricture (Fig. 52-8) if the cruciate incision has been employed.

In the postoperative course, nasogastric suction

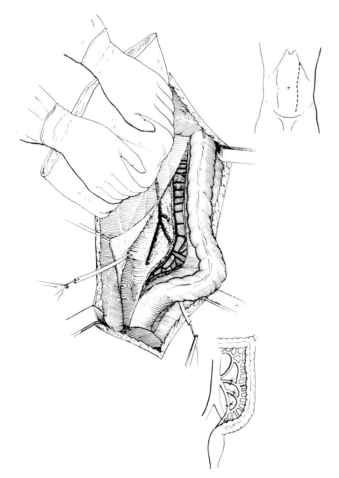

FIG. 52-3. Through the posterior peritoneal incisions, the vasculature of the mesocolon is identified and secured, permitting mobilization of the sigmoid. (Campos Freire JG, Góes GM: Annals XII Congress Soc Int Urologie, 1961)

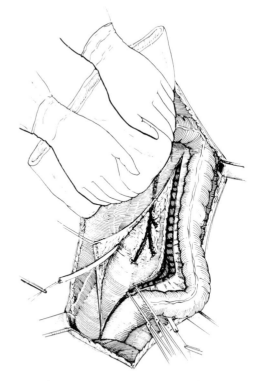

FIG. 52-4. The rectosigmoid is divided between intestinal clamps. (Campos Freire JG, Góes GM: Annals XII Congress Soc Int Urologie, 1961)

is used when indicated. Usually the patient is maintained on oral feeding beginning on the second postoperative day. Antibiotics are prescribed as indicated. Early ambulation is encouraged. As a rule the patient is mobilized on the third postoperative day. On the 8th or 10th postoperative day the sigmoid is trimmed under general or local anesthesia as previously described. The catheter draining the rectal bladder is removed on the eighth postoperative day. The patient is encouraged to resume a normal diet, and antibacterial drugs are given as indicated. Instructions are given to the patient for sphincteric exercises.

The patient's chemical profile is reviewed frequently to determine the level of Na^+, K^+, Cl^-, CO_2, and urea. Excretory urograms are made in order to evaluate the condition of the upper urinary tract. Cystograms are performed to check for reflux.

Barium enema is performed after 2 months in the supine and upright positions to check the continence of the anal sphincter and the capacity of the colon to evacuate normally.

HEITZ–BOYER TECHNIQUE

In Heitz–Boyer's technique (Fig. 52-9), the perineal pull-through sigmoidostomy is performed posterior to the rectum, and the perineal incision is carried out at the level of the anocutaneous verge with blunt dissection of rectal mucosa for 5 cm. The posterior wall fo the rectum is then incised to reach the retrorectal space which has already been dissected during the abdominal stage. Thus, a tunnel is made in which the sigmoid is pulled down and the distal stump is sutured to the mucocutaneous line with interrupted sutures.

DUHAMEL TECHNIQUE

In Duhamel's technique, the perineal incision is effected posteriorly at a distance of 1 cm from the anocutaneous margin (Fig. 52-9). The posterior part of the anal sphincter is dissected bluntly,

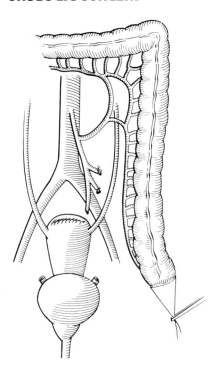

FIG. 52-5. Ureteral implantation into the closed bladder may be accomplished by end-to-side or direct anastomotic technique. (Campos Freire JG, Góes GM: Annals XII Congress Soc Int Urologie, 1961)

which results in its separation from the anal canal. When dissection reaches the superior margin of the external sphincter, the retrorectal space is entered. Then the tunnel is developed and the pull-through sigmoidostomy is performed. The sigmoid is sutured to the perineal incision as previously described.

MAUCLAIRE TECHNIQUE

The Mauclaire technique is reserved for patients in whom the pull-through is impossible owing to a short sigmoidal proximal stump, narrow retrorectal tunnel, or incompetent anal sphincter. The construction of rectal bladder by this technique follows the same steps as previously described. Instead of the pull-through of the sigmoid proximal stump to the perineum, the stump is brought to the skin of the abdomen as a terminal sigmoidostomy.

Complications

In the pull-through techniques, it is necessary that an excess of sigmoid be left outside of the perineal incision. This stump is further resected, usually at

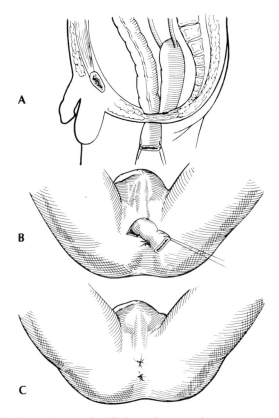

FIG. 52-6. Perineal pull-through sigmoidostomy. **(A)** The mobilized proximal sigmoid is brought down through the tunnel anterior to the rectal bladder and beneath the external sphincters. **(B)** Properly positioned, the sigmoid stump extends 6 cm to 10 cm beyond the incisional margin. **(C)** The ultimate appearance of the perineum with the anal opening of the rectal bladder posteriorly and the perineal sigmoidostomy 1 cm to 2 cm anteriorly (Campos Freire JG, Góes GM: Annals XII Congress Soc Int Urologie, 1961)

the 10th postoperative day. This avoids the possibility of retraction of the perineal sigmoidostomy.

In the Gersuny procedure, stenosis of the perineal sigmoidostomy may appear, necessitating additional surgical repair. Such stenosis is due to the retraction of the skin around the perineal sigmoidostomy. Sigmoid mobilization must be performed, and a new stoma should be created.

In patients operated on by Heitz–Boyer's technique, retraction of the perineal sigmoidostomy is common. The new anus remains located above the external sphincter. In these patients, spontaneous appearance of intestinal gas in the upper urinary tract may be observed in pyelographic studies. This indicates that the major objective of the surgery—namely, complete separation between urine and feces—has not been achieved. Often a secondary diversionary procedure such as an ileal conduit is

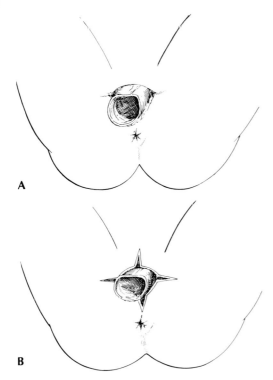

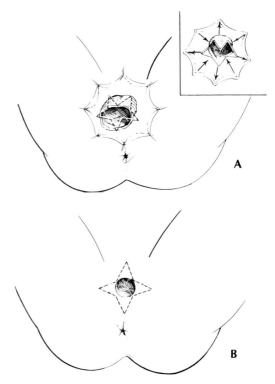

FIG. 52-7. The alternative perineal incisions include **(A)** the usual transverse anterior incision for a sigmoid pull-through, and **(B)** the alternative cruciate incision, employed to minimize stenosis of the perineal sigmoidostomy. (Campos Freire JG, Góes GM: Annals XII Congress Soc Int Urologie, 1961)

FIG. 52-8. Secondary revision of perineal sigmoidostomy at 8 to 10 days. **(A)** Stellate incisions are made in the protruding sigmoid colon and the surrounding skin with interposition of colon and skin flaps. **(B)** The final result of plastic perineal sigmoidostomy (Campos Freire JG, Góes GM: Annals XII Congress Soc Int Urologie, 1961)

FIG. 52-9. Comparison of perineal pull-through procedures. The Gersuny procedure involves sigmoid pull-through anterior to the rectal wall and beneath the sphincters, whereas the Duhamel procedure is similar but posterior to the rectal bladder. In the Heitz–Boyer or Hovelacque technique, the mobilized sigmoid is brought through the rectal wall and behind the rectal mucosa for a distance of approximately 5 cm. (Campos Freire JG, Góes GM: Annals XII Congress Soc Int Urologie, 1961)

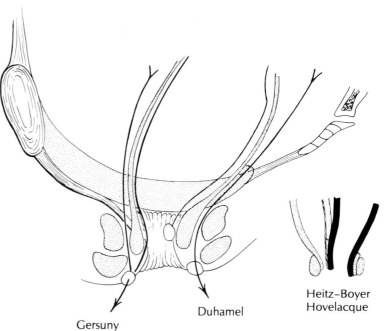

required. In the patient operated on by Duhamel's technique this complication is rare.

Rectal bladder has been tried in many centers but it is not yet generally accepted because of the possible complications. The major problems in the anterior perineal sigmoidostomy are retraction and stenosis of the stoma. In the posterior perineal sigmoidostomy, communication between the sigmoid stump and the rectum may transform both into a cloaca wherein all the advantages of the procedure are lost.

REFERENCES

1. BELT E, EBERT CF, SURBER AC: A new anatomic approach in perineal prostatectomy. J Urol 41:482, 1939

2. BRACCI M, TACCIUOLI M, LOTTI T: Rectal bladder: Indications, contraindications, and advantages. Eur Urol 5:100, 1979

3. BRICKER EM: The technique of ileal segment bladder substitution. In Meigs JV, Sturgis SH (eds): Progress in Gynecology, Vol. 3. New York, Grune & Stratton, 1957

4. CAMPOS FREIRE JG, MENEZES DE, GÓES G: Neo-rectal bladder with anterior intraspincteric perineal sigmoidostomy. Thirteenth Cong Soc Internat Urol 1:175, 1964

5. COFFEY RC: Transplantation of the ureters into the large intestine. Surg Gynecol Obstet 47:593, 1928.

6. CONSTANTINI A, LENZI R, SELLI C: Motion picture: Rectal bladder with Gersuny procedure after radical cystectomy. Trans Am Assoc Genitourin Surg 68:97, 1977

7. CORDONNIER JJ: Uretero-sigmoid anastomosis. Surg Gynecol Obstet 88:441, 1949

8. DEVINEAU G: La neo-vessie rectale. Thése de Doctorat de Médicine Faculté de Médicine et Pharmacie de Nantes, 1961

9. DORSEY JD, BARNES RW: Urinary diversion through an isolated rectal segment. J Urol 85:569, 1961

10. DUHAMEL MBH: Création d'une nouvelle vessie par exclusion du rectum et abaissement retro-rectale et transanal du colon (Rapport d M. Pierre Baissonnot). J Urol Med Chir 63:925, 1957

11. ENSOR RD, ATWILL WH, SECREST AJ et al: The modified Gersuny procedure for urinary diversion. J Urol 104:93, 1970

12. GARSKE GL, SHERMAN LA, TWIDWELL JA et al: Urinary diversion: ureterosigmoidostomy with continent pre-anal colostomy. J Urol 84:322, 1960

13. GERSUNY R: Quoted in Hinman F, Weyrauch HM, (eds): A critical study of the different principles of surgery which have been used in uretero-intestinal implantation. International Abstracts of Medicine 64:313, 1937

14. GOES GM: Contribuição para o estudo da neobexiga retal (estudo baseado em 39 casos). Tese apresentada à Faculdade de Medicina da Universidade de São Paulo

15. HANLEY HG: The rectal bladder. Br J Urol 39:693, 1967

16. HINMAN F, JR: Technique of ureterosigmoidostomy with perineal colostomy in vesical exstrophy. J Urol 81:126, 1959

17. HINMAN F, WEYRAUCH HM: A critical study of the different principles of surgery which have been used in uretero-intestinal implantation. International Abstracts of Medicine 64:313, 1937

18. LEADBETTER WF: Consideration of problems incident to performance or uretero-enterostomy: Report of a technique. J Urol 65:818, 1951

19. LOWSLEY OS, JOHNSON TH: Operation for creation of an artificial bladder with voluntary control of urine and feces. J Urol 73:83, 1955

20. MARSHALL VF: Current clinical problems regarding bladder tumors. In Brice M (ed): Bladder Tumors. A Symposium. Philadelphia, JB Lippincott, 1956

21. MAUCLAIRE, cited in Hinman F, Weirauch HM (eds): A critical study of the different principles of surgery which have been used in uretero-intestinal implantation. International Abstracts of Medicine 64:313, 1937

22. MAYDL K, quoted in Hinman F, Weyrauch HM (eds): A critical study of the different principles of surgery which have been used in uretero-intestinal implantation. International Abstracts of Medicine 64:313, 1937

23. NESBIT RM: Ureterosigmoid anastomosis by direct elliptical connection: A preliminary report. J Urol 61:728, 1949

24. STONINGTON OG, EISEMAN B: Perineal sigmoidostomy in cases of total cystectomy. J Urol 76:74, 1956

25. TRUC MM, LEVALLOIS M, HENRIET J: Néo-vessie rectale et colostomie perinéale trans-sphincterienne, assurant derivation separée et continence des urines et des matiéres. J Urol Med Chir 64:444, 1958

Urinary Undiversion

53

W. Hardy Hendren III

There are many patients who have undergone various types of urinary diversions in the past because it was felt that diversion was the best way of managing their problems at a given time. In recent years, however, advances in reconstructive urologic surgery have made it feasible to reassess those diverted patients. Many of them can indeed be reconstructed. It should be stressed that the surgeon assumes a large responsibility when suggesting undiversion to a patient who is getting along fairly well with a prior urinary diversion, because an undiversion procedure is usually a long and potentially risky operation. These patients, especially those with reduced renal function, cannot tolerate complications such as leaks, strictures, massive reflux, or loss of a kidney.

The remarks in this chapter derive from a personal experience in undiverting the previously diverted urinary tract in 113 patients from 1969 through 1981; some of the patients have been described previously.[5,11,12,14,15,16,17,18] The numbers and types of their diversions include 47 ileal loops (12 pyeloileal), 28 loop ureterostomies, 15 end ureterostomies, 16 cystostomies, and 7 nephrostomies. In 3 out of the 113 cases, the diversions were at Massachusetts General Hospital. The patients ranged in age from 1 to 24 years; there were 31 females and 82 males. Duration of their urinary diversions ranged from 1 to 18 years; 85 were permanent diversions and 28 were temporary diversions. Patients with diversions of long standing proved to be as good candidates for undiversion as those with diversion for only a few years. Of the 113 patients, 31 had been diverted for more than a decade. Thirty-three of the 113 patients had a solitary kidney.

Preoperative Assessment of Bladder Function

In considering an individual patient for possible urinary undiversion, it is important to look at why the patient was diverted in the first place. The most common causes we have seen include severe obstructive uropathy thought to be too advanced to repair, failed ureteral surgery with deterioration of the upper tracts, neurogenic bladder, urinary incontinence, urethral valves with severe upper tract changes, prune-belly syndrome, and urethral stricture with upper tract deterioration. Obviously, if the problem still remains for which diversion was done, it will require repair. For example, an appropriate procedure should be done to correct urinary incontinence, either as a first stage or during the undiversion operation.

It would be nice to be able to predict precisely how the bladder will function by urodynamic testing preoperatively. However, that has not been as helpful in our experience as doing some simple observations, starting with cystourethrography in the awake state with fluoroscopic monitoring. This will readily disclose the size of the bladder, its sensation, whether there are refluxing ureteral stumps, the contour of the urethra, and detrusor contractility. We have observed many different patterns, however, in long diverted bladders. In some patients, when the bladder is filled for the first time they will void on request as if they have never been diverted. Other patients cannot void at all initially. Some long diverted bladders are very small, and others may hold 200 ml to 300 ml despite disuse.

Cystoscopy under anesthesia is then performed to assess the anatomy. Temporary suprapubic cystostomy is established by the technique shown in Fig. 53-1. This has proven to be a great help in testing bladder function and continence, stretching up the size of small bladders, and preparing the patient for voiding once again.[22] In boys with urethral valves, the valves are destroyed with a cutting electrode at the time of suprapubic tube placement. Otherwise they would be unable to void during the period of physiologic bladder stretching and testing. Valves should never be fulgurated in a defunctioned urethra unless flow of urine or saline will begin immediately, because it can form an impermeable stricture. We have seen this happen in several cases.

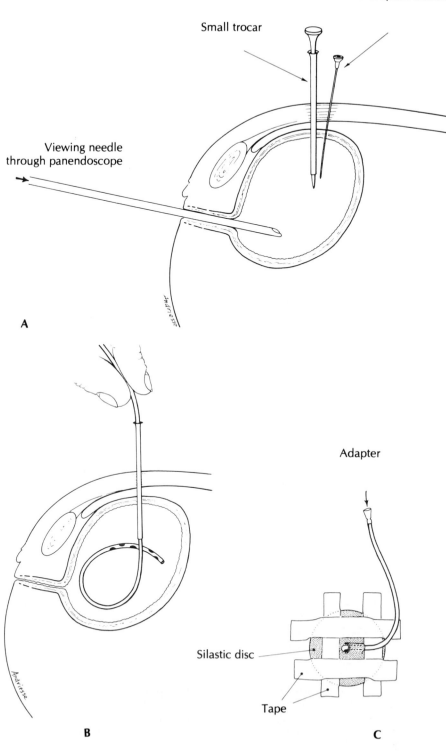

No. 22 spinal needle

Small trocar

Viewing needle
through panendoscope

A

Adapter

Silastic disc

Tape

B

C

FIG. 53-1. Percutaneous insertion of a Silastic catheter into a defunctioned small bladder (prior diversion), for preoperative testing and stretching. A Malecot catheter may be used instead; it has the advantage that it cannot pass down into the urethra as will occasionally happen with a straight catheter. **(A)** A No. 22 spinal needle is used to locate the correct position for a small trocar, which is then inserted below the needle. **(B)** The trocar is removed and the Silastic catheter is inserted through a cannula into the bladder. **(C)** A Silastic disc is glued to the skin, and an adapter is used to irrigate with saline.

FIG. 53-2. **(A)** The ureter is widely mobilized with all the periureteral tissue and the gonadal vessels. **(B)** The kidney is moved down 2 inches to 3 inches (5 cm to 7.6 cm) to allow long implantation of the ureter with a psoas hitch. The left colon is then reattached to cover the kidney and ureter. The gutter is drained. (Hendren WH: Some alternatives to urinary diversion in children. J Urol 119:652–660, 1978. © 1978, The Williams & Wilkins Co, Baltimore)

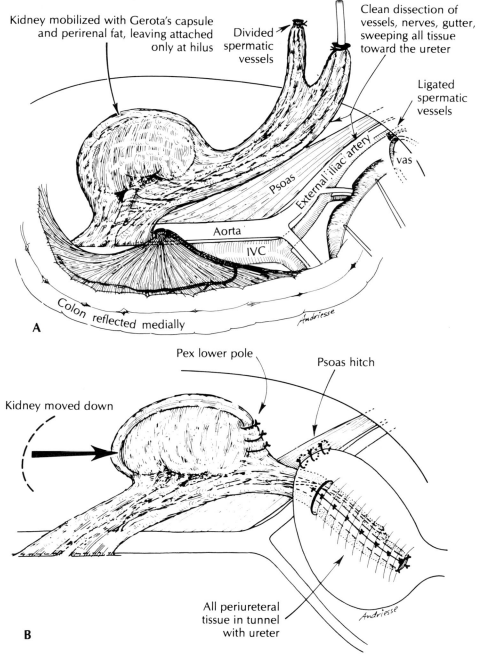

Some bladders will increase their capacity remarkably in a short time, but others will increase slowly. If a bladder is small at the outset and does not increase to a reasonable size despite hydrostatic stretching, it will probably require an augmentation procedure during undiversion. We did not appreciate that fully in our early experience, which made reoperation necessary on three patients.

Hydrostatic stretching of the long defunctioned bladder can be painful at first. It is accomplished by rapid-drip technique from a reservoir bottle 3 ft to 4 ft above the patient's bladder level, until the patient becomes accustomed to this. The patient is then taught to fill the bladder using a large syringe, increasing the pressure and the capacity a little each day if possible. Saline is used as the irrigating fluid. To it is added some 0.5% neomycin solution to prevent infection. No attempt should be made to forcibly stretch a long defunctioned bladder under anesthesia by applying high pres-

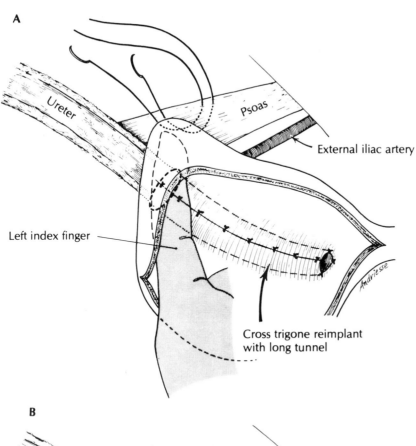

A

Ureter

Psoas

External iliac artery

Left index finger

Cross trigone reimplant
with long tunnel

Andriesse

FIG. 53-3. Technique of psoas hitch performed after completion of ureteral reimplant. Nonabsorable suture material is used, and care must be taken not to enter the bladder mucosa. (Hendren WH: Some alternatives to urinary diversion in children. J Urol 119:652–660, 1978. © 1978, The Williams & Wilkins, Baltimore)

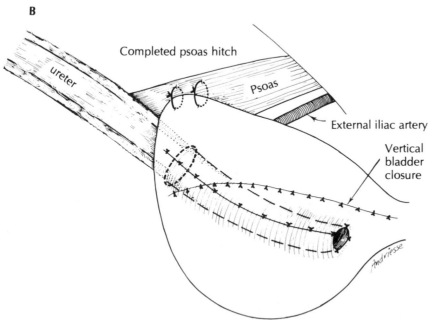

B

ureter

Completed psoas hitch

Psoas

External iliac artery

Vertical
bladder
closure

Andriesse

sure. A small, thin-walled bladder is easily ruptured. This occurred in two of our early cases; both were closed and later undiverted.

Patients with neurogenic bladders from myelodysplasia are the greatest problems in judgment on whether they should be considered for undiversion.[1,3,18,25] In these cases it is especially important to learn as much as possible about the patient's bladder function prior to the time of their diversion. A flaccid bladder with an intact urethra and bladder

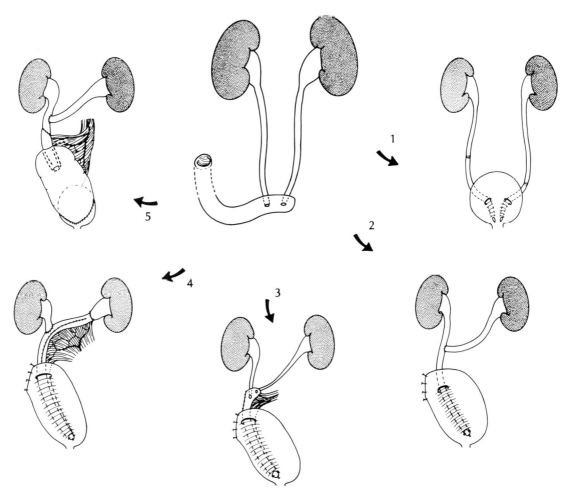

FIG. 53-4. Principal options available when undiverting a patient with previous ileal loop

neck may be manageable by intermittent catheterization after undiversion. A small, spastic bladder, however, may require a bladder-neck-narrowing procedure, together with bladder augmentation to allow management by intermittent catheterization. Artificial sphincters have been used in some of these patients in some centers. However, there is still a relatively high incidence of long-term failure in these devices, and so we have not used them yet in reconstructing previously diverted patients.

Urinary incontinence in the nonneurogenic bladder may be dealt with by a bladder-neck-narrowing procedure at the time of undiversion. In several female patients whose incontinence was based on lack of a urethra, the first step consisted in making a urethra and testing it by filling the bladder through the previously placed suprapubic tube. This technique has been described elsewhere.[19] In brief, a long urethral extension is created by tub-

ularizing the anterior vaginal wall and introitus. The sometimes hypospadiac urethra can be lengthened to the level of the clitoris. The new urethra is covered by a pedicle flap taken from the buttocks. This urethral extension can provide continence by giving more resistance through increased length. Introital muscle which surrounds the distal part of this urethral extension probably gives additional resistance.

Technical Principles in Undiversion Surgery

Some of the problems in undiversion surgery have been described recently in publications from several centers.[1–6,10–18,25,31] The cardinal principle is not to decide exactly how an individual case will be reconstructed until the anatomy is laid out on the operating table. Several options are often pos-

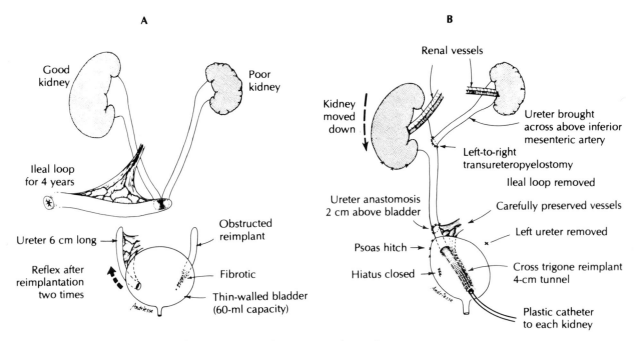

FIG. 53-5. Preoperative (**A**) and postoperative (**B**) anatomy of case 1

sible, and which is best should not be decided until all facts are at hand. For example, does the bladder stretch easily, or is it relatively small and inelastic? Is it feasible to reimplant two ureters into the bladder, or is it safer to reimplant only one with a long tunnel, draining the other by transureteroureterostomy (TUU)?[21]

Wide transabdominal exposure is needed in most cases. A vertical incision is made from the symphysis pubis to the xiphoid process. This gives ideal exposure for the bladder, both ureters, and the kidneys. Kidneys and ureters are exposed by reflecting the right and left colon medially. In mobilizing a ureter it is essential to do it in a manner that preserves the blood supply, as shown in Fig. 53-2. This entails mobilizing all periureteral tissue with it, as well as the gonadal vessels, which provide collateral blood supply. We have not seen ischemic loss of testes or ovaries from dividing their main blood supply and leaving them next to the ureter being mobilized. In dissecting the ureter away from retroperitoneal structures (*i.e.*, the peritoneum, vessels, nerves, and psoas muscle), they should be skeletonized as in a lymphadenectomy for cancer, retaining all of that tissue for the ureter. This will allow wide mobilization and reimplantation of ureters which would be doomed to failure by less thorough techniques. Many of these reconstructive procedures require doing a procedure at two or three levels of the same ureter. For example, the lower ureter is mobilized and reimplanted; the

midureter has the opposite ureter joined to it as a TUU; and the upper ureter has a kinked ureteropelvic junction which is resected and reanastomosed through a small opening in the periureteral adventitia. This can be done by carefully preserving all blood supply. A little extra length can be attained by mobilizing the kidney, also sliding it down and pexing it at a lower position.

Psoas hitch, shown in Fig. 53-3, is an important adjunct in these operations, whether one is implanting a ureter which is somewhat dilated or a tapered bowel segment for which an especially long tunnel is needed to prevent reflux.[26,32] For success it is necessary to obtain a tunnel-length-to-ureter-diameter ratio of about 5:1.

Transureteroureterostomy is an invaluable adjunct in undiversion surgery.[21,33] In a relatively small number of previously diverted bladders there is the option of simply reconnecting two ureters which have been divided or reimplanting two ureters which have been previously taken from the bladder. Much more often it proves more feasible to reimplant the better of two ureters, relying on TUU to drain the second one.[20] The ureter to be drained is mobilized widely, with all of its periureteral tissue and often its gonadal vessels. It is brought to the donor ureter so that there will be no tension. It should not be wedged beneath the inferior mesenteric artery, which can compress it.

Augmentation of the bladder should be per-

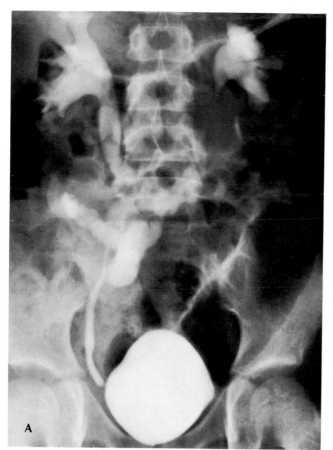 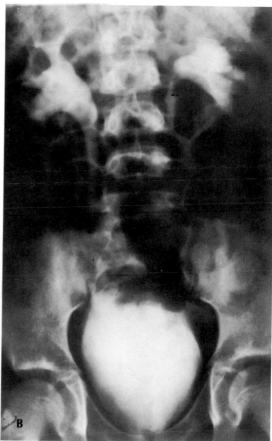

FIG. 53-6. Case 1 roentgenograms. **(A)** Simultaneous preoperative cystogram and loopogram. Note the reasonable size of the bladder in this case despite previous diversion, and the refluxing right ureteral stump. The ileal loop in midabdomen was discarded. **(B)** Intravenous pyelogram (IVP) 2 years after undiversion

formed when it is small, fibrous, and inelastic.[7,8,28,34] Augmentation can be performed with a patch of small intestine or colon, or using an ileocecal segment. The ileocecal junction can be altered to provide an antireflux mechanism, joining one or both ureters to the terminal ileum.

When there is no alternative, small intestine can be used as a substitute ureter. It is a better alternative than accepting tension between a short ureter and the bladder or attempting to reimplant a fibrotic, nonpliable ureter into the bladder with the false hope that it will not reflux. It is our experience in surgery that whatever appears questionable at the operating table generally proves unsuccessful postoperatively. When small bowel is substituted for a ureter in patients with stone disease, experience has shown that reflux does not seem to be a great problem.[9,29] These are generally adult patients, however, with relatively normal

bladders. In undiversion patients, whose bladders are often abnormal at the outset, we have found it to be very important to prevent reflux.[18] When we have failed, reoperation has been needed for recurrent infection and upper tract deterioration.

UNDIVERSION FROM ILEAL LOOP

There are several reconstructive options possible in undiverting the urinary tract of a patient with an ileal loop, as shown in Fig. 53-4. The technique suitable for an individual patient will depend on the length of ureters available to reconstruct and the suitability of the bladder. Obviously, it is best to drain kidneys into the bladder through ureters, when that is possible. Only when the ureters are not satisfactory for reconstruction should bowel be used. Some diverted bladders will have at least one ureteral stump intact which is long enough to

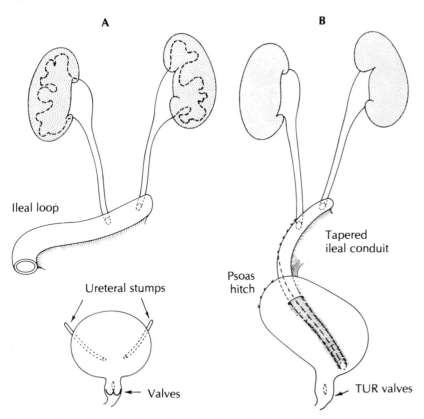

A

B

Ileal loop

Ureteral stumps

Valves

Tapered
ileal conduit

Psoas
hitch

TUR valves

FIG. 53-7. Preoperative **(A)** and post-operative **(B)** anatomy of case 2 (Hendren WH: Refunctionalizing the urinary tract after prior diversion. Contemp Surg, p 71, 1975. Reproduced with the permission of Contemporary Surgery)

use, with or without doing a ureteral reimplantation of the stump. Reflux into a usable ureteral stump in a diverted bladder does not necessarily mean that ureteral reimplantation will be necessary, because a normal ureterovesical junction can initially show reflux during cystography in a diverted bladder. When the bladder subsequently increases in capacity, the tunnel may lengthen and reflux may disappear. On the other hand, if there was known to be reflux before diversion, it will probably be there after undiversion. If at the time of operation the ureters are laterally placed, with absent tunnels, reimplantation is best to prevent reflux.

In 47 ileal loops that I have undiverted it was possible in only one to rejoin the upper tracts to existing ureteral stumps, which were both reimplanted. In ten patients one ureter could be reimplanted into the bladder (seven of those patients had a contralateral TUU). In 30 patients it was necessary to use the ileal loop to reestablish continuity of the upper tracts to the bladder. Twelve of those patients had pyeloileal conduits. In six patients the bladders were unsuitable for reimplantation of a tapered bowel segment; they were managed by ileocecal cystoplasty.

Four ileal loop undiversion cases illustrate the use of some of these technical options.

Case 1 (Figs. 53-5 and 53-6). A 10-year-old girl was referred with an ileal loop for undiversion. At age 4 internal urethrotomy had been performed for recurrent urinary infection and reflux. During her fifth year ureteral reimplantation was performed, followed by urinary extravasation, repeat reimplantation, nephrostomy, repeat urethrotomy, and finally ileal loop urinary diversion. Although previously twice reimplanted, the right ureter had sufficient length and blood supply to allow reimplantation for a third time. The useless left ureter was removed. By widely mobilizing the right kidney and its ureter, with all periureteral blood supply, direct ureter-to-ureter continuity on the right could be reestablished. The ileal loop was discarded. Transureteropyelostomy was used to drain the opposite kidney. The patient is well, six years following this reconstruction.

Comment: It cannot be decided preoperatively in many cases whether a ureteral stump will be suitable for use or not. That decision will depend on its length, degree of fibrosis, and whether it can be technically reimplanted if that is necessary. Some refluxing stumps do not require reimplan-

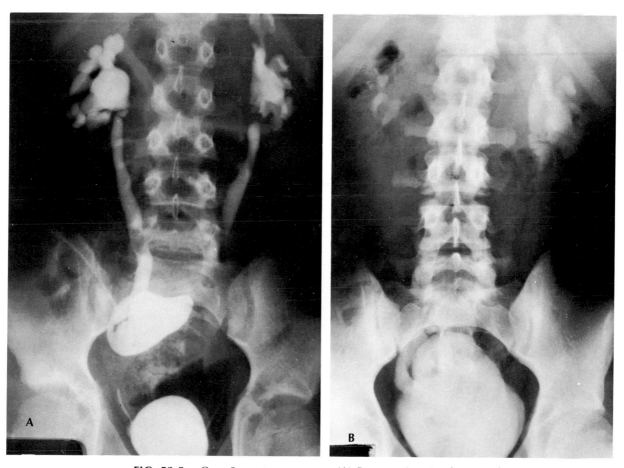

FIG. 53-8.   Case 2 roentgenograms.   **(A)** Preoperative simultaneous loopogram and cystogram. Note the small bladder and the nonusable short ureteral stumps.   **(B)** IVP 6 years following undiversion. Note the normal bladder size.

tation if the orifice is normal and there is a good submucosal tunnel. Reflux may disappear after refunctionalization of the bladder. In this child, however, there was reflux originally and a golfhole orifice with no submucosal ureteral segment. Reimplantation was mandatory. The option of ureter-to-ureter anastomosis depends on maintaining good blood supply for the ureter and attaining tension-free anastomosis. When that is not possible, it is better to use a bowel segment.

Case 2 (Figs. 53-7 and 53-8). An 11-year-old boy was referred with an ileal loop done 8 years previously. His original pathology was severe urethral valves. Prior surgery included suprapubic cystostomy at age 3 months, bilateral pyelolithotomy at 2 years, ileal loop urinary diversion at 3 years, and repeat left pyelolithotomy. Restoration of ureteral continuity was not possible, because there was a long gap between the upper ureters and short remaining stumps. The urethral valves

were destroyed endoscopically. The ileal loop was tapered and reimplanted with a long tunnel to prevent reflux. Now, 8 years following undiversion, the patient is well, stands 6 ft 2 in tall (188 cm) and weighs 172 pounds (78 kg).

Comment: The technique for tapering an ileal loop is shown in Fig. 53-9. Often its mesentery must be incised to straighten the segment. Megaloureter clamps can facilitate trimming the bowel segment but it can also be done freehand. It must not be made too narrow, lest stenosis be created. Catheters in the bowel segment and up both ureters will protect against inadvertently compromising the ureteral drainage into the bowel segment. The bowel is closed with two layers of catgut. The first is a running, inverting watertight closure. The second layer is interrupted seromuscular sutures. To prepare a bed for implantation of the tapered bowel segment, a long diagonal incision is made across the back wall of the bladder, laying back

(*Text continues on p. 538*)

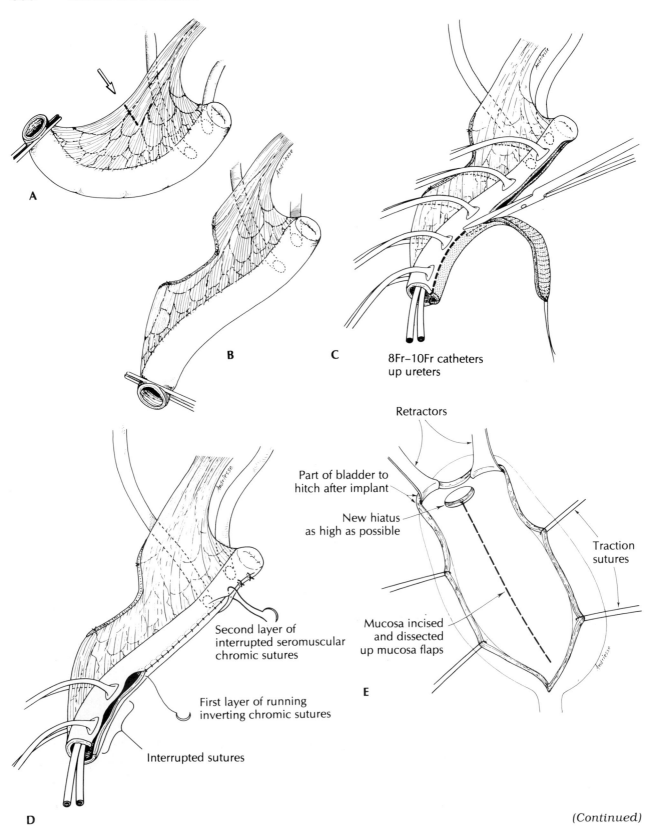

A

B

C

8Fr–10Fr catheters
up ureters

D

Second layer of
interrupted seromuscular
chromic sutures

First layer of running
inverting chromic sutures

Interrupted sutures

E

Retractors

Part of bladder to
hitch after implant

New hiatus
as high as possible

Mucosa incised
and dissected
up mucosa flaps

Traction
sutures

(Continued)

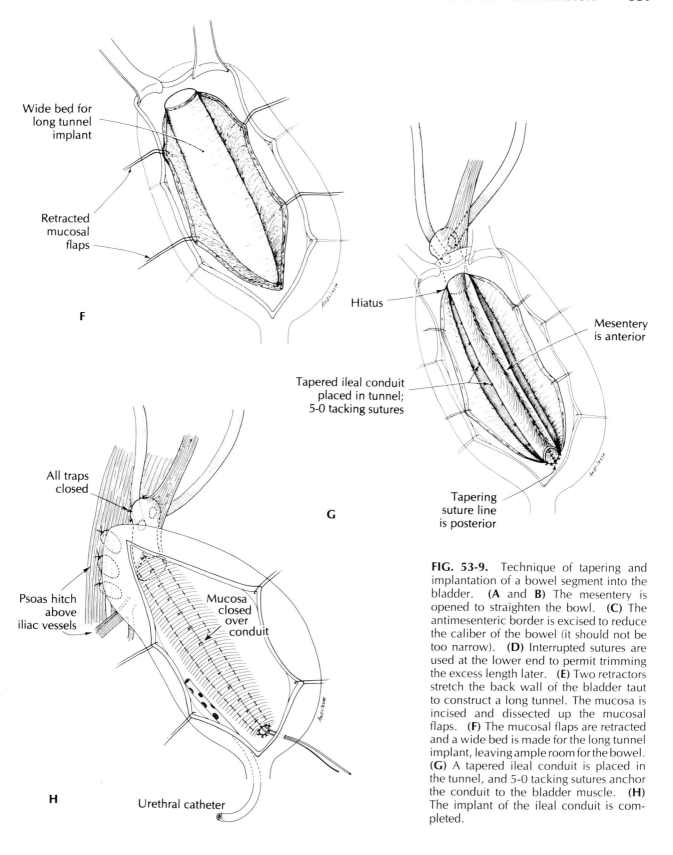

Wide bed for
long tunnel
implant

Retracted
mucosal
flaps

F

Hiatus

Mesentery
is anterior

Tapered ileal conduit
placed in tunnel;
5-0 tacking sutures

Tapering
suture line
is posterior

All traps
closed

G

Psoas hitch
above
iliac vessels

Mucosa
closed
over
conduit

H

Urethral catheter

FIG. 53-9. Technique of tapering and implantation of a bowel segment into the bladder. (**A** and **B**) The mesentery is opened to straighten the bowl. (**C**) The antimesenteric border is excised to reduce the caliber of the bowel (it should not be too narrow). (**D**) Interrupted sutures are used at the lower end to permit trimming the excess length later. (**E**) Two retractors stretch the back wall of the bladder taut to construct a long tunnel. The mucosa is incised and dissected up the mucosal flaps. (**F**) The mucosal flaps are retracted and a wide bed is made for the long tunnel implant, leaving ample room for the bowel. (**G**) A tapered ileal conduit is placed in the tunnel, and 5-0 tacking sutures anchor the conduit to the bladder muscle. (**H**) The implant of the ileal conduit is completed.

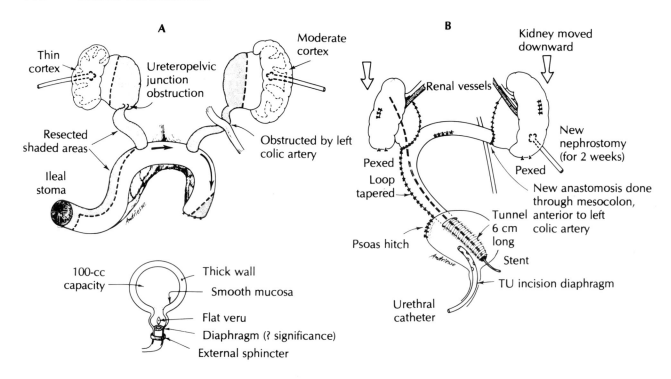

FIG. 53-10.   Preoperative (**A**) and postoperative (**B**) anatomy of case 3

mucosal flaps which will be closed later over the implanted bowel segment. Seldom is it possible to make a submucosal tunnel in one of these bladders as is customary in reimplanting a ureter. We know that in reimplanting ureters a 5:1 ratio of tunnel length to ureter diameter is desirable to stop reflux. The same is true in these tapered bowel segments, which measure 10 mm to 15 mm in diameter even after trimming their caliber. We strive to make the tunnel 8 cm to 10 cm long. When closing the mucosal flaps over the ureter it is important that there be no constriction of the bowel. It is futile to implant a tapered bowel segment into a scarred, contracted, bladder where only a short tunnel can be made. Psoas hitch is mandatory to keep the tunnel long. It also prevents angulation of the tapered bowel segment by fixing the bladder wall to the gutter near the entry of the loop.

Nineteen of 28 loops which were tapered and reimplanted into the bladder were successful initially. In two other patients the ileal loop was tapered and used as a substitute midureter with success. Nine patients required reoperation because of reflux. In six it was possible to create a longer tunnel and prevent reflux. These were basically good bladders, which were much larger than at the time of undiversion. It was possible to bring the bowel in at a higher point in the bladder

and make a longer tunnel. These were patients early in the series whose undiversions had been performed without first hydrostatically stretching the bladder. This reemphasizes the desirability of hydrostatically stretching bladders to a larger size when they are initially small. Three of the reoperative cases had poor bladders. It had been a judgmental error to attempt implantation of a tapered loop into them in the first place. Ileocecal cystoplasty was performed to solve the problem.

Patients with tapered bowel in their urinary tracts must be followed radiographically. In three of our cases there occurred late stenosis of a tapered bowel segment. In two this was dealt with by open operation, excising the stenotic segment. The third was managed endoscopically by passing a panendoscope up the tapered segment, incising a mucosa diaphragm with a cutting electrode, and eliminating the narrowing. Late stricture is a recognized complication of ileal loop urinary diversions. Our experience would indicate the same to be true when bowel is used to reconstruct the intact urinary tract.

Small bowel has been used to substitute for the ureter in stone-forming adult patients. If there is no outlet obstruction, reflux does not seem to be a significant problem, despite simple end-to-side anastomosis of the bowel segment to the back wall

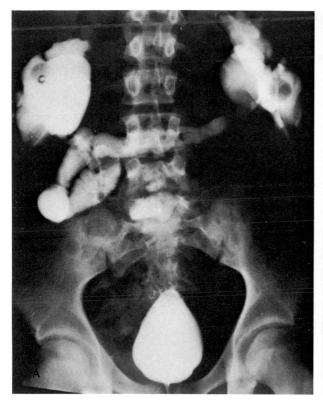 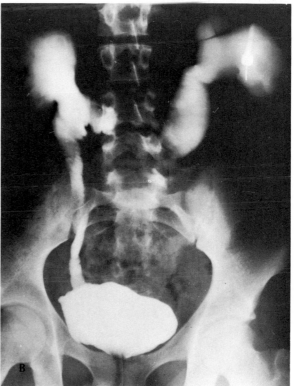

FIG. 53-11.   Case 3 roentgenograms.   **(A)** Preoperative simultaneous cystogram, loopogram, and bilateral nephrostogram. Drainage of the kidneys into the loop was obstructed bilaterally. **(B)** Antegrade pyelogram by means of a percutaneous needle in the left kidney (*arrow*) 3½ years after undiversion. Note the tapered bowel conduit implanted into the bladder. A cystogram showed no reflux.

of the bladder.[9,29] On the other hand, in our experience whenever there has been reflux after reimplantation of a tapered bowel segment in undiversion cases there has been urinary infection, which these patients can ill afford. It is my belief, therefore, that it is best, whenever possible, to use a tapering and tunneling technique to prevent reflux, particularly in a young patient with potentially long life expectancy.

Pyeloileal loop gained considerable popularity some years ago, allegedly as the best way to ensure good drainage of bad upper tracts. Long-term follow-up, however, showed that all ileal loop urinary diversions run a considerable rate of upper tract deterioration, particularly in patients with high loops for severe hydronephrosis.[24,27] Some of these patients should be considered for undiversion.

Case 3 (Figs. 53-10 and 53-11). A 15-year-old boy with the prune-belly syndrome was referred with bilateral nephrostomies since birth. There was also an ileal loop which never had drained, because

both ureters were blocked. The short segment of ureter on the left was obstructed by the left colic artery. On the right there was ureteropelvic junction obstruction. The conduit was rearranged as a pyeloileal conduit, tapering its distal segment, and implanting it with a long tunnel and psoas hitch. Seven years following undiversion, the patient leads a normal life, is free from urinary infection, and has diminished but stable renal function.

Comment: Patients like this with high loops often have poor renal function. They do not concentrate IVP contrast medium well, so their periodic anatomic reevaluation is best performed by antegrade percutaneous pyelography. It is also possible to use an endoscope to visualize the interior of a tapered bowel conduit. A long telescope can be passed from below all the way to the interior of the kidney. Two patients developed late narrowing of the ostium of the tapered bowel segment in the bladder. This was managed by endoscopically incising the edge of the orifice to enlarge its caliber.

Case 4 (Figs. 53-12 and 53-13). A 10-year-old

A

B

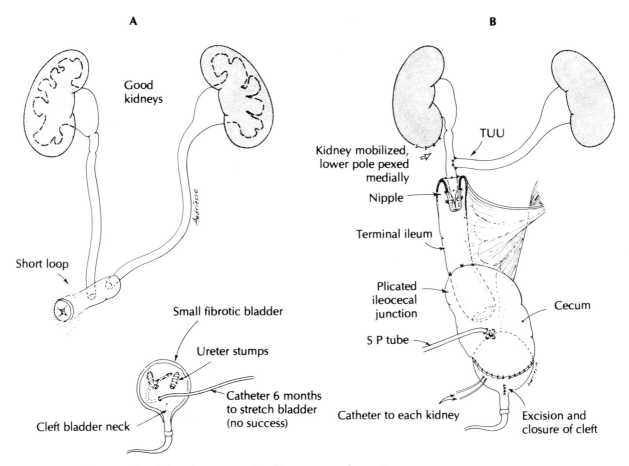

FIG. 53-12. Preoperative **(A)** and postoperative **(B)** anatomy of case 4

boy was referred for possible undiversion. After two failed ureteral reimplantations and partial cystectomy, ileal loop had been performed 3 years previously. Despite a trial of 6 months of hydrostatic stretching of the bladder, its maximal capacity remained at 50 ml. Ileocecal augmentation of the bladder was performed to increase its volume. The ileum was intussuscepted into the cecum to provide an antireflux mechanism. A nipple was made between the right ureter and the terminal ileum as a second defense against reflux. The left side was drained by transureteroureterostomy. The bladder neck, which had been opened previously by endoscopic resection, was excised and narrowed. Four years postoperatively, the patient has stable IVP, no reflux, urinary continence, and satisfactory bladder volume.

Comment: When the bladder is small, fibrotic, and nondistensible, urinary undiversion will be feasible only if an augmentation procedure is included in the reconstruction. Ileocecal bladder augmentation has proven essential in undiverting patients with a bladder that was too small and unsuited for reimplantation of a ureter or tapered bowel conduit. Patients whose external sphincter and bladder neck are competent void in a remarkably normal manner with cecal augmentation of the small bladder. The most troublesome technical problem in these cases in my experience has been obtaining a nonrefluxing ileocecal valve. A normal ileocecal valve will usually reflux at pressures of 10 cm to 15 cm of water. Plication of the cecal wall around the terminal ileum as described elsewhere can make the valve competent to pressures of over 60 cm on the operating table.[8,34] However, in our experience, this antireflux mechanism breaks down when the cecum is intermittently filled and emptied when serving as a substitute bladder. In several of these patients an actual intussuscepted nipple of terminal ileum was created. The mesentery was first removed from the segment to be intussuscepted. Seromuscular incisions were made in the bowel wall to promote adherence of the walls after creating a nipple. Even with reinforcing sutures

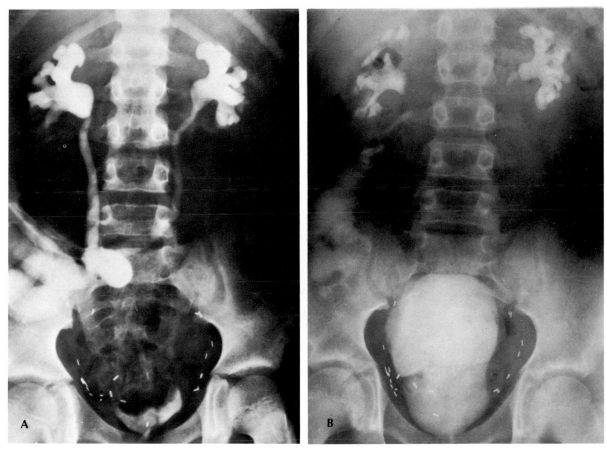

FIG. 53-13. Case 4 roentgenograms. **(A)** Preoperative cystogram and loopogram. The bladder did not increase in size with 6 months of attempted stretching. **(B)** IVP 3 years after undiversion. Note the normal size of the "bladder," which is mostly cecal augmentation, and the improved upper tracts. There is no reflux.

this did not prove to be uniformly effective. Some nipples spontaneously reduced and allowed reflux. In the most recent cases the nipple has been made as before but reinforced by stapling its walls with a gastrointestinal stapler. Whether this will prove reliable and whether stones will form on staples remain to be seen in time. The ureter-to-bowel nipple illustrated in this case is an appealing second line of defense against reflux. In our experience, however, it cannot be depended upon if there is any substantial back pressure in the bowel segment. The nipple will reduce and become incompetent.

Other Types of Undiversion

Patients with other types of temporary or permanent urinary diversions can be reconstructed using the same general principles outlined in this chapter. Cutaneous ureterostomy has been used extensively

in the past 25 years. It is an easy operation to perform, and this has probably contributed to its overuse. Forty-three patients presented with loop or end ureterostomy for undiversion.

Case 5 (Figs. 53-14 and 53-15). An 11-year-old girl presented with bilateral end ureterostomies for undiversion. During infancy she had undergone Y–V plasty to the bladder neck, partial cystectomy, and bilateral ureteral reimplants twice. Ureterostomies were performed at age 15 months. Both ureter stumps were unusable. The bladder was small despite 3 weeks of hydrostatic stretching, but was of adequate size to accomplish one good ureteral reimplantation. This was possible by sliding the right kidney down and hitching the bladder upward. TUU drained the second side. The bladder size increased slowly postoperatively to 300 ml. Now 3 years later the patient is continent, even during competitive roller skating.

Comment: It would be ideal to get two ureters

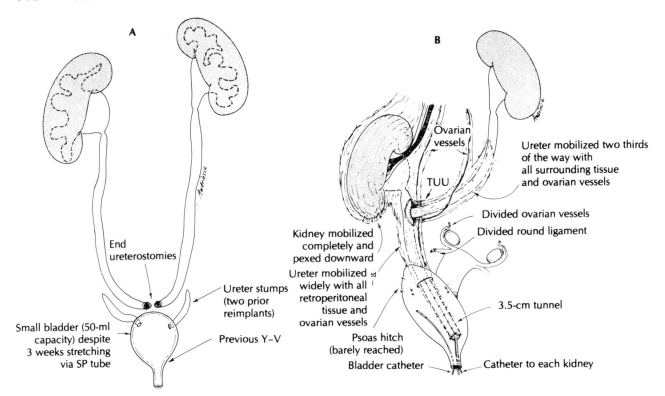

FIG. 53-14. Preoperative (**A**) and postoperative (**B**) anatomy of case 5

reimplanted into the bladder in every case, but that is usually impossible in undiversion cases and often not feasible in repeat ureteral reimplantation cases. Reimplanting the better ureter with a long tunnel and psoas hitch, relying on TUU for the second side, has proved to be an entirely satisfactory option.

Case 6 (Figs. 53-16 and 53-17). A 3½-year-old boy was referred with bilateral loop cutaneous ureterostomies and suprapubic cystostomy. Complete stricture of the prostatic urethra had occurred following abdominal–perineal pull-through anoplasty for imperforate anus. Loop cutaneous ureterostomy was performed to relieve bilateral hydronephrosis, but pyonephrosis developed. Suprapubic cystostomy was done for bladder washouts. Permanent ileal loop urinary diversion was then recommended. The parents refused and sought possible reconstruction. The urethral stricture, despite considerable length by urethrogram, proved reparable by mobilization and primary anastomosis. Hydrostatic testing of the bladder showed good function despite previous diversion and pyocystis. Undiversion was accomplished 2 months after repair of the stricture that had precipitated the

need for diversion in the first place. The patient has done extremely well in the 4 years since his undiversion.

Comment: In undiverting a patient with high loop ureterostomies, we have found it most satisfactory to do the entire undiversion in one procedure. This entails taking down ureterostomies and reimplanting the lower ureters, being very careful of the ureteral blood supply. If a ureter is reimplanted into the bladder while defunctioned from above, it is essential to keep a small stent in it until the ureterostomy is subsequently closed. A dry reimplant can quickly seal over. Closing the ureterostomy in the same sitting will prevent that complication. Further, a ureter can be tethered upward by a cutaneous ureterostomy. This can make it impossible to gain adequate mobility of the lower ureter to accomplish a tension-free ureteral reimplantation unless the ureterostomy is taken down. Autotransplantation of the kidney is another procedure which can be used to overcome a gap between the kidney and the bladder.[23,30] I have not thought that to be a feasible maneuver in any of the undiversion cases encountered to date, because so often these are already damaged

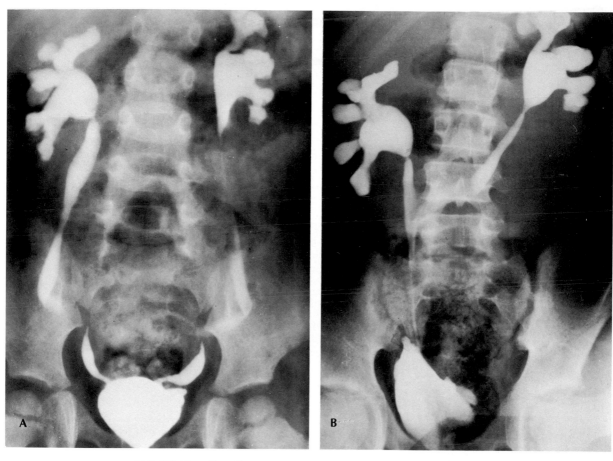

FIG. 53-15.   Case 5 roentgenograms.   **(A)** Preoperative simultaneous cystogram and bilateral ureterograms. The short, previously reimplanted ureteral stumps were not usable.   **(B)** Retrograde pyelogram 1 year postoperatively (allergic to IVP contrast medium)

kidneys with reduced renal function, in whom autotransplantation might offer undue additional risk.

Case 7 (Figs. 53-18 and 53-19). A 14-year-old boy presented with end cutaneous ureterostomies for undiversion. At cystoscopy, residual Type I urethral valves were opened up endoscopically. They had strictured almost completely closed from previous valve fulguration years before when the bladder was defunctioned. The bladder increased in size from 150 ml to 300 ml in just 10 days, after which undiversion was performed. All three renal segments were drained through the one good ureter, which was implanted with a long tunnel into the bladder. The patient has had an unremarkable course during 5 years postoperatively.

Comment: This case illustrates the extensive maneuvers that can be accomplished with a ureter if

its blood supply is carefully preserved by retaining all periureteral tissue and the gonadal vessels as collateral. The megaloureter to the lower pole of the right kidney was removed, draining the lower pole by pyeloureterostomy. Separating a large ureter like this from an adjacent smaller ureter can be accomplished without harming the blood supply of the smaller ureter if the dissection is done through a series of stair-step incisions in the periureteral tissue. The dissection is carried close on to the wall of the ureter to be removed. In duplex collecting systems with two ureters of normal size, double ureteral reimplantation is the best option. When one ureter is very large, however, it is best removed, relying on the smaller ureter to drain both segments. An alternative is to taper the lower end of the larger ureter. However, we have seen that lead to ureteral reimplantation failure of both the tapered ureter and the adjacent smaller ureter.

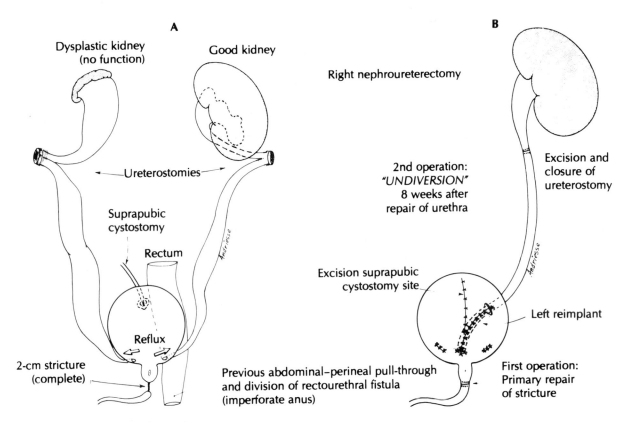

A

Dysplastic kidney (no function)

Good kidney

Ureterostomies

Suprapubic cystostomy

Rectum

Reflux

2-cm stricture (complete)

Previous abdominal–perineal pull-through and division of rectourethral fistula (imperforate anus)

B

Right nephroureterectomy

2nd operation: "UNDIVERSION" 8 weeks after repair of urethra

Excision and closure of ureterostomy

Excision suprapubic cystostomy site

Left reimplant

First operation: Primary repair of stricture

FIG. 53-16. Anatomy of case 6

In this boy's case the blood supply to the one good ureter was adequate despite mobilization of the lower ureter to reimplant it, separation of the adjacent megaloureter, pyeloureterostomy at its upper end, and transureteroureterostomy in the midureter.

Some Conclusions about Undiversion

Clearly urinary undiversion is a practical consideration for many patients whose urinary tract is diverted. Each case will differ from all others in some respects. The surgeon must have a broad-spectrum armamentarium of technical maneuvers to use in an individual case. If one adheres to the general principles enumerated in this chapter, success should be possible in most instances. These are long and arduous operations, requiring great attention to technical details. A leaking anastomosis, ischemic ureter, or obstructed ureter could prove catastrophic. Cases of this magnitude require expert anesthesia. Metabolic management of those patient with diminished renal function requires supervision by a knowledgeable nephrologist. There have been no operative deaths in this series. (One late death occurred in a patient at age 28, 11 years

after undiversion. His original pathology had been prune-belly syndrome, with one kidney with a staghorn calculus. Death came from sepsis during hemodialysis. His original creatinine clearance at the time of undiversion had been only 20% of normal.) Eight patients have subsequently undergone renal transplantation. Usually this followed a gradual decline of function with growth from childhood to adulthood, with an increased body mass too great for their initially low renal function to support. Twenty additional patients will likely require transplantation when they become older.

Undiversion has provided several distinct benefits. First it has greatly improved the quality of life, getting rid of bags. Bacilluria, which is so common in patients wearing a bag,[24,27] has proven much more easily controlled when the urinary tract is closed. Those patients whose undiversion was performed despite already failing renal function have been made better candidates for transplantation with a refunctionalized bladder, as compared to patients who present for transplantation with an established urinary diversion.

None of these patients required rediversion. In none was it thought that undiversion hastened the decline of already low renal function. However, patients with low renal function who have bowel

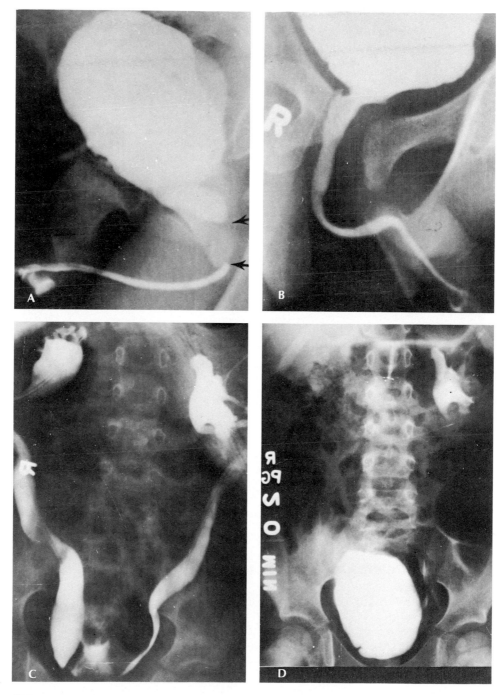

FIG. 53-17. Case 6 roentgenograms. **(A)** Preoperative cystourethrogram showing long stricture (*arrow*). **(B)** Cystourethrogram following repair of stricture by excision and anastomosis. **(C)** Preoperative ureterograms obtained by means of bilateral cutaneous loop ureterostomies; right kidney was nonfunctional. **(D)** IVP 1 year after undiversion. Note the normal bladder and the normal left ureter.

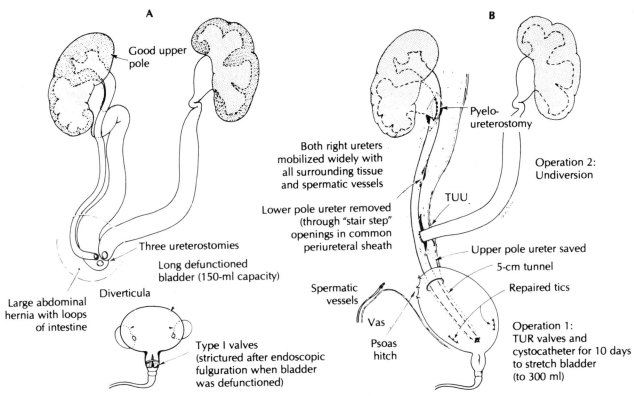

FIG. 53-18.   Preoperative **(A)** and postoperative **(B)** anatomy of case 7

incorporated into their urinary tract, especially cecal bladder augmentation, require special metabolic supervision because of serum electrolyte exchange across the bowel surface. One patient "ran out of his pills" and had a near catastrophe with severe weakness from hypokalemia until medication was restarted.

"Internal Diversion" of Patient with No Bladder

There is another group of patients who are wearing bags who should be considered for a possible reconstructive operation to remove their bags. These are patients who have undergone cystectomy for malignancy or an unreconstructable bladder exstrophy. Many such young individuals are living with ileal conduit diversions. It is possible to accomplish staged ureterocolic diversion of the urine in these patients if they have good upper tract function and normal rectal control.[13] Ureterocolic internalization of urine drainage should not be performed in patients who have very low renal function, whose kidneys are inadequate to reexcrete the obligatory reabsorbed solute load imposed by ureterosigmoidostomy.

Case 8 (Fig. 53-20). An 8-year-old girl had under-

gone ileal loop urinary diversion during infancy for a rudimentary exstrophic bladder, thought unsuited for functional reconstruction. Although both ureters and kidneys were originally normal, there was some dilatation of the right ureter which took place after ileal loop urinary diversion, despite two stoma revisions (Fig. 53-20A). The ileal loop was removed, substituting for it a sigmoid conduit with long, tunneled anastomoses of the ureters into the conduit to prevent reflux. The right ureter was tapered slightly to reduce its caliber. The right upper tract dilatation disappeared when drainage was switched from a refluxing ileal loop to a nonrefluxing colon conduit. Later loopogram showed no reflux of contrast medium to the kidneys. One year after conversion to the colon conduit, the conduit was taken down from the abdominal wall and implanted into the rectosigmoid at age 9, thereby accomplishing staged ureterocolic diversion of the urine. Now, 10 years following this internal diversion of the urine to the colon, the patient is well, has satisfactory control of continence of urine by rectum, and has stable IVP. There has been no clinical evidence of ascending urinary infection.

Comment: An ileal loop cannot be directly anastomosed to the colon, because it will reflux and

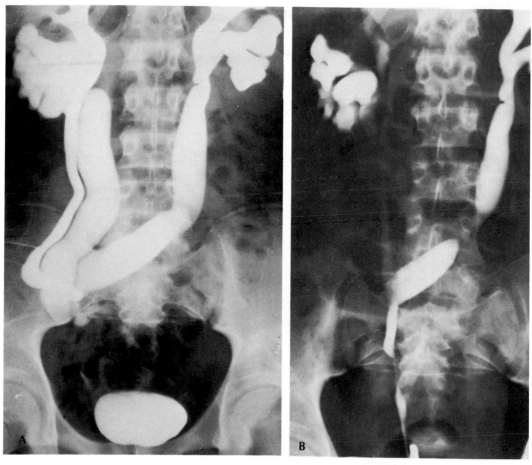

FIG. 53-19   Case 7 roentgenograms.   **(A)** Simultaneous preoperative cystogram and ureterograms.   **(B)** Retrograde study was done 1 year postoperatively.

cause pyelonephritis. Classic one-stage ureterosigmoidostomy will not prove feasible in most patients who have previously undergone an ileal loop urinary diversion, because the ureters are usually somewhat shortened. They may be dilated also, as in this patient, which is a contraindication to direct ureterosigmoidostomy. It is, therefore, safer in most cases to transfer the ureters first into an isolated colon conduit, to allow a period of observation to be certain that the ureterocolic anastomoses drain well and do not reflux, and later to connect the conduit to the intact colon. This method of staged ureterosigmoidostomy has been performed in 31 cases, including 27 former bladder exstrophy cases, 2 cases of cystectomy for tumors, 1 post trauma case, and 1 case of interstitial cystitis in an adult. Twelve patients had a primary colon conduit, which was subsequently reconnected to the rectosigmoid. All of their upper tracts were normal initially and none of them have had ascending urinary infection since hookup. Nineteen

other patients who first had ileal loops were switched to a colon conduit, which was later hooked to the colon. Some of those patients had preexisting dilated ureters and or calicectasis from previous ileal conduit diversion. Four of these 19 patients have had pyelonephritis from ascending infection. If pyelonephritis is suspected in a patient with ureterocolic internal drainage, percutaneous aspiration of the kidney with a 22-gauge spinal needle is performed to obtain a urine specimen for culture and sensitivities. If one ureterocolic anastomosis seems to be allowing ascending infection, and the other does not, transureteroureterostomy of the refluxing ureter into the nonrefluxing ureter is a possible solution to that problem. The increased flow of two kidneys through one competent ureterosigmoidostomy may further reduce the likelihood of ascending infection.

All patients with ureterocolic diversion of the urine should be warned of the increased incidence of carcinoma of the colon with that type of urinary

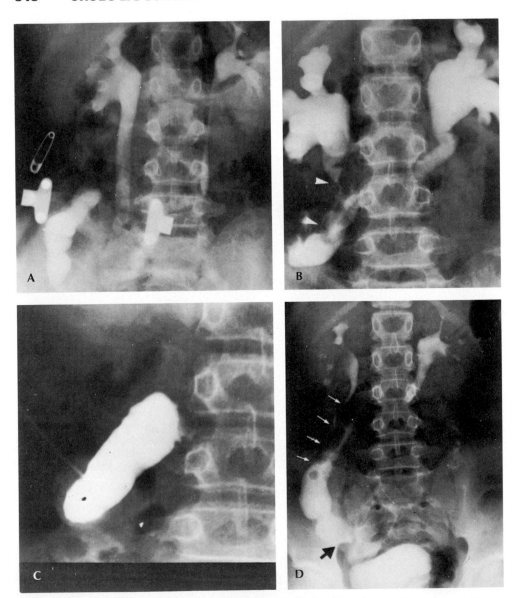

FIG. 53-20. Case 8 roentgenograms. **(A)** An IVP shows dilatation of the right side from ileoureteral reflux. There is no obstruction. **(B)** An IVP 10 days after the colon conduit operation shows edema surrounding the tapered right ureter, which has been implanted into the colon wall. Considerable temporary edema of the left side is also evident, but this receded completely as seen on an IVP 2 months later. Temporary edema in a defunctioned bowel loop creates no problem. If the loop were implanted in the colon with fecal material, this could result in early ascending pyelonephritis. **(C)** Retrograde filling of the loop, tamponading the stoma with a Foley catheter, shows no reflux even at pressures higher than 60 cm of water. It was judged feasible to implant the colon conduit into the rectosigmoid. **(D)** An IVP 2 years after anastomosis of the conduit to the rectosigmoid shows delicate upper tracts. The *small arrows* show the long intramural course of the right ureter in the wall of the conduit. The *large arrow* shows anastomosis of the conduit to the rectosigmoid. (Hendren WH: Urinary diversion and undiversion in children. Surg Clin North Am 56:437, 1976. © 1976, W B Saunders, Philadelphia)

drainage. They should be instructed to watch daily for blood in their combined urine and stool. They should also undergo periodic endoscopic assessment of the lower colon in the region of the ureterosigmoidostomies. It is our belief that the increased incidence of colon carcinoma, although real, should not as an isolated factor mitigate against use of ureterocolic diversion of the urine, when that is the only practical means for removing a bag when the patient has previously undergone cystectomy. Obviously, normal rectal control is a prerequisite for use of ureterocolic "internal diversion" of the urine, which obviates its use in most patients with myelodysplasia.

REFERENCES

1. AHMED S, CARNEY A: Urinary undiversion in myelomeningocele patients with an ileal conduit diversion. J Urol 125:847, 1981
2. ALLEN TD: Undiverting the ileal conduit. J Urol 124:519, 1980
3. BAUER SB, COLODNY AH, HALLET M et al: Urinary undiversion in myelodysplasia: Criteria for selection and predictive value of urodynamic evaluation. J Urol 124:89, 1980
4. CARCASSONNE M, MONFORT G, BENSOUSSAN A et al: Reconstruction of previously diverted urinary tract in children. J Pediatr Surg 10:741, 1975
5. DRETLER SP, HENDREN WH, LEDBETTER WF: Urinary tract reconstruction following ileal conduit diversion. J Urol 109:217, 1973
6. FIRLIT CF, SOMMER JT, KAPLAN WE: Pediatric urinary undiversion. J Urol 123:748, 1980
7. GIL-VERNET JM, JR: The ileocolic segment in urologic surgery. J Urol 94:418, 1965
8. GITTES RF: Bladder augmentation procedure in reconstructive surgery in urology. In Libertino J, Zinman I, (eds): Pediatric and Adult Reconstructive Urologic Surgery. Philadelphia, W B Saunders, 1977
9. GOODWIN WE, WINTER CC, TURNER RD: Replacement of the ureter by small intestine; clinical application and results of the "ileal ureter." J Urol 81:406, 1959
10. HENEY NM, ALTHAUSEN AF, PARKHURST EC: Ileal conduit undiversion: Experience with tunnelled vesical implantation of tapered conduit. J Urol 124:329, 1980
11. HENDREN WH: Reconstruction of previously diverted urinary tracts in children. J Pediatr Surg 8:135, 1973
12. HENDREN WH: Urinary tract refunctionalization after prior diversion in children. Ann Surg 180:494, 1974
13. HENDREN WH: Nonrefluxing colon conduit for temporary or permanent urinary diversion in children. J Pediatr Surg 10:381, 1975
14. HENDREN WH: Refunctionalizing the urinary tract after prior diversion. Contemp Surg, Nov 1975
15. HENDREN WH: Urinary diversion and undiversion in children. Surg Clin North Am 56:425, 1976
16. HENDREN WH: Complications of ureterostomy. J Urol 120:269, 1978
17. HENDREN WH: Some alternatives to urinary diversion in children. J Urol 119:652, 1978
18. HENDREN WH: Tapered bowel segment for ureteral replacement. Urol Clin North Am 5:607, 1978
19. HENDREN WH: Construction of female urethra from vaginal wall and a perineal flap. J Urol 123:657, 1980
20. HENDREN WH: Reoperative ureteral reimplantation: Management of the difficult case. J Pediatr Surg 15:770, 1980
21. HENDREN WH, HENSLE TW: Transureteroureterostomy: Experience with 75 cases. J Urol 123:826, 1980
22. KOGAN SJ, LEVITT SB: Bladder evaluation in pediatric patients before undiversion in previously diverted urinary tracts. J Urol 118:443, 1977
23. LILLY JR, PFISTER RR, PUTNAM CW ET AL: Bench surgery and renal autotransplantation in the pediatric patient. J Pediatr Surg 10:623, 1975
24. MIDDLETON AW, JR, HENDREN WH: Ileal conduits in children at the Massachusetts General Hospital from 1955 to 1970. J Urol 115:591, 1976
25. PERLMUTTER AD: Experiences with urinary undiversion in children with neurogenic bladder. J Urol 123:402, 1980
26. PROUT GR, JR, KOONTZ WW, JR: Partial vesical immobilization: An important adjunct to ureteroneocystostomy. J Urol 103:147, 1970
27. SHAPIRO SR, LEBOWITZ R, COLODNY AH: Fate of 90 children with ileal conduit urinary diversion a decade later: Analysis of complications, pyelography, renal function and bacteriology. J Urol 114:289, 1975
28. SKINNER DG: Secondary urinary reconstruction: Use of the ileocecal segment. J Urol 112:48, 1974
29. SKINNER DG, GOODWIN WE: Indications for the use of intestinal segments in management of nephrocalcinosis. J Urol 113:436, 1975
30. STEWART BH, HEWITT CB, BANOWSKY LHW: Management of extensively destroyed ureter: Special reference to renal autotransplantation. J Urol 115:257, 1976
31. SUNDAR B, MACKIE GG: Urinary undiversion, Montreal Children's Hospital experience. Urology 16:172, 1980
32. TURNER WARWICK R, WORTH PHL: The psoas bladder hitch procedure for the replacement of the lower third of the ureter. J Urol 41:701, 1969
33. UDALL DA, HODGES CV, PEARSE HM et al: Transureteroureterostomy; a neglected procedure. J Urol 109:817, 1973
34. ZINMAN L, LIBERTINO JA: Ileocecal conduit for temporary and permanent urinary diversion. J Urol 113:317, 1975

Cystostomy and Vesicostomy

54

Floyd A. Fried

Surgery of the urinary bladder received its initial impetus in conjunction with treatment of bladder stones, which were more prevalent prior to industrialization than they are now.[6] Reference to the surgical treatment of bladder stone can be found as early as 1400 B.C. in the Hindu Vedas. The lithotomy position, which was devised for perineal lithotomy, was first noted in the 13th century book, *Physicians of Midvay.* Pierre Franco is credited with performing the first "high operation," or suprapubic lithotomy, in 1561. However, the procedure was deemed by Franco as being too dangerous to repeat and was performed as a "last resort." By the 19th century newer methods for exposing the extraperitoneal anterior bladder wall were introduced. Most notable of these techniques was the Peterson colpeurynter, a large, distensible rubber bag which, when placed in the rectum and distended with "a pint," pushed the bladder anteriorly.[3] Guyon's maneuver of "rolling up" the perivesical fat together with the peritoneum and pushing these to the superior end of the wound became a popular practice and prevented entry into the peritoneal cavity. By the end of the 19th century the high operation was clearly indicated for the treatment of bladder stones that were too hard or too large for lithotrity.[7]

Anatomic Considerations

Excellent anatomic reviews of the bladder can be found elsewhere.[2,8,9] This discussion represents a summation of anatomic points that are relevant to the urologic surgeon.

The bladder is an extraperitoneal organ. In infants it is relatively more cephalad in position. Growth of the pelvic bones permits the bladder to descend to its adult intrapelvic location. In adults the superior surface is covered by the pelvic reflection of the peritoneum, which extends a short distance over the posterior aspect of the bladder. The anterior surface of the bladder is largely devoid of peritoneum except for the most superior aspect, which may be partly covered by it. The anteroinferior surface is devoid of peritoneum and is in relation to the pubis and anterior abdominal wall (Retzius space). In the male, the inferior surface of the bladder is in contact with the prostate gland and the posterior surface is separated from the rectum by the rectovesical space. In the female, the posterior aspect of the bladder is closely related to the uterus and upper vagina. In the empty state the fundus of the uterus rests upon the superior bladder surface.

The superior limit of the bladder is attached to the umbilicus by the middle umbilical ligament which is the urachal remnant. Inferiorly, the base of the bladder is moored to the deep fascia reflected over the pubic bone in the female, which forms the pubovesical ligaments. In the male, the prostate occupies this area and the reflected fascia from the pubic bones forms the puboprostatic ligaments through which passes the dorsal vein of the penis. Posteriorly, the bladder is attached to the sides of the rectum and sacrum by the rectovesical ligaments and fascia (Denonvilliers). This layer is a clinically important landmark in the performance of perineal prostatectomy. Denonvilliers' fascia also forms a barrier to contain extravasated urine and often prevents against the direct extension of prostatic and rectal tumors. Laterally, the lateral vesical ligaments anchor the base of the bladder to the levator ani muscles and the lateral pelvic wall. These ligaments contain the inferior vesical and vesicodeferential arteries, the vasa deferentia, the pudendal venous plexus, and the vesical neural plexus. They are understandably referred to as the neurovascular pedicle of the bladder.

The epithelial lining of the bladder is of the transitional variety, which is particularly well suited to the function of the bladder. The mucosa is attached to a layer of areolar tissue which permits the formation of folds in its contracted state. Deep to the submucosa areolar layer are a series of smooth muscle layers which are difficult to discern in the operating room. It is believed that the outermost fibers arise from the posterior surface of the body of the pubis, the adjacent prostate, and the capsule. These muscle fibers pass superiorly in a predominantly longitudinal fashion and form the detrusor muscle. A middle circular layer predominantly oriented transversely spirals inferiorly to the bladder base, where they are deposited in a circular fashion and continue with the muscular fibers of the prostate forming the vesical sphincter. The innermost layer of muscle takes a predominantly longitudinal direction. Bell's muscle is a band of muscle fibers emanating from the ureters and inserting on the posterior aspect of the prostate.

The arterial supply of the bladder comes from the paired superior, middle, and inferior vesical arteries, which branch from the internal iliac arteries. Small variable branches may come from the inferior gluteal and obturator arteries. In the female, other vessels may arise from the uterine and vaginal arteries. The venous drainage is by way of a plexus at the posterior inferior surface, in close relation to the prostate, which empties into the internal iliac veins. The lymphatic drainage is to the external, internal, and sacral nodes. The motor innervation arises from the second, third, and fourth sacral roots of the parasympathetic nervous system reaching the bladder by way of the pelvic nerve. Sympathetic innervation arises from the L1, L2, and L3 by way of the hypogastric nerve.

Indications

Urinary diversion at the vesical level can be conveniently categorized as intubated (cystostomy) and unintubated (vesicostomy). Intubated vesical diversion is indicated in a wide range of clinical situations such as urinary retention, either secondary to an impassable urethral stricture or in a patient with bladder neck obstruction whose general condition prevents immediate prostatic surgery. Cystostomy is also advocated in patients with certain types of bladder and urethral trauma. Its use as a means of long-term diversion in the spinal-cord-injured patient is, as are other forms of urinary diversion, being supplanted by pharmacologic and nonoperative means of management such as intermittent catheterization. The use of tubeless vesical diversion is helpful in the temporary management of infants with bladder-emptying problems associated with hydronephrosis and reflux.

Both vesicostomy and cystostomy have advantages and limitations, and the selection of the proper vesical diversion should be given careful consideration. When the general condition of the patient prevents any but the simplest of procedures, a cystostomy is appropriate. If the patient is stable and a longer-term period of bladder drainage is planned, a tubeless vesicostomy may be a better choice.

Insofar as possible, the functional state of the bladder should be considered. It is advisable, if possible, to first perform cystoscopy to look for clinically unsuspected lesions which may contraindicate the diversion procedure. If clinical evidence of infection is present, then the procedure should be performed under antibiotic coverage. The procedure of trocar cystostomy is contraindicated in patients with prior pelvic surgery and in small or empty bladders unless concomitant cystoscopic guidance is used.

Procedures

SUPRAPUBIC CYSTOSTOMY

Suprapubic cystostomy is indicated in situations in which effective urinary drainage is needed above the bladder neck. It is frequently performed in conjunction with other surgical procedures of the lower urinary tract and bladder, such as hypospadias repair, ureteral reimplantation, suprapubic prostatectomy, and repair of ruptured bladder. Simple cystostomy is also useful performed by itself as a means of draining an obstructed bladder.

If done by itself the procedure should be performed using a small 4-cm to 5-cm incision. A transverse incision is made 3 cm to 4 cm above the symphysis pubis (Fig. 54-1). After filling the bladder with sterile irrigating fluid, the incision is carried down to the anterior fascia of the rectus muscles. The fascial surface is cleaned of adipose tissue with a Kittner dissector, and a transverse fascial incision is made. The upper and lower fascial leaves are elevated from the body of the muscle to facilitate closure. The rectus abdominus muscles are separated at the midline by blunt dissection and retracted laterally, exposing the perivesical space. If the bladder is distended it should be easily palpable through the perivesical fascia.

The peritoneum should be identified and a vertical midline incision made in the perivesical fascia below the peritoneum. The peritoneum is dissected from the anterior wall of the bladder and retracted cephalad. This is easily accomplished with a sponge. The dissection should be limited to include only the area needed to open the bladder. More extensive peritoneal mobilization may result in infection or create pockets in which extravasated urine may become trapped. The bladder wall is examined for obvious vessels in the proposed line

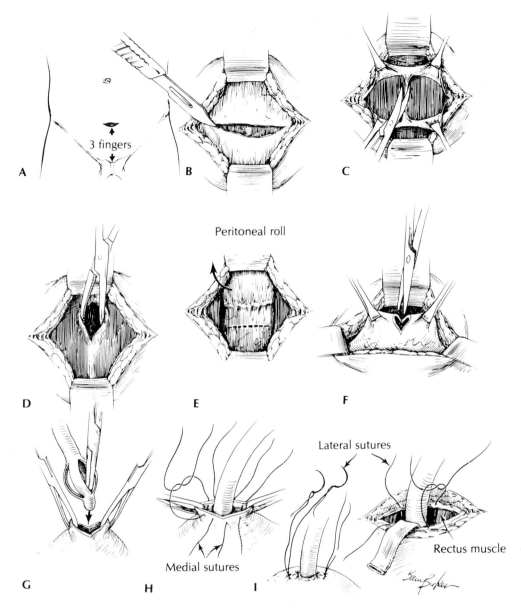

FIG. 54-1. Suprapubic cystostomy. **(A)** A small, high, transverse suprapubic incision is used. **(B)** The anterior rectus sheath is incised and retracted. **(C)** The rectus muscles are exposed. **(D)** The rectus muscles are separated at the midline. **(E)** The peritoneal roll is displaced upward, and the prevesical fascia is incised to expose the bladder. **(F)** The dome of the bladder is incised. **(G)** A Malecot catheter is inserted. **(H)** Medial sutures are placed very snugly around the catheter. **(I)** Lateral sutures are retained and passed through the anterior fascia, fixing the bladder anteriorly.

of incision. These can be lightly fulgurated prior to opening the bladder. If the operator is uncertain about the location of the bladder, aspiration with a 20-gauge needle is helpful.

The anterior bladder wall is grasped on either side of the midline with Allis clamps and a 2-cm to 3-cm incision is made between the clamps. The

Allis clamps should be repositioned after opening into the lumen of the bladder so that they now grasp the full bladder wall, including the epithelium. If more extensive intravesical surgery is planned, bladder-holding sutures of 2-0 or 3-0 chromic should be used in place of the Allis clamps to minimize trauma to the bladder wall. The bladder contents are aspirated and a 24Fr to 28Fr Silastic Malecot catheter with its flanges straightened by stretching the tip over a hemostat is introduced into the bladder. The catheter should exit from the superior aspect of the bladder incision, care being taken that the tip of it is not touching the trigone because this can provoke painful bladder spasms. The bladder should be closed snugly around the Malecot catheter with 2-0 chromic. The catheter should be irrigated to evacuate any blood clots in the bladder, to check the watertightness of the closure, and to ensure that the catheter is properly positioned within the bladder.

The suprapubic tube should be brought out by a separate stab wound 2 cm to 3 cm above the incision. A Penrose drain can be brought out through one end of the incision or through an additional stab wound. The rectus fascia is then closed with interrupted 2-0 chromic or polyglycolic acid sutures. The subcutaneous tissue is closed with interrupted 3-0 absorbable suture and the skin with 3-0 nonabsorbable suture of silk or nylon. The suprapubic tube must be adequately secured. This can be accomplished by using a 1-0 silk suture through the skin close to the exit site of the tube and tied around the catheter. The Penrose drain can usually be removed by the first postoperative day.

TROCAR CYSTOSTOMY

The trocar cystostomy, for inserting a suprapubic catheter, is easily performed and can be done at the bedside after local infiltration with lidocaine. It is a simple and effective method of diverting children undergoing hypospadias repair. It is contraindicated in patients who have had previous pelvic surgery, because loops of bowel adherent to the bladder may be inadvertently punctured. This procedure should be performed on patients with distended urinary bladders. It is often helpful to have cystoscopic visualization of the bladder during trocar insertion; this is especially important in the defunctionalized bladder. If there is any question concerning bladder distention in a patient with an impassable urethra, the procedure can be done with ultrasound monitoring.

A site 2 cm above the symphysis and in the midline should be suitably prepped. After making a 0.5-cm incision in the skin and rectus fascia, the trocar with the obturator in place is aimed posteriorly and pushed through the abdominal wall into the bladder lumen (Fig. 54-2). Removal fo the obturator should result in urine or previously instilled fluid flowing from the trocar. The catheter

of the proper size must be on hand and ready to use and is passed through the lumen of the trocar before the bladder is emptied of fluid. The retention balloon is inflated and the trocar is removed. Other options include the use of the Silastic "cystocath" or the trocar Malecot catheter set. The suprapubic catheter is secured as already described.

BLOCKSOM'S VESICOSTOMY

Blocksom's vesicostomy, first described in 1957, remains a simple and useful means of providing temporary unintubated bladder drainage.[1] Its virtues include its ease of performance and its ease of closure. Complications include stomal stenosis and bladder prolapse through the stoma.

Prior to surgery the site of the vesicostomy stoma should be selected, ideally in an area devoid of skin folds when the patient is in the sitting position. The bladder should be filled with approximately 300 ml of sterile water. A midline incision is made 3 finger-widths above the symphysis pubis (Fig. 54-3). The anterior rectus fascia is incised in the midline and the rectus abdominus muscles are retracted laterally, exposing the perivesical space. The perivesical fascia is incised and swept away from the midline of the bladder. The peritoneal reflection should be bluntly dissected from the anterior bladder wall and retracted cephalad. The bladder is entered through a high midline stab incision. The operator inserts an index finger into the bladder, elevating the bladder to the area of the abdominal wall previously selected to be the site of the stoma. In large bladders this is easily accomplished, but smaller bladders may require some blunt dissection of the surrounding bladder wall. The most superior portion of the bladder wall freed of peritoneum as it passes through the separated rectus muscles is sutured to the edges of the rectus fascia with interrupted suture of 2-0 chromic. Some authors recommend removing an ellipse of fascia. The margins of the bladder are sutured circumferentially to the skin. The completed stoma should easily admit an index finger. A sterile appliance can be fitted in the operating room at the end of the procedure.

LAPIDES VESICOSTOMY

Lapides described a vesicostomy procedure in 1960.[4] The main indication is for long-term vesical diversion in patients with neurogenic bladder dysfunction in whom bladder rehabilitative programs have failed. It was devised to resolve two problems encountered with Blocksom's procedure: the dif-

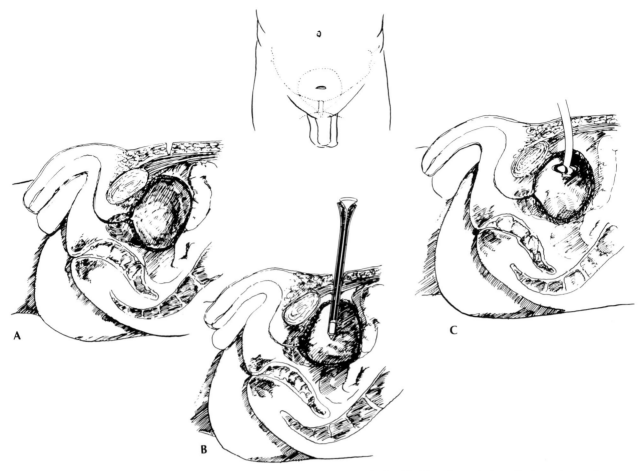

FIG. 54-2. Trocar cystostomy. **(A)** With the bladder distended to displace the peritoneum superiorly, an incision is made 2 cm above the symphysis. **(B)** The trocar with obturator is inserted directly into the bladder lumen. **(C)** The obturator is removed and an appropriate catheter is inserted through the lumen of the trocar.

ficulty of achieving adequate elevation of the bladder to the skin of the anterior abdominal wall and the occurrence of stricture at the vesicocutaneous anastomosis.[5] In Lapides's procedure, the difficulty of approximating the bladder to the skin is obviated by creating a flap of anterior bladder wall which is rotated upward to the abdominal wall. The tendency for stricture of the stoma is alleviated by forming a skin flap turned downward to the bladder defect, resulting in a vesicocutaneous channel.

The procedure is performed with the patient in the supine position. The bladder should first be filled with approximately 300 ml of fluid. A 10-cm to 12-cm transverse incision is made 3 cm to 4 cm above the symphysis pubis (Fig. 54-4A). The anterior rectus fascia is opened transversely and elevated from the underlying rectus muscles to the level fo the umbilicus. A skin flap measuring 3.2 cm at its base and 3.2 cm in length is planned so that the base of the flap is situated halfway between the incision and the umbilicus. It is important that the rectus fascia be pulled down to its original location prior to creating the flap. This is accomplished by grasping the fascia with Allis forceps and clasping it to the skin edges. After incising the skin and subcutaneous tissues, the flap is elevated from the anterior rectus fascia. A segment of rectus fascia thus exposed is excised. Excision of the posterior rectus fascia may also be necessary to create an unobstructed defect.

The bladder is next exposed through the previously made incision. The peritoneum is reflected superiorly. With the bladder filled with 300 ml, a flap of anterior bladder wall measuring 4 cm by 4 cm based superiorly is outlined (Fig. 54-4B). The outline of the vesical flap should be done with

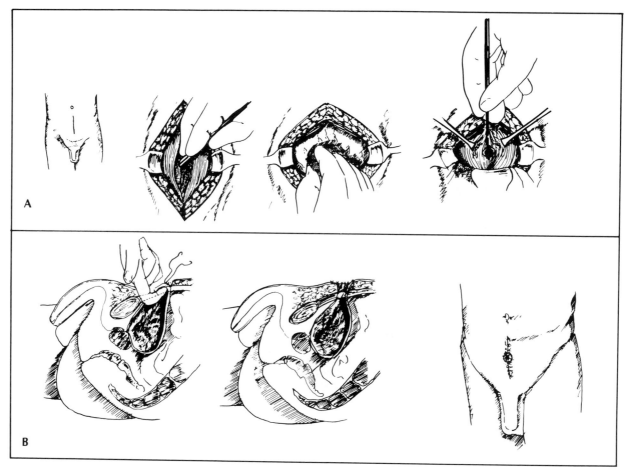

FIG. 54-3. Blocksom's vesicostomy. **(A)** A vertical midline incision is made, the recti are separated, the bladder is exposed, and a small incision is made through the bladder wall. **(B)** With a finger in the vesicostomy opening, the bladder wall is brought up to the abdominal wall and sutured in all diameters, creating a cutaneous vesicostomy.

sutures, because collapse of the bladder will make it difficult to adhere to the proper dimensions. Holding sutures of 3-0 chromic are placed in the end of the bladder flap. A hemostat passed through the skin flap defect is used to grasp the holding sutures, and the bladder flap is drawn through the abdominal wall defect. The end of the flap is anastomosed to the inverted-U skin margin with interrupted 2-0 chromic sutures. Using an Allis clamp passed from the inside to the outside through the skin flap defect, the end of the skin flap is grasped and pulled downward through the defect so that the skin surface of the skin flap faces the mucosal surface of the bladder flap. The adjacent margins of the skin and bladder flaps are approximated with interrupted sutures of 2-0 or 3-0 chromic. The remaining bladder defect is closed by approximating the edges in the midline (Fig. 54-4C).

At the conclusion of the procedure the stoma should admit a finger. There should be no tissue margins encroaching upon the lumen. If margins of fascia are palpated they should be incised. The perivesical space is drained with a Penrose drain, and the incision is closed with interrupted absorbable suture. The stoma is dressed with Vaseline gauze. Temporary bladder drainage should be accomplished with a urethral catheter. After the first few days a suitable ostomy appliance can be used.

Postoperative Care

In patients with suprapubic cystostomies care must be taken to adequately secure the catheter. Malfunction of the catheter should raise the suspicion of dislodgement from the bladder, and an immediate x-ray study should be obtained after intro-

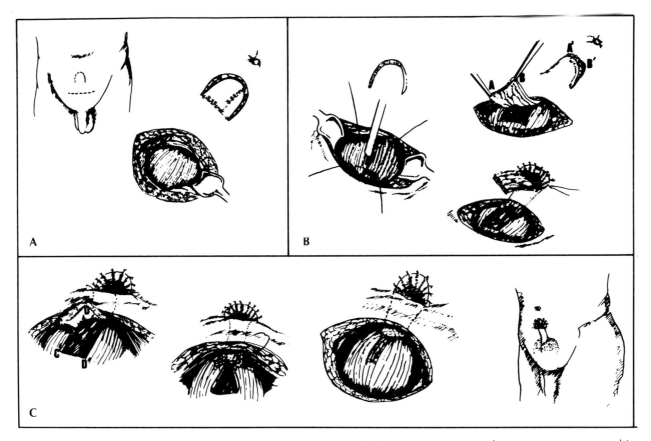

FIG. 54-4. Lapides's vesicostomy. **(A)** Two incisions are made, a transverse suprapubic incision and a horseshoe incision through the skin midway to the umbilicus. **(B)** Incision of the bladder wall creates a flap which is then brought up through the superior incision. **(C)** The skin flap is depressed inferiorly and thus a vesicostomy tube is created, composed of both skin and bladder wall.

ducing contrast media through the suprapubic catheter. The suprapubic catheter should not be changed until the third or fourth postoperative week, thereby allowing for the formation of a fibrous tract around the catheter. Patients with vesicostomy can usually have a sterile urinary appliance placed over the stoma at the conclusion fo the operative procedure. The patient and appropriate members of the family should be instructed in the care of the catheter or appliance prior to discharge.

REFERENCES

1. BLOCKSOM BH JR: Bladder pouch for prolonged tubeless cystostomy. J Urol 78:398, 1957
2. GOSS CM (ed): Gray's Anatomy of the Human Body, 28th ed. Lea Febiger, Philadelphia, 1966
3. KEYES EL: The Surgical Diseases of the Genito-urinary Organs Including Syphilis, p. 312, New York, D Appleton, 1892
4. LAPIDES J, AJEMIAN EP, LICHTWARDT JR: Cutaneous vesicostomy. J Urol 84:609, 1960
5. RINKER RJ, CAFFREY EL, WITHERINGTON R: Use of bladder pouch for tubeless drainage in permanent incontinence. J Urol 81:136, 1959
6. SUTOR DJ: The nature of urinary stones. In Finlayson B, Hench LL, Smith LH (eds): Urolithiasis: Physical Aspects p 43. Washington, DC, National Academy of Sciences, 1972
7. WHITE JW, MARTIN E: Genito-urinary surgery and venereal diseases, 4th ed, p 706. Philadelphia, JB Lippincott, 1900
8. WOODBURNE RT: Structure and function of the urinary bladder. J Urol 84:79, 1960
9. WOODBURNE RT: The ureter, ureterovesical junction and vesical trigone. Anat Rec 151:243, 1965

Vesical Diverticulectomy

55

Matthew S. Smith

A vesical diverticulum is a circumscribed sac of variable size which results from the herniation of bladder mucosa through the muscular wall of the bladder. Occasionally, histologic examination will demonstrate the presence of a variable amount of smooth muscle within the diverticular wall. These muscle bundles have been dragged along by the protruding mucosa and are most commonly seen in children with congenital lesions. A chronic inflammatory cell infiltrate secondary to urinary stasis and infection is often present in the wall of the diverticulum. A thick outer layer of fibrous tissue is often noted and is related to the degree of inflammation and the length of time the diverticulum has been present.

Bladder diverticula usually become manifest in either the first or seventh decades of life and can be either acquired or congenital. Acquired diverticula are secondary to lower urinary tract obstruction and can be seen in both adults and children. In the adult population, bladder diverticula are more commonly seen in men and are usually secondary to bladder outlet obstruction from either benign prostatic hyperplasia or urethral stricture disease. In children, acquired diverticula can result from anatomic obstruction (urethral valves, congenital urethral stricture, *etc.*) or functional obstruction as seen in patients with neurogenic bladder disease. A subset of the latter group includes patients with enuresis who have high intravesical tension secondary to incomplete bladder inhibition as a result of delayed neurologic maturation. Chronic high intravesical pressure due to distal obstruction results in bladder muscle hypertrophy. Cellules of bladder mucosa form between these thickened interlacing muscle bundles and, with time, these areas of mucosa protrude through the muscular wall to be diverticula of variable size. Acquired diverticula are often multiple in location.

Congenital diverticula are often large and solitary and are seen in the absence of bladder hypertrophy and trabeculation. The majority of bladder diverticula in children are not secondary to distal obstruction or neurologic disease but are due to a fetal developmental defect.[5] This has been substantiated by fluoroscopic voiding cystourethrograms[9] and by the documentation of normal voiding pressures in the absence of bladder trabeculation on cystoscopic examination.[7] Williams and Eckstein could demonstrate no evidence of infravesical obstruction in 23 of 49 children examined with bladder diverticula.[16] King noted that 50% of bladder diverticula in children were not associated with lower urinary tract obstruction.[7]

Congenital diverticula are usually located at or near the corner of the trigone immediately superior to the ureteral orifice. Decreased muscular development at the ureterovesical junction occurs as a result of the interface of trigone and detrusor musculature, which have different embryologic origins. This results in a weak hiatus through which bladder mucosa can herniate at normal voiding pressures. The presence of a supernumerary ureteral bud has been advanced as another explanation for solitary congenital lesions.

Evaluation and Presentation

Bladder diverticula are usually discovered during the evaluation of chronic lower urinary tract infection, incomplete bladder emptying, or bladder outlet obstruction. Excretory urography and voiding cystourethrography with anteroposterior, lateral, oblique, and drainage films are necessary as part of the initial evaluation. It has been reported that 80% of diverticula can be missed with excretory urography alone.[9] Cystoscopic examination of all bladder diverticula should be performed, and urine cytology specimens should be evaluated.

Ureters that enter a diverticulum often reflux. As the diverticulum initially forms in the vicinity of the ureterovesical junction, it can pull the ureteral orifice to an extravesical position and deprive it of its normal muscular backing, thus allowing it to reflux. Bladder diverticula can cause ipsilateral and contralateral hydroureteronephrosis from either ureteral compression or incomplete bladder emptying. Posterior urethral and rectal obstruction have also been reported from large bladder diverticula.[14]

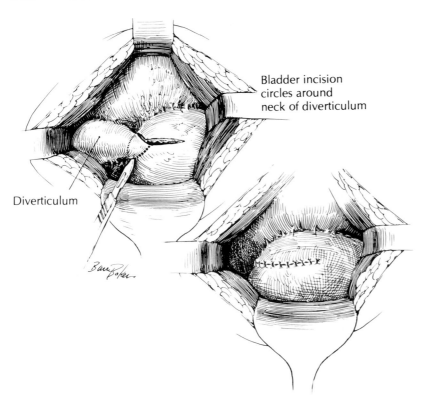

Diverticulum

Bladder incision
circles around
neck of diverticulum

FIG. 55-1. Extravesical diverticulectomy. It may or may not be necessary to open the bladder proper for exposure.

Bladder diverticula can give rise to multiple other urologic problems. Poorly emptying diverticula can be a source of chronic infection and stone formation. Ineffective bladder emptying can occur secondary to preferential filling of the bladder diverticulum during voiding, leading to high postvoid residuals and urinary frequency. A high incidence of bladder carcinoma in diverticula, ranging from 2% to 7% in various reports with an overall incidence of 3.6% noted by Peterson, makes the periodic inspection and treatment of bladder diverticula mandatory.[1,6,8,12] The presence of stagnant urine allows urinary carcinogens to complete hydrolysis and promotes chronic mucosal irritation secondary to infection and calculus formation. These factors predispose the urothelium to malignant degeneration. Squamous metaplasia is often seen,[12] and an increased incidence of squamous cell carcinoma has been noted.[6] Because these tumors are often of high grade and lack the protective backing of bladder musculature, bladder carcinomas arising in diverticula will readily spread into perivesical tissue and are associated with a high mortality rate. The prophylactic removal of all bladder diverticula with wide excision of surrounding bladder wall has been recommended.[6] At the very least, periodic cystoscopic inspection of all diverticula is necessary and, if neoplasia is

noted, preoperative irradiation, wide surgical excision, and unilateral node dissection should be performed. Transurethral biopsy is contraindicated.

In summary, surgery is indicated when the diverticula have small mouths and do not empty with voiding, when chronic infection or stone is present, when neoplasia is present, or when the diverticulum cannot be explored cystoscopically. In all cases of acquired bladder diverticula, it is necessary to identify and treat the cause of bladder outlet obstruction.

Surgical Technique

In 1849, Rokitansky first noted that bladder diverticula resulted from urethral obstruction.[13] Both Alexander (1884) and Czerny (1896) are credited with performing the first extravesical excisions of bladder diverticula during the latter part of the 19th century.[2,3] Hugh Hampton Young used suction to perform an intravesical inversion and excision of a diverticular sac during the early 1900s,[17] and, since that time, the intravesical inversion technique has been modified several times. In 1912, Lerche inserted a balloon attached to a ureteral catheter transurethrally to aid in the extravesical dissection of bladder diverticula.[10] Ten years later

FIG. 55-2. In intravesical inversion diverticulectomy, excision of the mucosal sac and approximation of the detrusor are followed by mucosal closure.

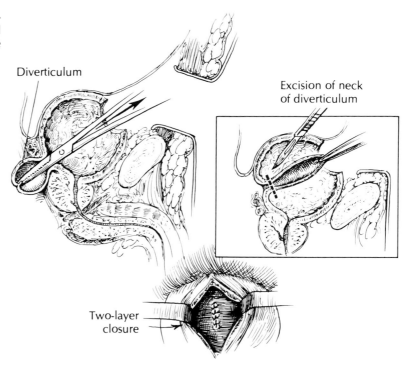

Diverticulum

Excision of neck of diverticulum

Two-layer closure

Geraghty recognized that a diverticulum was composed of an inner mucosal layer and an outer fibrous layer and that removal of the mucosa alone would allow obliteration of the fibrous sac.[4]

As with all major surgical procedures, preoperative preparation of the patient is important. In the past, vesical diverticulectomy has been associated with a high degree of morbidity. It is therefore imperative to treat urinary tract infection vigorously, to maximize renal function, and to correct other metabolic problems prior to surgery. In addition, perioperative antibiotics are required to reduce morbidity in vesical diverticulectomy.

The open surgical treatment of bladder diverticula can involve either an extravesical or intravesical approach, or a combination of both. Small diverticula are best handled by intravesical surgery, and large diverticula are best dealt with by either an extravesical or a combined approach.

The initial step in vesical diverticulectomy involves insertion of a Foley catheter and inflation of the bladder and diverticula with sterile normal saline. A routine midline (from pubic symphysis to umbilicus) or Pfannenstiel incision is then performed. The rectus muscles can be divided if additional exposure is needed. The peritoneum is swept cephalad, the perivesical retroperitoneal space is developed, and the anterior wall of the bladder is cleaned of fibroareolar tissue. A self-retaining retractor is then inserted.

In the extravesical approach (Fig. 55-1), the distended diverticulum is bluntly and sharply dissected free from the surrounding pelvic structures. The neck of the diverticulum is completely circumscribed at the level of the bladder and amputated. The diverticular sac is then removed. The bladder defect is closed in two layers. A running suture of 3-0 chromic catgut is used on the mucosa, and running 2-0 chromic catgut is used to close the muscularis-serosal layer. A ⅝ or GU needle often facilitates the mucosal closure. A large suprapubic tube (24Fr–26Fr) is brought out through a separate stab wound on the anterosuperior aspect of the bladder, secured with a pursestring suture of chromic catgut, and left in place for 7 to 10 days. Penrose drains are left perivesically and within the diverticular bed for 3 to 10 days.

If the diverticulum is located adjacent to or contiguous with a ureter, the bladder must be opened. A routine vertical cystotomy incision or an incision in the direction of the diverticulum is then made on the anterior bladder wall. The bladder contents are evacuated and a 5Fr ureteral catheter is passed up the ureter. For a large diverticulum, extravesical mobilization is begun after the diverticular cavity is distended with gauze packing, with a large Foley catheter balloon (secured at the mouth of the diverticulum with a pursestring suture),[6] or by the insertion of a finger in the manner of a hernia-sac excision. These

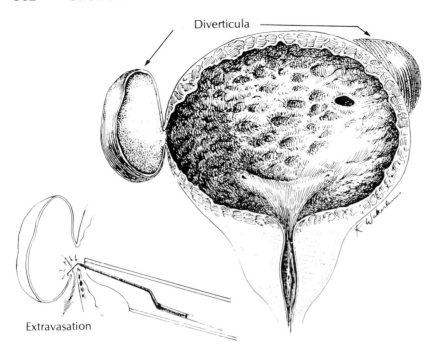

Diverticula

Extravasation

FIG. 55-3. Resection of the neck of the diverticulum of the bladder. Perforation and extravasation may result on rare occasion.

methods will help to prevent shredding of the diverticulum and to facilitate the dissection. The diverticulum composed of mucosa and surrounding fibrous tissue can then be mobilized and removed in its entirety and the bladder closed as previously described. If the diverticulum is adherent to surrounding tissue and not readily freed, one need only expose the anterior surface of the diverticulum, open it, and remove the inner lining of mucosa. This can be accomplished by a continuation of the initial cystotomy incision into the mouth and along the exposed surface of the diverticulum or by a separate extravesical incision into the diverticular cavity. The bladder is then closed in standard fashion and the fibrous lining of the diverticular bed is drained to the abdominal surface with a Penrose drain. Suprapubic catheter drainage is then used for 7 to 10 days.

If the diverticulum is small, a purely intravesical approach can be used (Fig. 55-2). After the initial vertical cystotomy incision, an Allis clamp is passed through the mouth of the diverticulum and the most extravesical portion of the diverticular wall is grasped and inverted into the bladder cavity. The whole diverticulum can then be amputated at its neck and the bladder closed in two layers. This method carries the risk of injury to adjacent structures which may be adherent to the fibrous covering. Alternatively, only the lining mucosa of the diverticulum need be removed, leaving the fibrous shell *in situ* and thus protecting the surrounding

viscera. This can be accomplished by circumscribing the bladder mucosa at the mouth of the diverticulum with a hot knife and placing circumferential silk holding sutures through the mucosa of the diverticulum.[4] Using scissor dissection, the mucosa is then freed from the overlying fibrous layer and the bladder defect is closed in two layers. The remaining fibrous cavity will spontaneously obliterate during the healing period. A urethral or suprapubic catheter is left to straight drainage for 7 days. A perivesical Penrose drain is optional.

In high-risk surgical patients with poorly emptying bladder diverticula, a circumferential transurethral diverticulotomy can be performed.[15] Very often the mouth of the diverticulum is surrounded by hypertrophied bundles of smooth muscle which act as a sphincter during voiding. Few reports of extravasation with this method have been noted (Fig. 55-3).

A recently described technique for management of bladder diverticula is the transurethral fulguration of the entire diverticular wall with the electrocautery.[11] Pure coagulation current is used. This method has been reported to shrink or obliterate bladder diverticula in 14 out of 17 cases.

It is often necessary to do a ureteral reimplantation when managing bladder diverticula that are intimately associated with the ureter. If the preoperative evaluation shows absent to markedly decreased ipsilateral renal function, a nephroureterectomy is indicated.

REFERENCES

1. ABESHOUSE BS, GOLDSTEIN AE: Primary carcinoma in a diverticulum of the bladder: A report of four cases and a review of the literature. J Urol 49:534, 1943

2. ESHO JO, CASS AS: Bladder diverticulectomy with aid of inflated Foley balloon catheter. Urology 3:38, 1974

3. FIRSTATER M, FARKAS A: Transvesical submucosal diverticulectomy: Experience with 48 cases. Urology 10:436, 1977

4. GERAGHTY JT: A simple procedure for the radical cure of large vesical diverticula. South Med J 15:54, 1922

5. JOHNSTON JH: Vesical diverticula without urinary obstruction in childhood. J Urol 84:535, 1960

6. KELALIS PP, MCLEAN P: The treatment of diverticulum of the bladder. J Urol 98:349, 1967

7. KING LR: Observations on vesical diverticulum in childhood. J Urol 116:235, 1976

8. KNAPPENBERGER ST, USON AC, MELICOW MM: Primary neoplasms occurring in vesical diverticula: A report of 18 cases. J Urol 83:153, 1960

9. LEBOWITZ RL, COLODNY AH, CRISSEY M: Neonatal hydronephrosis caused by vesical diverticula. Urol 13:335, 1979

10. LERCHE W: The surgical treatment of diverticulum of the urinary bladder. Ann Surg 55:285, 1912

11. ORANDI A: Transurethral fulguration of bladder diverticulum. New procedure. Urology 10:30, 1977

12. PETERSON LJ, PAULSON DF, GLENN JF: The histopathology of vesical diverticula. J Urol 110:62, 1973

13. ROKITANSKY K: A Manual of Pathological Anatomy, Vol 2, p 220. London, Sydenham Society, 1849

14. TAYLOR WN, ALTON D, TOGURI A et al: Bladder diverticula causing posterior urethral obstruction in children. J Urol 122:415, 1979

15. VITALE PJ, WOODSIDE JR: Management of bladder diverticula by transurethral resection: Re-evaluation of an old technique. J Urol 122:744, 1979

16. WILLIAMS DI, ECKSTEIN HB: Bladder disorders: Diverticula. In Williams DI (ed): Pediatric Urology, p 213. London, Butterworth, 1968

17. YOUNG HH: Young's Practice of Urology, Vol 2, p 338. Philadelphia, W B Saunders, 1926

Partial Cystectomy and Simple Cystectomy

56

William Brannan

Partial Cystectomy

Partial resection of the bladder has been an accepted modality in the treatment of transitional cell carcinoma for many years.[3,5,10] This approach has been advocated by several authors, each reporting variable success in survival and recurrence rates.[2,3,5,7,8,14] Others have espoused caution in choosing this form of treatment because of the relatively higher recurrence rate with which it is associated.[6]

INDICATIONS AND CONTRAINDICATIONS

If segmental resection is to prove successful as a treatment for primary transitional cell carcinoma, the physician must exercise strict patient selection and adhere to certain basic principles when choosing candidates for this procedure. First the lesion should be a solitary one; multiple lesions indicate a field change within the bladder mucosa and suggest that the involved bladder will continue to show neoplastic changes later in other areas. Second, the lesion should be a primary one—that is, restricted to the initial diagnosis of carcinoma of the bladder—because recurrent tumors usually continue to exhibit recurrences in other areas of the bladder mucosa. Third, the tumor should be one that cannot be removed transurethrally. This decision depends upon the ability of the particular surgeon and his experience in resecting bladder tumors transurethrally; it also depends upon the depth to which one can resect as well as the accessibility of the tumor.[13] Relatively low-grade lesions occasionally lie in the dome of the bladder and may coexist with some fixation of the prostatic urethra. Obesity may compound the difficulty in reaching relatively inaccessible areas. One may not feel confident about having removed such tumors in their entirety. Thus, very few low-grade noninvasive tumors can be handled to advantage with partial cystectomy.[12,14]

Invasive tumors (*i.e.,* B-2 or C lesions) may be appropriate candidates for partial cystectomy if they are primary tumors.[2,5] However, partial cystectomy must be reserved for the patient who has a documented residual tumor in the muscle at the base of the initial neoplasm on rebiopsy 6 to 8 weeks later. Our custom is to remove as much tumor as possible plus its underlying base at an initial transurethral resection. If deep muscle bites indicate muscle invasion, a rebiopsy is performed approximately 8 weeks postoperatively. At this time we take even deeper and wider pieces of tissue from the previously involved area. If a residual tumor is found within this deep muscle, these patients then become candidates for either partial or radical cystectomy. If the neoplasm is well localized and primary, the rate of survival for removing the involved area and a minimum of 2 cm of surrounding bladder should be the same as one would expect from removing the entire bladder. If one feels confident at the initial procedure that there is residual tumor, a waiting period with rebiopsy is unnecessary. Tumors that occur in a vesical diverticulum are at higher risks from penetration because most vesical diverticula are devoid of muscle fibers; one should proceed immediately to segmental resection of the bladder that includes a wide margin around the vesical diverticulum.

Certain patients who are poor operative risks because of pulmonary or cardiovascular disease and who might ordinarily be selected for radical cystectomy may be candidates for partial cystectomy, because the mortality from the latter procedure is quite low. However, this indication is becoming less supportable as the mortality rate from cystectomy steadily declines owing to better anesthesia, pre- and postoperative monitoring, and paraoperative care.

There are certain contraindications to partial cystectomy which must be recognized. Recurrent or multiple tumors should not be treated by partial resection. Tumors located so close to both ureteral orifices or the bladder neck that they prevent one from obtaining at least a 2-cm margin around the tumor are not candidates. The exception may be in male patients, if one is able to enucleate the prostate and resect a wide portion of the prostatic capsule and adjacent bladder neck for a tumor lying reasonably close to the trigone and the bladder neck. Invasion of the tumor into the prostatic urethra, however, should be an indication for more radical surgery. Tumors involving or lying close to one ureteral orifice can be managed by partial resection and reimplantation of the ipsilateral ureter if the other criteria are met. Tumors that involve obvious field change in the bladder, for example, carcinoma *in situ* and recurring or multiple high- or low-grade lesions, cannot be expected to respond to this therapy. Stage D disease is a contraindication for this therapy, as it is for most cases in which radical cystectomy is planned.

Bladders that can be anticipated to have a very poor capacity following partial removal are poor candidates for segmental resection. This group includes those patients in whom a neoplasm may require so extensive a resection that the residual bladder cannot be functional postoperatively and those in whom high doses of irradiation or other causative factors may preclude a functional bladder. Postoperatively, high-dose irradiation may also interfere with proper healing; therefore, one must use extreme caution in using this procedure as a salvage maneuver. Bush indicates that one can consider using some type of augmentation procedure together with a partial cystectomy only when high-dose preoperative irradiation has been avoided.[3]

OPERATIVE TECHNIQUE

The surgeon should approach segmental cystectomy much as he does radical cystectomy. He must obtain as wide a dissection as possible, beginning first with evaluation of the regional lymph nodes. Selective node biopsies or even unilateral pelvic node dissection should accompany this procedure. If positive nodes are found, one must reexamine the selection of this treatment unless it is assumed to be entirely palliative.

In most instances, the peritoneum and perivesical fat should not be disturbed, making this a transperitoneal approach (Fig. 56-1A). The perivesical dissection should be completed before opening the bladder; one may, however, elect to perform a combined maneuver when resecting neoplasms which involve the trigone or one ureteral orifice. If the tumor lies close to the trigone on one side or along the lateral wall, it may be helpful to ligate the superior vesical artery initially as one evaluates the pelvic nodes on that side. The bladder should be opened well away from the tumor-bearing area and multiple cystotomy incisions should be avoided. (Fig. 56-1B).

Assessment of the desired margins is made. The bulk of the tumor has been previously resected and the base widely fulgurated, permitting an accurate assessment of a 2-cm margin to the fulgurated lesion. Adherent perivesical fat and peritoneum are resected along with the full thickness of the bladder wall, keeping the ureteral orifices in view at all times (by means of indwelling ureteral catheters, if necessary). It may be helpful to obtain frozen sections of the resected margins. Blood loss may be reduced by using Allis forceps applied to the cut margins as one progresses. This also facilitates closure when the dissection has been completed.

If the surgeon elects to remove one ureteral orifice with the resected bladder the ureter should be isolated and divided precystotomy. This maneuver prevents any unnecessary manipulation of the intravesical orifice and distal ureter. In male patients, a portion of the prostatic capsule and bladder neck may be included in the resected tissue, allowing a much wider margin than could be accomplished in the female. If the surgeon elects to perform this maneuver, the prostatic enucleation should be done before the segmental resection procedure. It may be necessary to stent the undisturbed ureteral orifice for 2 to 3 days postoperatively if one anticipates edema of the trigone secondary to dissection and suturing. The reimplanted ureter should also be stented for a short period postoperatively, because urinary leakage following such wide dissection is not uncommon.

Closure of the bladder is done in a standard fashion using a two-layer closure (Fig. 56-1C). We prefer a continuous 4-0 polyglycolic acid suture in the mucosa and interrupted 2-0 or 1-0 polyglycolic acid suture interrupted in the muscularis. The use of a cystostomy tube is optional. Those condemning it feel that it may act as a tract for tumor recurrence of tumor seeding. We have not encountered this, and I think it can be avoided by meticulous removal of all vestiges of exfoliative tumor transurethrally before performing the partial resection of tumor-bearing muscle. If the surgeon feels that he has a water-tight closure, transurethral Foley catheter drainage may be adequate. If there is a question, a suprapubic cystostomy tube can be placed and brought out as far away from the symphysis pubis as possible. Allowing a suprapubic catheter to rest against the symphysis enhances the chances of a distressing late complication in the form of a vesicocutaneous fistula. The perivesical space is adequately drained postoper-

FIG. 56-1. Partial cystectomy. **(A)** The peritoneum over the involved area of the bladder and the ipsilateral nodes are incised and removed with the pelvic nodes and perivesical fat. The superior vesical artery is ligated. **(B)** A wide excision of the tumor-bearing area is accomplished with a minimum of 2-cm margin. **(C)** A two-layer closure is accomplished; suprapubic cystostomy is individualized.

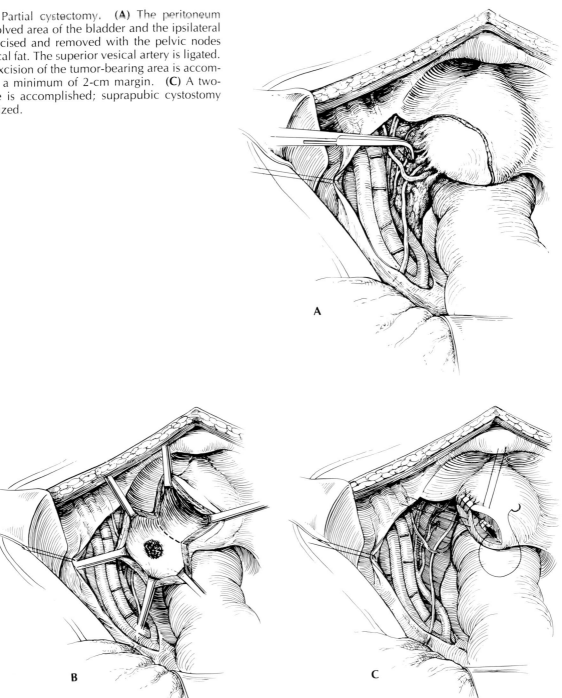

atively, and reperitonealization of the pelvis should be accomplished before wound closure by mobilizing the peritoneum after the segmental resection has been accomplished.

Continued or delayed postoperative urinary drainage can be seen following this procedure more frequently than after transvesical prostatectomy, vesical diverticulectomy, or simple cystostomy because of the longer suture lines and in some cases mobilization of the remaining bladder. Urethral or

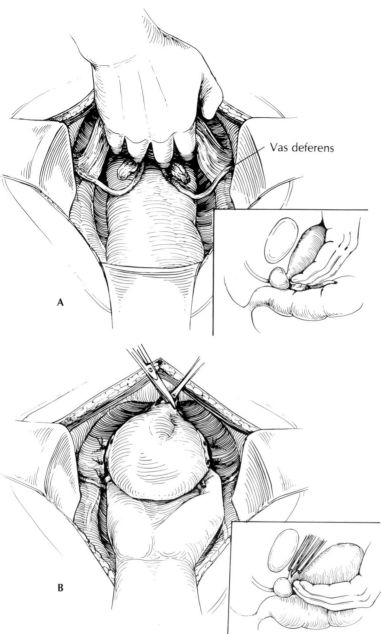

Vas deferens

A

B

FIG. 56-2. Simple cystectomy. **(A)** With the bladder emptied through an indwelling catheter, the peritoneum is dissected cranially. The plane between the bladder and rectum (or vagina) is developed by blunt and sharp dissection. **(B)** Transfixion sutures are used on the perivesical tissues containing the blood supply laterally. **(C)** The vesical neck is identified by bimanual palpation, and the bladder is incised circumferentially beginning anteriorly. Use of the Allis forceps facilitates exposure and controls bleeding. **(D)** The bladder neck is closed in two layers of heavy continuous absorbable suture. No drains are used.

suprapubic drainage must be continued until all vestiges of perivesical leak have stopped.

FOLLOW-UP

Patients can be reassured that their bladder capacities will return to normal within 3 to 6 months postoperatively if there is no previous irradiation cystitis or postoperative infection. Subsequent follow-up care with routine cystoscopy every 3 months postoperatively for at least 2 years is required. Urine cytology obtained at the time of cystoscopy is also mandatory even if the results of a cystoscopic examination are negative.

If the lesion being treated by segmental cystectomy has been completely removed, a recurrence, if it develops, is usually detected early and handled by less drastic means. The segmental cystectomy should not compromise the patient's chance for cure, either by subsequent cystectomy if needed

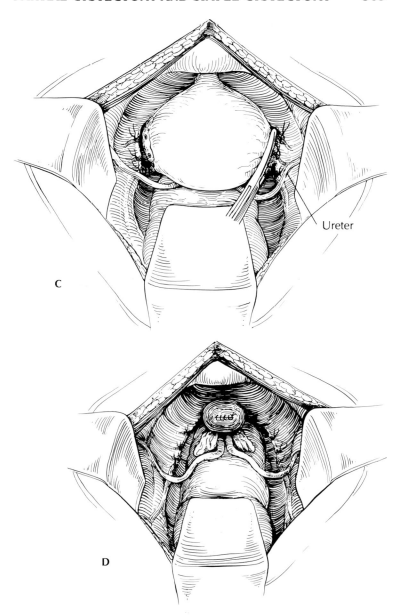

C

Ureter

D

or other suitable means. The question of whether a short course of preoperative irradiation should be prescribed is as yet unanswered. Such an approach may be helpful for the survival of the patients with high-grade invasive tumors and, therefore, should be considered as an adjunct in the patients being considered for segmental cystectomy just as it is for those who may undergo cystectomy.[4,11]

Simple Cystectomy

Simple cystectomy is defined as removal of the bladder without removal of all or part of the urethra. In the male patient, this procedure avoids removal of the prostatic urethra; in the female, it avoids removal of the entire urethra.

INDICATIONS

Simple cystectomy is not a procedure that one considers as a means of contemplated cure for a patient with carcinoma of the bladder. Rather, it is considered in patients who may have been relegated to a mode of therapy less drastic than radical cystectomy. This procedure can be used as a means of palliation for an incurable bladder neoplasm associated with a great degree of disability resulting from necrosis, continued bleeding, or other lower tract symptoms—*i.e.,* extreme frequency, dysuria, and uncontrolled infection.

Simple cystectomy is usually chosen to manage nonmalignant lesions of the bladder that produce many of the problems already mentioned. The procedure is indicated for bladders that have been subjected to many years of interstitial cystitis resulting in a markedly decreased bladder capacity and for changes involving the greater part of the bladder wall, including the trigone. It is appropriate therapy for postcyclophosphamide (Cytoxan) cystitis, which can cause uncontrollable and recurrent vesical bleeding. It also may be indicated for those patients with a persistent vesicovaginal or vesicocolonic fistula in which salvage of the bladder seems impossible. Lastly, it is used for cases of pyocystitis, in which a previous urinary diversion has preserved renal function in patients with neurogenic disease, but the remaining bladder continues to be infected and accumulates pyogenic material, causing fever, pelvic pain, urethral discharge, and other problems.

Simple cystectomy may be planned together with appropriate urinary diversion or its need may become apparent following diversion.[9] In our recent experience with one-stage cystectomy,[1] no mortality was encountered as result of simple cystectomy accomplished at the same time as urinary diversion except in one individual who had received Cytoxan therapy for a number of years and who died 1 month postoperatively from causes unrelated to her surgery. In most instances, we have performed ileal conduit urinary diversion and simple cystectomy together, doing the diversion first and then accomplishing the removal of the bladder.

OPERATIVE TECHNIQUE

The approach to simple cystectomy differs dramatically from either a segmental procedure or a radical one. If it is performed at the time of the diversion, the peritoneal cavity has already been opened. One begins the cystectomy by removing the peritoneum from the dome of the bladder and developing the lateral perivesical planes by blunt and sharp dissection (Fig. 56-2A). Once the peritoneum has been removed from the dome of the bladder, one should develop the plane between the rectum and the bladder in the man or the bladder and the uterus in the woman by blunt and sharp dissection until one reaches the bladder neck (Fig. 56-2B). This can be facilitated by draining the bladder with a Foley catheter, the balloon being

readily palpable bimanually. One can then stay as close to the bladder wall as necessary or comfortable, clamping and ligating the blood supply and perivesical tissues as one proceeds down each lateral wall.

Since we are not concerned with leaving any bladder mucosa behind near the bladder neck, the latter may be identified and opened anteriorly, again using the Foley catheter as a landmark or the prostatovesical junction as a line of incision. A transverse incision is made at the bladder neck, and the bladder neck or prostatic urethra is grasped with Allis forceps as sharp dissection proceeds around from the anterior to the posterior direction on each side until the distal trigone is reached bilaterally (Fig. 56-2C). With the bladder open, the bladder musculature may be incised from within posteriorly to identify the space between the bladder and seminal vesicles or bladder and anterior vaginal wall. It is not absolutely necessary to remove the entire thickness of the bladder wall in this area if one is fearful of entering the rectum or vagina, because we are not dealing with a "cancer operation" *per se.* Leaving a remnant of the bladder wall on the anterior wall of the vagina or uterus or, more importantly, the rectum, is not contraindicated. Once the bladder has been removed and its blood supply ligated with transfixion sutures of 1-0 synthetic absorbable material the prostatic urethra should be closed by oversewing with two layers of continuous 1-0 synthetic absorbable suture. This, in the case of pyocystis in the male, does not lead to impotence, and the patient retains any preexisting ability to ejaculate. The urethra in the female may be simply ligated using a transfixion suture of the same material. Troublesome venous bleeding from under the symphysis generally can be managed with transfixion sutures, and blood loss should be minimal.

If one obtains adequate hemostasis, drains are not necessary and, in most instances, are contraindicated. Should the bladder be badly infected before surgery, a small Penrose drain may be used for a brief period of time. In instances of pyocystis, the bladder can usually be sterilized before surgery by continuous irrigations with appropriate antibiotics or bactericidal agents such as iodophor solution. This must be accomplished before elective surgery is contemplated. In our experience, wound infection has been minimal since the use of drains in the vesical fossa was discontinued.

Wound closure is accomplished by reperitonealization of the pelvic floor if the peritoneum has been opened, and the abdominal incision is closed with a through-and-through figure-of-eight mattress suture of nonabsorbable material through all muscle and fascia layers, including the peritoneum (Fig. 56-2*D*). I prefer 2-0 stainless steel wire for this closure, but appropriate synthetic material may be selected. The only other suture needed is interrupted absorbable material in the subcutaneous tissue and subcuticular absorbable suture for the skin. These patients either have a preexisting abdominal stoma or will have a fresh one postoperatively, and this type of closure provides a flat and smooth abdominal wall to which the appliance can be attached. We have not encountered any complications with this closure, and the avoidance of stay suture has drastically reduced the problems with stomal adherence and has shortened the postoperative stay. If the use of postoperative pelvic drainage is necessary, it should be discontinued within 48 hr to 72 hr. Wound infections in this area usually become apparent from the 7th to the 14th postoperative day and usually occur because of contamination from the drain in this cavity rather than from the surgery itself.

REFERENCES

1. BRANNAN W, FUSELIER HA, JR, OCHSNER MG et al: Critical evaluation of 1-stage cystectomy—Reducing morbidity and mortality. J Urol 125:640, 1981
2. BRANNAN W, OCHSNER MG, FUSELIER HA, JR et al: Partial cystectomy in the treatment of transitional cell carcinoma. J Urol 119:213, 1978
3. BUSH IM, SADOUGHI N, GUINAN PD et al: Segmental cystectomy. In Whitehead ED, Leiter E (eds): Current Operative Urology, 2nd ed. Philadelphia, Harper & Row, 1983
4. CALDWELL WL: Radiotherapy: Definitive, integrated and palliative therapy. Urol Clin North Am 3:129, 1976
5. CUMMINGS KB, MASON JT, CORREA RJ, JR et al: Segmental resection in the management of bladder carcinoma. J Urol 119:56, 1978
6. FAYSAL MH, FREIHA FS: Evaluation of partial cystectomy for carcinoma of the bladder. Urology 14:352, 1979
7. JEWETT HJ, KING LR, SHELLEY WM: A study of 365 cases of infiltrating bladder cancer: Relation of certain pathological characteristics to prognosis after extirpation. J Urol 92:668, 1964
8. JOHNSON DE: Surgery of bladder carcinoma. Part I: Superficial (Stage O/A) disease. Weekly urology update series, p 2. Princeton, Biomedia, 1978
9. MATHUR VK, KRAHN HP, RAMSEY EW: Total cystectomy for bladder cancer. J Urol 125:784, 1981
10. MELICOW MM: Carcinoma in situ: an historical perspective. Urol Clin North Am 3:5, 1976
11. PROUT GR, JR: The surgical management of bladder carcinoma. Urol Clin North Am 3:149, 1976
12. ROWLAND RG, GRAYHACK JT: Evaluation and staging of bladder tumors. Weekly Urology Update Series, p 2. Princeton, Biomedia, 1978
13. UTZ DC, SCHMITZ SE, FUGELSO PD et al: A clinicopathologic evaluation of partial cystectomy for carcinoma of the urinary bladder. Cancer 32:1075, 1973
14. WHITMORE WF, JR: Surgical management of low stage bladder cancer. Semin Oncol 6:207, 1979

Cystoscopic Management of Bladder Tumors

57

William A. Milner

The management of vesical cancer would not present so great a problem if the urinary bladder were not so important a social and physiologic convenience. If there were any way of dealing with the storage and disposal of urine that would provide continence and maintain renal form and function, bladder tumors would much more frequently be treated by cystectomy, and transurethral surgery would play a diagnostic and relatively restricted therapeutic role. Currently, however, most bladder tumors are managed by transurethral surgery, and in view of the variations in activity and behavior of these neoplasms, it is a tribute to the refinements of endoscopic techniques and the skill of the endoscopic surgeon that so many tumors can be so well controlled in this fashion.

HISTORICAL BACKGROUND

Billroth was credited with having been the first surgeon to remove a bladder tumor suprapubically under visual control in 1874. After this, very few advances were made in the treatment of the disease until 1877, when Max Nitze presented his first cystoscope, which could be used in both sexes. Kelly cystoscopes with external reflected illumination were used in the United States for removing small polypoid, pedunculated tumors from around the vesical neck. With the introduction of the modern lens system, cystoscopic diagnostic examinations of the bladder became far more accurate.[1]

As early as 1901, Dees and Wolbarst stated in their textbook of urology that "bladder tumors are best treated by the transurethral approach." In 1910, Wappler became interested in this subject and began to develop instruments and electrodes that could be used through the cystoscope for the destruction of papillary vesical tumors. In 1930, an electrical cautery was developed that would cut satisfactorily under water, thus initiating the transurethral approach to bladder tumors. Much credit should be given to pioneers in the field before 1930, such as Keys, Buerger, Young, Beer, Squier, Bugbee, Barringer, Alcock, and Braasch.

I recall watching Joseph McCarthy use the resectoscope to resect a prostate in the fall of 1931; I was so impressed by the cutting ability of the instrument that I felt that the whole future of the treatment of bladder tumors as well as prostatism was about to change.

Results with suprapubic cystotomy and massive fulguration of bladder tumors during the early 1930s were attended by such morbidity and mortality that any new procedure was inviting. The 5-year follow-up on my own series of patients treated by this method was so discouraging that anything that could be done transurethrally would have seemed a great boon to the patient. As a result, starting early in 1932 an honest attempt was made to treat as many bladder tumors as possible by transurethral resection with or without fulguration of the base. Obviously, in the early years only the smaller tumors could be resected, but with added experience and marked improvement in the survival statistics, as well as the unusual decrease in both morbidity and mortality, larger and more malignant tumors were attacked by this method. By keeping good records and frequently checking statistics, it soon became apparent that transurethral resection was the treatment of choice in practically all bladder tumors.

It is interesting that as early as 1954 I predicted in a paper given at the British Urologic Society meeting in Dublin that cystectomy as a treatment for bladder tumors would soon be largely discarded.[6]

Etiology and Pathology

Very little is actually known about the etiology of bladder tumors. The relationship between certain aniline dyes and papillary tumors is well established. The tars associated with smoking are thought to be occasionally a causative factor, but proof is still not substantial. Long-standing chronic cystitis with associated bladder encrustations or calculus

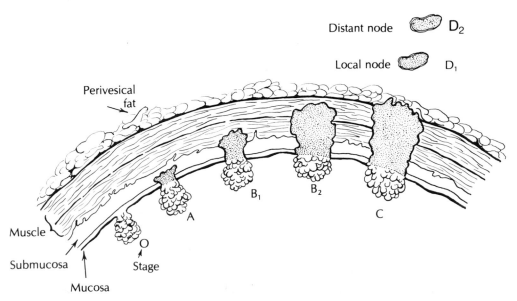

FIG. 57-1. The relationship between depth of infiltration and grade of malignancy is described by Marshall's modification of Jewett's original classification of the relationship of grade to stage. (Marshall VF: The relation of the preoperative estimate to the pathologic demonstration of the extent of visical neoplasms. J Urol 68:714, 1952)

has long been thought to be a causative factor in the development of bladder cancer. *Schistosoma* has been considered as a possible causative agent in papillary tumor formation. Recently, some studies have suggested that cyclamates might play a part in the production of bladder tumors.

Implants from renal tumors are relatively common. This is especially true of the transitional cell tumors of the renal pelvis or ureter. One case in my series was a clear-cell carcinoma implant from a similar kidney tumor, and one malignant melanoma was encountered as a metastasis. Only one rhabdomyosarcoma was seen in this series.

Most of the tumors are, of course, the usual transitional cell tumors, either papillary or solid. Adenocarcinomas are extremely rare, aside from extensions to the bladder from without.

The majority of tumors may be classified as follows:

Papillary noninfiltrating tumors
    Papillomas Stage O, Grade I
    Papillary cancer Stage A, Grade II (a few)
Papillary infiltrating tumors
    Stage A, usually Grade II (very few)
    Stage B_1, usually Grade II–III
    Stage B_2, usually Grade III–IV
Solid tumors
    Usually Stage B_2, Grade III–IV
    Stage C, usually Grade III–IV

Stage D_1, local metastasis Grade IV
Stage D_2, distant metastasis Grade IV

One can readily see that stage and grade of the tumors, as described by Jewett and Strong[2,3] and modified by Marshall,[4] are probably the most important factors in arriving at a reasonable prognostic evaluation (Fig. 57-1).

The efficacy of transurethral biopsy can best be illustrated by Figure 57-2. These are photomicrographs of tissue removed by resection and also the gross specimen removed from the same patient by either segmental resection or total cystectomy.[5] Figure 57-3 depicts the theoretic divisions between conservative treatment (transurethral) and radical treatment (surgery). It must be remembered that 65% of the B_2 tumors have metastasized when first seen.[4]

Preoperative Evaluation and Diagnosis

The patient usually comes to the urologist with a history of painless hematuria. Many times this has occurred as long as a year before but has stopped spontaneously, lulling the patient into a false sense of security so that he has sought no advice. Infection or dysuria is usually one of the later symptoms. Frequency and nocturia are usually associated with infection or advanced disease. Difficulty in voiding is occasionally associated with papillary pedunculated tumors located near the vesical orifice.

Duration of symptoms, physical findings, and the cystoscopic picture greatly help in determining the surgical course to follow. Bimanual examination under anesthesia is of inestimable value, and biopsy is mandatory. Preoperative flat plate and intravenous pyelograms are extremely important. They often show the character and extent of the tumor in the cystogram and also give a good idea of the extent of the upper urinary tract damage, if any (Fig. 57-4).

The method of obtaining and preparing the biopsy specimen is most important.[5] The specimen should be taken from the base of the tumor and should include some muscle fibers. If muscle fibers are not exposed, the biopsy probably is inadequate to give an accurate evaluation about depth of extension. Of course, if the entire muscle layer is involved, one may find tumor even in the deepest part of the cut, and great care must be taken to prevent bladder wall perforation.

At the time of the biopsy, a therapeutic resection is done, removing all the tumor possible in the hope that a cure may result. Thus, ample material is available for microscopic study. If for any reason the tumor extends beyond where the operator believes he can safely resect transurethrally, the remaining tumor area should be carefully mapped for radon-seed implantation, or more radical surgery may be considered.

The tissue removed for special study and involving muscle should be transfixed with a common pin placed vertically through the tissue (Fig. 57-5) so that the laboratory technician can mount the specimen in the paraffin blocks to obtain good vertical sections for microscopic study. Thus, the actual stage and grade of the tumor can be made with amazing frequency. In a series of over 200 consecutive cases, I diagnosed the tumor clinically by stage and grade at the time of surgery and my pathologist diagnosed them histologically. We were in exact accord in over 90% of the cases. I believe this proves the importance of the method.

Surgical Technique

I use the original Stern–McCarthy resectoscope because I believe that it gives the surgeon better control of the loop at all times. I use a high setting on the cutting current, 70 on the Bovie machine with the machine set on spark-gap cutting. Coagulation setting may be more optional but should be adequate. In using the resectoscope, one of the most important rules is always to use 12-gauge wire loops. These cut very accurately and with a minimum of coagulation. (If 10-gauge wire loops were available, I would probably prefer these to the 12-gauge loops because of their better cutting qualities. However, I do not know how long they would last, and 12-gauge loops are adequate.)

The size of the lesion and the degree of infiltration must first be estimated. The resection is then begun on the top of the lesion, always placing the loop at the posterior periphery of the lesion to begin the cut (Fig. 57-6A and B). The bladder should be filled with fluid sufficient to carry the normal bladder wall away from the lesion, thus reducing the chance of accidental perforation of the normal bladder wall. Because accurate visualization must be maintained throughout the operation, bleeding must be controlled as it occurs.

Accurate identification of the tissue by its gross appearance is mandatory. Tumor tissue usually appears as a homogeneous granular or sticky white tissue. Bladder muscle is arranged in definite fibrous bands and is more of a pink or dark shade. Fat has its usual glistening appearance. The serosa of the bladder shows up as a pearl gray or blue area because the loose areolar tissue around the bladder readily absorbs light.

In Stage O, A, and B_1 lesions, as resection is carried deeper into the tumor, muscle is exposed near the periphery of the base; as the operation progresses, the entire base is cleaned down to muscle fibers (Fig. 57-6C and D). In some B_2 lesions, the entire periphery of the base can be cleaned down to muscle fibers, but the center may still be penetrated by the homogeneous granular tumor tissue. Every attempt should be made to remove all tumor tissue. When all visible tumor tissue has been removed, the border of the resected area should be lightly resected and fulgurated (Fig. 57-6E). This destroys an additional 0.5 cm of tissue beyond the diseased area. If the resection is clean, there is no need to fulgurate the resected area itself, and in fact this only delays healing (Fig. 57-6F).

Multiple small tumors occurring in an area of perhaps 1 sq in (6.5 cm²) should be resected in continuity, because they sometimes recur in between the resected areas if they are removed separately. There may well be submucosal extensions in these cases. If a tumor is located over a ureteral orifice, it should be resected just as elsewhere. The cutting current does not cause stricture. Fulguration, however, should be avoided here. No tumor larger than 2 mm in diameter should be fulgurated. Accurate resection with the cutting current not only gives a better result, but also

(Text continues on p. 578)

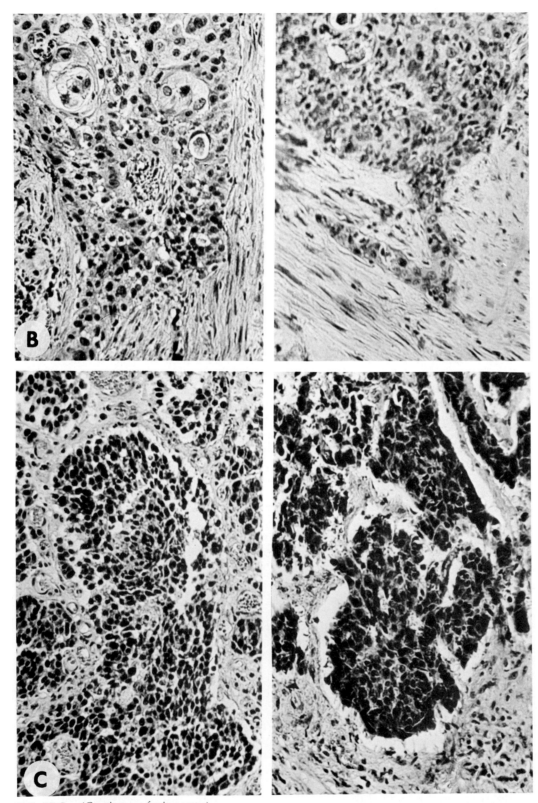

FIG. 57-2.   *(Caption on facing page)*

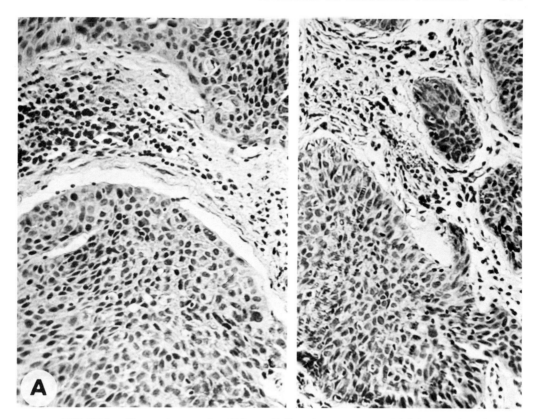

FIG. 57-2. Photomicrographs of biopsy (*left*) and gross anatomy (*right*) prove the adequacy of transurethral biopsy, as shown by the almost identical pathology seen both in the specimen removed by transurethral resection and in that taken from the gross specimen which was subsequently removed by radical surgery. (Milner WA: Transurethral biopsy: An accurate method of determining the true malignancy of bladder carcinoma. J Urol 61:917, 1949)

FIG. 57-3. The approximate division between conservative and radical surgery is shown by the *diagonal line*. Out of 50 patients, 36 (70%) could theoretically be treated by conservative transurethral methods.

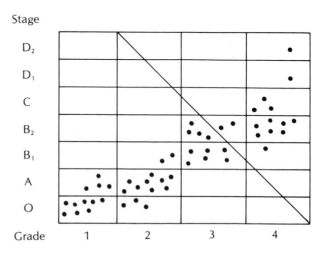

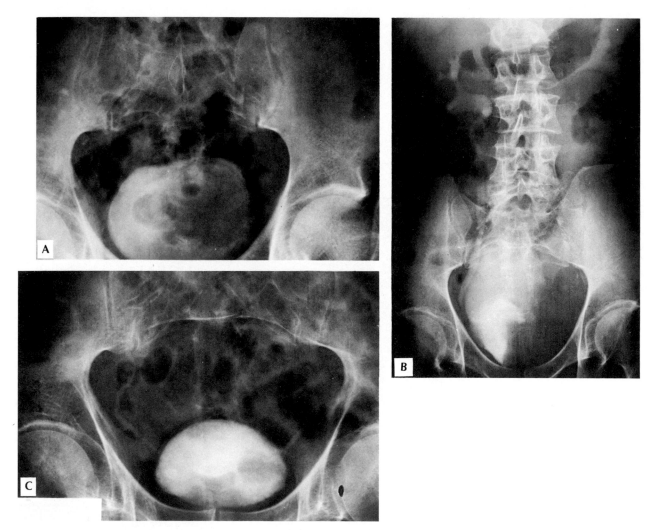

FIG. 57-4. Roentgenograms showing tumors. **(A)** A roentgenogram of an intravenous pyelogram shows a typical filling defect on the left wall of the bladder caused by a huge carcinoma of the bladder. **(B)** In a second case, the same type of defect is seen here on the left lateral wall. **(C)** The filling defect near the left ureteral orifice is caused by a small papillary tumor.

provides tissue for microscopic study. Large tumors should be resected systematically; early in the operation, one area of the tumor base should be cleaned down to bare muscle to serve as a guide in removing the balance of the lesion. As the base of the tumor is approached, the bladder should never be allowed to become overdistended, because this thins the wall and increases the chance of perforation. There is no nonresectable area in the bladder if one has an assistant to apply suprapubic pressure in the proper area (Fig. 57-7).

When tumor remains in the center of the base after as deep a resection as possible, either more radical surgery should be planned or the area

should be mapped for radon-seed implantation. In mapping a suspicious area for radon-seed implantation, it should be remembered that one 1.5-mc radon seed destroys only 1 cm of tissue. Hence the area should be measured in terms of planning to use the seeds only 1 cm apart or perhaps slightly less to ensure overlapping radiation. At the periphery of the suspicious area, seeds should be placed right at the edge so as to destroy at least 1 cm of tissue beyond the site of the disease.

The area to be radiated should be resected down to a thickness of less than 0.5 cm. The seeds are then placed 1 cm deep and at 1-cm intervals in the distended bladder. Flexible implanters are used through the 26Fr cystoscope, and irradiation can be accurately accomplished. Following the insertion of the seeds, a Foley catheter is inserted in the bladder, 1 oz (28.35 g) of sterile water is instilled in the bladder, and the catheter is clamped off. The nursing staff is instructed to empty the bladder once an hour and to instill 1 oz (28.35 g) of sterile water after each emptying. This protects the opposite bladder wall from radiation, which is the most common cause of bladder irritability with associated dysuria after the use of interstitial radiation. Most patients have a bladder capacity of 150 ml to 250 ml within 1 week from the time the radon is inserted.

After 1 hr of resection, if too much tumor seems to be left to remove in one sitting, the operation should be temporarily abandoned and a Foley catheter put into the bladder. In 5 to 7 days, the remainder of the tumor can be successfully removed with much greater safety to the patient.

Complications

Bleeding should be controlled as it occurs. The bleeding vessel should be visualized well. The bleeding can then be controlled by gentle pressure of the wire loop over the cut end of the vessel and the application of light coagulation. I call this "spot coagulation" in contrast to coagulation of a large area, which may be performed in the hope that the offending vessel may be controlled blindly.

Perforation of the bladder into the perivesical space is of no serious consequence if extravasation is avoided. If any tumor is left at the time this occurs, great care should be taken not to overdistend the bladder and to complete the resection of the tumor with the bladder only partially filled at all times. At the termination of the operation, a Foley catheter should be inserted; in this instance, it should be left in for a minimum of 4 to 5 days and the patient should be started immediately on adequate antibiotic therapy.

Intraperitoneal perforation results almost immediately in pain under the left diaphragm; if the patient is under spinal anesthesia, he will apprise the surgeon of this. It should be treated by immediate laparotomy to remove the intraperitoneal fluid and close the laceration in the bladder. If any tumor is found remaining, a segmental resection may be done at this time if the condition of the patient warrants a more extensive procedure. I believe that suprapubic drainage is advisable in these cases for at least 4 to 5 days. This complication, however, should rarely occur.

A strong obturator reflex that causes the bladder wall to jump toward the loop may cause complete

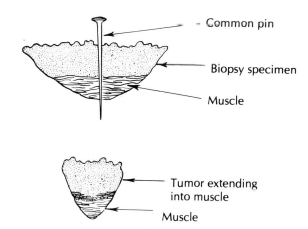

FIG. 57-5. A pin is inserted through a resected biopsy and set up in the paraffin block in such a way that vertical sections, from superficial to deep, can be obtained. This method improves the pathologist's ability to stage and grade tumors.

perforation and is to be strictly avoided. This occurs when the tumor is on the lateral wall and usually happens in the fully distended bladder. It is caused by stimulation of the obturator nerve by the cutting current and can be avoided by resecting in this area with the bladder as empty as good visualization will allow. Reducing the cutting current power also helps somewhat in avoiding this complication.

All the complications discussed here can be minimized if the resection is done as a gross histologic dissection, requiring that the gross histologic appearance of the tissue not only is well visualized but also is recognized at all times during the procedure.

Postoperative Evaluation and Follow-Up

The retrospective lens gives an excellent view of the resected area in most instances, and the various types of tissue can be readily recognized. Any elevation of the resected border should be resected more widely. All suspicious areas should be resected more completely. It is important to remove as much of the tumor as possible, because the first attempt is usually the best and the most curative, and there is no substitute for a meticulously performed operation.

Foley catheter drainage is used, except when the tumor measures 1 cm or less and has a small base not involving muscle. If the tumor is larger, the catheter is left in for 4 days; if it is small, the catheter is left in for 1 or 2 days.

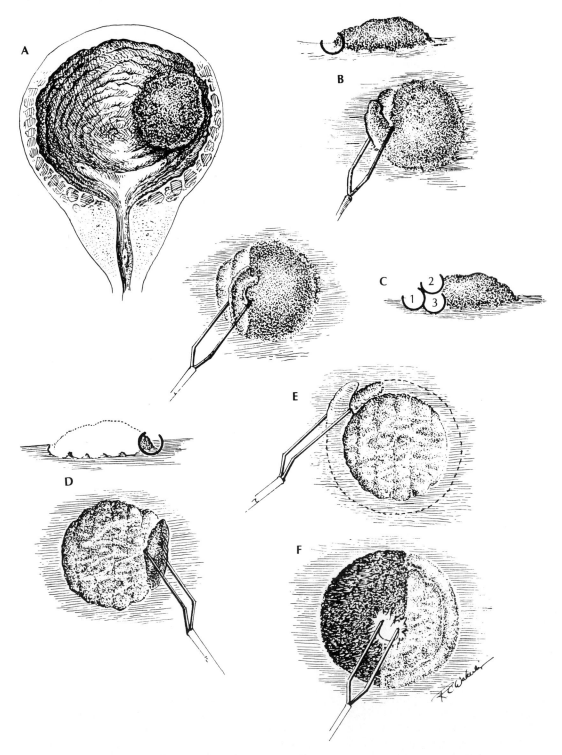

FIG. 57-6. **(A)** Tumor of posterior bladder wall. **(B)** Beginning of resection at posterior periphery of tumor. **(C)** Steplike resectional exposure of bladder muscle. **(D)** Completion of removal of visible tumor down to clean muscle. **(E)** Superficial resection and fulguration of visibly normal tissue around periphery of resected tumor base. **(F)** Complete cauterization of tumor base is unnecessary if clean muscle is exposed.

Cystoscopic reevaluation of the patient for possible recurrence is carried out at 3-month intervals for 2 years. This is then increased to 6-month intervals for 2 years and then yearly for life.

Most tumors adequately removed should be completely healed in 3 months. A few of the larger ones may take slightly longer. However, if there is any raised edge at the periphery of the resected areas it usually signifies unresected tumor, and the patient should be readmitted for reevaluation.

Overradiation or too much fulguration sometimes retards healing. Yet, in one interstitial radiation case—a Stage C tumor in a female that required 1 year to heal—the patient is alive and well 10 years after exposure to radiation.

Prognosis and Results

Stage O, A, and B$_2$ (Marshall classification) tumors can be eradicated by adequate transurethral resection. This has been well established statistically. Some B$_2$ tumors can be cured by transurethral resection followed by radon-seed implantation; of a group of 137 patients so treated in a series at Albany, 25.1% survived 5 years or longer. Stage C tumors or those that have metastasized often cannot be eradicated completely by any method of surgery, although a few C tumors have not recurred after transurethral resection and interstitial irradiation.

Palliation is important in treating some patients. A few patients have died of metastases, even though repeated cystoscopic checkups revealed a normal bladder before their deaths.

The results discussed in the following paragraphs are based on a study of 1000 patients treated 5 years or longer. Of these patients, 861 were treated by transurethral resection alone or with subsequent radon-seed implantation.

Of the 224 cases of Grade I tumors treated by resection alone, 131 cases were Stage O and 93 were Stage A (Table 57-1). Table 57-2 summarizes the results of the 137 cases that were treated by transurethral resection followed by radon-seed implantation. Most of these tumors were high-grade, and all but two were Stage B$_1$ tumors or greater. Thirty-four patients (25.1%) survived 5 years or longer. Thirteen patients (9.6%) survived 10 years or longer. Forty-nine patients (36.2%) seemed to have their disease eradicated; they died of other causes with no bladder tumors evident.

Transurethral resection alone was performed in 509 patients (Table 57-3). It must be appreciated

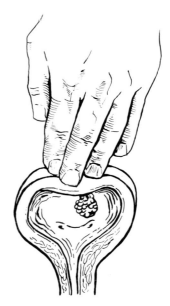

FIG. 57-7. An assistant depresses the posterior wall of the bladder to make the tumor more accessible.

TABLE 57-1.   224 Cases of Papillary Carcinoma Grade I (Treated by Transurethral Resection Alone) with Survival of 5 Years or Longer*

Years	Without disease	With disease	Years	Without disease	With disease
1	30	2	11	15	
2	13		12	8	
3	14		13	6	
4	9	1	14	5	
5	27		15	2	
6	21	1	16	5	
7	20		17	1	
8	14		18	3	
9	13		19	1	
10	12		20	1	

*18 cases were lost to follow-up before the 5-year period ended. The 224 patients included 159 men and 65 women, all with Grade I papillary carcinoma of which 131 were Stage O and 93 were Stage A. The survival rate was 67% (155) for 5 years or longer and 26.3% (59) for 10 years or longer.

that many of these patients were literally inoperable when first seen and were treated for palliation only. Two patients (0.35%) died as a result of the surgery; 225 (44.4%) survived 5 years or longer; 98 (19.2%) survived 10 years or longer; and 279 (54.8%) seemed to have had their disease eradicated.

On the basis of these statistical studies, it seems

TABLE 57-2.   137 Cases Treated by Transurethral Resection with Radon-Seed Implantation*

Years	Without disease	With disease	Years	Without disease	With disease
1	7	58	8	3	
2	4	12	10	1	
3	6	8		3	1
4	5	3	12	1	
5	6	4	13	1	
6	1		14	3	
7	5	2	15	2	
			21	1	

*The breakdown of cases by grade and stage is 31 in Grade II, 75 in Grade III, 29 in Grade IV, and 2 not graded; and 2 in Stage A, 52 in Stage B_1, 65 in Stage B_2, 6 in Stage C, 8 in Stage D_1, 2 in Stage D_2, and 2 not staged.

TABLE 57-3.   Results in 509 Cases Treated by Transurethral Resection Alone

Years	Without disease	With disease	Years	Without disease	With disease
1	31	164	13	8	2
2	11	24	14	11	1
3	20	10	15	6	
4	14	10	16	5	
5	27	4	17	3	
6	21	2	18		
7	25	4	19	3	
8	19		20	3	
9	23	2	21	1	1
10	20	1	22	2	
11	16	3	23	1	
12	8	2	24	1	

Grade II—254, Grade III, Grade IV, not graded—2; Stage O—3, Stage A—174, Stage B_1—171, Stage B_2—99, Stage C—24, Stage D_1—26, Stage D_2—2, not staged—10.

that some advances have been made in the treatment of bladder cancer. The extremely discouraging statistics of the 1930s have certainly been improved with more modern techniques. Careful analysis of the statistics suggests that conservative surgery in the form of transurethral resection, with or without radon-seed implantation as the case requires, offers perhaps a better than 5- and 10-year survival rate than more radical types of surgery. The age incidence of cancer of the bladder unfortunately precludes the possibility of a long-term follow-up.

It has long been established that whenever the urinary output is diverted from the spot where it was intended to go, the end result may not be all that is either anticipated or desired. To quote a phrase often used by the late Dr. Archie Dean: "A man with a bladder is much happier than the man without one."

REFERENCES

1. BEER E: Tumors of the Urinary Bladder. Baltimore, W Wood, 1935
2. JEWETT HJ: Carcinoma of the bladder: Influence of depth of infiltration on the 5-year results following complete extirpation of the primary growth. J Urol 67:672, 1952
3. JEWETT JH, STRONG GH: Infiltrating carcinoma of the bladder: Relation of depth of penetration of the bladder wall to incidence of local extension and metastasis. J Urol 55:366, 1946
4. MARSHALL VF: The relation of the preoperative estimate to the pathologic demonstration of the extent of vesical neoplasms. J Urol 68:714, 1952
5. MILNER WA: Transurethral biopsy: An accurate method of determining the true malignancy of bladder carcinoma. J Urol 61:917, 1949
6. MILNER WA: The role of conservative surgery in the treatment of bladder tumors. Br J Urol 26:375, 1954

Radical Cystectomy

58

David F. Paulson

Radical cystectomy, in men, removes the bladder and pelvic peritoneum, prostate, and seminal vesicles and, in women, the bladder, pelvic peritoneum, urethra, uterus, broad ligaments, and anterior third of the vaginal wall.[3,4,11] In addition, radical cystectomy includes pelvic lymphadenectomy of varying degree based on the extent of preoperative irradiation.[2,13] Cystectomy for control of bladder malignancy has been possible only since the development of satisfactory operative procedures for urinary diversion. Today, urinary diversion after cystectomy is accomplished by ureterosigmoidostomy or by a ureteroenteric diversion using either an ileal or colon segment. The method for urinary diversion is discussed in Chapters 48 through 52.

Presurgical Management

PREOPERATIVE IRRADIATION

Much debate exists regarding the necessity for preoperative irradiation. Most students of transitional cell carcinoma will recommend preoperative irradiation prior to radical cystectomy,[1,5,6,9,10,12,14] but the optimum dose level required for preoperative irradiation remains undetermined. There are strong proponents of both 2000 rads and 5000 rads. However, the few studies available would indicate that, although there is no significant survival benefit attached specifically to either high-dose or low-dose preoperative radiotherapy, preoperative radiotherapy does reduce the incidence of pelvic recurrence. It presently remains the choice of the clinician to assign the patient to either high-dose or low-dose preoperative radiotherapy.

High-dose preoperative radiotherapy supposedly controls microscopic nodal metastases and thus reduces the necessity for an extensive pelvic lymphadenectomy.[5,10] Formal extensive pelvic lymphadenectomy after high-dose preoperative radiotherapy carries the additional hazard of troublesome postoperative genital and lower extremity edema. Therefore, the clinician who adheres to 5000 rads preoperatively should modify his lymphadenectomy as indicated in the surgical discussion in this chapter. Low-dose preoperative radiotherapy supposedly devitalizes primary tumors of the bladder but does not control microscopic nodal metastases. Therefore, the surgeon who selects low-dose preoperative radiotherapy must do a formal pelvic lymphadenectomy in order to control microscopic nodal metastases.

SIMULTANEOUS URETHRECTOMY

The necessity for simultaneous urethrectomy in men undergoing radical cystectomy is debatable.[7,8,14] Only 7% of all patients subjected to radical cystectomy subsequently will develop urethral malignancy. However, this figure will double when diffuse *in situ* changes exist within the bladder or prostatic urethra or when the primary tumor is at the level fo the bladder neck. These patients should undergo simultaneous incontinuity urethrectomy with removal also of the fossae navicularis and the glandular meatus.

PREOPERATIVE BOWEL PREPARATION

Because the patient undergoing radical cystectomy will have the continuity of the bowel lumen disrupted during urinary diversion, it is appropriate that the patient undergo adequate preoperative cleansing of the bowel. This is best accomplished by giving the laxative of choice on the morning of the third preoperative day and on that day placing the patient on a clear liquid diet. The clear liquid diet should be maintained up through the evening prior to surgery. An antibiotic bowel preparation can be given to sterilize the bowel 24 hr prior to surgery.

Radical Cystoprostatectomy in the Male

The patient is placed supine and on spreader bars (Fig. 58-1). The pelvis can be opened by placing a

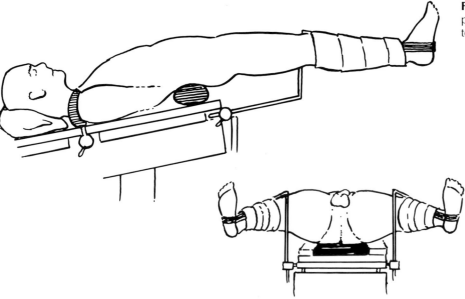

FIG. 58-1. Positioning of the patient for radical cystoprostatectomy

rolled towel beneath the sacrum to increase the pelvic tilt and provide better visualization of the pelvic structures.

The incision is made approximately 0.5 cm to 1 cm left of the midline, beginning at the level of the symphysis pubis and carried to the side of the umbilicus and into the upper abdomen for a distance of approximately 5 inches (12.6 cm) above the umbilicus. The incision is carried down to the level of the anterior rectus sheath, which is sharply incised beneath to the line of incision. The body of the left rectus muscle is mobilized in the midline and carried laterally. It is often convenient to enter the peritoneal cavity at the level of the umbilicus. The posterior aspect of the rectus sheath is incised, and the peritoneum is grasped with Halstead clamps. An opposing pair of Halstead clamps will permit the surgeon to palpate the anterior peritoneum with the thumb and the forefinger to determine that the bowel does not underlie the intended area of incision. The peritoneal cavity should be sharply incised between the Halstead clamps and an examining finger placed into the peritoneal cavity. Using this finger to provide tension, the anterior peritoneal surface should be lifted and sharply incised from the umbilicus to the upper aspect of the incision. The peritoneum is incised inferiorly to the level of the umbilicus.

Attention now is turned to preparing the anterior peritoneum for development of the anterior peritoneal flap. The intent is to provide an inverted "V," with the sharp point of the V based at the umbilicus and the upper arms of the V at the internal rings bilaterally just medial to the entrance of the testicular vasculature (Fig. 58-2). This is best accomplished by dissecting the peritoneum off the posterior rectus sheath. The urachus and the obliterated umbilical vessels now are grasped with a Kelly clamp just below the umbilicus, and an anterior peritoneal flap is developed. The incision is carried down toward the internal rings bilaterally, using the epigastric vasculature as the lateral margins of the distal aspect of the flap (Fig. 58-3).

The surgeon's finger can be passed beneath the peritoneum as it curves posteriorly. The incision is curved posteriorly and then a posterior peritoneal flap is developed as the peritoneum is incised posteriorly, this incision being carried up parallel and medial to the external iliac vasculature to a point approximately 2 cm above the bifurcation of the right and left common iliac (Fig. 58-4). During the course of this dissection the vas deferens will be encountered. The vas deferens should be divided, with the proximal end (the end closest to the testicle) being controlled either with metallic surgical clips or absorbable sutures and a long traction suture of either silk or chromic catgut being placed on the distal portion of the vas deferens, the portion that will be carried with the specimen.

The ureters will be identified above the bifurcation of the common iliac vasculature bilaterally, and they should be isolated and identified with surgical tapes. Division of the ureters should be delayed until it can be determined that radical cystectomy is appropriate for the patient.

PELVIC LYMPHADENECTOMY IN PATIENTS RECEIVING 2000 RADS PREOPERATIVELY

In patients receiving 2000 rads preoperatively, the adventitia and accompanying fibrofatty structures should be incised along the outer third of the external iliac vasculature, the incision being carried to a point approximately 1 cm to 2 cm above the bifurcation of the common iliac (Fig. 58-5). The external iliac vasculature can be lifted away from the pelvic floor, the assistant using appropriate retractors, and the lymphatic tissue can be passed behind the external iliac vasculature using a moist rolled sponge. This maneuver is relatively simple because penetrating vessels seldom are encountered on the posterior aspect of the external iliac vasculature. The anterior mass of lymphatic tissue should be pulled medially. The lymphatics distally should be controlled at their point of egress from the femoral canal either with metallic clips or absorbable suture prior to division of the lymphatic channels. This prevents continued drainage of lymph fluid into the pelvis and formation of a lymphocele or prolonged pelvic lymphatic drainage.

The external iliac vasculature should now be retracted superiorly and laterally. Just beneath the external iliac vein, the obturator nerve and its vessels will be encountered (Fig. 58-6). The obturator vessels should be divided and controlled either with surgical clips or absorbable sutures at their point of entrance into the obturator foramen. Dissection is then carried further medially to the reflection of the endopelvic fascia onto the prostate. This lymphatic package can then be elevated into the operative field and the dissection can be carried superiorly, carrying the lymph-node-bearing structures from around the external iliac vasculature, the obturator nerve, and the superficial lymphatic structures which accompany the hypogastric vasculature. As the bifurcation of the external iliac is approached, the node package can be released by ligation and division of the obturator vessels and the lymph node package can be removed. Dissection should be carried to a point approximately 2 cm above the bifurcation of the common iliac. It is not possible to do a complete node dissection around the hypogastric vasculature owing to the multiple posterior penetrating vessels which spring from both the hypogastric artery and vein. However, the anterior portion of the hypogastric vasculature can be cleaned sufficiently so that the vascular structures to the prostate and bladder can be identified.

After completion of this dissection, the superior bladder pedicle can be identified. The surgeon

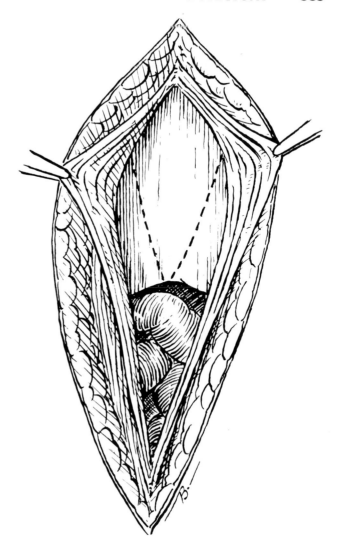

FIG. 58-2. Lines of incision for creation of the lower abdominal peritoneal flap

should be able to place a finger behind the superior, middle, and inferior vascular pedicles to the bladder. In those instances in which this is difficult to do because of significant pelvic scarring or inflammation reaction, the ureter can be elevated and a finger placed behind the ureter (Fig. 58-7). Tissues lateral to this finger will contain the vascular supply to the bladder and these can be controlled either with absorbable sutures or metallic clamps as the dissection proceeds.

PELVIC LYMPHADENECTOMY IN PATIENTS RECEIVING 5000 RADS PREOPERATIVELY

In patients receiving 5000 rads preoperatively, a formal lymphadenectomy encompassing the struc-

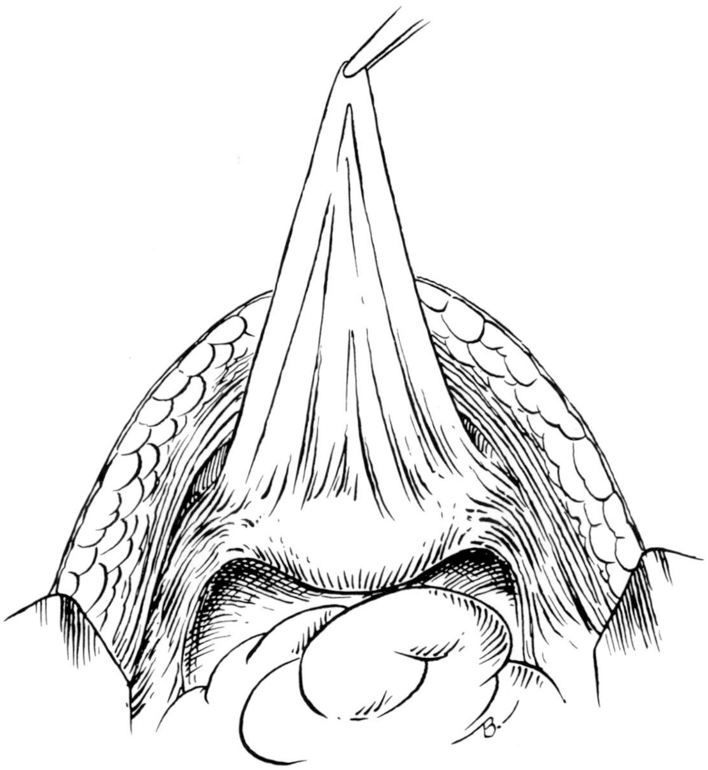

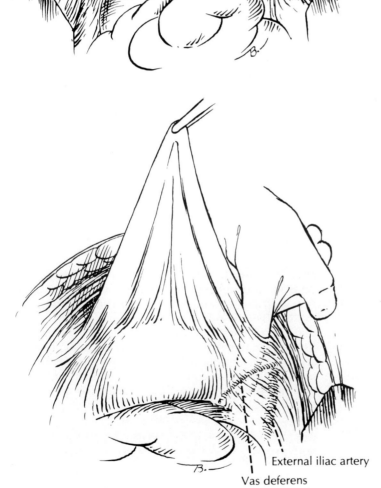

FIG. 58-3.   Creation of the anterior peritoneal flap

FIG. 58-4.   Mobilization of the peritoneum inferiorly and posteriorly to provide access to the pelvic vasculature and ureters

External iliac artery

Vas deferens

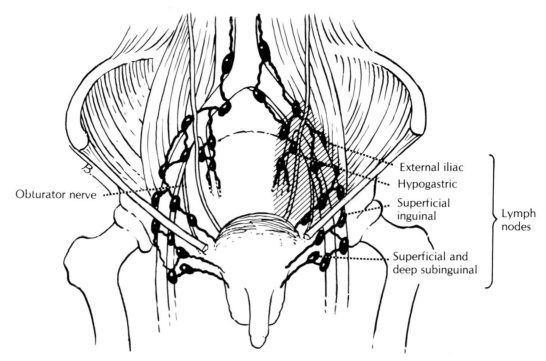

FIG. 58-5. Anatomic region to be encompassed during lymphadenectomy after 2000 rads preoperatively

tures that surround the external iliac vasculature is not done. This is because the high-dose preoperative radiotherapy is designed to control micrometastatic disease and, when extensive pelvic lymphadenectomy is conducted after high-dose preoperative radiation therapy, the incidence of debilitating postoperative genital and lower extremity edema is high. Subsequently, the lymphadenectomy is modified.

Following isolation of the ureter as already described, the dissection is begun at the bifurcation of the common iliac vasculature (Fig. 58-5). The lymphatic and fibrofatty tissue overlying the iliac vein is sharply incised, the incision being carried parallel to the iliac vein between the bifurcation and the pelvic floor. The iliac vein is then elevated with a vein retractor and the dissection is carried posterior to the pelvic floor. As the dissection is carried medially, the obturator nerve will be identified. The dissection then proceeds as with 2000-rads patients, except that the lymphatic structures surrounding the lateral portion of the iliac vein and the external iliac artery are not disturbed and the dissection is not carried above the common iliac bifurcation.

COMPLETION

After it has been determined that gross nodal metastases do not exist, one can proceed with the radical cystoprostatectomy. The endopelvic fascia on either side of the prostate should be incised from a point just inferior to the puboprostatic ligaments posteriorly to the inferior border of the prostate (Fig. 58-8). Once this has been accomplished, the surgeon may pass a finger between the prostate and the bony pelvis to the apex of the prostate.

The ureters should be divided deep in the pelvis. The proximal ureters should be tagged with a 3-0 black silk suture and packed behind the posterior peritoneum behind a moist sponge. This will protect the ureter from harm during completion of the dissection. The distal ureter should be tagged with a long chromic or silk suture. Traction on the distal ureter will assist in definition of the appropriate plane for control of the vascular pedicles.

The superior, middle, and inferior vascular pedicles can be controlled either by large metallic surgical clips or by absorbable sutures of either 2-0 chromic catgut or 2-0 Dexon. This should be carried as far distally as possible. With traction on the Kelly clamp previously placed on the obliterated urachus, the specimen now can be elevated in the pelvis. Digital palpation in the pouch of Douglas will reveal a ridge across the deep pelvis which identifies the appropriate line of incision for development of the posterior peritoneal flap. The peritoneum should be grasped in forceps and incised from side to side. Allis clamps should be

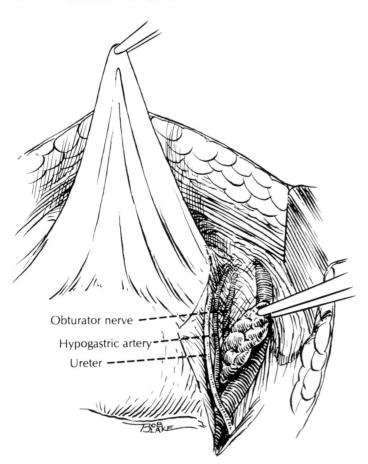

FIG. 58-6. Mobilization of the external iliac vasculature will permit exposure of the muscular pelvic floor and the obturator nerve and associated vascular structures

Obturator nerve

Hypogastric artery

Ureter

placed on the patient side of this flap, and the surgeon, with blunt digital dissection in the midline, can develop the appropriate plane behind the bladder and anterior to the rectum. This is best accomplished by moving the fingers in an anterior–posterior direction, sweeping the tissues away from the posterior aspect of the bladder, seminal vesicles, and prostate. The surgeon should be able to carry this dissection in the midline down to the apex of the prostate.

As the bladder is elevated from the pelvis, the surgeon will identify a fibrofatty fascial septum between the rectum and the bladder wall extending down to the apex of the specimen. Although this septum is frequently avascular, occasionally troublesome bleeding can be encountered, and it is best to divide this fibrofatty septum after control with either metallic surgical clips or absorbable suture material. This dissection can be carried down to the apex of the prostate.

The specimen should now be held in only by the urethra and by the puboprostatic ligaments superiorly. The rectum is protected by the hand of the surgeon behind the bladder and the prostate. With the specimen being elevated from this pelvis by the assistant, the surgeon can sharply divide the puboprostatic ligaments. Further elevation of the specimen will bring the membranous urethra from the muscular pelvic floor and it can be sharply divided and the specimen removed. A warm, moist pack should be placed in the pelvis and held in place with a curved Deaver retractor for approximately 5 minutes. During this time, the area of dissection lateral to the rectum and along the hypogastric vasculature should be inspected to be certain that adequate hemostasis has been established.

The pack now should be removed and the veins which accompany the urethra should be identified. The assistant can assist in visualization by placing a closed fist in the perineum and pushing inward. This will elevate the pelvic floor into the operative field and permit the surgeon to identify the venous bleeding points, which can be controlled by figure-of-eight sutures of 2-0 chromic catgut. In those instances in which diffuse venous bleeding is

FIG. 58-7.   Demonstration of avascular plane behind the ureter with definition of lateral vascular pedicles to the bladder

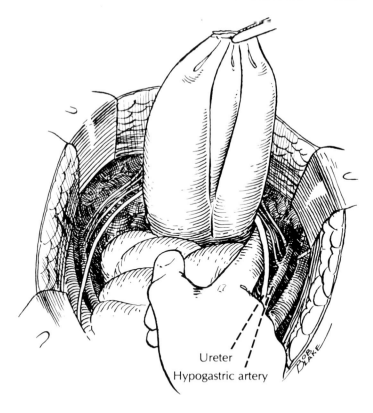

Ureter
Hypogastric artery

encountered and it is difficult to establish hemostasis, a small pack of absorbable Gelfoam can be placed in the midline and held firmly in place behind 1-0 chromic catgut sutures which have been passed into the muscular pelvic floor lateral to the urethra.

Radical Cystectomy in the Female

The woman is placed in a position similar to that of the man, and a similar line of incision into the abdomen is established. The anterior, inferior, and posterior peritoneal flaps are established as in the man; however, in the woman, as this line of incision into the peritoneum is established, both round ligaments will be encountered and should be divided. The tubes and ovaries should be carried with the specimen in the midline. The broad ligament should be incised and the ovarian vasculature divided and controlled with surgical clips. Lymphadenectomy is accomplished as in the man. After completion of the lymphadenectomy, the vascular supply of the bladder, the uterus, and the vagina can be identified. Vascular control can be established with surgical clips or absorbable sutures. The uterus is carried with the specimen, and the posterior peritoneal flap is developed across the base of the uterus at the level of the cervix.

Attention then should be turned to release of the bladder and the vagina. The vagina and the bladder are bound down around the rectum laterally by dense connective tissue which must be controlled with either absorbable sutures or metallic clamps and divided lateral to the rectum as dissection proceeds. The dissection should be carried from proximal to distal. Such a maneuver releases the tissue from the posterior pelvic wall, and rectum and dissection can be continued to the level of the bladder neck.

The assistant then can elevate the specimen by traction on the Kelly clamp, which has been placed across the urachus. The posterior portion of the vagina should be entered at the level of the cervix and the specimen released by incising the anterior third of the vagina moving from proximal to distal. As the bladder neck is reached, the incision in the vagina is moved more to the midline and carried parallel to the urethra and to the level of the urethral meatus. The urethra then can be released from either below or above and the specimen removed.

Extensive bleeding may be encountered from the margin of incision on the anterior third of the vagina. This can be moderated by grasping the vaginal tissue between Allis clamps. Following removal of the specimen, the vagina should be

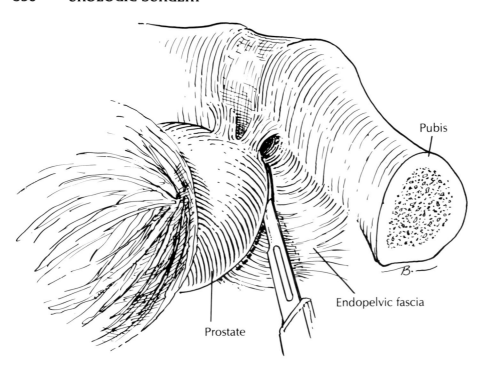

FIG. 58-8. Point of incision in the endopelvic fascia for mobilization of the prostate

Pubis

Endopelvic fascia

Prostate

closed by moving from distal to proximal with absorbable catgut sutures of 2-0 chromic or Dexon. A locking suture provides adequate vascular control.

Completion of the Cystectomy

In both men and women, following removal fo the specimen and after determining that hemostasis is secure, attention can be turned to the urinary diversion. After urinary diversion, the surgeon is ready to close the abdomen. No attempt is made to reperitonealize the pelvic floor. The omentum should be brought into the pelvis and used to line the pelvic floor. Mobilization of the omentum may be necessary to accomplish this. This is desirable because the omentum functions as an internal drain and also protects against adhesion and fixation of the bowel deep in the pelvis.

The abdominal incision is closed using figure-of-eight sutures of 2-0 Tevdek on the peritoneum and posterior fascia, with a second layer of figure-of-eight 2-0 Tevdek on the anterior fascia. The muscle is approximated in the midline with interrupted sutures. Subcutaneous tissues are loosely approximated with interrupted plain catgut. The skin margins are closed according to the preference of the surgeon.

The sump drains in the pelvis can be removed when the total drainage is less than 100 ml/day.

The pelvis should not be drained through the urethra in the man or the vagina in the woman. The bowel is decompressed by nasogastric suction until bowel activity returns. The patient then may be started on a liquid diet and the diet advanced as tolerated. Unless unforeseen complications occur, the patient may be discharged on the 8th to the 12th postoperative day.

REFERENCES

1. BLOOM HJF: Treatment of carcinoma of the bladder; A symposium. I. Treatment by interstitial irradiation using tantalum 182 wire. Br J Radiol 33:471, 1960
2. BOWLES WT, CORDONNIER JJ: Total cystectomy for carcinoma of the bladder. J Urol 90:731, 1963
3. CORDONNIER JJ: Cystectomy for carcinoma of the bladder. J Urol 99:172, 1968
4. KAUFMAN JJ: The management of tumours of the bladder. Practitioner 197:611, 1966
5. MILLER LS: Bladder cancer: Superiority of preoperative irradiation and cystectomy in clinical stages B2 and C. Cancer 30:973, 1977
6. MORRISON R: The results of treatment of cancer of the bladder: A clinical contribution to radiobiology. Clin Radiol 26:67, 1980
7. SCHELLHAMMER PF, WHITMORE WF, JR: Transitional cell carcinoma of the urethra in men having cystectomy for bladder cancer. J Urol 115:56, 1976
8. SCHELLHAMMER PF, WHITMORE WF, JR: Urethral mea-

tal carcinoma following cystourethrectomy for bladder carcinoma. J Urol 115:61, 1976

9. VAN DER WERF–MESSING B: Cancer of the urinary bladder treated by interstitial radium implant. Int J Radiat Oncol Biol Phys 4:373, 1978

10. WALZ BJ, PEREZ CA, RISCH J et al: Small dose preoperative irradiation in carcinoma of the bladder. Presented at the meeting of the American Society of Therapeutic Radiology, 1975

11. WHITMORE WF, JR: Bladder cancer: Combined radiotherapy and surgical treatment. JAMA 207:349, 1969

12. WHITMORE WF, JR, BATAT MA, HILARIA BS et al: A comparative study of two preoperative radiation regimens with cystectomy for bladder cancer. Cancer 40:1077, 1977

13. WHITMORE WF, JR, MARSHALL VF: Radical total cystectomy for cancer of the bladder: 230 consecutive cases in 5 years. J Urol 87:853, 1962

14. WOLINSKA WH, MELAMED MR, SCHELLHAMMER PF et al: Urethral cytology following cystectomy for bladder carcinoma. Am J Surg Pathol 1:225, 1977

Transurethral Surgery of Benign Bladder Conditions

59

Charles B. Brendler

This chapter discusses transurethral surgery of bladder conditions other than bladder tumors, which are covered in Chapter 57. It considers the transurethral management of bladder biopsy, bladder calculi, bladder diverticula, and ureteroceles. It also discusses ureteral meatotomy, which may be required in association with transurethral extraction of ureteral calculi.

Bladder Biopsy

Biopsy of bladder tumors is best accomplished with a resectoscope so that the lesion may be excised in its entirety and include a satisfactory muscle biopsy. For other suspicious bladder lesions, the cold cup biopsy forceps (Fig. 59-1) is ideal. The forceps is inserted through the cystoscope with the cups closed and is directed at the lesion to be biopsied. By varying the pressure exerted against the bladder wall, either a superficial or a deeper biopsy may be obtained. The forceps cups are opened and then closed to grasp the lesion, and the forceps is then withdrawn from the cystoscope, tearing away the biopsy specimen. Because of the minimal trauma to the bladder wall, bleeding is usually insignificant, and multiple biopsies may be obtained if necessary. Should hemostasis be required, it can easily be accomplished by means of coagulating electrode inserted through the cystoscope.

Bladder Calculi

Lithotripsy is defined as the operation of crushing a stone in the bladder or urethra. *Litholapaxy* refers to the combined operation of crushing a stone and washing out the fragments. For the sake of simplicity, in the following discussion all procedures will be referred to as litholapaxy. There are four methods of litholapaxy which are currently employed singly or in combination to remove bladder calculi: tactile, visual, electrohydraulic, and ultrasonic.

There are three major advantages of litholapaxy over cystolithotomy (open surgical removal of blad-

der calculi): shorter operating time, reduced length of hospitalization, and decreased morbidity and mortality.[2,24] Conversely, there are seven relative contraindications to litholapaxy where cystolithotomy may be preferable:[1,3,4]

A stone larger than 5 cm makes mechanical litholapaxy impractical, although it still may be possible to fragment the stone by electrohydraulic or ultrasonic litholapaxy.

Bladder calculi associated with a large obstructing prostate are best dealt with simultaneously through an open surgical approach.

Multiple diverticula represent a contraindication to litholapaxy because stone fragments may lodge in the diverticula.

A contracted or distorted bladder increases the risk of bladder perforation with litholapaxy, particularly with the tactile technique.

A dense urethral stricture may make litholapaxy impossible despite urethral dilation or urethrotomy

A foreign body in the bladder that acts as a nidus for stone formation may be adherent to the bladder wall and increase the risk of bladder perforation.

Stones in children, particularly boys, should be dealt with suprapubically to avoid injuring the urethra.

TACTILE LITHOLAPAXY

Introduced by Civiale in 1824, the blind lithotrite and technique of tactile litholapaxy were refined and perfected by Bigelow in the 1870s and have changed little to this day. Tactile litholapaxy has been abandoned by some in favor of other techniques, but it remains a valuable tool for those skilled in it.[7,17] The blind lithotrite is stronger than the visual lithotrite, allowing larger and harder stones to be crushed. The main contraindication to tactile litholapaxy is lack of experience with the technique, which greatly increases the risk of complications.

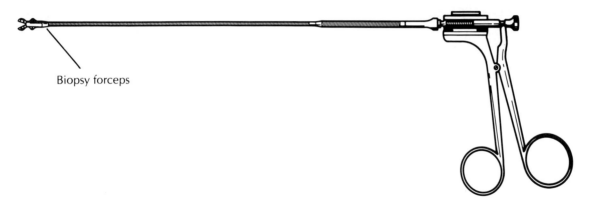

FIG. 59-1. Flexible cup biopsy forceps (Courtesy American Cystoscope Makers, Inc., Stamford, CT)

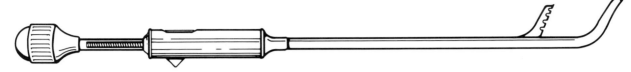

FIG. 59-2. Bigelow lithotrite (Courtesy American Cystoscope Makers, Inc., Stamford, CT)

Equipment

The Bigelow lithotrite (Fig. 59-2) for tactile litholapaxy comes in three standard sizes, 20Fr, 24Fr and 28Fr. The 20Fr lithotrite can grasp and crush a stone up to 2.5 cm, the 24Fr up to 4 cm, and the 28Fr up to 5 cm.

Technique

Adequate anesthetic relaxation is essential for tactile litholapaxy, which is performed with the patient in the lithotomy position. The urethra is calibrated and the correct size lithotrite is selected. The instrument is tested to be sure it is in working order. Cystoscopy is then performed to assess the number and size of the stones and to inspect for associated pathology such as tumors or diverticula. Following cystoscopy, approximately 150 ml of water is left in the bladder to keep the walls flattened out and away from the stone. The lithotrite is then lubricated and passed through the urethra into the bladder. The instrument has a sharper right-angled bend than an ordinary urethral sound, and one should be gentle while negotiating the bulbar urethra.

Once in the bladder, it is a mistake to try and locate the stone by poking at it with the lithotrite; doing so may injure the bladder wall. The lithotrite is depressed into the posterior wall fo the bladder (Fig. 59-3A); having too much water in the bladder may make this maneuver difficult. The jaws of the lithotrite are opened and the stone is allowed to roll between them, the male blade being moved up and down until the stone is engaged (Fig. 59-3B). The lithotrite is then elevated off the posterior bladder wall and moved gently from side to side to ensure that the bladder wall has not been grasped (Fig. 59-3C). Without withdrawing the lithotrite, the entire procedure is repeated until all the stone fragments have been reduced to a size that can be evacuated through a resectoscope sheath. The lithotrite is then removed, the resectoscope sheath is introduced, and the stone fragments are washed out with the Ellik evacuator. This is continued until cystoscopy confirms that all the stone fragments have been removed. At times it may be necessary to reintroduce the lithotrite to further crush fragments that are too large to evacuate. When all the stone fragments have been removed, an irrigating three-way Foley catheter is inserted into the bladder and left for 24 hr or until the urine is clear.

If transurethral prostatectomy is to be performed at the same time as litholapaxy, it is generally better to carry out litholapaxy first, because the prostate provides support for the lithotrite. However, if there is a sizable median lobe, it may be advisable to resect this first to facilitate litholapaxy.[4] Alternatively, the lithotrite may be rotated so that the jaws point toward the bladder floor in order to grasp the calculus.[7] If there is a bladder tumor

FIG. 59-3. Tactile litholapaxy. **(A)** With the lithotrite in the bladder, the blades are opened. **(B)** The lithotrite depresses the bladder base, allowing the calculus to roll between the jaws. **(C)** The lithotrite is moved to ensure that the bladder has not been grasped. **(D)** The calculus is fragmented as the jaws are closed.

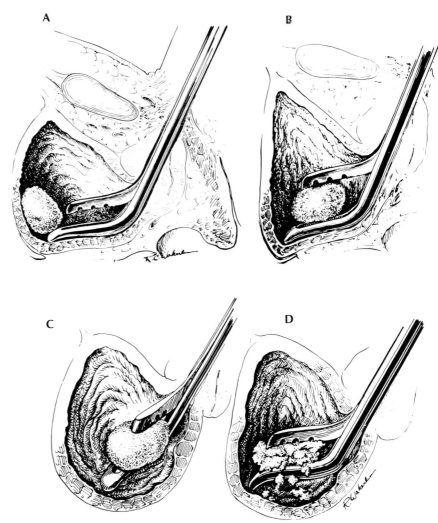

along with a stone, it is best to resect the tumor first to avoid grasping it with the lithotrite. Finally, if a stone is located in a diverticulum, it may be possible to dislodge it with the resectoscope.

Complications

Bladder laceration and perforation usually result from tactile litholapaxy when the jaws of the lithotrite are tightened without first moving the instrument from side to side to ensure that it has not grasped the bladder wall. Bladder injury is most likely to occur when the stone is adherent to the bladder wall, as when associated with a tumor or foreign body. Hemorrhage following litholapaxy usually is due to incidental prostatic trauma and will generally subside after irrigation and drainage. Persistent bleeding should arouse suspicion of bladder laceration or perforation, and a cystogram should be obtained. Finally, because most patients

with bladder calculi will have infected urine, it is prudent to obtain urine culture and sensitivities preoperatively. Antibiotic coverage should be initiated the night before surgery and continued for 24 hr to 48 hr postoperatively to reduce the possibility of sepsis associated with instrumentation.

VISUAL LITHOLAPAXY

Visual litholapaxy has the advantage of optical control and is often safer than tactile litholapaxy, particularly in the hands of those inexperienced with the blind lithotrite. However, stone fragments and bleeding may reduce visibility to the point that the procedure may become quite difficult. Furthermore, visual litholapaxy is limited by the width of the jaws to stones less than 2 cm in diameter. Despite these limitations, visual litholapaxy is an effective way of dealing with smaller

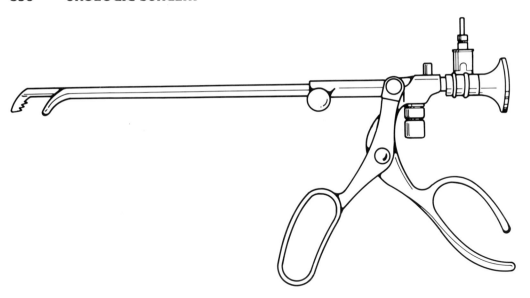

FIG. 59-4. Hendrickson lithotrite (Courtesy American Cystoscope Makers, Inc., Stamford, CT)

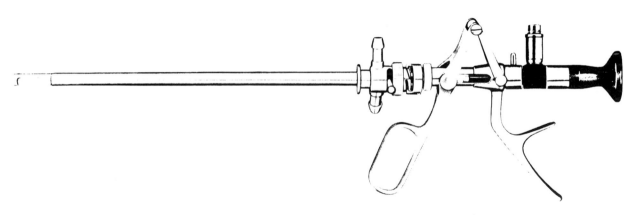

FIG. 59-5. Mauermayer stone punch (Courtesy Karl Storz Endoscopy-America, Inc., Culver City, CA)

stones, and is valuable in further reducing fragments of larger stones that have been crushed initially by other means.

Equipment

The visual lithotrite most commonly used today is the Hendrickson (Fig. 59-4).[10] This is a 26Fr instrument designed for use with a 30-degree Foroblique lens. It is well designed and reliable. Another visual lithotrite which has only recently been developed and marketed is the Mauermayer stone punch (Fig. 59-5). This is a 24Fr instrument designed for use with a 0-degree lens, which may enhance stone visualization. The design of the instrument may also facilitate crushing of harder stones.

Technique

The visual litholapaxy technique is similar to tactile litholapaxy. Care must be taken when advancing the Hendrickson lithotrite into the bladder to avoid traumatizing the bulbar urethra. Once the stone has been visualized and engaged, the instrument is moved slightly from side to side to ensure that the bladder wall is lying clear. The lithotrite handles are then squeezed to crush the stone, and the fragments are washed out with the Ellik evacuator.

FIG. 59-6 SD-1 electrohydraulic stone disintegrator (Courtesy Northgate Research Corp., Plattsburgh, NY)

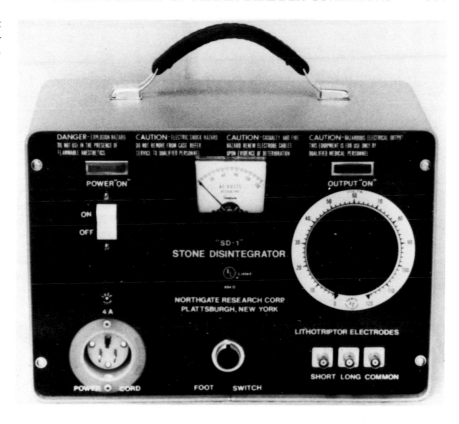

ELECTROHYDRAULIC LITHOLAPAXY

Electrohydraulic litholapaxy is based on the principle that high-voltage sparks generated in water will produce hydraulic shock waves which can crack stones. The technique was developed in the Soviet Union around 1960, and the Soviet-made Urat-1 pulse generator became popular in Europe toward the end of that decade.[21,22] Several years later, the instrument was tested successfully in the United States, and further clinical trials have supported its value.[5,16,20,26] Electrohydraulic litholapaxy is easy to learn, can be used to shatter stones of any size or composition, and appears to have a low incidence of complications.

Equipment

Electrohydraulic litholapaxy equipment consists first of a pulse generator, which contains the electronic circuitry. The generator currently manufactured in the United States is the SD-1 (Fig. 59-6). It operates on standard 120-volt, 60-hertz (Hz) current and transforms alternating current into high-voltage, low-amperage direct current. The current is discharged in bursts at the tip of a 9Fr coaxial lithotriptor electrode. The electrode is connected to the SD-1 by a cable and is inserted into the bladder through a 24Fr cystoscope. The voltage generated is variable and is controlled by a dial on the generator. The rate and duration of the discharge are regulated by a footswitch.

Technique

Topical anesthesia may be satisfactory for electrohydraulic litholapaxy in a patient with small stones and a normal prostate. If the stones are large or transurethral resection is required, regional or general anesthesia is preferable. The patient is placed in lithotomy position. The 24Fr cystoscope with a deflector is inserted into the bladder, and the bladder is filled with 150 ml to 200 ml of water. The lithotriptor electrode is then advanced through the cystoscope and the tip of the electrode is placed in contact with the stone, using the deflector to manipulate the electrode if necessary. The current is discharged with the foot switch in bursts of 1- to 5-seconds duration using the lowest voltage setting necessary to fracture the stone. The initial rough crushing is followed by further disruption of all stone fragments to a size which can be

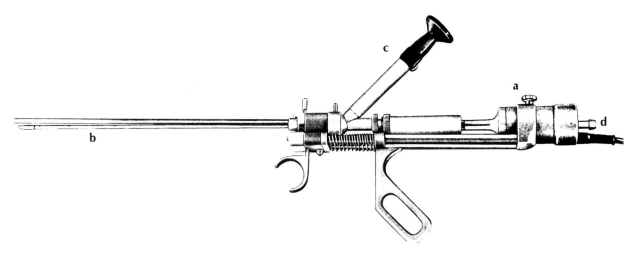

FIG. 59-7. Ultrasonic lithotriptor: (**a**) ultrasound converter; (**b**) ultrasonic probe; (**c**) endoscope; (**d**) connector to vacuum pump (Courtesy Karl Storz Endoscopy-America, Inc., Culver City, CA)

removed through the cystoscope with an Ellik evacuator.

Complications

In clinical series, the reported complications of electrohydraulic litholapaxy have been minimal. However, in experimental animals there has been a report of significant bladder and intestinal injuries associated with the technique.[28] If possible, the stone should be kept between the electrode and the bladder wall, and the electrode should never be discharged closer than 0.5 cm from the bladder wall. Shattering of the lens system may also occur if the electrode is not advanced far enough beyond the cystoscope.

ULTRASONIC LITHOLAPAXY

Ultrasonic litholapaxy uses high-frequency ultrasound to create vibrations sufficient to disrupt calculi. *In vitro* studies within the past decade have demonstrated the effectiveness and safety of the technique, and clinical trials subsequently have confirmed these experimental findings.[6,11,14,15,25] High-frequency ultrasound apparently causes no damage to the bladder even if the ultrasound probe makes contact with the bladder wall. Furthermore, there is no danger of stone fragments piercing the bladder wall, because stone destruction is achieved by vibration rather than by electrohydraulic explosion. It would appear that the main disadvantage of the procedure is the cost of the equipment, but this may well be justified for improved patient care, particularly in areas where bladder calculi are common.

Equipment

The ultrasonic lithotrite consists of three parts: an ultrasonic converter, an ultrasonic probe, and a cystoscope with a 0-degree lens (Fig. 59-7). The converter is powered by a generator which produces ultrasound of 26.5 KHz. The energy is delivered to the stone by the hollow steel ultrasonic probe. The lumen of the probe is connected to a vacuum pump; the stone is held against the probe by suction. The generator and vacuum pump are controlled independently by footswitches. A schematic drawing of the entire apparatus is shown in Figure 59-8.

Technique

Anesthesia for ultrasonic litholapaxy may be local, regional, or general, depending on the size of the stone and whether or not transurethral resection is necessary. Although safer, ultrasonic litholapaxy has been found to be somewhat slower than electrohydraulic litholapaxy; thus, a regional or general anesthetic may be preferable.[15] The patient is placed in lithotomy position. The lithotrite is advanced into the bladder through a 23Fr cystoscope sheath, and the bladder is filled with 150 ml to 200 ml of water. The ultrasonic probe is advanced toward the stone by squeezing the handles of the lithotrite. When the probe has made contact with the stone, the ultrasound generator and vacuum pump are activated by footswitches. The suction not only holds the stone against the probe, but also evacuates the loose stone fragments. A hole is drilled into the stone until the stone fractures; sometimes several holes must be drilled to disrupt the stone.

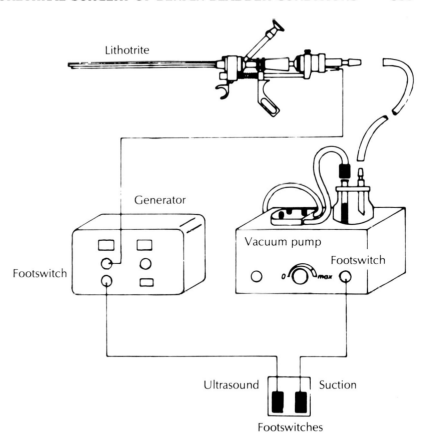

The stone fragments are individually reduced until they can be evacuated through the cystoscope sheath. The bladder is then inspected to be sure all the stone has been removed, and a 24Fr three-way irrigating Foley catheter is inserted for 24 hr.

Complications

Other than incidental trauma to the prostatic urethra and bladder due to irritation from the instrument, no significant complications have been reported with ultrasonic litholapaxy.

Bladder Diverticula

The ideal treatment of bladder diverticula is open diverticulectomy (Chapter 55). Transurethral resection of the neck of the diverticulum may decrease urinary stasis and infection, but it does not appear to reduce the incidence of subsequent carcinoma in the diverticulum, which ranges from 4% to 7%.[12,13] Because these tumors tend to be high grade and rapidly penetrate the thin wall of the diverticulum, vesical diverticulectomy is recommended in reasonably healthy patients under 70 years old.[19] However, transurethral manage-

ment may be appropriate in older or less fit individuals with poorly draining diverticula, such as older men undergoing transurethral resection of the prostate.

There are two transurethral techniques that have been employed to manage diverticula; both use standard resectoscope equipment. The first technique is transurethral resection of the diverticular neck to effect drainage of the diverticulum. This was described many years ago with good results,[8] but has never been widely accepted because of the fear of bladder perforation. The technique has been reevaluated recently, and no cases of perforation or extravasation were reported.[29]

The technique is straightforward (Fig. 59-9). The loop of the resectoscope is inserted through the ostium of the diverticulum, and the muscle fibers at the neck of the diverticulum are resected circumferentially. If the ostium is too narrow to admit the loop electrode, a Colling's knife may be used initially to incise the neck. After resection has been completed, meticulous hemostasis is achieved and a catheter is left indwelling for 3 to 5 days.

The second technique is transurethral fulguration of the diverticulum itself. Orandi has reported

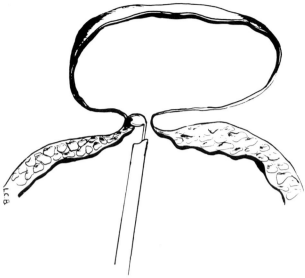

FIG. 59-9.   Resection of the neck of a bladder diverticulum

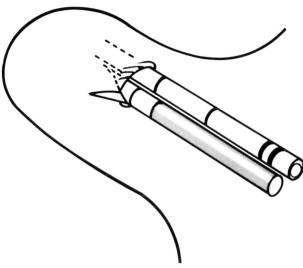

FIG. 59-11.   Ureteral meatotomy with the cystoscopic scissors

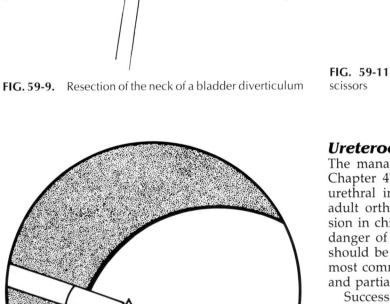

FIG. 59-10.   Incision of a ureterocele with the cystoscopic scissors

that thorough fulguration of the diverticular surface using a wide-loop electrode results in shrinkage or disappearance of the diverticulum.[18] To date his results have not been confirmed by others, but the technique would seem to merit further evaluation.

Ureteroceles

The management of ureteroceles is discussed in Chapter 47. It is enough to say here that transurethral incision is justified only in obstructing adult orthotopic ureteroceles. Transurethral incision in children is never indicated because of the danger of producing reflux.[9] Ectopic ureteroceles should be managed by open surgical techniques, most commonly by upper pole heminephrectomy and partial ureterectomy.

Successful transurethral resection of orthotopic ureteroceles has been reported.[30] However, it has not been shown to have any significant advantage over transurethral incision, and would seem to carry increased risks of creating reflux and damaging an associated normal ureter in a duplicated system. Transurethral incision is performed transversely along the distal base of the ureterocele to minimize the risk of creating reflux. A Colling's knife or the cystoscopic scissors may be used. If the ureteral orifice is located distally in the ureterocele, the tip of the scissors or the electrode may be inserted into the orifice to start the incision (Fig. 59-10). If a calculus is lodged in a ureterocele, the same incision is made until the stone can be milked out, crushed if necessary, and evacuated.

Following incision, serial intravenous pyelograms should be obtained to confirm that the obstruction has been relieved and that it does not recur. Bridging of the cut mucosal surfaces of the ureterocele can occur, and repeat snipping with the cystoscopic scissors may be required.[27]

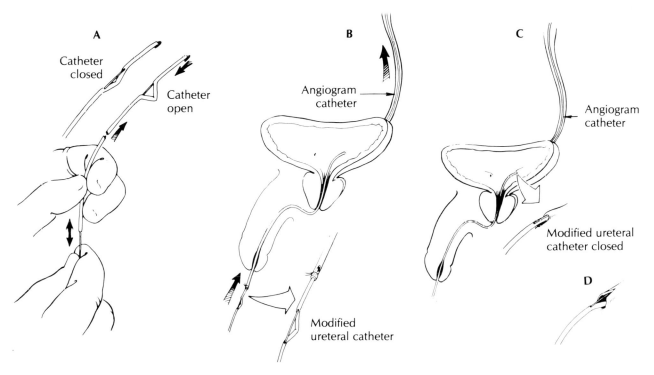

FIG. 59-12. Controlled ureteral meatotomy. **(A)** Modified ureteral catheter with steel stylet. Traction on the stylet angulates the catheter. **(B)** The ureteral catheter with the steel stylet is sutured into the lumen of an angiogram catheter and drawn into position. **(C)** The ureteral catheter is in position with the exposed portion of the stylet adjacent to the stricture. **(D)** Traction is applied to the stylet, and the stricture is incised with the cutting current. (Smith AD, Lange PH, Miller RP et al: Controlled ureteral meatotomy. J Urol 121:587. Baltimore, The Williams & Wilkins Co., 1979)

Ureteral Meatotomy

Ureteral meatotomy may be required in association with transurethral extraction of ureteral calculi (see Chap. 38). It also may be necessary when ureteral meatal stenosis results from previous transurethral resection or fulguration. If ureteral obstruction exists and scarring of the orifice is severe, formal ureteroneocystostomy may be required. In cases of obstruction with less severe scarring, ureteral meatotomy may suffice to relieve the obstruction.

The cystoscopic scissors, Colling's knife, or a steel ureteral stylet may be employed for meatotomy. If possible, a ureteral catheter is inserted from below to delineate the ureteral lumen and help prevent a false passage. The scissors or knife is then inserted alongside the catheter, and the stricture is incised longitudinally (Fig. 59-11). The ureteral catheter is left in place for 24 to 48 hr to allow drainage until postoperative edema subsides.

Often it is not possible to catheterize the ureter retrograde, and attempts to do so may result in

the catheter buckling or creation of a false passage. A new technique has been described to deal with this problem (Fig. 59-12).[23] An angiogram catheter and guidewire are inserted anterograde through the stricture by means of a percutaneous nephrostomy. Once through the stricture, the guide-wire is withdrawn, and the angiogram catheter is grasped with a cystoscopic forceps and drawn through the urethra. A 5Fr ureteral catheter is then modified by cutting two side holes in the catheter 1.5 cm apart. A steel stylet is inserted through the ureteral catheter so that it exits the catheter through one side hole and reenters the catheter through the second side hole. The tip of the stylet is bent over one end of the ureteral catheter so that traction on the other end of the stylet results in angulation of the catheter. The ureteral catheter and stylet are then inserted into the angiogram catheter and sutured in place. The angiogram catheter and attached ureteral catheter and stylet are then withdrawn back into the bladder. Under cystoscopic control, the exposed part of the steel stylet is positioned against the ureteral stricture. Traction on the other end of the stylet results in angulation of the ureteral catheter and direct contact between the stylet and the stricture. Cutting current is applied to the stylet, and the stricture is incised. The modified ureteral catheter is withdrawn and replaced by a Silastic stent. This stent exits through the previous percutaneous nephrostomy site, and is left in place to provide drainage during the period of postoperative healing.

REFERENCES

1. BAPAT SS: Endoscopic removal of bladder stones in adults. Br J Urol 49:527, 1977
2. BARNES RW, BERGMAN RT, WORTON E: Litholapaxy vs cystolithotomy. J Urol 89:680, 1963
3. BLANDY JP: Benign conditions of the bladder. In Operative Urology, p 109. Oxford, Blackwell Scientific Publications, 1978
4. BRITO RR, BORGES HJ, ALBUQUERQUE J et al: Litholapaxy: 385 cases. Endoscopy 7:142, 1975
5. EATON JM, JR, MALIN JM, JR, GLENN JF: Electrohydraulic lithotripsy. J Urol 108:865, 1972
6. FAHIQ SE, WALLACE DM: Ultrasonic lithotriptor for urethral and bladder stones. Br J Urol 50:255, 1978
7. HADLEY HL, BARNES RW, ROSENQUIST RC: Tactile litholapaxy—Safe and efficient. Urology 9:263, 1977
8. HARTUNG W, FLOCKS RH: Diverticulum of the bladder: A method of roentgen examination and the roentgen and clinical findings in 200 cases. Radiology 41:363, 1943
9. HENDREN WH, MITCHELL MD: Surgical correction of ureteroceles. J Urol 121:590, 1979
10. HENDRICKSON FC: A visualizing lithotrite. J Urol 60:656, 1948
11. HOWARDS SS, MERRILL E, HARRIS S et al: Ultrasonic lithotripsy: Laboratory evaluations. Invest Urol 11:273, 1974
12. KELALIS PP, MCLEAN P: The treatment of diverticulum of the bladder. J Urol 98:349, 1967
13. KNAPPENBERGER ST, USON AC, MEYER MM: Primary neoplasms occurring in vesical diverticula: A report of 18 cases. J Urol 83:153, 1960
14. LUTZEYER W, POHLMAN R, TERHORST B et al: Die Zerstörung von Harnsteinen durch Ultraschall I: Experimentelle Untersuchungen. Urol Int 25:47, 1970
15. MARBERGER M: Ultrasonic destruction of bladder stones. In Resnick MI, Sanders RC (eds): Ultrasound in Urology, p. 371. Baltimore, Williams & Wilkins, 1979
16. MITCHELL ME, KERR WS, JR: Experience with the electrohydraulic disintegrator. J Urol 117:159, 1977
17. NESBIT RM: Litholapaxy. J Urol 70:594, 1953
18. ORANDI A: Transurethral fulguration of bladder diverticulum. New procedure. Urology 10:30, 1977
19. PICONI JR, HENRY SC, WALSH PC: Rapid development of carcinoma in diverticulum of bladder: A pitfall in conservative management. Urology 2:676, 1973
20. RANEY AM: Electrohydraulic cystolithotripsy. Urology 7:379, 1976
21. REUTER HJ: Electronic lithotripsy: Transurethral treatment of bladder stones in 50 cases. J Urol 104:834, 1970
22. ROUVALIS P: Electronic lithotripsy for vesical calculus with "Urat-1." Br J Urol 42:486, 1970
23. SMITH AD, LANGE PH, MILLER RP et al: Controlled ureteral meatotomy. J Urol 121:587, 1979
24. SMITH JM, O'FLYNN JD: Transurethral removal of bladder stone: The place of litholapaxy. Br J Urol 49:401, 1977
25. TERHORST B, LUTZEYER W, CICHOS M et al: Die Zerstörung von Harnsteinen durch Ultraschall. Urol Int 27:458, 1972
26. TESSLER AN, KOSSOW J: Electrohydraulic stone disintegration. Urology 5:470, 1975
27. THOMPSON IM: Transurethral surgery. In Glenn JF (ed): Urologic Surgery, 2nd ed, p 470. Hagerstown, Harper & Row, 1975
28. TIDD MJ, WRIGHT HC, OLIVER Y et al: Hazards to bladder and intestinal tissues from intravesical underwater electrical discharges from a surgical electronic lithoclast. Urol Res 4:49, 1976
29. VITALE PJ, WOODSIDE JR: Management of bladder diverticula by transurethral resection: Re-evaluation of an old technique. J Urol 122:744, 1979
30. WINES RD, O'FLYNN JD: Transurethral treatment of ureteroceles: A report on 45 cases mostly treated by transurethral resection. Br J Urol 44:207, 1972

Urachal Abnormalities

60

Richard M. Ehrlich

Urachal anomalies occur rarely and are usually manifest in childhood. Symptomatic adult presentation is even less frequent. They are twice as common in male as in female patients. Fewer than 350 cases have been reported in the literature.

A full grasp of the embryology of this unique structure is essential to understanding developmental anomalies,[1,3,10,27] but this is beyond the purview of this chapter. Four anatomic variants of the normal urachus have been described and are helpful in understanding congenital variations and surgical approaches.[3]

A distinct fascial layer invests the urachus anteriorly and posteriorly. This fascia extends to the border of the obliterated umbilical artery laterally and inferiorly over the dome of the bladder to the internal iliac arteries. There is thus formed a distinct space separate from the peritoneal cavity which serves to contain leakage and infection within its borders.

Congenital Abnormalities

Five separate clinical anomalies have been described: patent urachus, urachal cyst, urachal sinus draining predominantly to the umbilicus, alternating sinus draining to both the bladder and umbilicus, and vesicourachal diverticulum.[1] These anomalies are depicted in Figures 60-1 and 60-2.

PATENT URACHUS

In the newborn period the diagnosis of patent urachus is most often made when leakage of urine is seen at the time of cord separation. Prior to cord ligation, reflux of urine through the urachus may lead to dilatation of the cord, mimicking an umbilical hernia.[8,26] The flow of urine through the fistula varies from a few drops to a strong stream and usually commences at the time of urethral voiding. Somewhat less than half of these cases will have a "red tumor" at the opening, which represents urachal mucosa. In others a minimal ooze may not be at first recognized and only a mild dermatitis appears, which is markedly different from the skin sloughing associated with bowel content leakage from a patent omphalomesenteric duct.

The diagnosis is most often obvious. Periumbilical and suprapubic pressure promotes urinary drainage, and confirmation of urine can be obtained by analyzing the fluid for creatinine. Other diagnostic aids, such as injecting methylene blue or indigo carmine through the fistula, the urethra, or a vein, can be employed. Voiding cystography, including oblique and lateral views, is essential and not only demonstrates the communication but also reveals concomitant lower urinary tract obstruction if it exists (Fig. 60-3).[19] Endoscopy is usually not necessary in the neonate unless an enigmatic situation exists, but cystoscopy is prudent in the adult.

Prompt treatment for patent urachus is recommended to forestall the development of severe ammoniacal dermatitis, infection, and sepsis. Local cauterization or ligation of the patent channel most often fails. Thus, complete operative resection of the urachus is recommended.[4,11,15,20] The operation is best performed by an extraperitoneal approach, with total removal of the urachus and layered closure of the bladder dome with absorbable suture material. Purulent wounds are first treated with incision, drainage, and packing, with a staged complete resection at a later date. Any lower tract pathology can be treated simultaneously or prior to the urachal surgery.

In neonates and younger children an infraumbilical incision affords satisfactory access to perform a complete excision of both the bladder and umbilical portions of the patent urachus (Fig. 60-4). In older children an incision midway between the umbilicus and symphysis is recommended.[27] All urachal elements should be carefully removed and the umbilicus spared if possible for cosmetic reasons. Complete removal is stressed to prevent the possibility of future sarcomatous degeneration of urachal elements.[9]

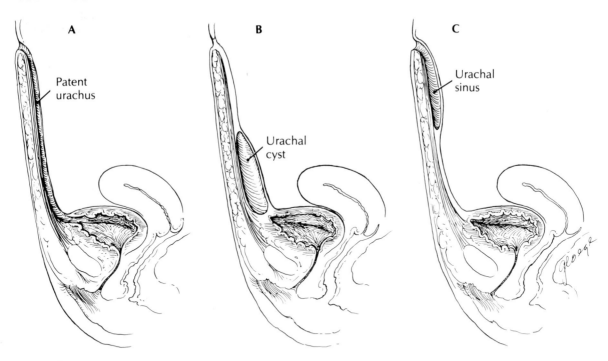

FIG. 60-1. Urachal anomalies include **(A)** patent urachus, **(B)** urachal cyst, and **(C)** urachal sinus (see also Fig. 60-2).

FIG. 60-2. Urachal anomalies also include **(A)** alternating sinus and **(B)** vesicourachal diverticulum.

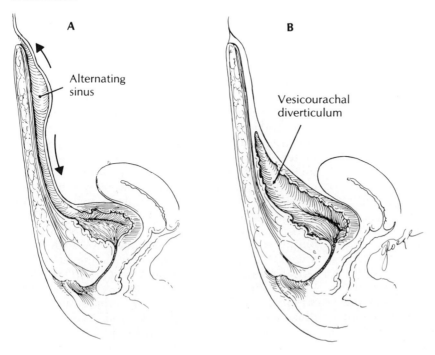

URACHAL CYSTS

Most cysts develop in the inferior third of the urachus and are uncommon congenital anomalies. They are usually asymptomatic unless a communication develops through the umbilicus, or they may become infected and enlarge (Fig. 60-5). An infected cyst usually presents as a tender palpable low midline mass with systemic signs of infection.[20] If left untreated it will eventually drain through the umbilicus or into the bladder, in which case urinary infection will become evident. The former situation mimics omphalitis, patent omphalomesenteric duct, or granuloma. Intraperitoneal rupture is also a possibility.[1,20]

The differential diagnosis includes bladder diverticulum, vitelline cyst, umbilical hernia, or ovarian cyst.[1] It is rarely considered in the adult. A voiding cystourethrogram with lateral projections may be helpful, but a B-mode gray scale ultrasound scan is the best, most cost-effective study, because the lesions are cystic and located in the anterior abdominal wall far from interference with intestinal gas.[22] Computed tomography (CT) is rarely necessary.

The treatment of a pyourachal cyst is surgical. Complete excision can be accomplished safely if

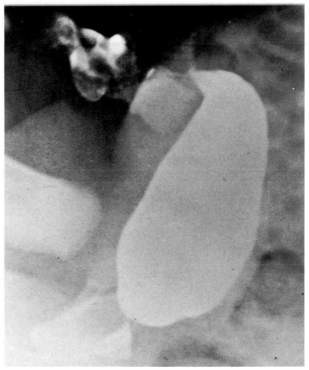

FIG. 60-3. Umbilical injection of contrast through patent urachus

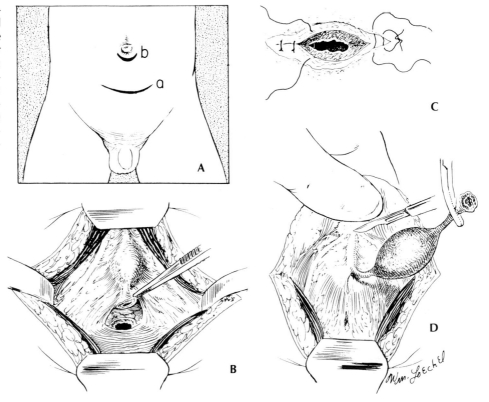

FIG. 60-4. Surgical considerations for benign urachal abnormalities: **(A)** preferable incision in **(a)** children or young adults and **(b)** infants; **(B)** urachal cyst being mobilized from the bladder dome; **(C)** two-layer closure with absorbable suture material; **(D)** complete removal of the urachal attachment at the umbilicus

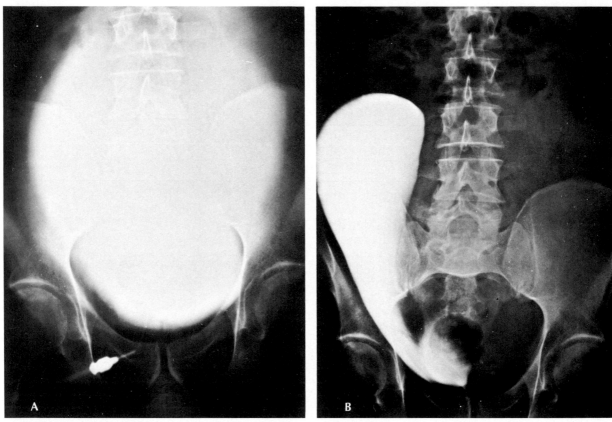

FIG. 60-5. **(A)** A huge urachal cyst is injected percutaneously with contrast. **(B)** A cystogram shows the bladder pushed laterally and out of the pelvis by the urachal cyst. (Courtesy Dr. Zoran Barbaric and Dr. Robert Davis)

the infection is within the cyst. If the cyst has ruptured, causing peritonitis or purulent drainage, antibiotic coverage and delayed secondary total extirpation with ligation of each end of the urachal remnant is recommended.

URACHAL SINUS

A blind urachal sinus may present as lower abdominal tenderness, fluctuation, fever, and purulent discharge from the umbilicus. It may drain into the bladder as well (See Fig. 60-2A), leading to urinary infection and symptoms.[12] The differential diagnosis must, as in urachal cyst, include a draining omphalomesenteric duct remnant, patent vitelline duct, or Meckel's diverticulum.[27] Fistulography may delineate the extent of the lesion, as may gentle probing. Ultrasonography may also be helpful in establishing the proper diagnosis.

As in the aforementioned urachal anomalies, complete surgical excision is required after antibiotic therapy. Excision of the umbilicus and sinus

and complete resection of the urachus with a bladder cuff is indicated in most instances. A bowel prep is a good precautionary measure because peritoneal contents may be involved.

VESICOURACHAL DIVERTICULUM

Vesicourachal diverticulum is most often seen with the prune-belly syndrome without obstruction,[7] and in conjunction with urethral obstruction.[11,25] If asymptomatic, no therapy is usually needed. If urinary infection or residual problems occur, which is unusual, resection is indicated.[28]

Adenocarcinoma

Adenocarcinoma of the bladder is rare, accounting for 1% of all bladder neoplasms. Of these only 35% qualify as urachal in origin,[23] and fewer than 200 cases have been reported in the world literature.[6]

The normal lining of the urachus is transitional

FIG. 60-6. Surgical treatment for carcinoma of the urachus. **(A)** The incision excises the umbilicus and extends to the pubis. **(B)** *En bloc* segmental resection of the bladder, the urachus, and the umbilicus. **(C)** If the rectus is infiltrated with tumor, portions of the muscles may need to be resected.

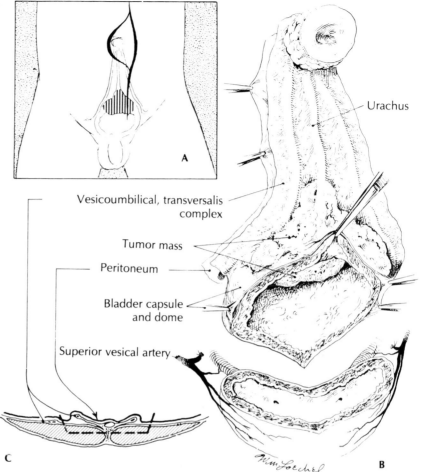

Urachus

Vesicoumbilical, transversalis complex

Tumor mass

Peritoneum

Bladder capsule and dome

Superior vesical artery

C

B

epithelium, but the histology of urachal carcinoma is mucin-producing adenocarcinoma, which is thought to represent a metaplastic transformation.[2,18,29] Transitional cell and squamous cell carcinomas of the urachus have been reported but are extremely rare.[16,17]

Criteria for distinguishing between urachal carcinoma and primary or secondary bladder adenocarcinoma include the following.

1. Position in the dome or anterior wall of the bladder
2. Intramural or suprapubic mass
3. Normal mucosa adjacent to or over a tumor with deep ramification in the bladder wall
4. No evidence of primary tumor elsewhere and
5. Absence of cystitis glandularis or cystica[16,21]

Vesical adenocarcinoma arising in the urothelium without urachal remnants may show a signet-ring cell pattern within a mucinous tumor.[13]

Urachal carcinoma occurs more commonly in male patients as opposed to the previously described benign conditions, which show a predilection for female patients. Most neoplasms occur in the fifth to seventh decades.

Because of the extravesical origin of urachal carcinoma, bladder symptoms are infrequent and late, leading to diagnostic delay. Early symptoms are usually vague and nonspecific. Cystoscopic examination will most likely be unrewarding at this stage until the mucosa is penetrated, at which time hematuria and passage of mucinous and necrotic debris is likely. A midline suprapubic mass, blood, or necrotic debris from the umbilicus may also be the first presenting sign.[21]

Both ultrasonography and CT are extremely helpful in establishing the diagnosis, visualizing extension to surrounding structures, and preoperative staging.[14,21] It may be that early employment of these modalities will improve the overall prognosis of this disease. The prognosis has been exceedingly poor, with 5-year survival ranging from 6% to 15%.[23,24]

Transurethral resection or radiation therapy alone has no place in the management of this neoplasm.[17] An aggressive *en bloc* surgical resection of the bladder dome and urachus is preferred by most authors (Fig. 60-6).[5,17,27] The role of preoperative or postoperative radiation therapy or chemotherapy, and the desirability of lymphadenectomy, have not been delineated, but there is some suggestion that aggressive surgery and postoperative radiation therapy is helpful.[29] Large, bulky tumors may require more radical exenterative procedures.

REFERENCES

1. BAUER SB, RETIK AB: Urachal anomalies and related umbilical disorders. Urol Clin North Am 5:195, 1978

2. BECK AD, GAUDIN HJ, BONHAM DG: Carcinoma of the urachus. Br J Urol 42:555, 1970

3. BLICHERT–TOFT M, KOCH F, NIELSON OV: Anatomic variants of the urachus related to clinical appearance and surgical treatment of urachal lesions. Surg Gynecol Obstet 137:51, 1973

4. BLICHERT–TOFT M, NIELSON OV: Diseases of the urachus simulating intra-abdominal disorders. Am J Surg 122:123, 1971

5. BOURNE CW, MAY JE: Urachal remnants: Benign or malignant? J Urol 118:743, 1977

6. Case Records of The Massachusetts General Hospital 304:469, 1981

7. COOPER EA, KINTZEN W: Patent urachus associated with abdominal muscle deficiency. Can Med Assoc J 87:27, 1962

8. ENTE G, PENZER P, KENIGSBERG K: Giant umbilical cord associated with patent urachus. Am J Dis Child 120:82, 1970

9. GENIESER NB, BECKER MH, GROSFELD J, KAUFMAN H: Draining umbilicus in infants. NY State J Med 74:1821, 1974

10. GRIFFITH GL, MULCAHYJJ, MCROBERTS JW: Umbilical anomalies. South Med J 72:981, 1979

11. HINMAN F, JR: Surgical disorders of the bladder and umbilicus of urachal origin. Surg Gynecol Obstet 113:605, 1961

12. HINMAN F, JR: Urologic aspects of the alternating urachal sinus. Am J Surg 102:339, 1961

13. JAKSE G, SCHNEIDER HM, JACOBI GH: Urachal signet-ring cell carcinoma; A rare variant of vesical adenocarcinoma: Incidence and pathological criteria. J Urol 120:764, 1978

14. KWOK–LIU J, ZIKMAN JM, COCKSHOTT WP: Carcinoma urachus: The role of computed tomography. Radiology 137:731, 1980

15. LATTIMER JK, USON AC: Abnormalities of the lower urinary tract. In Mustard WT (ed): Pediatric Surgery, 2nd ed, p 1154. Chicago, Year Book Medical Publishers 1969

16. LIN RY, RAPPOPORT AE, DEPPISCH LM et al: Squamous cell carcinoma urachus. J Urol 118:1066, 1977

17. LOENING SA, JACOBO E, HAWTREY CE et al: Adenocarcinoma of the urachus. J Urol 119:68, 1978

18. LOENING S, RICHARDSON JR, JR: Fibroadenoma of the urachus. J Urol 112:759, 1974

19. MCCAULEY RT, LICHTENHELD FR: Congenital patent urachus. South Med J 53:1138, 1960

20. MACMILLAN RW, SCHULLINGER JN, SANTULLI TV: Pyourachus: An unusual surgical problem. J Pediatr Surg 8:387, 1973

21. MEKRAS GD, BLOCK NL, CARRION HM et al: Urachal carcinoma: Diagnosis by computerized axial tomography. J Urol 123:275, 1980

22. MORIN ME, TAN A, BAKER DA et al: Urachal cyst in the adult: Ultrasound diagnosis. American Journal of Radiology 132:831, 1979

23. MOSTOFI FK, THOMSON RV, DEAN AL, JR: Mucous adenocarcinoma of the urinary bladder. Cancer 8:741, 1955

24. NADJIMI B, WHITEHEAD ED, MCKIEL CF, JR et al: Carcinoma of the urachus: Report of two cases and review of the literature. J Urol 100:738, 1968

25. NEY C, FRIEDENBERG RM: Radiographic findings in anomalies of the urachus. J Urol 99:288, 1968

26. NIX JT, MENNILLE JG, ALBERT M et al: Congenital patent urachus. J Urol 79:264, 1958

27. PERLMUTTER AD: Urachal disorders. In Glenn J (ed): Urologic Surgery, 2nd ed, p 393. Hagerstown, Harper & Row, 1975

28. WALDEN TB, KARAFIN L, KENDALL AR: Urachal diverticulum in a 3-year-old boy. J Urol 122:1979

29. WHITEHEAD ED, TESSLER AN: Carcinoma of the urachus. Br J Urol 43:468, 1971

Vesicovaginal and Vesicointestinal Fistulas

61

R. Keith Waterhouse

The causes of vesicovaginal fistulas and vesicointestinal fistulas are rather different. Vesicovaginal fistulas are almost always due to surgical or obstetric misadventure, whereas vesicointestinal fistulas are almost always due to disease, either diverticulitis or carcinoma of the colon. It is, however, appropriate for these two conditions to be discussed together, because the successful management of both illnesses requires strict adherence to established principles of preoperative examination, preoperative preparation, selection and performance of operation, and postoperative management. Failure to close the fistula usually occurs because of failure to give proper attention to one of these steps, not because of some inherent quality in the fistula that prevents its closure. There are some fistulas which cannot be closed and these should be carefully sought. "It is important for the surgeon to learn to recognize failure staring him in the face,"* because it is a disservice to the patient to attempt closure when the appropriate operation is urinary diversion.

Vesicovaginal Fistulas

The patient suffering from vesicovaginal fistula complains of being wet. The degree of wetness may be so mild as to suggest the possibility of a watery discharge or so severe that the patient never urinates and the whole urinary output is lost uncontrollably through the vagina.

In North America and Western Europe, the most common antecedent history in patients with vesicovaginal fistula is the performance of hysterectomy some 7 to 21 days before the onset of vaginal urinary drainage. Fistulas of obstetric origin are now rare, as are fistulas following irradiation. Unfortunately, fistulas due to recurrent carcinoma of the cervix are still seen. These are not amenable to surgical closure, and urinary diversion is usually needed if the patient's life expectancy is thought to be long enough to justify surgical intervention.

---

* Marshall VF: Personal communication

PREOPERATIVE EXAMINATION

In addition to the usual preoperative general assessment, the patient should have a careful study made of the urinary tract, any remaining internal genitalia, and the external genitalia. An excretory urogram is essential to look for concomitant ureterovaginal fistulas. The possibility that the ureteral fistulas may be bilateral must be borne in mind. Patients with long-standing fistulas may have developed stone disease.

Radiologic study of the bladder using contrast material is rarely of much value except in cases of vesicouterine fistula. In these patients the film made after emptying the bladder may show contrast material in the uterine cavity, cervical canal, or vagina.

Cystoscopic, vaginal, rectal, and abdominal examination should be carried out under general anesthesia. It is usually best to begin with a speculum examination of the vagina. This may show an obvious fistula, or the fistula may be so small that it is not seen until the bladder is filled with diluted methylene blue. Cystoscopic examination will show the site and number of fistulas. Vaginal, rectal, and abdominal examination will reveal the general state of the tissues and the condition of the adnexa. Urine specimens should be sent for culture and sensitivity.

Particular attention should be paid to estimating the competence of the urethral sphincteric mechanism, because in some patients repair of the sphincters is required at the time of repair of the fistula. There is nothing more disappointing, for both the patient and the surgeon, than to close successfully a vesicovaginal fistula only to find that the patient has severe stress incontinence which could easily have been corrected at the time of fistula closure.

PREOPERATIVE PREPARATION

The urine must be freed of infection by giving appropriate antibiotics preoperatively. If the vagi-

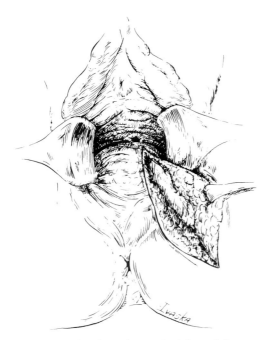

FIG. 61-1. Schuchardt's relaxing incision of the postero-lateral vaginal wall and adjacent musculature.

nal mucosa is ulcerated, local treatment with antiseptic douches and, in older patients, the use of diethyl stilbestrol is helpful. Some authors have recommended preoperative cortisone to reduce inflammation and allow earlier repair of the fistula.[3] We have not found this useful and no longer use it.

Patients coming from other countries may be iron deficient and have poor general nutrition. This needs attention preoperatively.

Some fistulas may heal with the aid of an indwelling catheter. We prefer a Malecot catheter rather than a Foley catheter because the bladder is kept completely dry with the former. A clinical trial of drainage is appropriate, and if the patient is made dry by the catheter then the fistula may heal. If loss of urine through the vagina continues after insertion of the catheter, then healing is unlikely.

Fulguration of small fistulas has been recommended. We have never had a personal success with the method and rarely use it. Marshall makes the same observation.[11]

In patients with large fistulas, keeping the patient reasonably dry during preparation for surgery presents a serious problem. A home-made device consisting of a Malecot catheter sealed, with rubber cement, into a perforation made in a contraceptive diaphragm is probably the best solution.[26] If pos-

sible the patient should wear diapers at night to avoid ulceration of the vagina.

SELECTION AND PERFORMANCE OF OPERATION

Inherent in the selection of operation is the matter of the timing of the surgical intervention. The very rare laceration of the base of the bladder occuring during forceps delivery may be repaired immediately through the vagina using 2-0 chromic catgut sutures full thickness through the bladder and the vagina. The bladder is drained suprapubically for 10 days. Because the tissues are fresh and there is no necrosis, *per primam* healing will almost always occur. We have had two examples of this injury and both healed uneventfully.

In the more common posthysterectomy fistula, there is a considerable element of inflammation and necrosis. Until recently, the general opinion has been that there should be a delay of between 3 and 6 months between the occurrence of the fistula and the attempted repair, and we concur with this view.[11,16] The case for early repair has been presented by Persky.[18] If early repair is attempted it would seem appropriate to use the transvesical transperitoneal route and to support the repair with omentum.[8,23] Following Persky's lead we have recently preformed early repair with satisfactory results. The selection of the route of operation depends on the site of the fistula, the size of the fistula, the condition of the perineum, and the timing of the operation.

In general, small posthysterectomy fistulas can be repaired through the vagina. Large fistulas are better repaired by a transvesical or combined transvaginal–transvesical approach.

Vaginal Repair

The vaginal route should be chosen when the vagina is capacious and not scarred by previous operation. Exposure may be improved by the use of Schuchardt's relaxing incision. This incision is started at about 4 o'clock from the introitus and carried posteriorly to a point 1 finger-width medial and posterior to the ischial tuberosity (Fig. 61-1). The vaginal route is particularly suitable for small, low-lying fistulas which are "mature," that is to say, fistulas in which 3 or 4 months has passed since they developed. Large series of posthysterectomy fistulas managed by this route have been presented. The Mayo Clinic series of 262 cases managed by this route was presented in 1964.[14] Further experience by this group of surgeons has confirmed their excellent figures.[20] Falk and Bulkin

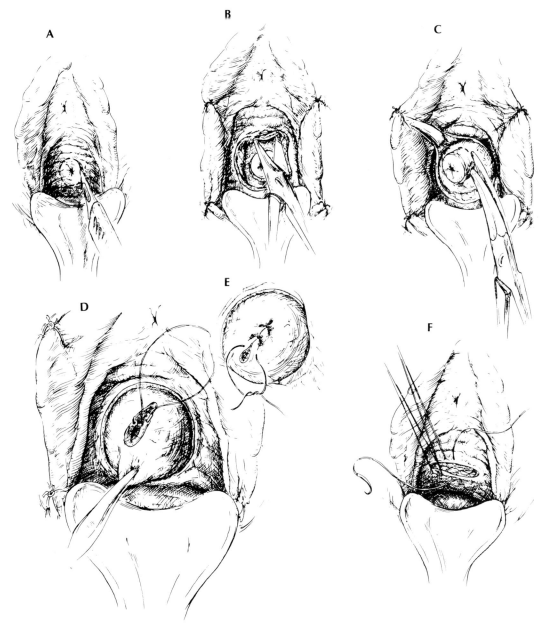

FIG. 61-2. Vaginal closure of vesicovaginal or urethrovaginal fistula: **(A)** circumferential incision; **(B)** mobilization of surrounding vaginal mucosa and adjacent bladder; **(C)** excision of fistulous tract; **(D)** closure of bladder wall, shown completed in **E; (F)** transverse closure of vaginal wall

reported on only 9 patients in 1951,[5] but in the course of his long experience with Latzko's operation[10] Falk successfully treated over 140 patients.[6] Tancer, using Latzko's operation, had 40 primary cures in 43 patients (93%) and 3 failures, each of which was cured by a second Latzko operation.[23]

The technique of closure used by the Mayo Clinic surgeons is fistulectomy and separate layered closure of the bladder and vagina. The Latzko technique is the performance of a partial colpocleisis. Although either technique can give excellent results, Latzko's operation is only suitable for patients who have had the uterus removed.

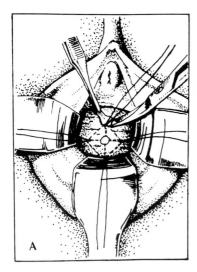
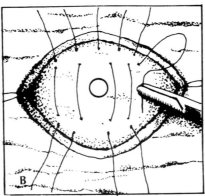
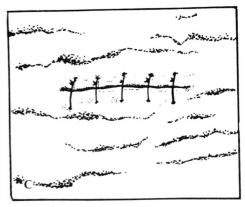

FIG. 61-3.   Technique of partial colpocleisis (Latzko's operation): **(A)** removal of diamond-shaped area of vaginal mucosa; **(B)** insertion of first layer of interrupted 2-0 chromic catgut sutures; **(C)** vaginal closure with 2-0 chromic catgut sutures

Fistulectomy With the fistulectomy technique, the patient is placed in the lithotomy or modified Kraske's position. The fistulous opening is widely excised, carrying the excision to normal bladder tissue (Fig. 61-2*A*, *B*, and *C*). The adjacent bladder is widely mobilized as is the vagina. The bladder is closed in two layers with 2-0 chromic catgut sutures. The vagina is then closed separately, again in two layers with 2-0 chromic catgut sutures (Fig. 61-2*D*, *E*, and *F*). In posthysterectomy fistulas, Symmonds opens the vaginal vault and enters the peritoneal cavity. This allows him to mobilize a flap of peritoneum, which he sutures over the bladder repair before closing the vagina. This greatly strengthens the repair.[20] Other techniques of strengthening the repair are the interposition operations of Ingleman–Sundberg and Martius.[7,13] These operations are particularly useful in patients who have been irradiated. We reported our own series of 18 interposition operations in 1980.[17]

Urethral catheter drainage is maintained for 2 weeks after fistulectomy.

Partial Colpocleisis (Latzko's Operation)
With the partial colpocleisis technique (Latzko's operation), the patient is placed in lithotomy position and an 18Fr indwelling catheter is placed in the bladder through the urethra. Using a weighted speculum posteriorly and lateral vaginal retractors, the fistula is exposed. Silk stay sutures (1-0) are placed approximately 2 cm from the fistula at 12, 3, 6, and 9 o'clock. Using sharp dissection, the vaginal mucosa is denuded as shown in Figure 61-3.

It is better to remove the lower segments of mucosa first, to diminish the loss of visibility from blood oozing over the field if the upper segments are removed first. The bladder is not entered, and the fistula is not excised. A partial colpocleisis is then performed using 2-0 chromic catgut on a round-bodied needle (Fig. 61-3). Two or three transverse rows of sutures are inserted and then the vaginal mucosa is closed. Prior to closing the vaginal mucosa and usually after the second layer of transverse sutures has been inserted, the bladder is filled with sterile milk to make certain that the closure is watertight.

We leave the catheter in place for 5 days, but Tancer removes it after 48 hr. This is an excellent operation in suitable cases. In the past 7 years we have selected it 23 times in 43 patients presenting with vesicovaginal fistulas.

Suprapubic Closure should be selected in high-lying fistulas, when the introitus is narrow or scarred and when it has been decided to close the fistula soon after its development. The operation we recommend is that described by Vincent O'Conor in 1957.[15] This operation was reported on subsequently in 1980 by Vincent O'Conor, Jr., who described 42 patients.[16] There were three failures in the first 20 patients and two failures in the second 22. The two failures in the second 22 were both cured by reoperation incorporating the interposition of a pedicled omental flap. It is our practice to use such a flap routinely, and we have had no failures in 20 cases.

Transvesical Repair

Transvesical repair is more easily performed through a midline transperitoneal incision but may be carried out through a transverse incision if the patient so wishes. The bladder is opened extraperitoneally and the fistula is identified. A ball retractor as described by Fagerstrom is used.[4,9] It is a sponge-rubber ball approximately 3.5 cm and obtainable in any dime store. Wire sutures are passed through in both directions and fixed so that they cannot slide when traction is applied in one direction to lift up the fistula and the other direction to remove the ball from the vagina at the completion of the closure. A No. 5 ureteral catheter or infant feeding tubes are inserted into both ureteral orifices to identify the orifices and the ureters. The back of the bladder is inspected transperitoneally, and any adherent bowel is dissected away so that the vesicorectal pouch is empty. A midline incision is made in the posterior wall of the bladder (Fig. 61-4A) and continued to the fistula. Stay sutures of 1-0 chromic catgut placed opposite one another as the bladder is incised are useful. The fistula is circumscribed (Fig. 61-4B) and then excised (Fig. 61-4C). The vagina is then closed with 2-0 chromic catgut and the bladder is closed with a suprapubic tube in the prevesical space.

The repair may be buttressed with either a piece of mobilized peritoneum or a pedicled omental flap.[8,23] We much prefer the latter and use it routinely, however simple the case may seem to be. The use of omentum to separate the two suture lines has in our view greatly improved the reliability of the O'Conor operation.

A Penrose drain is placed in the prevesical space and is removed after 72 hr. The suprapubic tube should remain in place for 10 days and then be removed, and a Foley catheter should be placed through the urethra to allow the suprapubic sinus to close. This ordinarily takes 48 hr.

Transvaginal–Transvesical Approach

In difficult cases the technique of simultaneous transvaginal–transvesical or transpubic–transvesical approach may be invaluable.[2,19,22] We always use a pedicled omental flap to buttress these repairs so as to diminish the possibility of refistulization.

Marshall and Twombley have described a useful modification of Latzko's operation combining a transvesical and transvaginal approach.[12] They have used this technique to cure a number of radiation fistulas.

POSTOPERATIVE MANAGEMENT

Vesicovaginal fistula is such a psychologically debilitating illness that all efforts should be made to effect a cure on the first attempt. For this reason we are in no hurry to remove the indwelling catheters until we are sure that the suture lines are well healed.

The urine should be kept sterile with suitable antibiotics and should be checked postoperatively for recurrence of infection.

Patients should not have sexual intercourse for 12 weeks following a successful repair. Patients with obstetric fistulas must inform their gynecologists if they become pregnant because vaginal delivery may be contraindicated.

Vesicointestinal Fistulas

In a study of 148 patients with vesicointestinal fistulas, Williams found 23 to be due to diverticulitis, 54 to carcinoma of the colon or rectum, 10 to carcinoma of the bladder, 8 to Crohn's disease, 22 to trauma, and 11 to miscellaneous other causes.[25] In a personal series of 18 cases, Ward and coworkers found diverticulitis of the colon to be the cause in all but two patients.[24] In these two the cause was carcinoma of the colon. In Ward's series, the most frequently recorded symptoms were fecaluria (15 patients), recurring urinary tract infections (12 patients), and pneumaturia (10 patients).

In some patients the diagnosis is obvious and the fistula can be demonstrated by cystography or barium enema and seen at cystoscopy. In other patients the diagnosis is much more difficult to prove but should always be suspected in patients (particularly male) with recurring bouts of urinary tract infection.

The fistula will rarely close spontaneously, but if it is small there may be long, symptom-free periods. If the patient's general condition warrants attempt at surgical closure, then the important decision is whether to perform one-stage bowel excision, intestinal reanastomosis, and closure of the bladder; or a multistage surgical repair. Carson, Malek, and Remine, in reviewing 100 cases treated at the Mayo Clinic, found that a one-stage bowel resection and closure of the fistula was performed in 66% of patients with diverticulitis.[1]. The remainder had mostly a two-stage procedure, namely bowel resection, fistula repair, and a diverting

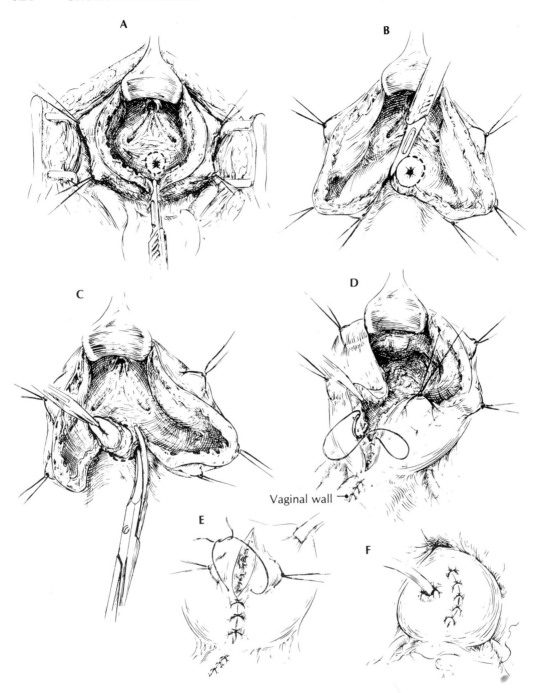

Vaginal wall →

FIG. 61-4. Suprapubic repair of vesicovaginal fistula: **(A)** fistula exposed and bladder opened posteriorly; **(B)** circumferential incision; **(C)** excision of fistula tract; **(D)** vaginal wall closed and posterior bladder closure initiated; **(E)** second layer of bladder closed; **(F)** cystostomy drainage

colostomy followed by restoration of bowel continuity. Patients with colonic malignancy more often underwent multistage than single-stage operation (44% vs 33%), but 25% had only fecal diversion because of an inoperable malignancy.

Preoperatively, patients should have the urine and bowel contents sterilized with appropriate antibiotics. Malnutrition, if present, should be corrected. The abdomen is opened through a long midline incision, and a complete examination is made of the contents of the peritoneal cavity. Only then can a final decision be made as to whether to perform a single-stage or a multistage operation. If there is a walled-off abscess associated with the fistula or a very large inflammatory mass, preliminary fecal diversion by transverse colostomy may be wise. If the surgical situation looks relatively simple, bowel excision, closure of the fistula, and diversion of the urine by suprapubic cystostomy may be performed. Use of a pedicled omental flap is often desirable. The decision of whether to perform a protecting transverse colostomy after bowel excision and closure of the fistula should be made by the surgeon in the course of the operation.

REFERENCES

1. CARSON CC, MALEK SR, REMINE WH: Urologic aspects of vesicoenteric fistulas. J Urol 119:744, 1978
2. CLARK DH, HOLLAND JB: Repair of vesicovaginal fistulas: Simultaneous transvaginal–transvesical approach. South Med J 68:1410, 1975
3. COLLINS CF, PENT D, JONES FB: Results of early repair of vesicovaginal fistula with preliminary cortisone treatment. Am J Obst Gynecol 80:1005, 1960
4. FAGERSTROM DP: Use of a ball retractor in the repair of vesicovaginal fistula. J Urol 62:717, 1949
5. FALK HC, BULKIN IA: Management of vesicovaginal fistula following abdominal total hysterectomy. Surg Gynecol Obstet 93:404, 1951
6. FALK HC, KURMAN M: Repair of vesicovaginal fistula: Report of 140 cases. J Urol 89:226, 1963
7. INGELMAN–SUNDBERG AG: Pathogenesis and operative treatment of urinary fistulae in irradiated tissue. In Youssef AF (ed): Gynecological Urology, p 263. Springfield, Illionis, Charles C Thomas, 1960
8. KIRICUTA I, GOLDSTEIN AMB: The repair of extensive vesicovaginal fistulas with pedicled omentum: A review of 27 cases. J Urol 108:724, 1972
9. LANDES RR: Simple transvesical repair of vesicovaginal fistula. J Urol 122:604, 1979
10. LATZKO W: Postoperative vesicovaginal fistulas; Genesis and therapy. Am J Surg 58:211, 1942
11. MARSHALL VF: Vesicovaginal fistulas on one urological service. J Urol 121:25, 1979
12. MARSHALL VF, TWOMBLEY GH: Further experiences with an operation for the repair of vesicovaginal fistula caused by radiation. Cancer 5:429, 1952
13. MARTIUS H: Die gynäkologischen Operationen. Stuttgart, Georg Thieme Verlag, 1954
14. MASSEE JS, WELCH JS, PRATT JH et al: Management of urinary–vaginal fistula. Ten-year survey. JAMA 190:902, 1964
15. O'CONOR VJ: Suprapubic Closure of Vesicovaginal Fistula, Springfield, Illinois, Charles C Thomas, 1957
16. O'CONOR VJ, JR.: Review of experience with vesicovaginal fistula repair. J Urol 123:367, 1980
17. PATIL U, WATERHOUSE RK, LAUNGANI G: Management of 18 difficult vesicovaginal fistulas with modified Ingelman–Sundberg and Martius operations. J Urol 123:653, 1980
18. PERSKY L, HERMAN G, GUERRIER K: Non-delay in vesicovaginal fistula repair. Urology 13:273, 1979
19. SHARMA SK, BAPNA BC, GUPTA CL et al: Pedicled omental graft in repair of large, difficult vesicovaginal fistulae. Int J Gynaecol Obstet 17:556, 1980
20. SYMMONDS RE: Vaginal repair of vesicovaginal fistula. Presentation at Annual Meeting Clinical Society of Genito-Urinary Surgeons, Mayo Clinic, February 1980
21. TANCER ML: The post-total hysterectomy (vault) vesicovaginal fistula. J Urol 123:839, 1980
22. TAYLOR JS, HEWSON AD, RACHOW P et al: Synchronous combined transvaginal–transvesical repair of vesicovaginal fistulas. Aust NZ J Surg 50:23, 1980
23. TURNER WARWICK RT: Use of omental pedicle graft in urinary tract reconstruction. J Urol 116:341, 1976
24. WARD JN, LAVENGOOD RW, JR, NAY HR et al: Diagnosis and treatment of colovesical fistulas. Surg Gynecol Obstet 130:1082, 1970
25. WILLIAMS RJ: Vesicointestinal fistula and Crohn's disease. Br J Surg 42:179, 1954
26. WOLFF HD, JR, GILLILAND NA: Vaginal diaphragm catheters. J Urol 78:681, 1957

Reduction and Augmentation Cystoplasties

62

Sheridan W. Shirley

During the early 20th century surgeons recognized the potential use of bowel segments as a partial or total "bladder substitute" to relieve severe lower urinary tract symptoms in patients with diseased and contracted urinary bladders. Patients with incapacitating symptoms had previously been treated surgically by creating vesicovaginal, intestinal, and cutaneous bladder fistulas for symptomatic relief. A review of the literature by Hinman in 1936 described a number of ingenious experimental and clinical surgical procedures using bowel segments for bladder substitute with generally poor results.[10] As newer surgical techniques, developed and antimicrobial agents became available, a more rational surgical use of isolated bowel segments ensued. Since 1936 many surgeons, including Bruce, Gil–Vernet, Kuss, Goodwin and Winter, and Turner Warwick, have successfully used all portions of the large and small bowel to replace part or all of the urinary bladder.[1,2,6,7,8,12,13,14,22]

Even though the bowel musculature is not ideal as a substitute detrusor and mucous production is undesirable, the functional results of partial, subtotal, and total enterocystoplasty can now be recommended for humans without reservations. Studies by Weinberg and Waterhouse and others give conclusive evidence through long-term follow-up that patients with enterocystoplasties have normal renal function and no metabolic or electrolyte imbalance.[24] Because of painful symptoms, the patient often becomes a urinary bladder cripple and a recluse when he fails to get adequate relief from medical therapy and has to have urinary diversion, which in the past was the only alternative. The use of reduction and augmentation cystoplasty to relieve severe urinary symptoms in patients with diseased and contracted urinary bladders now offers new hope for a significant number of patients to live an active and productive life.

Etiologic Factors in Treatment

Chronic interstitial cystitis and tuberculous cystitis with contracture prompted the early urologic surgeons to use segments of bowel as a substitute bladder after partial and total cystectomy.[3,6,7,9] Today in the United States, tuberculous cystitis has become a rarity and chronic interstitial cystitis, a disease primarily of women, is the most common cause of bladder contracture. From 1960 to 1980 we operated on 80 patients with diseased and contracted urinary bladder by performing enterocystoplasties for bladder augmentation. We achieved an overall success rate of 80% (50% excellent and 30% good). Table 62-1 summarizes the etiology of these cases.

We do not recommend enterocystoplasties for the primary surgical treatment of bladder cancer. Women with chronic interstitial cystitis rarely develop cancer of the bladder, but men with severe interstitial-cystitis-type symptoms must be highly suspect of having underlying cancer of the bladder.[17] Utz and Zincke have concluded that men with chronic interstitial-cystitis-type symptoms may have carcinoma *in situ* and need random biopsies with careful follow-up.[23] Because chronic interstitial cystitis accounted for the majority of our patients with severe incapacitating bladder symptoms, we agree with Hunner's thesis, alluded to in 1915 when he stated, "Severe ulcerative bladder disease is often given prolonged and painful medical treatment when more drastic measures are demanded for good results."[11] Since DMSO (dimethylsulfoxide) instillation therapy for chronic interstitial cystitis was introduced by Stewart in 1967,[18,21] the overall good-to-excellent results have been approximately 50%. Those who fail to get relief may be candidates for reduction and augmentation enterocystoplasty. DMSO instillation therapy has proven to be an excellent adjunct during the recovery period as well as for those who experience relapses after cystoplasty.

Surgical Considerations and Technique

Walsh and others advocate total cystectomy as the preferred procedure for the bladder contracted by chronic interstitial cystitis. They often fail, how-

TABLE 62-1. Etiology of 80 Enterocystoplasties, 1960–1980

Etiology	Patient Data			
	AGE	MALE	FEMALE	TOTAL
Chronic interstitial cystitis (typical or atypical)	19–78	9	40	49
Tuberculous cystitis	20–40	6	4	10
Radiation cystitis	54–70	5	5	10
Neuropathic bladder	55–72		6	6
Pericystitis related to trauma	25–35	2		2
Undiversion	7–34	1	2	3
Total		23	57	80

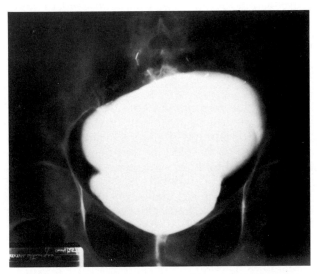

FIG. 62-1. Cystogram in patient with patch augmentation colocystoplasty. Note absence of reflux.

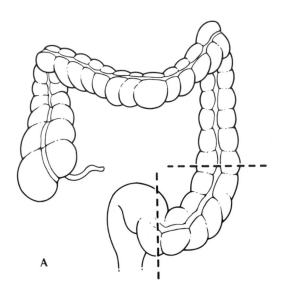

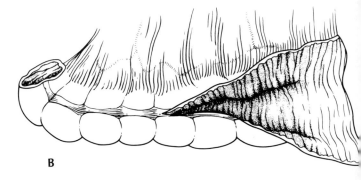

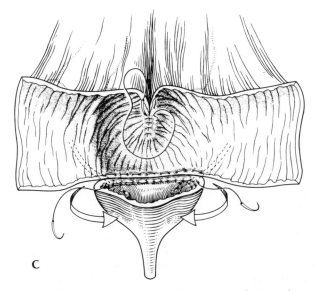

FIG. 62-2. Technique of augmentation colocystoplasty. **(A)** The upper sigmoid colon is selected. **(B)** The colon is opened along the teniae coli, preserving the mesenteric attachment. **(C)** The opened colon is joined and attached to the remaining bladder.

ever, to reveal the high incidence of significant residual urine and recurrent infections. The inability to empty presents a new problem of infection and stone formation which necessitates self-catheterization several times a day. Not only is self-catheterization a very disappointing inconvenience to the patient, but also many patients do not tolerate self-catheterization and experience a higher incidence of recurrent irritation and infections. Our best results have been in those patients with severe symptoms of frequency, urgency, and suprapubic pain who have a good bladder capacity under anesthesia (300 ml–500 ml) but experience severe pain when distended to 100 ml to 150 ml without anesthesia.[17] If medical treatment fails, we advise a reduction and augmentation ileocystoplasty before fibrotic contracture becomes severe and more difficult to cure. Even though there is no unanimity of opinion on how much bladder should be removed in patients with chronic interstitial cystitis, we have found that it is not necessary to remove all of the bladder down to the trigone to obtain a good functional result. Our experience clearly indicates, however, that when most of the bladder is removed, the more likely incomplete emptying results.

During the early 1960s in Birmingham, Alabama, we first used isolated segments of ileum and rectosigmoid to enlarge the contracted bladder after minimum reduction. We chose to use 20-cm segments with a T-type augmentation after closing both ends. The segment was then opened on the antimesenteric border and sutured to the dome of the remaining bladder in a T-type fashion. We found, as did Hanley, that such constructed segments often retained urine in the lateral "horns" of the T, and one patient developed stones from urinary stasis. We have since revised four patients and modified our technique by opening the segments of large and small bowel after removing the diseased portion of the bladder and fashioning it into a patch-type enterocystoplasty to give a better surface area (Figs. 62-1 to 62-4).

During the early 1970s, we began using ileocecal segments for more severely diseased and contracted bladders (Table 62-2). When all but the trigone with intact ureters must be removed, we have used an ileocecal pouch created by opening the terminal ileum through the ileocecal valve and into the antimesenteric side of the cecum to fashion a large pouch (Figs. 62-5 and 62-6).

When the entire bladder and lower ureters are involved by severe inflammatory disease, such as tuberculosis, all of the bladder (including the lower ureters) must be removed for a good result.[1,4,5,7,9]

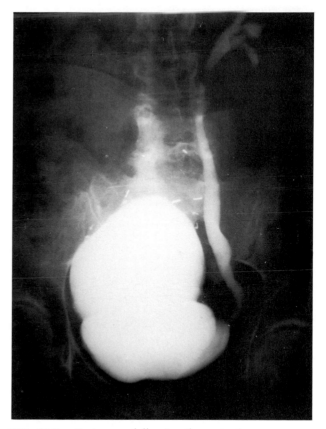

FIG. 62-3. Cystogram following ileocystoplasty

We have successfully operated on 13 patients using an intact ileocecal segment (Fig. 62-7) by suturing the ureters to the terminal ileum using antireflex technique and the distal colon-cecum to the bladder neck. Ten had long-term good to excellent results; two had fair results and one had a poor result. Many authors indicate they prefer using colon, rectosigmoid, and ileocecal segments for total bladder replacement.[*,1,3–6a,8,12,14,22] Most have had experiences similar to ours, with incomplete emptying in a varying number of patients. A low bladder outflow resistance is necessary to allow emptying of a totally colonic bladder, and Turner Warwick advises selective sphincterotomy to enhance emptying.[22] Intermittent self-catheterization is necessary in many of these patients and in our experience is superior to sphincterotomy, which may result in an incontinent patient.

In our experiences as reported by others, the etiology of bladder contracture did not seem to affect the overall success rate.[3,20] We have also had about equal success with each bowel segment used

---

* Walsh A: Personal communication, 1978

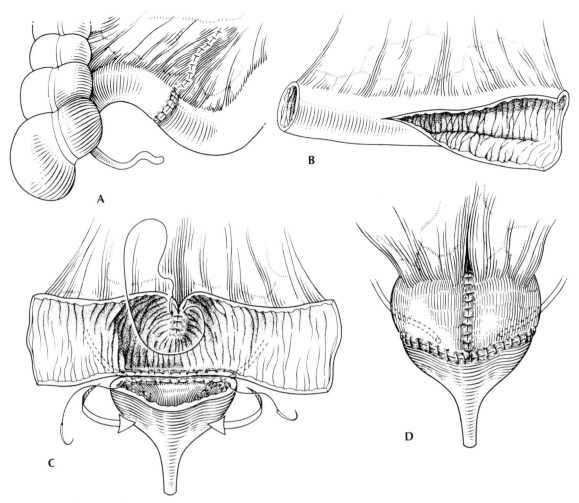

FIG. 62-4. Technique of ileocystoplasty. **(A)** After isolating a segment of the terminal ileum, the continuity of the small bowel is reestablished. **(B)** The ileum is opened along the anterior surface. **(C)** The ileal patch is constructed and anastomosed to the bladder. **(D)** The cystoplasty is completed.

TABLE 62-2.   Types of Segments Used in 80 Cases

Etiology	Type of Segment		
	RECTOSIGMOID	ILEOCECAL	ILEUM
Chronic interstitial cystitis (typical or atypical)	13	2	34
Tuberculous cystitis		10	
Radiation cystitis	5		5
Neuropathic bladder	2		4
Pericystitis related to trauma	1		1
Undiversion (same segment)		1	2
Total	21	13	46

TABLE 62-3.   Results by Type of Bowel Segment

Result	Type of Bowel Segment		
	RECTOSIGMOID	ILEOCECAL	ILEUM
Excellent*	10	7	20
Good	6	3	15
Fair	3	2	6
Poor	2	1	3
Total	21	13	44

* Pain-free, minimal nocturia, 300-ml or greater capacity, volitional control, no incontinence, no infection, and able to live normal active life.

(Table 62-3). The choice of bowel segment depends upon the degree of bladder disease and the experience of the surgeon.

Complications

No deaths have been attributed to our reduction and augmentation enterocystoplasties. There is no doubt, however, that the colon segments are more prone to wound infection and abscess. Such complications have been minimized by thorough preoperative mechanical cleansing of the bowel as well as by oral nonabsorbable antibiotics. Since 1976 we have almost eliminated wound infection and abscess by preoperative bowel cleansing and judicious use of antibiotic irrigating solutions during the procedure. We intermittently irrigate the pelvis and bowel segments with separate solutions of bacitracin, neomycin, kanamycin (Kantrex), and gentamicin (Garamycin). At the end of the procedure we thoroughly lavage the pelvic and bladder with normal saline. We have had a total of eight pelvic abscesses and wound infections; colon seg-

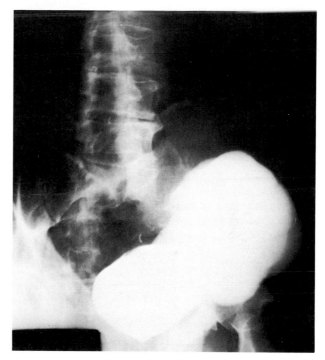

FIG. 62-5.   Cystogram in patient with ileocecal cystoplasty

ments were used in seven and ileal segments in one. Table 62-4 summarizes the complications of our reduction and augmentation enterocystoplasties.

Urinary fistulas were one of our early complications. It has been completely eliminated since we discontinued the use of suprapubic tubes through the bowel segments and started using three-way continuous irrigating urethral catheter during the first 7 to 10 days of the postoperative period. A sump drain is routinely left in the retropubic space until it can be clearly established that the bladder has sealed. We use a single layer of continuous

TABLE 62-4.   Complications

Early	No.	Late	No.
Abscesses	8	Intestinal obstruction	8
Fistulas	5	Urinary retention with acute infection	10
Ischemic atrophy (ileum)	1	Urinary retention with recurrent infection	8
Renal failure (transient)	3	Stone formation	1
Prolonged ileus	5	Reoperation Y–V plasty	6
		Urinary diversion	5
Total	22		38

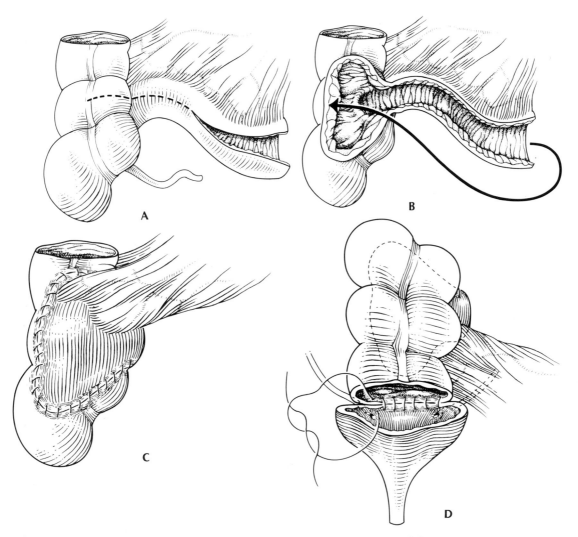

FIG. 62-6. Technique of ileocecal cystoplasty. **(A)** The isolated ileum and the cecum are opened along the anterior surface. **(B)** The ileum is closed over the cecal opening, creating a large pouch **(C)**, which is then rotated 180 degrees for anastomosis to the bladder **(D)**.

inverting chromic catgut for watertight enterocystoplasty closure. Nonabsorbable sutures and clips must never be used, even as a second layer, because they often erode into the urinary system and cause infection and stone formation. We have had only one ischemic atrophy following the use of an isolated segment of ileum in 1961. This was due to a compromised blood supply when closing the peritoneum.

Prolonged ileus and transient renal failure has been a problem in eight patients and pelvic hematomas, in five patients. During the early 1970s we were influenced by Moulder and Meirowsky and others to employ presacral neurectomy, fifth lumbar sympathectomy, and selected (S2, S3, S4)

sacral neurotomy in conjunction with reduction and augmentation enterocystoplasties, in an effort to reduce bladder pain and hypertonicity and to increase capacity.[15] This procedure is not only time consuming but also was the complicating factor in pelvic hematomas. After comparing our results on 15 patients with and 15 patients without presacral and lumbar sympathectomy and sacral neurotomy, there has been no discernible long-term functional difference. At best, the combined cystoplasty and neurosurgery approach gives temporary and transient additional relief; we have abandoned this approach.

Intestinal obstruction, as a late complication, has happened 3 to 18 months following cystoplasty

FIG. 62-7. Bladder augmentation with an intact ileocecal segment. **(A)** The ureters are implanted into the terminal ileum and the segment is rotated 180 degrees to join the bladder base. **(B)** A cystogram reveals reflux in this patient with ileocecal cystoplasty.

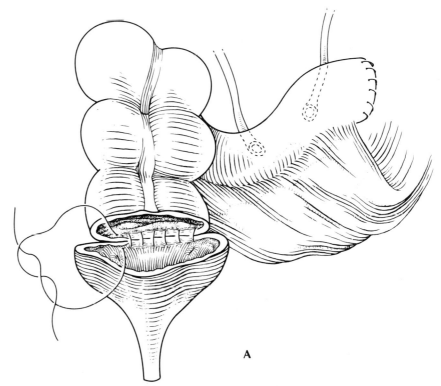

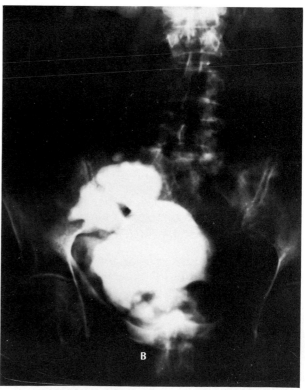

using ileum in eight patients. Six cases have been related to the metal clip autosuture. The etiology is not entirely clear. The autosuture people attribute it to adhesiveness between the raw mucosal edges, but if this is true, why is there such a delayed contracture? We have not entirely abandoned the autosuture for ileoileal reapproximation but prefer a handsewn two-layer closure (inner catgut, outer silk).

Varying degrees of urinary retention, with acute or recurrent infections, have been our most frequent problem after enterocystoplasty. Eighteen patients have experienced this problem, and six have required a second operation (Y–V plasty) to restore emptying ability. Fortunately, four have totally reverted to complete emptying, and most recurrent infections have been cured with short- and long-term antimicrobials. Eight patients are satisfactorily controlled on intermittent self-catheterization. Why, at times, some fail to empty, and yet void without residual at other times, is difficult to understand but may be due to overindulgence in tranquilizers and analgesics. Mucous excess has not been a problem as we first anticipated. Mucous production in the early healing stages (4–6 weeks) is only a minor problem. If excessive mucous production is experienced later, it indicates bacterial infection.

A hysterectomy should be done at the time of reduction and augmentation cystoplasty because the uterus is a mechanical deterrent and may lead to displacement and encroachment on the blood supply of the isolated bowel segment, although successful pregnancies and deliveries have been reported after enterocystoplasties. One must take care to suspend the posterior vagina adequately to the round ligaments and lateral pelvic wall to prevent the bowel segment from dropping into the cul-de-sac and retaining urine. If the patient has had a previous bladder neck suspension for incontinence, it is wise to release the bladder neck and urethra to prevent postoperative retention in most patients.

We prefer a midline incision for better exposure and use a continuous 1-0 Prolene lateral mattress fascial closure. The peritoneum around the newly constructed bladder is best left partially open, but the omentum should be tucked around the fornices to prevent the small bowel from contacting any raw surface.

One must view with caution patients with severe lower urinary tract symptoms suggestive of nonspecific chronic cystitis who carry varying amounts of residual urine and have ill-defined neuromuscular dysfunction of the urinary bladder. They are generally poor candidates for augmentation cystoplasty. Even though some patients may gain considerable relief of their symptoms and may become completely cured, they often do not empty and require self-catheterization. Augmentation cystoplasty for the neuropathic bladder[19,20] may still be more favorable than urinary diversion and proved to be satisfactory, but not excellent, in four of six patients with bladder neuropathy. Six of our patients have come to total cystectomy and urinary diversion because of failure of reduction and augmentation cystoplasty to adequately relieve their painful bladder symptoms.

Our goal is to maintain volitional control of urination and to alleviate severe disabling symptoms so that the patient may live a more normal life.

REFERENCES

1. BRUCE PT: Colocystoplasty: Bladder replacement after total cystectomy. Aust NZ J Surg 43:270, 1973
2. BRUCE PT, BUCKHAM GJ, CARDEN ABG et al: The surgical treatment of chronic interstitial cystitis. Med J Aust 1:581, 1977
3. CHAN SL, ANKENMAN GJ, WRIGHT JE et al: Cecocystoplasty in the surgical management of the small, contracted bladder. J Urol 124:338, 1980
4. CHARGHI A, CHARBONNEAU JR, GAUTHIER GE: Colocystoplasty for bladder enlargement and bladder substitution: A study of late results in 31 cases. J Urol 97:849, 1967
5. DOUNIS A, ABEL BJ, GOW JG: Cecocystoplasty for bladder augmentation. J Urol 123:164, 1980
6. GIL–VERNET, JM, GOSALBEZ R: Colocystoplasty versus ileocystoplasty to increase bladder capacity. J Urol 63:466, 1957
7. GIL–VERNET, JM et al: A functioning artificial bladder: Results of 41 corrective cases. J Urol 86:825, 1962
8. GOODWIN WE, WINTER CC: Technique of sigmoidocystoplasty. Surg Gynecol Obstet 108:370, 1959
9. HANLEY HG: Ileocystoplasty: A clinical review. J Urol 82:317, 1959
10. HINMAN F, WEYRAUCH HM, JR: A critical study of the different principles of surgery which have been used in ureterointestinal implantation. Trans Am Assoc Genitourin Surg 29:15, 1936
11. HUNNER GL: Bladder ulcerations in female patients. Boston Med Surg J 172:600, 1915
12. KUSS R: Colo-cystoplasty rather than ileo-cystoplasty. J Urol 82:587, 1959
13. KUSS R, BITKER M, CAMEY M et al: Indications and early and late results of intestino-cysto-plasty: A review of 185 cases. J Urol 103:53, 1970
14. MORALES PA, ONG G, ASHNARI S et al: Sigmoidocystoplasty for contracted bladder. J Urol 80:455, 1958
15. MOULDER MK, MEIROWSKY AM: The management of Hunner's ulcer by differential sacral neurotomy: Preliminary report. J Urol 75:261, 1956

16. ROBLEJO PG, MALAMENT M: Late results of an ileo-cystoplasty: A 12-year follow-up. J Urol 109:38, 1973

17. SHIRLEY SW, MIRELMAN S: Experiences with colocystoplasties and ileocystoplasties in urologic surgery: 40 patients. J Urol 120:165, 1978

18. SHIRLEY SW, STEWART B, MIRELMAN S: Dimethyl sulfoxide in treatment of inflammatory genitourinary disorders. Urology 11:215, 1978

19. SMITH RB: Use of ileocystoplasty in the hypertonic neurogenic bladder. J Urol 75:125, 1975

20. SMITH RB, VAN CANGH P, SKINNER DG et al: augmentation enterocystoplasty: A critical review. J Urol 118:35, 1977

21. STEWART BH, SHIRLEY SW: Further experience with intravesical dimethyl sulfoxide in the treatment of interstitial cystisis. J Urol 116:36, 1976

22. TURNER–WARWICK RT, ASHKEN MH: The functional results of partial, subtotal, cystoplasty with special reference to uretero cecocystoplasty, selective sphincterotomy of cystocystoplasty. Br J Urol 39:3, 1967

23. UTZ DC, ZINCKE H: The masquerade of bladder cancer in situ as chronic interstitial cystitis. J Urol 111:160, 1978

24. WEINBERG S, WATERHOUSE K: Function of bladder after ileocystoplasty, III. J Urol 82:80, 1959

Vesical Trauma

63

Jack W. McAninch

Bladder ruptures occur in 8% to 10% of patients sustaining pelvic fractures from blunt trauma.[4,7] Penetrating injuries, largely from gunshot wounds, may rarely traverse the bladder.[5,6] If they are unrecognized, injuries from pelvic operations such as hysterectomy, bowel resection, surgical intervention for cancer, hernia repair, and transurethral procedures may result in major complications.[1,2,3]

Surgical Anatomy

The anterior bony pelvis protects the bladder to a large degree. When rupture occurs from blunt trauma, anterior pubic rami fractures are commonly noted and, if extraperitoneal injury is present, spicules of bone have perforated the bladder wall. When the bladder is full, its position is more intra-abdominal; this position makes injury more likely from lower abdomen blows. The bladder dome is covered by peritoneum, which accounts for intra-peritoneal rupture, a condition occurring when the bladder is full. The bladder receives its blood supply from branches of the hypogastric artery—the superior, middle, and inferior vesical branches. Venous drainage corresponds with arterial supply and may be ruptured during injury, causing heavy bleeding and pelvic hematoma.

The major continence mechanisms are in the bladder neck and trigone areas: should injuries occur in this area, meticulous repair must be done to ensure postoperative continence. The ureteral orifices insert in the lateral trigone and attach to deep underlying trigonal muscles. Extensive injury may result in reflux and other abnormalities. Para-sympathetic nerve supply S2, S3, and S4 courses through a plexus through the posterior aspect of the bladder and allows proper function. Extensive posterior and lateral dissections can cause functional problems from the nerve damage.

Assessment of Injury

Bladder rupture should be suspected in any case of pelvic fracture. Such patients have lower abdominal injury and pain. Voiding is difficult and catheterization reveals grossly bloody urine in most cases. Before catheterization the urethral meatus should be carefully inspected for blood, and urethral injury should be suspected if a blood discharge is observed. Urethrography will enable diagnosis of the injury. A urethral catheter should not be passed if there is urethral trauma.

Cystography is diagnostic. Gravity filling of the bladder with 300 ml of contrast material is done. This volume of contrast medium allows complete bladder expansion and extravasation in areas of disruption. Two films are important: a full bladder film and a drainage film. The full film will demonstrate all areas of extravasation in most cases. In intraperitoneal rupture (25% of cases) there will be free contrast in the peritoneal cavity highlighting bowel loops (Fig. 63-1). The drainage film should be done with the bladder completely empty and will detect residual extravasation from extraperitoneal rupture. Extraperitoneal ruptures (75% of cases) are seen frequently after pubic rami fracture (Fig. 63-2).

Intraoperative bladder injuries can be detected by filling the bladder with saline colored with Indigo Carmine or methylene blue and noting areas of extravasation. Cystography may also be of diagnostic benefit.

An excretory urogram will ensure that no injury to the kidneys and ureters has occurred.

Operative Approach and Repair

A lower abdominal midline incision should be used. This incision provides easy access to full abdominal exploration for possible associated visceral injuries. A small peritoneotomy is carried out, and if free blood is present, full abdominal exploration should be done. If there is no intra-abdominal injury, attention is directed to the bladder. A vertical midline incision well above the bladder neck provides access to the bladder lumen. The surgeon should stay in the midline and avoid lateral dissection into the pelvic hematoma. Opening into the hematoma removes any tamponade effect, thus heavy bleeding may develop.

Damage can be assessed from inside the bladder.

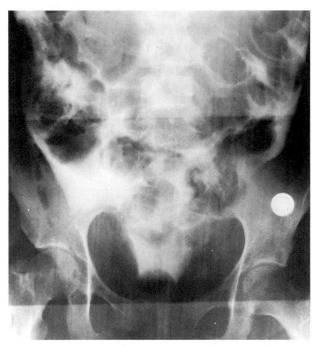

FIG. 63-1. In intraperitoneal rupture of the bladder, free contrast within the peritoneal cavity outlines bowel loops.

FIG. 63-2. In extraperitoneal rupture of the bladder, contrast fills the pelvic cavity around the bladder.

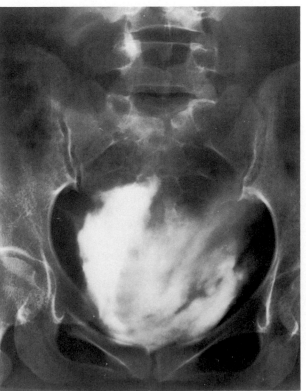

Extraperitoneal perforations are closed from within by 3-0 polyglycolic acid or chromic sutures. Sutures are placed interrupted and require a single layer to include the muscle and mucosa. Extensive lacerations may be closed in two layers, but this is usually unnecessary. Intraperitoneal ruptures require multilayer closure—the peritoneum, the bladder muscle, and the mucosa, all in separate layers.

The ureteral orifices should be carefully observed for bloody efflux. If efflux is present, ureteral catheterization and exploration are indicated to ascertain that ureteral injury has not occurred.

Lacerations extending into the bladder neck area require careful, detailed repair to avoid postoperative incontinence or bladder neck contractures. Precise reconstruction with interrupted sutures will usually prevent such complications.

A suprapubic cystostomy (28Fr Malecot catheter) should be used in most cases. It will avoid catheter obstruction from blood clots in the postoperative period. In cases with bladder neck lacerations, a urethral catheter may also be desirable to remove pooled urine from the bladder floor and to stent the injury. Catheters are left in place for 7 to 14 days, depending upon the extent of injury. Penrose drains are left in for 48 to 72 hr, then removed. Leaving drains in place for prolonged periods increases the chance of infecting the pelvic hematoma. In many cases with watertight bladder closures no drains are necessary.

The cystotomy incision is closed in two layers by 3-0 polyglycolic acid suture. Fascial layers and skin are approximated in routine fashion.

Massive injuries to the pelvis can result in heavy bleeding from pelvic vessels even though the pelvic hematoma has not been violated. Packing the pelvis with laparotomy tapes usually controls the problem; should bleeding persist, the tapes can be left in place, the wound closed, and the tapes removed in 24 hr at reoperation. Embolization of pelvic vessels with Gelfoam or skeletal muscle under angiographic control is helpful to control arterial bleeding.

Penetrating injuries to the bladder can be repaired in a similar manner. Débridement of nonviable tissue must be done in cases of high-velocity missile injury. Special care should be taken to evaluate the ureters because they are more at risk. Free efflux of clear urine, use of Indigo Carmine, and ureteral catheterization will ensure that no ureteral injury has occurred. Occasionally, bullets or other objects may penetrate the rectum and lower sigmoid below the peritoneal reflection without suggesting obvious bowel injury. If there is any question about bowel injury, a sigmoidoscopy should be done on the operating table and a proximal colostomy should be carried out. Unrecognized perforations of the low large bowel show a high incidence of morbidity and mortality.

Nonoperative management of extraperitoneal bladder perforations by urethral catheter drainage has been suggested. This approach should not be used for perforations from blunt or penetrating trauma. The degree of extravasation noted on cystogram correlates poorly with the number and extent of perforations. The possibility of pelvic hematoma infection exists in this type of management.

Surgical injuries should be documented in the operating room by injection of Indigo Carmine into the bladder. The area of injury should be repaired in two or more tissue layers, using 3-0 absorbable suture. Diversion by urethral or suprapubic catheter for 7 to 10 days is usually adequate. Perforations from transurethral operation can be managed usually by 7 to 10 days of catheter drainage. Heavy bleeding or massive fluid extravasation may require open operation, repair, and drainage.

Spontaneous bladder rupture has been reported but it is a rare problem. When it occurs, the patient is generally in urinary retention and a questionable history of minor trauma can be obtained. Often these patients are chronic alcoholics and medical histories are unreliable. Urethral catheter drainage combined with Penrose drains in the Retzius space is sufficient therapy, because most cases have single, small perforations.

Complications

Once repaired, the bladder has extraordinary healing ability. Complications seldom develop. Voiding becomes normal rather quickly. Bladder neck and trigone injuries may be accompanied by temporary incontinence but usually improve to normal control after meticulous repair. Prolonged dysfunctional voiding and fistulas are rare. Unrecognized injury at operation is the most common cause of vesicovaginal fistulas. Pelvic abscess from hematoma infection requires prolonged care, but eventually a good result can be expected.

REFERENCES

1. DEL VILLAR RG, IRELAND GW, CASS AS: Management of bladder and urethral injury in conjunction with immediate surgical treatment of the severe trauma patient. J Urol 108:581, 1972
2. MCANINCH JW: Traumatic injuries to the urethra. J Trauma 2:291, 1981
3. MCANINCH JW, MOORE CA: Diagnosis and treatment of urologic complications of gynecologic surgery. Am J Surg 120:542, 1970
4. MONTIE J: Bladder injuries. Urol Clin North Am 4:59, 1977
5. OCHSNER TG, BUSCH FM, CLARK BG: Urogenital wounds in Vietnam. J Urol 101:224, 1969
6. SALVATIERRA O, JR: Vietnam experience in 252 urological war injuries. J Urol 101:615, 1969
7. WEEMS WL: Management of genitourinary injuries in patients with pelvic fractures. Am Surg 189:717, 1979

The Vesical Neck

64

Bradford W. Young

In a discussion of surgery of the vesical neck, it is traditional to think primarily of obstruction. For the purposes of this discourse, a slight shift in point of view should provide the parallax necessary to contemplate the vesical neck in its full dimensions. The surgical management of incompetence of the vesical neck is of equal importance. The same basic anatomic and functional principles apply to both types of surgery and need to be carefully observed in all the surgical techniques to be described.

The vesical neck is the internal portion of the sphincteric urethra. During resting continence, urine within the bladder is arrested at the vesical neck. The smooth musculature of the vesical neck is at the same time a continuation of the detrusor muscle and part of the sphincteric urethra. The vesical neck is subject to various anatomic and functional disturbances which can result in rigid obstruction or lax incompetence. In either case, its sphincteric function is compromised to some degree. The vesical neck cannot be lightly regarded; nor should it be overestimated. It is simply an integrated, anatomic portion of the sphincteric urethra with certain capabilities and limitations which are dependent upon the composition of its tissues.

Anatomy and Function

The careful definitive description of the histotopographic anatomy of the sphincteric urethra by S. Gil–Vernet emphasizes the importance of smooth muscle detrusor loops as the functional anterior arc of the internal portion of the sphincteric urethra.[10,11] A posterior (or trigonal) loop curves upward beneath the superficial trigonal muscle and interdigitates with fibers of the detrusor loop ventrolaterally. These two intersecting loops constitute what we regard as the *internal sphincter* (Fig. 64-1). This is not an isolated muscle. The studies of Gil–Vernet, Hutch, Lapides, Manley, Tanagho and Smith, Umhlenhuth and associates, and Woodburne, as well as my own work, should

be consulted for the controversial details (Fig. 64-2).[10,11,14,15,21,26,39,44,46,49]

Two other symmetrical structures of great importance in vesical neck surgery are the *pubovesical bundles,* surgically referred to as the *puboprostatic* or *pubovaginal ligaments.* These are bundles of anterior longitudinal smooth muscle of the detrusor which insert into the periosteum on the undersurface of the pubis, providing support to the vesical neck and fixation for the anterior contractility of the detrusor. The insertion of these muscles into the periosteum, more importantly, marks the distal limit of ablative vesical neck surgery. The intraurethral landmark for the distal limit of vesical neck incisions is the superior margin of the verumontanum in the male.[3,7] The external portion of the sphincteric urethra lies just distal to these landmarks. Damage to both the internal and external portions of the sphincteric urethra results in incontinence.

On both gross and histotopographic examination of the detrusor musculature of the lower third of the bladder, it is possible to demonstrate the anterior longitudinal muscle bundle and the heavier and more important posterior longitudinal bundle (posterior bandelette). These two bundles have broad musculotendinous insertions into the apogees of the detrusor and trigonal loops. These longitudinal detrusor bundles are responsible for much of the sphincteric function of the vesical neck.

The smooth musculature of the vesical neck and sphincteric urethra can be considered to be composed of two antagonistic functional groups, the *retentive* and the *expulsive* (Fig. 64-3). The muscle bundles and connective tissue elements responsible for retentive function are the detrusor loops and the trigonal loop acting as obliquely opposed arcs at the vesical neck; the arcuate ventral smooth muscle of the membranous urethra; the intrinsic striated sphincter; the dense dorsal elastic submucosal arc (Pennington's arc) in the membranous urethra; and the submucosal mesh of collagen, elastic fibers, and vascular spaces throughout the

631

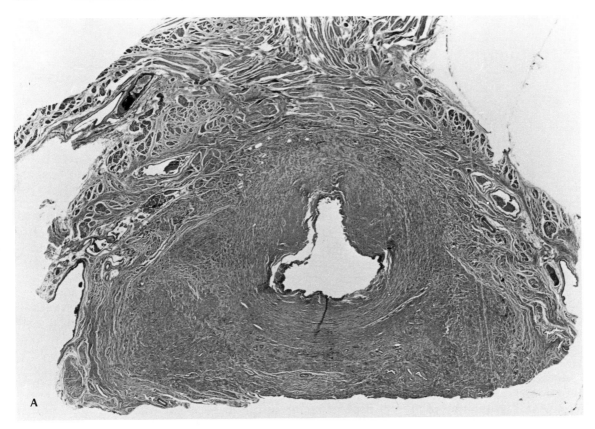

A

FIG. 64-1. *(Caption on opposite page)*

sphincteric urethra which transmit the periurethral muscular forces to the lumen and effect a cushioned coaptation of the mucosa. The expulsive group— those muscular elements responsible for the initiation and maintenance of urination—includes the detrusor; the longitudinal continuations of the detrusor into the sphincteric urethra, namely, the posterior longitudinal bundle (bandelette), the anterior longitudinal bundles of the detrusor, the vesicocervical, vesicoprostatourethral and prostatourethral systems (and their analogues in the female, the vesicourethral and cervicourethral systems); the transverse precervical arc; and the inner anterior longitudinal bundle.[11,49]

The onset of micturition is dependent, first, upon detrusor contraction. At the moment of contraction, the longitudinal extensions of the detrusor throughout the sphincteric urethra actively draw aside the arcuate muscle bundles of the vesical neck to form the funneled internal urethral orifice.[27,28] (Fig. 64-4). At the end of micturition the vesical neck closes (detrusor and trigonal loop) as the contraction of the detrusor diminishes and dies away over a few seconds. With the cessation of active contraction of the posterior longitudinal

bundle, the bladder base in the adult resumes its resting, right-angled relationship to the internal urethral orifice. The lumen is occluded and the resting length of the urethra is restored.

In such a brief stylized description, it should be evident that a great deal of anatomy and physiology of micturition, both real and speculative, has been omitted. For the purposes of the surgical procedures to be described, however, these are the most essential concepts.

Vesical Neck Obstruction

Obstruction to the outflow of urine at the bladder neck without apparent cause has been the subject of much concern and empiric surgery for more than 100 years. The great 19th century French urologists, Civiale, Mércier, and Guyon ("Prostatisme sans prostate") struggled as vigorously with this intellectual paradox as with one another. Marion,[30] in 1933, swept aside all previous theories, including the so-called "prostatiques" of Guyon, to proclaim his own theory of the "maladie du col vesical." Marion identified the internal sphincter as the site of obstruction and described four causes

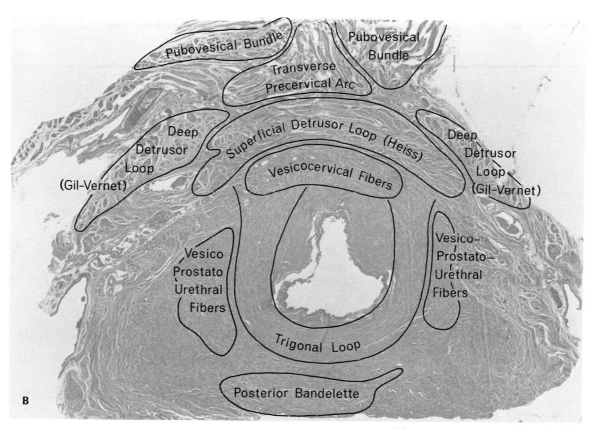

FIG. 64-1. A transverse histotopographic section of the vesical neck in a 2-year-old boy shows normal distribution of the internal sphincteric urethral musculature. The section is taken at the level of the insertion of the posterior longitudinal bundle into the cranial lobe of the prostate. **(A)** Photomicrograph. **(B)** Photomicrograph with overlaid tissue map. (Verhoeff–van Gieson stain, original magnification × 15) (Yung BW: Lower Urinary Tract Obstruction in Childhood. Philadelphia, Lea & Febiger, 1972)

for the observed phenomenon: hypertonicity, hypertrophy, inflammatory sclerosis, and sclerosis associated with glandular proliferation. Time and subsequent studies have somewhat elaborated Marion's original classification. We now recognize a possibly congenital, fibroelastic variant in children, fibrosis secondary to electroresection, functional neurogenic obstruction, and mesenchymal dyplastic disease of the detrusor and sphincteric musculature as additional causes of this syndrome.[12]

Dyskinesia of the vesical neck, a term proposed by Beer in 1915,[1] and *dyssynergic bladder neck occlusion,* as recently described by Turner Warwick and associates,[43] reflect the unimpressive histology of surgically removed tissue from the vesical neck. These two terms, reminiscent of Marion's *hypertonicity,* suggest a functional autonomic, or perhaps somatic, neuromuscular dysfunction in certain cases. Although these terms indicate our insufficient

awareness of the underlying cellular pathophysiology, for the present we must deal surgically with the clinical manifestations of these subtle obstructions as they present themselves.

Once the normal anatomy and functional principles of the vesical neck are clear, the surgical indications and limitations and the technique and the operative variations become more obvious. The principle of ablative vesicourethroplasty is simply the weakening of the internal portion of the sphincteric urethra by dividing its anterior or posterior arcs (the detrusor or trigonal loops). The principle of reconstructive vesical neck surgery is fortification of the normal musculature of the vesical neck, while preserving its connections with the anterior and posterior longitudinal muscle bundles of the detrusor. Reconstructive operations are primarily tubularization procedures or wrapped-flap techniques applied to either the detrusor or trigonal loops. (*Text continues on p. 636*)

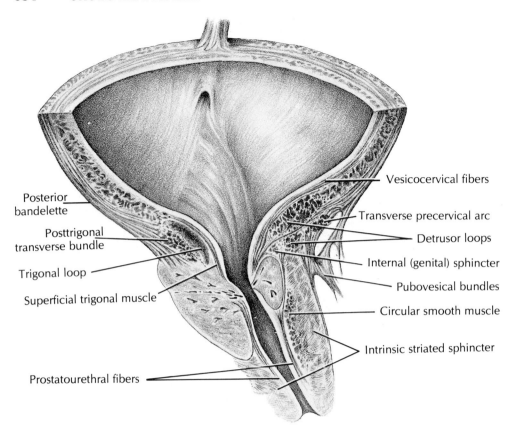

Posterior bandelette

Posttrigonal transverse bundle

Trigonal loop

Superficial trigonal muscle

Prostatourethral fibers

Vesicocervical fibers

Transverse precervical arc

Detrusor loops

Internal (genital) sphincter

Pubovesical bundles

Circular smooth muscle

Intrinsic striated sphincter

FIG. 64-2. Course and insertions of the principal muscle bundles of the male sphincteric urethra (Young BW: Lower Urinary Tract Obstruction in Childhood. Philadelphia, Lea & Febiger, 1972)

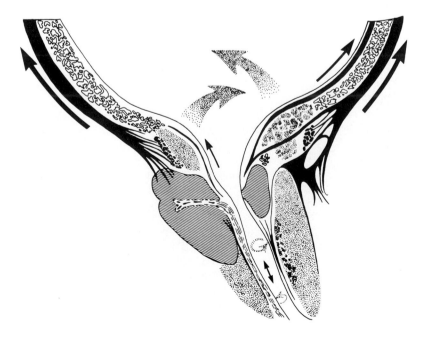

FIG. 64-3. Presumed function of the various muscle bundles of the sphincteric urethra. The direction of contraction and relative strength are indicated by the size and orientation of the *arrows*. The muscle groups representing forces of expulsion are indicated in *black*. Those representing arrest of urination are *stippled*. (Young BW: Lower Urinary Tract Obstruction in Childhood. Philadelphia, Lea & Febiger, 1972)

FIG. 64-4. (A) Oblique voiding cystourethrogram in a 6-year-old boy. Detrusor contraction produces an irregular configuration of the fundus of the bladder. The base of the bladder is widely funneled and smooth in luminal outline. (B) Note the slight decrease in density of the contrast medium and the indentations of the lumen at the sites of the most dense circular arcuate muscular (vesical neck and membranous urethra). (Young BW: Lower Urinary Tract Obstruction in Childhood. Philadelphia, Lea & Febiger, 1972)

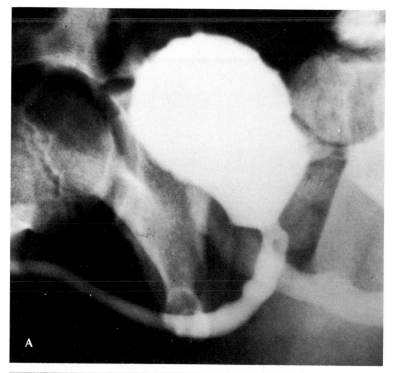

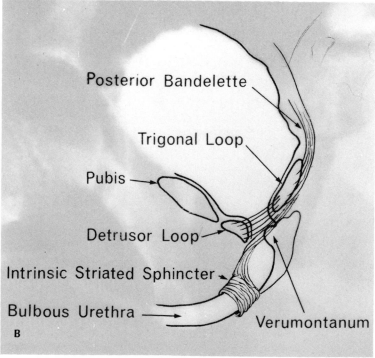

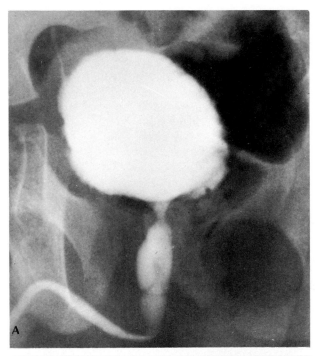

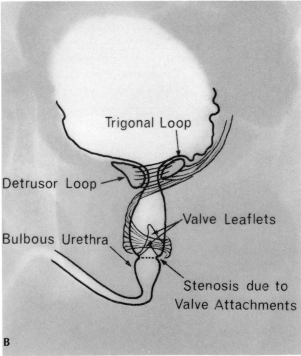

FIG. 64-5. Oblique voiding cystourethrogram in a 7-year-old-boy with urethral valvular obstruction. **(A)** Note the annular obstruction at the distal insertions of the valvular folds. **(B)** Hypertrophy of the detrusor (including the vesical neck) and trabeculation are secondary changes. (Young BW: Lower Urinary Tract Obstruction in Childhood. Philadelphia, Lea & Febiger, 1972)

Ablative Vesical Neck Surgery

INDICATIONS

Pure ablative vesical neck surgery (internal sphincterotomy) is rarely indicated as a solitary surgical procedure. It has become evident that what we formerly regarded as primary contracture of the vesical neck in children (congenital fibroelastosis, submucosal fibrosis) is a somewhat rare and perhaps familial condition.[17,18,36,49]

Internal sphincterotomy is not an indiscriminant panacea for recurrent infection, urinary frequency, urgency, enuresis, or dysuria. It is not a substitute for urethral meatotomy or hymenotomy in infant girls or young women with recurrent lower urinary tract infection.

There are three primary indications for ablative internal sphincterotomy: fibrosis of the vesical neck due to postoperative scarring, chronic bacterial or parasitic infection, or congenital fibroelastosis; secondary obstructive hypertrophy of the detrusor loop accompanied by detrusor hypertrophy in cases of distal urethral obstruction (primarily valves or bulbomembranous stenosis in males;[4,31,32] and neurogenic bladder, in which an attempt at balance of the hypertrophied detrusor and sphincteric urethra is planned.

DIAGNOSIS

It is evident that partial destruction of the internal portion of the sphincteric urethra is likely to be of advantage in diminishing residual urine only within the bladder. There is no question that destroying the function of the vesical neck alone has provided clinical improvement in children with ureteral reflux,[23,24,47] but this should be considered an indirect effect of the operation and may be accounted for either by reduction of intravesical voiding pressures or by allowing an unimpeded maturation of the ureterovesical junctions. A freely refluxing ureter with a severely damaged or congenitally incompetent ureterovesical junction is not likely to improve following vesical neck surgery alone.

The urologic findings of most value in planning vesical neck surgery to relieve obstruction include voiding cystourethrographic evidence of stenosis or obstruction at the vesical neck alone, persistent infected bladder residual urine without an obvious distal obstructive lesion, and cystoscopic or hydrodynamic evidence indicating obstructive dysfunction of the vesical neck.

Cystourethroscopy is essential for two reasons: to eliminate obstructive lesions of the distal urethra in the female and the inframontane urethra in the male, and to verify definite trabeculation of the bladder wall. The actual estimate of the size of rigidity of the vesical neck is notoriously difficult endoscopically and, except in cases of severe fibrosis, glandular or fibromuscular median bar formation is of little value. Moderate to marked trabeculation and cellule formation can be taken as supportive evidence of *any* outflow obstruction and merely represents detrusor hypertrophy with some degree of decompensation. It should be remembered that there may be a neurogenic component responsible for this finding in some cases. The cause and functional implications of trabeculation should be considered carefully in each case.

In practice, a most valuable specific study is a high-volume excretory urogram producing adequate bladder concentration to permit voiding cystourethrography (Fig. 64-5). The combination of this study with intravenous radionuclide techniques for the demonstration of residual urine and ureteral reflux provides much of the pertinent structural and functional information necessary to make the surgical decision[5,13] (Fig. 64-6).

OPERATIVE TECHNIQUES

Transurethral

Simple transurethral dilation of the vesical neck or sphincteric urethra is not an effective method of management for either primary or secondary contractures of the vesical neck. It is at best an extremely temporary measure, which does nothing to correct the basic lesion and may even aggravate it by further tissue destruction and scar formation.[29,33,38,42]

Transurethral electroresection of the vesical neck or cold-punch resection for fibromuscular hyperplasia (median bar), small middle lobe glandular hyperplasia, or inflammatory fibrosis in adults produces an excellent result and is probably the procedure of choice. This approach is not entirely suitable in infants and children. Here, the anatomic requirements are not met. The vesical neck is indiscriminantly widely funneled circumferentially; and healing occurs by reepithelialization and fibrosis. McDonald, in his transurethral approach, satisfies the anatomic requirements more closely by resecting the vesical neck deeply anteriorly (ventrally) in children to the point of extravasation.* In so doing the detrusor loops are completely divided and, despite the fact that healing occurs by fibrosis, an impressive anterior sphincterotomy is accomplished. Turner Warwick performs an equally effective full-thickness endoscopic "dorsolateral" internal sphincterotomy with the resectoscope knife electrode, making two deep incisions through the vesical neck which are extended to the verumontanum in the 4 o'clock and 8 o'clock positions.[43] The use of the cold 21Fr optical urethrotome (Sachse knife) might be even more appropriate; with electrocoagulation minimized. Histotopographically,

---

* McDonald HP: Personal communication, 1968

FIG. 64-6. An intravenous radionuclide voiding urogram demonstrates gross bilateral ureteral reflux and a small amount of residual bladder urine. Computer analysis applied to specific areas of interest can detect subvisual degrees of reflux and permits noninstrumental measurement of residual urine volumes. (Courtesy Hirsch Handmaker)

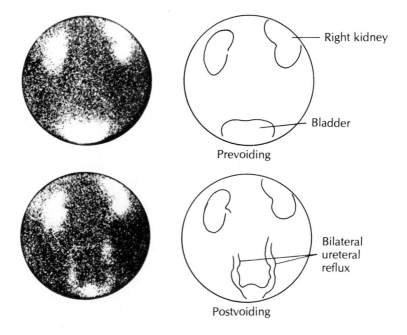

Right kidney

Bladder

Prevoiding

Bilateral ureteral reflux

Postvoiding

this corresponds to severing the lateral limbs of the trigonal loop (Fig. 64-1). This procedure destroys the function of the posterior half of the internal sphincter mechanism. An alternate method, accomplishing the same purpose, is the conventional midline vesical neck incision with the Colling's knife. In retropubic surgery, "wedging of the posterior lip" of the vesical neck is the anatomic analogue of these endoscopic procedures.

The transurethral approach is exceptionally well suited to the critical demonstration of inframontane valvular folds in children and their pinpoint destruction, preferably with a single, fine wire electrode. Valvular folds should never be resected deeply with the loop, because this may lead to incontinence from damage to the underlying delicate musculature of the external portion of the sphincteric urethra.

Transvesical

The vesical neck has been approached transvesically with direct excision of a collar (Marion's rim; of musculature or fibrosis under direct vision. This is the operation originally described by Marion[29] and has little to recommend it from an anatomic standpoint. Portions of a fibrotic vesical neck have been ronguered out transvesically,[38] and cuneiform (wedge) resection of the posterior lip of the vesical neck (trigonal loop) can be carried out when necessary.[50]

Retropubic (Y–V Vesicourethroplasty)

In children and adults with severe fibrotic contracture of the vesical neck, Y–V vesicourethroplasty provides a direct open surgical approach, permitting a thorough evaluation fo the bladder, ureterovesical junctions, and the obstructive lesion.[50] Surgical correction can be carried out with minimal damage to the surrounding sphincteric musculature.[25] The two structures to be attacked are the detrusor and the trigonal loops, comprising the internal portion fo the sphincteric urethra. A V-shaped incision on the anterior bladder wall is made so that the apex is immediately above the detrusor loops. The distal limb of the Y is then made by dividing the loops with the scissors (Fig. 64-7). The incision is closed as a V, which interposes longitudinal detrusor muscle between the cut edges of the detrusor loop and destroys its function.

Alternate Vesicourethral Incisions

Longitudinal incision fo the detrusor loops with transverse closure,[7,48] adapted from the Heineke–Mikulicz procedure for pyloroplasty, is a simple and effective operation which satisfies all the an-atomic demands. It may be perfectly safe in men. Due to the rigidity of the proximal sphincteric urethra reinforced by the prostate, the finished suture line is not exactly transverse. In effect, the anterior longitudinal musculature is drawn down to fill the urethral defect, giving a somewhat irregular U-shaped closure. In women this has some potential danger. The very short external portion of the sphincteric urethra can be deformed by the tension of the transverse closure, leading to incontinence. DeWeerd has reported an excellent experience with the incision, and suggests that it may have been too hastily abandoned.[7] A transverse supracervical incision (above the detrusor loop) described by Bonnin, with a distal limb to provide a T–V shaped incision, is an excellent variation and provides somewhat wider exposure of the interior of the bladder.[2] A modification of this incision by Kaplan and King[17] facilitates a more tailored closure by trimming the sharply angled dog ears from the edges of the incision (Fig. 64-8). A U-shaped supracervical incision prior to the division of the detrusor loops has been advocated by G. W. Leadbetter, Jr. This incision has the advantage of eliminating the angular, potentially necrotic, tip of the V-shaped flap, while maintaining an adequate, well-fitting, mobile flap of anterior longitudinal musculature to insert between the divided ends of the detrusor loop.

There are occasions when the flap of anterior longitudinal musculature to be inserted into the urethral defect presents a marked disproportion in the thickness of the bladder wall to that of the urethra. In this situation, the adventitia and superficial longitudinal muscle bundles can be filleted away from the mucosal surface to provide a more exact fit of the tissues to be coapted.

Reconstructive Vesical Neck Surgery

The incompetent vesical neck has received less surgical attention than bladder neck obstruction, because vesical neck incompetence alone does not produce urinary tract infection, obstruction, or even incontinence.

Considerable ingenuity has been displayed in refashioning the internal portion fo the sphincteric urethra in cases of congenital or acquired urinary incontinence. In dealing with total urinary incontinence it must be assumed that the entire sphincteric urethra is defective. Not only is the vesical neck or internal portion of the sphincteric urethra incompetent, but also the external portion (membranous urethra in the male, and midurethra in the female) is involved. The surgical landmarks

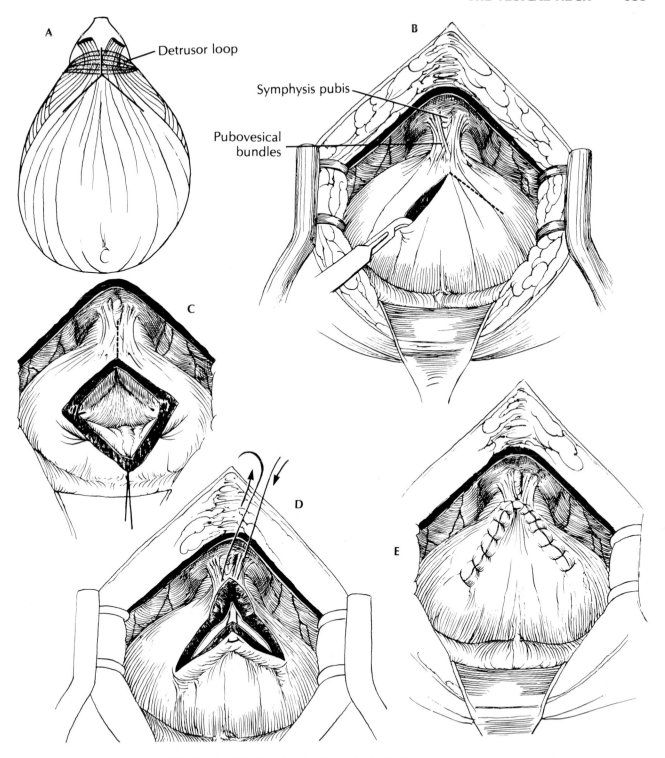

FIG. 64-7. **(A)** Functional principal of ablative vesical neck surgery. In this instance, Y–V vesicourethroplasty is shown as an example of operations designed to prevent normal arcuate contractile function of the detrusor loop.   **(B** and **C)** Note that the loop is completely divided. **(D** and **E)** A tongue of anterior longitudinal bundle muscle fibers is interposed between the cut ends of the loop. A similar principle applies to the transvesical division of the trigonal loop.

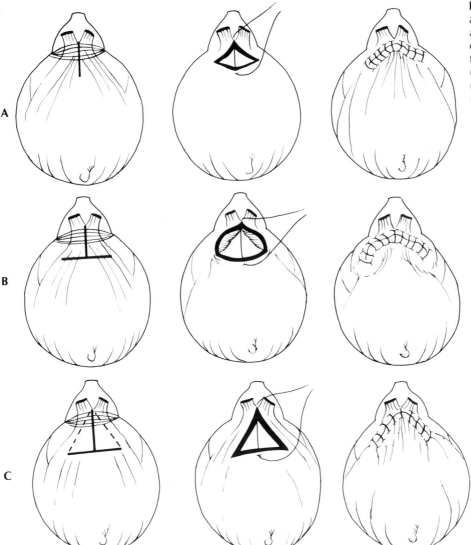

FIG. 64-8. Alternate anterior ablative vesical neck incisions, all of which rely upon division of the detrusor loop and abolition of its contractile function: (**A**) B. W. Young and DeWeerd, (**B**) Bonnin and Youngblood, (**C**) Kaplan and King

useful in cautious ablative surgery of vesical neck obstruction are valueless; in fact, they often are missing or distorted. In this situation more daring dissection is not only indicated but advisable.

Previously, operations for the control of urinary incontinence have been directed toward supporting or reconstructing the external sphincteric urethra. Recently, due to a renewed awareness of the detrusor and trigonal loop systems at the vesical neck, the internal portion of the urethral sphincter has been found to be a more attractive structure for surgical reconstruction. An appreciation of the arcuate nature of the muscle bundles at the vesical neck underlies all of the more successful techniques.

TRIGONAL TUBED FLAPS

Vesical tubed flaps of the trigone, incorporating the arcuate fibers of the trigonal loop and the deep transverse trigonal muscle, have been used in operations to relieve incontinence following prostatectomy. Ian Thompson's operation provides a limited trigonal tubed flap with a reduction in luminal diameter, combined with a cranial displacement of the detrusor loop.[41] The operation of G. W. Leadbetter, Jr. is a more extensive trigonal tubularization, extending from the urogenital diaphragm to a point 1 cm to 2 cm above the interureteric ridge.[22] The full thickness of bladder wall (*i.e.*, the entire trigone) is mobilized, but no attempt

FIG. 64-9. Two procedures to reconstruct the vesical neck by trigonal tubularization (the detrusor loop is not used in either of these procedures): **(A)** I. M. Thompson operation; **(B)** G. W. Leadbetter operation, which is more extensive and provides a long tube of full-thickness circular trigonal muscle

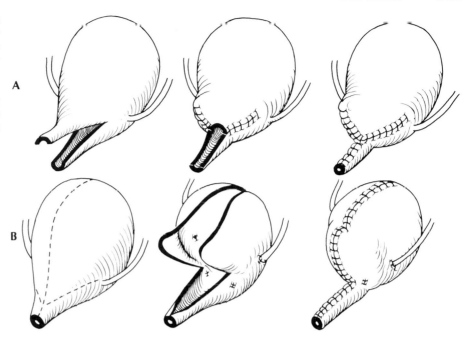

is made to narrow its lumen. The major reliance for resting continence in this operation is placed upon the circular disposition of the muscle fibers and the considerable length of the tube. This operation usually requires reimplantation of both ureters to the posterior wall of the bladder, well above the newly formed internal urethral orifice (Fig. 64-9).

TRIGONAL LOOP PLICATION

The trigonal loop can be approached transvaginally. This is the basis for an operation described by King and Wendel in 1969.[19] In this operation, useful in female epispadias, the posterior aspect of the trigone is exposed by a longitudinal incision on the anterior vaginal wall. A row of plicating silk sutures is placed directly into the trigonal loop musculature and tied down to infold the trigonal loop, thus tightening the posterior half of the vesical neck. Urethroscopic control to ensure adequate closure is carried out during the procedure. A second layer of plicating sutures can be placed to provide further occlusion of this portion of the internal sphincter, if necessary. This procedure has the advantage of not interfering with subsequent detrusor loop reconstructions. Female epispadias is exceedingly difficult to correct and the addition of an anterior reconstruction is usually required. The principle of the operation is sound, and keeping in mind the function of the posterior longitudinal bundle in drawing aside the trigonal loop

during micturition, it might well be more widely applied in cases of female incontinence from other causes, when the detrusor loop is intact.

Transvesical plication of the trigonal loop and deep transverse trigonal muscle has been advocated by F. D. Stephens in a technique which he describes as "bipennation and keeling" of the trigone.[37] Through the opened bladder a midline, full-thickness longitudinal incision is made in the trigone, through the interureteric ridge and carried to the verumontanum in the male, but just through the vesical neck in the female. The lateral wings of trigonal musculature thus created are plicated, first with a 4-0 chromic gut running suture in the deep trigonal muscle, and then with interrupted 4-0 chromic gut sutures in the trigonal loop to form a thick keellike bundle (Fig. 64-10). Not only does this effectively reduce the arc of the trigonal loop, but also the deep trigonal suture may have an indirect effect in increasing the tension of the detrusor loop fibers which anatomically appear to be continuous with it (*e.g.*, the superficial detrusor loop of Heiss).

DETRUSOR LOOP TUBED FLAPS

The central portion of the detrusor loop has been successfully used as a surrogate sphincter by incorporating its arching fibers into a tubed muscular flap, which can then be anastomosed to the distal urethra.[9,40] Flocks and Boldus have recently described a spiral bladder flap vesical neck recon-

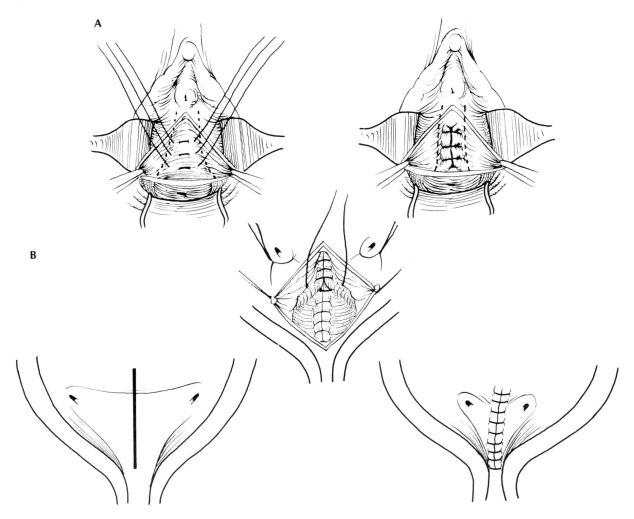

FIG. 64-10.   Reconstruction of the vesical neck by trigonal plication.   **(A)** An extravesical (transvaginal) approach.   **(B)** Transvesical bipennation and keeling operation of F. D. Stephens has the advantages of a more extensive trigonal plication and applicability to male patients.

struction for use in cases of postprostatectomy incontinence (Fig. 64-11).[8] This operation takes advantage of the arcuate muscular distribution of both the trigonal and detrusor loops. A further interesting addition to this reconstruction is a cleverly conceived interference with the opening mechanism of the detrusor loop, accomplished by a transverse division of the anterior longitudinal bundle of the detrusor. This incision is made well above the detrusor loops; when it is closed longitudinally, the function of the anterior longitudinal bundle is destroyed. The reconstituted detrusor loop, unable to be withdrawn, retains its retentive position during micturition, thus partially impeding the normal funneling of the vesical neck.

Restoration of the arcuate contractility of the detrusor loop, in cases of previous cicatricial damage, can sometimes be accomplished by wedge or elliptic excision of the anterior vesical neck and snug closure around a small urethral catheter in the manner of H. H. Young.[51] The Dees modification of the Young operation incorporates tightly tubularized triangular flaps of denuded trigonal muscle around a central strip of trigonal mucosa, in addition to the anterior reapproximation of the detrusor loop.[6]

Innes William has described an interesting variation of the anterior tubularized flap, useful in urogenital sinus abnormalities resulting in a short, wide urethra with a deficient bladder neck.[16] The

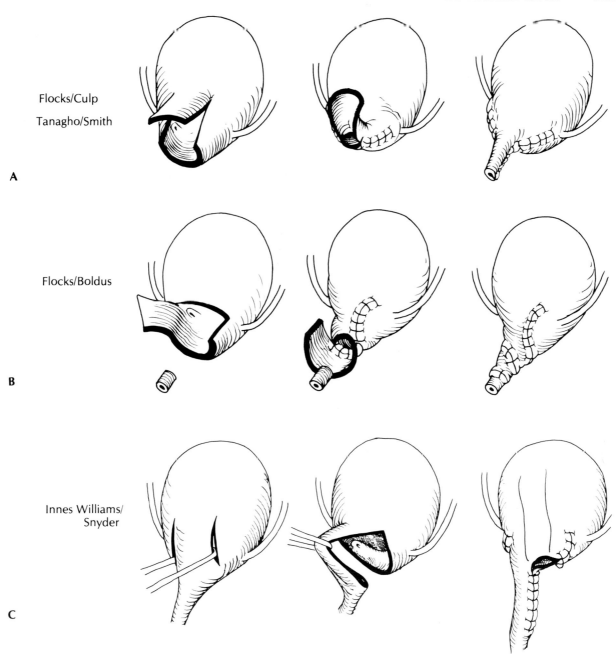

Flocks/Culp
Tanagho/Smith

A

Flocks/Boldus

B

Innes Williams/
Snyder

C

FIG. 64-11.   **(A)** Reconstruction of the vesical neck with a detrusor loop flap. The anterior flap is tubularized and approximated to the distal urethra.   **(B)** The spiral flap technique may incorporate more circular fibers into the final reconstruction.   **(C)** The anterior tubularized urethral strip in continuity takes advantage of the heavy detrusor loop fibers and preserves the blood supply.

modification (Fig. 64-11C) consists of tubularization of an anterior bladder ''strip'', maintaining its continuity at both ends to ensure an adequate blood supply, transverse division of the trigone as in the Tanagho–Smith procedure, and transverse closure of the posterior defect. In effect, this is an anterior variation of the trigonal tubularization of Ian Thompson.

To conclude, the looped musculature of the vesical neck, together with the anterior and posterior longitudinal detrusor muscle bundles, presents the urologic surgeon with two functionally antagonistic muscle groups whose functions are importantly concerned with the arrest and expulsion of urine. Balancing the sphincteric musculature against the detrusor by weakening the obstructing vesical neck appears to be a solidly established principle. This can be achieved by any of the techniques described appropriate to a given case. The possibilities for imaginative surgical reconstruction of this unique anatomic system are only beginning to be explored.[35] Successful techniques must be carefully planned to conform to the delicate underlying structure of the sphincteric urethra. The prospect for control of certain types of incontinence using these principles appears bright indeed.

REFERENCES

1. BEER E: Chronic retention of urine in children. JAMA 65:1709, 1915
2. BONNIN NJ: Plastic reconstruction of the bladder neck and prostatectomy: An operation suitable for all types of nonmalignant bladder neck obstruction. Aust NZ J Surg 27:161, 1957–1958
3. BRUÉZIÈRE J, FIRMIN F: Maladie du col vésical chez l'enfant. Étude clinique, diagnostique, thérapeutique. Ann Urol 4:169, 1970
4. COBB BG, WOLF JA JR, ANSELL JS: Congenital stricture of the proximal urethral bulb. J Urol 99:629, 1968
5. CONWAY JJ, KING LR, BELMAN AB: Detection of vesicourethral reflux with radionuclide cystography. Am J Roentgenol 115:720, 1972
6. DEES JE: Congenital epispadias with incontinence. J Urol 62:513, 1949
7. DEWEERD JH: Heineke–Mikulicz principle applies to retropubic revision of the vesical neck. J Urol 95:368, 1966
8. FLOCKS RH, BOLDUS R: The surgical treatment and prevention of urinary incontinence associated with disturbance of the internal sphincter mechanism. J Urol 109:279, 1973
9. FLOCKS RH, CULP DA: A modification of technique for anastomosing membranous urethra and bladder neck following prostatectomy. J Urol 69:411, 1953
10. GIL–VERNET S: Patologia Urogenital. Tomo I. Barcelona, Miguel Servet, 1944
11. GIL–VERNET S: Patologia Urogenital. Tomo II. Madrid, Paz Montalvo, 1953
12. GLENN JF, MONTGOMERY WG: A clinical classification of bladder outlet obstruction. J Urol 91:232, 1964
13. HANDMAKER H, MCRAE J, BUCK EG: Intravenous radionuclide voiding cystography: An atraumatic method of demonstrating vesico-ureteral reflux. Radiology 108:703, 1973
14. HUTCH JA: A new theory of the anatomy of the internal sphincter and the physiology of micturition. Invest Urol 3:36, 1965
15. HUTCH JA: The internal sphincter: A double loop system. Trans Am Assoc Genitourin Surg 62:30, 1970
16. INNES WILLIAMS D, SNYDER H: Anterior detrusor tube repair for urinary incontinence in children. Br J Urol 48:671, 1976
17. KAPLAN GW, KING LR: An evaluation of Y–V vesicourethroplasty in children. Surg Gynecol Obstet 130:1059, 1970
18. KEITZER WA, BENAVENT C: Bladder neck obstruction in children. J Urol 89:384, 1963
19. KING LR, WENDEL NM: A new application for transvaginal plication in the treatment of girls with total urinary incontinence due to epispadias or hypospadias. J Urol 102:778, 1969
20. KIRCHHEIM DR, TREMANN JA, ANSELL JS: Transurethral urethrotomy under vision. J Urol 119:496, 1978
21. LAPIDES J: Structure and function of the internal vesical sphincter. J Urol 80:341, 1958
22. LEADBETTER GW, JR: Surgical correction of total urinary incontinence. J Urol 91:261, 1964
23. LEADBETTER GW, JR, LEADBETTER, WF: Diagnosis and treatment of congenital bladder–neck obstruction in children. New Engl J Med 260:633, 1959
24. LEADBETTER GW, JR, LEADBETTER WF: Ureteral reimplantation and bladder neck reconstruction. JAMA 175:349, 1961
25. LICH R, JR, MAURER JE: Surgical relief of vesical neck obstruction in children. Southern Surgery 16:127, 1950
26. MANLEY CB, JR: The striated muscle of the prostate. J Urol 95:234, 1966
27. MARBERGER H: Blasenhalsplastik. Helv Chir Acta 28:768, 1960
28. MARBERGER H: Hydrodynamische Probleme in der Urologie von Heute. Z Urol 58:871, 1965
29. MARION G: Surgery of neck of bladder. Br J Urol 5:351, 1933
30. MARION G: In Report Fifth Congress, Société International d'Urologie, 1933
31. MOORMAN JG: Angeborene Enge der bulbären Hanröhre als Ursache der Erkrankungen des urogenitalen Grenzgebietes. Urologe 11:157, 1972
32. MOORMAN JG: Pathogenese und klinik der blasenhalshypertrophie. Urologe 11:267, 1972
33. NANSON EM: Marion's disease or bladder neck stenosis. Aust NZ J Surg 20:215, 1951
34. SCOTT FB, BRADLEY WE, TIMM GW: Treatment of urinary incontinence by an implantable prosthetic urinary sphincter. Urology 1, No. 3:252, 1973
35. SCOTT FB, MADERSBACHER H: The twelve o'clock sphincterotomy: Technique, indications, results. (In press)
36. SPENCE HM, MURPHY JJ, MCGOVERN JH et al: Urinary tract infections in infants and children. J Urol 91:623, 1964
37. STEPHENS FD: Form of stress incontinence in children: Another method for bladder neck repair. Aust NZ J Surg 40:124, 1970

38. STEWART CM: Congenital bladder neck obstruction: Diagnosis by delayed and voiding cystography and surgical removal by use of a new cold-crush cutting punch. J Urol 83:679, 1960

39. TANAGHO EA, SMITH DR: The anatomy and function of the bladder neck. Br J Urol 38:54, 1966

40. TANAGHO EA, SMITH DR: Clinical evaluation of a surgical technique for the correction of complete urinary incontinence. J Urol 107:402, 1972

41. THOMPSON IM: Incontinence following prostatectomy. J Urol 86:130, 1961

42. THOMPSON IM, BAKER JJ: The histologic effects of dilation and internal urethrotomy on the canine urethra. J Urol 103:168, 1970

43. TURNER WARWICK R, WHITESIDE CG, WORTH PHL et al: A urodynamic view of the clinical problems associated with bladder neck dysfunction and its treatment by endoscopic incision and transtrigonal posterior prostatectomy. Br J Urol 45:44, 1973

44. UHLENHUTH E, HUNTER DT, JR, LOECHEL WF: Problems in the Anatomy of the Pelvis. Philadelphia, J B Lippincott, 1953

45. WOODBURNE RT: Structure and function of the urinary bladder. J Urol 84:79, 1960

46. WOODBURNE RT: The sphincter mechanism of the urinary bladder. Anat Rec 141:11, 1961

47. WOODROW SI, MARSHALL VF: Y–V enlargement of the vesical outlet in ordinary cases of vesicoureteral reflux. J Urol 105:301, 1971

48. YOUNG BW: The retropubic approach to vesical neck obstruction in children. Surg Gynecol Obstet 96:150, 1953

49. YOUNG BW: Lower Urinary Tract Obstruction in Childhood. Philadelphia, Lea & Febiger, 1972

50. YOUNG BW, GOEBEL JL: Retropubic wedge excision in congenital vesical neck obstruction. Stanford Med Bull 12:106, 1954

51. YOUNG HH: An operation for the cure of incontinence associated with epispadias. Surg Gynecol Obstet 28:48, 1919

52. YOUNGBLOOD VH, TOMLIN EM, CROSSLAND DB: Contracture of bladder neck: Experience with Bradford Young operation. South Med J 51:1516, 1958

Exstrophy and Epispadias

65

Julian S. Ansell

This chapter deals with primary surgical closure of the exstrophied bladder and correction of epispadias. Several advances in the surgical treatment of this difficult complex of congenital anomalies have been introduced by Cohen, Devine and Horton, Duckett, Jeffs, and Johnston.[8,12,14,19,21] The unkept promise of avoiding renal damage from obstruction, infection, and stones by means of diversion through ileal conduits has provided added stimulus to those of us whose efforts have been directed to primary closure of ectopia vesicae. In the long run, a mediocre bladder may function better than an excellent segment of gut as a substitute.[3,27] Newly developed pharmacologic adjustments for treatment of the neuropathic bladder, a variety of effective antibiotics to prevent and control infection, salvage of the incompetent detrusor by means of intermittent catheterization, and the reward of the continent child with normal upper urinary tracts have all spurred on those of us who are proponents of primary closure.

Even that ultimate congenital urologic horror, cloacal exstrophy, is beginning to yield to surgical correction. Successes notwithstanding, this multistaged procedure is not to be undertaken lightly. The first stage creates a complete epispadias in the male, closes the female, and may be sufficient in a few. Usually secondary procedures will be required to repair groin hernias, correct reflux, or further tighten the bladder neck. Epispadias repair can be frustrating, requiring as many as three or more separate staged procedures months apart.[10,13] Parents must be fully informed about the need for multiple procedures over a period of years before deciding on attempted reconstruction, or they will fail to cope with the emotional, financial, and other strains imposed.

HISTORY

Attempts to close exstrophic bladders using flaps of abdominal skin, fascia, or both go back at least to the 1850s.[5] The concept of approximating the midline structures to a more nearly normal position was proposed by Trendelenburg, who disarticulated the sacroiliac joints to allow the pubes to swing toward each other. His principle of "closing the open book" was rediscovered by Schultz, who reported his and Schwartzmann's use of iliac osteotomies for this purpose in 1958.[35] They closed the bladder and pubes 2 weeks after the iliac osteotomies were done. Almost all subsequent workers are indebted to the principles of Young and Dees in fashioning a bladder neck[11] Their techniques were extended by Leadbetter's maneuver of reimplanting the ureters further cephalad to allow a longer bladder neck. This principle has been carried as far as possible by Arap, who rolls the entire bladder into a tube for passive control and uses colon as a detrusor with ureters implanted into it in antireflux fashion.[4]

In 1960, Lattimer and associates suggested that osteotomies and bladder closure be carried out at one sitting.[26] Cook, Leslie, and Brannon cut across the pubic and ischial rami to accomplish midline abdominal wall closure at the time of bladder reconstruction.[9] Closure in the first few weeks postpartum was suggested by Swenson,[39] and Rickham first wrote that closure was easiest in the newborn.[33] Bairov wrote the same in 1966.[6] Dees's procedure for repair of epispadias required two separate stages,[11] and most series describe multiple unplanned or planned stages.[28] Jeffs adds suspension of the bladder neck and uses intraoperative intravesical pressure measurements to help establish correct resistance to flow at the bladder neck.[19,20] Hinman was the first to recognize the complexity of epispadias repair and the need for interposition flaps of skin.[18] Michalowski and Modelski used a Z-plasty for lengthening the epispadiac urethra.[31] Duckett devised an elegant means of providing skin needed to bridge the urethral defect following release of the epispadiac chordee by swinging paravesical flaps, which are also said to contribute to urinary control by allowing the bladder neck to migrate cephalad to a more normal intrapelvic location.[14] Johnston devised a practical method for

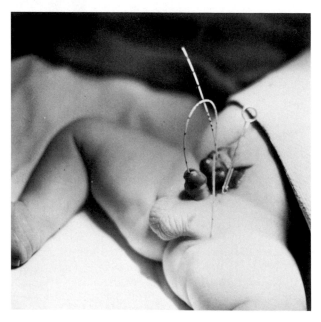

FIG. 65-1 Newborn with superior vesical fissure. Note that the penis is normal except for the ventrally displaced foreskin.

FIG. 65-2. Smooth bladder in a newborn female, probably of the hypotonic neuropathic variety

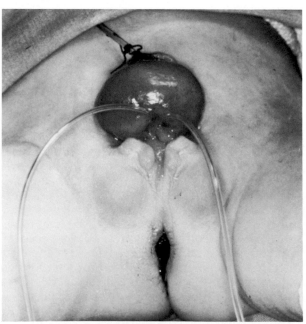

improving phallic length while minimizing the danger of damaging pudendal nerves and vessels.[21,22] Cohen's crossed trigonal ureteral implants are ideal for exstrophic bladders.[8] The Devines's full-thickness tube graft for bringing the urethral

channel to the meatus is a useful adjunct in what can be a most difficult surgical exercise, the repair of the epispadias.[12]

Ambrose, Fonkelsrud and Linde, Gravier, Johnston and Penn, Koontz and associates, Markland and Fraley, Rickham, Soper and Kilger, Spencer, Tank and Lindenauer, and others have made contributions to surgical correction of the most severe of all the exstrophic anomalies, the cloacal variety.[2,15,16,23,25,29,34,37,38,41] The concept of an artificial sphincter, which has been brought a long way by Scott and associates is appealing,[36] but the extent and the amount of scarring encountered at the bladder neck or penile urethra in a failed exstrophy is such that one wonders if there is enough flexibility in these tissues to allow a hydromechanical device to succeed. In one female patient, I have converted incontinence following five failed procedures to control following elevation of the bladder base by injection of powdered Teflon in a glycerin base.[7]

Exstrophy

The exstrophic complex is a spectrum of diseases which can vary from simple involvement of the glans creating a spade penis to ectopia splanchnica with complete absence of the external genitalia. Marshall and Muecke describe many varieties between these extremes.[30] Each child with the problem has similarities to other children with exstrophy, but few cases are identical. The surgeon who attempts to tackle such problems must anticipate individual variations and be prepared to tailor the procedure accordingly.[40] The following brief case histories illustrate this point:

1. A child with superior vesical fissure (Fig. 65-1) does well with simple excision of the fistula and closure of the bladder and abdominal wall in layers.

2. A 13-year-old incontinent girl with intact abdominal wall but separated pubes, solitary kidney, and imperforate vagina has a simple diamond excision from the bladder neck and urethra and remains incontinent. A bladder neck suspension leaves her with suprapubic drainage for a year because of inability to void. On a combination of bethanechol chloride (Urecholine) and phenoxybenzamine hydrochloride (Dibenzyline), she succeeds in emptying her bladder and goes off drugs 2 years after bladder neck suspension. She is continent but has infections once every 2 years which respond to antibiotics.

3. A boy with classical exstrophy is continent after simple midline closure as a newborn.

4. A boy with classical exstrophy fails to gain control after six procedures in 5 years and is diverted.

5. A 4-year-old with cloacal exstrophy and colonic segment excised became continent after a Young–Dees repair aided by iliac osteotomies.

The large smooth bladder (Fig. 65-2) generally is said to be more amenable to closure than the small knobby one (Fig. 65-3). I believe the smooth bladder tends to hypotonic neuropathy and the knobby tends to hypertonic neuropathy. These concepts must be weighed when constructing the bladder neck.

Table 65-1 summarizes the results in our 42 cases of various types of exstrophy. Failure are unfortunately inevitable, but success does come to a significant portion of those children whose surgeons and parents are willing to devote much time and effort.

CLASSICAL EXSTROPHY AND MINOR VARIANTS

Stage I

I agree with Rickham and Bairov that closure in the newborn period is easiest. Most, but not all, classical cases can be closed within 48 hr postpartum without the need for iliac osteotomies. If one can push the medial edges of the pubes together by pinching the greater trochanters between the thumb and forefinger of one hand, osteotomies probably will not be required. A few of our primary closures without osteotomies have undergone dehiscence during the first 10 days after surgery. We have then done osteotomies and redone the closure immediately in such newborns.

Theoretically, according to the embryologic model of Muecke and Marshall, exstrophy is caused by overgrowth of the cloacal membrane keeping the mesodermal structures from the midline without deleting any parts.[32] Therefore, if one can bring the structures together surgically in the midline, continence should be obtained. Clearly the problem is not that simple, but this is the model followed.

It is important to bring the muscles of the urogenital diaphragm toward the midline to provide support for the urethra and bladder neck (Fig. 65-4). Those who have observed retropubic anatomy during radical prostatectomy will realize that the skeletal muscles of the urogenital diaphragm and levators remain slightly ajar anteriorly. Therefore, we make an effort to "close the open book"

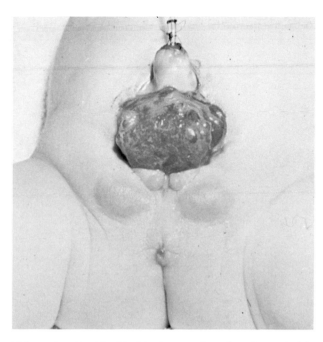

FIG. 65-3. Knobby bladder in a newborn female, probably of the hypertonic neuropathic type

but do not try to obtain tight approximation anteriorly. The objective of Stage I is to create a complete epispadias.

In the newborn, the entire body below the costal margins is prepared. The legs are wrapped individually in sterile stockinettes to the thighs for placement in the sterile field. The child is placed supine. Plastic feeding tubes (5Fr or 3½Fr) are passed into the lumbar ureters and anchored to the trigonal mucosa with 5-0 chromic gut fixation sutures (Fig. 65-5A). With a No. 15 blade or cutting electrocautery knife, incisions are made at the mucocutaneous junction, starting where the bladder joins the urethra (Fig. 65-5B). The incision is continued cephalad, with particular care taken to avoid cutting into the umbilical vessels or peritoneum as the umbilicus is approached. The incisions are then extended along the urethra to the corpora in the male or the divided clitoris in the female.

The dissection is carried down to subcutaneous fat at the bladder neck. By palpation, the medial edge of either pubic ramus is then identified (Fig. 65-5C). This is the most important landmark of the procedure, because it is the key to exposure of the medial borders of the rectus muscles and bladder neck or prostate tissues. The medial borders of the recti along with the medial edges of the pubes must be dissected free to enable placement of the sutures, which when tied will bring these struc-

TABLE 65-1. Summary of Experience with Exstrophy Syndrome

	Male	Female	Too early	Continent	Incontinent	Diverted
Classical						
DP		X				X
KA		X				X
ML	X					X
CG	X					X
AJ		X				X
DC	X			X		
MR	X					X
EA	X			X		
OB	X					X
CB		X				X
LT		X				X
SR		X		X		
GP		X				X
JB	X				X	
EF	X					X
CT	X				X	
TL	X			X		
BV	X			X		
AD	X			X		
ZD	X			X		
TV		X	X			
DE		X		X		
KM		X	X			
BV	X			X		
CP	X			X		
TA		X	X			
NA		X	X			
Complete epispadias						
AM		X		X		
SL	X			X		
JR	X			X		
BA	X				X	
Fissure-fistula						
JW	X			X		
WF	X			X		
Cloacal						
FC*	X					X
CP	X					X
MK*	X				X	
JA		X		X		
SL		X				
MD	X		X			
SG	X		X			
Other variants						
GD	X			X		
DM		X		X		
Total 42	26	16	6	18	4	13

* Died

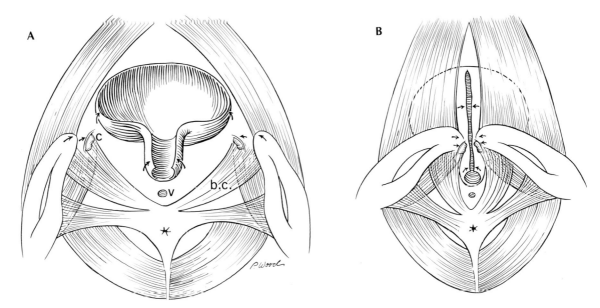

FIG. 65-4. Closure of exstrophy. **(A)** In association with the exstrophy, there is wide separation of the musculature and the skeleton. **(B)** Effective closure must include all involved structures. **C**-clitoris, **v**-vagina, **b. c.**-bulbocavernosus

tures to the midline and close the "open book." After the medial pubic ramus is identified by palpation, dissection is carried out sharply and directly to it through the subcutaneous fat. It does no harm to cut through the periosteal tissues into the cartilage. The perichondrium will appear pearly gray.

After the medial edge of the pubic bone has been identified, dissection is directed cephalad to the insertion of the rectus to expose its entire infraumbilical medial border (Fig. 65-5D). The bladder edge also is freed as dissection proceeds cephalad. The same dissection is completed on the opposite side. The bellies of the recti are identified, and enough rectus fascia is exposed for easy placement of sutures. The paraurethral incisions are deepened to expose periurethral muscles and corpora. Care is taken to avoid the pudendal nerves and vessels. A 8Fr feeding tube is then sutured in place to the trigonal mucosa, making a total of three catheters—two ureteral and one urethral—to be brought out through the urethra for drainage (Fig. 65-5D).

The ureteral catheters are essential for diversion. In two of our early patients in whom we did not drain the ureters, the tissue edema and pressure associated with closure were enough to obstruct the ureters, rendering the infants anuric for 72 hr. The urethra is transected a few millimeters distal to the verumontanum and freed from the corpora

distally. We have done Duckett's paravesical flaps (Fig. 65-6A to I) or Michalowski and Modelski's urethral Z-plasty (Fig. 65-7). The Duckett flaps are sewn to each other in the midline. To fill the gap left by the retraction of the urethra, the flaps are sutured in place. The bladder closure is begun. In this and subsequent steps, tension while tying sutures can be relieved by having an assistant push on the newborn's greater trochanters to bring the midline structure together. Interrupted Prolene 5-0 sutures are then placed to approximate the bladder muscle and serosa (see Fig. 65-5E). Mucosa is avoided.

Prolene sutures (5-0) are placed in the rectus bellies and fascia to close these structures in the midline down to the level of the pubes (see Fig. 65-5F). Two interrupted figure-of-eight 2-0 or 3-0 Prolene sutures are placed through the pubes on a cutting needle. These pubic sutures include cartilage and periosteal and other associated structures (see Fig. 65-5G). No attempt is made to approximate the distal male urethra at this time. The subcutaneous tissues and skin are brought together with Prolene sutures (see Fig. 65-5H). A complete epispadias has been created.

If the child is older than 48 hr, the procedure is started with bilateral iliac osteotomies, making sure both tables of the ilium are broken (my orthopedic consultants do this for me). The sacral incisions are closed, the infant is placed supine, and the

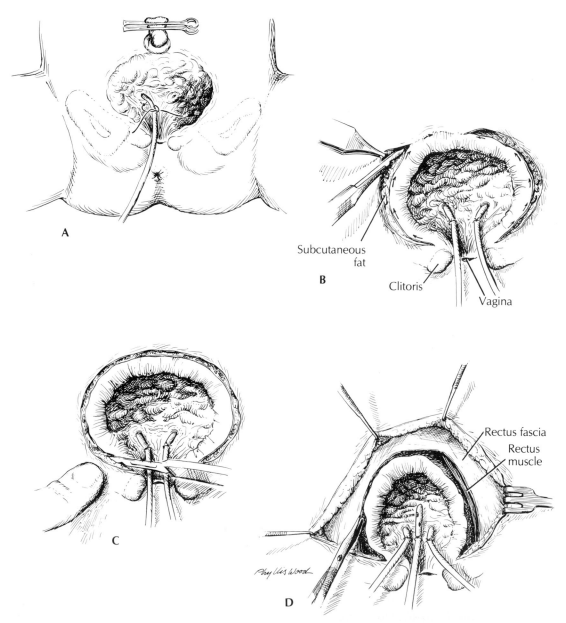

FIG. 65-5.   Primary closure of exstrophy in the infant.   **(A)** No. 5 plastic feeding tubes are inserted in the ureters and anchored with No. 5 chromic gut.   **(B)** The vesicocutaneous junction is separated.   **(C)** The medial edge of the symphysis is palpated and exposed by sharp dissection.   **(D)** A No. 8 plastic feeding tube is anchored to the trigonal muscle. The exposed symphysis is a guide to the dissection of the rectus fascia and muscles.   **(E)** The bladder is closed.   **(F)** The rectus fascia and muscles are sutured.   **(G)** Two figure-of-eight sutures approximate the pubic rami.   **(H)** The subcutaneous tissue and skin are approximated.

steps described previously for bladder closure are carried out.

The child's pelvic girdle is wrapped with half a length of 2-in (5-cm) Ace bandage immediately after the procedure. The bandage is rewrapped

once a day or more often as desired for airing the skin and cleansing. The parents are given a supply of Ace bandages to take home; they are encouraged to continue wrapping outside the diaper for at least 6 months in the hope that the procedure will

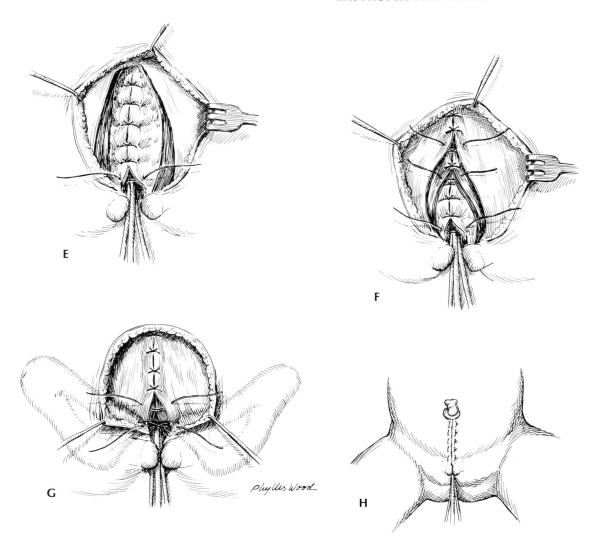

E

F

G

H

Phyllis Wood

help to mold the pelvic girdle together at the symphysis.

In two boys and one girl in our series, a continent bladder was created in a single stage, but most patients require additional surgery. All of our boys have had groin hernias repaired. All of our patients are followed periodically with radioisotope renography for individual renal function and assessment of obstruction, cystograms, and intravenous pyelograms. They are cystoscoped at age 6 months and every 1 or 2 years thereafter because of concern about malignant degeneration. Diaper rashes are common early but respond to Mycolog ointment.

Stage II

When does one reintervene if the child remains incontinent? If there is a continuous dribble from an empty or near-empty bladder, a secondary procedure will usually be required. I tend to do secondary bladder surgery later now than I used to, sometime between 3 to 4 years of age. This is in the hope that the child will have reached an age at which it can cooperate by "pushing" to empty the bladder with a Valsalva maneuver at parental request or on his own. If not, a good closure may require that the parents learn intermittent catheterization to empty the child's bladder two or three times a day. If iliac osteotomies have not been done, they are now carried out. If iliac osteotomies have been done, secondary closure may be performed (Fig. 65-8 shows an alternative). The secondary bladder procedure is done through a midline incision. I use Jeffs's version of the Young–Dees–Leadbetter procedure with Cohen cross-trigonal reimplants (Fig. 65-9) and bladder neck

(Text continues on p. 656)

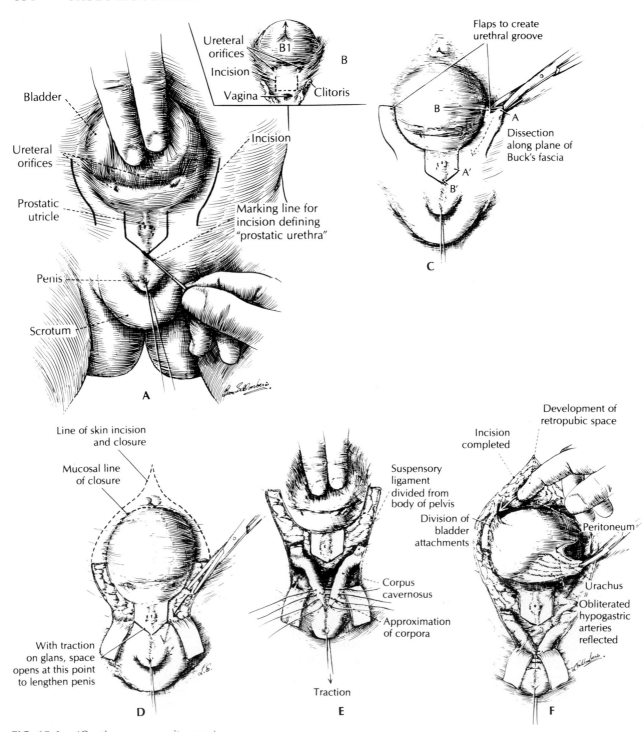

Bladder

Ureteral orifices

Prostatic utricle

Penis

Scrotum

Ureteral orifices

Incision

Vagina

B1

Clitoris

B

Incision

Marking line for incision defining "prostatic urethra"

A

Flaps to create urethral groove

B

A

Dissection along plane of Buck's fascia

A'

B'

C

Line of skin incision and closure

Mucosal line of closure

With traction on glans, space opens at this point to lengthen penis

D

Suspensory ligament divided from body of pelvis

Division of bladder attachments

Corpus cavernosus

Approximation of corpora

Traction

E

Incision completed

Development of retropubic space

Peritoneum

Urachus

Obliterated hypogastric arteries reflected

F

FIG. 65-6. (*Caption on opposite page*)

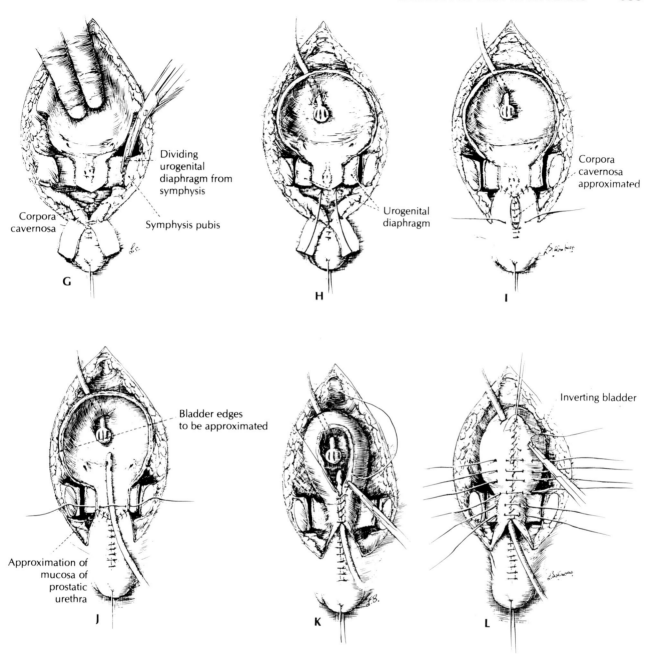

FIG. 65-6. Jeffs's closure of bladder exstrophy including Duckett's paraurethral flaps for urethral lengthening (Jeffs RD: Closure of bladder exstrophy including Duckett paraurethral flaps for urethral lengthening. In Harrison, Gittes, Perlmutter et al (eds): Campbell's Urology, 4th ed, Vol 2, p. 1682. Philadelphia, W B Saunders, 1979) (*Illustration continues on p. 656*)

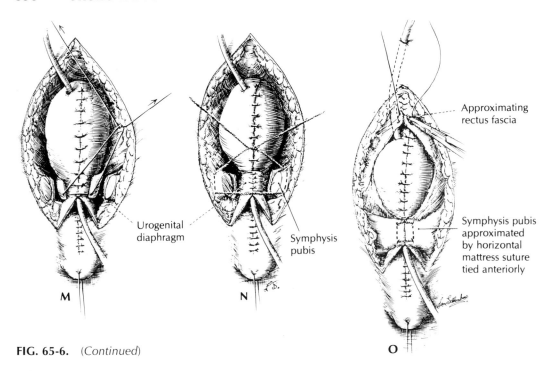

Urogenital
diaphragm

M

Symphysis
pubis

N   L.S.

Approximating
rectus fascia

Symphysis pubis
approximated
by horizontal
mattress suture
tied anteriorly

O

FIG. 65-6.   *(Continued)*

suspension sutures. Unless this stage goes very easily and quickly (it rarely does), I prefer to do the epispadias repair separately, as described later in this chapter.

Arap describes a staged procedure in which he diverts the ureters in antireflux fashion to an isolated segment of colon as a conduit. At the same time, the entire bladder is closed as a tube in Young–Dees fashion. In a subsequent stage, the two are connected. I have not done this procedure but plan to use it as a means of undiversion in some of our patients with failed primary repairs and ileal conduits whose bladders seem suitable. Of our 27 classical closures, there are 15 boys and 12 girls. Ten are continent and two are incontinent. Eleven have been diverted. In four it is too early to predict outcome.

Cloacal Exstrophy

Cloacal exstrophy appears to arise embryologically before the urogenital septum of the cloaca has reached the perineum. As Johnston has depicted, this results in abnormal colon being situated between two bladder halves.[23] Such children almost always have short gut, vertebral anomalies, and omphalocele. They also have meningomyeloceles, hydrocephalus, paraplegia, renal anomalies, vascular abnormalities, talipes equinovarus, divided or absent phallus, and undescended testes. It is

the gut, with its rapid transit time and poor absorption or perhaps obstructed by an atretic segment, that proves to be the greatest threat to the child's survival. Because difficult decisions will have to be made rapidly, surgeons who deal with this problem must be prepared to inform the parents of their options so they can make knowledgeable decisions. If the child has meningomyelocele with paraplegia, most feel surgical treatment should be withheld. I agree, but some will survive anyway and then the surgeon must do whatever can be done to improve the situation. The team approach to such individuals has proved invaluable.[17] Decisions as to sex of rearing will be obvious in the absence of phallic structures but more difficult in the diphallic male. Some of these structures appear to undergo remarkable metamorphosis when they are brought to the midline, joined, and straightened in association with iliac osteotomies.

Excision of the omphalocele and disposition of gut is the primary problem. In our patients, the blood supply to ileum, colon, tail gut, and bladder has all come from branches of the superior mesenteric artery. This has created difficulty in saving colon segments when trying to divert the fecal stream. Our choice has usually been to excise the rudimentary colon. Duckett feels that this is an error and saves all he can. The bladder halves are usually quite generous. They are sewn together in the midline. Triangular portions of mucosa from

(Text continues on p. 660)

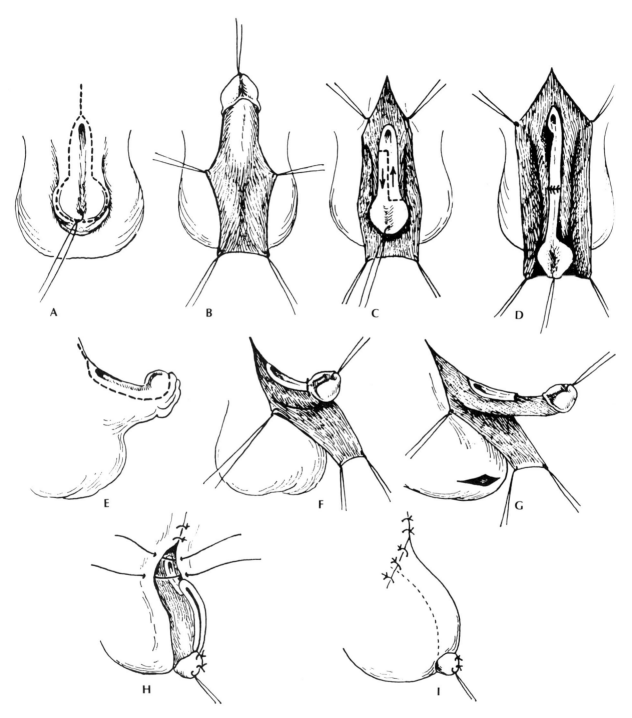

FIG. 65-7.   Michalowski and Modelski's method of urethral Z-plasty for urethral lengthening (Michalowski E, Modelski W: The surgical treatment of epispadias. Surg Gynecol Obstet 117:465, 1963)

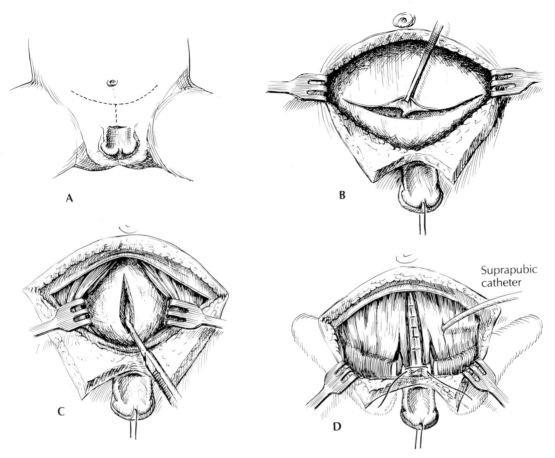

FIG. 65-8. Secondary reconstruction of the bladder outlet and the urethra, an alternative method of decreasing the interpubic distance. **(A)** Pfannenstiel's incision with a "T" is made. **(B)** The rectus fascia is elevated to the umbilicus and the pubes. **(C)** The rectus muscles are separated and the bladder is incised and examined. **(D)** The medial 5 mm of pubes are separated and sutured in the midline.

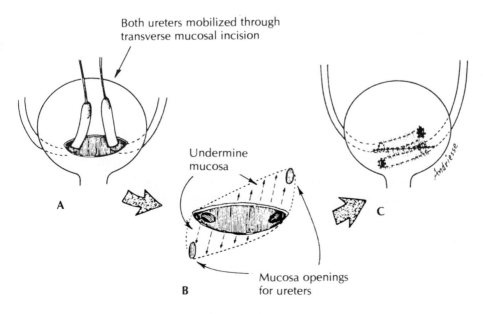

Both ureters mobilized through transverse mucosal incision

Undermine mucosa

Mucosa openings for ureters

FIG. 65-9. Cohen's cross-trigonal reimplantation (Hendren, WH: Complications of ureteral reimplantation and megaureter repair. In Smith RB, Skinner DG (eds): Complications of Urologic Surgery, p. 168. Philadelphia, WB Saunders, 1976)

FIG. 65-10. Penopubic epispadias with continence: **(A)** typical presenting appearance and **(B)** postoperative result (Dees JE: Congenital epispadias with incontinence. J Urol 62:518, 1949)

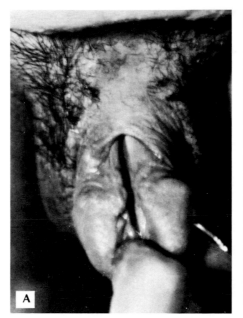

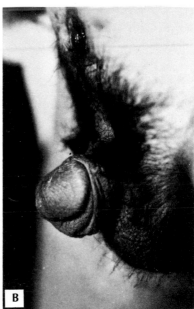

FIG. 65-11. Correction of chordee and creation of a distal urethra in the male.

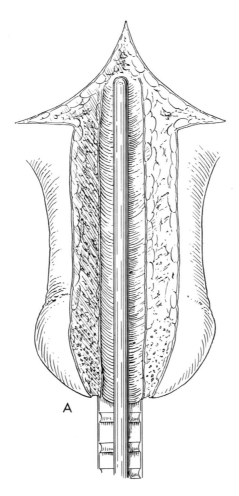

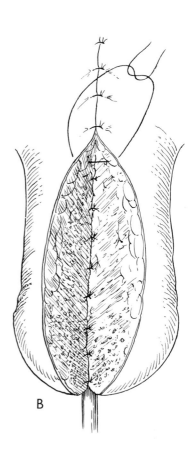

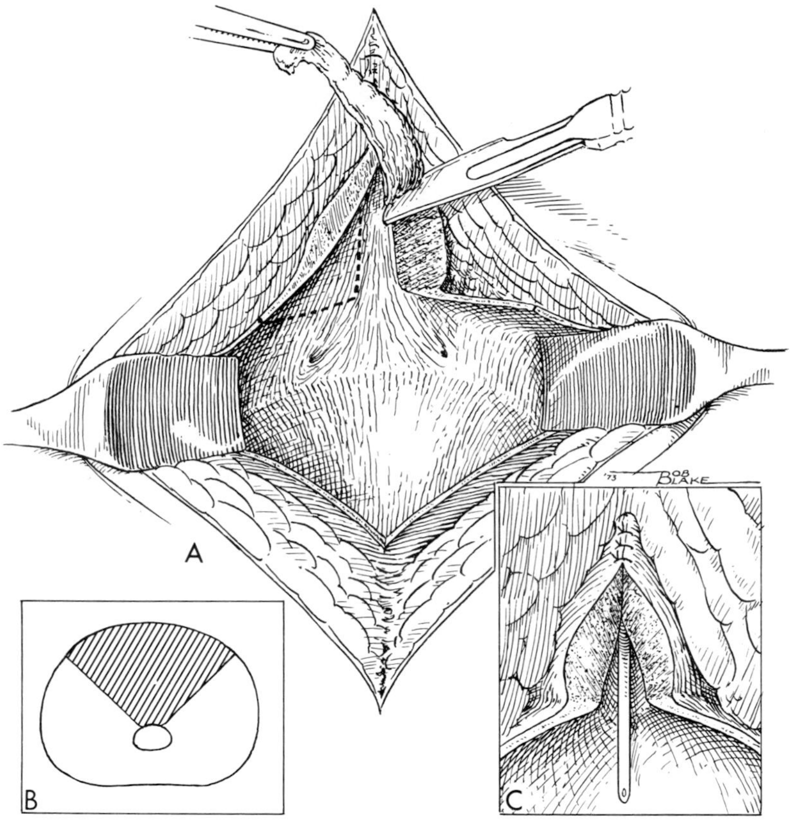

FIG. 65-12. Creation of a new posterior urethra in the male

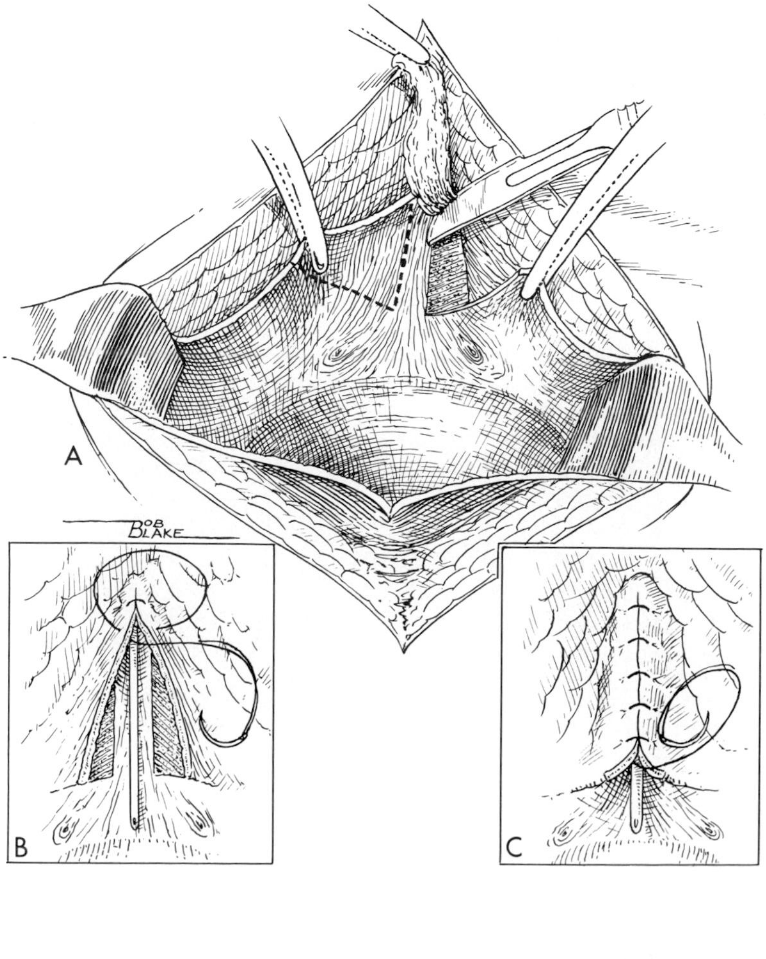

FIG. 65-13. Creation of a new posterior urethra in the female

each half of the bladder neck are excised in Young–Dees pattern, and the bladder is closed. The ureters are splinted with feeding tubes and one is also used for bladder drainage. The pubes are exposed and the abdominal wall is closed, creating a complete epispadias. Subsequent procedures to correct phallic and genital anomalies are done as indicated. Of seven children with cloacal exstrophy in our experience, one was not treated at parental request and died. One child died suddenly at age 2, probably of inadequate fluid replacement and electrolyte imbalance. The rest survive; four are ambulatory and one is wheelchair bound. One is currently continent, one is training, and it is too early to know what will happen with the last two. In summary, results of surgical treatment of the worst of the varieties of exstrophy have been unexpectedly rewarding and are but a reflection of recent progress in the entire field.

Epispadias

As a rule, few procedures in exstrophic children are truly easy and correcting epispadias follows that rule. Tactically, most of the armamentarium for correction of hypospadias is used but in the reverse direction (*i.e.*, ventral to dorsal). Although the maneuvers are similar, the degree of difficulty in performing them creates a qualitative difference. If one wishes to inflate the corpora, for example, two needles must be placed, one in each corpora, because of lack of communication between them. The chordee is so much more extensive than that ordinarily encountered in hypospadias that the dissection required to correct it often extends from corona to the crura. In cloacal exstrophy, I have encountered chordee which bound each separated corporal half into a tight S shape. When the epispadiac corpora have been lengthened and straightened, it may be necessary to rotate inguinal flaps to cover the defect at the base, something almost never necessary in hypospadias.

For purposes of discussion the repair of epispadias should be divided into two categories: incomplete and continent (Fig. 65-10) and complete and incontinent. Treatment of the relatively rare incomplete varieties depends in part on the degree of chordee and location of the meatus. The glandular varieties can usually be closed by freeing up the broad urethral strip from the splayed glans, closing it, and then approximating the wings of the glans over it (Fig. 65-11).

In shaft epispadias, once the chordee has been corrected, skin is transferred ventral to dorsal, and a urethral tube is created and covered by any

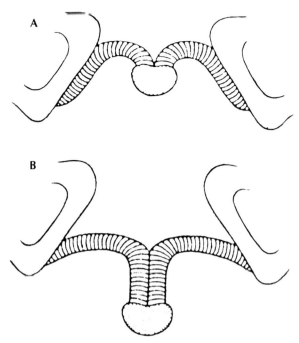

FIG. 65-14. Johnston's method of penile lengthening. **(A)** The corpora cavernosa are of nearly normal length but do not contribute to the penile shaft because of the pubic separation. **(B)** Lengthening is obtained by detaching the crura from the puboischial rami, thus allowing the corpora to be advanced into the shaft. (Johnston JH: The genital aspects of exstrophy. J Urol 113:701, 1975)

of the several procedures used for hypospadias. I frequently rotate inguinal flaps as described by Allen, Spence, and Salyer to cover the dorsal defect created by correction of chordee,[1] but I may stagger them as in a Z-plasty as suggested by Williams to avoid contraction of straight suture lines along the entire length of the penis.[42] Procedures specially designed for epispadias repair are Hinman's technique, Khanna's technique of shaft burial beneath a scrotal flap, Michalowski and Modelski's Z-plasty, Williams's V–Y plasty, and the scrotal break technique.[18,24,31,42]

Generally, the continent epispadiacs are far less difficult to deal with than the incontinent varieties, which take on most of the characteristics of classical exstrophy. If during initial examination, on spreading the proximally displaced meatus, one can see the verumontanum, incontinence is almost a certainty and will have to be corrected. Incontinence has in the past been easier to correct in complete epispadias than in classical exstrophy.[10] Endoscopic assessment of the external sphincter area and the proximal urethra may provide important diagnostic clues to the extent of repair necessary

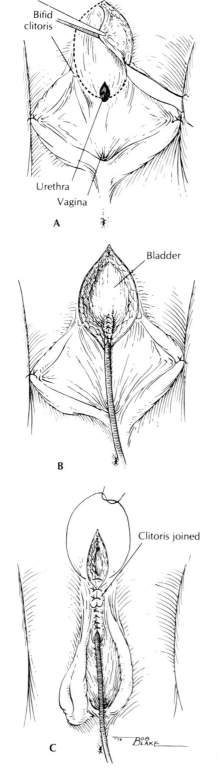

FIG. 65-15. Creation of a distal urethra and correction of the defect in the external genitalia of the female

to establish control. In some, the sphincter area will contain irislike folds posteriorly but will be smooth from 10 o'clock around 12 to 2 o'clock, indicating a defect that will require correction in that area. The prostatic fossa may likewise show evidence of anterior defect or be more broadly flattened and foreshortened. The greater the anterior defect, the flatter the prostatic urethra, the more major the reconstruction that will need to be performed. For minor defects, resection of the malfunctioning segment and reapproximation done through a pubis-splitting incision may suffice. One may wish to transect the urethra, release the chordee, and swing Duckett flaps to cover the defect at the same time. More extensive abnormalities will require Young–Dees–Leadbetter reconstruction through an abdominal incision (Figs. 65-12 and 65-13) in addition to urethral and chordee release with the aid of paravesical flaps. I prefer to complete the repair of the pendulous urethra as a separate procedure. The chordee is corrected by Johnston's procedure (Fig. 65-14).

We have treated three boys and one girl with complete epispadias. The girl and two of the boys are continent. Distal urethral reconstruction in the female patient is depicted in Figure 65-15; this is the Dees method.

REFERENCES

1. ALLEN TD, SPENCE HM, SALYER KE: Reconstruction of the external genitalia in exstrophy of the bladder. J Urol 111:830, 1974
2. AMBROSE SA: The repair of genital defects associated with persistent cloaca. Trans Am Assoc Genitourin Surg 65:58, 1973
3. ANSELL JS: Surgical treatment of exstrophy of the bladder with emphasis on neonatal primary closure: Personal experience with 28 consecutive cases treated at the University Hospital from 1962 to 1977; techniques and results. J Urol 121:650, 1979
4. ARAP S, GIRON AM, DEGOES GM: Initial results of the complete reconstruction of bladder exstrophy. Urol Clin North Am 7, No. 2:477, 1980
5. AYERS cited in Gross SD: North American Surgical Review:709, 1895
6. BAIROV GA: Reconstructive plastic surgery of bladder exstrophy in newborn infants. Vestnik Khirugii Imeni II Grekova Moskow 97:85, 1949
7. BERG S: Polytef augmentation urethroplasty. Arch Surg 107:379, 1973
8. COHEN SJ: Ureterozystoneostomie: Eine neue Antireflux Technic. Aktuelle Urologie 6:1, 1975
9. COOK FE, JR, LESLIE JT, BRANNON EW: Preliminary report: A new concept of abdominal closure in

infants with exstrophy of the bladder. J Urol 87.823, 1962

10. CULP OS: Treatment of epispadias with and without urinary incontinence: Experience with 46 patients. J Urol 109:120, 1973

11. DEES JE: Congenital epispadias with incontinence. J Urol 62:513, 1949

12. DEVINE CJ, HORTON CE: Hypospadias and epispadias. Clin Symp 20:24, 1972

13. DEVINE CJ, HORTON CE, SCARFF JE, JR: Espispadias. Urol Clin North Am 7:465, 1980

14. DUCKETT JW, JR: Epispadias. Urol Clin North Am 5:107, 1978

15. FONKELSRUD E, LINDE LM: Successful management of vesicointestinal fissure: Report of 2 cases. J Pediatr Surg 5:309, 1970

16. GRAVIER L: Exstrophy of the cloaca. Am Surg 34, No. 5:387, 1968

17. HAYDEN PW, CHAPMAN WH, STEVENSON JK: Exstrophy of the cloaca. Am J Dis Child 125:879, 1973

18. HINMAN F, JR: A method of lengthening and repairing the penis in exstrophy of the bladder. J Urol 79:237, 1958

19. JEFFS RD: Exstrophy and cloacal exstrophy. Urol Clin North Am 5:127, 1978

20. JEFFS, RD, CHARROIS R, MANY M et al: Primary closure of the exstrophied bladder. In Scott B (ed): Current Controversies in Urologic Management, p 235. Philadelphia, WB Saunders, 1972

21. JOHNSTON, JH: The genital aspects of exstrophy. J Urol 113:701, 1975

22. JOHNSTON JH, KOGAN SJ: The exstrophic anomalies and their surgical reconstruction. Curr Prob Surg August, 1974

23. JOHNSTON JH, PENN IA: Exstrophy of the cloaca. Br J Urol 38:302, 1966

24. KHANNA NN: Techniques of epispadias repair. Plast Reconstr Surg 52:365, 1973

25. KOONTZ WW, JOSHI VV, OWNBY R: Cloacal exstrophy with the potential for urinary control: An unusual presentation. J Urol 112:828, 1974

26. LATTIMER JK, DEAN AM, JR, DOUGHERTY LJ et al: Functional closure of the bladder in children with exstrophy. J Urol 83:647, 1960

27. LATTIMER JK et al: Long-term follow-up after exstrophy closure. Late improvement and good quality of life. J Urol 119:664, 1978

28. LATTIMER JK, SMITH MJV; Exstrophy closure: A Follow-up of 70 cases. J Urol 95:356, 1966

29. MARKLAND C, FRALEY EE: Management of infants with cloacal exstrophy. J Urol 109:740, 1973

30. MARSHALL VF, MUECKE EC; Variations in exstrophy of the bladder. J Urol 88:766, 1962

31. MICHALOWSKI E, MODELSKI W: The surgical treatment of epispadias. Surg Gynecol Obstet 117:465, 1963

32. MUECKE EC, COOK GT, MARSHALL VF: Duplication of the abdominal vena cava associated with cloacal exstrophy. Trans Am Assoc Genitourin Surg 63:135, 1971

33. RICKHAM PP: Incidence and treatment of ectopia vesicae (abridged). Proceedings of the Royal Society of Medicine 54:389, 1961

34. RICKHAM PP: Vesico-intestinal fissure. Arch Dis Child 35:97, 1960

35. SCHULTZ WG: Plastic repair of exstrophy of the bladder combined with bilateral osteotomy of the ilia. J Urol 79:453, 1958

36. SCOTT FB, BRADLEY WE, TIMM, GW: Treatment of urinary incontinence by an implantable prosthetic urinary sphincter. J Urol 112:75, 1974

37. SOPER RT, KILGER K: Vesico-intestinal fissure. J Urol 92:490, 1964

38. SPENCER R: Exstrophia splanchnica. Surgery 57:751, 1965

39. SWENSON O: Changing trends in the management of exstrophy. Surgery 42:61, 1957

40. SWENSON O: Changing trends in the management of exstrophy. Surgery 42:281, 1960

41. TANK ES, LINDENAUER SM: Exstrophy of the cloaca. Am J Surg 119:95, 1970

42. WILLIAMS DI, KEETON JE: Further progress with reconstruction of the exstrophied bladder. Br J Surg 60:203, 1973

Female Urinary Incontinence

66

George D. Webster

Urinary incontinence is the involuntary loss of urine, and it is one of the most distressing problems in urologic practice. For the purposes of this chapter, we will discuss loss of urine through the urethra; however, the possibility of leakage through a fistula tract should always be considered. Successful storage of urine demands that the bladder not contract inappropriately (remain stable) and that the sphincter mechanism be competent. These two criteria separate nonsurgical incontinence (detrusor or urgency incontinence) from surgical incontinence (genuine stress incontinence). The main thrust of the evaluation of the incontinent patient is to identify the underlying pathophysiologic cause, on which treatment selection is totally dependent.

Classification

GENUINE STRESS INCONTINENCE

Genuine stress incontinence is the involuntary loss of urine due to a sudden rise in intra-abdominal pressure. It is an exceedingly common condition, and even normal women at some time, and under certain stress, leak a small amount of urine. Indeed, between 40% and 50% of young, healthy nulliparous women admit to occasional mild stress incontinence; however, at least 80% of stress incontinence patients are in the perimenopausal age group and are multiparous.[38] Raz has suggested that the female urethral continence mechanism is dependent on the interaction of four urethral factors: urethral closing pressure, urethral length, urethrotrigonal anatomy, and urethral reception of intra-abdominal pressure.[24]

The urethral closing pressure is predominantly a result of the interaction of smooth and striated muscle sphincter activity, but there is also some contribution by nonmuscular urethral factors such as the submucosal vascular plexus, the elastin and collagen content of the urethral tissues, and a sphincter like effect of the mucosa. There has been considerable diversity of opinion regarding the anatomic structure and the innervation of the urethral sphincters, and the interested reader is referred to the reference literature for a more detailed discussion of this subject.[12,14,30]

Lapides and associates have stressed the importance of urethral length in the maintenance of continence in the female.[18] However, although it certainly interacts with other factors to contribute to continence, a short urethra alone will not produce incontinence. Urethral length varies considerably in normal women, and women with proven genuine stress urinary incontinence do not invariably have urethral shortening.

Urethrotrigonal anatomy, which can be demonstrated by lateral cystourethrography, should fulfill certain criteria. The bladder base should lie above the level of the inferior ramus of the symphysis, and with straining should not descend more than 1.5 cm.[29] There should be a normal urethrotrigonal alignment with an angle normally less than 100 degrees, and the urethral axis should be approximately 35 degrees from the vertical. In the hypermobile situation loss of all of the normal anatomic features may occur, a radiologic finding that correlates with the clinical finding of cystourethrocele. However, clinical experience has shown that the coexistence of cystourethrocele and incontinence does not predict that the incontinence is of a genuine stress variety.

The transmission of intra-abdominal pressure to the intra-abdominal portion of the proximal urethra is also important in the maintenance of continence. This is a passive phenomenon, and is the result of the normal anatomic configuration just described. Whenever there is a rise in intra-abdominal pressure during such stresses as coughing or straining, the pressure is transmitted not only to the bladder but also to the proximal urethra, with resultant increase in the closing pressure, and prevention of leakage. If the urethral axis is altered, rotational descent will drop the proximal urethra and bladder base from its intra-abdominal location, and will obviously impair such pressure transmission. It is my opinion that repositioning of the proximal urethra and bladder neck within the abdomen is the factor primarily responsible for the correction of stress incontinence by the currently available surgical techniques. Correct repositioning not only will raise the proximal urethra into the abdomen, but also will tend to correct anatomic abnormalities and lengthen the urethra.

URGENCY (DETRUSOR) INCONTINENCE

The normal bladder is stable, that is, it contracts only when the patient voluntarily voids. The unstable bladder, however, contracts inappropriately with resultant active incontinence. Bladder instability may be idiopathic, and it is estimated that some 10% of the population exhibit this abnormal activity.[32] Uninhibited detrusor activity may also occur in the neurologically impaired patient. In such cases the bladder instability is termed *detrusor hyperreflexia,* and it results in reflex neurogenic incontinence. In most cases it is not possible to differentiate idiopathic bladder instability from neurogenic bladder hyperreflexia, and it therefore behooves the physician to seek out a neurologic cause in patients with this condition.

A majority of adults with idiopathic bladder instability are symptom-free, although some may exhibit an increased frequency of micturition and some might rise to void at night. In women with normal sphincter mechanisms, bladder instability will not necessarily lead to incontinence. The uninhibited bladder contraction will result in bladder neck opening, but continence can be maintained by an adequate distal sphincter mechanism. Once this distal mechanism weakens with progressing age, incontinence may result, and in most patients will be associated with a sensation of urgency to void.

The stimulus making the detrusor contract is varied; however, it is important to note that in some patients cough and straining may be the cause. Hence, cough/strain-provoked urinary leakage is not always diagnostic of genuine sress incontinence.

Genuine stress incontinence and urgency (detrusor) incontinence frequently coexist, and in such cases careful evaluation is essential to determine the relative contribution of each component.

Patient Evaluation

HISTORY

A careful history is crucial in identifying the etiology of incontinence, and the circumstances surrounding the urine loss must be carefully questioned. The object of careful history taking is to separate patients with urgency incontinence from those with genuine stress incontinence, and whereas this cannot invariably be achieved by the history alone, those cases most deserving of further evaluation can be identified. The symptoms of the unstable bladder are frequency of micturition, nocturia, urgency to void, and episodes of urgency incontinence. Obviously, these symptoms are not exclusive to bladder instability, and for this reason Bates and associates introduced the concepts of *sensory urgency* and *motor urgency.*[2] Motor urgency is the occurrence of these symptoms in the presence of uninhibited bladder contractions. Sensory urgency describes these same symptoms associated with bladder-irritative phenomena but with a stable detrusor. Any bladder-irritative state, including urinary tract infections, the urethral syndrome, interstitial cystitis, and carcinoma *in situ,* may be responsible. Very careful history taking can often differentiate between these two types of urgency; but objective testing by cystometry, as will be discused later, is the final arbiter.

Farrar and associates published an interesting study of the presenting symptoms of 570 females with micturition disorders, and correlated the symptoms with the function of the detrusor on urodynamic testing (Fig. 66-1).[10] The data gleaned from this study are invaluable in the assessment of the incontinent patient, because they identify those symptoms most likely to be associated with abnormal detrusor activity. The study showed that those patients who were incontinent, but only leaked urine on stress, invariably had stable bladders. If in addition to the stress leakage the patient also had frequency and nocturia, then the incidence of an unstable bladder was 45%. If urgency and episodes of urgency incontinence accompanied the stress leakage, then the bladder was noted to be unstable in approximately 80% of cases. In those patients who had only frequency, nocturia, urgency, and urgency incontinence without any stress component, all patients were found to have an unstable bladder. It is also interesting to note that 15 patients complained of urinary incontinence on "getting out of the chair" and the incidence for instability in this group was also 80%, as it was in those patients who complained of "always being wet" regardless of their other associated symptoms.

The importance of careful evaluation of those patients with apparent stress incontinence who also have symptoms of bladder instability (frequency, nocturia, urgency, or urgency inconti-

FIG. 66-1. Incidence of bladder instability by symptom groups in incontinent women (After Farrar DJ, Whiteside CG, Osborne JL et al: A urodynamic analysis of micturition symptoms in the female. Surg Gynecol Obstet 141:875, 1975. By permission of Surgery, Gynecology & Obstetrics)

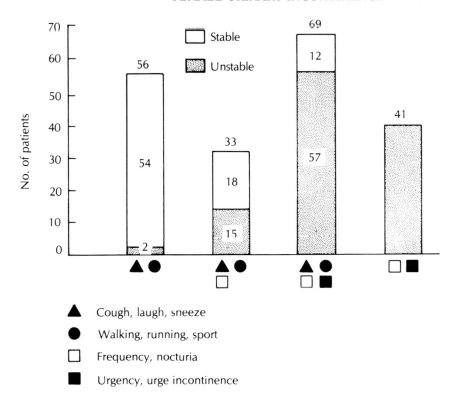

▲ Cough, laugh, sneeze

● Walking, running, sport

□ Frequency, nocturia

■ Urgency, urge incontinence

nence) is that those with unstable urinary incontinence enjoy an exceedingly poor success rate from surgical repair. The failure rate is four times higher than for those with stable bladders.[1] This does not indicate that surgical correction is absolutely contraindicated in the face of an unstable bladder, but the actual contribution of genuine sphincter weakness to the problem must be identified by appropriate urodynamic and other objective testing. Also, the patient should be adequately counseled preoperatively to ensure that she understands that only the stress component is likely to be completely corrected by surgery, and that frequency, urgency, and some urgency incontinence will persist.

Figure 66-1 shows that 55% of women with apparent stress incontinence and associated frequency and nocturia will have stable bladders. These are women with sensory urgency due to hypersensitive bladders in whom surgical correction is entirely justified. In some, it has been suggested that the bladder hypersensitivity symptoms are due to distortion of the trigone and bladder base as a result of cystourethrocele and, as such, may improve following suspension surgery. In this group with sensory urgency, the success rate of suspension surgery equals that of patients with pure genuine stress incontinence.

PHYSICAL EXAMINATION

The general physical examination should pay particular attention to neurologic and gynecologic systems. Patients with neurogenic incontinence will generally manifest obvious symptoms and signs of their neurologic disease, but in a few cases subtle changes may elude the cursory examination. Overflow incontinenmce may masquerade as stress urinary leakage, and identification of the distended bladder is important. If there is any doubt, catheterization to measure the postvoid residual should be done.

Gynecological examination includes digital and speculum examination. The finding of vaginal prolapse does not correlate well with the presence of genuine stress incontinence; however, it is still important to identify it in the incontinent patient, because its presence does somewhat dictate the type of surgical procedure necessary. As will be seen later, cystourethrocele is corrected by some of the suspension procedures, but associated enterocele or rectocele might require concomitant vaginal surgery. Significant uterine decensus or other uterine abnormalities may justify simultaneous hysterectomy.

In the patient who is strongly suspected of having true stress incontinence and who does not have evidence of a vaginal anatomic abnormality, confirmatory radiographic and urodynamic studies should be performed. The Marshall test is useful to determine whether incontinence is likely to be true stress urinary incontinence, and whether it can be improved by correction of the anatomic abnormality. The test is ideally performed with the patient's bladder moderately full. Should stress induce urinary leakage, one should note whether the leakage is transient and occurring simultaneously with the cough, in which case it is likely to be due to sphincter weakness. If it occurs momentarily after the cough and is of a more prolonged nature, it may be due to an uninhibited bladder contraction precipitated by the stress. If continence cannot be precipitated during supine testing, the patient should be reexamined erect. When cough-induced incontinence occurs, two fingers are introduced into the vagina and the anterior wall is elevated, taking care not to compress the urethra. If elevation corrects the incontinence the Marshall test is positive, and suspension surgery may be successful.

UROLOGIC WORK-UP

The urologic work-up may include urinalysis, radiographic studies, endoscopy, and urodynamics.[34]

Because bladder instability symptoms may be mimicked by urinary infection and other bladder-irritative phenomenon, urinalysis takes on great significance. Bacteriuric urinary infections occur in a significant number of multiparous women who might also have stress urinary incontinence, and such infections should be identified and treated before surgical correction. In those patients who have bladder-irritative symptoms due to hypersensitive bladders, the urinalysis and culture are generally unremarkable.

There is some disagreement about the role of radiographic studies in the evaluation of the incontinent female. I routinely perform excretory urography preoperatively; however, it might be acceptable to reserve such study for those patients who have symptoms or signs requiring further elucidation. One important role of the preoperative excretory urogram is to identify preexistent abnormalities of the upper tracts, lest the surgery be held responsible for them should they become apparent at a later date. The role of cystourethrography in the investigation of the incontinent female is controversial. Static cystography films will identify the posterior vesicourethral angle, bladder neck competence, and urethral axis. More valuable information is obtained if these studies are performed under fluoroscopy, at which time anatomic changes under various conditions of stress may be seen. These preoperative radiographic studies of the urethrovesical junction are by no means necessary in all cases; but they might add valuable information in the complicated case, particularly in the patient who has had previous repairs, and in whom examination suggests recurrent stress incontinence but in whom anatomic support is good. In such instances, the lateral cystograph might show whether better forward and upper displacement of the urethrovesical junction can be achieved.

Endoscopy is not routinely indicated in the preoperative evaluation of the incontinent woman; but I prefer to perform it, particularly in the patient with bladder-irritative symptoms or abnormalities on urinalysis. It might provide further information on anatomic support of the urethra and bladder base, but one should not attempt to interpret sphincter competence endoscopically. In patients who have undergone multiple previous repairs, gross scarring of the bladder neck and urethra may be evident, and in hormone-deficient women mucosal atrophy may be seen. Such findings may significantly influence the choice of therapy.

URODYNAMIC STUDIES

Urodynamic studies are the only functional method for evaluating the incontinent patient. These studies are not necessary in all cases, and careful history taking will identify those deserving of study. Patients who have recurrent incontinence following a previous failed repair have a 76% incidence of instability.[1] Identification of this instability might avoid unnecessary further surgery, and so all women deserve urodynamic evaluation before reopertion. Urodynamic study is also indicated in patients who, in addition to apparent stress incontinence, have associated bladder instability symptoms. Women who have urinary incontinence and void inefficiently also should have urodynamic evaluation. In some the problem is due to a urethral distortion phenomena resulting from bladder base and uretrhal descent during voiding. Others have detrusor dysfunction, which might be adversely affected by a surgical procedure which increases outlet resistance. Women who have associated neurologic problems, no matter how subtle, should have urodynamic evaluation prior to attempted surgical correction of urinary incontinence. Asymptomatic bladder hyperreflexia and uninhibited striated sphincter relaxation can occur in this group, and will not be improved by surgery.

Urodynamic studies performed on the incontinent patient are aimed at identifying alterations in detrusor and sphincter function. The detrusor is ideally evaluated by cystometry, but it is noteworthy that simple supine cystometry may fail to identify subtle detrusor instability, and, therefore, various provocative measures are used to unmask abnormal detrusor activity.[35] The urodynamic tools available for evaluation of the urethra and sphincter give far less interpretable information. Sphincter electromyography studies only electrical activity in the striated distal sphincter mechanism. It may identify uninhibited striated sphincter relaxation, which is seen in a few women with apparent stress incontinence and which may actually be the precipitating cause of urine loss. Urethral pressure profile studies have failed to convincingly differentiate stress from urge incontinence. Newer technology using microtransducer-tip catheters facilitates the measurement of pressure at various points within the urethra during rest and stress, and in this way it is possible to ascertain whether intra-abdominal pressure is transmitted to the proximal urethra, a determination which may prove important in the selection of cases for reoperation.

Micturition studies are indicated in patients who demonstrate voiding inefficiency. Simple uroflowmetry is a useful screening study to identify inefficient voiding but is never diagnostic. Should an abnormal peak flow rate be obtained, or significant residual urine be identified, a micturition study monitoring bladder pressures, sphincter electromyography, and urine flow rate during the act of voiding best elucidates the problem further. It is important to identify those patients who have poor detrusor contractility; they are likely to have significant voiding problems following surgical repair because such repairs invariably increase outlet resistence.

Video urodynamic studies offer the most elaborate tool for the functional evaluation of the lower urinary tract.[36] The study includes multifunction urodynamic testing together with the intermittent fluoroscopic screening of the bladder and outflow tract during both provocative cystometry and voiding.

Nonoperative Management

STRESS INCONTINENCE

It is useful to grade the severity of stress urinary incontinence in order to logically select appropriate treatment, and so that the results of treatment may be assessed and compared. I follow a four-category grading system:[37]

Grade 1—Mild urinary leakage with moderate stress, but no protection needed

Grade 2—Moderate urinary leakage with moderate stress, and protection necessary with exesssive activity

Grade 3—Severe urinary leakage with mild stress, constant protection needed except during rest

Grade 4—Incontinence at rest, requiring constant protection

Surgical intervention is rarely justified in patients with Grade 1 stress incontinence. They respond best to nonoperative forms of management. As one progresses through the more severe grades, surgical intervention becomes more essential. Nonoperative therapy may be considered in four parts: correction of local and general adverse factors, exercises to improve pelvic muscle tone, mechanical devices, and pharmacologic treatment.

General conditions that tend to accentuate stress incontinence include obesity and chronic pulmonary problems. Every effort should be made to correct these before embarking upon operative treatment. Urinary tract infections occur in up to 10% of women with stress urinary incontinence, and because they might aggravate the symptoms and compromise the success of surgery, these infections should be corrected preoperatively. Very mild stress urinary incontinence may occur in the woman with the urethral syndrome or abacteriuric urethrotrigonitis. These patients rarely have an anatomic defect on physical examination, and may benefit from simple urethral dilatation. Atrophic urethritis occurs in the postmenopausal woman with senile atrophy of the vaginal mucosa due to hormone deficiency. Estrogenic suppositories or creams applied to the vagina and introitus may significantly improve the vascularity and muscular tone of the vagina and perineal tissues in these patients.

Kegel exercises will also improve minimal stress urinary incontinence.[16] These exercises of the levator muscles probably achieve elevation of the urethrovesical junction in the same manner as surgical suspension. Obviously, the degree of elevation achieved by improvement in muscle tone is minimal, and only mild incontinence will be corrected.[15] Success with this method demands a highly motivated patient with a minimal anatomic abnormality, who is prepared to perform the exercises at least ten times each 30 minutes during the day, holding the elevated perineal position for 3 seconds each time.

A variety of mechanical devices (pessaries) have been designed to improve the anatomic abnormality that exists in most stress-incontinent women, by elevating the urethrovesical angle.[7,9] This technique is not always aesthetically acceptable to the patient; but it is a useful and safe maneuver in the older, poor-risk patient in whom surgical intervention may be contraindicated. The addition of electrical stimulation to the pelvic floor through the pessary device has also been explored, but these devices await refinement.[8]

Pharmacologic therapy for stress incontinence is limited by the fact that the drugs do not produce cure and must be used continuously to have the desired result. The medications available improve only the mildest incontinence and are not without side-effects. Because the nerve supply to the periurethral musculature is of the alpha-adrenergic system, drugs with this activity will improve sphincter tonus and hence improve continence. Drugs with a predominantly alpha-adrenergic mode of action include ephedrine, which is used in a dosage of 25 mg orally (PO) three or four times daily.[5] Phenylpropanolamine has similar action but with fewer side effects. This drug may be administered as Propadrine in a dosage of 50 mg b.i.d., or in Ornade spansules b.i.d.[28] None of these medications enjoy Food and Drug Administration approval for use in the treatment of bladder dysfunction, and the patient must be well counseled regarding the rationale for their use.

URGENCY INCONTINENCE

Urinary incontinence due to detrusor instability is not a surgical disease. As outlined earlier, however, detrusor instability frequently coexists with genuine stress incontinence, and in these patients surgical correction of the stress component is justified, the bladder instability being controlled conservatively after surgery. Therapy for the unstable bladder is most unsatisfactory, probably reflecting our poor understanding of the exact etiology of the condition. It is most likely that instability of the bladder is the final common manifestation of a variety of pathologies, and for this reason diverse therapeutic regimens are likely to be necessary. Treatments range from simple pharmacologic manipulation of detrusor and urethral function to surgical denervation of the bladder and urinary diversion.

A variety of pharmacologic agents have been identified as useful in this condition. Because the bladder is predominantly a parasympathetically innervated organ with acetylcholine as the neurotransmitter, anticholinergic agents are used. Oxybutynin chloride (Ditropan), propantheline bromide (Pro-banthine), methantheline bromide (Banthine), and flovoxate hydrochloride (Urispas) are the usual choices. A variety of other pharmacologic agents are also in the experimental stage, and their widespread use should await better identification of their role.

Frewen suggests that idiopathic bladder instability causing urinary incontinence in females is of psychosomatic origin.[11] He and others have reported objective remission in over 80% of these cases using a combination of a bladder drill, sedation, simple psychologic counseling, and detrusor inhibitory drugs. Biofeedback therapy and psychotherapy have also been reported with some success for the treatment of the urgency-incontinent woman.[4,13] These therapies require a highly motivated patient and the input of highly trained personnel. Bladder distention therapy and electrical stimulation to inhibit the spinal cord detrusor nucleus are also described, as are surgical denervation operations performed either at the level of the spinal motor root or at the peripheral bladder level.[6,20,31] These aggressive procedures do not enjoy invariable success, and their role in the management of the urgency-incontinent patient is limited.

Surgical Management

There is no single operation appropriate for all cases of genuine stress urinary incontinence. A philosophic diversity of opinion exists between gynecologists and urologists regarding the ideal management of such cases. Historically, the gynecologist has approached the problem with a primary vaginal repair, reserving suprapubic or retropubic procedures for vaginal failures. The anterior vaginal repair using the Kelly plication[17] had the merit of being able to correct coexistent anterior vaginal wall prolapse, which is found in at least 50% of patients with genuine stress incontinence. The procedure had low morbidity, and also facilitated concomitant vaginal hysterectomy and rectocele repair, if indicated. The disadvantage of this approach was the poor long-term success rate. The procedure is still widely performed, and Green suggests that it is still justified, provided that the vaginal approach is reserved for cases in which incontinence is accompanied by an anatomic defect in which the posterior urethrovesical angle is lost, but urethral axis is normal. I contend that retropubic and needle suspension procedures enjoy more universal and sustained success regardless of the type of anatomic abnormality causing the stress incontinence, and are a more logical first choice. Associated cystourethrocele is often corrected by the retropubic or needle-suspension procedure, and associated enteroceles or rectoceles can be repaired through a separate incision. Hysterectomy is by no means indicated in all cases of female stress urinary incontinence, and, indeed, the same indications for hysterectomy should exist in the incontinent woman as exist in the general female population.

Undoubtedly the best chance for success in the surgical management of stress urinary incontinence is the first operation. Each subsequent procedure contends not only with the abnormal anatomy, but also with operative scarring of the urethral tissues and sphincter mechanism, adverse healing factors, abnormal anatomic fixation of tissues, and possibly denervation phenomena incurred during the prior surgical procedure. The object of all operations should be correct fixation of the proximal urethra and bladder neck within the intraabdominal pressure zone, and the concurrent repair of other abnormalities such as cystourethrocele, rectocele, or significant uterine descensus. All of the currently performed procedures successfully achieve these ends, and procedure selection revolves predominantly around the surgeon's familiarity and expertise with a particular operation, and the local factors requiring correction.

MARSHAL–MARCHETTI–KRANTZ CYSTOURETHROPEXY

The Marshall–Marchetti–Krantz (MMK) cystourethropexy is best performed with the patient in the supine position with the legs abducted on spreader bars to give access to the vagina during the procedure.[19] An 18Fr Foley catheter is inserted, and the abdomen is entered through a Pfannenstiel or lower abdominal midline incision. The rectus muscles are separated in the midline, and the anterior peritoneal reflection is swept off the bladder to give access to the retropubic space. The space is carefully dissected, teasing away retropubic fat and identifying retropubic veins, which are cauterized and severed. The bladder neck, anterior vaginal wall, and urethra as far as the urethral meatus are dissected in this manner. The bladder neck is generally easy to identify, but confirmation is obtained by gentle traction on the Foley catheter, to observe where the Foley balloon impacts. In patients who have had previous vaginal or retropubic operations, the dissection may be lengthy and difficult. In a previous failed repair,

it is important to take down all old retropubic adhesions. If difficulty is encountered, the bladder may be opened to identify its limits, and an assistant's examining finger in the vagina may help to identify the vaginal wall.

Chromic catgut sutures (2-0) on a Mayo needle are used to suspend the paraurethral anterior vaginal wall to the back of the symphysis pubis. Marshall describes three pairs of sutures being placed on each side of the urethra; the most proximal pair being at the level of the bladder neck (Fig. 66-2). Each suture takes a double bite through the paraurethral fascia and anterior vaginal wall close to but not through the urethra, and each suture is passed into an appropriate portion of the back of the cartilaginous portion of the symphysis.

FIG. 66-2. Marshall–Marchetti–Krantz procedure: **(A)** suture placement between the paraurethral tissue and the synchondrosis of the pubic bone; **(B)** bladder neck suspension after completion

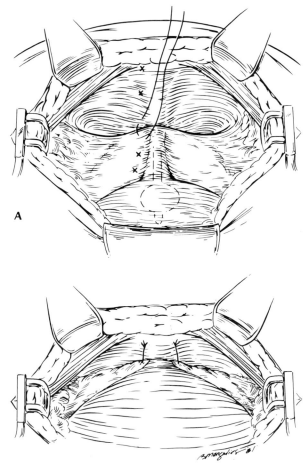

A

B

All six sutures are inserted, and while an assistant elevates the anterior vaginal wall, each suture is individually tied, starting with the more distal pair. The proximal or bladder neck suture frequently needs to be passed through the insertion of the rectus abdominis muscle. In some cases the synchondrosis of the pubis is poorly developed, in which case sutures are passed through the periosteum. This is often difficult to achieve, and should this problem be encountered it might be more appropriate to select a Burch procedure, which ensures more secure suspension. Some describe a further pair of sutures placed through the anterior bladder wall just above the bladder neck, suspending this area from the fibrous insertion of the rectus muscle.

A suction drain is placed in the retropubic space, and the abdominal wall is closed in the routine fashion. The patient is mobilized the day after surgery, and the Foley catheter is removed on the third to fifth postoperative day. The suction drain is generally removed on the second or third day.

The most frequent postoperative problem encountered is that of delayed return of voiding. A postvoid residual urine check is routinely made following removal of the catheter, and should the volume be significant (more than 100 ml), a postvoid intermittent catheterization program is instituted until voiding efficiency improves. In most cases this is achieved within 7 days of operation, and the patient is generally discharged by this time. Should voiding be delayed longer, bethanechol in a dosage of 25 mg or 50 mg PO three or four times daily is prescribed. The patient is taught self-catheterization and then discharged from the hospital. Providing one is careful to exclude patients who had preexistent voiding difficulties, it is unusual for postoperative urinary retention to be prolonged. Urinary antiseptics are continued until 2 days following catheter removal or discontinuation of intermittent catheterization, and a urine culture is routinely checked at the first postoperative visit. During the immediate postoperative period, the patient is warned to avoid all energetic activities, and heavy lifting and similar activities should be avoided for at least 3 to 6 months.

With good patient selection, taking care to avoid those with detrusor incontinence, and good operative technique, most authors report an 80% to 90% long-term success rate with the MMK procedure. Failures generally reflect either improper patient selection or technical problems resulting in a failure to achieve adequate vesicourethral suspension and restore anatomy to normal (Fig. 66-3). These technical problems generally stem from failure to identify landmarks during suture placement, or suture failure. Nonabsorbable sutures are not advisable because of the danger of these being inadvertently passed through the bladder with resultant stone formation or vesicovaginal fistula. Dexon is a good alternative choice. Placement of sutures through the anterior bladder wall rather than the periurethral fascia and vagina not only fails to achieve correct suspension, but may, in fact, hold open the bladder neck by suspending its anterior lip, leaving the posterior lip to be pulled inferiorly by the cystocele. Overcorrection of the urethral axis by overzealous elevation of the urethra and vaginal wall can result in permanent urinary retention. This can usually be identified by physical examination, endoscopy, and lateral cystography, and genrally requires surgical revision.

BURCH RETROPUBIC COLPOSUSPENSION

The Burch retropubic colposuspension, a modification of the MMK procedure, has many attractive features making it more universally applicable.[3] The supine spreader bar position is again optimal, and the procedure is similar to the MMK operation except for the extent of dissection and the suture placement (Fig. 66-4). It is important to identify the lateral limits of the bladder as it reflects off the vaginal wall, because it is only in this manner that one can avoid inadvertent suturing of the bladder itself. Using careful technique, and sometimes by incision of the endopelvic fascia, the lateral bladder wall may be "rolled off" the vaginal wall, venous bleeding from the large vaginal veins being controlled by suture ligature. To aid in this identification of the lateral margin of the bladder, it is helpful to displace the balloon of the Foley catheter into the lateral recess of the bladder, where it can be easily palpated through the bladder wall. This degree of extensive dissection is not always necessary; but in reoperated cases it does ensure correct suture placement for ideal suspension.

Cooper's (iliopectineal) ligaments are identified beneath the lateral margins of the incision, and their examination confirms that they will give very good support for the suspension suture. Adipose tissue on the lateral pelvic wall is teased away because it does not promote adhesion of the elevated vagina, which is necessary for the prolonged success of the operation. Because of the risk of sutures traversing the bladder wall, and also inadvertent ligation of a ureter, some advise routine opening of the bladder by midline cystotomy and placement of ureteral catheters. Sutures are of No.

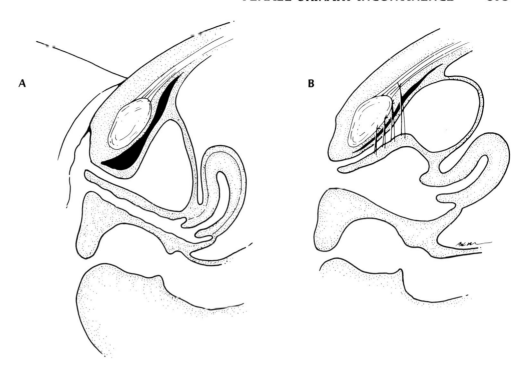

FIG. 66-3.   **(A)** Preoperative cross section of the pelvis in stress incontinence.   **(B)** Correction of the anatomic defect by the MMK procedure.

1 Dexon, and their placement is facilitated by the assistant elevating the dissected anterolateral vaginal wall into the field. The bladder is retracted to the opposite side using a narrow-blade Deaver retractor. Four sutures are placed on each side, each suture taking a good bite of fascia and vaginal wall, taking care not to pass through the vaginal mucosa. The most distal suture is at the level of the midurethra and is placed approximately 2 cm lateral to the urethra. This suture cannot be brought through Cooper's ligament, and instead picks up pubic periosteum and the fibrous insertion of the rectus muscle. The second suture is at the level of the bladder neck but somewhat lateral to it, and picks up the commencement of Cooper's ligament. The two subsequent sutures are proximal to the level of the bladder neck as shown in Figure 66-4, and each picks up an adjacent portion of Cooper's ligament.

The highly vascular vaginal wall bleeds profusely during suture placement, and often large vaginal veins need to be undersewn with 2-0 chromic catgut, but most bleeding ceases once the sutures are tied and the vagina is suspended from the anterior pelvic wall. To facilitate tying the sutures, the assistant elevates the appropriate portion of the vaginal wall as each suture is tied,

commencing with the more distal pair. It is important to note that no attempt is made to tie these sutures tightly. In most cases the anterolateral vaginal wall will not approximate Cooper's ligament, and free suture material will be seen between the vagina and ligaments. The object of the operation is to approximate this vaginal wall to the lateral pelvic wall where it will heal and "stick," hence the importance of removing fat from this area. Once the sutures have been tied, a broad support for the urethra and bladder neck is seen to have been created; however, the urethra, although suspended, is not compressed behind the symphysis pubis, and one can usually insert an examining finger between it and the synchondrosis of the pubis.

A suction drain is left in the retropubic space, to be removed on the second postoperative day. The 18Fr Foley catheter remains until the third of fifth postoperative day, and the same program as is used with the MMK operation of checking for residual urine and intermittent catheterization is instituted if necessary until residual urine is less than 100 ml. The patient is mobilized from bed the day following surgery, and restrictions on activity are similar to those described for the MMK operation.

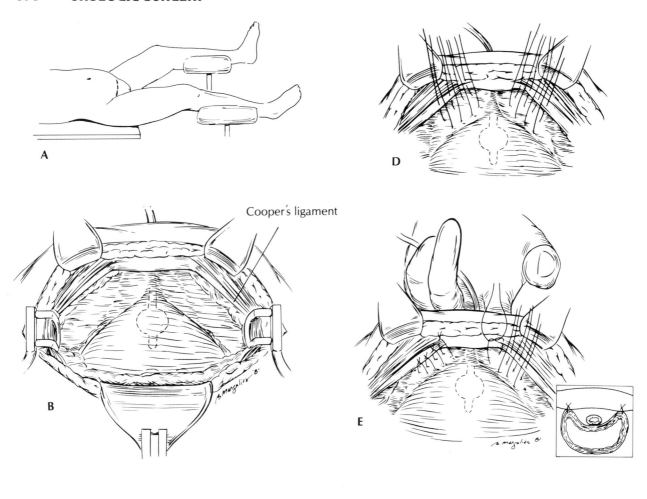

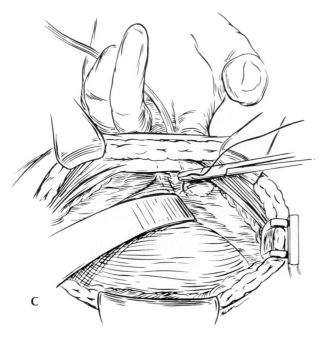

Cooper's ligament

FIG. 66-4. Burch retropubic colposuspension. **(A)** Ideal operating position. **(B)** Initial exposure of the retropubic space, showing Cooper's ligament. **(C)** The bladder is mobilized from the anterior vaginal wall. Suture placement into the vaginal wall is directed by the examining finger in the vagina. **(D)** Each of the four sutures traverses Cooper's ligament and the vaginal wall without penetration of the vaginal mucosa. Note that the suture placement differs from the MMK procedure. **(E)** The sutures are tied while elevating the anterior vaginal wall. No attempt is made to approximate the vaginal wall to Cooper's ligament (*inset*). A vaginal sling is created for the urethra. The urethra is not compressed against the symphysis pubis.

An advantage of the Burch procedure is that it simultaneously corrects cystourethrocele. It corrects urinary incontinence by repositioning of the vesicourethral region within the abdomen but in no way compresses the urethra. It is my operation of choice in patients who have had multiple previous failed procedures, but in such cases it is important that the adhesions from the previous repairs be taken down so that resuspension in better anatomic positions can be achieved. In some women who have undergone many previous vaginal operations, digital vaginal examination will confirm fixation of the anterior vaginal wall and an inability to elevate it to the pubis. This situation may be resolved by commencing the operation with the patient in the lithotomy position and incising the vaginal mucosa in the midline over the proximal urethra and bladder neck. Once the vaginal flaps have been mobilized laterally, it is seen that the anterior vaginal wall can be elevated, and the patient is repositioned and the routine colposuspension completed. No attempt is made to suture the anterior vaginal wall.

Stanton and Cardoza reported an 84.2% cure rate using the colposuspension operation for patients who had undergone previous incontinence surgery, and an overall cure rate of 86% at 2 years.[27] They also noted that in their series simultaneous hysterectomy did not improve the cure rate for incontinence, and they advised reserving this procedure for patients with significant uterine pathology. The possible complications of the Burch procedure have been alluded to. Delayed voiding is less common, but the risk of vesicovaginal fistula and ureteral ligature are ever present. The anterior suspension of the bladder might also weaken the posterior vaginal wall and predispose to enterocele formation, which might require subsequent vaginal correction; however, if this potential is appreciated at the time of surgery the pouch of Douglas can be closed with successive pursestring sutures in the pelvic peritoneum in this area, thereby closing and protecting this weak region.

MODIFIED PEYRERA NEEDLE SUSPENSION PROCEDURE

Originally introduced by Peyrera in 1959, the Peyrera needle suspension procedure has been further revised by Peyrera and Lebherz.[21,22] A number of other variations including that of Stamey have also been reported.[26] The operation is most ideally suited to previously unoperated cases who have only moderate cystourethrocele, although successes are reported even after multiple previous surgical failures. The operation achieves success by precise relocalization of the proximal urethra and bladder neck into the intra-abdominal pressure zone. Avoiding open pelvic surgery, the procedure has low morbidity, and unlike the suprapubic procedures, it is not significantly more difficult in the obese woman. Proponents of this procedure do not consider the presence of cystocele or rectocele to be a contraindication, because they may be simply repaired in the same operative field.

The patient is operated upon in the lithotomy position. The labia are sutured laterally, and a weighted speculum is inserted into the vagina to expose the anterior vaginal wall. An 18Fr Foley catheter with a 5-ml balloon is inserted, and the anterior vaginal wall is infiltrated with normal saline to establish the correct plane between urethra and vagina. An inverted-U or midline vaginal incision is made, and the vaginal wall is dissected from the overlying urethra using Metzenbaum scissors (Fig. 66-5). The dissection is carried laterally a good distance from the urethra and superiorly to above the level of the bladder neck, which is noted by gentle traction on the Foley catheter and identification of the balloon. In the lateral margins of the vaginal dissection, only the musculofascial tissues of the urethra and vagina and the endopelvic fascia separate the vaginal lumen from the retropubic space. Using the Metzenbaum scissors, this tissue in the anterolateral vaginal wall is sharply dissected onto the pubic bone. The index finger can then be inserted into the retropubic space, and the periurethral and perivesical tissues are bluntly dissected off the posterior pubis digitally. This dissection is accomplished keeping close to the pubic bone. Careful rotation of the finger within the retropubic space will break down adhesions. Even following previous operative procedures these adhesions can generally be broken down, but, if they are extensive, judicious scissor dissection may be accomplished through the vaginal incision, or alternatively through a small suprapubic incision. Bleeding is surprisingly mild and can generally be stopped by a short period of gauze packing.

A narrow Deaver retractor placed through the lateral vaginal incision into the retropubic space and retracted laterally identifies the musculofascial tissue bordering the urethra. This tissue may be grasped with an Allis forceps and presented into the wound. A No. 1 Prolene suture anchors this musculofascial vaginal tissue by picking up three spiral loops approximately one-half inch (1.3 cm) deep and a quarter of an inch (0.6 cm) apart, the more proximal suture being at the level of the

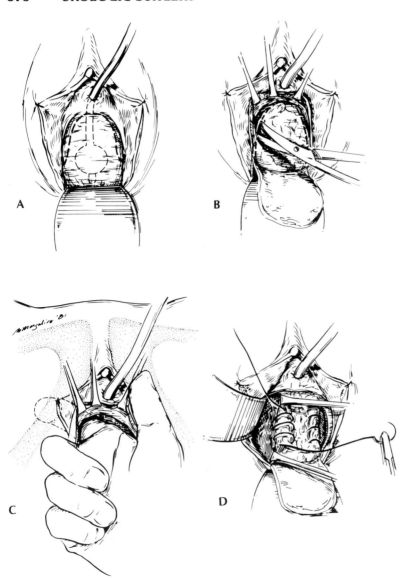

FIG. 66-5. Peyrera needle suspension procedure. **(A)** An inverted-U vaginal incision is made. **(B)** The vaginal musculofascial tissue and the endopelvic fascia are dissected into the retropubic space. **(C)** The retropubic space is dissected digitally. **(D)** A suspension suture picks up the musculofascial vaginal tissue adjacent to the urethra. **(E)** A small suprapubic incision is made, and a Peyrera needle is directed through the rectus fascia onto the retropubic finger and guided into the vagina. **(F)** The Peyrera needle picks up the suspension sutures. **(G)** The suspension sutures are transferred to the suprapubic region. The sutures from the right and left sides are tied, suspending the urethra.

bladder neck. During placement of these sutures, care is taken to avoid injury or encroachment upon the urethra or bladder. This same maneuver is repeated on the opposite side, and then a small 2.5-cm transverse abdominal incision is made just at the upper border of the symphysis pubis. It is carried down to the fascia overlying the rectus muscle, at which point the index finger of the left hand is introduced through the vaginal incision, along the dissected retropubic space to the inferior border of the deep surface of the rectus tendon. The Peyrera ligature carrier needle is passed through the rectus fascia and muscle onto the fingertip, and then guided through the retropubic space and vaginal incision out into the vagina itself. The two

loose ends of the Prolene suture are picked up by the needle and transferred suprapubically.

Because the needle is directed under digital control, there is little danger of injury to the bladder; however, after the sutures have been transferred suprapubically, cystoscopy is accomplished to ensure that no injury has resulted. While an assistant elevates the Prolene suspension sutures, one may endoscopically assess the success of suspension. Once the cystoscopy has been completed, and it has been confirmed that hemostasis is satisfactory, the retropubic space is thoroughly irrigated with saline or antibacterial solution, and the vaginal wall is closed with interrupted 3-0 Dexon sutures. Should the vaginal wall not be

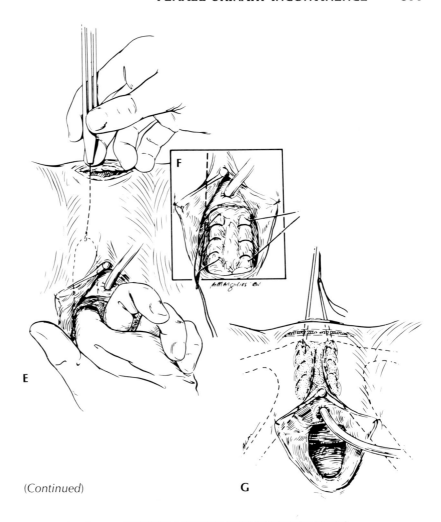

(*Continued*)

E

F

G

closed before the elevating sutures are tied, the vaginal incision becomes most inaccessible for closure later. A 18Fr Foley catheter is inserted, the weighted speculum is removed, and the Prolene sutures, exiting through separate holes in the rectus fascia, are tied together with six knots while the assistant elevates the vagina with an examining finger. A Foley catheter is inserted for 48 hr, and the vagina is packed for 24 hr. Most patients are able to void immediately following catheter removal, but if they are not, an intermittent catheterization program as previously described is instituted.

The advantage of this procedure is its simplicity, low morbidity, and apparent success. Raz reports success rate of over 90% in 100 cases, some of whom had previous failed repairs.[23] Modifications and refinements to this Peyrera technique are described; but the final arbiter of the merits and demerits of the different modifications must await the test of time.

OTHER OPERATIVE PROCEDURES

Few patients with genuine stress incontinence alone will fail to be corrected by a well-performed suspension procedure. Some women, however, who have had multiple previous repairs exhibit such scarring of the urethra and bladder neck that anatomic repositioning alone is insufficient to provide continence. In such cases, an operative procedure providing extrinsic compression of the urethra may be necessary. Fascial sling operations find their place here. The Brantley–Scott Model 792 sphincter prosthesis is also appropriate in these very adverse circumstances, and Scott and associates report an 87% success rate in 15 cases of this sort.[25]

The Brantley–Scott sphincter prosthesis has undergone considerable modification and refinement in recent years, and the current prosthesis (Fig. 66-6) is superior in that the pressure exerted against the tissues by the cuff can be regulated

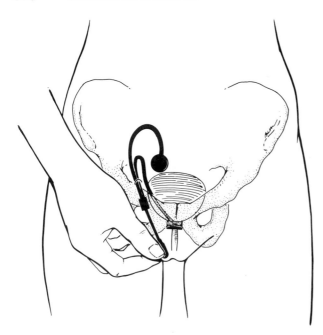

FIG. 66-6. Brantley–Scott Model A S 792 sphincter prosthesis

according to the surgeon's choice of balloon pressure. In many instances the prosthesis is inserted in a deactivated state. This is particularly the case when it is necessary to open the bladder to facilitate dissection around the bladder neck, or should there by any suspicion of inadvertent injury to the urethra during this dissection. During a 6-week interval a protective pseudocapsule forms around the implanted prosthesis, and a further minor procedure is necessary to activate the device by connection of the control assembly. The obvious complications include mechanical failure, which is uncommon; erosion of the cuff through the urethra; and infection of the prosthesis. Careful case selection and surgical technique can avoid these problems.

REFERENCES

1. ARNOLD EP, WEBSTER JR, LOOSE H et al: Urodynamics of female incontinence: Factors influencing the results of surgery. Am J Obstet Gynecol 117:805, 1973
2. BATES CP, WHITESIDE CG, TURNER–WARWICK R: Synchronous cine/pressure/flow/-cystourethrography with special reference to stress and urge incontinence. Brit J Urol 42:714, 1970
3. BURCH JC: Urethrovaginal fixation to Cooper's ligament for correction of stress incontinence, cystocele and prolapse. Am J Obstet Gynecol 81:281, 1961
4. CARDOZA LD, ABRAMS PD, STANTON SL et al: Idiopathic bladder instability treated by biofeedback. Br J Urol 50:521, 1978
5. DIOKNO AC, TAUB M: Ephedrine in treatment of urinary incontinence. Urology 5:624, 1975
6. DUNN M, SMITH JC, ARDRAN GM: Prolonged bladder distension as treatment for urgency and urge incontinence of urine. Br J Urol 46:645, 1975
7. EDWARDS LE: Incontinence of urine. In JP Blandy (ed): Urology. Oxford, Blackwell, 1976
8. EDWARDS LE, MALVERN J: Electronic control of incontinence; A critical review of the present situation. Br J Urol 44:467, 1972
9. ENDSLEY LG, HAWTREY CE, VERVAIS P et al: Treatment of urinary incontinence in women using an intravaginal tarsette. J Urol 114:50, 1975
10. FARRAR DJ, WHITESIDE CG, OSBORNE JL et al: A urodynamic analysis of micturition symptoms in the female. Surg Gynecol Obstet 141:875, 1975
11. FREWEN WK: Urgency incontinence: Review of 100 cases. J Obstet Gynecol Br Commwlth 79:77, 1972
12. GOSLING J: The structure of the bladder and urethra in relation to function. Urol Clin North Am 6:31, 1979
13. HAFNER RJ, STANTON SL, GUY J: A psychiatric study of women with urgency incontinence. Br J Urol 49:211, 1977
14. HUTCH JA, RAMBO OA, JR: A new theory of the anatomy of the internal urinary sphincter and the physiology of micturition: III. Anatomy of the urethra. J Urol 97:696, 1967
15. JONES EG: Nonoperative treatment of stress incontinence. Clin Obstet Gynaecol 6:220, 1963
16. KEGEL AH: Physiologic therapy for urinary stress incontinence. JAMA 146:915, 1951
17. KELLY HA, DUNN WM: Urinary incontinence in women without manifest injury to the bladder. Surg Gynecol Obstet 18:444, 1914
18. LAPIDES J, AJEMIAN EP, BRUCE HS et al: Physiology of stress incontinence. Surg Gynecol Obstet 111:224, 1960
19. MARSHALL VF, MARCHETTI AA, KRANTZ KE: The correction of stress urinary incontinence by simple vesico-urethral suspension. Surg Gynecol Obstet 88:590, 1949
20. MERRILL DC, CONWAY C, DEWOLF W: Urinary incontinence treatment with electrical stimulation of pelvic floor. Urology 5:67, 1975
21. PEYRERA AJ: A simplified surgical procedure for the correction of stress incontinence in women. Western Journal of Surgery 67:223, 1959
22. PEYRERA AJ, LEBHERZ TB: The revised Peyrera procedure. In Buchsbaum HJ, Schmidt JD (eds): Gynecologic and Obstetric Urology. Philadelphia, W B Saunders, 1978
23. RAZ S: Modified bladder neck suspension for female stress incontinence. Urology 17:82, 1981
24. RAZ S, MAGGIO AJ, KAUFMAN JJ: Why Marshall–Marchetti operation works or does not. Urology 14:154, 1979
25. SCOTT FB, LIGHT JK, FISHMAN I et al: Implantation of

an artificial sphincter for urinary incontinence. Contemporary Surgery 18:11, 1981

26. STAMEY TA: Urinary incontinence in the female. In Harrison JH, Gittes RF, Perlmutter AD et al (eds): Campbell's Urology, 4th ed. Philadelphia, W B Saunders, 1979

27. STANTON SL, CARDOZA LD: Results of the colposuspension operation for incontinence and prolapse. Br J Gynecol 86:693, 1979

28. STEWART BH, BAROWSKY LHW, MONTAGUE DK: Stress incontinence: Conservative therapy with sympathomimetic drugs, J Urol 115:558, 1976

29. TANAGHO EA: Simplified cystography in stress urinary incontinence. Br J Urol 46:295, 1974

30. TANAGHO EA, SMITH DR: Mechanism of urinary continence. I: Embryologic, anatomic and pathologic considerations. J Urol 100:640, 1968

31. TORRENS M, HALD T: Bladder denervation procedures. Urol Clin North Am 6:283, 1979

32. TURNER–WARWICK R: Observations on the function and dysfunction of the sphincter and detrusor mechanisms. Urol Clin North Am 6:13, 1979

33. WEBSTER GD: The unstable bladder. In Raz S (ed): Female Urology. Philadelphia, W B Saunders, 1982

34. WEBSTER GD: Urinary incontinence. In Resnick MI, Older RA (eds): Diagnosis of Genitourinary Disease. New York, Grune & Stratton, 1982

35. WEBSTER GD: Urodynamic studies. In Resnick MI, Older RA (eds): Diagnosis of Genitourinary Disease. New York, Grune & Stratton, 1982

36. WEBSTER GD, OLDER RA: Video urodynamics. J Urol 16:106, 1980

37. WILLIAMS TJ: Urinary stress incontinence in the female. Surgical Rounds 18:40, 1981

38. WOLEN LH: Incontinence in young healthy nulliparous women. J Urol 101:545, 1969

Female Urethral Disorders

67

Peter L. Scardino

The female urethra is vulnerable to a variety of diseases, a number of which are treated by urethral dilatation, meatotomy, Richardson urethrolysis, or urethral diverticulectomy. Indications for the application of one or more of these useful techniques are incorporated in the following discussions. With the exception of urethral diverticulectomy, the several procedures are directed most frequently to the relief of that poorly understood phenomenon, the urethral syndrome.[4]

Female Urethral Stenosis

INFANCY AND CHILDHOOD

Hesistancy; stranguria; a slow, narrow, or interrupted urinary stream; enuresis; and recurrent urinary tract infections (cystitis, pyelonephritis) may be related to congenital urethral stenosis and spasm of the striated external sphincter. The cause of the stenosis is an inelastic urethral ring (Lyon's), not present at birth or puberty but present in the in-between years, perhaps due to the absence of estrogens.

The meatal or submeatal stenosis may best be diagnosed on a voiding cystourethrogram if the proximal urethra is dilated (Fig. 67-1). The diagnosis is substantiated with a bougie à boule (Fig. 67-2). These instruments, preferable to metal sounds, are inserted into the urethra starting with the smallest bougie and gradually increasing the size until a hanging sensation is felt at the urethral meatus as the bougie is withdrawn. Any size less than 22Fr in children and 26Fr in adults is considered abnormally small. Treatment consists of overdilatation of the meatus with sounds of up to 32Fr to 36Fr, or preferably an internal urethrotomy using the Otis urethrotome (Fig. 67-2).

In the adult, dyspareunia, suprapubic discomfort, low backache, easy fatigability, urgency, dysuria, frequency, recurrent urinary tract infections, dribbling, and loss of urinary stream size and force are common complaints in a rather confused and somewhat bizarre entity, the urethral syndrome. Recent data imply a low-grade infectious etiology of organisms numbering less than 100,000 which have been obtained by suprapubic aspirations.[4] An increase of collagenous tissue and a loss of elasticity at the urethral meatus or the distal musculature of one fourth of the urethra has been suggested as the cause of adult urethral stenosis, without a more definitive etiologic basis. It has been postulated that, unlike normal micturition in which the elastic urethra and meatus dilate allowing free urine flow, the inelastic, abnormal urethra has a small stream resulting in back pressure, turbulent flow, and perhaps incomplete emptying of the bladder.

In an effort to overcome the complaints and the implied pathology of the urethra, the following techniques in treatment are suggested: urethral dilatation, meatotomy/urethrotomy, and Richardson urethrolysis.

URETHRAL DILATATION

The most popular method of treatment of female urethral syndrome or stenosis is periodic urethral dilatation with Van Buren metal sounds, sizes 36Fr to 38Fr. Dilatation is usually performed under local, topical, jelly anesthesia instilled in the urethra and allowed to remain 10 minutes before the dilatation is undertaken. Occasionally a mild analgesic or an antispasmodic such as a flavoxate is prescribed. Irregular dilatations are usually required once this form of therapy has started. However, repeated dilatations may be avoided in some patients if urethrotomy is performed.

MEATOTOMY/URETHROTOMY

In meatotomy/urethrotomy, the urethra is calibrated as demonstrated in Figures 67-3 and 67-4. If a definite meatal or submeatal stenosis is demonstrated with the bougie à boule, the urethrotome (Fig. 67-5) is inserted and positioned to cut at 11 o'clock and 1 o'clock to provide a urethral size of 28Fr to 32Fr in children and adults. The urethro-

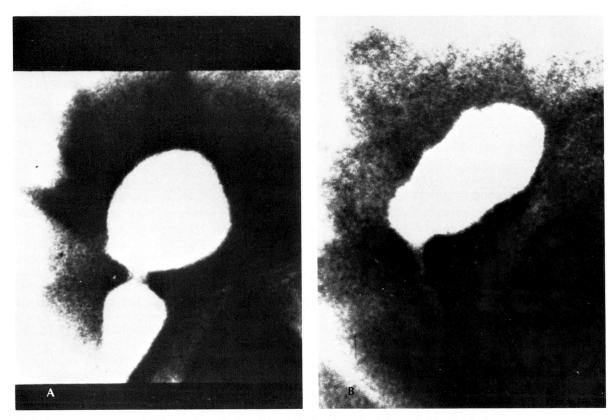

FIG. 67-1. Voiding cystourethrograms in a patient with distal urethral stenosis (Lyon's ring): **(A)** preoperative voiding cystourethrogram with marked dilation of the urethra and **(B)** postoperative study following interal urethrotomy

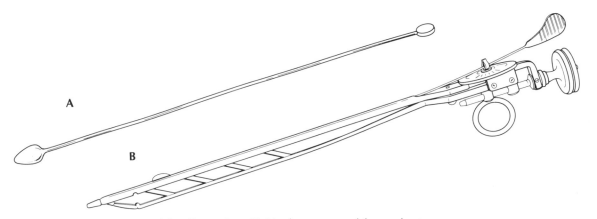

FIG. 67-2. **(A)** Bougie used for diagnosis. **(B)** Urethrotome used for urethrotomy

tome is opened sufficiently to prevent its slipping out of the urethra. No actual cutting is performed such as might occur if the opened instrument were withdrawn. Rather, a dull urethrotome is thought simply to cut those inelastic areas by blade pressure. The urethra is recalibrated after the initial cut. If bougie à boule size 32Fr cannot pass, a second cut is made again at the same positions, 11 and 1 o'clock.

The control of bleeding may require indwelling catheter for 24 hr postoperatively. The patients are advised to return to the office for outpatient follow-

FIG. 67-3. Bougie and meatal stenosis: restriction of the instrument and blanching of the stenotic inelastic urethral meatus

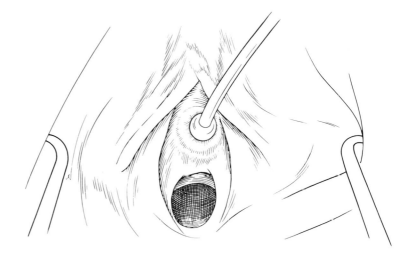

up and two to three dilatations over the course of 3 months. Urinary incontinence is not encountered. Urethrovaginal fistula is precluded by avoiding incisions at the 4 to 8 o'clock position of the urethra. With this treatment urinary tract infections clear and ureterovesical reflux is controlled or reversed in those children who have had the urethral stenosis corrected and who have normal trigone and ureteral orifices and tunnels. Children with abnormal trigonal anatomy continue to reflux and eventually require surgical correction of more than the urethral meatus.

RICHARDSON URETHROLYSIS

If the basis of decreased urine flow rate is connective tissue constriction of the distal urethra, Richardson's technique of freeing the urethra from the collagenous fibrotic obstruction may be a valid and useful operative technique, albeit one with which I have had no personal experience (Fig. 67-6). A Van Buren sound large enough to produce blanching of the adjacent urethral mucosa is inserted into the female urethra. A posterior meatotomy is performed using a midline incision at the 6 o'clock position. The incision made vertically from below upward is taken through the vaginal mucosa, subcutaneous tissue, and urethral mucosa for about 1 cm, depending on the degree of stenosis. Larger sounds are passed until the distal urethra hugs the sound snugly (30Fr). The urethra is drawn away from the symphysis by retraction on the sound. A vertical, midline, anterior vaginal incision permits reflection of the vaginal mucosa laterally to expose the posterior portion of connective tissue surrounding the distal urethral segment. The tissue is grasped and excised with little regard for Skene's

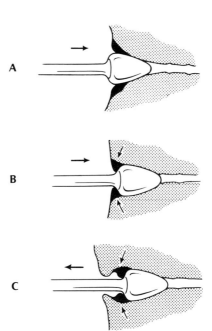

FIG. 67-4. Diagnosis of urethral stenosis. **(A)** The bougie is inserted. **(B)** The "shoulders" of the bougie are hung up on the meatal stenosis. **(C)** The shoulders of the bougie are hung up on the submeatal stenosis (Lyon's ring).

glands. The vaginal mucosal edges are reapproximated with three or four interrupted 3-0 chromic catgut sutures. The sound is removed. The meatal incision is sutured transversely with 3-0 chromic catgut sutures. If meatotomy is unnecessary, the submucosal connective tissue is excised using a T (vaginal mucosal) incision.

If failure occurs, the procedure may be repeated. No catheter is used postoperatively. Bleeding has not been a problem.

Urethral Diverticulectomy

Urethral diverticula should be considered in the differential diagnosis of any female patient who complains of recurring cystitis, dribbling after voiding, dyspareunia, or a palpable, tender, cystic swelling on the undersurface of the urethra, or who notices a recurrent urethral discharge. The correct diagnosis can be acccomplished by applying pressure on the vaginal swelling, which produces pus at the urethral meatus, and can be substantiated by cystourethroscopic and urethrographic studies. In the absence of a mass, the diagnosis may be difficult.

After a thorough urologic history and a good physical examination, radiologic and endoscopic efforts may be required to locate the elusive diverticulum. Often helpful is the injection of methylene blue into the urethra, which may aid in identifying diverticular tracts. The diverticulum may be filled with a liquid plastic agent such as might be prepared for coagulum pyelolithotomy. Special catheters have been designed to occlude the urethra at the meatus and bladder neck, permitting the filling of the urethra with contrast media and thereby outlining the diverticulum.

Stone or neoplasm may be found inside the diverticulum. Diverticula may extend beyond the urethra to the bladder base or anteriorly where the diagnosis may be quite difficult. Treatment of a urethral diverticulum with neoplasm is radically different from the treatment of a simple diverticulum but does not fall within the scope of this chapter.

The surgical treatment of diverticula includes transurethral incision of shallow pockets and small

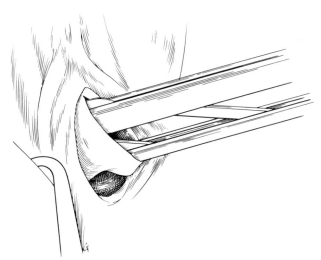

FIG. 67-5. A urethrotome cuts the stenotic urethral meatus at 11 o'clock.

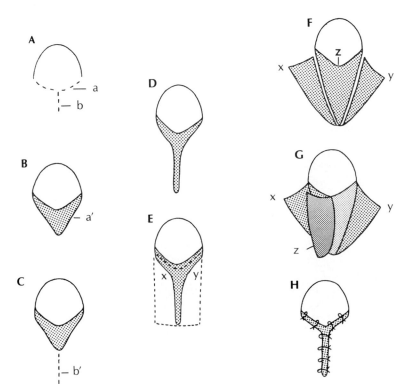

FIG. 67-6. Richardson urethrolysis and external urethroplasty procedure. **(A)** The incisions are outlined: **(a)** Transverse incision only and **(b)** T-shaped incision. **(B)** The transverse incision is shown gaping open, exposing the suburethral connective tissue. **(C)** The proposed T-incision is outlined **(b').** **(D)** The T-shaped incision is completed, exposing the suburethral connective tissue. **(E)** The vaginal flaps **(x, y)** are turned outward **(F)**, exposing the suburethral connective tissue **(z).** **(G)** The submucosal connective tissue **(z)** is excised. **(H)** Closure of the anterior vaginal wall is completed.

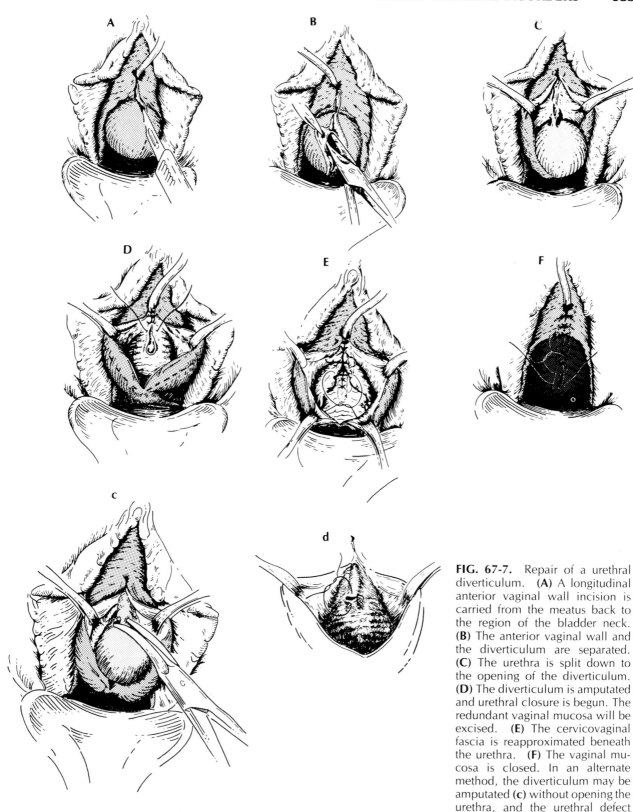

FIG. 67-7. Repair of a urethral diverticulum. **(A)** A longitudinal anterior vaginal wall incision is carried from the meatus back to the region of the bladder neck. **(B)** The anterior vaginal wall and the diverticulum are separated. **(C)** The urethra is split down to the opening of the diverticulum. **(D)** The diverticulum is amputated and urethral closure is begun. The redundant vaginal mucosa will be excised. **(E)** The cervicovaginal fascia is reapproximated beneath the urethra. **(F)** The vaginal mucosa is closed. In an alternate method, the diverticulum may be amputated **(c)** without opening the urethra, and the urethral defect may be closed transversely **(d)**.

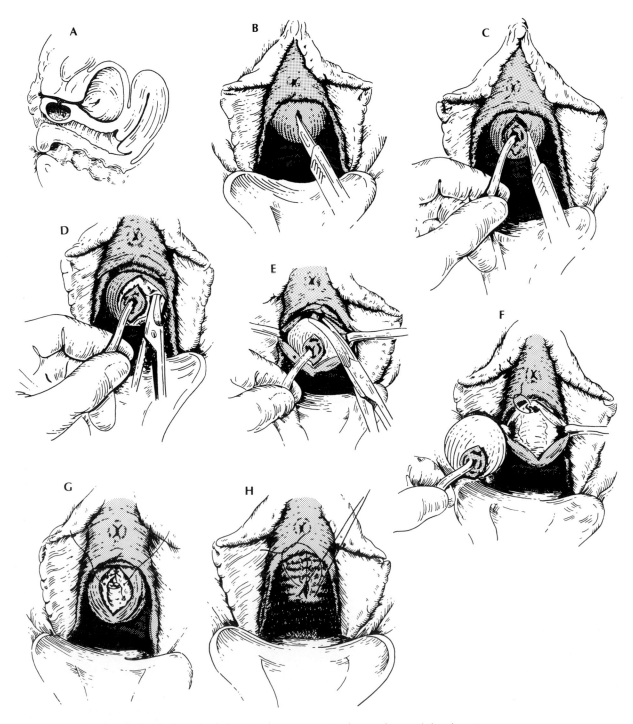

FIG. 67-8. Moore's method of urethral diverticulectomy. **(A)** The urethra and the diverticulum are seen in vaginal section. **(B)** A stab wound is made into the diverticulum for introduction of a Foley catheter. **(C)** A pursestring suture is placed around the catheter, and elliptic incision is made into the vaginal mucosa. **(D)** The diverticulum is freed from the vaginal wall. **(E)** The urethral connection is divided. **(F)** The urethra is closed transversely. **(G)** The cervicovaginal fascia is closed. **(H)** The vaginal mucosa is closed.

infective crypts, or complete removal of the lesion and healing without the complication of vesicovaginal fistula. The four procedures to be discussed here are the technique of Spence and Duckett, the transmeatal–vaginal procedure, a procedure similar to the transmeatal–vaginal procedure but without urethral meatal splitting, and the technique of T. D. Moore.

Spence and Duckett introduced an ingenious technique for the treatment of large urethral diverticula.[3] The basic feature of their procedure is a division of the distal urethral floor between the external meatus and the orifice of the diverticulum. A midline incision is made in the diverticulum and the underlying vaginal wall. The sac is saucerized. A running, locking suture of 3-0 chromic catgut is used to approximate the margins of the incised diverticulum and the adjacent vagina. The bladder neck and the urethra proximal to the orifice are untouched. An indwelling catheter and iodoform packs are employed for a few days. If the diverticulum is very large, the redundant folds are excised. No attempt is made to dissect the residual sac, whose margins are sutured to the contiguous vaginal mucosa.

Kropp's technique for repair of urethral diverticula is quite popular.[1] The usual vaginal preparation is completed with the application of surgical drapes. A Foley catheter is introduced into the bladder through the urethra. The cervix is pulled downward with a tenaculum. A vaginal incision is made to expose and carefully separate the proximal urethra and bladder from the anterior vaginal wall (Fig. 67-7). Small diverticula are treated by an incision through the vaginal mucosa from the urethral meatus to the bladder neck region or to the initial transverse incision. The bladder and urethra having been separated from the cervix, the cervicovaginal fascia is separated bilaterally from the vaginal mucosa. The diverticulum becomes clearly visible and is easily separated from the vaginal mucosa. The urethral catheter is removed. The urethra is incised along the posterior midline from the meatus down to the opening of the diverticulum. With one third of the urethra exposed, the diverticulum with its urethral attachment is excised. A Foley catheter is reinserted. Reapproximation of the urethral edges and subsequently the vaginal mucosa is accomplished with interrupted 3-0 chromic catgut sutures. The urethral catheter is removed after 2 weeks.

In the modification of Kropp's technique (Fig. 67-7), the diverticulum is divided at its opening into the urethra after the sac has been mobilized. The urethra is not split, but the opening that results after dividing the neck of the diverticulum is closed transversely with interrupted sutures of 3-0 chromic catgut. The cervicovaginal fascia and vaginal mucosa are approximated over the urethra with similar interrupted sutures. Usually small rubber drains are placed on either side of the urethral repair and brought through a lateral stab wound.

The Moore's technique was introduced in 1952 (Fig. 67-8).[2] Transvaginally a stab wound is made deliberately in the diverticulum. A small Foley catheter with the part distal to the bag removed is inserted into the diverticulum. The bag is inflated. A pursestring suture is placed around the diverticulostomy. A second Foley catheter is inserted through the meatus into the bladder and inflated. It is now easy to deal with this solid mass diverticulum. Using an elliptic incision around the catheter and a pursestring suture, the diverticulum is freed to its origin from the urethra, and the urethral neck is transected. After closure of the urethral opening with a pursestring suture of 3-0 chromic catgut, the cervicovaginal fascia is reapproximated with interrupted 3-0 chromic catgut suture. A final layer of vaginal mucosa is managed with 3-0 chromic sutures also. A vaginal pack which is inserted is removed in 24 hr. The urethral catheter is removed in 2 weeks.

REFERENCES

1. KROPP, KA: The female urethra. In Glenn JF (ed): Urologic Surgery, 2nd ed, p 755. Hagerstown, Harper & Row, 1975
2. MOORE, TD: Diverticulum of female urethra; An improved technique of surgical excision. J Urol 68:611, 1952
3. SPENCE HM, DUCKETT JW: Diverticulum of the female urethra: Clinical aspects and presentations of a simple operative technique for cure. J Urol 104:432, 1970
4. STAMM WE, WAGNER KF, AMSEL R et al: Causes of the acute urethral syndrome in women. N Eng J Med 303:409, 1980

Urethral Stricture Surgery

68

Richard T. Turner-Warwick

Many different techniques are available for the resolution of urethral strictures in the male. Some have a higher restricture and complication rate than others, and some can be regarded as general urologic procedures, but a high success rate with the more complex definitive procedures requires some special training and experience.*

Most of the operative procedures that were in use 10 years ago for the reconstruction of the male urethra have now been superseded or greatly modified; standards have also changed within this time. A success rate in the region of 75% to 80% was previously regarded as reasonable, but now even a 10% failure of a definitive reconstructive procedure should call into question either the selection of a procedure or the technique of its performance.

Procedures and Principles of Urethral Stricture Surgery

Three basic procedures are available for the restoration of an epithelialized urethral lumen:

1. Regeneration procedures. These depend upon the regenerative proliferation of uroepithelium to complete part of the circumference of the urethral lining. The resolution of a stricture by urethral dilatation or internal urethrotomy relies entirely upon this principle, and success depends upon whether the epithelialization can occur before restenosis develops. Internal urethrotomy regeneration procedures leave much to be desired in terms of a long-term, stricture-free success rate, but they have the great ad-

---

* The avoidance of complications is personal to a surgeon and consequently many of the views expressed in this chapter are essentially personal; references to personal publications have been made to substantiate statements, but no one is more aware than I am of the contributions of many friends and colleagues across the world who are interested in this most intriguing field of surgery and many others who have generously referred challenging cases.

vantage of being relatively simple general urologic procedures.

2. Anastomosis procedures. These consist of excision of the stricture with end-to-end anastomosis as a circumferential one-stage procedure or as a part of a "combination" procedure; they are the only definitive stricture procedures with a success rate approaching 100%. However, relatively few strictures are suitable for management.

3. Substitution procedures. Because no substitute for the urethra is as good as the urethra itself, all epithelial (skin) substitutes and all techniques for their use have some shortcomings and, consequently, an inherent failure rate. To reduce the incidence of substitution-graft failure, techniques of "combination" urethroplasty have been developed using anastomosis, free-patch grafts, and pedicle inlays in paired combinations. With these, a high stricture-free success rate of approximately 95% has been achieved during the past 7 years.[19,22]

The fundamental decision relating to the treatment of a stricture is whether to try internal urethrotomy or proceed to a definitive reconstruction. However, it is most important to recognize that *any* failed surgical attempt to resolve a stricture usually makes a subsequent definitive procedure more difficult. Furthermore, damage to the distal urethral sphincter mechanism is virtually irreparable.

STRICTURE LOCATION AND URETHRAL RECONSTRUCTION

Four different parts of the male urethra—the glans–meatus, the penile, the bulbar, and the posterior sphincter-active urethra—present distinct anatomic features that affect a reconstructive procedure (Fig. 68-1).

The repair of posterior (prostato–membranous) strictures is complicated not only by problems of surgical access but especially by the fact that the

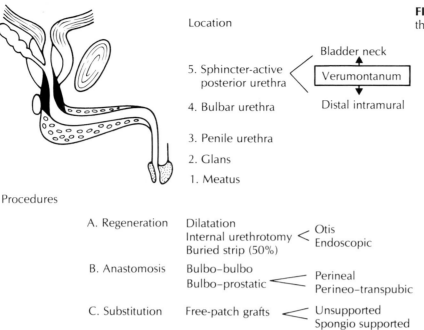

Location

5. Sphincter-active posterior urethra

Bladder neck

Verumontanum

Distal intramural

4. Bulbar urethra

3. Penile urethra

2. Glans

1. Meatus

FIG. 68-1. Principles and types of urethral reconstruction

Procedures

A. Regeneration   Dilatation
                  Internal urethrotomy — Otis
                  Buried strip (50%)   Endoscopic

B. Anastomosis   Bulbo–bulbo
                  Bulbo–prostatic — Perineal
                                     Perineo–transpubic

C. Substitution   Free-patch grafts — Unsupported
                                        Spongio supported

                  Pedicle grafts — Penile foreskin
                                     Scrotal skin

whole length is sphincter active. Strictures of the anterior (bulbo–penile) urethra present the relatively simple challenge of reconstructing a stricture-free conduit of reasonably even caliber, lined by stable epithelium. The penile urethra is very much easier to reconstruct than the bulbar urethra because it is pendulous and self-draining.

The essence of good reconstructive surgery is to adjust the procedure to the findings at the time of operation. Just as tennis players cannot predict the next stroke before they see how the ball is coming, even surgeons with an in-depth experience of the various urethral reconstruction techniques are often unable to predict the procedure they will use to reconstruct a difficult bulbar urethra before the extent of the stricture and the state of the periurethral tissues are seen and felt at the time of the operation. Unlike the bowel or the ureter, the urethra is not an easy or "forgiving" tube to reconstruct. Even a simple anastomotic repair has a distinct tendency to restenose unless special techniques are used to prevent it.

URETHRAL HEALING AND DEVELOPMENT OF STRICTURES

The urethral lining is sometimes loosely referred to as "mucosa" when in fact it is modified squamous epithelium. In the posterior urethra the uroepithelium is based directly on the muscle of the inner layer of the urethral sphincter mechanism; however, throughout the anterior urethra it is based directly upon the underlying spongy tissue.

Normal urethral spongy tissue provides a very good vascular bed for a graft; however, its inflammatory response to the loss of its delicate protective epithelial lining is the rapid development of "spongiofibrosis."

The loss of any portion of the circumference of the urethral lining, whether from internal trauma, external trauma, or infection, usually results in a commensurate narrowing of the lumen during healing. The narrowing occurs because the margins of the residual circumferential epithelium are approximated by the natural urethral closing pressure; the defect forms a cleft, which tends to be overbridged by reepithelialization (Fig. 68-2).

The natural process of bridge healing of a uroepithelial defect is rapid when it is not disturbed by the passage of urine. This can be observed directly when the bulbar urethra is marsupialized during the interval stage of a two-stage inlay urethroplasty; under these circumstances, healing is often complete within 2 or 3 days. However, in the absence of an effective proximal diversion, distension of the urethra by the passage of urine

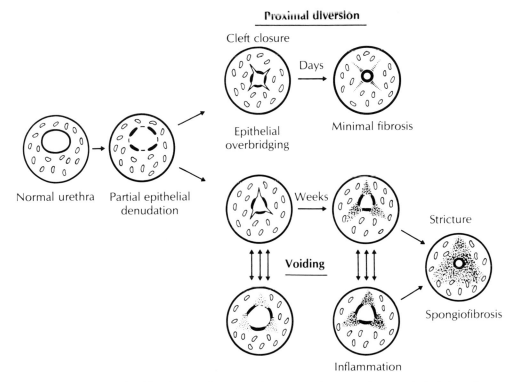

FIG. 68-2.   Urethral healing and stricture formation after partial uroepithelial denudation

every few hours opens the clefts repeatedly. Although uninfected urine is a relatively mild tissue irritant, repeated separation and exposure of the vascular spaces of the spongy tissue lead to a gradual increase in the spongiofibrosis, and the lumen gradually diminishes until the epithelium approximates.

The speed with which a urethral stenosis recurs varies greatly. Stenosis seems to be particularly rapid in the following circumstances: when effective cleft opening is reduced by a poor voiding flow rate due to posterior urethral obstruction (bladder neck or prostatic); when the urethral closing pressure is increased (by inflammatory swelling or extensive periurethral fibrosis); or when it is located in the sphincter-active distal posterior urethra.

To be successful, a definitive urethral reconstruction must take into account the inherent characteristics of urethral healing that result in a tendency to cross-adhesion of adjacent or opposing areas of granulation tissue or suture lines. The plane of a spatulated anastomotic repair should be arranged horizontally, not side-to-side, so that the opposing suture lines can be anchored laterally to prevent them from approximating and cross-adhering.[15]

SPONGIOFIBROSIS AND "GREY" URETHRA

A urethral stricture itself is impalpable; any thickening that is felt clinically or at surgery must represent surrounding spongiofibrosis. Proximal and distal to almost every urethral stricture (with the possible exception of one that is truly congenital and untreated), there is a length of unstrictured urethra surrounded by spongiofibrosis which immediately underlies the epithelium (Fig. 68-3) and gives it a somewhat greyish-yellow color; there may be other abnormalities resulting from urethritis, such as cavitation of the dorsal urethral glands of Littre or lineal scars resulting from epithelial splitting due to previous dilatations or urethrotomy.

To emphasize the tendency of the unstrictured spongiofibrotic urethra to stenose in response to minimal additional trauma, we have termed it the *grey urethra*.[22] The longitudinal extent of mild but significant spongiofibrosis may not be apparent until a sufficient length of the urethra is opened for comparison with normal, supple urethra, the lining surface of which appears pink because the underlying vascular spongy tissue is seen through the translucent uroepithelium. The methylene blue

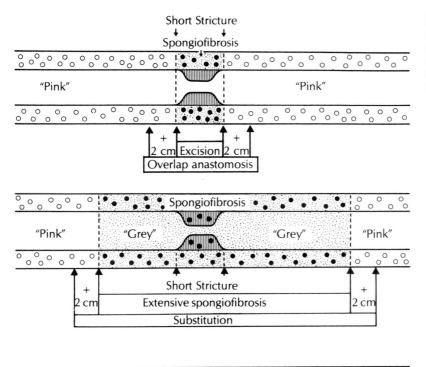

Short Stricture
Spongiofibrosis

"Pink"   "Pink"

+
2 cm Excision 2 cm
Overlap anastomosis

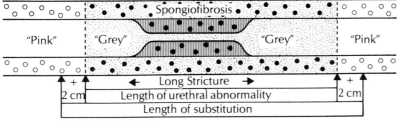

Spongiofibrosis

"Pink"   "Grey"   "Grey"   "Pink"

+   +
2 cm   2 cm
Short Stricture
Extensive spongiofibrosis
Substitution

Spongiofibrosis

"Pink"   "Grey"   "Grey"   "Pink"

+   +
2 cm   2 cm
Long Stricture
Length of urethral abnormality
Length of substitution

FIG. 68-3. The "grey" unstrictured area of abnormal urethra, resulting from spongiofibrosis that extends proximally and distally from the identifiable stricture, cannot always be identified accurately from radiographic appearances

test provides differential staining only where the urethral epithelium is deficient. Therefore, it underestimates the full extent of epithelialized grey urethra. Besides graft failure and poor surgical technique, the most common cause of restenosis of a definitive urethral repair is failure to extend the repair proximally and distally into normal pink urethra and, thus, failure to reconstruct the whole length of the urethral abnormality rather than just the stricture itself.

URETHROGRAPHY

The information provided by urethrography generally is fundamental to the management of urethral injury or stricture; the radiologic procedure must be appropriate to the clinical problem and it must be meticulously performed. Full distension of the urethra is very important; this is generally easier to obtain with gel contrasts. However, gel contrasts should never be used for evaluation of

acute injuries, because the extravasation that identifies a rupture does not dissipate rapidly and the consequent tissue reaction is a potent cause of spongiofibrosis. For acute-injury urethrography, which is often important for management, dilute aqueous contrast should be used and the volume of the extravasation should be reduced to the minimum required for diagnosis.

The length of a stricture is sometimes underestimated radiographically when attention is focused upon the length of a severely stenosed segment rather than upon the total length of the marginally narrowed lumen. Features such as cavitation of Littre's glands or ectasia of Cowper's duct indicate the probability of extensive spongiofibrosis. The true extent of a posterior bulbar stricture cannot be assessed accurately by retrograde urethrography when its luminal narrowing merges with that caused by the distal sphincter activity, but the distensibility of the sphincter may by apparent on appropriate voiding studies. Urethrography usually provides the basis for the primary decision, whether to treat an anterior urethral stricture by a trial of internal urethrotomy or to proceed to a definitive repair.

Synchronous retrograde and voiding urethrographic studies, the "up-and-down-agram," are particularly important in the repair of posterior urethral strictures, especially those resulting from pelvic fracture injuries. Without these studies, important features such as false passages, fistulous tracks, and bladder neck incompetence are often difficult to identify at operation. Whereas a stricture may thus be identified as complex and consequently in need of a synchronous transpubic repair, it is impossible to predict reliably the suitability of a simple perineal excision and anastomosis for an apparently short pelvic-fracture stricture, because exploration may reveal unexpectedly extensive hematoma fibrosis requiring a retropubic or a transpubic extension (see Fig. 68-27).

TERMINAL AND SUBTERMINAL STRICTURES

Terminal and subterminal strictures developing after instrumentation or use of an indwelling catheter are usually the result of abrasion-denudation of the uroepithelial lining. Hence, the development of a stricture of the meatus can usually be prevented by recalibrating it to a size at least 6Fr larger than the instrument or the catheter by a combination of dorsal and ventral Otis urethrotomy.

Simple subterminal strictures resulting from uroepithelial denudation can often be resolved by the simple regeneration procedure of overdilatation or internal urethrotomy, provided the strictures are not associated with an extensive spongiofibrosis. After 2 or 3 months of repeated dilatations to a normal caliber, the lumen may become re-epithelialized so that dilatations can be discontinued.

A simple inferior meatotomy resolves a terminal stricture into a hypospadiac urethral situation that does not require subsequent dilatation, provided it extends sufficiently proximally into the normal urethra. This rather crude procedure may be a reasonable expedient for the elderly.

Although a glans-tip meatus can be reconstructed by an inturned foreskin flap or a glans flap, it tends to be very imperfect, flared, or trumpet-shaped and not only looks abnormal but also creates a sprayed voiding stream.

A short subterminal stricture associated with a significant spongiofibrosis can usually be resolved by a simple one-stage, inrolled, wide-based pedicled island graft of foreskin or anterior penile skin.

This procedure is generally reliable and is particularly satisfactory when the last few millimeters of the urethra and the meatus are relatively normal.

NEOMEATOPLASTY

A normal-shaped meatus is situated terminally; its lips are smooth and sharp edged, forming a vertical slit that creates a clean, spray-free voiding stream. With meticulous attention to detail it is possible to construct a meatus that approximates very closely to normality positionally, functionally, and cosmetically. The common indications for this procedure are hypospadiac malformations and meatal strictures, including those known as balanitis xerotica obliterans.

A simple study of the normal relationship of the terminal urethra and meatus to a normal glans provides the basic format for a satisfactory reconstruction (Fig. 68-4).[21] If a normal glans is opened ventrally by a midline incision, it can be spread flat, exposing the normal terminal urethra as an epithelial strip some 2.5 cm in width in the adult, with a relatively thin layer of spongy tissue between it (the roof of the fossa navicularis) and the dorsal surface of the glans. The glans, the urethra, and the meatus can be restored simply by reclosing the incised spatulated glans. Thus, the construction or reconstruction of a normal terminal urethra and meatus involves bivalving the glans by a deep ventral midline incision and grafting a neourethral lining onto the exposed surface of the spongy tissue of the glans cleft.[16,21]

Hypospadias

In the past, the correction of terminal hypospadiac malformations has usually been limited to the correction of chordee of the penile shaft and extension of the foreshortened urethra to the coronal sulcus. There is a growing awareness that a subcoronal urethral meatus is an unacceptable standard of reconstruction. However, many current procedures that endeavor to achieve a glans-tip extension, such as simple skin tube extension or the V-shaped glans flap, result in a meatus that is less than perfect.

An additional deformity associated with many hypospadiac malformations is the ventripositioned "globular" glans, which few reconstruction techniques attempt to correct. However, the deep glans-clefting procedure does just this.[21] After closure, a split-glans meatoplasty should result in a meatus that is virtually normal in appearance; margins should be sharp and slitlike with a slight

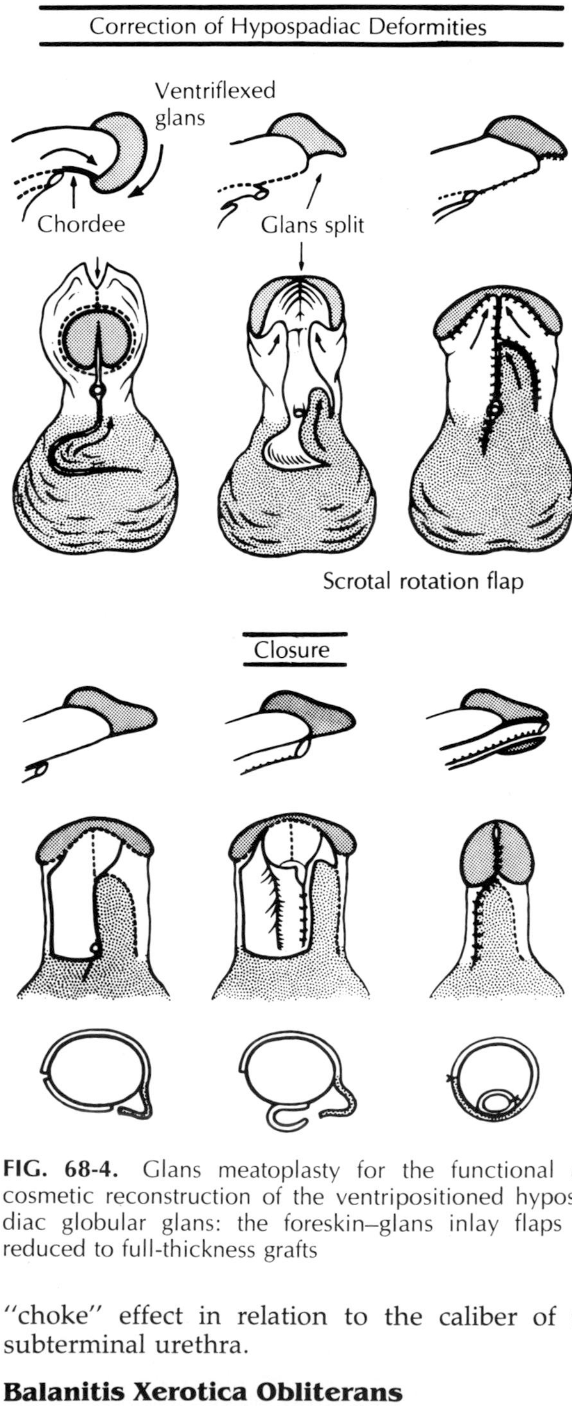

Correction of Hypospadiac Deformities

Ventriflexed glans

Chordee

Glans split

Scrotal rotation flap

Closure

FIG. 68-4. Glans meatoplasty for the functional and cosmetic reconstruction of the ventripositioned hypospadiac globular glans: the foreskin–glans inlay flaps are reduced to full-thickness grafts

"choke" effect in relation to the caliber of the subterminal urethra.

Balanitis Xerotica Obliterans

Although the etiology of balanitis xerotica is obscure, it is easily recognized by the characteristic dense spongiofibrosis in the substance of the glans and the terminal urethra. The principle of bivalved glans meatoplasty for this condition is essentially the same as that for simple hypospadiac deformity. The dense spongiofibrosis is excised, a reasonably vascularized graft bed is provided, and, of course, the graft is observed and adjusted during the interval stage before the final closure.[22]

Penile Urethral Strictures

The treatment of penile urethral strictures by internal Otis or endoscopic **urethrotomy** is less likely to result in a stricture-free urethra than similar treatment of bulbar strictures. However, inasmuch as urethrotomy is a relatively simple general urologic procedure, the attempt may be worthwhile. Any failed attempt to resolve a stricture by internal urethrotomy results in some extension of the surrounding spongiofibrosis, but rarely this compromises the subsequent definitive resolution of a stricture in the penile area.

One-stage **excision and reanastomosis** rarely is appropriate in the penile area, both because short strictures with a minimal extent of spongiofibrosis are most unusual in this area and because there is relatively little excess elasticity in the penile urethra during an erection. Even when the penile urethra is quite extensively mobilized, an overlap anastomosis is likely to result in a curvature chordee.

SUBSTITUTION RECONSTRUCTION

Compared with reconstruction of the bulbar urethra proximally and the glans meatus distally, penile urethral reconstruction is simple; however, it is usually done in association with one of these procedures because isolated penile strictures are unusual.

Penile skin provides a very satisfactory substitute for the urethra. It is smooth, almost hair free, and well vascularized by its uniquely mobile subcutaneous tissue so that it is easy to roll in on a lateral pedicle extending throughout its length, either as a one-stage island skin graft or as a two-stage procedure.[8,13,14]

The whole circumference of the penile urethra can be reconstructed from a 3-cm (30-mm or 30Fr) inrolled strip; an oversized, irregular reconstructed urethral lumen in the penile area does not retain urine because it is pendulous and free draining. The skin defect on the penile shaft may be covered with scrotal skin, which is a relatively poor substitute for urethra but a satisfactory one for penile skin.[13]

In general, when the penile urethra is reconstructed on a two-stage basis, it is best to rotate the skin-replacement scrotal flap onto the penile shaft at the first stage to reduce the incidence of fistulas by wide separation of the closure suture lines (Fig. 68-5).

FIG. 68-5. First-stage penile urethroplasty. **(A)** the entire length of the abnormal "grey" urethra is opened with an inlay of scrotal drop-back; **(B)** a scrotal flap rotated onto the penile shaft to provide additional skin for subsequent closure; **(C)** final appearance of scrotourethral redeployment; **(D)** sequential steps in overlapping penile urethral tube closure and scrotal overclosure with widely separated suture lines

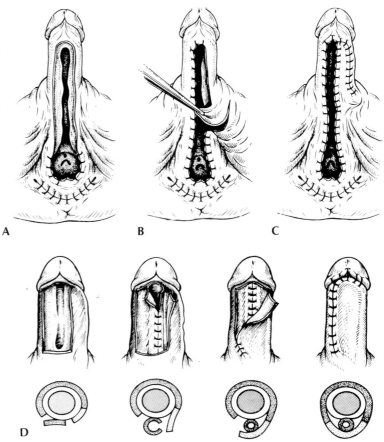

"BURIED STRIP" TUBE RECONSTRUCTION

The principle of reconstructing a tube by burying a strip of skin is based upon the fact that tissues do not adhere to an epithelial surface; hence, if a strip is not free to roll up, the circumference of the lining will be completed by epithelialization of the opposing surface of the overlying tissue.[21]

Hamilton Russell devised the buried-strip principle in 1912 for short strictures of the bulbar urethra.[9] Denis Browne used this principle as an economy measure for penile urethral reconstruction, to overcome the paucity of circumferential skin on the penile surface; by burying a flat strip of skin 1.5 cm wide, he was able to obtain a normal lumen of 30Fr (30 mm = 15 mm + 15 mm). It is important to appreciate that this principle only works as a partial regeneration procedure if the buried strip is *fixed flat*, by sutures if necessary, so that its lateral margins cannot roll up.

The lumen of a urethra that has been reconstructed by a Denis Browne buried-strip procedure has a grossly irregular caliber. This method of penile reconstruction would never have been adopted if the potential complications of stagnation of urine in sacculated irregularities of hair-bearing skin had not been avoided naturally by its pendulous self-drainage. The Denis Browne buried-strip urethroplasty is not commonly used because the incidence of cutaneous fistulae is unacceptably high compared with that of formal two-stage tube closure reconstructions.

Strictures of the Bulbospongy Urethra

Although the primary characteristics of strictures involving the bulbar urethra usually relate to their etiology, the identifying features of long-established strictures may be altered by treatment and by superimposed complications. Furthermore, although the history may be helpful, it is often unreliable, especially when it relates to minimal trauma. However, apart from the need to identify active urethritis, carcinoma, and schistosomiasis and to treat these appropriately, the definitive resolution of a bulbar urethral narrowing relates to its extent and that of the surrounding fibrosis.

Congenital strictures are rare but do occur in the younger age group in the absence of a history of instrumentation, significant external trauma, or infection.

External urethral injuries are caused by identifiable accident situations and commonly result in a short segmental injury to both elements of the bulbar urethra, a short stricture surrounded by a well-localized spongiofibrosis. If both the urethral element and the spongy element immediately proximal and distal to a short stricture prove to be essentially normal at operation, repair by excision and anastomosis is indicated.

During the acute stage of urethritis, the inflammatory changes commonly extend throughout the length of the bulbar urethra and into the penile urethra. Thus, spongiofibrosis due to inflammation often extends distally into the penile urethra; proximally, it is sometimes associated with slight narrowing of the membranous urethra, though competence of the intramural distal sphincter mechanism is rarely compromised by urethritis alone.

SPONGIOPLASTY

The bulbospongy urethra has two functional elements, the uroepithelial conduit and the spongy tissue. Although these two elements are integral, it is helpful to regard them as distinct entities, not only because they tend to be affected differently by stricture-generating pathologic processes, but also because there sometimes is an advantage in separating them surgically and redeploying them individually in the course of bulbar urethral reconstructions.

The urethral element of the bulbar urethra is eccentrically positioned within the bulb so that most of the spongy tissue lies posterolaterally, and it is only 2 mm to 3 mm thick on the dorsal aspect of the urethra. The procedure for separating the bulk of the posterolateral spongy tissue from the relatively thin layer required to support and vascularize the urethral element is conveniently referred to as *spongioplasty*. A posterior-flap spongioplasty is a contributory feature of bulbo–bulbar and bulbo–prostatic urethral anastomosis.[15] A bilateral posteriorly based redeployment spongioplasty is fundamental to the "combination" procedures for bulbo–urethral reconstruction (see Fig. 68-11).[18,22]

INTERNAL STRICTUROTOMY

Although endoscopic urethrotomy has an advantage, in that it can sometimes be used when the Otis urethrotome cannot be passed, the endoscopic appearances of the immediate result are virtually indistinguishable; success depends upon epithelial regeneration.

Urethrotomy. The basic principle of stricturotomy is to carry the incision through the rigid stricture into a layer of tissue that is sufficiently supple to open up and reepithelialize before the cleft closes and epithelial bridge healing occurs. The supple layer may be either relatively normal spongy tissue surrounding the spongiofibrosis or the adventitial tissue outside it.

As soon as an endoscopic stricturotomy extends into a supple tissue layer, the pressure of the irrigation fluid expands the lumen. However, it is often impossible to find an adequate supple spongy-tissue layer in the 12 o'clock position in the bulbo–penile urethra for several reasons: (1) the penile urethra is only a few millimeters thick, (2) it may be spongiofibrotic, and (3) its natural adhesion to the undersurface of the corpora in this area may prevent its lateral expansion even when its full thickness is transected. The dorsal adhesion between the relatively thin walls of the penile urethra and the penile corpora is somewhat broader, between 10 o'clock and 2 o'clock. Thus, lateral or inferior incisions may be necessary to expose a supple layer of spongy tissue in the bulbar urethra and the periurethral tissue plane in the penile urethra.

Urethrotomy Healing. When the pressure of the endoscopic irrigation fluid is released, the urethra collapses and the incisional clefts tend to close. Attempts to delay the urethrotomy cleft closure and to increase the extent of circumferential healing of the lumen by reepithelialization have met with only limited success. Many surgeons have increased the period of indwelling catheter stenting without definitive success, possibly because even the smoothest catheter surface tends to erode the proliferating epithelial margins and because the drainage of the exudates from the denuded areas tends to be obstructed by the catheter so that they accumulate, become infected, and increase the inflammatory reaction.

Urostatic distension (interrupting the voiding stream by digital compression of the terminal urethra) has also been advocated for cleft opening in an attempt to delay restenosis. Reduction of the spongiofibrotic reaction of the bare areas by the local application of steroids is not strikingly effective. The use of temporarily located, urethra-expanding cage splints and endourethral skin grafting is currently under evaluation.

Indications and Contraindications. A particularly critical decision is required when a stricture appears short radiographically and the history strongly suggests that it is either congenital or traumatic. Such strictures are ideal for one-stage anastomotic repair which, in appropriate cases and experienced hands, carries a success rate approaching 100%. Although such cases usually are easy to treat by endoscopic incision, few surgeons would claim a success rate much greater than 70% with the technique and secondary fibrosis associated with failure is likely to preclude a simple anastomotic resolution. However, when a bulbar urethral stricture clearly will require a substitution procedure if a definitive reconstruction is advised, little is lost by a trial of internal urethrotomy.

Complications of Urethrotomy. In treating a stricture of the penile urethra by internal urethrotomy, it is important to avoid incising too deeply in the dorsal position, because exposure of the cavernous tissue may result in the formation of a secondary Peyronie-like cavernosis and can cause a ventral-curvature chordee. Destruction of the distal sphincter mechanism by internal urethrotomy is an avoidable disaster. As shown in Figure 68-6, the problem commonly arises when a posterior bulbar stricture extends up to the distal margin of the membranous urethra; it is often difficult or impossible to distinguish endoscopically where the stricture ends and the sphincter begins. Because the distal external sphincter mechanism is located entirely withing the 3- to 4-mm thickness of the wall of the membranous urethra, it should not be incised (see Fig. 68-16). Failure of internal urethrotomy can be attributed to recurrent fibrosis (Fig. 68-7).

EXCISION AND ANASTOMOSIS

Any failure to obtain a stricture-free result after the treatment of a short stricture by excision and reanastomosis must call into question the selection either of the procedure or of the surgical technique. When the total length of the urethral abnormality (the stricture and the grey urethra) is sufficiently short to enable a good overlap anastomosis to be achieved between the spatulated ends of entirely normal urethra, the introduction of the complication rate inherent in a substitution reconstruction is generally inadvisable. Thus, when the radiologic appearances indicate that the length of a bulbar stenosis is less than 1 cm, the decision whether to use an anastomotic or a substitution procedure must depend upon the additional length of the proximal and distal "grey" spongiofibrotic urethra found at the time of operation.

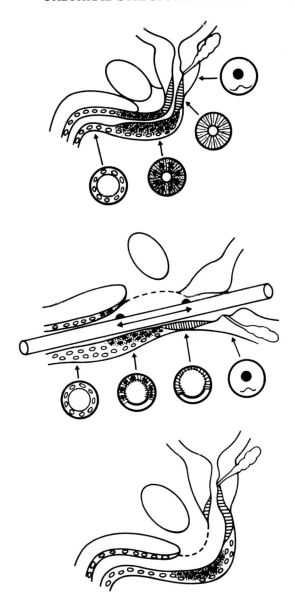

FIG. 68-6. The potential disaster of internal urethrotomy of a posterior bulbar stricture: the incision extends into the membranous urethra and divides the full thickness of the intramural distal sphincter mechanisms

URETHRAL MOBILIZATION AND CHORDEE

The factor limiting the length of a bulbar urethral abnormality that can be resolved by excision and anastomosis is the extent of the elastic lengthening that can be obtained by mobilizing the residual bulbar urethra between the stricture and the membranous urethra proximally and the base of the penis distally. In practice, the maximum length of a bulbar urethra that can be excised and reconsti-

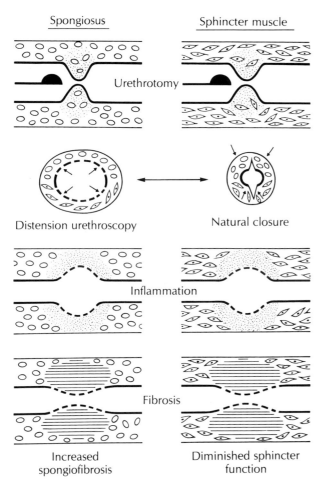

Spongiosus   Sphincter muscle

Urethrotomy

Distension urethroscopy   Natural closure

Inflammation

Fibrosis

Increased   Diminished sphincter
spongiofibrosis   function

FIG. 68-7. Partial-thickness internal urethrotomy of the spongy bulbo–penile urethra and the membranous urethral sphincter: secondary extension of the spongiofibrosis is relatively unimportant compared with the fibrosis of the intramural distal sphincter

tuted by a 2-cm spatulated overlap anastomosis is only about 1 cm. Attempts to excise a longer segment may result in a chordee that significantly alters the angle of an erection; however, it should not create a curvature chordee of the penile shaft if this part of the urethra has not been mobilized.

For simple mechanical reasons, angulation chordee is likely to be increased when the base of the penis is well elevated by a short suspensory ligament. It is wise to reduce this by dividing the ligament through the perineal incision by retracting the base of the penis to one side. The suspensory ligament is not a fundamentally important structure.

BULBAR URETHRAL POOLING AND HAIR-BEARING SUBSTITUTION

The normal bulbar urethra is emptied completely after voiding by the closing pressure created by the combination of the surrounding spongy tissue and bulbospongiosus muscle. Furthermore, tumescence of the bulbar spongy tissue during erection increases the urethral closing pressure and transmits the contractions of the bulbospongiosus muscle, which converts the sustained prostatovesicular emission into an intermittent forceful ejaculation.

After the age of 40 it is not uncommon for men to develop a postmicturition dribble, which urodynamic evaluation proves to be the result of bulbar pooling.[1,20] Saccular irregularities of the lumen of a reconstructed bulbar urethra are also a common source of a small-volume postmicturition dribble. They can usually be resolved by finger pressure in the perineum after voiding.

Occasional hairs growing in a scrotal-graft, bulbo–urethral reconstruction do not usually create problems unless the lumen is strictured or sacculated with retained stagnant urine, predisposing to encrustation, stone formation, infection, and secondary strictures. In certain patients a particularly profuse growth of hairs in a scrotal-skin reconstruction may cause obstruction, even without a significant encrustation. This emphasizes the importance of careful epilation of a neourethral scrotal pedicle graft, the advisability of using a two-stage procedure to provide access for this when using a hair-bearing skin substitution, and the advantages of "combination" substitution procedures.

SUBSTITUTION BULBAR URETHROPLASTY

Substitution reconstruction of the posterior bulbar urethra is considerably more difficult than that of the penile urethra for a number of reasons:

1. The only skin that easily reaches the posterior urethra on a pedicle basis is that of the scrotum and the perineum, and both of these have serious shortcomings as urethral substitutes.

2. The bulbar urethra is not pendulous and self-draining. Once the normal evacuative pressure of the surrounding spongy tissue and bulbospongiotic muscles is lost, it is often impossible to restore.

3. It is important that the lumen of a reconstructed bulbar urethra should have a normal and even caliber.

FIG. 68-8. (A) unsupported and (B) spongiosupported free skin graft urethral reconstructions with schematic indication of the exudate-drainage routes

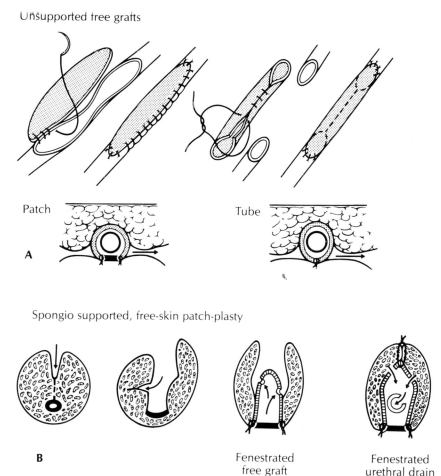

Unsupported free grafts

Patch   Tube

A

Spongio supported, free-skin patch-plasty

B   Fenestrated free graft   Fenestrated urethral drain

Unfortunately, no substitute for the urethra is as good as the urethra itself. The options lie between free-patch grafts of penile or foreskin and pedicle inlay grafts of scrotal skin, both of which have inherent shortcomings that result in a significant incidence of recurrent stricture.

Free Full-Thickness Skin Patch Grafts

The pioneer work of Devine and Horton showed full-thickness skin to be superior to split-skin grafts for urethral reconstruction; foreskin or anterior penile skin is preferred.[4] Meticulous plastic surgical technique determines the success rate; it is particularly important to remove all the subcutaneous tissue adherent to the graft (so-called defatting) to ensure close contact between the basal epidermal cells and the vascular graft bed. Long free skin patch grafts are naturally less successful than short ones; unlike pedicle grafts, if the length of a free graft is doubled, the risk of failure is also doubled. The survival of free patch grafts is compromised

when the graft-bed tissue is densely fibrotic or infected.

Free urethral patch grafts can be unsupported or supported (Fig. 68-8). An unsupported graft is either a partial-circumference patch plasty or a total-circumference tube plasty. The graft is applied to the urethral defect around a stenting catheter with a regular shaft. The bulbar spongy tissue is not overclosed, so the graft bed is formed by the subcutaneous tissues of the perineum and scrotum and the exudates that might otherwise accumulate and separate the graft from its bed can escape into the lateral wound space (Fig. 68-8A).

A supported graft or patch spongioplasty is used to reepithelialize the inner surface of the bulbospongy tissue. Normal spongy tissue is a particularly good graft bed and the end result approximates the normal pink urethra. In one-stage procedures graft-bed exudates are drained by fenestrating both the graft and the urethral catheter shaft (Fig. 68-8B).

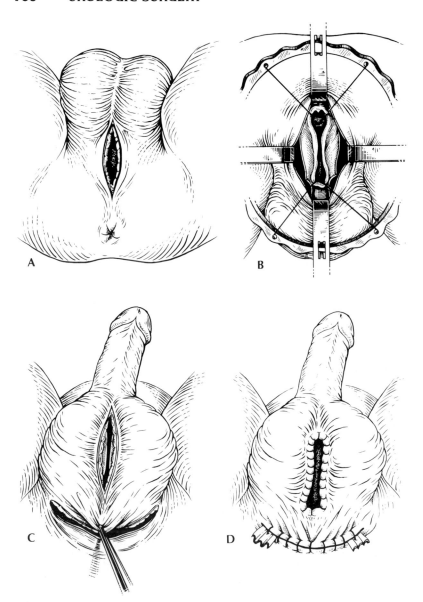

FIG. 68-9. First-stage, drop-back scrotourethral inlay: **(A)** vertical perineal incision; **(B)** incision of the whole length of the abnormal bulbar urethra; **(C)** secondary scrotal-inlay incision in front of scrotal drop-back; **(D)** scrotourethral inlay and horizontal closure of the primary incision

The success rate of a one-stage, unsupported free patch graft urethroplasty depends considerably upon the circumstances of the case and the experience of the surgeon with this specialized form of plastic reconstruction. Few can claim an overall success rate much in excess of 80% stricture-free cases on the basis of a 5-year follow-up, and in many series the results are much less satisfactory.

Scrotal Pedicle Grafts

Although the characteristic mobility of the subcutaneous tissues of the scrotum facilitates a scrotourethral inlay to the bulbar urethra, the scrotal skin itself is not a good substitute for urethral epithelium both because it is hair-bearing and because it sometimes develops an eczematous inflammatory reaction when it becomes urine soaked. These inherent shortcomings do not contraindicate the use of scrotal skin as a urethral substitute but they compromise its reliability; the "two stage" inlay procedure was developed specifically to enable these shortcomings to be overcome. The term *two-stage* is, to some extent, a misnomer because it is the meticulous management of the *interval stage* that is the key to success with this procedure.

Johanssen's original scrotal-tunnel procedure for bulbo–membranous strictures was superseded by

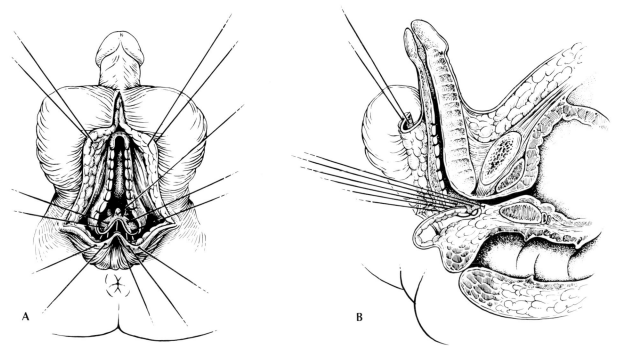

FIG. 68-10. First-stage posterior flap scroto-urethral inlay urethroplasty. If the membranous urethra is opened too widely back to the level of the verumontanum, the function of the distal sphincter mechanism may be compromised so that continence depends upon the bladder neck mechanism

a posteriorly placed scrotal inlay that provided access for direct observation and revision.[12] Such a posteriorly placed funnel can be achieved either by a scrotal drop-back procedure (Fig. 68-9) or by a posteriorly based perineoscrotal flap (Fig. 68-10).[2,6,12,13] In most cases the choice between these procedures is simply a matter of the surgeon's preference. There are a few particular indications and contraindications for each; for instance, a posterior flap is particularly useful in children when the scrotum is small, but it is compromised by infection associated with a "wateringcan perineum."

The success of a scrotal urethral inlay depends upon the management of the interval stage. Provided the epilation of the neourethral area of the scrotal inlay has been carried out properly, and provided the inlay has been proven to be stricture free over a period of 8 to 12 months before closure, the stricture-free success rate in a consecutive series of cases over a 5- to 10-year follow-up period should be better than 90%.[11] Because both free-patch graft procedures and pedicled scrotal grafts result in an unacceptably high long-term complication rate when used as circumferential urethral

substitution procedures, we have developed "combination procedures" that avoid using either for replacement of more than half of the urethral circumference in any area.

"COMBINATION" BULBAR URETHROPLASTY PROCEDURES

Fixed-Flat Roof Strip

The basic principle of a "combination" urethroplasty is the creation of an epithelialized roof strip that is at least 1.5 cm wide and is definitely fixed flat by lateral sutures anchoring its margins to the undersurface of the crura; a laterally anchored roof strip is unlikely to contract (Fig. 68-11).[22] After a redeployment spongioplasty, an epithelialized roof strip can be created in several ways (Fig. 68-12):

1. Rearrangement of a strictured bulbar urethral element by side-to-side overlap anastomosis after a full-length bulbar urethral mobilization

2. Multiple longitudinal incisions into a narrowed urethral element, which are held open by its lateral fixation so that they heal be regeneration epithelialization

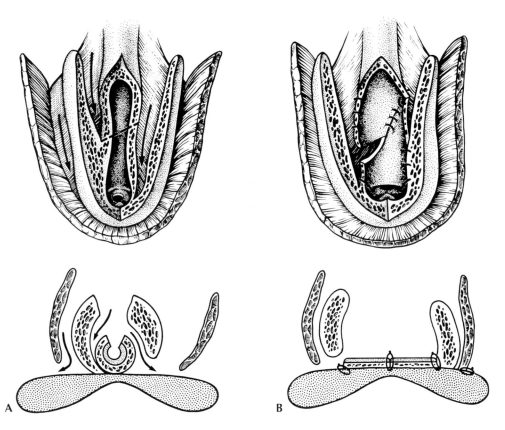

FIG. 68-11. Combination urethroplasty and redeployment spongioplasty: **(A)** separation of the lateral spongiosum from the urethral element; **(B)** redeployment lateral to the fixed-flat urethral roof strip

FIG. 68-12. Combination urethroplasty procedures for creating a fixed-flat bulbar roof strip: **(A)** excision of stricture and reanastomosis of the urethral element; **(B)** multiple overlapping longitudinal incisions and lateral spread; **(C)** augmentation by free skin graft; **(D)** substitution free skin graft

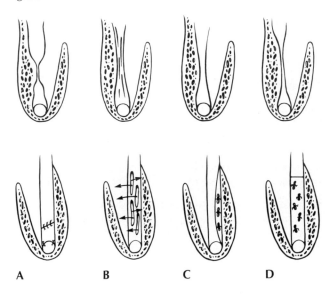

3. Augmentation of a urethral roof strip with a free-patch graft
4. Complete replacement of the urethral roof strip by a free patch graft

After the creation of a fixed-flat roof strip, the posteriorly based flaps of spongy tissue are resutured to the lateral margins of the roof strip for subsequent overclosure (lateral redeployment spongioplasty), as previously discussed.

The decision whether to complete a fixed-flat urethral roof strip in the bulbar area by a one-stage or a two-stage procedure depends upon the assessment of its quality. If a really satisfactory full-width roof strip has been created by a clean oblique anastomotic urethral rearrangement, it may be appropriate to complete it by a one-stage, free skin patch plasty or even by an inert absorbable patch with or without redeployment spongioplasty support (Fig. 68-13). A two-stage operation is necessary if the bulbar urethral roof strip is imperfect as a result of inflammatory changes or of a somewhat precarious rearrangement procedure, or if the roof strip has required augmentation by multiple longitudinal incisions or a patch-graft. In such circum-

FIG. 68-13. Completion of combination root-strip urethroplasty: **(A)** one-stage spongiosupported free skin graft; **(B)** observational scrotourethral inlay to urethral redeployment roof-strip; **(C)** observational scrotourethral inlay to free skin substitution roof-strip

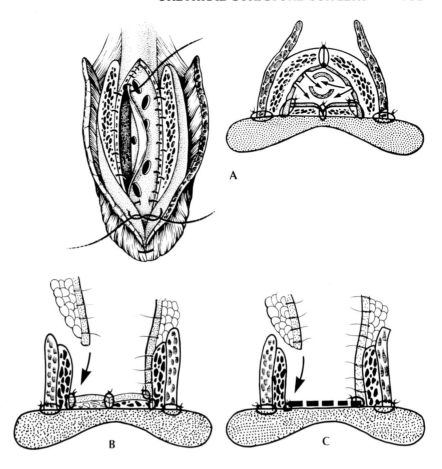

stances, a scrotal drop-back inlay is sutured to the margins of the roof strip (Fig. 68-13*B* and *C*).

Many advantages accrue from the use of a combination procedure for the reconstruction of complex bulbar strictures, particularly those associated with extensive spongiofibrosis:

1. Restricturing due to partial failure of free patch grafts to "take" is obviated, even when long grafts are used to create the whole length of the bulbar and part of the penile urethra roof strip. Furthermore, these grafts can often be based in residual normal spongy tissue after excision of areas of spongiofibrosis. Occasionally a redeployment patch spongioplasty can be created that is sufficient to receive a free graft 3 cm to 4 cm wide, so that it forms the whole circumference of a spongiosupported patch-plasty urethra.

2. As soon as the satisfactory healing of a fixed-flat roof strip has been verified and any tendency to recurrent narrowing of the posterior inlay meatus has been excluded, the closure stage

can be considered. Thus, the interval stage is often reduced to 6 to 10 weeks as compared with the 8 to 12 months required to verify the stability of a circumferential scrotourethral substitution.

3. Because the roof strip of a combination procedure is fixed flat by lateral suturing, it is unlikely to contract once its reepithelialization is firmly established. Although it is preferable to complete the circumference of the urethral lining by an appropriate overclosure of a narrow strip of epilated scrotal inlay skin, the reconstructed lumen would probably be satisfactory on the basis of the Denis Browne, buried-strip regeneration principle, even if the scrotal skin should prove unstable.

Full-Length Anterior Urethroplasty

The procedures of glans meatoplasty, penile urethral reconstruction, and combination bulbar urethral reconstruction can be used together to reconstruct the whole length of the anterior urethra from

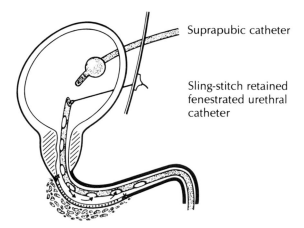

Suprapubic catheter

Sling-stitch retained
fenestrated urethral
catheter

FIG. 68-14. Safe catheter management after urethral reconstruction by patch-plasty is ensured by positive drainage of the pericatheter urethral space, a catheter-gram that identifies extravasation, a sling-stitch preventing premature removal, and no balloon-risk to the graft

the sphincter mechanism to the external meatus. The development of a recurrent stricture distal to any urethral reconstruction almost always represents a failure to recognize the full anterior extent of the spongiofibrotic abnormality of the unstrictured ''grey'' urethra and consequent failure to ensure that the substitution should extend into 2 cm of normal pink urethra (Fig. 68-3).

Urinary Drainage and Catheter Management

The procedure for urinary drainage and stenting catheters after a one-stage reconstruction of the final closure of a two-stage procedure is important. We never use a balloon-retained catheter after a urethral reconstruction for several reasons:

1. Balloon failure may result in premature loss of the catheter.
2. Partial deflation of the balloon may result in its slipping, while still oversize, into the reconstruction and dislocating it.
3. Severe inadvertent traction may pull a fully inflated balloon into the reconstructed area.
4. Even if it is properly deflated, residual corrugations of an overstretched balloon may be sufficient to disturb a free-patch graft.

Thus, if a urethral catheter is used there are many advantages in retaining it with a sling-stitch to a button on the abdominal wall.

A standard-shaft catheter indwelling in a reconstructed (or injured) urethra often obstructs the urethral drainage, and the increased exudates tend

to become infected and compromise the reconstruction; consequently we never use a standard-shaft indwelling catheter in overclosed urethral reconstructions. Drainage of reconstruction exudates along the urethra can occur passively if there is no indwelling catheter; however, a stenting catheter is particularly important to the success of an unsupported free-patch graft urethral reconstruction.

Positive drainage of the urethral lumen can be achieved by a fenestrated catheter.[15] Although some urine may drain through a fenestrated catheter, the catheter is used primarily to remove exudates from the urethra; it always is used in conjunction with a suprapubic catheter, which provides the main urinary drainage route (Fig. 68-14). Fenestrated catheters are best made from plastic because these are relatively thin walled and consequently the lumen is relatively larger than latex or silicone catheters.[5] The catheter holes extend through the bulbar urethra and into the proximal penile urethra but not into the distal penile urethra, because urine may discharge around the catheter. A fenestrated catheter is best retained by an abdominal wall sling-stitch. A simple technique for the synchronous insertion of the sling-stitch and a suprapubic catheter is illustrated in Figure 68-15.

Gentle irrigation of the pericatheter space by urine passing along a fenestrated catheter has not resulted in any attributable complications over a large series of cases. A fenestrated catheter aids verification of the state of healing of a reconstruction by a ''cathetergram''; contrast introduced into a fenestrated catheter naturally flows into the pericatheter space, so extraurethral extravasation can be excluded radiographically.

Catheter Strictures

Catheter strictures commonly develop as a result of uroepithelial abrasion or urethritis. Mechanical abrasion of the urethral lining is particularly prone to occur at points where a relatively large catheter is gripped tight: at the meatus, in the membranous urethra, and at the peno–scrotal junction in children. This can usually be prevented by the use of relatively small catheters for urinary drainage or by oversize recalibration of the urethra by internal urethrotomy when larger catheters have to be used for drainage of hematuria clots.

Catheter urethritis is usually the result of infection of exudates trapped in the pericatheter space. When the formation of urethral exudates is greatly increased by urethral injury, it is best to avoid using an indwelling catheter.

In the adult, the risk of abrasion strictures and

infection strictures can be virtually eliminated by using an indwelling 12Fr to 14Fr plastic urethral catheter. Its relatively large lumen is quite adequate for simple urinary drainage, and the normal output of urethral exudates can drain freely around it. The development of a stricture after a 20Fr urethral catheter has been used as a nursing convenience (*e.g.*, after coronary bypass or orthopedic surgery) should be an avoidable disaster.

Strictures of the Sphincter-Active Posterior Urethra

Reconstruction of a bulbo–penile urethra is a relatively simple surgical challenge compared with the resolution of strictures of the sphincter-active posterior urethra. The bulbo–penile urethra is subcutaneous, so access is easy. All that is required is the reconstruction of a full-length conduit of appropriate and uniform caliber. Compared with this, not only is access to the posterior urethra relatively restricted, but its all-important intramural sphincter mechanism, already damaged to some extent by the trauma that created the stricture, is at further risk during surgery. Thus, posterior urethral surgery requires an accurate knowledge of the anatomy of the sphincter mechanism, an understanding of its functional characteristics, appropriate video-urodynamic preevaluation, special instrumentation and surgical technique.

FUNCTIONAL CONSIDERATIONS: CONTINENCE AND INCONTINENCE

The whole length of the posterior urethra in the male is sphincter active; all injuries to it involve some element of sphincter damage and all operations upon it involve some aspect of preservation, ablation, or restitution of sphincteric function. The feasibility of many posterior urethral surgical procedures depends upon the independent function of the proximal and the distal mechanisms, each of which is normally competent and able to maintain continence in the absence of the other. However, in spite of this functionally effective duplication, neither sphincter should be ablated unneccessarily.

Bladder Neck Sphincter Mechanism

The bladder neck mechanism is functional from the internal urethral meatus down to the level of the verumontanum. In the male the bladder neck is almost invariably competent when the detrusor is at rest but opens when the detrusor contracts. Consequently, in the absence of a distal sphincter

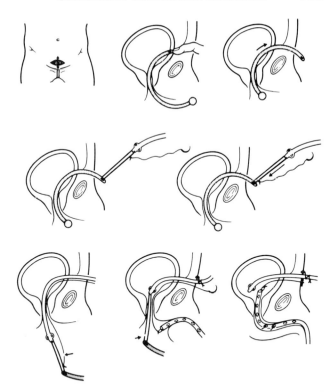

FIG. 68-15. A technique for synchronous insertion of suprapubic catheter and urethral catheter sling-stitch

mechanism, a patient's continence is additionally dependent upon the stability of the detrusor mechanism; patients naturally tend to leak if they develop involuntary unstable bladder neck opening contractions. The competence of the bladder neck mechanism is compromised as a prostate enlarges upward through it, and it is almost invariably functionally incompetent after any prostatectomy procedure, even when it supposedly is preserved.[23] The distal sphincter mechanism should be conserved whenever possible, even if the proximal posterior urethra is normal at the time of operation, both because one cannot predict prostatic enlargement before it occurs, and because, if prostatectomy does become necessary at a later date, continence depends upon it.

Distal Sphincter Mechanism

The distal sphincter mechanism is functional from the verumontanum down to the lower margin of the membranous urethra, but its major functional activity is located in its distal two thirds. Although textbook illustrations commonly suggest otherwise, the functionally effective element of the distal sphincter mechanism is located entirely within the 3- to 4-mm thickness of the wall of the membranous

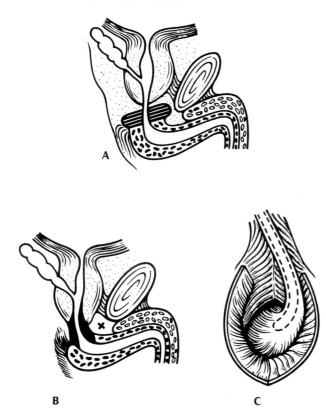

FIG. 68-16. The distal urethral sphincter mechanism: **(A)** erroneous concept of urogenital diaphragm and periurethral external sphincter; **(B)** sectional representation of intramural distal sphincter mechanism; **(C)** subpubic space anterolateral to the membranous urethra, viewed during perineal mobilization

and supramembranous urethra; a longitudinal incision into it will divide it completely (Fig. 68-16).[23]

The common description of a urogenital diaphragm that encloses a bulk of external striated sphincter muscle encircling the membranous urethra is extraordinarily inaccurate.[3,23] There is no urogenital diaphragm or periurethral musculature immediately anterior or lateral to the membranous urethra, only a space that will admit a fingertip. The only periurethral muscles that relate directly to the membranous urethra insert into the perineal body adherent to its posterior surface (the pubourethral element of the levator ani, the transverse perinei, and the bulbospongiosus), and these are incapable of any sustained occlusion of the lumen except in spastic neuropathic states. The "external sphincter" was so-called because it was external to the internal sphincter at the bladder neck; it does not refer to muscles outside the urethra. It has been further confused by using it to denote the outer (as distinct from the inner) of the two layers of the intramural distal sphincter.

BULBO–MEMBRANOUS STRICTURE MANAGEMENT

A bulbo–membranous stricture is commonly the result of a severe bulbar urethral inflammation caused either by a specific urethritis or by an indwelling catheter. The surrounding fibrosis usually extends up to the distal margin of the membranous urethra; occasionally it results in a narrowing of the membranous urethra but rarely in significant impairment of the function of its intramural sphincter mechanism. However, impaired elasticity of the membranous urethra often limits its calibration to about 20Fr to 22Fr, and the subepithelial spongiofibrosis extends imperceptibly into the sphincter area, making it difficult or impossible to distinguish a transition point between the stricutre and the distal sphincter mechanism.

Potential Disaster: Internal Urethrotomy for Bulbo–Membranous Stricture

The greatest caution is required in the treatment of a bulbo–membranous stricture by internal urethrotomy both because of the difficulty in distinguishing the transition point between the spongiofibrotic stricture and the sphincter, and because incision 3 mm to 4 mm into the wall of the membranous urethra can transect the functionally effective distal urethra mechanism and render it incompetent (Fig. 68-17). There can be no doubt that this is a real risk: when a definitive reconstruction is undertaken for a bulbar stricture persisting after an extensive urethrotomy, the membranous urethra is sometime so lax that the verumontanum can be seen easily without a posterior urethral retractor. A patient in such condition is almost certain to become disastrously incontinent should he later require a prostatectomy.[20,23]

Substitution Bulbo–Membranous Urethroplasty

When no normal pink urethra intervenes between a bulbo–membranous stricture and the sphincter mechanism, it is necessary to extend a substitution urethroplasty through the sphincter mechanism into the distal prostatic urethra to find the 2 cm of normal urethra required to reduce the incidence of proximal substitution urethroplasty restenosis.

Trans-Sphincteric Urethroplasty

The technique of deeply incising or overstretching the distal sphincter mechanism, which is sometimes advocated to enable a posteriorly based perineoscrotal flap to be advanced up to the level of the verumontanum and sutured into position without special instruments, is obviously as potentially damaging to its sphincteric competence as an endoscopic urethrotomy transection. A conservative trans-sphincter inlay that endeavors to minimize both the risk of recurrent proximal stenosis and distal sphincter damage is based on the fact that oversize dilatation of a reasonably normal distal sphincter mechanism to 36Fr does not seem to impair its competence significantly. (A damaged sphincter mechanism associated with a rigid membranous stricture, on the other hand, may be rendered incompetent by recalibration to a normal size.)

The position of the membranous urethra is relatively easy to identify externally when it is exposed by perineal dissection. It is recalibrated gently by stretching to 36Fr. The epithelium is encouraged to split posteriorly by a minimal superficial incision that expands to an inverted V-shaped defect with its apex extending just to below the verumontanum. Special instruments are required to suture a pedicle inlay or a free-patch graft to the margins of this defect within a caliber of 36Fr. Retraction can be achieved by the tapered groove of a Teale's probe-pointed gorget or by a T–W calibrating posterior urethral retractor for the posterior sutures. The blades of the latter are 9 mm wide, so when they are separated by an equivalent distance, the posterior urethra calibrates to $4 \times 9 = 36$Fr (Fig. 68-18). A fully curved posterior urethral needle facilitates the insertion of the posterior, interrupted, deep-bite 3×0 polyglycolic acid sutures. Alternatively the sutures can be inserted by Chalmer's technique with an atraumatic needle bent into a spoon shape, which is pushed on, up the urethra, and withdrawn after the suture bites have been taken.

Postoperative Management of a Trans-Sphincter Urethral Inlay. It is not easy to establish a stricture-free urethral substitution in the sphincter-active urethra, but there are considerable advantages in using a temporary scrotourethral inlay to provide direct access for supervision during the healing period. An indwelling, regular-shaft balloon catheter inserted through the inlay urethrostomy provides immediate postoperative urinary drainage. For the first 2 months it is advisable to pass a 32Fr to 34Fr straight meatal sound through the posterior inlay meatus every week or so reduce the chance of cross-adhesion of the suture-line granulations where they are approximated by the sphincter activity. Any residual tendency to narrow to a caliber of less than 30Fr thereafter should be treated either by repeated oversized 32Fr to 34Fr dilatation or by a local rearrangement of the inlay as a definitive interval procedure.

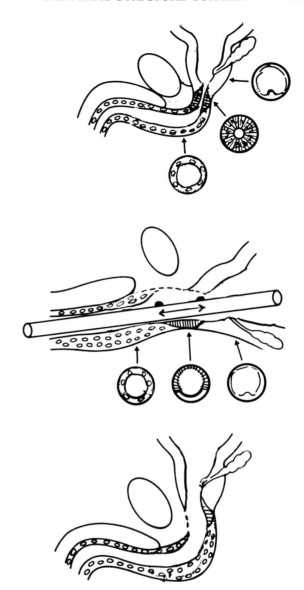

FIG. 68-17.   The disaster of internal urethrotomy of postprostatectomy membranous urethral strictures: transection of the residual intramural distal sphincter

Subsphincter Urethral Expansion by Spongioplasty Fixation

During the creation of a fixed-flat, roof-strip combination bulbar urethroplasty associated with a lateral redeployment spongioplasty, the incidence of subsphincter stenosis can be reduced by urethral expansion. The posterior bulbar urethra is incised posteriorly up to the distal sphincter mechanism; the lateral margins of the subsphincter posterior bulbar urethra can then be spread open gently and anchored laterally to the inner surface of the crura after exposing this by dissection from the overlying

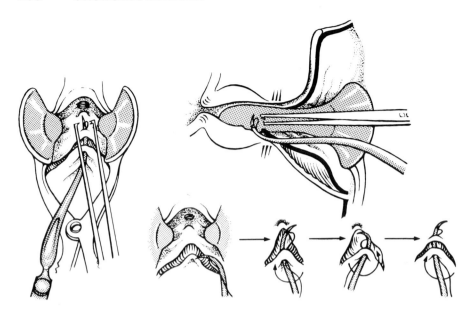

FIG. 68-18. Instrumentation for inlay suturing of trans-sphincteric urethroplasty within the caliber of 36Fr: 4 blades of the posterior retractor, each measuring 9 mm; 4 × 9 = 36Fr. A fully curved posterior urethral needle rotates within this

layer of bulbospongiosus muscle. The effect is to funnel what is left of the circumference of the posterior bulbar urethra to form a fixed-flat roof strip to which the margins of a free-patch graft or an inlay graft may be sutured. Care must be taken not to extend into the distal sphincter mechanism so that it will not be functionally immobilized by the lateral anchoring sutures (Fig. 68-11).

POSTPROSTATECTOMY SPHINCTER STRICTURES

Postprostatectomy strictures in the distal sphincter mechanism may result from both transurethral and enucleation procedures. They are much the most difficult of all strictures to manage satisfactorily, for the following reasons:

1. The stricture is located in the only sphincter mechanism that remains after a prostatectomy.
2. The preoperative or postoperative trauma that injured the sphincter-active area of the urethra also damaged its functional competence.
3. Strictures in the sphincter-active area of the urethra tend to recur particularly rapidly.
4. Any form of treatment of a stricture in the sphincter-active urethra carries some risk of further impairment of its functional competence.

It follows that the prime consideration in the management of a postprostatectomy stricture in the distal sphincter mechanism must be the preservation of its residual sphincteric function, rather than the definitive resolution of the stricture itself.

Extent of Coincident Sphincter Damage

There is a wide variation in the extent of sphincter damage associated with strictures in the sphincter-active area of the urethra (Fig. 68-19). On the one hand, the sphincter mechanism may be almost undamaged and supple, the stricture itself resulting largely from a simple denudation of the epithelial lining in this area as a result of abrasion during transurethral surgery or the tight gripping of an indwelling urethral catheter postoperatively. On the other, densely fibrotic membranous urethral strictures are usually associated with severe damage of the intramural sphincter mechanism and tend to result from a more positive urethral injury during the course of an enucleation procedure or a loop resection; the sphincter damage in such cases may be so severe that, had a stricture not developed, the patient would be simply incontinent.

Residual Sphincter Function

Urethral pressure profilometry may give some indication of residual sphincter function but clinically it is rather unreliable. In practice, the best evaluation probably is obtained by simple observation of the results of progressive dilatation. When a membranous stricture is associated with severe sphincter damage, simple recalibration by dilatation to a size as small as 16Fr to 18Fr may render it temporarily incontinent. On the other hand,

FIG.   68-19. Postprostatectomy sphincter strictures: (**A**) supple epithelial denudation stricture with surviving sphincter mechanism; (**B**) rigid stricture with intramural sphincter damage. Supple strictures may be converted to sphincter-damage strictures by aggressive management

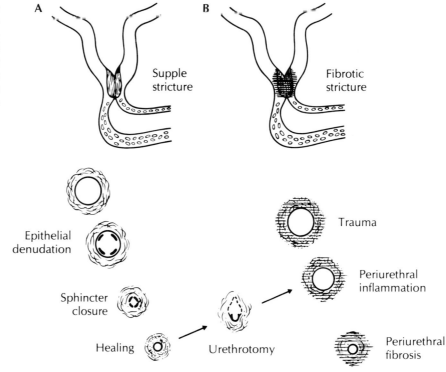

oversize dilatation of a supple stricture with minimal sphincter damage to a caliber of 36Fr to 38Fr results in no significant diminution of urinary control. A trial recalibration can be achieved by a simple passage of dilators when the membranous urethra is exposed by an inlay urethrostomy. The potential dangers of treating postprostatectomy sphincter strictures by internal endoscopic or Otis urethrotomy have already been emphasized.

The definitive resolution of a postprostatectomy sphincter stricture can be considered when the sphincter mechanism has been proven to be functionally efficient by over dilatation or when the indications are increased by a moderately impaired sphincter stricture that proves particularly difficult to manage conservatively by frequently repeated dilatation.

"Push-In" Bulbo–Urethral Resleeving Procedure

When the bulbar urethra is normal, our procedure for the surgical resolution of urethral sphincter is the relatively simple bulbar "push-in" sleeve. It must not be undertaken without most careful consideration and only if the patient accepts that he may be one of the small percentage that becomes incontinent. The push-in operation achieves epithelialization of a supple membranous urethral

stricture with a short sleeve of bulbar urethral uroepithelium supported by a thin cuff of spongy tissue (Fig. 68-20).[18]

Substitution Procedures

When the bulbar urethra is normal, the bulbar sleeve reepithelialization procedure of sphincter stricture is so satisfactory that it is rarely necessary to introduce the additional complication rate inherent in substitution procedures. In general, it is best to avoid two-stage trans-sphincter inlay procedures for sphincter strictures when the bladder neck mechanism is known to be incompetent, because there is always some risk of incontinence, and urinary leakage from a perineal urethrotomy is very difficult to collect.

POSTPROSTATECTOMY BULBO– MEMBRANOUS STRICTURES

Occasionally, a postprostatectomy stricture in the sphincter-active urethra is associated with a stricture of the bulbar urethra resulting from previous urethritis or a postoperative indwelling catheter. The presence of the additional bulbar stricture anteriorly may make the passage of dilators difficult. In such cases a trial of internal urethrotomy for the bulbar element of the stricture may be

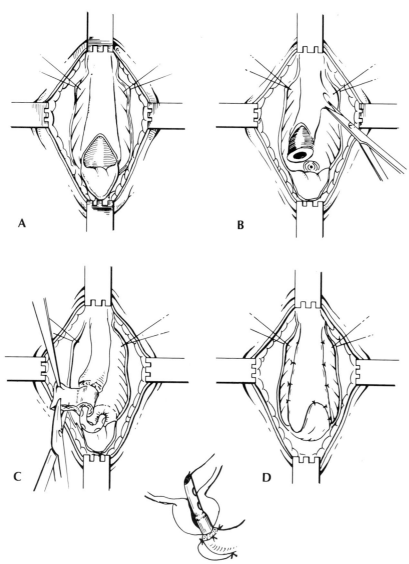

FIG. 68-20. Sphincter-preserving repair of supple sphincter strictures by push-in sleeve reconstruction: **(A)** posterior flap spongioplasty; **(B)** transection and mobilization of bulbar urethra: dilatation of supple sphincter stricture; **(C)** trimming of spongiosum to form urethral sleeve push-in graft; **(D)** transsphincteric sleeve pushed in and retained by spongy-collar sutures and posterior flap spongioplasty. No attachment to sling-stitch–retained fenestrated urethral splint

worthwhile. Inasmuch as it needs to be selective and not to extend into the sphincter-active stricture, it should be achieved endoscopically rather than by the Otis instrument. Even if the bulbar stricture does recur after this procedure, it may facilitate the frequent passage of dilators required for the conservative management of a precarious sphincter stricture.

The bulbar element of a combined bulbar and membranous postprostatectomy stricture is unsuitable for internal urethrotomy if it is associated with periurethral inflammation. In such cases it may be best to proceed to a definitive two-stage scrotourethral inlay combination repair of the *bulbar* element of the stricture, specifically avoiding extending this into the sphincter-active urethra so

that the sphincter element can be reassessed by overdilatation during the interval stage, thus avoiding the immediate risk of incontinence.

PELVIC FRACTURE STRICTURES

In the adult male about 10% of pelvic fractures have a coincident urethral injury that is almost always located in the 2 cm of sphincter-active segment distal to the apex of the prostate. All but the most minor pelvic fracture injuries to the subprostatic urethra destroy its sphincteric competence; the majority of partial tears and virtually all complete ruptures result in a stricture.

Simple Strictures. However, most pelvic fracture injuries do not result in wide separation of

FIG. 68 21. Development of pelvic fracture urethral strictures

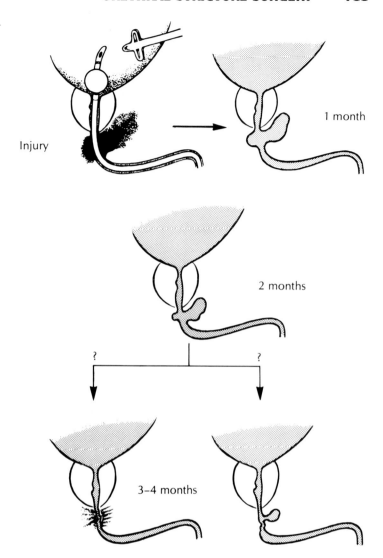

Injury

1 month

2 months

?   ?

3–4 months

the ruptured urethral ends; hence, the common end result, after healing, is a short stricture, 1 cm to 1.5 cm long. Furthermore, the periurethral hematoma associated with a minimal dislocation tends to be confined by the boundaries of the preurethral subpubic-arch space; its upward extension is often limited by intact puboprostatic ligaments (Fig. 68-21). Such urethral strictures associated with a well-localized hematoma fibrosis are conveniently designated as "simple" because they can usually be resolved conservatively or by a definitive one-stage excision and anastomosis through a perineal approach.[15]

In summary, the end result of a minimal pelvic fracture urethral injury may be as follows (Fig. 68-22):[15]

1. No stricture and no sphincter injury

2. Distal sphincter damage without stricture formation (not an unusual result of a partial urethral injury) with the patient likely to become incontinent after subsequent prostatectomy

3. A short simple stricture almost invariably associated with loss or severe impairment of sphincter function

Complex Strictures. Pelvic fracture injuries may result in severe prostatic-dislocation injuries and development of a large hematoma between the widely distracted urethral ends. If this is not reduced appropriately, the common end result of healing is likely to be the formation of a complex stricture (*inserts,* Fig. 68-22) with one or more of the following characteristics, the definitive resolution of which requires a transpubic approach:[15,19]

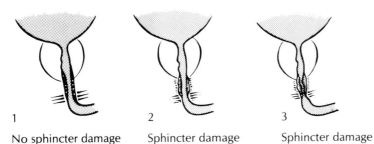

1 — No sphincter damage / No stricture

2 — Sphincter damage / No stricture

3 — Sphincter damage / Short stricture

4 / Complex strictures

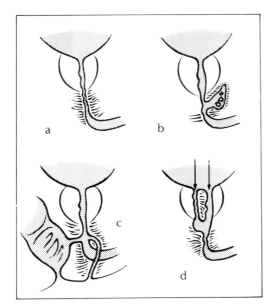

FIG. 68-22. End results of pelvic fracture urethral injuries

1. A long stricture surrounded by dense hematoma fibrosis
2. A periurethral cavity that frequently contains calculi
3. Rectal or cutaneous fistulas into the perineum or suprapubic area
4. False passages into the bladder base
5. Incompetence of the only remaining sphincter mechanism at the bladder neck, which may result either from coincident or incidental damage or from simple tethering due to an extensive retropubic hematoma fibrosis

Management of Simple Strictures

Simple, short, pelvic fracture strictures do not necessarily require a definitive surgical repair. Some can be resolved by internal urethrotomy but when they are longer than about 1 cm, they are characteristically surrounded by a commensurate thickness of dense hematoma fibrosis. Because this fibrosis does not tend to ''open up'' when it is incised by a knife, a carefully localized transurethral resection using a small loop is more likely to succeed.

A subprostatic pelvic fracture urethral stricture can almost always be repaired by a one-stage bulbo–prostatic anastomosis if the bulbar urethra is normal. Simple strictures can be repaired by a perineal procedure, whereas the complicating fractures of a complex stricture require a synchronous retropubic or transpubic approach. Even for complex strictures, the results of anastomotic repair can be so good, and the stricture recurrence rate so low, that the additional complications inherent in a substitution repair are difficult to justify.[15,19]

Management of Complex Strictures

Preoperative Evaluation and Considerations. The basic investigation for a posterior urethral stricture is a synchronous voiding cystogram and a retrograde urethrogram. Properly performed, this combination outlines most of the features that identify a complex pelvic-fracture

FIG. 68-23. Technique of fixed-flat spatulated bulboprostatic anastomosis

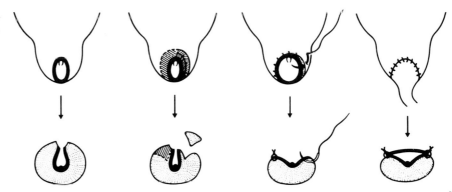

stricture. However, a stricture that appears short and simple on preoperative radiography may prove to require a retropubic or transpubic procedure when it is assessed at operation. It invites disaster to embark upon a perineal procedure for an apparently simple stricture without proper preparation for an immediate abdomino–perineal procedure, because mobilization of the bulbar urethra is more than likely to compromise an appropriate transpubic procedure performed at a later date.

Because the 2-cm portion of prostatic urethra distal to the verumontanum seems to be protected from injury by the adult prostatic tissue, this section of the urethra is almost always available for a definitive anastomosis to the mobilized urethra without compromising the bladder neck sphincter mechanism proximal to the verumontanum. In our experience, based on the resolution of more than 350 pelvic fracture strictures, it is almost invariably possible to achieve a stricture-free, one-stage anastomotic repair if the bulbar urethra is not badly damaged. The remarkable reliability of this procedure, which far exceeds that of substitution procedures, depends upon a number of principles and techniques and the ability of the surgeon to adjust the procedure appropriately according to the findings at the time of operation.

The success of a bulbo–prostatic anastomotic procedure depends upon the following:

1. A spatulated 2-cm overlap of normal-ends caliber; the opposing suture lines are spread apart to prevent cross-adhesion during healing.
2. Preparation of the distal prostatic urethra for anastomosis; irrespective of whether the bulbo–prostatic anastomosis is achieved from above or below, the spatulation of its distal segment requires a small wedge resection of the lateral apical tissue before its lateral fixation (Fig. 68-23).[15]
3. Spatulation of the posterior bulbar urethra for

anastomosis. Because the posterior bulbar urethra lies eccentrically within the spongy tissue, its spatulation requires the removal of the excess of spongy tissue on its posterolateral surface. This tissue is best separated and left *in situ* as a posteriorly based spongioplasty flap that can be used as an overclosure layer to support the bulbo–prostatic anastomosis.[15]

4. Mobilization of the bulbar urethra. About 3 cm to 4 cm of elastic lengthening can be obtained by mobilizing a normal bulbar urethra and this is sufficient for the anastomotic repair of almost all pelvic fracture strictures. Long strictures may require a transpubic rerouting of the mobilized bulbar urethra over one crus to enable it to reach a high-lying prostate. The urethra receives its main blood supply from the bulbar vessels entering posteriorly; however, if its collateral spongy-tissue vascular communications with the penile urethra and glans are intact, it can be divided at the bulbo–membranous junction without compromising its survival. Mobilization of the penile urethra anterior to the bulbopenile junction may compromise its retrograde blood supply and tends to result in a penile-curvature chordee, owing to its lack of excess elasticity during an erection.

5. Whether it is achieved by the perineal or the transpubic route, a spatulated overlap anastomosis between a 30Fr bulbar urethra and the apical prostatic urethra of similar caliber produces an anastomotic caliber of about 60Fr; hence, a satisfactory postoperative urethrogram shows a characteristic anastomotic dilatation that overtly excludes anastomotic narrowing (Fig. 68-24). The anastomosis is best achieved by 3 × 0 polyglycolic-acid sutures which include an anchor bite of lateral periurethral tissue to spread the tissue apart; the knots are tied on the lumen, when possible, so that they fall off and are voided.

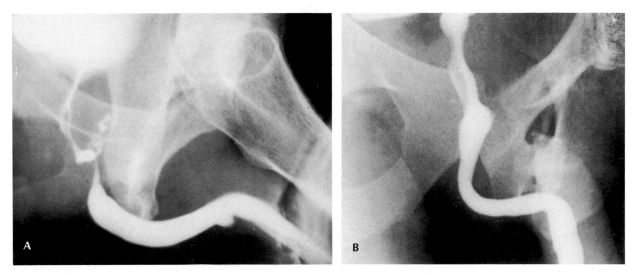

FIG. 68-24.   Pelvic fracture stricture **(A)** before and **(B)** after a spatulated bulboprostatic repair. Note the increased anastomotic caliber created by 30Fr + 30Fr overlap spatulation

FIG. 68-25.   Mobilization of omental pedicle graft for supporting abdomino–perineal anastomotic repair of pelvic fracture strictures: **(A)** long apron is separated from the mesocolon.   **(B)** moderate apron is mobilized by dividing left pedicle vessels.   **(C)** short apron is mobilized on right gastro–epiploic vessels

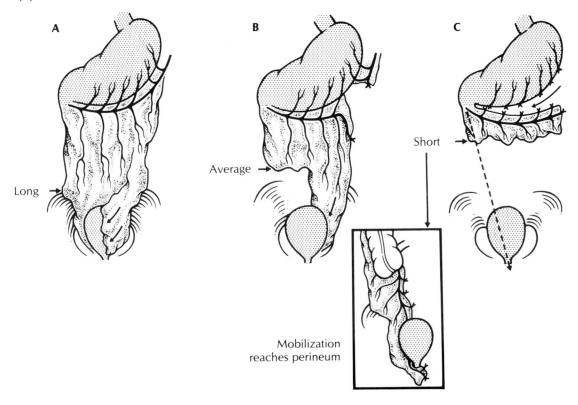

6. Removal of the periurethral hematoma fibrosis and obliteration of the para-anastomotic dead space. In our opinion it is important to remove the anterior and distal paraprostatic hematoma fibrosis and any contained fistulous tracts associated with a complex stricture; this inevitably leaves a fibro-osseous perianastomotic dead space that is an obvious source of infection, postoperative fistula, and recurrent stricture formation. Obliteration of this space with an omental pedicle graft is important in avoiding postoperative complications (Fig. 68-25).[17] Formal mobilization of the omental vascular pedicle is necessary when its apron is not long enough to reach the pelvis; the access for this requires a midline abdominal incision and the technique, which requires meticulous care, is detailed elsewhere.

7. Postoperative catheter management. It is recommended that, in conjunction with a suprapubic catheter, a sling-stitch–retained, 16Fr fenestrated plastic catheter be used routinely after an anastomotic repair to ensure positive drainage of the exudates and to facilitate postoperative contrast verification of anastomotic healing before its removal.

Positioning the patient in the flat legs-apart table position (Fig. 68-26)[15] enables the surgeon to move from the perineum to the abdomen and back as often as necessary in the course of an operation, making this position as ideal for the resolution of a pelvic fracture stricture as it is for a vesico–vaginal fistula. A combined abdomino–perineal approach is often required for the resolution of a pelvic fracture stricture and it is rarely possible to rule out the need for it even when the stricture is short, because the periurethral hematoma fibrosis may prove unexpectedly extensive at operation.

Perineal Procedure. A simple midline perineal incision provides the best access for exploration of an apparently simple bulbo–prostatic pelvic fracture stricture and bulbar urethral mobilization. Posterolateral horseshoe extensions behind the apex of the prostate may increase the risk of impotence, because the nervi erigentes lie in the perineal body in close posterolateral proximity to the membranous urethra. When repair is achieved by a perineal procedure, cystoscopy is important to identify and remove any intravesical calculous debris that might otherwise impact in the urethra. A descending sound may be helpful for the unequivocal identification of the prostatic urethra.

The feasibility of a perineal procedure cannot finally be assessed until the bulbar urethra has been mobilized and detached; the anterior peri-

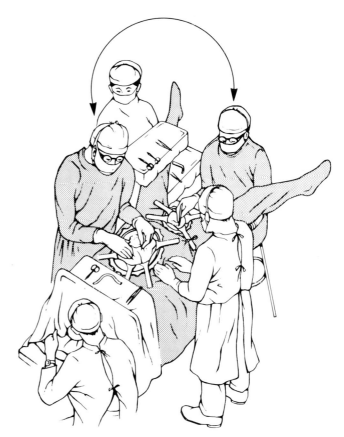

FIG. 68-26. Positioning of patient for repair of posterior urethral strictures

urethral fibrosis, excised; and the apical prostatic urethra, spatulated. If this results in a perineal tunnel that extends to supple paraprostatic tissue and that is not too capacious to be filled by the inlaid bulbar urethra, then a perineal procedure alone is appropriate.

After the completion of a perineal anastomosis, oblique tension-relieving sutures should be inserted between the sides of the mobilized bulbar urethra and the crura to prevent distraction of the anastomosis by a postoperative erection. A tight sensory ligament may be divided to reduce the tendency toward angulation chordee.

Retropubic Procedure. The retropubic procedure has been developed for the resolution of short strictures associated with unexpectedly extensive retropubic fibrosis.[22] After preparation for a perineal anastomosis, the retropubic fibrosis is removed through a midline abdominal incision, but no pubic resection is required for access to the prostatic apex because the anastomosis is achieved from below. After the removal of the retropubic fibrosis, the omental apron is mobilized so that it

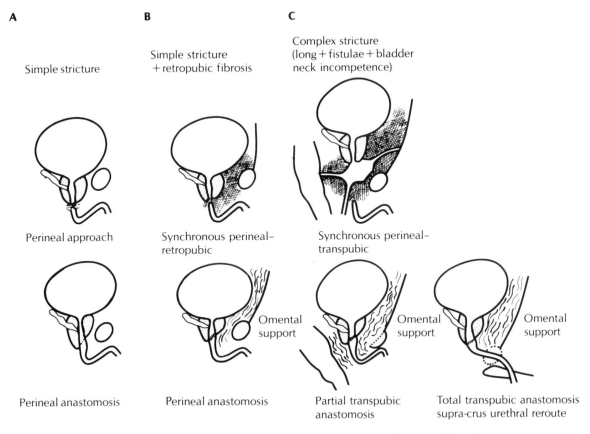

A   Simple stricture

B   Simple stricture
+ retropubic fibrosis

C   Complex stricture
(long + fistulae + bladder
neck incompetence)

Perineal approach

Synchronous perineal–
retropubic

Synchronous perineal–
transpubic

Perineal anastomosis

Perineal anastomosis

Partial transpubic
anastomosis

Total transpubic anastomosis
supra-crus urethral reroute

Omental
support

Omental
support

Omental
support

FIG. 68-27. Anastomotic repair of pelvic fracture strictures: **(A)** perineal repair of simple strictures; **(B)** retropubic repair of short strictures with extensive retropubic fibrosis with omental support; **(C)** partial and total transpubic repair of complex strictures with omental support

can be interposed and pulled through to support the perineal anastomosis. This retropubic procedure is a relatively simple extension of a perineal bulbo–prostatic method which has improved the resolution of the intermediate simple/complex procedures (Fig. 68-27*B*).

Transpubic Procedure. Our preferred technique for the resolution of complex pelvic fracture strictures (Fig. 68-27*C*) differs in some details from that described by Waterhouse and colleagues:[15,24]

1. An abdomino–perineal position is used, rather than the frog-leg abdominal approach; the operation is always started, and often completed, from the perineum.
2. A wide access to the apex of the prostate is obtained by partial removal of the upper and posterior border of the pubis using a Capener's double-curved gouge; this is preferred to the V-shaped access obtained by removing the whole pubis with a Gigli saw. Removal of the whole

pubis is sometimes necessary, particularly when the bulbar urethra has to be rerouted over one crus to reach a particularly high prostate. However, this further extension is also easily achieved with the Capener's gouge.

3. The whole extent of the hematoma fibrosis anterior, lateral, and distal to the prostate is excised rather than bypassed.
4. The fibro-osseous dead space around the anastomosis is filled with omental pedicle graft, and we believe that the reliability of the procedure is fundamentally improved in this way.[15,17]

The variations of a complex fracture stricture are such that there can be no predetermined, set procedure. The removal of the hematoma fibrosis and any fistulous tracts or abscess cavities in it is relatively straightforward. A synchronous repair of a rectal fistula does not complicate the procedure significantly. The point of entry into the rectum is usually quite small and, once the main track has

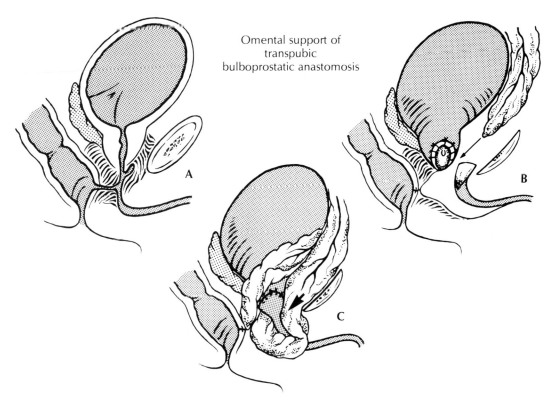

Omental support of
transpubic
bulboprostatic anastomosis

FIG. 68-28. Simultaneous anastomotic repair of pelvic fracture stricture and closure of an associated rectal fistula with omental pedicle graft

been opened widely into the paraprostatic transpubic cavity, formal closure is rarely required; the omental graft supporting the anastomosis closes it and the procedure is covered postoperatively by a colostomy (Fig. 68-28). Narrow false passages into the bladder base usually close after simple curettage; but those that are wider or associated with abscess ramifications require formal exposure and closure.

Subprostatic Strictures with Anterior Urethral Abnormalities

Abnormalities of the bulbo–penile spongy tissue may critically compromise the resolution of a subprostatic pelvic fracture stricture by bulbo–prostatic anastomosis because of impairment of the tissue's distal collateral blood supply. It is unusual for an anterior urethra to be damaged at the time of a pelvic injury; more often a compromising spongiofibrosis is the result of a preexisting urethritis, a catheter stricture, or previous surgical attempts to resolve the stricture. Vascular continuity between the glans and the penile urethra is congenitally absent in all but the mildest forms of hypospadias.

Abnormalities of the anterior spongy tissue are not an absolute contraindication to bulbo–prostatic anastomosis; each case must be assessed on its merits. However, particular caution relating to the extent of bulbar urethral mobilization is necessary. Remobilization of the anterior urethra after a previous failure of an anastomotic procedure can be very difficult. It can be disastrous to attempt a potentially reliable subspecialist procedure without appropriate training and experience.

All substitution procedures carry an inherent failure rate, quite apart from the difficulties of establishing any graft on dense fibrous tissue. However, a variety of *ad hoc* combination procedures may be useful, including the pedicled urethral island bladder graft technique, which specifically avoids compromising an intact bladder neck mechanism.[14]

Evaluation of Success— Calibration versus Flow Rate

Two distinct criteria are used for the evaluation of the results of operative procedures for urethral strictures: A truly successful urethral reconstruc-

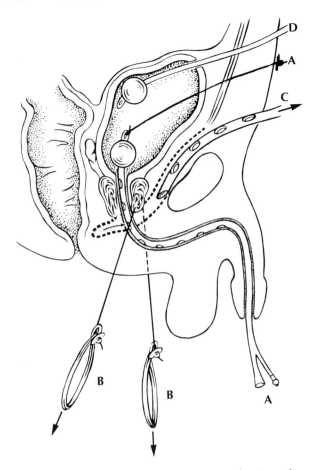

FIG. 68-29. The immediate operative reduction of severely dislocated pelvic fracture urethral injuries after retropubic evacuation of hematoma: fenestrated urethral catheter stenting drain retained with abdominal wall sling-stitch (**a**), elastic band traction on nylon prostato–perineal reduction sling-stitch (**b**), retropubic suction drainage (**c**), suprapubic catheter (**d**)

tion should recreate a tube of even caliber that calibrates to normal size; such a state of affairs cannot be proven urodynamically because a recording flowmeter, while an important instrument for the evaluation of patients both before and after urethral reconstruction, is only appropriate as a screening test for the identification of bladder outlet obstruction. A rigid stricture can stenose to a caliber of about 10Fr before it impairs the voiding flow rate significantly.[10] Furthermore, a patient's stricture may not be the only cause of outlet obstruction. Therefore, retrograde urethrography is important in the diagnosis and the follow-up of all cases, especially when flow studies identify a significant outlet obstruction in the absence of a rigid urethral stenosis.

IMPOTENCE

Impotence may result from a pelvic fracture injury even if the urethra was not injured; the incidence is higher if the urethra is injured, and higher still if the prostate and bladder base are greatly dislocated.

The studies of Moorehouse and associates showed that impotence is more frequent in patients with pelvic fracture urethral injuries treated by primary repair; this is one good reason for avoiding such a procedure in the management of minimal dislocation injuries. However, a major dislocation injury is almost always associated with impotence and usually results in a complex stricture. In our opinion such a situation is best treated by early repositioning (not a primary repair), maintaining urethral reapproximation around a fenestrated urethral stent by an elastic anchoring of a single stitch (Fig. 68-29). This usually avoids the development of a complex stricture situation and is unlikely to increase the already high chance of impotence in such cases.

The results of treating pelvic fracture impotence by insertion of a penile prosthesis are generally satisfactory, because orgasm usually survives the injury and ejaculation is usually restored by resolution of the subprostatic stricture. However, special care is necessary in the insertion of these prostheses, particularly if the urethra has been rerouted over the crus. One crus, and sometimes both, may be damaged or destroyed by the pubic fracture injury; it is important to anticipate this possibility, both because some prostheses cannot be foreshortened to penile length without exposing their core material and because the cavernosal space, once developed, will obliterate if an appropriate "keeper" is not available. All that is necessary in this circumstance is a simple Silastic rod of penile length, irrespective of the type used on the "normal" side.

Conclusion

Few strictures are resolved, in the long term, by simple dilatation. Nevertheless, intermittent dilatation may be the best form of treatment for some strictures and some patients.

Some strictures, particularly those located in the bulbar urethra, may be resolved or dilated more easily after the general urologic procedure of internal urethrotomy. Provided that the potential disasters of extending the urethrotomy into the sphincter-active area of the membranous and supramembranous urethra are avoided, patients have little to lose and sometimes much to gain by a trial of this approach.

Strictures in the sphincter-active urethra require special consideration, but almost all urethral strictures can be resolved by some form of definitive urethroplasty with the expectation of a dilatation-free result. However, a failed surgical attempt to resolve a stricture, whether by internal urethrotomy or a definitive procedure, almost always makes a subsequent definitive procedure more difficult, and damage to the distal urethral sphincter mechanism is virtually irreparable.

The problems of urethral stricture surgery should not be underestimated. A surgeon interested in urethral reconstruction must adopt a variety of procedures to meet a wide range of problems and must have an aptitude for the minutiae of plastic surgical techniques, an appropriate period of specialist training, personal experience and understanding of video-urodynamic sphincter evaluation, and the opportunity for an ongoing, in-depth practice.

Unfortunately, it is all but impossible to convey surgical technique and judgment meaningfully in a written description.

REFERENCES

1. ARNOLD EP: Bladder Outlet Obstruction in the Male: A Urological Analysis of the Detrusor Response, Ph.D. thesis, London University, 1980; and in Turner Warwick R, Whitcorde CG (eds): Urol Clin North Am, Vol 6, 1979
2. BLANDY JP, SINGH M, TRESSIDER GC: Urethroplasty by scrotal flap for long urethral strictures. Br J Urol 40:261, 1968
3. CHILTON CP, TURNER WARWICK RT: The relationship of the distal sphincter mechanism to the pelvic floor musculature. Br J Urol (to be published)
4. DEVINE CJ, HORTON CE: One-stage hypospadias repair. J Urol 85:166, 1961
5. GIBBON NOK: A new type of catheter for urethral urinary drainage. Br J Urol 30:1, 1958
6. GIL–VERNET JM: Chirurgie de retrecissement de l'urethre. In Auvigne J (ed): Encyclopedie Medico Chirurgicale. Paris, Presse Medicale, 1967
7. MOREHOUSE DD, BELITSKY P, MACKINNON KJ: Rupture of the posterior urethra. J Urol 107:255, 1972
8. ORANDI A: One-stage urethroplasty: Four year follow-up. J Urol 107:977, 1972
9. RUSSELL RH: The treatment of urethral stricture by excision. Br J Surg 2:375, 1914
10. SMITH J: The measurement and significance of urinary flow. Br J Urol 30:701, 1966
11. STEPHENSON TP, TURNER WARWICK RT: A long term follow-up of 100 consecutive cases of scroto-urethral inlay urethroplasty. Br J Urol (to be published)
12. TURNER WARWICK RT: A technique for posterior urethroplasty. J Urol 83:416, 1960
13. TURNER WARWICK RT: The repair of urethral strictures in the region of the membranous urethra. J Urol 100:303, 1968
14. TURNER WARWICK RT: The use of pedicle grafts in the repair of urinary tract fistulae. Br J Urol 44:644, 1972
15. TURNER WARWICK RT: The management of traumatic urethral strictures and injuries. Br J Surg 60:775, 1973
16. TURNER WARWICK RT: The complications of urethral surgery in the male. Smith RB, Skinner DG (eds): Complications of Urologic Surgery. New York, WB Saunders, 1976
17. TURNER WARWICK, RT: The use of the omental pedicle graft in urinary tract reconstruction. J Urol 116:341, 1976
18. TURNER WARWICK RT: The sphincter preserving "push in sleeve" bulboprostatic anastomosis. In Rob G, Smith R, Innes Williams DI (eds): Operative Surgery, 3rd ed. London, Butterfield, 1977
19. TURNER WARWICK RT: Complex traumatic strictures. J Urol 118:564, 1977
20. TURNER WARWICK RT, WHITESIDE G: Clinical urodynamics. Urol Clin North Am 6:13, 1979
21. TURNER WARWICK RT: Observations upon techniques for reconstruction of the urethral meatus, the hypospadias glans deformity of the penile urethra. Urol Clin North Am 6:643, 1979
22. TURNER WARWICK RT: Lower urinary tract reconstruction. In Bevan G (ed): Reconstructive Surgery. London, Blackwell, 1981
23. TURNER WARWICK RT: The sphincter mechanisms; their relation to prostatic enlargement and its treatment. In Hinman F, Chisholm GD (eds): Benign Prostatic Hypertrophy. Berlin, Springer-Verlag, 1982
24. WATERHOUSE K, ABRAMS J, GRUBER H et al: Transpubic approach to the lower urinary tract. J Urol 109:486, 1973

Urethral Fistula and Diverticula

69

Kenneth A. Kropp

The surgical treatment of urethral diverticula and fistulas will be dealt with in this chapter following an initial discussion of certain anatomic considerations. Because the etiology, symptoms, diagnostic tests, and treatment are different in the male and female and in adults and children, each disease entity will be discussed as it relates to the male, the female, and children. The size and the complexity of the lesions differ from patient to patient. We will try to discuss the simplest approach first, followed by a more complex approach to the more complex problem. The operations described in the text are listed in the references and do not constitute a complete list. Some procedures have been performed by our staff; others have not. For more exact details of each procedure, the reader is referred to the original article.

Anatomy

A thorough knowledge of the anatomy of the male and the female urethra and perineum is essential when performing surgery in this area. The female perineum can be conveniently divided into an anterior urogenital triangle and a posterior anal triangle (Figs. 69-1 and 69-2).[3] The urogenital part of the perineum contains the urethra and vaginal opening. The urethral meatus is a vertical slitlike or irregularly ovoid opening about 4 mm to 5 mm in diameter located 2 cm to 3 cm below the clitoris. About the orifice are several minute cryptlike openings, the minor vestibular glands, which are homologues of Littre's glands in the male urethra. Numerous paraurethral ducts empty into the distal one third of the urethra. These ducts and their terminal divisions form an extensive branching mass of tubular channels and glandular elements which are widely distributed in the tissue about the urethral canal and open into it. In most individuals the orifices of two large paraurethral ducts (Skene's ducts) will be found near the meatus at the 3 and 9 o'clock positions.

The length of the urethra varies between 3 cm and 5 cm and assumes an angle of about 15 degrees upward with the meatus. The lower two thirds of the urethra is difficult to separate from the anterior vaginal wall because of the lack of the pubocervical vesical fascia. The urethra is held in position beneath the pubic symphysis by several important structures, the first and most superficial of which is the urogenital diaphragm. The urogenital diaphragm lies in the same plane as the pubic rami at the pelvic outlet. This diaphragm is composed of a superficial and deep layer of fascia attached to the inner aspect of the pubic arch, and enclosing a slitlike compartment termed the deep perineal compartment. In this compartment, between the two fascial layers, lies the deep transverse perineal muscle (sometimes called the sphincter urethra) and pudendal nerves and vessels. The superior fascia of the urogenital diaphragm arises from the pubic bone and forms bilateral bands that narrow somewhat and spread out upon reaching the urethral wall. These bands insert firmly into the urethra and might well be called the pubourethral ligaments. They hold the urethra firmly attached to the undersurface of the pubic symphysis. These bands bound a tiny cul-de-sac anterior to the urethra through which the perineal veins communicate with the pelvic venous plexus. This cul-de-sac, oval in outline, about 1.5 cm in width and about 0.8 cm in length, constitutes a retropubic hiatus of the urogenital diaphragm.

The deep transverse perineal muscle is the arbitrarily separable posterior part of the musculature of the urogenital diaphragm which is situated deep to the superficial transverse perinei muscle (Fig. 53-1B). The deep transverse perinei muscle passes across the perineum behind the vaginal orifice and then sends muscle fibers into the rectum and posteriorly behind the rectum into the coccyx. The other muscular structure, which is the arbitrarily separable anterior portion, is termed by some investigators the sphincter urethra. This muscle arises from the inner surface of the ischiopubic rami and passes medially. It sends muscle slips into the urethral wall and into the vagina, the anal

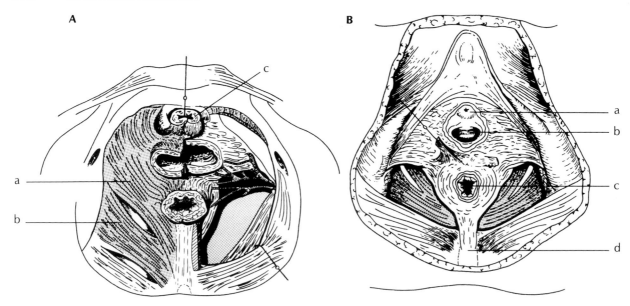

FIG. 69-1.   **(A)** The female pelvis is viewed from above. The pubococcygeus **(a)** and the iliococcygeus **(b)** muscles have been removed from the right half of the drawing, and the urogenital diaphragm is exposed. The urethra **(c)** is being drawn forward and demonstrates the attachments of the pubococcygeus to it.   **(B)** The urogenital diaphragm is viewed from below. The superficial transverse perineal muscle has been removed and is being held upward by a hook. The urogenital diaphragm is demonstrated with its fibers inserting into the urethra **(a)**, the vagina **(b)**, the rectum **(c)**, and the coccyx **(d)**. A portion of the pelvic diaphragm is seen beneath the inferior edge of the urogenital diaphragm.

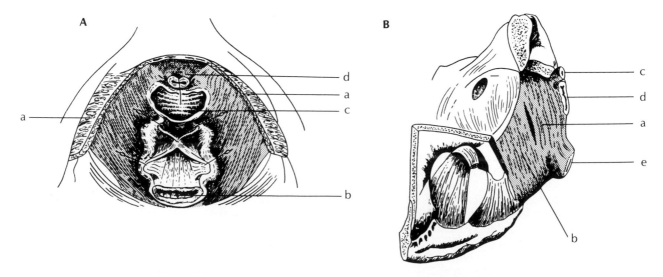

FIG. 69-2.   **(A)** The female perineum is viewed from below. The urogenital diaphragm **(a)** has been removed except for a narrow strip of attachment on both ischiopubic rami. The pelvic diaphragm has been incised in the midline from the anal **(b)** to the vaginal **(c)** canal. Note how the urethra receives special fibers from the pelvic diaphragm (at **d**).   **(B)** The superior pubic ramus and the body of the ischium have been removed to expose the pubic and ischial attachments of the pubococcygeus **(a)** and the iliococcygeus **(b)** muscles. Note how these fibers insert into the urethra **(c)**, the vagina **(d)**, and the rectum **(e)**.

canal, and the coccyx. The term sphincter urethrae implies that this muscle might encircle the urethra in a ringlike manner and serve a sphincteric function. The outline of the urogenital diaphragm is then quadrangular and not triangular, although the muscular fibers surround and insert into the urethra, the vagina, and the anal canal and may serve a sphincter function. The main function of this urogenital diaphragm seems to be supportive.

The pelvic diaphragm, lying deep to the urogenital diaphragm and in a slightly different plane, is the most important structure providing support. The pelvic diaphragm is composed of superior and inferior fascial layer with an interposed layer of muscle. The pelvic diaphragm divides the pelvic cavity above from the perineum below. The muscular layer is composed of two pairs of muscles: the levatores ani and the coccygei. From the pelvic wall on either side these muscles pass downward toward the midline, there to meet each other and to fuse, or to surround the terminal portions of the rectum, the vagina, and the urethra. The pubococcygeus portion of the levator ani muscle arises along the bone and tendinous arch and inserts not only into the coccyx as its name implies, but also into the urethra, the vagina, and the rectum. The muscular slips that pass into the urethra do so on its posterolateral aspect and intermingle with the urethral wall. The muscle is deficient only in an area immediately behind the pubic symphysis where there is a retropubic hiatus for the transmission of the dorsal clitoral vessels.

The urethra itself is of endodermal and mesodermal origin. Hutch has shown that the female urethra is made up primarily of components represented in the bladder.[7] The deep trigonal musculature rolls into a tube and continues down the urethra as the middle circular muscle layer of the urethra (Fig. 69-3). The middle circular muscle layers of the bladder terminate at the bladder neck in a thickened ring to form what has been termed the fundus ring (Fig. 69-4). At the base of the bladder this middle circular layer is fused with the deep trigonal musculature. The trigone, which is derived from mesonephric (wolffian) duct structures, can easily be divided into a superficial and deep layer. The tubularization of the deep trigone in the region of the proximal urethra is incomplete arteriorly for about 0.1 cm to 0.5 cm, and it is at this point where the detrusor loop of middle circular muscle fibers comes into position.

These smooth muscle components of the urethra are also mixed with a striated muscle component from the urogenital diaphragm. In addition, longitudinally oriented periurethral striated muscle,

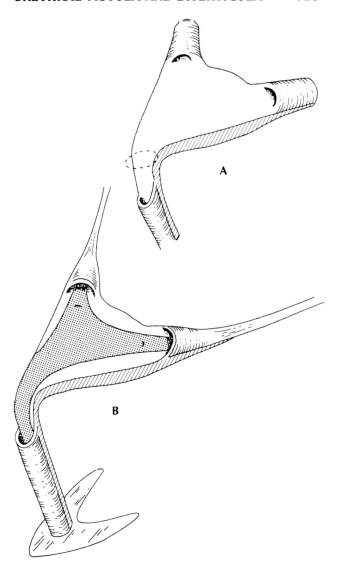

FIG. 69-3. A deep trigone rolls into a tube at its craniolateral borders (Waldeyer's sheath) and its caudal end (core structure of the urethra). **(A)** The *dotted line* is the bladder neck. A superficial trigone (*stipled area*), a continuation of the ureteral smooth muscle, lies on top of the trigone in **B**.

probably originating from the deep transverse perineal or pubococcygeus musculature, can be demonstrated. The striated muscle inserts into and mixes with the smooth muscle and connective tissue structures of the urethra only about halfway anteriorly, but can be identified to the bladder neck posteriorly. This posterior component, however, is quite thin and is difficult to identify on dissection.

The bladder is surrounded by endopelvic fascia which is continuous with the superior fascia of the

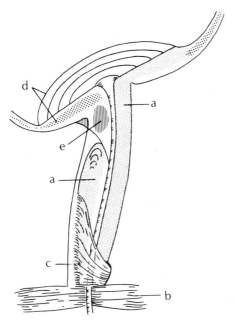

FIG. 69-4. Midsagittal section. **(a)** A deep trigone makes up the core structure of the urethra. **(b)** and **(c)** The external sphincter and paraurethral striated muscles are shown. **(d)** The fundus ring is actually the thickened middle circular bladder muscle above the bladder neck. **(e)** Just below the bladder neck are additional circularly oriented smooth muscle bundles derived from the posterior outer longitudinal muscle layer of the bladder—the detrusor loop.

pelvic diaphragm. The proximal one third of the urethra will remain separate from the anterior vaginal wall by the continuation of the loose connective tissue which actually envelops the vagina and rectum and is called the pubocervical vesical fascia or the cervico vaginal fascia. Recognition of the intimate association of the urethra and the vaginal wall leads to a better understanding of how vaginal and other gynecologic problems, including hormonal influences on the vaginal wall, may also affect the urethra and produce difficult-to-explain symptoms.

Although the urethra receives its blood supply in segments, there is a free anastomosis between each source. The proximal urethra receives its primary blood supply from anastomotic vessels in the bladder wall. The distal urethra receives direct branches from the inferior vesical artery as it courses along the superior lateral aspect of the vagina supplying both the urethra and the anterior vaginal wall. Distal blood supply to the urethral wall comes from the ischiocavernosus, bulbocavernosus, and clitoral arteries. The venous drainage

is proximal through the inferior, middle, and superior vesical veins and distal through the clitoral venous plexus.

Nerves supplying the urethra originate from the hypogastric plexus. Lymphatic drainage of the urethra is also segmental and drains primarily into four main trunks. Drainage from the anterior two thirds is into the vestibular plexus and then into the superficial and deep inguinal nodes. The proximal urethra has three directions of flow. The anterior superior portion lymphatics course into the anterior bladder wall and the external iliac chain. The lateral regions drain into the internal iliac, external iliac, and obturator group. The posterior region drains into the posterior surface of the bladder and ureters.

Bulbocavernous muscles lie lateral to the urethra at the external meatus. They originate from the central tendinous line and mix with fibers of the ischiocavernosus muscles. The latter muscles arise along the medial aspect of the ischiatic ramus and ensheath the crus of the clitoris anteriorly and superiorly, whereas inferiorly they course over the urethra in the midline. The urethra contains three types of epithelium: squamous at its meatus, pseudostratified columnar through its middle portion, and transitional at the bladder neck and proximal urethra. A beautiful anatomic description of the paraurethral glands is provided by Huffman.[6] These glands extend almost back to the bladder neck, but usually open into the distal urethra. The paired Skene's glands lying on either side of the urethra have their ducts opening at the 3 and 9 o'clock positions and can be easily identified in most individuals.

The anatomy of the male urethra and perineum is much less controversial than that of the female, and the reader is referred to a standard anatomic text for a description. As an aid to surgery and for ready reference, Figures 69-5 and 69-6 demonstrate the anatomically surgical important structures that need to be reviewed prior to operations on the male urethra.

Urethral Diverticula

MALES

Male urethral diverticula are nearly always acquired. They can occur in the distal penile urethra, usually at the penoscrotal junction, or in the deep urethra (Fig. 69-7A). They are commonest in the paraplegic patient or those who are required to wear an indwelling Foley catheter. In these in-

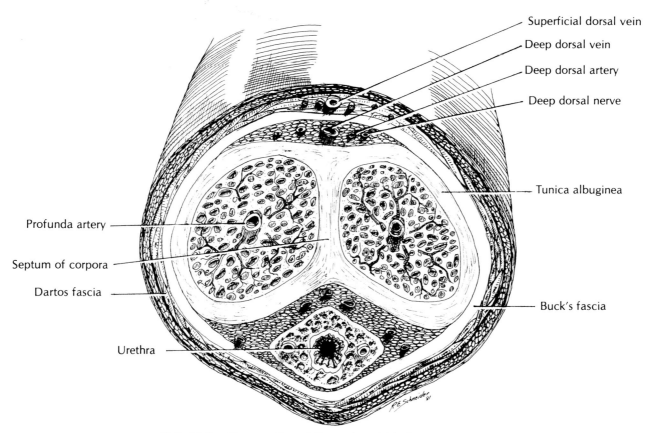

FIG. 69-5. Cross section of the penis, midshaft

FIG. 69-6. Superficial and deep structure of the male perineum

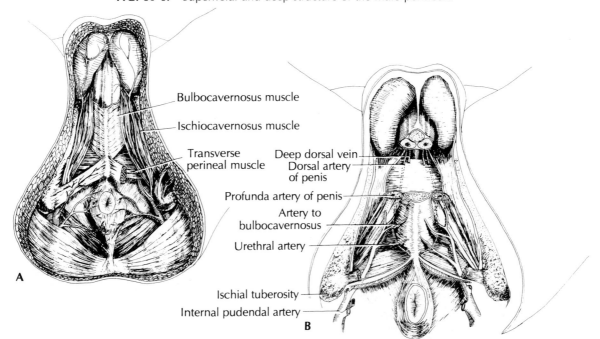

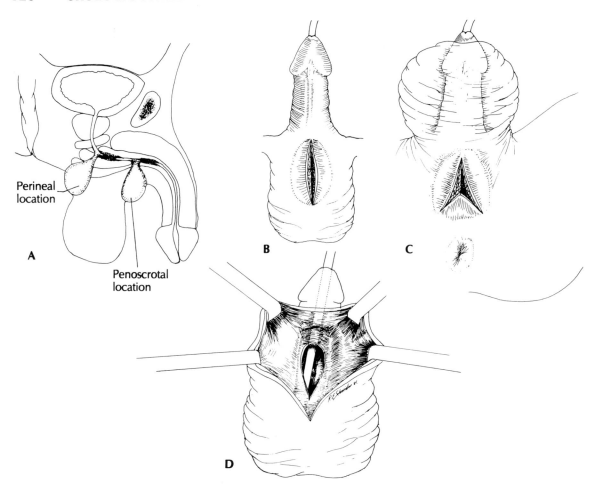

FIG. 69-7. **(A)** Penoscrotal and perineal diverticula. **(B)** A longitudinal incision is made over the penoscrotal diverticulum. **(C)** Either a midline or an inverted-Y incision can be made over the perineal diverticulum. **(D)** The diverticulum has been excised, and the urethral defect is closed with the interrupted absorbable sutures.

stances, because of the S-shaped bend of the male urethra, catheters that are taped to the thigh produce pressure necrosis of the urethral epithelium at the penoscrotal junction and subsequent urinary extravasation. From this a periurethral abscess may form. Drainage outward will result in a urethrocutaneous fistula, whereas drainage back into the urethra will create a urethral diverticulum. Other common causes of urinary extravasation leading to abscess, which causes diverticulum formation are stricture diseases, use of the Cunningham clamp, external condum catheters, and trauma.

The diverticular cavities can be lined with either urethral epithelium or infected granulation tissue. When the condition is diagnosed in the acute stages, they present exactly as does a periurethral

abscess, with pain and swelling over the infected diverticulum and a drainage of purulent material from the urethral meatus. If seen at a later time, the patient will frequently complain of a bulging on the undersurface of the penis or in the perineum after urination, along with postmicturition dribbling. On physical examination a bulging mass can be detected on the undersurface of the urethra, and many times urine or purulent material can be expressed from the mass and collected at the urethral meatus. The diagnosis is confirmed by retrograde or antegrade urethrography or endoscopic visualization of the diverticular opening.

Treatment of acquired diverticula of the male urethra should first involve antibiotics to sterilize the urine and to decrease the inflammatory response around the urethra. Once this has been

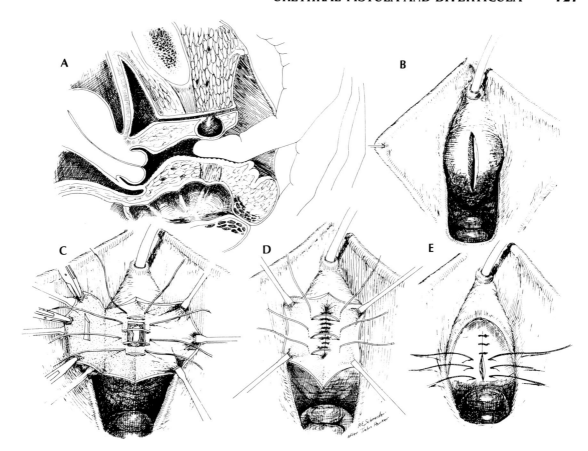

FIG. 69-8. Repair of a female urethral diverticulum. **(A)** The diverticulum is palpated vaginally. **(B)** A midline vaginal incision has been made over the diverticulum. **(C)** The diverticulum has been excised, leaving a small defect in the urethra. The urethral mucosa is closed with inverting mattress sutures. **(D)** The pubovesical cervical fascia is closed over the urethral mucosa. The excess vaginal mucosa has been trimmed equally. Alternatively, the vaginal mucosal flaps can be trimmed on one side only, which avoids placing the suture lines in oppostion. **(E)** The vaginal mucosa is closed.

accomplished, which is not always possible, the patient is ready for surgery. The surgical objectives are to eliminate distal obstruction and to remove the diverticulum.

For maximum surgical exposure, the patient is placed in the lithotomy position. It is extremely helpful to distend the diverticulum, which can be done by filling the urethra with either a viscous lidocaine (Xylocaine) or surgical jelly and applying a urethral clamp to the distal urethra. This allows distention of the urethral diverticulum and makes dissection easier. With the penis on stretch, a midline skin incision is made over the bulging mass and deepened through the dartos layer of fascia. If the diverticulum is in the perineum, the next structures encountered are the bulbocavernosus muscles, which are divided in the midline

and gently dissected off the diverticulum. If the diverticulum is in the anterior or pendulous portion of the urethra immediately beneath the superficial dartos layer, Buck's fascia may be encountered or the diverticulum may have separated Buck's fascia. The urethral diverticulum is separated from the surrounding structures by sharp dissection down to its attachment to the urethra. At this point the urethral diverticulum is amputated, and the urethra is closed with interrupted or continuous 5-0 chromic suture. A drain is placed through a stab wound on either side of the incision and sutured to the skin. Buck's fascia is reapproximated over the closure, or, in the case of a perineal diverticulum, the bulbocavernosus muscles are reapproximated in the midline with interrupted sutures of fine chromic. The dartos layer is then reapproxi-

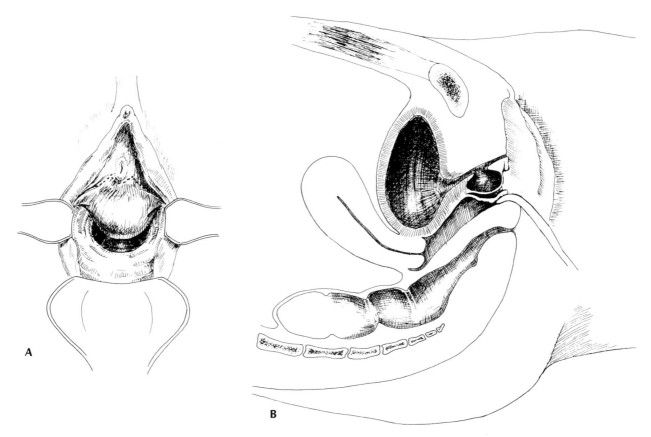

FIG. 69-9. Repair of a female diverticulum. **(A)** A suburethral meatal incision has been made. **(B)** A plane of cleavage has been developed between the diverticulum and the vaginal mucosa.

mated and the skin is closed with a subcuticular suture of 4-0 chromic or 4-0 Vicryl. An indwelling Foley catheter is taped to the abdomen, and a compression dressing is applied. We find it best to remove the compression dressing in 48 hr and to begin applying a heat lamp to the perineum for 15 minutes, four times a day. The Foley catheter is removed on the 10th to 14th day, and the patient is allowed to urinate.

FEMALES

The incidence of female uretheral diverticula is directly related to the enthusiasm of the surgeon for uncovering the lesion. Although female urethral diverticula can be divided into congenital and acquired types, the latter is far more common. Huffman described the anatomy of the paraurethral glands using wax model reconstruction from injected urethrae and found numerous paraurethral glands and ducts.[6] Some of them were considerably dilated. It is tempting to reconstruct the probable

events leading to the development of a urethral diverticulum in the female as follows: an initial meatal or distal urethral stenosis, infection of the paraurethral glands, periurethral abscess, then spontaneous drainage of the infected abscess back into the urethra with eventual epithelialization of the cavity.

The classic symptoms of a urethral diverticulum in the female are dysuria, dribbling, and dyspareunia. Other symptoms include localized pain and swelling and a persistent urethral discharge. Physical examination usually confirms the presence of a bulging suburethral mass, which produces a discharge at the urethral meatus. The diagnosis is sometimes suggested by the presence of a soft tissue mass at the floor of the bladder seen on excretory urography.[5] Distal urethral diverticula are identified by voiding excretory urography, voiding cystourethrography, or positive pressure urethrography using such devices as a Trattner, Hyams, or Davis model urethrographic catheter. A Foley catheter can be modified by tying a silk

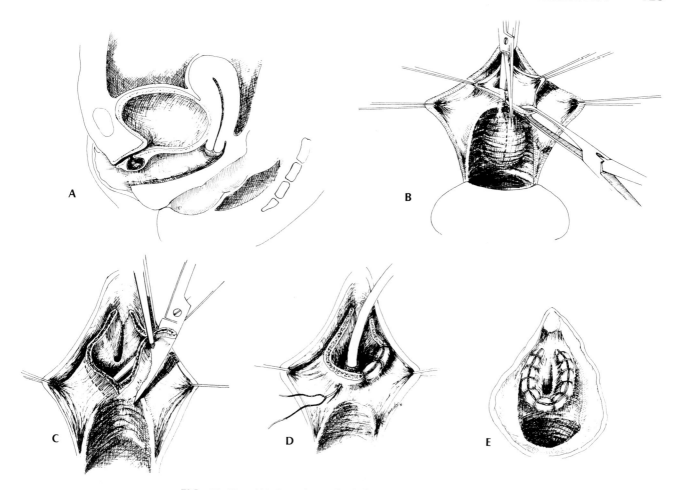

FIG. 69-10. **(A)** Female urethral diverticulum. **(B)** An incision is made from the urethral meatus back into the diverticulum. **(C)** The redundant vaginal mucosa and the diverticulum are excised. **(D)** The vaginal mucosa is sutured to the urethra, creating a generous meatotomy. **(E)** Closure is completed.

suture at the tip of the catheter beyond the Foley balloon and creating a opening in the side of the catheter opposite the inflation channel.[10]

Surgical treatment of a urethral diverticulum is directed at complete removal of the lesion and healing without the development of a urethrovaginal fistula. Surgical failures are usually caused by incomplete removal of the sac, and this problem has led to several techniques for converting the flabby, indiscreet, thin-walled mass into a firm, solid, and easily definable structure that remains so during the dissection. In 1938, Young suggested passing a sound through the urethra into the orifice of the diverticulum to aid in recognizing the sac beneath the anterior vaginal wall.[16] Hyams and Hyams advised packing the sacs transurethrally with a strip of gauze,[8] and Cook and Pool sug-

gested the insertion of a small urethral catheter through the urethra, allowing it to coil in the sac.[2] We have used the firm fibrin clot made with cryoprecipitate, thrombin and $CaCl_2$ as used in the coagulum pyelolithotomy. This clot is injected thru a modified Foley catheter,[10] with the urethral meatus occluded by a pursestring suture. The coagulum fills the diverticulum and solidifies.

There are several important points to remember in excision of a urethral diverticulum. First, the distal two thirds of the urethra is not easily separable from the anterior vaginal wall. Second, any mechanism that converts the diverticulum into a firm, well-defined structure should be used. Third, the neck of the diverticulum and urethral edges should be clearly demarcated and identified. Fourth, the urethral opening should be carefully closed.

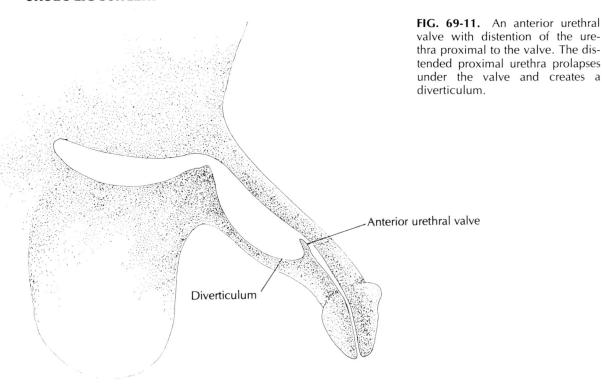

FIG. 69-11. An anterior urethral valve with distention of the urethra proximal to the valve. The distended proximal urethra prolapses under the valve and creates a diverticulum.

Anterior urethral valve

Diverticulum

Fifth, if at all possible, urethral and vaginal suture lines should not be in apposition.

After vaginal prepping, preparation, and draping, a Foley catheter is introduced into the bladder and the diverticulum is filled by whatever means is appropriate. If the diverticulum is large, the cervix can be grasped with a tenaculum and pulled downward. This exposes the undersurface of the anterior vaginal wall and the diverticulum. The initial incision is in the midline, extending from the urethral meatus back to the bladder neck region (Fig. 69-8). Following separation of the proximal urethra and bladder from the cervix, the pubocervical vesical fascia is separated bilaterally from the vaginal mucosa. This then frees the proximal urethra in the midline and makes the diverticulum more clearly visible and demonstrable. By working distally, the diverticulum is carefully dissected from the vaginal mucosa. The small defect created in the urethral mucosa is then closed with 5-0 chromic suture, the pubocervical vesical fascia is closed over the urethral mucosa with interrupted 4-0 chromic sutures, and any excess vaginal mucosa is trimmed away. This trimming can be done asymmetrically so that the vaginal closure does not overlie the urethral closure. A vaginal pack is placed for 48 hr and the urethral catheter is left indwelling for 10 to 14 days.

An attractive technique which is designed to eliminate overlying suture lines is advocated by Sholem, Wechsler, and Roberts (Fig. 69-9).[11] In this technique, a U-shaped incision is made in the vaginal mucosa just proximal to the meatus from 3 to 9 o'clock, and a plane of cleavage is developed between the anterior vaginal wall and the diverticulum. After removal of the diverticulum, the anterior vaginal wall is brought forward and resutured.

An alternate approach has been advocated by Spence and Duckett (Fig. 69-10).[12] In this procedure a deliberate division of the floor of the distal urethra between the urethral meatus and the orifice of the diverticulum is first accomplished. In essence, this constitutes a deep and very long ventral urethral metaotomy extending into the diverticulum sac. Any redundant flaps are trimmed flush, and a running suture is used to coapt the margins of the sac with the overlying vaginal mucosa. No attempt it made to close the urethra, and an indwelling Foley catheter is left for 48 hr. It would seem that the loss of this considerable amount of urethral length would result in incontinence. However, the authors reported complete continence in seven of the nine patients and mild incontinence in two.

One must always be careful that a carcinoma does not occupy a urethral diverticulum. The majority of these lesions are transitional cell, but adenocarcinomas and epidermoid carcinomas have

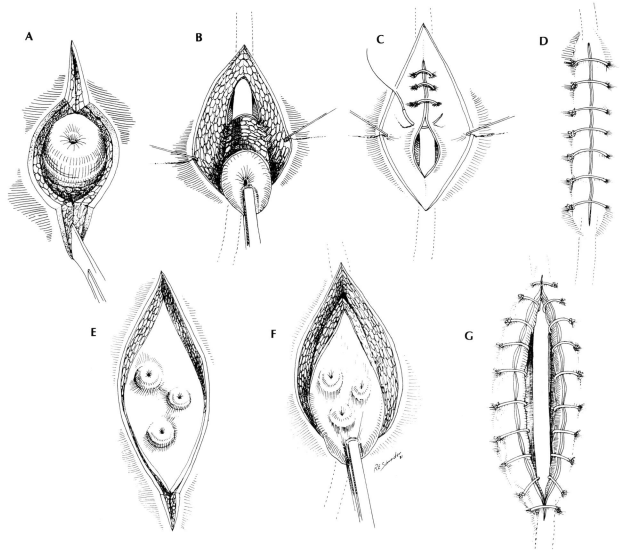

FIG. 69-12. **(A** to **D)** Repair of a simple urethrocutaneous fistula. **(A)** An elliptic incision is made around the fistula. **(B)** The fistula is dissected off the urethra. **(C)** The urethra is closed over an indwelling Silastic catheter. The dartos and the skin **(D)** are closed in layers. **(E** to **G)** Repair of more extensive or multiple fistulas. **(E)** An elliptic incision is made. **(F)** The fistulas and infected tissue are excised along with the urethra. **(G)** The urethral mucosa is sutured to the skin as in a first-stage Johanson.

occurred. Of course, the treatment of these would be different, with wide excision of the involved urethra, diverticulum, cancer, and anterior vaginal wall.

CHILDREN

Urethral diverticula in children occur primarily in males. Although the etiology can be secondary to distal meatal stenosis with infection, most of them are congenital in origin. Williams describes four types: a wide mouth diverticulum with a distal valvular flap, a narrow neck diverticulum with no urethral obstruction, megalourethra with deficiency of the corpus spongiosum, and an acquired diverticulum secondary to trauma or indwelling Floey catheter drainage with infection.[14] The diverticulum associated with anterior urethral valves is probably the commonest type (Fig. 69-11). Posterior urethral valves are seven times more common

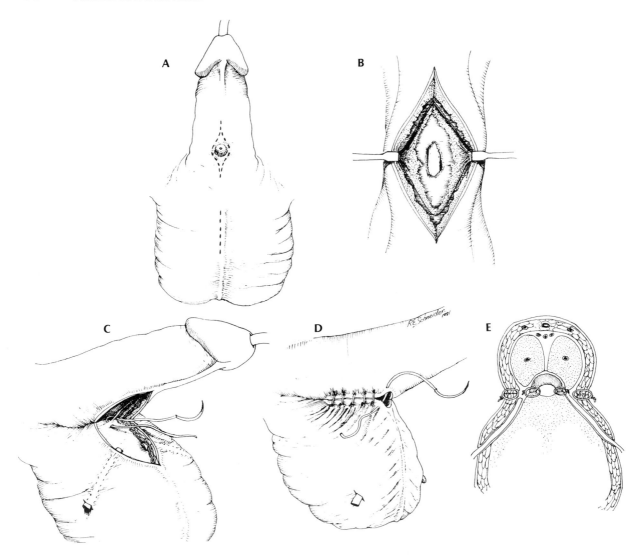

FIG. 69-13. Repair of a male urethrocutaneous fistula using a modified Cecil urethroplasty. **(A** and **B)** The fistulous tract and the surrounding inflammatory tissue is excised. **(C)** A corresponding longitudinal apposing incision is made in the scrotum, and the urethral mucosa is sutured to the dartos layer of the scrotum. **(D)** The penile and scrotal skin is approximated. **(E)** Drains are placed laterally through separate stab wounds and up to the urethral–dartos suture line.

than anterior urethral valves. The anterior urethral valve can exist as a cusp or an iris diaphragm configuration in the distal urethra. Often these anterior urethral valves are associated with proximal urethral distention, which has been termed an anterior urethral diverticulum. At times this obstruction can be so severe that it causes upper tract damage.

Anterior urethral valves may present with either an absent urinary stream or a poor voiding system.

Following voiding, a urethral swelling can be appreciated on the undersurface of the penis. Following termination of urination, there is dribbling of urine from the urethra. Associated symptoms can include those related to urinary tract infection. The diagnosis of anterior urethral valves is made with anterograde urethrogram, which shows the typical proximal bulging and the leaflet of the valve coming up from the ventrum of the urethra. The opening of the urinary channel is dorsal. The diagnosis is

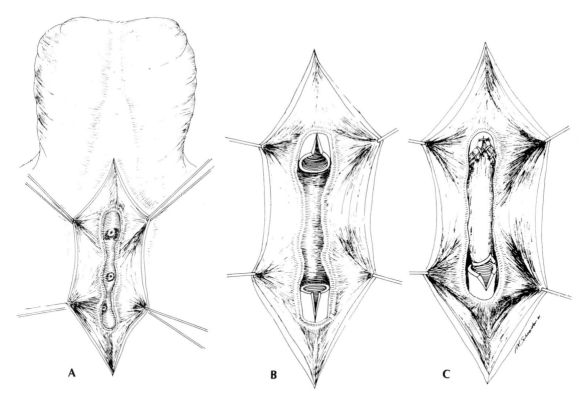

FIG. 69-14.   Repair of urethrocutaneous fistulas.   **(A)** Multiple perineal fistulas are explored by a midline elliptic incision around the fistulas.   **(B)** The fistulas along with the urethra are excised back into normal tissue.   **(C)** The urethra is replaced with a full-thickness tubed skin graft. (After Horton and Devine)

confirmed at the time of urethroscopy by identifying small leaflets with either a Bugbee electrode or the loop of the pediatric resectoscope.

The treatment of anterior urethral valves is fulguration with either the Bugbee electrode or the resectoscope loop. The urethral diverticulum disappears with the elimination of the obstructing valve.

Urethral Fistulas

MALES

Urethral fistulas in adult men are nearly all acquired. They frequently occur secondary to an indwelling Foley catheter which causes erosion of the urethral mucosa, paraurethral infection, and drainage to the skin. Urethrocutaneous fistulas can also occur as a result of distal urethral obstruction secondary to severe stricture disease with infection. The most common urethrocutaneous fistulas that we see are those developing after urethroplasty for stricture or hypospadias repair.

The diagnosis is easily made by noting a history of leakage of urine proximal to the urethral meatus at the time of urination. The fistulous tract is easily identified by inspection and, depending on its size, can be further identified by the placement of an indwelling Foley catheter or a urethral sound. Those fistulas associated with urethral stricture disease may have several openings (watering pot perineum) and can be identified by the injection of methylene blue through the urethral metaus.

The treatment of a urethrocutaneous fistula either can be done in stages or can be attacked primarily following the elimination of infection.[15] If the fistulous tract is small and inflammation is not a problem, an incision can be made in the midline encircling the fistulous tract. The dissection then proceeds by elevating dartos and Buck's fascia laterally off the fistulous tract and surrounding inflammatory tissue to its attachment to the urethra (Fig. 69-12*A* to *D*). The urethra is opened at the base of the fistulous tract, and the fistulous tract is removed. The urethra is then carefully reapproximated with interrupted fine chromic catgut or Vicryl suture over an indwelling Foley catheter.

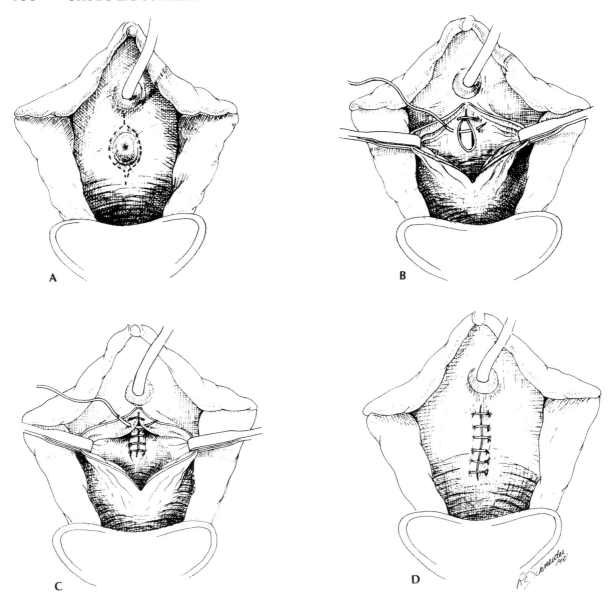

FIG. 69-15.   Repair of a female urethrovaginal fistula.   **(A)** A midline elliptic incision is made around the fistula.   **(B)** The fistulous tract is excised from the urethra.   **(C)** The urethra is closed with interrupted sutures.   **(D)** The pubocervical vesical fascia is closed over the urethra, and the vaginal mucosa is approximated.

The fascial layers are closed over the urethra with interrupted fine chromic, and the skin is approximated with a subcuticular suture of Vicryl, chromic, or interrupted nylon for removal at a later date. In larger fistulas or with multiple fistulous tracts, the first stage is really a first-stage Johanson and consists of an excision around the urethrocutaneous fistula in the midline and dissection of the skin and Colles' fascia beginning in the midline and extending laterally until the fistulous tract and inflammatory tissue around the fistulous tract have been isolated (Fig. 69-12*E* to *G*). This block of tissue containing the urethral fistula is then excised from its attachment with urethra, and the urethra is marsupialized by suturing the skin edges to the remaining normal urethra. A second stage urethroplasty is done 3 to 6 months later.

A modified Cecil urethroplasty can be used to close large or recurrent fistulas in the pendulous urethra as suggested by Malament (Fig. 69-13).

FIG. 69-16. Repair of a large female urethrovaginal fistula. **(A)** The labia majora are sutured laterally to aid in exposure. **(B)** The vaginal mucosa is developed laterally. **(C)** The urethra is closed with interrupted absorbable sutures. **(D)** The labia majora are retracted medially and an incision is made. **(E)** The bulbocavernous muscle is dissected and transected at its insertion into the perineal body. **(F)** A tunnel is developed beneath the labia minora and the bulbocavernous is drawn through the tunnel. **(G)** The muscle is used to cover the urethra. **(H)** The vaginal mucosa is reapproximated. (Redrawn from Wheeless CR, Jr: Atlas of Pelvic Surgery, p 88. Philadelphia, Lea & Febiger, 1981)

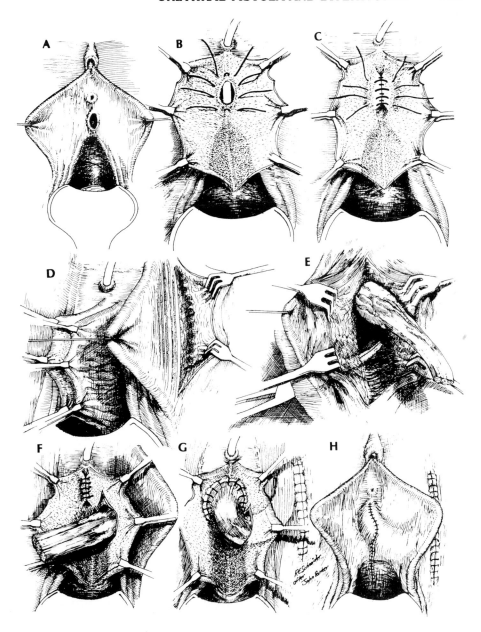

The urethrocutaneous fistula is excised down to the urethra. A longitudinal incision is then made in the scrotum corresponding to the length of the incision in the penile urethra. The scrotal incision is carried down through the dartos layer with dissection laterally to free up dartos and scrotal skin separately. The urethral rim is then sutured to the dartos layer in the scrotum with interrupted 4-0 to 5-0 chromic suture, and the penile skin is approximated to the scrotal skin using 4-0 chromic subcuticular or 4-0 nylon. Drains can be placed laterally and brought out through separate stab incisions to be removed at a later date. The second stage of this procedure requires freeing the penis from the scrotum 6 weeks to 3 months later. When the penis is separated from the scrotum, the scrotal incisions are made wide enough so as to use scrotal skin which has now become revascularized by penile skin to close over the previous repair. The defect in the scrotum is then closed separately. The free full-thickness tube graft (Horton and Devine) technique can also be used. (Fig. 69-14).[4]

FEMALES

Female urethrovaginal fistulas are usually acquired. They can be secondary either to paraureth-

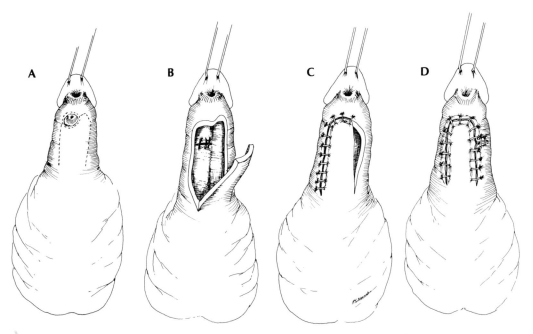

FIG. 69-17. A method of fistula closure after Belman and King. **(A)** The incisions are outlined and the fistula is excised. **(B)** The urethra is closed horizontally and the skin is elevated. **(C)** The skin is closed. (Redrawn from Belman and King. In Clinical Pediatric Urology, Vol. 1, p 593. Philadelphia, WB Saunders, 1979)

ral infection with drainage into the vagina or to surgical or obstetric trauma. In most instances, a urethrovaginal fistula is associated with no complaints. However, distortion of the urinary stream and voiding into the vagina can be troublesome for some patients. A urethrovaginal fistula located in the proximal urethra can be associated with incontinence.

Urethrovaginal fistula can easily be diagnosed by either inspection or retrograde injection of saline or Xylocaine and viewing the discharge of fluid into the vagina. The patient is placed in the lithotomy position and the vulva and vagina are prepped and draped. A midline elliptic incision is made in the vaginal mucosa, which can be dissected off the underlying pubocervical vesical fascia (Fig. 69-15). The fistulous communication with the urethra is then excised, and the urethra is closed with 4-0 or 5-0 chromic suture. The overlying pubocervical vesical fascia is sutured over the utethra, and the vaginal mucosa is closed in the midline. An alternative to this is to develop a plan of cleavage asymmetrically on one side of the urethra so that the vaginal closure can be lateral to the midline closure of the urethra. For larger fistulas, Wheeless advocates that a pedicile of bulbocavernosus muscle be dissected free and brought over the repair. The vaginal mucoas is then closed over the top of this vascularized muscular pedicle (Fig. 69-16).[13]

CHILDREN

Urethral fistula in children can be congenital or acquired. The congenital variety is usually associated with imperforate anus, with a communication between the urethra and the rectum being a part of this congenital abnormality. Congenital urethrocutaneous fistulas are exceedingly rare and usually associated with duplication of the urethra. Acquired urethrocutaneous fistulas in children are common following hypospadias repair. These fistulas are usually small and located at the junction of the new and the old urethras.

Urethrocutaneous fistulas are usually best managed when initially identified with cauterization of the tract or secondary closure and, if this is not successful, closed at 3 to 6 months after the initial hypospadias repair. These procedures can usually be done on an outpatient basis. If the fistulous tract is small, it can simply be excised using a small longitudinal incision over the fistulous tract and inversion of the urethral mucosa with several interrupted sutures.[1] In larger fistulas, a simple closure will usually compromise the urethral lumen. In this situation it is best to construct a flap

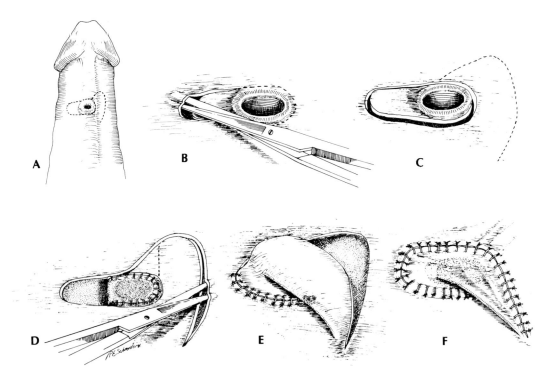

FIG. 69-18. Wise's closure method for urethrocutaneous fistula following hypospadias repair. **(A)** The skin incision is outlined. **(B and C)** The edges of the flaps are developed and mobilized. **(D)** The skin flap is turned over the fistula and sutured. **(E and F)** The lateral skin flap is mobilized and sutured into place over the closure. No narrowing of the urethra occurs with this method. (Redrawn from Wise HA II, Berggren RB: Another method of repair for urethrocutaneous fistulae. J Urol 118:1054, 1977)

and to secure this skin flap in the urethral defect with fine interrupted sutures (Figs. 69-17 and 69-18). If possible, a second layer of suture can be placed over this to cover this urethral suture line. Skin flaps can then be mobilized laterally for coverage. Rarely, insufficient skin remains.

REFERENCES

1. BELMAN AB, KING LR: In Clinical Pediatric Urology, Vol 1, p 593. Philadelphia, WB Saunders, 1976
2. COOK EN, POOL TL: Urethral diverticulum in the female. J Urol 62:495, 1949
3. CURTIS AH, ANSON BJ, MCVAY CB: The anatomy and urogenital diaphragms in relation to urethrocele and cystocele. Surg Gynecol Obstet 68:161, 1939
4. DEVINE CH: Surgery of the penis and urethra. In Campbell's Urology, Vol 3, 4th ed, p 2425, 2427. WB Saunders, Philadelphia, 1979
5. DRETLER SP, VERMILLION CS, MCCULLOUGH DC: The Roentgenographic diagnosis of female urethral diverticulum. J Urol 107:72, 1972
6. HUFFMAN JW: Detailed anatomy of the paraurethral ducts in adult human female. Am J Obstet Gynecol 55:86, 1948
7. HUTCH JA: Anatomy and physiology of the bladder, trigone and urethra. New York, Appleton-Century-Crofts, 1972
8. HYAMS JA, HYAMS NM: New operative procedure for treatment of diverticulum of the female urethra. Urol Cutan Ref 43:573, 577, 1939
9. MALAMENT M: Repair of the recurrent fistula of the penile urethra. J Urol 106:704, 1971
10. REDMAN JF, TAYLOR JN: A technique for urethrograms in female patients. J Urol 108:91, 1972
11. SHOLEM SL, WECHSLER M, ROBERTS M: Management of the urethral diverticulum in women: A modified operative technique. J Urol 112:485, 1974
12. SPENCE HM, DUCKETT JW, JR: Diverticulum of the female urethra: Clinical aspects and presentation of a simple operative technique for cure. J Urol 104:432, 1970
13. WHEELESS CR, JR: Atlas of Pelvic Surgery, p 88. Philadelphia, Lea & Febiger, 1981
14. WILLIAMS DI: Urology in Childhood, p 222. New York, Springer-Verlag, 1974
15. WISE HA II, BERGGREN RB: Another method of repair for urethrocutaneous fistulae. J Urol 118:1054, 1977
16. YOUNG HH: Diverticulum of the female urethra. South Med J 31:1043, 1938

Lower Urinary Tract Trauma

70

James M. Pierce, Jr.

Trauma is no respecter of specialty lines or organ systems. One of the cardinal rules in the management of trauma is to think of all possibilities of injury such as vascular injury, bony injury, bowel injury, and injury to other viscera such as liver, spleen, or lung.

Injuries to the lower urinary tract have three etiologies. The first is external blunt trauma, the second is penetrating injury such as gunshot or stabs, and the third is injury occurring at the time of operative procedures. This chapter deals primarily with blunt trauma and penetrating injuries; operative complications resulting in injury to the lower urinary tract are dealt with in other parts of the text.

SURGICAL ANATOMY

Figure 70-1 shows certain aspects of the basic anatomy of the bladder and male urethra. The urinary bladder is protected by the bony pelvis and has the rectum behind it in the male; in the female, the genital tract and the rectum lie posterior. The bladder and prostate, as well as the proximal urethra in the female, are extraperitoneal. The dome of the bladder is covered by peritoneum; thus, ruptures in this area are intraperitoneal. The prostatic urethra tends to be fixed in position because the prostate is attached to the pubic symphysis by the pubovesical ligaments; in the female, the proximal urethra is similarly attached by the pubourethral ligaments. The membranous or intradiaphragmatic urethra in the female is very short, perhaps only a few millimeters in length because of the thinness and delicacy of the urogenital diaphragm in the female. In the male, however, it is about 1½ cm thick. The membranous or intradiaphragmatic portion of the male urethra, which is a fixed portion of the urethra, is a centimeter or so in length. The distal urethra is extrapelvic and thus is susceptible to more injuries.

Types of Injury

INJURY OF THE URINARY BLADDER

Blunt Trauma Blunt trauma injury to the bladder is of two types: intraperitoneal rupture and extraperitoneal rupture. The former is more likely to occur when the bladder is full and the distribution of pressure when the patient falls or is hit is such that the bladder blows out at the point of least resistance, the dome, producing extravasation of urine into the peritoneal cavity. Figure 70-2 shows an intraperitoneal rupture of the bladder with contrast material visualized in the left colic gutter.

Extraperitoneal rupture of the urinary bladder secondary to blunt trauma (Fig. 70-3) is often associated with fracture of the bony pelvis, especially the pubic and ischial rami.[2,10] This type of injury may produce a bony spicule that, during the motion of the bone broken at the time of injury, lacerates the extraperitoneal portions of the bladder wall. This injury can also be associated with injury to the prostatomembranous urethra in the male or the proximal urethra in the female.[1] These latter injuries are important to remember. On one occasion, this author saw dismemberment of the right ureter just above the bladder following blunt trauma to the pelvis, probably due to motion of a bony fragment. This is a rare injury in blunt trauma but should be kept in mind.

Penetrating Injuries Involving the Urinary Bladder Penetrating injuries in this society are primarily gunshot or stab wounds.[11] The point of entrance and exit, if any, of the wound should be noted, to get an idea of what various organs might be injured. Small bowel, rectum, distal ureters, pelvic blood vessels, and bony structures can all be damaged in these injuries (Fig. 70-4). In gunshot wounds in the area of the base of the bladder, one must be sure to ascertain that the ureter was not

739

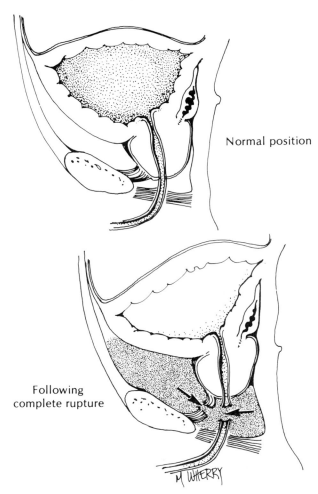

Normal position

Following
complete rupture

M WHERRY

FIG. 70-1. Normal anatomy with demonstration of prostatomembranous disruption. Note severance of puboprostatic ligament and supramembranous urethra. (© Royal Victoria Hospital)

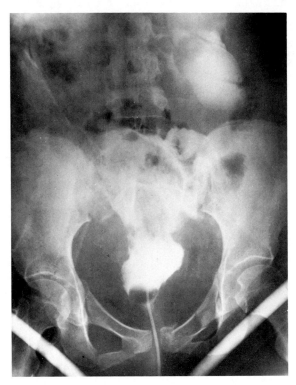

FIG. 70-2. Retrograde cystogram. Cystogram in case of intraperitoneal rupture of bladder with collection of dye in both paracolic gutters

FIG. 70-3. X-ray appearance of extraperitoneal rupture demonstrated by retrograde cystogram. Note that dye has extravasated to the labiae as well as pre- and perivesical space

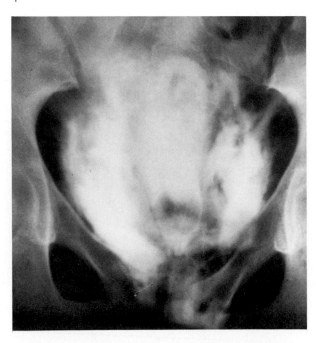

blown off with the injury (Fig. 70-5). It can be catastrophic if this injury is not picked up at the time of the original exploratory operation.

INJURY TO THE URETHRA

Injury to the urethra is divided into two types. The first is injury to the proximal urethra which, in the male, constitutes the membranoprostatic portion of the urethra; the second is to the distal urethra, which is that portion inferior to the urogenital diaphragm.

Injury to the Membranoprostatic Urethra is almost always associated with pelvic crushing injuries, and Figure 70-2 shows a diagram of the most common point of dismemberment in a pelvic crushing injury due to movement of the bony fragments and rupture of the puboprostatic ligaments. Figure 70-6, from Pokorny and co-workers, shows what happens when the different types of forces are applied acutely to the pelvis with movement of the symphysis and rupture of the puboprostatic ligaments.[10] Figure 70-7, also from Pokorny and co-workers, shows the typical "collar injury," which usually involves all four fragments of the pelvis. The fragments are downwardly displaced, stretching out the membranous urethra between the urogenital diaphragm and the prostate by rupturing the puboprostatic ligaments; as the urethra gets stretched, it also ruptures. Figure 70-8 shows the stretching of the supradiaphragmatic portion of the urethra after rupture of the puboprostatic ligament without dismemberment; we have seen this type of situation in seven or eight patients when reviewing pelvic fractures in general (Fig. 70-9).

Figure 70-10 demonstrates a retrograde urethrogram in a patient with a crushed pelvis and dismembered membranoprostatic urethra above the urogenital diaphragm. Figure 70-11 shows an intravenous urogram and retrograde urethrogram in one of these patients. Occasionally, one sees a gunshot injury of the prostatic membranous urethral area; this often involves the rectum (Fig. 70-12).

The Distal Urethral Injury most commonly is a straddle injury in which the force pushes the bulbous urethra up against the inferior arch of the pubis, causing it to crush and perhaps explode, and thus producing the rupture (Fig. 70-13).[8] There are other injuries of the male distal urethra such as stab wounds, gunshot wounds, and results of sexual aberrations such as sticking the penis in the hose of a tank vacuum cleaner.[12]

Diagnosis

Many emergency rooms in this country are staffed by full-time emergency room physicians, and larger centers are often staffed by trauma surgeons. It is important that these people be educated to recognize the signs and symptoms of urinary tract trauma so that the injuries are not unrecognized or mistreated. Any patient with a pelvic crush with fractures to the bony pelvis, patients with hematuria after injury, patients who cannot void after lower abdominal or pelvic injury, and patients with penetrating wounds of the lower abdomen and pelvis—especially when associated with hematuria—should be investigated. The same is true for injuries of the lower thorax and upper abdomen

(*Text continues on p. 744*)

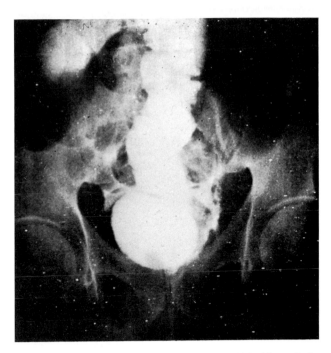

FIG. 70-4. Gunshot wound of rectum and bladder. Bladder wound closed transvesically; suprapubic cystotomy and colostomy

FIG. 70-5. Gunshot wound and ruptured bladder. The right ureter was blown off at the entrance to the bladder

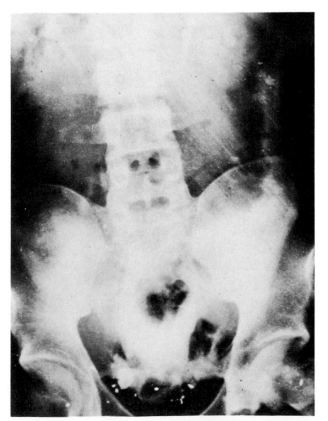

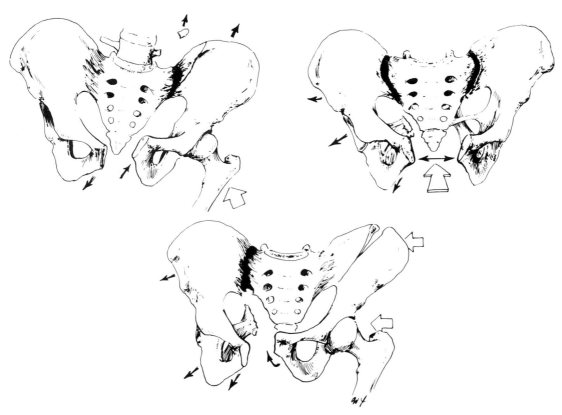

FIG. 70-6. Dynamics of various injuries producing dismemberment of membranoprostatic urethra. *Large arrows* indicate direction of force

FIG. 70-7. Classic "collar" injury

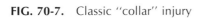

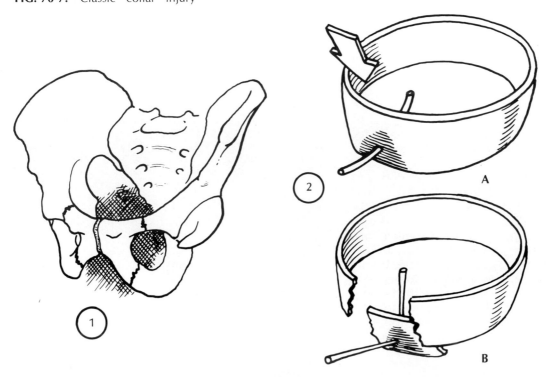

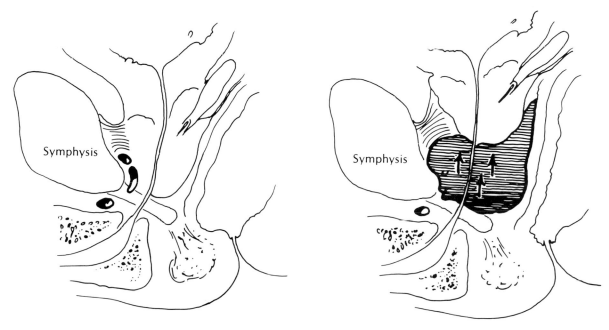

FIG. 70-8.   Stretching of posterior urethra short of rupture

FIG. 70-9.   Stretching of posterior urethra without rupture with extraperitoneal bladder rupture

FIG. 70-10.   Retrograde urethrogram. Urethrogram in case of supramembranous rupture. Dye extravasation is typical of that seen with this type of injury.

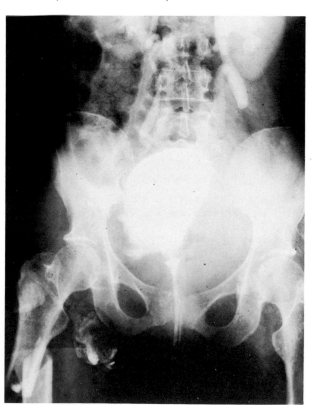

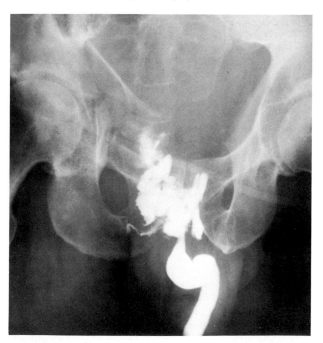

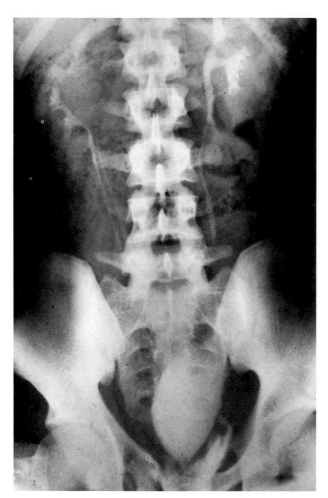

FIG. 70-11. Excretory urogram combined with retrograde urethrogram. Note elevation of bladder, tear-drop deformity, and extravasation

when renal or ureteral injury is a possibility. All these patients should have drip infusion pyelography and retrograde urethrocystography.

Mitchell had great concern over retrograde urethrography and cystography in injuries to the lower urinary tract because of the fear of causing infection and further damaging the structures.[4] Most people, including this author, have used retrograde urethrocystography for years with no known complications resulting. A 20% solution of organic iodide radiographic compound is usually used; in the male, it can usually be injected through the urethral meatus without catheterizing the patient and gradually the bladder can be filled. If the urethra is normal, a catheter can be passed and the bladder filled. If there is a urethral injury, it is noted and treated accordingly. When the bladder is filled, views should be taken in both oblique

angles and the anteroposterior projection. A post-drainage film should be taken also, because sometimes the extravasation cannot be seen when the bladder is full.

In penetrating trauma especially, one may not see an extravasation of contrast material beyond the confines of the bladder itself. However, extensive hematuria and perivesical hematoma indicated by displacement of the bladder into a parachute shape or to the opposite side of the pelvis should suggest that there is a penetrating injury of the bladder. The injury does not show because it functions like a self-sealing gas tank; it causes bleeding in the bladder wall that seals off the injury, and sometimes a hematoma in the extravesical position seals off the extravasation.[7] In this type of situation, we may endoscope the patient or treat the patient as though he had a ruptured bladder. Again, one must be aware of the possibility of a dismembered ureter, and injuries to other viscera such as the rectum or small bowel must be considered.

Treatment

RUPTURED BLADDER

In the case of a ruptured bladder, if the patient is in poor condition, it is often sufficient to put a urethral catheter in place in the bladder with dependent drainage. If the patient is in decent condition, one may elect to do an exploration of the bladder with débridement of the edges of the tear and closure of the bladder in three layers. If the wound is clean and the closure seems good, a urethral catheter is left in for 24 to 48 hours and then removed.

At the time of exploration, one should make a vertical midline incision and look in the peritoneal cavity for evidence of any bowel or vascular injury or injury to other viscera such as liver or spleen. If the bladder injury is severe and a closure may not be considered competent, a cystotomy tube is left in. A drain may also be left in place if the urine is infected and the closure is not competent.

MEMBRANOPROSTATIC URETHRAL INJURY

These injuries are diagnosed by the presence of the fractured pelvis, an inability to urinate, and the inability to pass a catheter. If such injury is suspected, I would recommend that a retrograde urethrogram be done first by the technique mentioned above and then the decision be made to intervene operatively (Fig. 70-10). Again, a vertical midline incision is used to make sure no other viscera are involved in the injury; ordinarily, this author recommends that only a suprapubic cystotomy be done.[4,5] However, in certain institutions in this country and certainly in many European institutions in which one, two, or three surgeons take care of all these injuries for large population areas, a primary reapproximation of the ends of the dismembered membranoprostatic urethra may be recommended.[3,6]

In this country, with its generalized dissemination of trauma care, most urologists see none, or at most one or two, of these patients in their professional lives. Therefore, they do not get experience in managing these problems, and the patient is much safer to have a cystotomy with management of any obliterative stricture that may occur, by someone who does these procedures. Figure 70-14 shows the use of the interlocking sounds to try to approximate the ends of the urethra. These should never be forced because they may end up compounding the injury, especially in the area of the urogenital diaphragm.[9]

If primary approximation can be effected at the time of the injury without difficulty, such as with two passes of instruments from the bladder and distal urethral ends, then a catheter plus a cystotomy tube can be left indwelling. The catheter should never be put on tension. This may result in an incontinent patient because the distal membranoprostatic urethral continence mechanism is destroyed with the injury, and injury to the vesical neck or primary continence mechanism can be produced by ischemia from prolonged traction on a urethral catheter. This leads to an incompetent vesical neck and thus to incontinence, a catastrophic event which, unfortunately, does occur.

On the other hand, some form of Vest sutures through the prostate and out through the perineum, with the sutures tied over thyroid packs or buttons, can be used to put gentle traction on the prostate to aid its being held down close to the urogenital diaphragm. However, it should be stated strongly that unless the individual has had a lot of experience in deciding when to try a primary reapproximation at the time of injury, the patient is best treated a simple cystotomy as recommended by Mitchell and Morehouse and MacKinnon.[4,5] The possibility of producing impotence by overmanipulation in an attempt to reapproximate the urethra has been emphasized by Morehouse and MacKinnon and should be kept in mind.[5]

After simple cystotomy treatment of this injury, in 4 to 6 months the hematoma gradually absorbs in the pelvis and the prostate and bladder settle

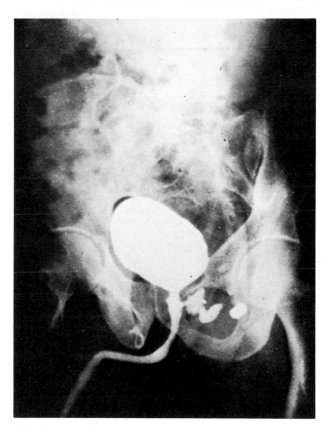

FIG. 70-12. This gunshot wound of the prostatic urethra was treated successfully with suprapubic cystotomy

FIG. 70-13. Ruptured bulbous urethra from straddle injury. Note bullet from previous encounter

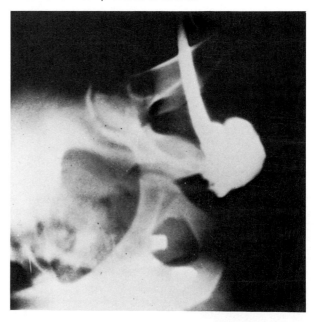

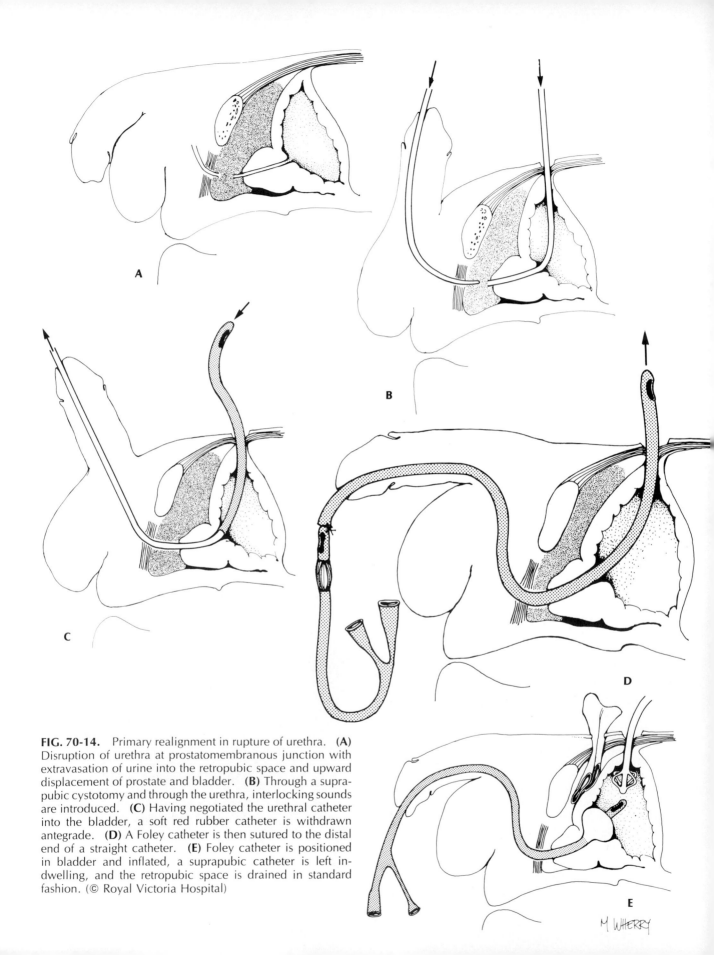

FIG. 70-14. Primary realignment in rupture of urethra. **(A)** Disruption of urethra at prostatomembranous junction with extravasation of urine into the retropubic space and upward displacement of prostate and bladder. **(B)** Through a suprapubic cystotomy and through the urethra, interlocking sounds are introduced. **(C)** Having negotiated the urethral catheter into the bladder, a soft red rubber catheter is withdrawn antegrade. **(D)** A Foley catheter is then sutured to the distal end of a straight catheter. **(E)** Foley catheter is positioned in bladder and inflated, a suprapubic catheter is left indwelling, and the retropubic space is drained in standard fashion. (© Royal Victoria Hospital)

down so that the separation is usually no more than 3 mm to 5 mm, which then allows the surgeon to repair these injuries effectively.

INJURIES TO THE DISTAL URETHRA

Blunt trauma is usually from a straddle injury, whose mechanism was mentioned above. Usually there is blood dripping from the urethra in these individuals, and there may be a perineal hematoma. A urethrogram is done; if there is extravasation of contrast material, this author recommends a suprapubic cystotomy and, at the end of 3 weeks, a voiding cystourethrogram to see if there is any evidence of difficulty.[12] Frequently, the urethra is normal.

There has been discussion of attempts at primary repair of straddle injuries, and it is this author's experience that in most of these attempts the result is not as good as if one were to do a simple cystotomy. The problem with primary repair is that, because of the crushing nature of the injury, there is hematoma dissecting into the walls of the urethra. The hematoma discolors the urethra, making it soggy and difficult to repair. Under these circumstances, the attempt to repair may extend the injury to the urethra and cause more damage than if one just diverted the urinary stream with a suprapubic cystotomy. If there is just a small extravasation of the urethra, then perhaps the use of an indwelling catheter for 10 days is all that is required. The use of the inlying urethral catheter always raises the risk of urethritis; if any suggestion of this occurs, perhaps a cystotomy is indicated.

More esoteric distal urethral injuries occasionally occur. The gunshot or stab wound has to have individualized treatment. If it is a small wound, especially a knife wound, it can be operated upon and repaired if there is no great loss of tissue. If there is loss of tissue, sometimes the treatment can be an exteriorization of the urethra at this time, followed by second-stage urethroplasty at a later date. More severe injuries are best treated with suprapubic cystotomy with time allowed for the injured area to clean out and heal; then a decision can be made about management of any stricture or defect that may have resulted.

Finally, it cannot be overemphasized that in the acute management of crushing pelvic injuries, overzealous attempts to restore urethral continuity may lead to an increased incidence of impotence and, in some individuals, may result in even greater urethral damage. In inexperienced hands, suprapubic cystotomy is the best treatment.

REFERENCES

1. BELIS J, RECHT K, MILAM D: Simultaneous traumatic bladder perforation and disruption of the prostatomembranous urethra. J Urol 122:412, 1979
2. CASS A, IRELAND G: Bladder trauma associated with pelvic fractures in severely injured patients. J Trauma 13:205, 1973
3. DEWEERD JH: Immediate realignment of posterior urethral injury. Urol Clin North Am 4:75, 1977
4. MITCHELL JT: Injuries to the urethra. Br J Urol 40:649, 1968
5. MOREHOUSE D, MACKINNON J: Urologic injuries associated with pelvic fractures. J Trauma 9:479, 1969
6. MYERS R, DEWEERD J: Incidence of stricture following primary realignment of the disrupted proximal urethra. J Urol 107:265, 1972
7. NOWAK A, ZIEBRISKI J: Difficulties in bladder rupture diagnostics. Eur Urol 3:351, 1977
8. PERSKY L: Childhood urethral trauma. Urology 11:608, 1978
9. PIERCE JM: Management of dismemberment of prostatic membranous urethra and ensuing stricture disease. J Urol 107:259, 1972
10. POKORNY M, PONTES JE, PIERCE JM: Urologic injuries associated with pelvic trauma. J. Urol 121:455, 1979
11. PONTES JE: Urologic injuries. Surg Clin North Am 57:77, 1977
12. PONTES JE, PIERCE JM: Anterior urethral injuries: Four years experience at the detroit general hospital. J Urol 120:563, 1978

Internal Urethrotomy

71

Dieter Kirchheim

Internal urethrotomy in the treatment of urethral strictures is one of the oldest urologic operations.[1] Ferri of Naples in 1530 first used a cutting sound.[4] At the end of the 17th century and in the early 18th century several different fixed-blade urethrotomes were designed. Jean Civiale and Guillon were the first to introduce a blind urethrotome with retractable blades.[5] This instrument cut strictures from the proximal to the distal urethra. The best-known further improvements or modifications of this urethrotome were the Otis and Maisonneuve urethrotomes.[9,11]

In 1972 Sachse presented his first results with a new visual urethrotome and a cold knife, which he had developed together with Storz.[12,13] Other urologists applied and further developed the technique of endoscopic internal urethrotomy using the Sachse urethrotome. They reported a number of advantages and improved results with this technique.[7,8,10,14,15] Most instrument makers are now manufacturing visual (endoscopic) urethrotomes. The following chapter will describe the technique of internal urethrotomy, using such visual urethrotomes. The technique has been named optical urethrotomy, transurethral urethrotomy, and endoscopic internal urethrotomy (EIU), but the latter term is probably the most descriptive.

Indications and Contraindications

The main indication for internal urethrotomy is urethral stricture. Soft and resilient strictures may respond to a few dilations. Dense, unresilient strictures frequently get worse after urethral dilatations. If urethral dilation is not successful or tears the tissue, the stricture is cut with less tissue irritation and more effectively by EIU. Most urethral strictures that contain a bridge of mucosa between the proximal and distal end of the stricture can be treated by EIU. Because many strictures are relatively avascular and free of sensory nerve fibers, anterior and shorter strictures may be done under local anesthesia.

EIU may also be used prior to transurethral prostatic resection or other transurethral procedures if the urethra does not calibrate to an adequate caliber owing to either an existing stricture or a small-caliber urethra.[2,3] Cutting the urethra by EIU to an adequate lumen of 26Fr to 28Fr can be easily done with the Sachse urethrotome, and results in a smoother urethra and fewer injuries to other tissues than when done by blind urethrotomy with the older nonvisual instruments.

Experience in patients under 18 years of age is still limited. American Cystoscope Makers makes a pediatric endoscope urethrotome which I have used with good results, but further long-term follow-up and a larger number of patients will have to be evaluated. In patients under 18 years of age, EIU should probably only be used for shorter and anterior strictures.

Contraindications are the same as for any transurethral surgical procedure: patients with uncorrectable bleeding tendencies or infections, especially in the presence of cardiac valvular lesions or other high-risk diseases. Patients with traumatic strictures in the membranous urethra after primary suprapubic cystostomy are better treated by open urethroplastic procedures, especially after total tear of the membranous urethra unless the patient is a poor risk for major surgery. Internal urethrotomy should not be performed in the presence of periurethral infection or abscess or urethral fistula. Every effort should be made to sterilize the urine prior to EIU.

The majority of strictures seen today can be transformed into a functional urethra by EIU. If failure occurs even after one or two repeat EIUs, an open urethroplasty can be done without difficulties. Cold knife EIU is usually less painful and tissue disruptive than dilations of small-caliber dense strictures. Failures after EIU and also after open urethroplasties are amenable to another internal urethrotomy, especially if only a short residual stricture is remaining.

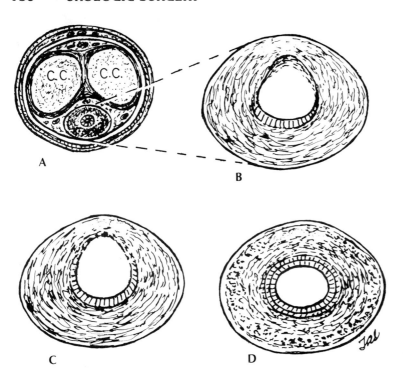

FIG. 71-1. Regeneration of the urethra following EIU. **(A)** Urethra with stricture. **(B)** Urethra after cutting. **(C)** Beginning regeneration (critical stage at 3–6 months). **(D)** Regeneration completed. c.c. = corpora cavernosa.

Surgical Anatomy and Rationale

Urethral strictures are characterized by a great diversity and extent, possible multiplicity, and variable etiology. They may be complicated by urinary tract infection and periurethral infection or fistula. We rarely see strictures today that are complicated by urethral abscess, fistula, or hydronephrosis. At present the history of a previous transurethral instrumentation accounts for over 50% of all strictures. The remainder of the patients give a history of gonorrhea, urinary tract infections, or trauma, or else the strictures are congenital or unexplained.

The normal urethral wall structures become replaced by scar tissue, which progressively contracts the urethral lumen. Voiding or retrograde urethrograms show the length of the narrowed lumen, but not the extent and depth of the stricture. A clear realization of the extent and depth of the scar tissue can only be realized by open exposure or when the stricture is inspected and cut with the 0-degree lens and the straight forward urethrotome. The stricture seen at first by urethroscopy or retrograde urethrogram is only the intraluminal "tip of the iceberg" of the whole stricture (Figs. 71-1 and 71-3). The scar tissue frequently extends all the way through the corpora spongiosum and always further proximally and distally than the area of the intraluminal stricture. An understand-ing of this fact is most important for adequate cutting in depth and length to avoid recurrent stricture formation at the margins.

The rationale of internal urethral cold knife cutting lies in the ability of the cut urethra to regenerate mucosa and urethral wall structures and to form a functionally adequate lumen.[16,17,18] Cold knife cutting appears to cause less interference with regeneration than electric surgical knife cutting, and it is also easier to control in regard to the proper depth of the cutting. Internal urethrotomy under direct endoscopic vision permits complete transection of the scar tissue ring, preferably at the 12 o'clock position, and selective cutting throughout the extent of the stricture.

Preoperative Preparation and Anesthesia

Preoperative preparation is similar to that for transurethral surgery. Every effort should be made to sterilize the urine, and the patient should be in optimal condition. Shorter and especially anterior strictures can frequently be cut under local anesthesia with premedication. More extensive strictures are better treated under a short spinal or general anesthesia. Pre-, intra-, and postoperative antibiotic screen is advisable because of the possibility of bacterial contamination from the anterior urethra. This is mandatory in patients with cardiac valvular lesions.

Operative Technique and Instruments

EIU is performed under the same aseptic conditions and preparations as is any transurethral operative procedure. Nonhemolyzing fluids are used. The instrument used consists of the following components:

Urethrotome sheath (20Fr) with round, blunted aperture to allow straightforward urethroscopy. A side arm allows introduction of a 4Fr ureteral catheter through the stricture for guidance if needed.

Obturator for introduction into the meatus

Lens (0-degree angle) for urethroscopy

Working element from the resectoscope of the urologist's preference. A flat, cold knife blade is inserted at the usual site for the loop.

Fiberoptic light cable

Inflow for nonhemolyzing irrigating solution.

The original Sachse endoscopic urethrotome manufactured by Storz is depicted in Figure 71-2.

The 20Fr sheath with its obturator is inserted into the meatus and navicular fossa. The obturator is withdrawn. The instrument is advanced into the urethra under direct vision with the 0-degree-angle lens until the distal end of the stricture is seen (Fig. 71-3). The flat knife is extended to a convenient position outside the sheath and introduced into the lumen of the stricture with the blade directed toward the 12 o'clock position. The cutting is done by moving the whole instrument in a short arc upward and backward, making short and shallow incisions to avoid perforations. The fulcrum is where the left hand holds the end of the penis with the urethrotome sheath inside the urethra (Fig. 71-3). The first incisions are done through the distal portion of the stricture. The lumen of the urethra opens progressively after each cut (Fig. 71-4). Gradually the whole length of the stricture or several strictures are cut to a 20Fr caliber. The instrument can be passed into the bladder and urine can be evacuated and sampled. The prostatic urethra, the vesical neck, and the bladder can be inspected, and other lesions, such as stones, cystitis, vesical neck contracture, or tumors in the bladder or prostate can be recognized. The urethrotome is then withdrawn and the entire strictured area is reviewed.

Deeper cutting is now done, in a gradual progressive fashion, all the way through the scar tissue. The direct vision lens permits clear recognition of scar tissue and normal tissue. When the usually grayish white, frequently not very vascular, scar tissue has been transected, one can see softer, normal-appearing tissue which bleeds more easily, especially if the irrigating pressure is decreased. At this stage no deeper cutting should be done to avoid perforation, extravasation, and bleeding. Proximally and distally the cutting is extended beyond the margin of the stricture for about 0.5 cm into normal urethra, with the exception of the area of the external sphincter. This creates a smooth tapered transition from the normal urethra into the area of the cut urethral stricture and should result in a relatively smooth, circularly contoured urethra of about 24Fr to 28Fr caliber. Any uneven protrusions are smoothed out at the end of the urethrotomy to allow an unobstructed free urinary flow afterward.[7]

On rare occasions, as in one of our impalement injuries to the bulbous urethra, there may be more scar tissue posteriorly. In such cases, one may consider also making a cut at the 6 o'clock position, but one has to be careful not to create a urethrocutaneous fistula.

After termination of the procedure, a 24Fr Silastic Foley catheter is placed into the bladder and irrigated until clear. The Foley catheter is removed, as it is after transurethral prostatic resection, when there is no more significant hematuria, usually on the first or second postoperative day. Prolonged indwelling catheterization only results in urinary tract infection. A clean-catch midstream urine specimen should be obtained about a week after surgery. A urinalysis, and if necessary, a culture and sensitivity, should be done to make absolutely sure that the healing takes place without the presence or urinary tract infection. At the same time the urinary flow can be measured.

Postoperative Care

Careful and long-term follow-up of patients treated with EIU cannot be overemphasized. Initially, we used hydraulic urethral distention, but some patients felt discomfort and its effect was questionable. Patients are seen as outpatients 2 weeks after EIU and then at monthly intervals or whenever they notice any slowing of urinary flow or any indication of infection or other problems. If there is evidence of infection or reduction of urinary flow rate, the urethra should be calibrated in order to gently separate any adhesions between the cut surfaces of the stricture. In the majority of the

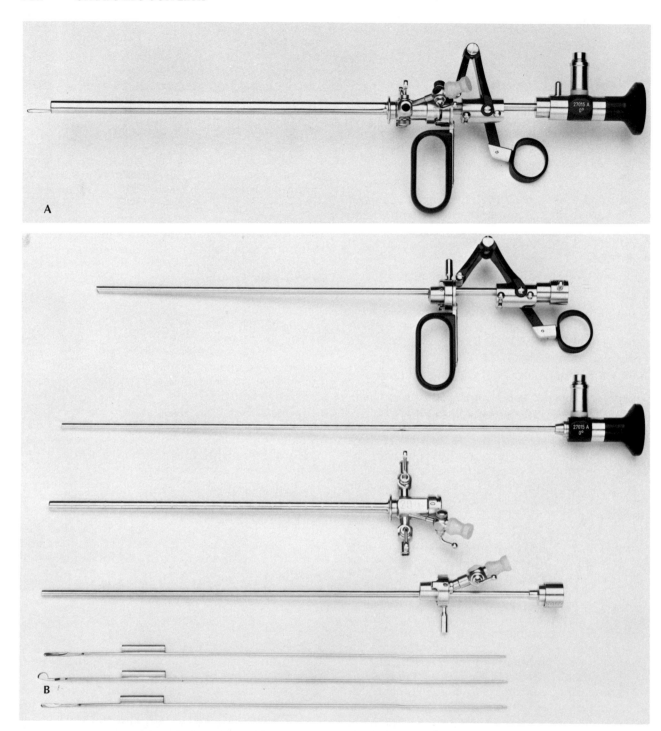

FIG. 71-2. Sachse endoscopic internal urethrotome. **(A)** Assembled Sachse optical ure-throtome. **(B)** Components include (top to bottom) working element, 0-degree lens, sheath, bridge assembly, and various knife blades. (Courtesy Karl Storz Endoscopy-America, Inc., Culver City, CA)

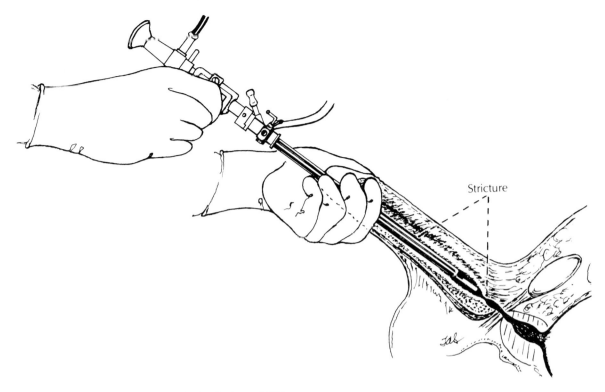

FIG. 71-3. Sagittal view of EIU

patients, good hydration and forceful urination appear to keep the urethra open and allow satisfactory regeneration of the urethra (see Fig. 71-1). In patients with extensive and long-standing chronic strictures, we have used periodic office calibration or have given cooperative patients a straight, 20Fr or 24Fr steel sound in order to self-calibrate their urethras during the critical postoperative regeneration time. This lasts from 2 to 6 months depending on the type of stricture. We try to have the patient come for final checkup about 1 year after EIU, because it is known the strictures may recur at a later stage. Bougie à boules are the most reliable calibrators to detect recurrent stricture formation.

Improved technique and careful long-term postoperative follow-up (more than 1 year) have improved our initially reported good results from 75% to over 85% in 57 patients.[6] These were all small-caliber strictures (less than 14 Fr) and more than 2 cm in length. Twelve percent of the strictures had a second or third urethrotomy, usually at the margin of the previous stricture. The incidence of recurrence could be decreased by cutting initially further proximally and distally to avoid such marginal strictures. Such recuts can usually be done

in the office, because recurrent strictures are often of short length.

Failures, which are patients with recurrent urinary complaints or decreasing urinary flow rate, can be treated by periodic urethral dilatations or preferably by open urethroplasty.

Complications

As far as I know, no mortality has been reported after EIU. Perforation with extravasation and hematoma are rare complications and decrease with increasing experience of the surgeon. If perforation and extravasation occur, and are recognized early, any serious scrotal swelling can be prevented by applying a pressure dressing around the penis or by manual pressure from the perineum against the urethra, compressing it against the public bone.

We have not encountered any significant urethral bleeding. This is usually venous in origin and can be controlled by compression dressing around the penis and the indwelling 24Fr Foley catheter. When doing the operation after the urine has been sterilized, and when operating under an antibiotic screen, infection should also be extremely rare.

We have not observed any urinary incontinence

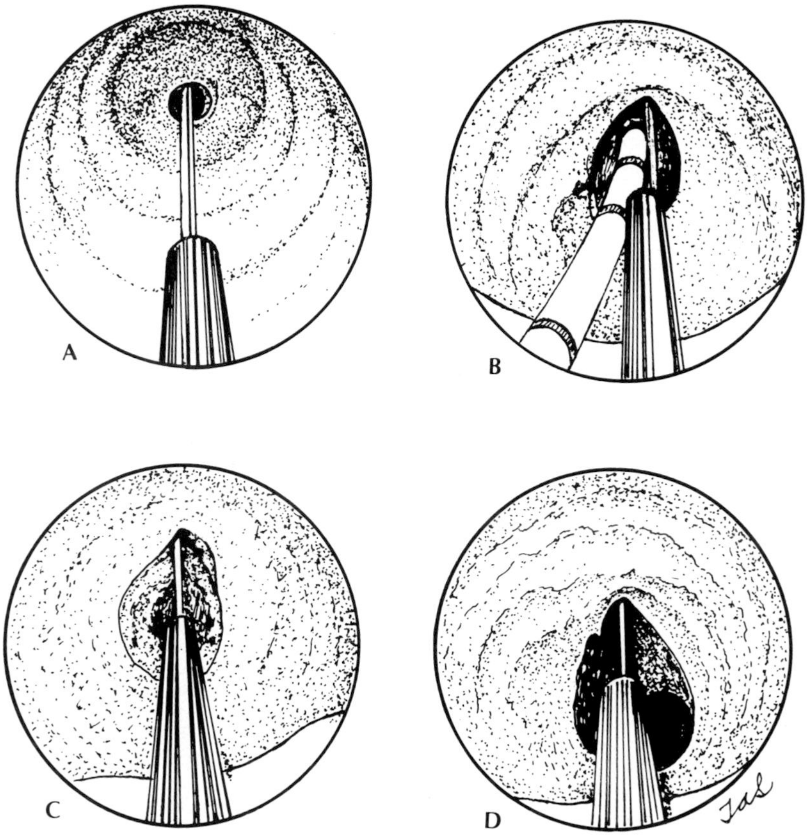

FIG. 71-4. Urethroscopic view of cut stricture at 12 o'clock

or chordee. One of our patients with a severe 4Fr to 6Fr stricture extending from the navicular portion to the membranous urethra, with a 16-year history of periodic filiform urethral dilatations, reported decrease in his potency after EIU. This has been improving and it is very difficult to tell whether psychologic factors are involved. None of the other patients has noticed any problems with potency. It is probably wise not to cut all the way through the membranous urethra, and especially not deep into the underlying tissues at that location, because of the danger of incontinence.

Urethrostomy

The main indication for doing a urethrostomy is usually severe anterior urethral stricture or small caliber urethra. In such cases, one can do a perineal urethrostomy to allow passage of the resectoscope or any other transurethral instrument, in order to bypass the anterior urethra.[2]

If it is possible, one can pass a small steel sound into the bulbous urethra and then make a short (1 cm–1.5 cm) longitudinal incision into the bulbous urethra. Bleeders can be fulgurated or ligated with fine suture material. If it is temporarily necessary to keep the stoma open, the urethral mucosa can be sutured to the skin with a few interrupted 4-0 Vicryl sutures. If the perineal urethrostomy is used only to allow passage of an endoscopic instrument, one can close the stoma by reapproximating the layers and by avoiding any protrusion of suture material into the lumen of the urethra. If a permanent perineal urethrostomy is indicated, possibly because the patient is too old or too poor a risk for EIU or urethroplasty, then the mucosa should be sutured to the skin with interrupted fine suture material to keep it permanently open. Frequently the stoma has a tendency to recontract and may require periodic dilatation.

We rarely use this procedure now because EIU can be done more readily and with fewer complications.

REFERENCES

1. ATTWATER HL: The history of urethral stricture. Br J Urol 15:39, 1943
2. BISSADA NK, REDMAN JF, WELCH LT: Transurethral

resection of prostate via perineal urethrostomy. Urology 7:70, 1976

3. EMMETT JL, KIRCHHEIM D, GREENE LF: Prevention of postoperative stricture from transurethral resection by preliminary internal urethrotomy: Report of experience with 447 cases. J Urol 78:456, 1957

4. FERRI A: De caruncula sive callo qual cervici vesical innascitur. Lugd Bat 1553

5. GUILLON G: De la stricturotomie Soc Med Practique 1831

6. KIRCHHEIM D: Results of endoscopic internal urethrotomy with improved postoperative care. Presented at the 75th annual meeting of the American Urological Association, San Francisco, May 1980

7. KIRCHHEIM D, TREMANN JA, ANSELL JS: Transurethral urethrotomy under vision. J Urol 119:496, 1978

8. LIPSKY H, HUBMER G: Direct vision urethrotomy in the management of urethral strictures. Br J Urol 498:725, 1977

9. MAISONNEUVE J: Catheterism a la suite. Bull Acad Med 1845

10. MATOUSCHEK E, MICHAELIS WAE: Internal urethrotomy of urethral strictures in men under endoscopic control. Urol Int 30:266, 1975

11. OTIS FN: The treatment of stricture of the urethra. Br Med J 1:251, 1876

12. SACHSE H: Ärztliche Fortbildungstagung. Praxis Kurier 36:85, 1972

13. SACHSE H: Zur Behandlung der Harnröhren-striktur. Die transurethrale Schlitzung unter Sicht mit scharfem Schnitt. Fortschr Med 92:12, 1974

14. SACKOFF EJ, KERR WS, JR: Direct vision cold knife urethrotomy. J Urol 123:492, 1980

15. WALTHER PC, PARSONS CL, SCHMIDT JD: Direct vision urethrotomy in the management of urethral strictures. J Urol 123:497, 1980

16. WEAVER RG, SCHULTE JW: Experimental and clinical studies of urethral regeneration. Surg Gynecol Obstet 115:729, 1962

17. WEAVER RG, SCHULTE JW: Clinical aspects of urethral regeneration. J Urol 93:247, 1965

18. YELDERMAN JJ, WEAVER RG: Behavior and treatment of urethral strictures. J Urol 97:1040, 1967

Urethrectomy

72

Harry W. Herr

The potentially multifocal nature of transitional cell carcinoma places the entire urothelium at risk in the patient with bladder cancer. The possibility of urethral recurrence in the male patient raises the question of the advisability of total urethrectomy in conjunction with cystectomy. Autopsy evidence of *in situ* urethral cancer was found by Gowing in 6 of 33 (18%) and by Hendry and associates in 19 of 101 (19%) patients who had died of bladder cancer.[2,4] Wallace cited a 12% incidence of urethral or perineal tumor recurrence after cystectomy for posterior urethral or multifocal tumors.[11] The incidence of overt urethral cancer subsequent to cystectomy for bladder carcinoma has been reported to be 4%, 7%, and 12%.[1,2,7,9] Such patients often have a poor prognosis because recurrent urethral cancer may cause local perineal tumors or inguinal lymph node metastases.[5,9] Schellhammer and Whitmore found unrecognized severe epithelial atypia or *in situ* urethral carcinoma in 12.5% of 110 male patients in whom urethrectomy was performed prophylactically during total cystectomy for bladder cancer.[9] The incidence of urethral lesions was greatest in patients with multiple low-stage tumors.

Surgical techniques for urethrectomy have been described by Johnson and Guinn and by Whitmore and Mount.[6,12] The penile inversion technique devised by Whitmore provides a safe and simple method for the incontinuity excision of the urothelium of the male urethra distal to the prostate while preserving the normal appearance of the male genitalia. Of practical importance is the observation that carcinoma may occur in the glandular urethral remnant after subtotal urethrectomy;[10] this is further evidence of tumor multicentricity and emphasizes the importance of including the fossa navicularis and urethral meatus when performing urethrectomy.

Indications

Urethrectomy in conjunction with total cystectomy is indicated when the bladder tumors are multifocal, associated with flat carcinoma *in situ*, or located near the bladder neck, or when they involve the posterior urethra or prostate; and when the prognosis, considering tumor stage and grade and the age and general condition of the patient, is favorable enough to render the risk of urethral recurrence significant. Cystourethrectomy, by allowing incontinuity removal of the bladder and urethra, may improve the margin of resection and reduce the hazard of local implants from tumor cell spillage occurring during transection of the membranous urethra at cystectomy.

Close follow-up by urethral biopsy or cytology and a high index of suspicion are indicated if incontinuity urethrectomy is not performed at the time of cystectomy.[3,8] Urethrectomy may be performed as an isolated procedure if these investigations indicate the presence of malignant cells or if the patient develops a bloody urethral discharge. Secondary urethrectomy may be a less adequate operation than primary urethrectomy, because the perineal scarring and proximity of the small bowel to the urogenital diaphragm after radical cystectomy renders complete excision of the membranous portion of the urethra more difficult and less certain.

Operative Technique

A modified lithotomy position is used for urethrectomy, with hips and knees gently flexed and the lower limbs abducted in foot stirrups. When urethrectomy is to be performed in conjunction with cystectomy, the anterior abdominal wall, external genitalia, and perineum are prepared and included in the operative field, excluding the anus posteriorly. A Foley catheter is introduced.

When bladder mobilization has been completed, except for division of the puboprostatic ligaments, it is helpful to incise the endopelvic fascia at the basal margins of the prostate on either side and to mobilize completely the lateral and posterior aspects of the prostate and membranous urethra from the urogenital diaphragm and rectum proper

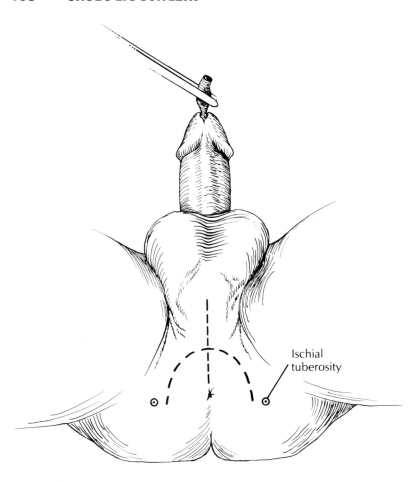

FIG. 72-1. A midline or inverted-U perineal incision between the ischial tuberosities (or a combination thereof) is used to expose the urethral bulb.

Ischial tuberosity

before beginning the perineal dissection. Temporary packing is then placed in the pelvis, and the Foley catheter is cross clamped and divided just distal to the urethral meatus. The catheter is kept securely clamped to facilitate the urethrectomy and to prevent potential tumor spillage from the urethra.

A 4-cm to 5-cm midline or inverted-U perineal incision may be used (Fig. 72-1). The latter affords easier access to the urethral arteries and greater exposure of the urethral bulb and urogenital diaphragm. Subcutaneous tissues and the bipennate bulbocavernosus muscle are divided in the midline and retracted (Fig. 72-2) to expose the corpus spongiosum, which is then isolated. A small tape is passed around the urethra and traction is applied to facilitate sharp dissection of the urethra distally, thus separating the corpus spongiosum from the adjacent corpora cavernosa (Fig. 72-3).

As dissection proceeds, the penis becomes inverted as the corpora cavernosa become bowed and the glans recedes into the phallus as it follows the line of traction on the urethra (Fig. 72-4). In

this manner, the penis is turned inside out onto the perineum and dissection is completed to the base of the glans (Fig. 72-5). To excise the meatus and glandular urethra, the penis is replaced in the anatomic position and an incision is made around the meatus and extended on either side down the ventral aspect of the glans (Fig. 72-6A). The distal urethra is then freed from its investments within the glans penis using sharp dissection (Fig. 72-6B). The isolated pendulous urethra may now be delivered onto the perineum and the filleted glans penis is reapproximated to minimize blood loss.

Proximal sharp dissection of the urethral bulb is completed to the level of the perineal membrane and inferior fascia of the urogenital diaphragm. Further sharp and blunt dissection is used to enlarge the urethral hiatus and to free the urethra above the level of the urogenital diaphragm, all or a portion of which may be included with the specimen. Vigorous traction on the urethra during this perineal phase of the operation should be avoided to prevent tearing or avulsing the urethra at the prostatomembranous junction.

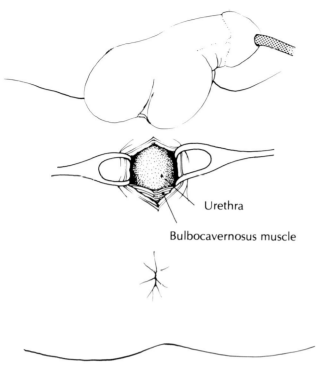

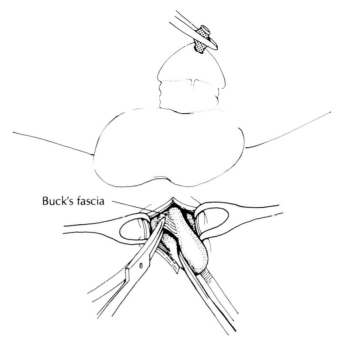

FIG. 72-2.   The bulbocavernosus muscle is retracted, demonstrating the underlying urethral bulb. (© Royal Victoria Hospital)

Urethra

Bulbocavernosus muscle

FIG. 72-3.   Sharp dissection of Buck's fascia with traction on the urethra separates the corpus spongiosum from the corpora cavernosa.   (© Royal Victoria Hospital)

Buck's fascia

FIG. 72-4.   Schematic representation of catheterized pendulous urethra **(A)** prior to dissection and **(B)** with penis inverted at completion of distal dissection to glans penis (© Royal Victoria Hospital)

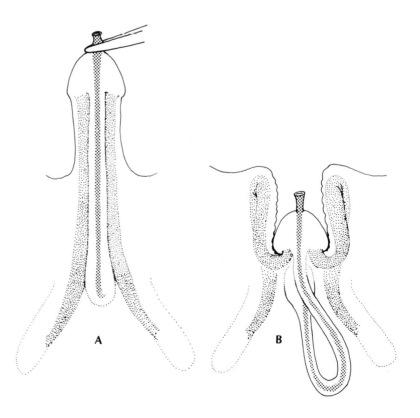

A

B

The large urethral branches of the internal pudendal arteries are isolated, ligated, and divided as they enter the bulb at 4 and 8 o'clock, just inferior to the perineal membrane (Fig. 72-7). Blunt and sharp division of the puboprostatic ligaments completes the mobilization, and the specimen is removed through the anterior abdominal incision.

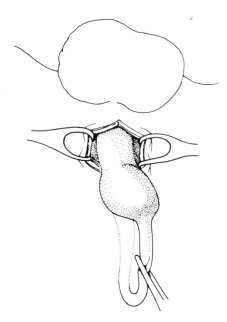

FIG. 72-5. Completion of distal dissection to the undersurface of the glans penis (© Royal Victoria Hospital)

Closure of the bulbocavernosus muscle, subcutaneous tissue, and skin with interrupted absorbable sutures completes the procedure. A light pressure dressing is applied. A small Penrose drain exiting near the frenulum is used to drain the urethral bed. It is removed on the first postoperative day. Pelvic or deep perineal drainage is not routinely employed.

A similar technique may be used when urethrectomy is performed as an isolated procedure after cystectomy. Care must be exercised in completing the proximal dissection in this situation in view of the possible postcystectomy adherence of intestine to the superior surface of the urogenital diaphragm.

Complications

The corpora cavernosa undergo acute angulation at the suspensory ligament level and again as they abut against the undersurface of the glans during the course of the dissection (see Fig. 72-4). Although some degree of corporal congestion is thus induced, detumescence is immediate on restoring the anatomic position of the penis.

Hemorrhage can be minimized during the dissection if anatomic planes are followed and if conventional techniques of clamp and ligature are used. On occasion, however, the procedure may result in blood loss of up to an additional 2 units. Division of the dorsal vein of the penis prior to urethrectomy should be avoided, because this may induce an unusual degree of corporal venous congestion and increase bleeding.

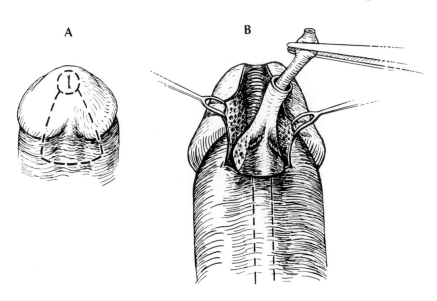

A   B

FIG. 72-6. **(A)** Incision used for **(B)** dissection of the urethral meatus and the glandular urethra. Note that the penis has been placed in its normal anatomic position.

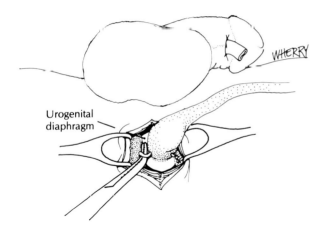

Urogenital
diaphragm

WHERRY

FIG. 72-7. Isolation and division of the artery to the urethral bulb, with a drain in the bed of the corpus spongiosum (© Royal Victoria Hospital)

The frequent superficial hematoma and edema along the penile shaft during the early postoperative period quickly resolve, although on occasion serous drainage continues for 6 to 10 days.

Unlike perineal prostatic surgery, rectal continuity is not in jeopardy during this procedure, because dissection is well anterior to the rectum at the level of the urogenital diaphragm. Caution should be exercised in patients undergoing "salvage cystourethrectomy" after prior definitive irradiation or with tumor involvement of the prostate, because in these circumstances otherwise normal tissue planes may be obliterated.

No instance of ischemia of the penis has been encountered. Edema of the wound and minor wound separation are fairly common. Superficial perineal infections are seen occasionally, but they usually drain spontaneously and pose no special problems. Serious perineal abscess is rare.

The urethrectomy may be completed in 30 to 45 minutes and adds little potential morbidity to a cystectomy.

REFERENCES

1. CORDONNIER JJ, SPJUT HJ: Urethral occurrence of bladder carcinoma following cystectomy. Trans Am Assoc Genitourin Surg 53:13, 1961
2. GOWING NFC: Urethral carcinoma associated with cancer of the bladder. Br J Urol 32:428, 1960
3. GRABSTALD H: Resectoscope loop for urethral biopsy following cystectomy in the male patient. J Urol 124:605, 1980
4. HENDRY WF, GOWING NFC, WALLACE DM: Surgical treatment of urethral tumors associated with bladder cancer. Proc Roy Soc Med 67:304, 1974.
5. HERR HW: Cis-diaminedichloride platinum II in the treatment of advanced bladder cancer. J Urol 123:853, 1980
6. JOHNSON DE, GUINN GA: Surgical management of urethral carcinoma occurring after cystectomy. J Urol 103:314, 1970
7. POOLE–WILSON DS, BARNARD RJ: Total cystectomy for bladder tumors. Br J Urol 43:16, 1971
8. RICHIE JP, SKINNER DG: Carcinoma in-situ of the urethra associated with bladder carcinoma: The role of urethrectomy. J Urol 119:80, 1978
9. SCHELLHAMMER PF, WHITMORE WF, JR.: Transitional cell carcinoma of the urethra in men having cystectomy for bladder cancer. J Urol 115:56, 1976
10. SCHELLHAMMER PF, WHITMORE WF, JR.: Urethral meatal carcinoma following cystourethrectomy for bladder carcinoma. J Urol 115:61, 1976
11. WALLACE D: Cancer of the bladder. Am J Roentgenol 102:581, 1968
12. WHITMORE WF, JR, MOUNT BM: A technique of urethrectomy in the male. Surg Gynecol Obstet 131:303, 1970

Periurethral Abscess

73

D. Patrick Currie

Periurethral abscess, with or without urinary phlegmon (extravasation), is a life-threatening emergency requiring surgical intervention. Prior to the advent of antibiotics, the mortality of those afflicted with this disease was greater than 50%, but with the currently available antibiotics capable of controlling gonorrhea and other infections, the mortality and incident rates have greatly decreased. Successful treatment of the initial periurethral abscess as well as the later reconstruction of the urethra require a thorough knowledge of the pathophysiology and anatomy of the lower urogenital tract and perineum.

Periurethral abscess is almost always a disease of men and will be so considered in this chapter. It occurs in all age and socioeconomic groups, but most commonly in patients from 40 to 60 years of age and in large indigent populations. Approximately 80% of periurethral abscesses are secondary to urethral strictures. Other causes are primary urethritis, common mainly in patients infected with *Neisseria gonorrhoeae*; trauma, usually from a straddle-type injury, with urethral damage, urinary phlegmon, and subsequent infection; urethral cysts or diverticula; urethral calculi, which usually occur secondary to strictures; indwelling urethral catheters; and trauma from instrumentation.[1,4,6,8]

Pathophysiology

Whether stricture, trauma, urethritis, or instrumentation, the basic offending mechanism injures the urethral epithelium and produces inflammation and suppurative periurethritis.[16] These processes may resolve, or they may intensify, developing into an abscess. In turn, this necrotizing infection causes localized vascular thrombosis and ischemia, and these conditions, influenced by the hydrostatic force of the urine during micturition, may extend through the corpus spongiosum and the tunica albuginea. The infection may be contained there by Buck's fascia, or, as it more commonly does, it may penetrate Buck's fascia. It could then occupy the space between Buck's fascia and Colles' fascia

in the perineum (Fig. 73-1), the space between Buck's fascia and the dartos fascia around the penis, the space between the dartos and the external spermatic fascia in the scrotum, or even the space between Scarpa's fascia and the deep fascia over the aponeurosis of the external oblique muscle of the abdomen.[18] Although any of these fascial barriers may be effective against uninfected urine, this is not the case when the urine is infected.[15]

Eventually the abscess may rupture through the cutaneous layer, usually of the perineum, draining pus and urine. This rupture may be in the form of a single fistula or multiple fistulas, creating the "watering pot perineum" (Fig. 73-2). The initial periurethral abscess may rupture into the urethra, thus forming a periurethral diverticulum with its inherent stasis and infection. Finally, the abscess may fail to rupture but instead spread subcutaneously. Urinary phlegmon from periurethral abscess has been seen subcutaneously as high as the nipples and axillae, down into the upper aspects of the thighs and into the buttocks.[2,3,5,7,10,13,20]

Presentation and Diagnosis

All gradations of signs and symptoms of infection can be seen with periurethral abscess. The patient may have only a mild perineal swelling and fever with a history of diminished urinary stream and dysuria, or he may be quite ill and moribund with the general signs of sepsis—high fever, chills, and dehydration—and uremia. There may be marked or mild penile and scrotal pain and swelling, depending on the direction in which the infection has spread. The symptoms may be chronic, but if phlegmon occurs, are usually abrupt and severe.[14] Pus and urine may be seen on the surface of the perineum or scrotum if fistulas have formed (Fig. 73-2A).

The diagnosis of periurethral abscess is usually evident from the history and physical examination and is supported by studies of blood chemistries revealing dehydration, uremia, and leukocytosis. Urine and blood cultures are also helpful. Gentle

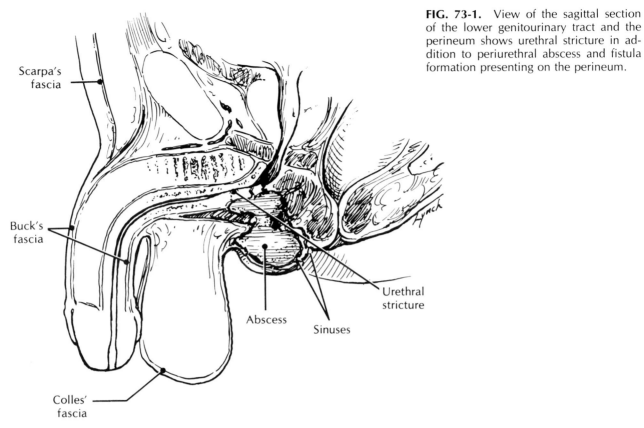

Scarpa's fascia

Buck's fascia

Colles' fascia

Abscess

Sinuses

Urethral stricture

FIG. 73-1. View of the sagittal section of the lower genitourinary tract and the perineum shows urethral stricture in addition to periurethral abscess and fistula formation presenting on the perineum.

FIG. 73-2. "Watering pot perineum" of urethral stricture and fistulas. **(A)** Extravasation, necrosis, slough, and abscess formation. **(B)** Retrograde urethrogram in patient with watering pot perineum

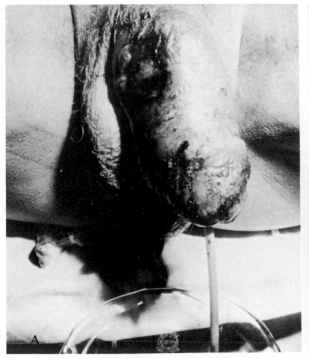

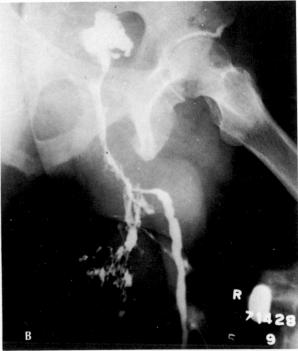

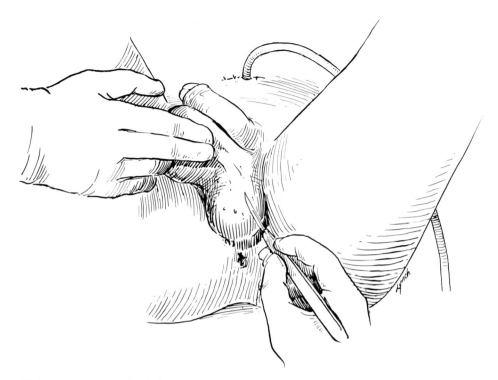

FIG. 73-3. Periurethral abscess presenting on the perineum. A lateral incision is made for drainage after suprapubic vesical diversion.

instrumentation with a catheter or sound can be helpful in diagnosing urethral stricture. Other tests of value in diagnosis are a retrograde urethrogram (Fig. 73-2*B*), a voiding cystourethrogram, and injection of fistulas with radiopaque material.[9,19] If time permits, intravenous pyelography is beneficial in evaluating obstructive uropathy and other upper tract abnormalities. Occasionally, massive scrotal and perineal edema, streptococcal cellulitis, or perirectal abscess can be confused with periurethral abscess.[17]

Treatment

Periurethral abscesses require surgical drainage and débridement as well as urinary diversion. Preoperative supportive medical measures include appropriate antibiotic therapy in high doses, rehydration of the patient, correction of electrolyte imbalances, and attention to any chronic medical conditions.

If the disease process is mild, one can dilate the urethra, usually using filiforms and Le Forte urethral sounds, and divert the urinary stream by inserting a urethral catheter. The abscess can then be drained. Usually, however, the process is much more severe and requires urinary diversion through an intubated perineal urethrostomy or by suprapubic vesical diversion (Fig. 73-3).[12] The suprapubic diversion can be performed by the usual open cystotomy or by trocar intubation.

The abscess is best drained through multiple incisions lateral to the midline and with multiple through-and-through drains. In addition to draining the abscess, the devitalized and severely diseased tissue must be debrided, preserving as much viable perineal and scrotal skin as possible for future urethroplasty. If the periurethral abscess has drained spontaneously, creating a urethrocutaneous fistula, then fistulectomy would be the primary operation.[11] This can be accomplished by excising the fistulous track, or tracks, and by performing some type of urethroplasty. The simplest procedure would be to "core out" a single fistulous track and to close the urethra primarily (Fig. 73-4). In the patient with a watering pot perineum, a block of perineal tissue containing the numerous sinus tracks, along with the ventral urethra, should be excised and a first-stage Johanson urethroplasty accomplished (Fig. 73-4). Inherent in most of these procedures is subsequent reconstructive surgery. The particular form of urethroplasty (Chap. 68) should be individualized to fit each case.

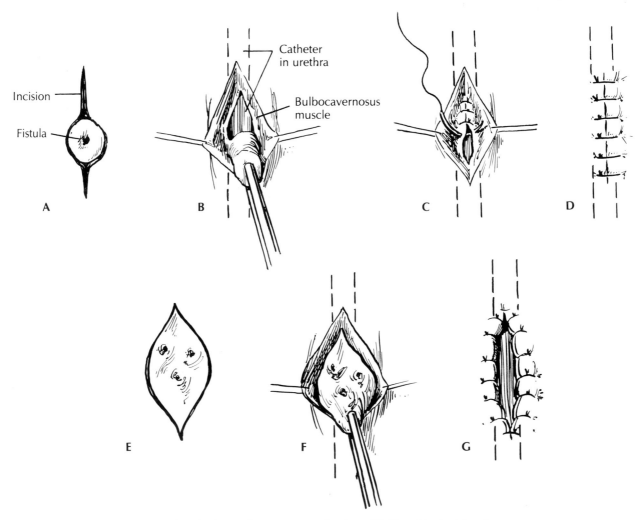

Incision

Fistula

Catheter
in urethra

Bulbocavernosus
muscle

A

B

C

D

E

F

G

FIG. 73-4. **(A** to **D)** Repair of a single urethrocutaneous fistula. **(A)** The skin incision is made. **(B)** The instrumented fistulous tract is cored out with a urethral catheter in place. **(C)** The urethra is closed over the diverting catheter. **(D)** The skin is closed. **(E** to **G)** Repair of multiple urethrocutaneous fistulas or watering pot perineum. **(E)** The skin incision is made. **(F)** The block containing the fistulous tracts and the urethra is removed. **(G)** The skin edges are sutured to the remaining normal urethra with catheter diversion either transurethrally or through urethrostomy.

REFERENCES

1. ABESHOUSE BS: Diverticula of the anterior urethra in the male: A report of four cases and a review of the literature. Urol Cutan Rev 55:690, 1951
2. ALLEN TD: Periurethral phlegmon: Posterior rupture through Colles' fascia. Br J Urol 37:335, 1965
3. BAKER WJ, WILKEY, JL, BARSON LJ: An evaluation of the management of peri-urethral phlegmon in 272 consecutive cases at the Cook County Hospital. J Urol 61:943, 1949
4. BLANDY JP, SINGH M: Fistulae involving the adult male urethra. Br J Urol 44:632, 1972
5. CAMPBELL MF: Periurethral phlegmon (urinary extravasation). A study of one hundred and thirty-five cases. Surg Gynecol Obstet 48:382, 1929
6. CAMPBELL MF: Complications of gonorrhea: Periurethral abscess, stricture, arthritis. Am J Surg 12:277, 1931
7. FINESTONE EO: Urinary extravasation (periurethral phlegmon); Pathogenesis and experimental study. Surg Gynecol Obstet 73:218, 1941
8. GOLDBERG HW, GROVE JS: Acquired diverticulum of the male urethra with calculi formation. Chicago Medical School Quarterly 24:30, 1964

9. LANG EK: Periurethral abscess. J Indiana State Med Assoc 63:352, 1970

10. LURIA J, EVANS AT: Periurethral phlegmon. J Urol 106:384, 1971

11. MALAMENT M: Repair of the recurrent fistula of the penile urethra. J Urol 106:704, 1971

12. MEHAN DJ, BERSON J: One stage management of periurethral abscess complicating urethral stricture. South Med J 63:1179, 1970

13. RIEKERT JG: Management and mortality of periurethral phlegmons. J Urol 61:424, 1949

14. SINGH M: Emergency treatment of impassable urethral strictures in the tropics. Proc Roy Soc Med 60:871, 1967

15. SMITH HS, FINTON RE: Urinary extravasation from urethra, with analysis of 151 cases. Urol Cutan Rev 45:481, 1941

16. STONE HH, WILLIS TV, JR: Periurethral abscess in patients with major burns. Am Surg 38:318, 1972

17. TASHIRO S, HINMAN F, JR: Periurethral and perirectal infections; Pathological and clinical differentiation. J Urol 57:338, 1947

18. UIILENHUTH E, SMITH RD, DAY EC et al: A re-investigation of Colles' and Buck's fasciae in the male. J Urol 62:542, 1949

19. VEIGA–PIRES JA, ELEBUTE EA: Urethrocystography in the male. Br J Urol 39:194, 1967

20. WILKEY JL, BARSON LJ, PORTNEY FR: Urinary extravasation and periurethral phlegmon: Clinical analysis of 100 cases. J Urol 82:657, 1959

Megalourethra

74

Jorge L. Lockhart

Anomalies of the male urethra other than hypospadias are uncommon, and megalo-urethra is rare. As described by Nesbitt, megalourethra is a distinct anomaly, readily differentiated from urethral diverticulum.[2]

The male urethra is derived from the urogenital sinus, and the erectile tissue of the corpora cavernosa and the corpus spongiosum represent differentiation of mesodermal columns during the seventh week of fetal life. Thus, very early failure of mesenchymal development may be incriminated as the cause of megalourethra.[1] This anomaly is usually associated with others. One of these other anomalies, severe renal dysplasia, may be incompatible with life.

As defined by Stephens and elaborated by Williams, there are two types of megalourethra.[4,5] Both forms probably represent a portion of the spectrum of mesodermal defects which includes the prune-belly syndrome. The first and most severe is the complete or fusiform type. In such instances there is total failure of development of erectile tissue. The urethra becomes massively dilated, filling and distending the flabby penile structure, which consists of skin, subcutaneous tissue, and scanty fascial elements. Although Belman documents successful management of one patient with fusiform megalourethra,* it is suggested that there might be justification for sex reassignment in the neonatal interval. The second type of megalourethra is the incomplete or scaphoid form (Fig. 74-1), which has a better prognosis. In this situation, the corpora cavernosa are intact, but there is congenital absence of the distal portion of the corpus spongiosum, permitting rather dramatic dilatation of the terminal portion of the urethra, which balloons during voiding.

When first seen, these patients may need urinary decompression. The problem can usually be solved with a meatotomy, but occasionally a cutaneous vesicostomy is required to improve bladder and upper tract drainage. Reconstruction should occur at approximately 1 year of age, and Nesbitt's reductive urethroplasty using general principles of

---

* Belman AB: Unpublished data

FIG. 74-1. Incomplete or scaphoid megalourethra, involving distal portion of penile urethra only. **(A)** Patient voiding with demonstration of ballooning of distal urethra. **(B)** Voiding cystourethrogram, showing massive cystic dilatation of distal penile urethra

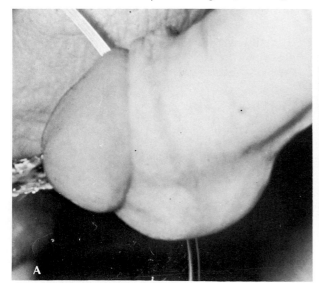
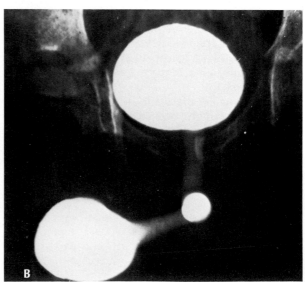

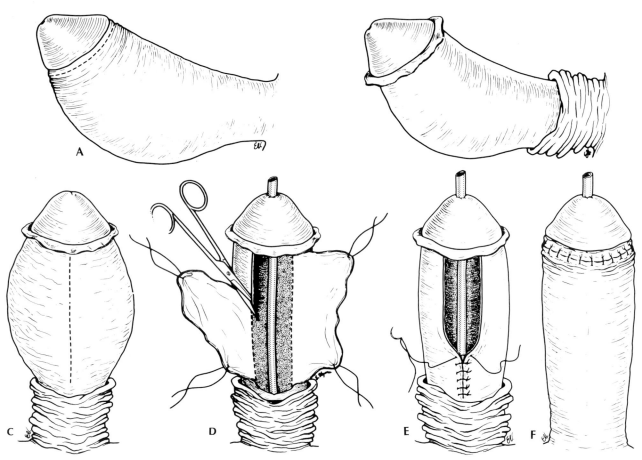

FIG. 74-2. Nesbitt procedure for correction of incomplete megalourethra. **(A)** A circumferential incision is made proximal to the glans. **(B)** The penile skin is mobilized to expose the corpora and the urethra. **(C)** The line of incision into the dilated urethra is shown. **(D)** With an indwelling catheter as a guide, the redundant excess urethral tissue is excised. **(E)** The urethra is reconstructed with multiple interrupted absorbable sutures; a second running layer of absorbable suture may also be employed, bringing together elements of fascia for further support. **(F)** The penile skin is replaced, using multiple interrupted absorbable sutures.

hypospadias repair achieves good functional and cosmetic results. Vesical diversion in the form of a vesicostomy or a temporary suprapubic cystostomy is advisable.

A collar incision is made in the skin around the corona and brought back to the base of the penis (Fig. 74-2A and B). The redundant, dilated urethra is incised from the base of the glans up to the proximal extension of the sac. The redundant lateral wings of urethra are excised, leaving a strip of normal urethra of approximately 1.5 cm in width. The lateral margins of the strip are sutured over an 8Fr plastic feeding tube with submucosal, interrupted 6-0 chromic sutures. After the penile skin is brought back over the shaft, the excess is removed and its free margin is sutured to the coronal mucosa.

An alternative to this repair, particularly in cases of severe infection, would be a two-stage Johansson type of urethroplasty.[3]

REFERENCES

1. LOCKHART JL, REEVE HR, KRUEGER RP et al: Megalourethra. Urology 12:51, 1978
2. NESBITT TE: Congenital megalourethra. J Urol 73:839, 1955.
3. SHROM SH, CROMIE WJ, DUCKETT JW, JR: Megalourethra. Urology, 17:152, 1981
4. STEPHENS FD: Congenital Malformations of the Rectum, Anus and Genito-Urinary Tract, p 226. London, Livingstone, 1963
5. WILLIAMS DI: The male bladder neck and urethra. In Pediatric Urology, p 272. London, Butterworths, 1968

Urethral Valves

75

Guy W. Leadbetter, Jr.

Urethral valves, because of their obstructive nature, may cause the death of infants and children. If the obstruction is minimal, the valves may not be discovered until childhood or later.[2,5] Diagnosis and proper treatment are extremely important.[1,9] The newborn with posterior urethral valves may present with uremia and all its complications. Later in childhood or adolescence the patient may present with only nocturnal or diurnal enuresis. In any case, diagnosis of urethral valves may be considered. The preferred treatment is primary destruction of the valves, but temporizing drainage to the upper urinary tract may be necessary if the patient's condition warrants.[3]

Classification and Diagnosis

Most authors agree that Young's classification of valves is incorrect. Type 2 valves probably do not exist, but are mucosal folds mistaken for valves. Type 1 valves are common. Type 3 valves are rare and diaphragmatic in appearance. A Type 3 valve is considered a severe form of Type 1 valve, which consists of mucosal folds attached at the distal apex of the verumontanum and extending posterolaterally to be fastened on the urethral wall proximal to the external sphincter.

The voiding cystourethrogram (VCU) is a *sine qua non* for the presence or absence of valves (Fig. 75-1). If "valves" are observed only during cystoscopy and obstruction is not demonstrated by VCU, the diagnosis of valves is incorrect, these "valves" being normal urethral folds or plicae colliculi.

Preparation for Surgery

If the patient is in good condition, primary valve resection is the treatment of choice, and mild azotemia is not a contraindication to this procedure.

As a rule, no special preparation is needed preoperatively. However, if the neonate presents with uremia, acidosis, dehydration, or sepsis, care must be directed to correcting fluid imbalance, sepsis, and drainage of the urinary tract.

Often drainage may be accomplished by passing a 5Fr or 8Fr infant feeding tube through the urethra to the bladder. If after 72 hr the child's condition is no better and not satisfactory for surgery, temporary vesicostomy (Duckett) may be performed. If sepsis persists, higher drainage through open or percutaneous nephrostomy or high ureterostomy should be done. If high diversion is performed, renal biopsy should be done to document the prognosis and the current state of the kidney. Because of ureteral coiling secondary to obstruction, low ureterostomy should not be done; good drainage does not result.

Operative Techniques

Open operative procedures and techniques for destroying valves by retrograde passage of sounds through a suprapubic cystotomy, retropubic re-

FIG. 75-1. VCU illustrates posterior urethral valves

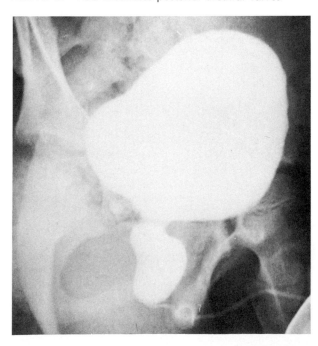

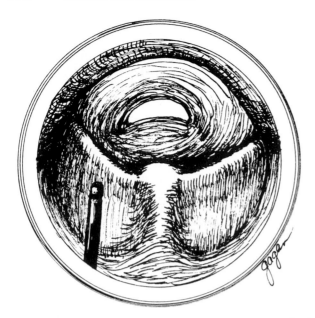

FIG. 75-2. Bugbee electrode and intact posterior urethral valves

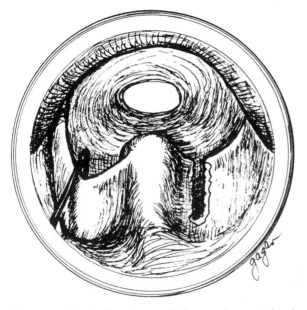

FIG. 75-3. Ureteral catheter with bent stylette. Left valve is incised.

moval through the anterior commissure of the prostate, or removal through the perineum should be considered of historical interest. Proper therapy is transurethral identification and obstruction of valves using a pediatric endoscopic instrument (8Fr, 10Fr, and 12Fr). The lens and light systems of these instruments are so clear that identification

and destruction of the valves can be performed much more easily than previously.

ENDOSCOPIC RESECTION OR FULGURATION OF VALVES

Using endoscopic instruments in a newborn and young boy requires great care. Even though the instruments are small, the irritation by the instrument of the urethra may cause rapid swelling and edema with subsequent stricture formation. This occurs particularly when the instrument is slightly large and tight in the urethra. However, with miniature endoscopes, this will not occur if the procedure is carried out with care and expeditiousness. In an unusual case, if the urethra is too small a perineal urethrotomy should be performed and a resection carried out using this route.

PERINEAL URETHROTOMY

Perineal urethrotomy is most easily performed by inserting a 5Fr or 8Fr feeding tube through the urethra into the bladder, incising into the bulbous urethra over the catheter, pulling the catheter out of the opening, placing sutures in the edges of the urethra, and removing the catheter through the opening and inserting the endoscope. Postoperatively the catheter is left in the urethra for 3 to 4 days. Perineal urethrostomy is a frequent cause of urethral stricture.

In infants the endoscope is used with a Bugbee electrode or an ureteral catheter with the stylet inserted and bent at right angles at the tip. The valves are visualized running from the distal end of the verumontanum posterolaterally toward the urethral wall. Valves may be either resected or excised with the cutting current, or fulgurated (Fig. 75-2 and Fig. 75-3). With either technique, care must be taken not to injure the external sphincter, which is closely adjacent to the valves. Because of this, I prefer to push the cutting instrument from distal to proximal toward the bladder neck. If the urethra is large enough to use the infant resectoscope, the loop is used to divide the valves at their base where they are attached to the verumontanum. Usually it is only necessary to free this attachment because the valves are made nonobstructing (Fig. 75-3). If they are not free enough to accomplish this, the valves should be destroyed. Confirmation of valve destruction and an unobstructed urinary flow may be demonstrated by postoperative voiding cystourethrogram. It certainly is better to do too little and perform a second-stage procedure than to do too much and injure

FIG. 75-4. Anterior urethral valves. Open excision will be done.

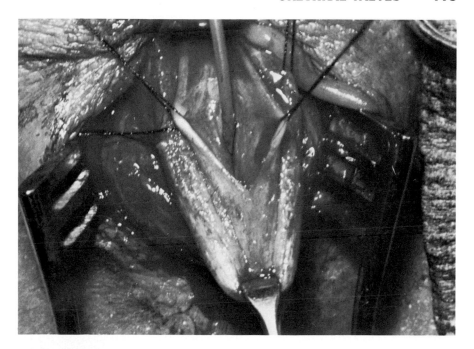

FIG. 75-5. Voiding cystourethrogram illustrates anterior urethral valves with diverticulum.

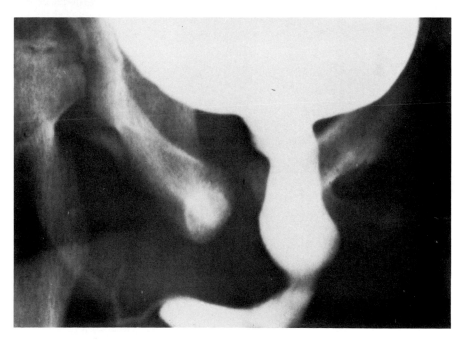

the external urethral sphincter. In most cases, with experience, enough valve can be destroyed to accomplish a nonobstructive urinary flow. The Bugbee electrode and ureteral catheter with an angled stent can be used in the 8Fr or 10Fr endoscope. Following destruction of the valves, an urethral catheter is left in place for 3 to 4 days.

One must be aware that after relief of obstruction there may be a large loss of fluid and electrolytes. These must be replaced. In most cases, following surgery, the dilated upper urinary tract will resolve toward normal and nothing further will need to be done.[7,8] If diversion has been performed preoperatively, closure may be done at any convenient time.

Anterior urethral valves are rare (Fig. 75-4). When present they are distal to the posterior urethra and often near the penoscrotal junction.[4,6] Radiologic appearance is usually that of a diverticulum in the midurethra (Fig. 75-5). Valves of this nature may be fulgurated as described. If the leaflets are thick, as they often are, the valves may be excised by open urethrotomy.[10] I prefer open excision and repair of the diverticulum. Both the valves and the excess urethral tissue forming the diverticulum are sharply excised. The urethra and surrounding tissue are closed in layers, and the urethral catheter is left in place for several days.

A word of caution is indicated. I remember a patient with posterior urethral structure secondary to an anal repair for imperforate anus. The stricture was repaired successfully, but the patient continued to have mild symptoms and developed intermittent urinary tract infections. Follow-up VCU demonstrated anterior urethral valves, overlooked because of the more proximal urethral stricture. The valves were treated successfully by open repair.

REFERENCES

1. CORNIL C: Endoscopic diagnosis of posterior urethral valves. In Bergsma D, Duckett JW (eds): Urinary System Malformations in Children. New York, Alan R Liss, 1977
2. DUCKETT JW: Current management of posterior urethral valves. Urol Clin North Am 1:471, 1974
3. DUCKETT JW: Cutaneous vesicostomy in infants and children. Urol Clin North Am 1:484, 1974
4. FIRLIT CF, KING LR: Anterior urethral valves in children. J Urol 108:972, 1972
5. HENDREN WH: Posterior urethral valves: Management J Urol 110:682, 1973
6. KELALIS PP: Anterior Urethra. In Kelalis PP, King LR, Belman AS (eds): Clinical Pediatric Urology, p 328. Philadelphia, W B Saunders. 1976
7. WHITAKER RH: Methods of assessing obstruction in dilated ureters. Br J Urol 45:15, 1973
8. WHITAKER RH: The ureter in posterior urethral valves. Br J Urol 45:395, 1973
9. WHITAKER RH, KEETON JE, WILLIAMS DI: Posterior urethral valves: A study of urinary control after operation. J Urol 108:167, 1972
10. WILLIAMS DI, RETIK AB: Congenital valves and diverticula of the anterior urethra. Br J Urol 41:228, 1969

Chordee and Hypospadias

76

Charles J. Devine, Jr.

Normal development of the external genitalia in the male is the result of the reaction of the local tissues to circulating testosterone produced by the developing testes. Incomplete development of the penis and urethra results in hypospadias with the urethral meatus on the underside of the shaft of the penis. Mesenchymal tissue distal to the urethral meatus develops in a dysgenetic fashion, forming a fan-shaped fibrous band of tissue with its apex surrounding the urethral meatus and its base inserting into the underside of the glans penis. This band causes chordee, a ventral bend of the penis. Except in cases with a very distally placed meatus, the tissues of this band must be resected to straighten the penis. Normal development of the prepuce begins in the ventral midline proximal to the corona of the glans after development of the urethra in the glans.[2,5] In hypospadias the prepuce becomes a dorsal hood deficient on the ventral side the width of the insertion of the fibrous band causing chordee (Fig. 76-1).

Treatment of hypospadias depends upon the location of the urethral meatus and the presence or absence of chordee. Over the course of the last 25 years, surgical techniques have been developed that allow the surgeon to correct the chordee and place the urethral meatus at the tip of the penis in one stage with a complication rate of under 15%. Multistaged surgical procedures and those not concerned with getting the meatus into the glans are described adequately in older publications and will not be discussed here.[11] However, these procedures should not be dismissed because from time to time they will be valuable in rescuing what otherwise might be a disastrous situation.

We prefer to do operations for hypospadias when the child is 2 years old. The penis is large enough to operate upon comfortably and the psychologic effects of the genital surgery are minimized. At this age the child is going through a phase of attachment to his mother, so it is important that she stay with him during the period of hospitalization. Some have recommended earlier or later times for the surgery,[1] but we have found that at this age the child's attention span is longer than at 1½ or 3 years and that he is more easily distracted, thus easier to manage in the hospital.

Delicate instruments, fine suture materials, and, when necessary, optical loupes are all important in this type of surgery.* We retract tissues with fine hooks and make skin incisions with knife blades rather than scissors. We dissect in deep tissue by engaging the tips of the scissors in the tissue and spreading them apart, opening tissue planes with minimal cutting. We electrofulgurate bleeding vessels, not large clumps of tissue, and avoid ligatures and suture ligatures. We use fine Vicryl suture for subcutaneous tissue and 6-0 or 5-0 chromic for the epithelium. We drain the operative area with small suction drains† and usually do not apply pressure dressings. When a pressure dressing is needed for more than an hour or two postoperatively, this amount of pressure will damage tissue and delay healing.

Postoperatively we place a Xeroform patch to cover the repair and then wrap the penis with

---

* The following instruments are available from Snowden Pencer Instruments, Parke, Davis & Co., Medical–Surgical Division, Detroit, MI:

Needle Holder Derf (400) 7000 insert 2 ratchet, adjusted to apply pressure without locking (like the third ratchet was there). Devine modification.

Scissors (700) Strabismus curved B.B.

Iris (705) slightly tipped blunt like PAR. Devine modification.

Iris straight (706) S.S. (used with suture).

Iris (705) S.S. shortened thicker blade. Devine modification.

Metz (711) stock item.

Devine–Horton Adson (500) 1 × 2 rat tooth with 7000 insert.

5-0 and 6-0 Vicryl and 5-0 and 6-0 chromic sutures are available from Ethicon, Inc., Somerville, NJ.

† The "minivac" has been a valuable adjunct. We cut the Luer hub off a 16-gauge or smaller butterfly needle and cut holes in the side of the tube so that blood and serum will drain, leaving the plastic tube long enough so that the needle end will reach the abdominal wall from the wound. The tip of this tube with the side holes is left in the wound. Plugging the needle at the other end into a sterilized Hemovac blood collection tube provides suction drainage.

absorbent cotton (a practical, short-fiber, bleached 4 by 5 cotton that is easily autoclaved or gas sterilized) cut into 1 × 4 inch (2.5 cm by 10.2 cm) strips. We keep this wet with cold saline solution for the first 3 days after the surgery and keep the child in bed with his feet elevated. Our nurses and the child's mother keep the patient amused. The saline solution is dripped on the dressing every 15 to 30 minutes during the first day, and the cotton is changed when it becomes too sodden to remain in place. The frequency of irrigations is decreased on the second and third days. As these dressings are changed we are able to evaluate the penis, looking for hematoma, excessive swelling, and

evidence of infection or of ecchymosis or necrosis in the flaps. Care of postoperative complications has been discussed elsewhere.[4,9]

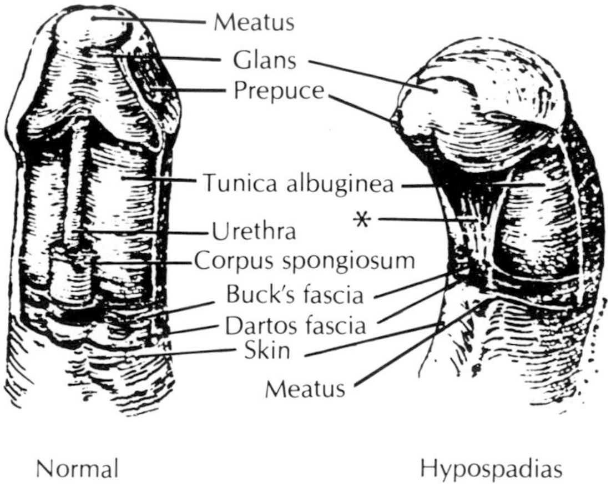

Distal Hypospadias

The glans penis is not firmly attached to the ends of the corporal bodies; and in very distal hypospadias, when the urethral meatus is on the glans or at the corona, the glans will tilt ventrally as the penile skin is retracted owing to the loose prepuce on the dorsal side (Fig. 76-2). The artificial erection enables us to evaluate the status of chordee prior to surgery and to select a procedure designed to correct the condition.[10,13] When there is no actual bend to the shaft of the penis (Fig. 76-3), circumcision to remove the unsightly hood is all that is necessary (Fig. 76-3D).

When we demonstrate chordee prior to surgery, we plan the skin incisions necessary to do what we have called our flip-flap operation. We make incisions and reflect the skin from the shaft of the penis, often cutting fibrotic bands of dartos fascia to accomplish this, (Fig 76-4). If an artificial erection then shows a straight penis (Fig. 76-4C), the residual mesenchyme plays no part in the clinical picture and we do not need to dissect beneath the urethra. We feel that it is necessary to advance the urethra into the glans. If the meatus is proximal to the corona, we do a modification of our flip-flap operation in which we incise on each side of the grooved midline strip of glans mucosa and mobilize the lateral wings of glans tissue (Fig. 76-5). This dissection can be accomplished without a lot of bleeding by using strabismus scissors and keeping their tips against the surface of the tunica albuginea of the corpora cavernosa.

FIG. 76-1. Anatomy of the normal penis and that in hypospadias. The fan-shaped band of fibrous tissue marked with an asterisk is the structure that holds the penis in chordee. (Same as Fig. 82-7, used permission of W.B. Saunders)

Normal — Meatus, Glans, Prepuce, Tunica albuginea, Urethra, Corpus spongiosum, Buck's fascia, Dartos fascia, Skin, Meatus — Hypospadias

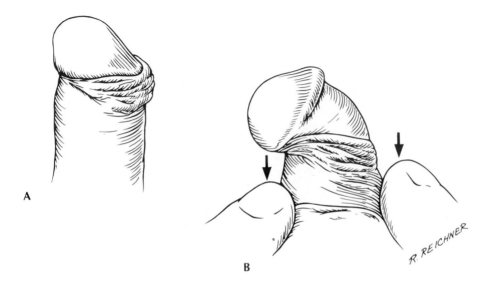

FIG. 76-2. **(A)** Distal hypospadias with dorsal hood of prepuce. **(B)** Traction of the skin toward the base causes ventral tilt of the glans.

R. REICHNER

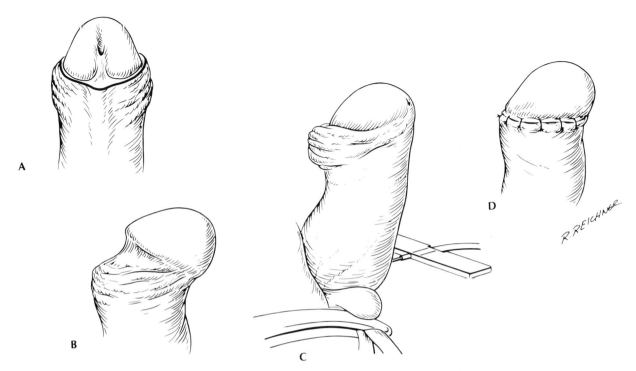

FIG. 76-3. Distal hypospadias: **(A)** ventral view; **(B)** lateral view traction on the skin has caused the glans to tilt; **(C)** artificial erection shows that the penis is straight; **(D)** dorsal hood of prepuce removed

FIG. 76-4. **(A)** The erection that occurred during induction of anesthesia demonstrates chordee. **(B)** As the skin is reflected, bands of fibrous dartos fascia may be excised. **(C)** Penis is straight and redundant prepuce will be excised.

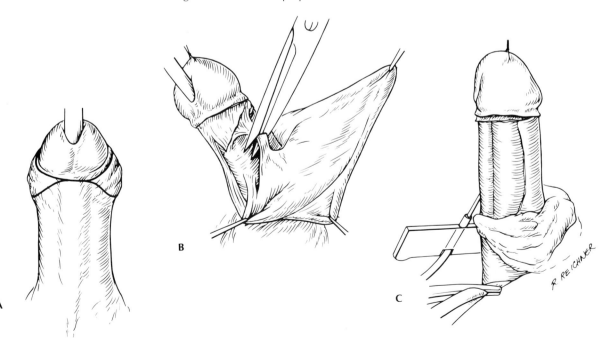

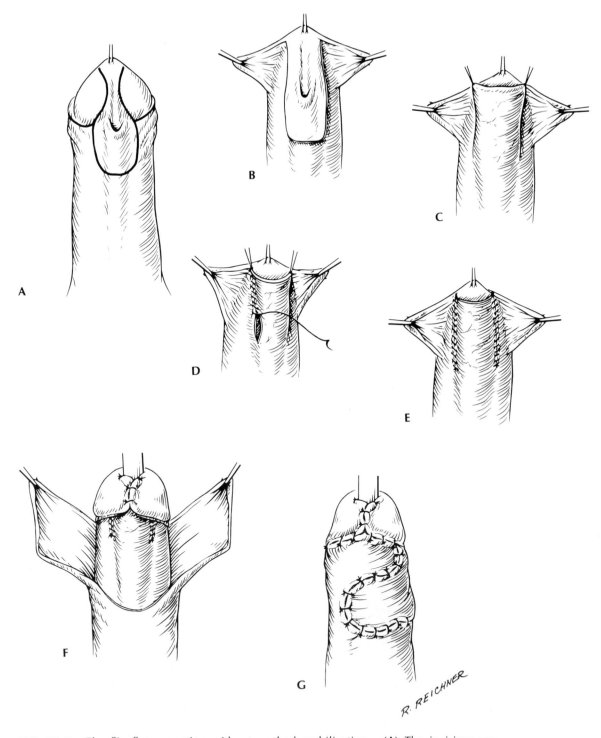

FIG. 76-5. The flip flap operation without urethral mobilization. **(A)** The incisions are marked out. **(B)** Incision and mobilization of the flip flap and the glans wings are performed. **(C)** The flap planned to form the ventral aspect of the neourethra is secured with distal holding stitches. **(D)** The lateral defect is closed with running subepithelial sutures, burying the edges. **(E and F)** Mobilized glans are wings approximated ventral to the neourethra. **(F and G)** Penile skin is transposed to the ventral side utilizing interrupted 6-0 chromic gut.

◀**FIG. 76-6.** Meatal advancement and glans plasty (MAGPI). **(A)** Erection has demonstrated no chordee; circumcising incision is marked. **(B)** Lateral pull with skin hooks elevates a fold of the midline urethral groove. **(C and D)** Fold is incised in the midline, creating a transverse defect. **(E)** The edge of the urethra is sutured to the edge of the skin of the glans, creating a large meatus. **(F)** A hook in the skin edges at the ventral midline is pulled distally, bringing the lateral edges of the skin together. **(G)** Several chromic sutures approximate these edges, bringing glans tissue ventral to the meatus. **(H)** The penile skin can usually be directly replaced, but making a dorsal incision and moving skin to the ventrum can secure a loose ventral penile surface.

its neocirculation from the covering tissues. If we use a graft we obtain it from the distal skin of the opened-up prepuce and sew it in place with interrupted sutures of chromic gut, trying to stay outside the lumen and also turning the epithelium in.

Hodgson's second procedure also fits this situation (Fig. 76-10).[11] After dissecting and sewing the glans flap to the urethra we approach the prepuce, which has not previously been unfolded, and isolate a patch of innerface epithelium by excising the rest of the epithelium from around it. We make a hole in the outerface skin proximal to this flap and stretch the hole, enlarging it so that the glans can be drawn through. We sew the edges of the preputial flap to the urethra and the glans flap; we excise the excess of the outerface skin,

(*Text continues on p. 784*)

FIG. 76-7. Distal hypospadias with urethral mobilization. **(A)** Incisions for flip flap operation are outlined. The glans incisions have not yet been marked. **(B)** After completion of mobilization of penile skin, the chordee is still present. **(D)** A dysgenetic band deep and distal to the meatus is dissected out and excised. **(D)** An artificial erection now reveals the penis to be straight.

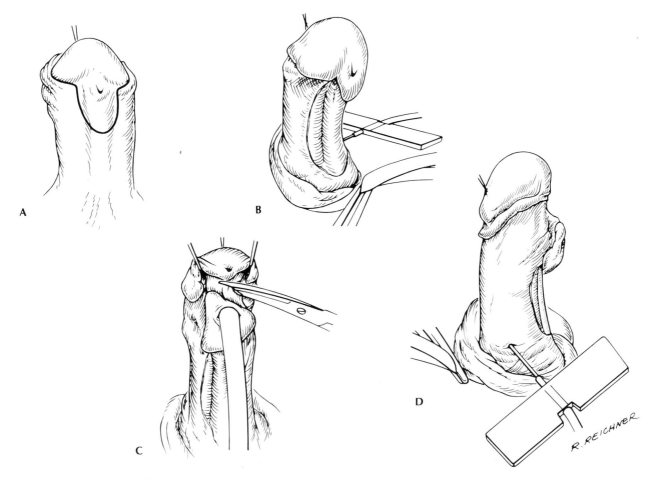

A

B

C

D

R. REICHNER

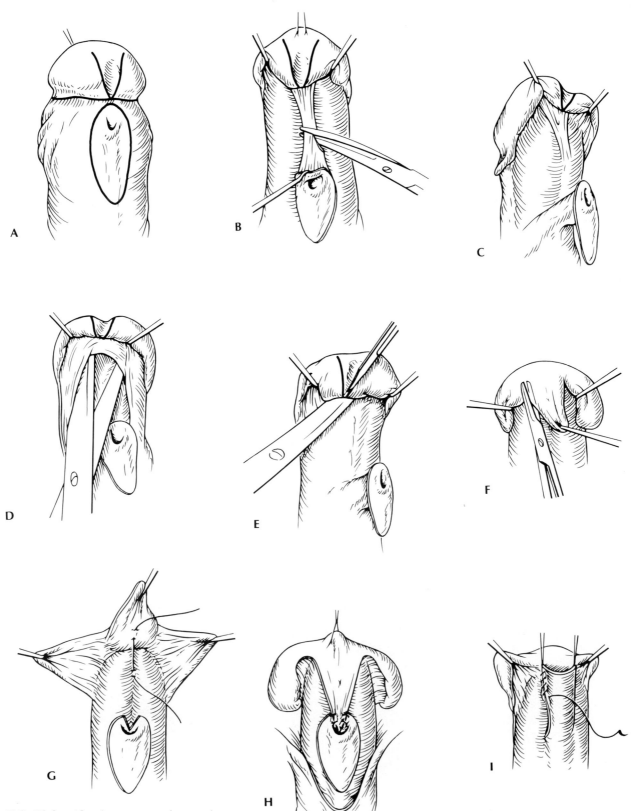

FIG. 76-8.   *(Caption on opposite page)*

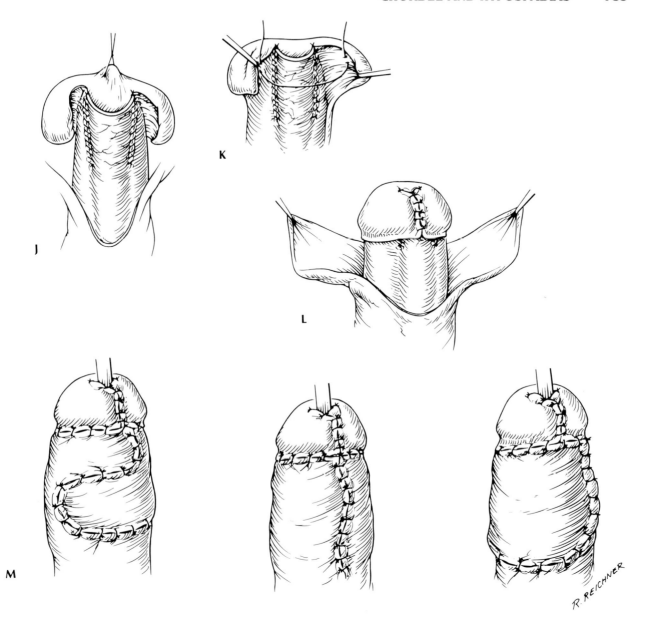

FIG. 76-8. Flip flap repair of distal hypospadias. **(A)** Incisions marked: circumcising incision is 3–5 mm proximal to the corona. The flip flap is based on the urethral meatus and the glans flaps is developed later. **(B)** The skin has been retracted and the dysgenetic band causing the chordee is being cut. **(C)** Hooks placed beneath the edge of the glans lift it to expose corpora. **(D)** Tips of iris scissors can be passed into the space between the glans and the corpora. **(E)** Epithelium of the glans is cut with a knife, using the scissors for counterpressure. **(F)** Midline flap is thinned by cutting subcutaneous tissue with the scissors. **(G)** After mobilizing the lateral wings the tips of the corpora cavernosa are exposed and the midline glans flap is secured to the midline of the corporal bodies with a subepithelial suture. **(H)** When the flap meets the urethral meatus, it is set into a dorsal meatotomy incision. **(I)** The edges of the flip flap are sutured to the edges of the glans flap. **(J)** When flaps are secure, the glans wings are brought ventral to the neourethra. **(K)** A suture through the erectile tissue takes tension off the epithelial edges. **(L)** A dorsal midline incision allows the hood of prepuce to be brought to the ventral surface. **(M)** Flaps are approximated as they fit best and excess tissue is excised.

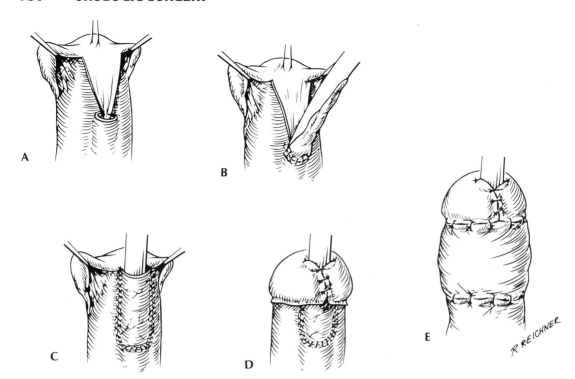

FIG. 76-9.   Patch graft repair for distal hypospadias.   **(A)** The midline glans flap meets the urethra and the flip flap is not feasible.   **(B)** A patch graft has been obtained from the prepuce and attached to the urethra by interrupted chromic sutures over a stenting catheter.   **(C)** Anastomosis is completed and glans wings are ready to be brought ventral to the neourethra.   **(D)** Glans wings are approximated.   **(E)** Skin closure is complete.

tailoring it to fit the defect in the ventral penile skin, and bring the glans wings around the neourethra, approximating the skin edges.

Midshaft Hypospadias

When the urethral meatus is more proximally located on the penile shaft, dissection to release the chordee is the same as in the more distal operations; but sometimes we will find that removing all of the tissue from the tunica will not straighten the penis. In these cases there is a defect in the tunica itself.[12,14] In the past we have made multiple transverse incisions in the tunica but recently have found that a deep incision into the midline structures will accomplish straightening with less trauma (Fig. 76-11). While the penis is still filled with saline, using a No. 15 blade we incise through the tunica into the fibers of the midline septum. If this is done with care, it can be accomplished without getting into the erectile tissue which is contained within its own sheath. The incision may have to be made the full length of the penis. If this procedure is not sufficient, as in

patients who have undergone multiple operations and have a lot of scarring of these layers, we make a transverse incision or excise the scar to place a dermal graft.[6] However, because we are unable to place a tube graft on the dermal graft, in virgin hypospadias cases we proceed to the ventral aspect of the penis where we excise a segment of tunica and, by sewing the tunica edges together, shorten the dorsal aspect of the penis to correct the bend. Although this basically accomplishes what the Nesbit plication does (Fig. 76-12), it is not simply a plication.[15] We mobilize the dorsal band of Buck's fascia containing the blood vessels and nerves; then, carefully retracting this band so that we do not traumatize the dorsal arteries which supply blood to the glans penis, we mark out and excise an ellipse of tunica about 1 cm in width at the center line. We then approximate the edges with one 5-0 Prolene suture at the midline and running sutures of 5-0 Vicryl from the midline to the lateral ends.

If, when the penis is straight, the midline glans flap will not meet the urethral meatus, we must

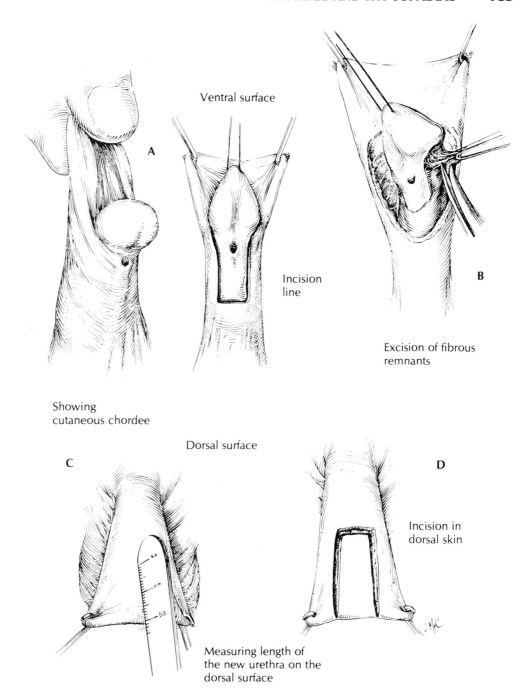

Ventral surface

Incision line

A

Showing cutaneous chordee

B

Excision of fibrous remnants

Dorsal surface

C

Measuring length of the new urethra on the dorsal surface

D

Incision in dorsal skin

FIG. 76-10.   Hodgson Type II procedure.   **(A to D)** Mobilization of foreskin and incision of dorsal skin.   **(E to J)** Reconstruction of urethra and ventral closure. (Urologic Procedures, Vol. 1, No. 4, Warner–Chilcott, 1972)

devise a tube to bridge the defect between the urethra and the glans. The tube graft procedure reported in another publication is our procedure of choice for this repair (Fig. 76-13).[3] We remove a full-thickness strip of skin from the distal end of

the unfolded prepuce. In a 2-year-old child this should be about 1.5 cm in width and as long as is necessary to bridge the gap. We remove all of the subcutaneous tissue from this skin and form it into a tube over a 12Fr red rubber catheter, leaving a

(*Text continues on p. 792*)

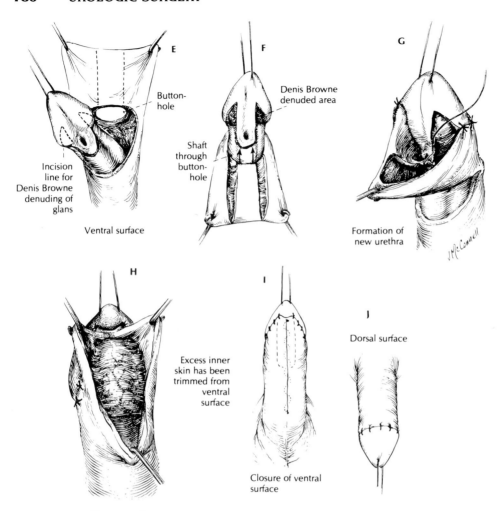

FIG. 76-10.   (Continued)

FIG. 76-11.   Midshaft hypospadias.   **(A)** After excising the subcutaneous layer of dysgenetic fibrous tissue, chordee may persist, indicating an abnormality in the corpora cavernosa.   **(B)** With the erection maintained, incision in the tunica albuginea in the midline carries the dissection into the septum between the erectile bodies.   **(C)** As the edges of the incised tunica move apart, the penis is straightened.

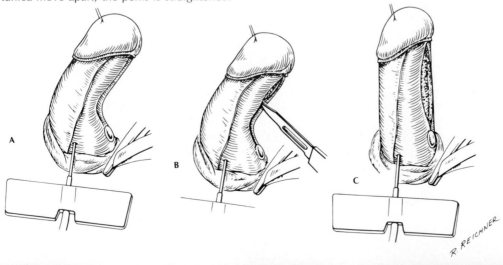

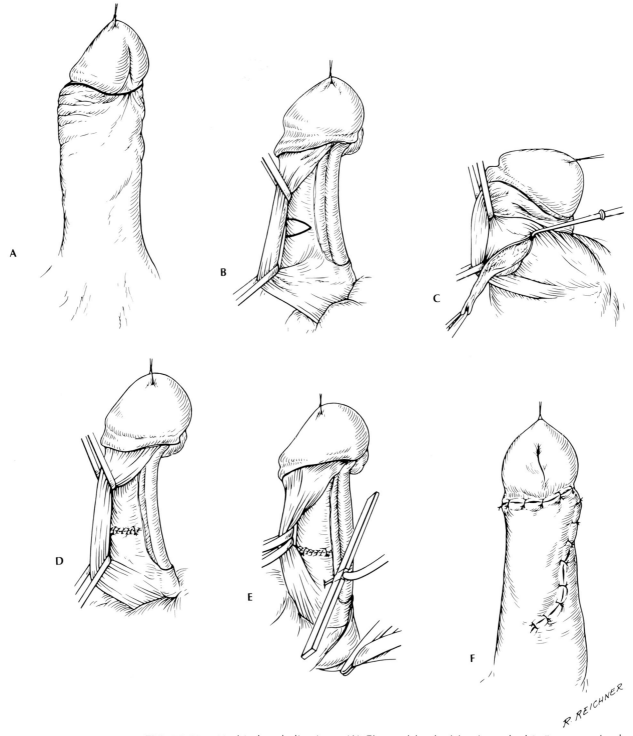

FIG. 76-12. Nesbit dorsal plication. **(A)** Circumcising incision is marked 3–5 mm proximal to the corona. **(B)** At the conclusion of the dissection, chordee persists. Dorsal bundle of Buck's fascia with the vessels and nerves is mobilized and segment of the tunica to be excised is marked. **(C)** The tunica is excised. **(D)** The edges of this defect are approximated. **(E)** An artificial erection shows the penis to be straight. **(F)** After the urethroplasty, the skin is approximated.

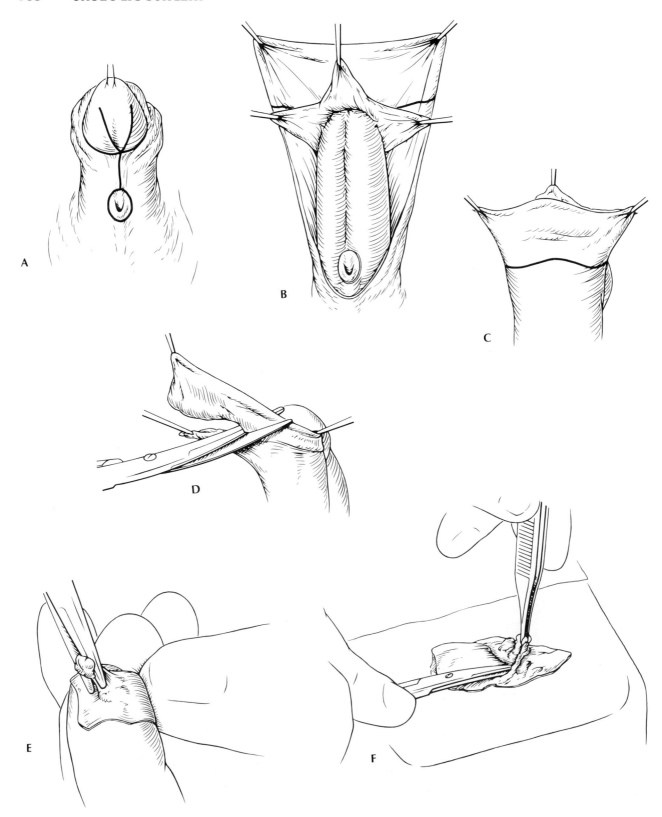

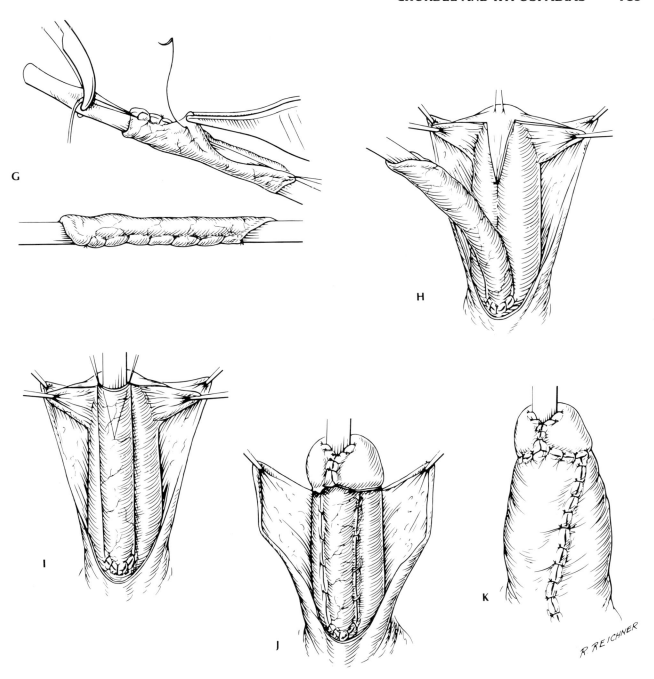

FIG. 76-13.   Tube graft repair of hypospadias.   **(A)** Incisions are marked around the urethral meatus and on the glans to develop the glans flaps.   **(B)** Chordee has been released and the glans flaps mobilized.   **(C)** The distal prepuce has been unfolded and the graft is marked. **(D)** Treputial graft is taken.   **(E)** Subcutaneous tissue is removed with the skin laid out over the top of a finger or **(F)** with the skin held flat on double-faced dermatome tape.   **(G)** The skin is formed into a tube over a red rubber catheter.   **(H)** The anastomosis of the proximal end is completed with interrupted sutures.   **(I)** The distal anastomosis has been completed in the same fashion and the glans wings are mobilized ventral to the neourethra.   **(J)** The glans construction is complete and the skin graft has been fixed to the shaft with interrupted chromic sutures.   **(K)** Repair is completed, approximating the skin with interrupted chromic sutures.

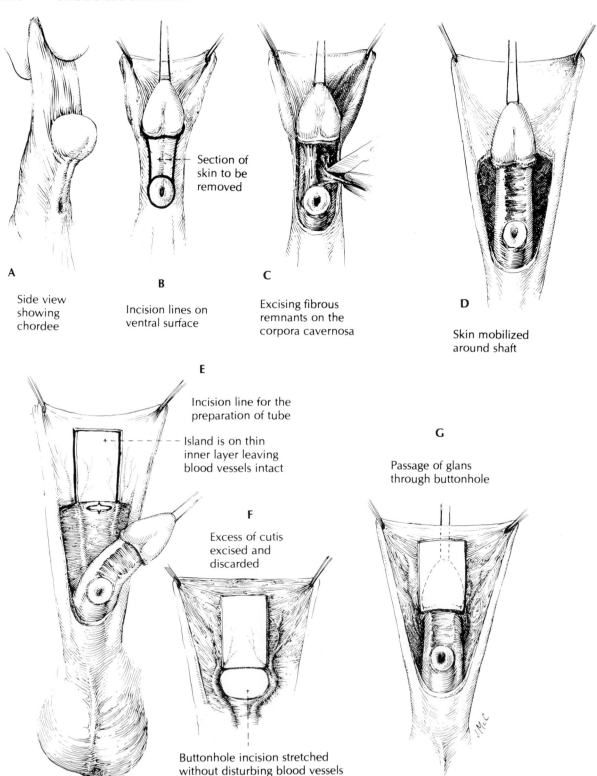

A

Side view
showing
chordee

B

Incision lines on
ventral surface

Section of
skin to be
removed

C

Excising fibrous
remnants on the
corpora cavernosa

D

Skin mobilized
around shaft

E

Incision line for the
preparation of tube

Island is on thin
inner layer leaving
blood vessels intact

F

Excess of cutis
excised and
discarded

G

Passage of glans
through buttonhole

Buttonhole incision stretched
without disturbing blood vessels

FIG. 76-14.   Hodgson Type I repair.   **(A to G)** Incision and mobilization of dorsal and ventral skin.   **(H to M)** Island tube urethroplasty and closure (Urologic Procedures, Vol. 1, No. 4, Warner-Chilcott, 1972)

FIG. 76-14.   *(Continued)*

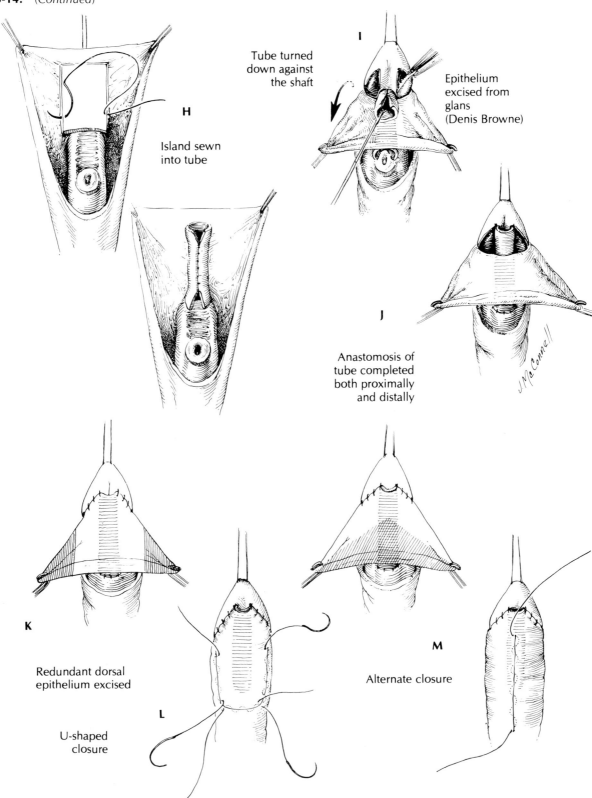

H   Island sewn into tube

I   Tube turned down against the shaft

Epithelium excised from glans (Denis Browne)

J   Anastomosis of tube completed both proximally and distally

K   Redundant dorsal epithelium excised

U-shaped closure

L

M   Alternate closure

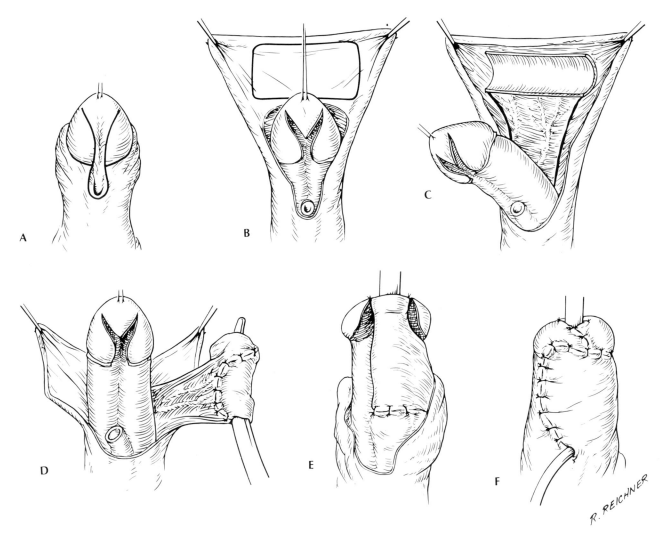

FIG. 76-15. Transverse preputial island flap. **(A)** Incision is marked to mobilize the skin and urethra and release the chordee. **(B)** Dissection is complete and the penis is straight. There is a measured area of innerface. Preputial skin is marked for incision. **(C)** Transverse flap of prepuce is isolated on its vascular pedicle. The rest of the prepuce is supplied with blood by vessels in the skin. **(D)** The flap has been formed into a tube lumen and transferred to the ventral surface on its pedicle. **(E)** The tube has been attached to the urethra at its proximal end and to the glans flap distally. **(F)** The glans wings have been closed over the neourethra and the skin of the prepuce has been brought ventrally to cover the penis.

gap at the distal end to fit the midline glans flap and a tongue on the proximal end to fit into an incision in the ventral side of the urethral meatus. Thus, we are sure to form long elliptic anastomoses at each end of this full-thickness tube graft neourethra.

We divert the urine with either a perineal urethrostomy or a suprapubic tube. In the past we

have not favored a suprapubic tube because of the difficulty of placing it; but now with readily available plastic tubes placed percutaneously or by cutting down on the tip of a sound with a hole in the tip and pulling a small Foley catheter into the bladder, we use the suprapubic tube for the more distal cases and the perineal catheter for the more proximal ones.

We make the anastomosis between the full-thickness skin graft tube and the urethra with interrupted sutures of 5-0 or 6-0 chromic gut, turning the epithelium into the lumen but allowing the sutures to penetrate the full thickness. At the distal end, we sew the midline glans flap to the tunica of the corpora cavernosa with several sutures of 5-0 or 6-0 Vicryl before the anastomosis. We then bring the glans wings around the neourethra and make a midline dorsal incision in the remaining preputial hood, bringing the flaps around laterally and trimming them to fit the defect on the ventral side. When the urethral meatus is located at the penoscrotal junction or the perineum, we do not have to make this incision because the skin will usually fit nicely.

Hodgson's first operation will also be useful when a tube is necessary for the neourethra (Fig. 76-14). The prepuce should not be unfolded, and more of the innerface epithelium than in his Type II is left *in situ* while the residual epithelium is excised. Without mobilization, this tissue is formed into a tube and the glans is drawn through a hole created at the proximal end of the flap. The distal end of the tube then becomes the proximal end of the neourethra and is sutured with multiple chromic sutures to the patient's own urethra. The now distal end of the neourethra is approximated to the midline glans flap. This part of the procedure differs from the illustrations of the repair done in Hodgson's classic fashion, and are like the procedure of Toksu. We would bring the glans wings around the neourethra and then close the skin to cover the defect without leaving unsightly tags.

Duckett has modified the flap-type repair by mobilizing the innerface epithelium on a vascular pedicle and bringing the tissue to the ventrum, where it is formed into a tube and approximated proximally and distally (Fig. 76-15).[8] We have used our glans reconstruction with this type of island flap, although Duckett brings the distal end of the tube through a tunnel in the glans to put the meatus at the tip. The dissection to release this flap must be done meticulously so as not to devitalize the remaining penile skin, which will be used for coverage of the ventral shaft. We make an incision, isolating a transverse section of the innerface preputial mucosa, and dissect between the skin (which has its own blood supply that can be visualized) and the pedicle in the dartos containing the blood vessels that come out to the preputial flap. Dissection should be carried back only as far as it is necessary to free up this flap so that it can be brought easily to the ventral side of the penis.

The urine must be diverted, and we do not recommend inserting a tube for drainage during the period of healing because a lot of edema develops in this flap. We leave a small stent through the repair and remove it on the first postoperative day, but we do not allow the patient to void through the neourethra until the seventh postoperative day. If there is a fistula we will open the diversion for a longer period of time. Because of this possibility we prefer a suprapubic tube to divert the urine in this repair.

We do not recommend constricting dressings because blood supply to the covering flaps may be somewhat tenuous. Fortunately, the urethra is not affected by the loss of a flap or a part of a flap, but should this occur the devitalized tissue must be excised immediately and a thin full-thickness graft applied. This island pedicle flap requires more meticulous surgical technique than other types of hypospadias repair and therefore should be attempted only by a surgeon who is thoroughly familiar with handling these delicate tissues.

For more proximal hypospadias cases, Hodgson has devised yet another procedure in which a flap of skin left *in situ* is carried to the required location by moving the skin of the penis (Fig. 76-16). To make a longer tube, he uses the outer skin of the dorsum of the penis, measuring the length of the defect and incising a strip of skin wide enough to make a satisfactory tube. A hole is made at the proximal end of this tube at the base of the penis, and the penile shaft is drawn through the hole. This places the tube in position so that it can be anastomosed to the urethra proximally and to the glans reconstruction distally. The ventral penile skin can then be mobilized to cover the dorsal shaft, and the excess preputial hood can be trimmed to cover the distal defect.

Perineal Hypospadias

For perineal hyposadias we continue to use our tube graft (Fig. 76-17). There is often suitable hairless tissue between the two halves of the cleft scrotum, so that the proximal end of the neourethra can be made by forming this into a Thiersch-type tube which moves the urethral meatus out to the penoscrotal junction. We construct the urethra from that point to the glans with a full-thickness tube graft obtained from the distal prepuce. In these cases we often use a suprapubic tube for urinary diversion because of the short length of urethra proximal to the meatus. We leave the stent tube for 6 to 7 days and do not let the patient void through the neourethra until the 10th day.[6]

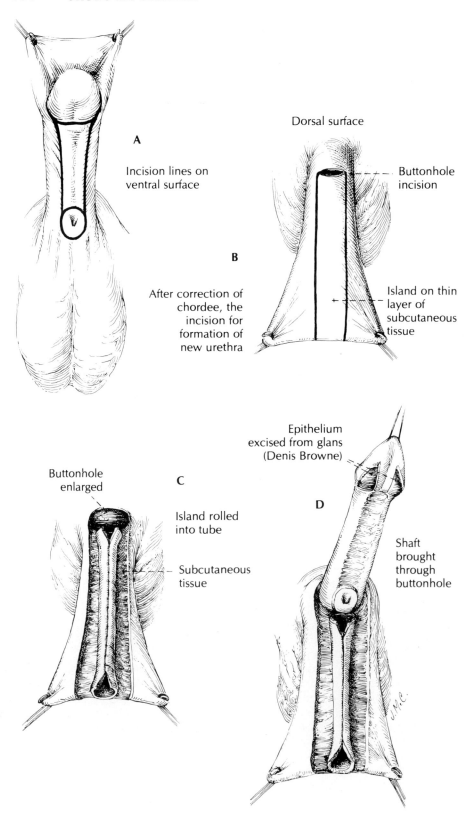

A

Incision lines on
ventral surface

B

After correction of
chordee, the
incision for
formation of
new urethra

Dorsal surface

Buttonhole
incision

Island on thin
layer of
subcutaneous
tissue

C

Buttonhole
enlarged

Island rolled
into tube

Subcutaneous
tissue

D

Epithelium
excised from glans
(Denis Browne)

Shaft
brought
through
buttonhole

FIG. 76-16.   *(Caption on opposite page)*

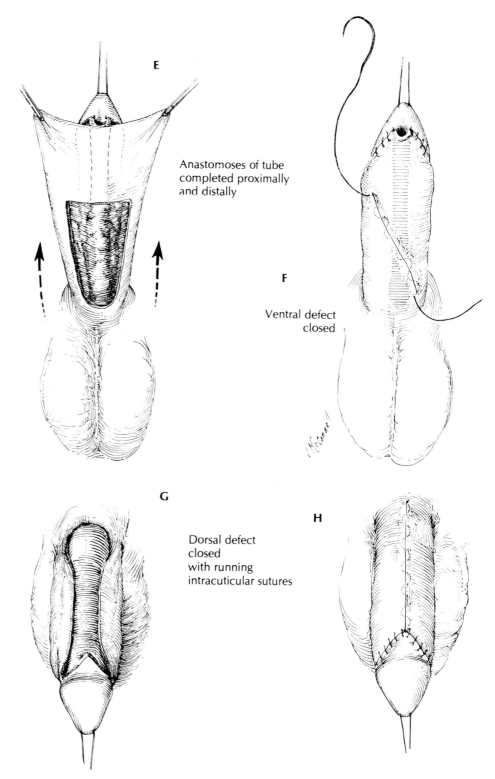

FIG. 76-16. Hodgson Type III procedure. **(A to D)** Incision and mobilization of penile skin. **(E to H)** Ventral and dorsal closures (Urologic Procedures, Vol. 1, No. 4, Warner-Chilcott, 1972)

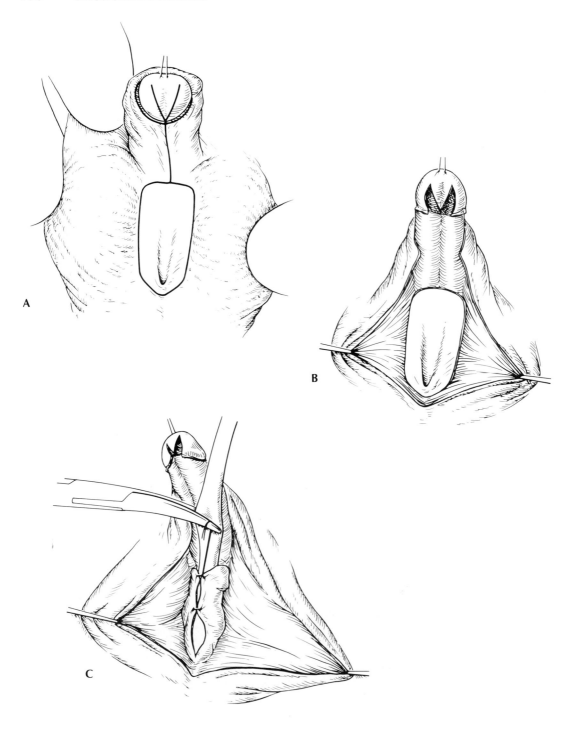

FIG. 76-17.   *(Caption on opposite page)*

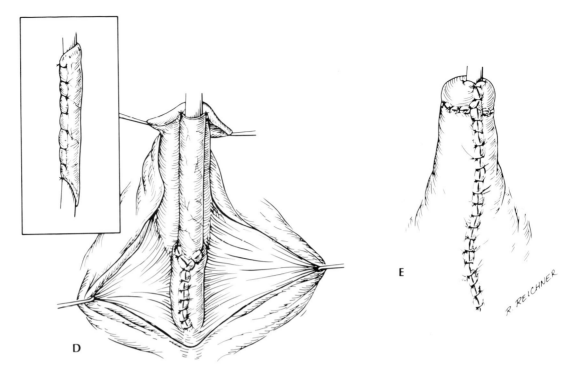

FIG. 76-17.   Repair of perineal hypospadias.   **(A)** Incisions marked for development of glans flaps, mobilization of penile skin, and release of chordee. The area of smooth skin outlined between the halves of the scrotum is used to form a tube extending the urethra to the penoscrotal junction.   **(B)** Chordee is released and skin flaps are mobilized.   **(C)** Intrascrotal skin is formed into a tube, turning the epithelial edges into the lumen.   **(D)** Skin graft tube, formed from skin of the prepuce, is attached to the graft proximally at the penoscrotal junction and distally to the midline glans flap. A stenting tube is in place.   **(E)** The glans wings are brought ventral to the neourethra, mobilizing the skin to cover the ventral aspect of the penis. The halves of the cleft scrotum are brought to the midline.

REFERENCES

1. American Academy of Pediatrics, Recommendations of: The time of elective surgery on genitalia of male children with particular reference to undescended testes and hypospadias. Pediatrics 56:479, 1975

2. DEVINE CJ: Embryology of the genitourinary tract. IN Hohenfellner R (ed): Urologie in Klinik und Praxis. Stuttgart, Georg Thieme Verlag (in press)

3. DEVINE CJ, HORTON CE: A one stage hypospadias repair. J Urol 85:166, 1961

4. DEVINE CJ, HORTON CE: Hypospadias. In Goldwyn RM (ed): The Unfavorable Result in Plastic Surgery: Avoidance and Treatment, p 531. Boston, Little Brown & Co, 1972

5. DEVINE CJ, HORTON CE: Chordee without hypospadias. J Urol 110:264, 1973

6. DEVINE CJ, HORTON CE: Hypospadias repair. J Urol 118:188, 1977

7. DUCKETT JW: Magpi (meatoplasty and glanuloplasty): A procedure for subcoronal hypospadias. Urol Clin North Am 8:513, 1981

8. DUCKETT JW: The island flap technique for hypospadias repair. Urol Clin North Am 8:503, 1981

9. DUCKETT JW, KAPLAN GW, WOODARD JR et al: Panel: Complications of hypospadias repair. Urol Clin North Am 7:443, 1980

10. GITTES RF, MCLAUGHLIN AP: Injection technique to induce penil erection. Urology 4:473, 1974

11. HODGSON NB: Hypospadias. In Glenn JF and Boyce WH (eds): Urologic Surgery, p. 656, 2nd ed. Hagerstown, Harper & Row, 1975

12. HORTON CE, DEVINE CJ: Hypospadias cripples. In Horton CE (ed): Plastic and Reconstructive Surgery of the Genital Area, p 235 Boston, Little, Brown & Co, 1973

13. HORTON CE, DEVINE CJ: Simulated erection of the penis with saline injection, a diagnostic maneuver. Plast Reconstr Surg 59:138, 1976

14. KAPLAN GW, LAMN DL: Embryogenesis of Chordee. J Urol 114:769, 1975

15. NESBIT RM: Congenital curvature of the phallus: Report of 3 cases with description of corrective operation. J Urol 93:230, 1965

Circumcision

77

Stephen A. Kramer

The indications for surgery on the foreskin include phimosis, paraphimosis, preputial neoplasms, balanitis, and posthitis unresponsive to conservative therapy. The necessity for routine circumcision has been questioned in recent years but will not be debated in this discussion. Circumcision is contraindicated in boys with hypospadias. Furthermore, in boys with chordee without hypospadias, circumcision should be deferred until after the penis has been straightened, because surgical correction may require division of the urethra or may result in a urethrocutaneous fistula (Chap. 76).

Phimosis is the condition in which the distal opening in the prepuce is so contracted that the visceral surface of the foreskin cannot be retracted back over the glans. This condition occurs in the young infant, secondary to physiologic congenital adhesions between the glans and the foreskin. Recurrent local irritation may result in balanitis, ulcerative balanoposthitis, or urethral meatal stenosis.

Paraphimosis occurs when the foreskin is retracted forcibly behind the glans penis and is not promptly reduced. The foreskin then becomes entrapped in the coronal sulcus by the secondary swelling of the glans. Paraphimosis may be reduced frequently by gentle but firm glandular compression (Fig. 77-1A). However, if the condition is neglected, continued swelling of the glans may render manual reduction impossible. In this situation, a longitudinal incision through the constricting ring may be necessary to allow the paraphimosis to be reduced (Fig. 77-1B). Edema and inflammatory changes make it advisable to postpone definitive circumcision until a later date.

Circumcision, particularly in children, is not a trivial procedure that can be performed within a few minutes by an inexperienced surgeon. Significant complications have included denuded penile shaft, buried penis secondary to inadequate removal of skin, necrosis of the glans, urethrocutaneous fistula secondary to removal of excessive ventral tissue, and amputation.[2,4] A properly performed circumcision requires a careful meticulous technique and good anesthesia to ensure a safe and satisfactory cosmetic result.

In adults, circumcision may be accomplished with local anesthesia using 1% lidocaine without epinephrine. The injection is performed through a cutaneous wheal at the base of the penis in the dorsal midline, with deeper infiltration subcutaneously around the circumference of the penile shaft. Particular care is directed to generous infiltration of the dorsal midline and the angles between the corpus cavernosum and the corpus spongiosum on either side. In younger children and infants more than 6 weeks old, general anesthesia is preferred. In neonates, circumsion may be performed without anesthesia or with augmentation of a "whiskey nipple."

Adequate hemostasis is mandatory to prevent postoperative hemorrhage or hematoma, with breakdown of the suture line. Postoperative edema occurs uniformly, and therefore sutures must be tied securely but loosely enough to avoid cutting through the skin edges.

Sleeve Resection Technique

Although several techniques of circumcision are available, the sleeve resection technique (Fig. 77-2) allows uniformly good results with adequate visualization of the glans throughout the procedure. With the prepuce in its usual position and without applying tension, the coronal junction on the skin is outlined with a marking pencil and is incised circumferentially, care being taken to follow the "V" of the frenulum on the ventral surface (Fig. 77-2A). The foreskin is then retracted proximally over the glans penis, and adhesions between the prepuce and the glans are thoroughly broken by retracting the foreskin over the shaft of the penis. The visceral prepuce should be stretched until the deep purple proximal corona is completely visualized. A circumferential incision is outlined approximately 1 cm proximal to the coronal sulcus on the mucosal surface of the prepuce. The incision

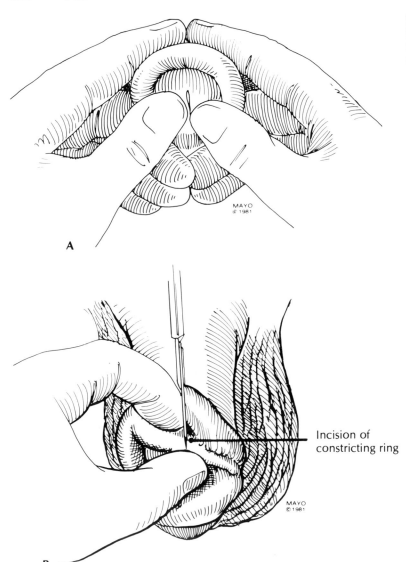

FIG. 77-1. **(A)** Reduction of paraphimosis by firm compression against the glans penis. **(B)** Incision is made through the constricting ring when manual reduction is unsuccessful.

Incision of
constricting ring

is straight across the base of the frenulum, which allows the frenulum to retract up into the V of the glans (Fig. 77-2*B*). This sleeve of skin between these two incisions is then excised, and bleeding sites are electrocoagulated or ligated with fine absorbable sutures (Fig. 77-2*C*). The skin edges are reapproximated with interrupted 4-0 or 5-0 chromic catgut, and a compressive dressing of Vaseline strip and sterile gauze is applied (Fig. 77-2*D*).

Dorsal Slit Procedure
The dorsal slit procedure may be used to promote healing of a refractory balanitis, to allow removal of preputial calculi, to expose the glans for biopsy, and to correct an irreducible paraphimosis. In the

dorsal slit procedure, the edges of the prepuce are secured with two clamps at the dorsal midline, and the prepuce is divided between them from its free end to within a few millimeters of the corona of the glans. Bleeders are fulgurated or ligated, and the severed edges are approximated with interrupted sutures of 4-0 chromic catgut. Circumcision may be performed electively after resolution of the balanitis or balanoposthitis.

Gomco Clamp Procedure
Circumcision in the neonate or young infant can be performed with a Gomco clamp. The foreskin is retracted, and adhesions between the foreskin and underlying glans penis are manually broken.

FIG. 77-2. Sleeve resection technique of circumcision. **(A)** The coronal junction on the skin is outlined and incised circumferentially following the "V" of the frenulum on the ventral surface. **(B)** The foreskin is retracted, the adhesions are thoroughly broken, and a circumferential incision is made in the mucosal skin just proximal to the coronal sulcus. **(C)** The sleeve of the skin between the two incisions is excised. **(D)** The skin edges are reapproximated, giving a good cosmetic result.

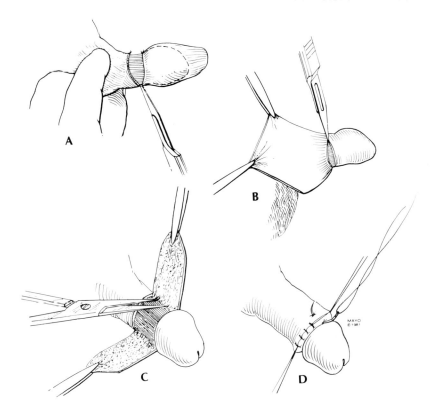

The appropriate-sized bell is placed over the glans, and the prepuce is drawn forward over the bell and clamped in position. Appropriate tension is necessary in advancing the foreskin over the bell to prevent an inadequate or overzealous circumcision. The clamp is applied as tightly as possible to ensure adequate hemostasis, and compression is maintained for several minutes. The skin distal to the clamp, at the junction of the clamp and bell, is cut away sharply with a scalpel (not by cautery).

Although this technique can provide an expedient and satisfactory result, the surgeon must have experience and confidence in using this mechanical device to avoid serious sequelae. The most common surgical complication is bleeding secondary to inadequate vascular compression. The vessels must be completely occluded by compression. In older boys, larger vessels prohibit the use of these clamps because the vessels are not easily sealed by compression, and vigorous bleeding may result. Inappropriate application of the Gomco clamp may result in clipping off the tip of the glans or in taking too little or too much skin. If excess skin has been removed, causing the shaft of the penis to be denuded, Allen recommends conservative management with local wound care.[1] In his experience, regeneration of penile skin affords complete coverage of the shaft defect. Alternatively, Devine recommends either immediate split-thickness skin grafting or burying the penis in the scrotum temporarily to obtain skin coverage.[3]

REFERENCES

1. ALLEN TD: Disorders of the male external genitalia. In Kelalis PP, King LR, Belman AB (eds): Clinical Pediatric Urology, Vol 2, p 638. Philadelphia, W B Saunders, 1976
2. BELMAN AB: Complications of circumcision. In: The Penis. Urol Clin North Am 5:25, 1978
3. DEVINE CJ, JR: Surgery of the penis and urethra. In Harrison JH, Gittes RF, Perlmutter AD et al (eds): Campbell's Urology, 4th ed, Vol 3, p 2401. Philadelphia, W B Saunders, 1979
4. SHULMAN J, BEN–HUR N, NEUMAN Z: Surgical complications of circumcision. Am J Dis Child 107:149, 1964

Priapism

78

Chester C. Winter

The term *priapism* is derived from Greek mythology and comes directly from the name of the Greek god Pria or Priapus. He is known as the son of Aphrodite, the Greek goddess of sexual love, beauty, and feminine fertility, and, in some descriptions, seduction and rape. This mythical god was called upon to enhance not only fertility but also agriculture production, good hunting, and generally good results from whatever occupation was practiced. The father of Priapus was believed to be Dionysus or Bacchus, god of fruitfulness, vegetation, and wine. The female worshipers of Priapus sought to become assimilated to him by wild nocturnal dancing.

Priapism is a penile erection that will not become flaccid. It is terminated only by appropriate medical or surgical therapy because it rarely goes into spontaneous remission.[2] It is uncomfortable and unaccompanied by sexual desire. If intercourse is attempted, it is usually found to be painful. In such a state, the patient either has considerable difficulty in urination or is unable to urinate and may require catheterization. The condition can occur at any age, but the incidence of etiologic factors varies at different ages. It is seen more often before puberty in patients with leukemia or sickle-cell disease. The idiopathic form occurs most often after puberty, particularly between the ages of 16 and 45. When the condition is caused by a neoplasm, it is most apt to affect the older man.

In a lifetime of practice many physicians may never encounter a patient with priapism; but urologists, because of their referral-type practice, usually see a few examples of the disease. Large medical centers encounter several such patients each year. A scattering of single case reports are to be found in the literature, but most articles are based upon discussion of a handful of patient examples. The largest series in the literature to date is that published by Winter, giving data on experience with 69 patients.[10] Twenty percent of these cases occurred in the pediatric age group.

Anatomy

Because the anatomy and physiology of the penis are so intimately involved with priapism and its management, a brief review of these basics is appropriate as an introduction to the pathology and treatment of priapism.

The penis is composed of three columnar bodies, a pair which are larger and dorsally located and extend the length of the penis. They contain cavernous-vascular spaces and are called the corpora cavernosa; they intercommunicate. The third columnar body in the midventral position, the corpus spongiosum, is smaller in diameter; it has less vascular tissue but more connective tissue and includes the urethra. Normally it does not have vascular communications with the corpora cavernosa. The bulbous enlarged end of the corpus spongiosum is known as the glans penis and is more vascular and sensitive than the main body. Each of these long cylindrical bodies is encased by a tunica albuginea fascia, and all are surrounded by Buck's fascia, which is fibrous and tough. Buck's fascia is continuous with Colles' fascia and the urogenital diaphragm (transverse ligament), and anteriorly it forms a suspensory ligament. This ligament not only holds the proximal penis firmly in place but also serves as a limiting membrane for infections and urinary extravasation. The skin, which rests on a more superficial and thinner fascia, normally protrudes over the glans penis as a fold called the prepuce or foreskin. A superficial smooth muscle layer is closely applied to the skin of the penis, which is similar to the dartos of the scrotum, and between the muscle layer and Buck's fascia is a loose layer of areolar connective tissue.

Between the superficial fascia and Buck's fascia in the dorsal midline resides a formidable group of vessels known as the dorsal arteries and vein. Smaller but important penile vessels also course between the corpora. A large central artery and vein form the ingress and egress, respectively, of the corpora, and the vein drains into the venous complex beneath the pubic arch and thence into the venous plexus of the pelvis.

The penis extends from the urogenital diaphragm and is supported and surrounded at its base by the paired ischiocavernosus muscles. These muscles arise from the inner surface of the tuberosity of each ischium and support the erect penis; they are innervated by the perineal nerves. The bulbocavernous or ejaculatory urinae muscle arises from the central perineum and moves to surround the bulb, and some fibers also surround the corpora cavernosa.

The arterial blood of the penis originates from the paired hypogastric (internal iliac) arteries, which are major branches of the external iliac arteries. The primary branches from the hypogastric arteries are the paired pudendal arteries, which give rise to the dorsal arteries of the penis, running beneath Buck's fascia on either side of the deep dorsal vein of the penis, and terminate in anastomosing branches surrounding the corona of the glans penis. A branch of the internal pudendal artery enters the crura on either side of the corpora cavernosa and runs lengthwise as the main blood supply. Additional branches enter the corpus spongiosum on either side and course along the entire length of the urethra. Only the skin and subcutaneous tissues derive blood from elsewhere, and they receive their supply from the superficial and deep external pudendal branches of the femoral arteries. The veins of the penis are paired, and the superficial group from the skin return through the superficial dorsal vein which empties into the saphenous and the superficial external pudendal veins of the abdomen. The deep veins are the tributaries emerging from the erectile tissue to form the deep dorsal vein, which passes beneath Buck's fascia anteriorly to the urogenital diaphragm, empties into Santorini's plexus, and continues to the hypogastric veins.

The lymphatic drainage of the superficial and deep channels of the skin and from the urethral meatus is into the superficial inguinal lymph nodes. The deeper vessels from the urethra and corpora pass into the iliac nodes.

The nerve supply to the penis is derived from both the cerebrospinal and the autonomic nervous systems. The dorsal nerves of the penis come from the cerebrospinal outflow and supply the skin in a paired fashion. The autonomic nervous system innervates the erectile bodies, whereas the hypogastric plexus supplies branches accompanying the arteries to the cavernosa–spongiosum bodies, which are comparable to the nervi erigens of animals. Additional cutaneous innervation is supplied at the base of the penis by branches of the ilioinguinal nerves.

Physiology

The physiology of penile erection and ejaculation is complex. Stimuli to the penis are received from the brain, reflexly from the spinal cord or through local stimulation of the glans penis. The impulses, carried through the autonomic nervous system, produce relaxation of the smooth muscles in the arteries carrying blood to the corpora cavernosa. Thus, the inflow vessels are widely patent during sexual excitement, and the vascular channels draining the corpora are constricted.

Vascular shunts are thought to exist between the arterial inflow and venous outflow systems, allowing bypass of the corpora cavernosa bodies. It is believed that these collateral vessels are constricted when the venous outflow channels of the corpora are closed during the erect state of the penis but become patent along with the venous outflow channels during the period of penile flaccidity (Fig. 78-1).

When the sexual stimulus is at its peak, orgasm occurs and the ejaculatory structures are activated. This system includes the epididymides, vasa deferens, ejaculatory ducts, seminal vesicles, prostate, bladder neck (internal urethral sphincter), external urinary sphincter, and the urethra. They undergo rhythmic contractions, and sperm, seminal fluid, and glandular secretions are expressed through the distal urethra in spurts. During orgasm, the bladder neck (internal sphincter), if intact and functional, is closed by tonic contraction and keeps the semen from entering the bladder.

Some physiologists believe that during sleep, dreaming of sexual activity stimulates the penis to be maintained in an erect posture. Men often awake in the morning with an erect penis, thought to be secondary to dreaming or from the stimulus of a full bladder. Ejaculation can also occur during sleep (nocturnal emission).

The normal male (dependent upon age and physical and mental health) will maintain an erection for many minutes to several hours during sexual activity or continuous erotic stimulation. Any prolongation of the erection beyond this time and unrelated to sexual stimulation is considered abnormal and would be included within the definition of priapism if the penis does not become flaccid. In disease states such as paraplegia or quadriplegia, or even in the man who has been hung by the neck, the penis may become erect and remain so for abnormally long periods of time,

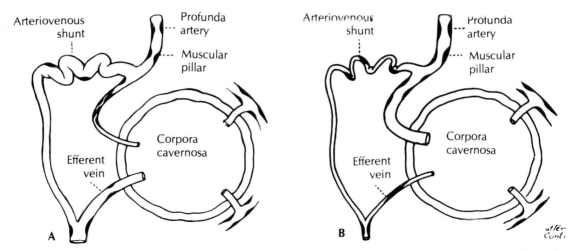

FIG. 78-1. **(A)** Flaccid state. The arteriovenous shunt is open, allowing blood to bypass the corpora cavernosa. **(B)** Erect state. The shunt is closed and the arterial system is open, allowing blood to enter the corpora cavernosa while the efferent veins are closed. This enables the patient to have an erection. (Farrer, Goodwin: J Urol 86:769. Baltimore, The Williams & Wilkins Co., © 1961)

but this is related to the reflex nerve activity rather than to the abnormality known as priapism.

Pathology

During a sustained erection beyond the duration of a normal period of time, the blood in the corpora cavernosa begins to lose oxygen and accumulates carbon dioxide. The viscosity of blood increases and its color becomes much darker. Sludging of the cellular elements within the blood may occur, and eventually edema and thrombosis of the vascular channels will result from stasis of blood. Finally, in the terminal state, fibrosis of the corpora cavernosa can occur so that the penis has a woody and indurated consistency to palpation and remains enlarged. In some instances, the phenomenon of sickle-cell trait may cause rouleau formation of the red blood cells and subsequent blockage or thrombosis of the venous outlet channels. In other instances, trauma or primary thrombosis is a cause of priapism, and in still others, neoplastic infiltration or faulty nervous mechanisms produce the vascular changes in priapism.

Etiology

Idiopathic Causes

The majority (60%) of the patients with priapism do not have a known cause of the disease.[9] Their history frequently indicates that commencement occurred during excessive sexual stimulation. Such activity may have been heightened by stimulatory drugs. Thus, actual mechanical manipulation of the penis in a prolonged or traumatic manner is thought to be commonly responsible for the idiopathic variety of priapism.

Sickle Cell-Disorders

Many instances of priapism are due to sickle-cell disease or the presence of the trait in the black male. This may occur in childhood as well as in adulthood. The abnormal red blood cells tend to form in rouleau and cause a thrombosis of the venous channels, blocking the outflow of blood from the penis and causing it to be maintained in an erect state. Sickle-cell trait causes about an equal incidence of priapism as do idiopathic causes in the black adult, but the disease is the major cause of priapism in children. The treatment is similar to that for the idiopathic variety in the adult, but exchange transfusions are used in children.

Leukemia

The patient with leukemia may have cellular infiltration of the corpora cavernosa and vessels, or cellular debris may involve the venous outlet channels and cause sustained erection. The priapism may resolve as the leukemia is successfully treated.

Neoplasia

Primary or, more often, metastatic lesions of cancer can cause blockage of the outflow of blood from

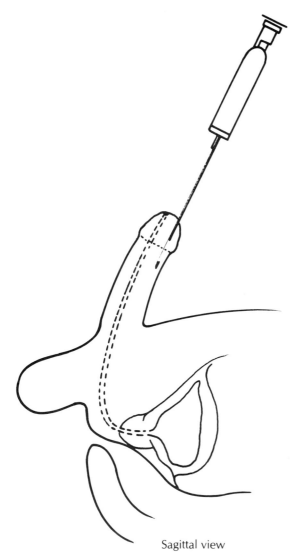

Sagittal view

FIG. 78-2. After the glans penis is anesthetized with lidocaine solution, a Travenol Tricut biopsy needle is inserted in the dorsal glans in order to remove a button of tissue between the glans and corpus cavernosum.

the penis and this cause priapism. Metastatic prostatic neoplasm would be a prime example. I encountered one patient with complete blockage from carcinoma of the sigmoid colon. Treatment is directed toward the cancer.

Neurogenic Causes

The nerve supply of the penis is all-important in the maintenance of the erectile state and for the achievement of flaccidity of the penis. If nervous stimulation is excessive and continuous, as in paraquadriplegia, and prolonged erection of the penis is maintained, then this can lead to priapism rarely.

Other Causes

Trauma to the penis or urethra (by sounds or cystoscopy) and diseases such as tularemia and Rocky Mountain spotted fever have been associated with priapism. Paradoxically, heparin and warfarin have been documented as a cause of priapism.[3] The exact mechanism is unknown but it is speculated that low heparin cofactor, antiheparin factor, action on vascular smooth muscle, and a rebound phenomenon may be causative factors.

Diagnostic Measures

The diagnosis of priapism is quite obvious, because the patient has marked prolonged erection of the penis which is accompanied by some tenderness or discomfort. He is uninterested in sexual activity. Urination may be so difficult and painful as to require catheterization, but this does not relieve the priapism. The penis may be somewhat inflamed and edematous as time goes on, but with the idiopathic variety there is no involvement of the corpus spongiosum or glans penis, which have a normal consistency; the latter may be flattened out.

A corporogram can be made to note if there is trapping of the blood. This is performed by placing a needle into the distal corpus cavernosum on one side and slowly injecting 10 ml of 30% diatrizoate sodium (Hypaque). Both corpora should fill with the contrast material because they intercommunicate, but the material cannot escape through the veins of Santorini. Usually the corpus spongiosum is not involved, and a lateral view will demonstrate this.[4]

A careful historical search for evidence of one of the known etiologic factors should be made, and a detailed sexual history should be taken. A complete physical examination, especially neurologic testing, should be done. It may be necessary to perform additional diagnostic tests directed at some particular organ system, such as the urologic system or the lower intestinal tract, to detect certain neoplasms. If metastatic lesions are suspected, one should also check out any system which the history suggests might be a primary site. The past history may reveal previous episodes of short-lived priapism that have resolved spontaneously or have been managed early enough to relieve the condition. A complete blood count and a battery of screening tests are performed in most hospitals and should be carefully evaluated. Sickle-cell preparations are one of the first tests to be performed in the black patient. Leukemia should be ruled out.

Treatment

MEDICAL MANAGEMENT

Many modes of nonsurgical therapy have been attempted in the management of priapism in the past, and few have been successful. Ganglionic blocking agents, spinal anesthesia, hypotensive anesthesia, fibrinolysins, diethylstilbestrol, and anticoagulation therapy have been tried with an insignificant success rate. Anticoagulants are particularly to be avoided, because a number of patients have developed priapism while on continuous anticoagulation therapy for cardiac and thromboembolic disease. These agents, therefore, may incite priapism, although the exact mechanism is not clear.

The prostate should be massaged at once and the secretion examined. Massage subsequently can be carried out in an opposite direction (*i.e.*, caudad to cephalad direction) in order to milk the major egress veins of the penis. This has been known to relieve the situation rarely. However, there is no solid evidence to incriminate prostatitis as an etiologic factor. Hot enemas and rectal diathermy have been reported in the literature to be successful, and I know of one instance in which a warm enema was effective after a few hours of priapism.

ASPIRATION AND IRRIGATION

I advocate immediate aspiration and irrigation of the corpora cavernosa as the initial measure.[7] The penis should be cleaned and draped. Lidocaine (1% Xylocaine) is used to anesthetize the glans penis and septum between glans and corpora; general or spinal anesthesia is an alternative. An 18-gauge needle is placed in one corpus, and the cavernosa are irrigated with saline solution (10% heparin may or may not be added). This allows the dark, viscid, trapped blood to be washed out by injecting the solution into the proximal end of one corpus cavernosum and allowing it to egress by squeezing or milking the penis. This should be repeated many times until the penis is completely flaccid. When the dark blood is fully cleared from the venous channels (no clots will be obtained), a favorable prognostic sign is the appearance of bright red blood, indicating that blood is getting into the penis although it may not escape.

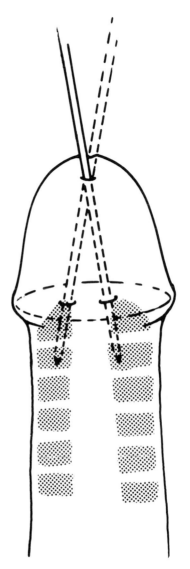

Dorsal view

FIG. 78-3. Several fistulas are created with the biopsy needle: usually two into each corpus cavernosum using the same entry site on the glans.

SURGICAL MANAGEMENT

Glans Spongiosum—Corpora Cavernosa Shunt

Following aspiration and irrigation of the penis, shunts should be made from the corpora cavernosal system. This is easily done by removing the irrigation needle from the glans and introducing a Travenol Trucut biopsy needle (Figs 78-2 and 78-3). Several cores of tissue that include the septum between the glans and the cavernosal bodies should be removed and sent for histologic examination

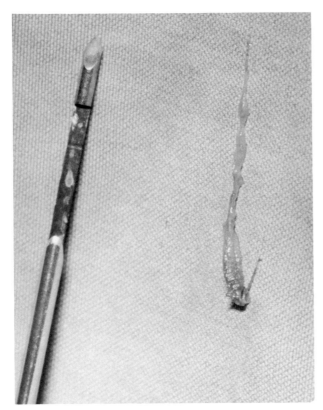

FIG. 78-4.   An example of the core of tissue removed from the septum between the glans penis and corpus cavernosum with the Travenol biopsy needle

(Fig. 78-4). Be sure to rotate the needle 360 degrees to break off the septal tissue. A Kerrison rongeur will remove larger pieces but requires use of a scalpel in glans and septum to enlarge the entry site.

After the needle or rongeur are removed the entry site is closed with a figure-of-eight 3-0 absorbable suture. There will be no hematomas or bleeding, because no other needle has been introduced. The penis should be kept flaccid by having the patient squeeze it every few minutes. As an alternative, the penis can be wrapped with a pediatric blood pressure cuff which is inflated to 200 mm Hg every few minutes for an instant using an automated device. This should be continued for 12 hr. In most cases the penis will stay flaccid or nearly so. If the penis is more than 50% erect after 12 hr to 24 hr, these procedures should be repeated or one may proceed to a different shunt. Great care and experience will prove this method to be highly successful. It is not indicated for children with sickle-cell disease. It is also not indicated for those in whom no blood can be

aspirated or the penis cannot be made flaccid, because this means thrombosis or fibrosis has occurred and so shunts will not work.

Anastomosis of Corpus Cavernosum to Corpus Spongiosum

Another operative procedure that is highly successful is the removal of a window of fascia and tunica albuginea from the base of one corpus cavernosum to allow the blood to egress into the corpus spongiosum.[8] The spongiosum does not have the same tough, thick, fibrous cover of the cavernosum and one must be careful, therefore, not to remove too much tissue from the spongiosum to avoid traumatizing the urethra. Fistula, stricture, gangrene, and generalized sepsis have been encountered after this operation.

It is better to approach the spongiosum in the perineum than more distally. A catheter should be present in the urethra during this procedure, acting as a guide as to the depth of the spongiosum dissection. The operation is not difficult nor time consuming. It is carried out as illustrated in Figure 78-5, with two semicircular sutures of 5-0 or 6-0 absorbable suture. After the skin closure is made with appropriate suture material, the penis should be wrapped with a gauze dressing. An infant-sized blood pressure cuff should be applied, and the pressure should be brought up to 200 mm Hg momentarily every 20 minutes for 12 hr to 24 hr. If this operation is unsuccessful or only temporarily so, then one may proceed to the saphenous vein–corpus cavernosum shunt.

Anastomosis of Saphenous Vein to Corpus Cavernosum

Another successful method of treating priapism that has been proved in many patients and in many institutions is the anastomosis of the saphenous vein to one corpus cavernosum.[1,5] This allows the blood to be released from both corpora and to bypass the venous obstruction. It is recommended that this be performed if lesser surgical measures have been unsuccessful. However, it is believed that priapism is reversable by surgical therapy if applied within a 72-hr period in most subjects, although isolated instances of success after 6- or 7-day delays have been described. If anastomosis of one saphenous vein to the corpus cavernosum is not completely rewarding or only temporarily so, then the contralateral saphenous vein may be anastomosed to the adjacent corpus.

The operation is performed by making two incisions. One incision is over the saphenous vein, which is mobilized down to the midthigh, where

FIG. 78-5. Incision at the base of the penis. **(A)** Site of the incision at the lateral posterior base of the penis. It is better to go further toward the perineum to avoid injury to the urethra. **(B)** The corpus spongiosum and the corpus cavernosum with their tunica albuginea covers are exposed. **(C)** A running suture is placed between the fascia of the two corpora. **(D)** A window of tunica albuginea is cut away from the corpus cavernosum. **(E)** A window of tissue is cut away from the corpus spongiosum with great care to avoid injury to the urethra. **(F)** Two windows between the corpora are anastomosed, allowing blood to flow from the corpus cavernosum into the corpus spongiosum.

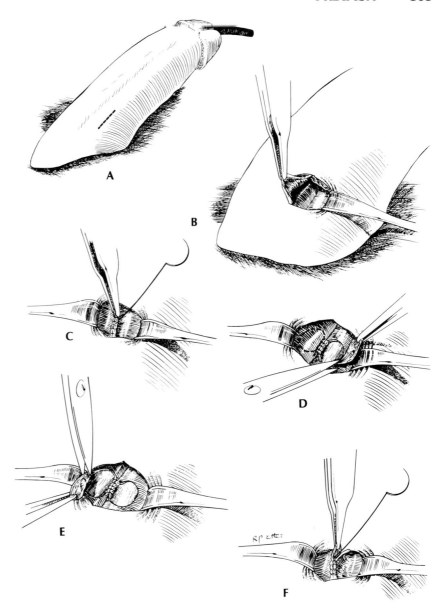

it is divided and the proximal end tied. The vein is then dissected to its junction with the femoral vein. It is brought to the penis through a subcutaneous tunnel made with blunt dissection. A second incision is made at the base of the penis, and a window of tissue is removed from the fasciae and albuginea covering the corpus cavernosum. The vein is then anastomosed to the corpus with two semicircular running sutures of 5-0 silk (Fig. 78-6). The penis should be wrapped with gauze and an infant-sized blood pressure cuff, and the pressure should be raised to 200 mm Hg every 20 minutes (for only a moment) to keep the blood flowing through the penis and out into the sa-

phenous system. This may be kept up for 12 hr to 24 hr as the clinical situation requires.

Other Procedures

Microsurgical anastomosis of dorsal veins to the corpora cavernosa is a tedious, time-consuming procedure that has been shown to work but is not within the armamentarium of most urologists. It is, therefore, rarely used.

The success and failure of ligation of the internal pudendal artery in reducing arterial inflow and thus relieving priapism have been reported. I prefer not to use this method for fear of producing impotence. One investigator even advocated an-

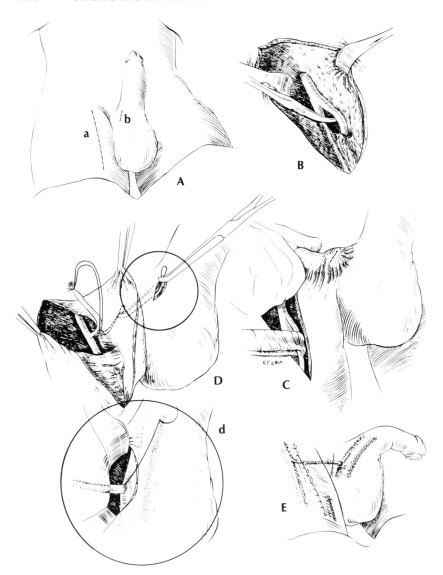

FIG. 78-6. Anastomosis of the saphenous vein to the corpus cavernosum. **(A)** Two incisions are made over the saphenous vein **(a)** and the lateral base of the penis **(b)**. **(B)** The saphenous vein is mobilized from its insertion into the femoral vein toward midthigh. **(C)** A tunnel is made in the subcutaneous tissue between the saphenous vein and the base of the penis by blunt dissection. **(D)** The saphenous vein has been divided in midthigh and the proximal end has been tied. The vein is pulled through the subcutaneous tissue to the base of the penis. **(d)** The saphenous vein is anastomosed to one corpus cavernosum with two semicircular running sutures of fine silk. **(E)** The skin incisions are closed and the saphenous vein–corpus cavernosum shunt is demonstrated to be working, with the penis becoming flaccid.

astomosis of the inferior epigastric artery to the corpus cavenosum to increase blood inflow.[6]

MEDICOLEGAL FACTORS

Impotence is often a sequela of priapism, especially the longer the disease is present. The patient and his wife, relative, or close friend should be so informed, and it is advisable to have the patient sign an informed consent acknowledging this fact. If the patient is a minor, his parents should be fully informed and sign the informed consent. The consent will then allow the urologist to proceed to aspiration, irrigation, or one of the shunting procedures as he sees fit. One of the chief purposes of such an informed signed consent is to obviate

legal action toward the surgeon in case the patient or his parents, relatives, or friends believe that it is the surgery that has produced the impotence. It must be fully impressed upon the patient that it is the disease and not the treatment that produces impotence. The shunting procedures in themselves may make it difficult to produce erections but usually this is temporary.

FOLLOW-UP

The patient should return to the physician's office as frequently as necessary depending on the therapy carried out. The surgeon may wish to perform a corpus cavernosogram after the patient is fully recovered to demonstrate the outflow tracts in the quiescent stage. It is probable that the anastomosis between the corpus cavernosum and spongiosum will close spontaneously in a variable period of time. One would also expect the saphenous vein to become blocked at a variable time interval after that type of shunting procedure; otherwise the patient would be unable to obtain an erection without compressing the saphenous vein with his finger or some other device. In my experience, all the shunts have closed and the patient's own normal venous outlet channels have become patent or recanalized in some manner, allowing the patient to maintain a flaccid penis, and the majority of the patients have regained some degree of their potency. About 40% of patients will still have some degree of impotence 1 year postoperatively regardless of type of management. Nearly 100% of untreated priapism will result in loss of potency.

REFERENCES

1. BURT FB, SCHIRMER HK, SCOTT WW: A new concept in the management of priapism. J Urol 83:60, 1960

2. CONTI G: L'erection du penis humain et ses bases morphologico-vasculaires. Acta Anat (Basel) 14:217, 1952

3. DUGGAN ML, MORGAN C, JR: Heparin: A cause of priapism? South Med J 63:1131, 1970

4. FITZPATRICK TJ: Spongiosograms and cavernosograms: A study of their value in priapism. J Urol 109:843, 1973

5. GRAYHACK JT, MCCULLOUGH W, O'CONOR VJ, JR et al: Venous bypass to control priapism. Invest Urol 1:509, 1964

6. GRUBER H: The treatment of priapism: Use of the inferior epigastric artery: A case report. J Urol 108:882, 1972

7. NELSON JH, WINTER CC: Priapism: Evolution of management in 48 patients in 22 years. J Urol 117:455, 1977

8. QUACKELS R: Cure of a patient suffering from priapism by cavernospongiosa anastomosis. Acta Urol Belg 32:5, 1964

9. WINTER CC: Cure of idiopathic priapism. A new procedure for creating fistula between glans penis and corpora cavernosa. Urology 8:389, 1976

10. WINTER CC: Priapism: A review. Urol Surv 28:163, 1978

Penoscrotal Trauma

79

David A. Culp

The incidence of penoscrotal trauma is considerably lower than injuries to other anatomic areas.[5] This low incidence is attributable to the mobility of the genitalia, which protects them from injury except from high-speed missiles. Injuries are much more prevalent during combat, particularly with land mine fragmentation devices. However, in civilian life genital injuries have become more common than in the past as a result of industrial, farm, and automobile accidents and athletic contests.[12] In addition, self-mutilation and malicious assault account for a few of the genital injuries encountered.[15]

These injuries may be classified much the same as wounds to other areas of the body. There are nonpenetrating or contusion-type injuries; penetrating injuries such as incisions, lacerations, or punctures; avulsions, or the loss of skin covering; burns of thermal, chemical, or electrical nature; radiation injuries; and traumatic amputation.[11,13]

Nonpenetrating Injuries

Nonpenetrating injuries are due to a crushing force that does not break the epithelial surface but does produce considerable damage to the underlying tissues. Hemorrhage and edema are unlimited because of the elastic nature of the underlying or subcutaneous tissue of the genitalia. In this respect, injuries differ from other areas of the body where mounting tissue pressure limits hemorrhage and edema.

Extravasated blood and edema may extend into the perineal and abdominal region limited by attachments of Colles' and Buck's fascia and are accompanied by pain and inflammation. Early management consists in elevating and immobilizing the genitalia and applying ice packs to reduce the hemorrhage and edema. Surgical exploration in a nonpenetrating injury is prompted when the hemorrhage and edema cannot be controlled or if there is trauma to the underlying organs such as the corporal bodies of the penis or the testes and the cord in the scrotum.

Access to nonpenetrating penile shaft injuries is best achieved through a circumferential coronal incision, bluntly dissecting the skin coverage from the underlying tissues (Fig. 79-1). Oftentimes the accumulated blood, urine, and edema fluid dissect along the fascial planes of the penile shaft, facilitating this step in the operative repair. Extravasations confined beneath Buck's fascia are limited to the penile shaft. Those confined by Colles' fascia extend from the genital area into the perineum and abdomen. The general location of bleeding vessels in the loose elastic tissue can be identified easily by the bulging, localized, dark red discoloration of the tissue, but the accurate localization of the bleeding vessel is often difficult because of this same discoloration and local tissue reaction.

Defects in the tunica albuginea of the corpora cavernosa are repaired with interrupted 3-0 Prolene sutures to minimize penile deformities and to provide adequate functional capacity (Fig. 79-1C). The degree of repair required for urethral disruption is dependent upon the extent of the injury. Partial disruption without devitalization can be repaired by simply closing the defect with 3-0 or 4-0 chromic catgut sutures. Complete urethral disruption or disruptions with devitalized tissue require freshening of the defect prior to the repair. All urethral injuries should be repaired with absorbable sutures supported by urethral stent, adequately drained with tissue drains, and defunctionalized by urinary diversion.

Suspected trauma to the scrotal contents from crushing injuries by blunt objects that impinge the testis between the force and bone is an indication for immediate surgical exploration. Frequently, rupture of the tunica albuginea occurs with hemorrhage and extravasation of the intracapsular contents. Exposure of the ruptured testis is achieved through a scrotal incision (Fig. 79-2). Unless the testis has been completely morcellated, repair should be attempted by excising the extravasated testicular tissue and reapproximating the fragmented segments with 3-0 Prolene sutures. Both spermatogenic and hormonal functions will survive testic-

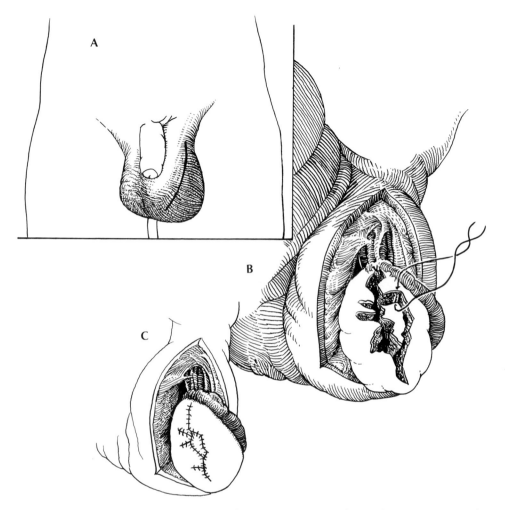

FIG. 79-1.   Repair of nonpenetrating penile injury: **(A)** circumferential incision proximal to the corona; **(B)** mobilization of the skin of the entire penile shaft; **(C)** repair of defects in the tunica

ular injury as long as sufficient blood supply remains to prevent subsequent atrophy. Bleeding vessels should be identified and ligated, hematomas evacuated, and Penrose drains inserted before closing the wound with interrupted 3-0 chromic catgut sutures. Pressure dressings are used only when bleeding cannot be controlled by other means. Ordinarily, a loose, fluffy dressing is all that is required.

Pain is controlled with analgesics or narcotics. Trauma can lead to rather extensive fulminating infections. Prophylactic antimicrobial therapy should be administered even though the skin surface is not broken, because this area is very frequently the source of anaerobic infections.

The late management of nonpenetrating injuries consists primarily in changing the cold applications which were used to control hemorrhage and exudation in the early stages to heat applications for absorption of edema and extravasated blood. Incision and drainage of unresolved fluid and blood or abscesses are necessary in the late stages.

Penetrating Injuries

Penetrating injuries, such as lacerations, incisions, and puncture wounds, are all potentially infected. Any time the skin surface is broken, organisms may be deposited into the depths of the wound. Therefore, their management consists in well-defined measures to control the infection and reduce the effects of the trauma.

All penetrating wounds should be washed thoroughly. Lavage should be carried out as early as

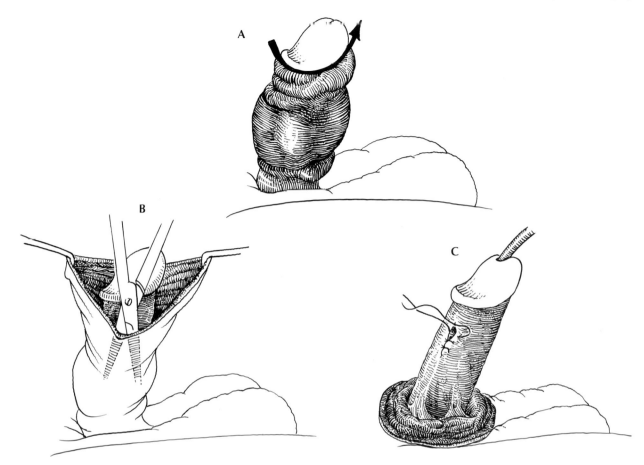

FIG. 79-2. Repair of ruptured testis: **(A)** transscrotal surgical approach; **(B)** débridement and reapproximation of fragments; **(C)** reapproximation of fragments with 3-0 Prolene sutures

possible, because within 6 hr to 8 hr a wound may be contaminated but not infected. An incubation time is necessary for organisms to produce an infected wound. If they can be washed away prior to the incubation period, the wound will be contaminated but not necessarily infected. Generous washing of the area around the wound as well as the wound itself with surgical soaps and water is indicated. Large quantities of nonirritating solutions such as sterile normal saline should be flushed through the wound. Antimicrobial solutions are of little value, because the main advantage of lavage is the mechanical washing of the wound, and antimicrobial solutions do not remain in contact with the wound or the organisms long enough to produce a specific effect.

The next step in the management of penetrating injuries is the removal of nonviable tissue or, débridement. All foreign bodies should be removed. Puncture wounds should be opened and

explored to the depth of their penetration to be certain that no foreign material has been carried into the depths of the wound. Hemostasis should be obtained. All extravasated blood should be washed away. The open vessels should be secured by incorporating as little tissue as possible, because this will also act as a foreign body. Underlying tissue destruction should be repaired and restored to as normal a relationship as possible. This is particularly true of a ruptured testis. It should be incorporated within its tunica albuginea and returned to the scrotum whenever possible. The area should be drained with tissue drains so that further collections of unwanted edema, serum, blood, and infected material have access to the surface. The wound should be closed primarily unless it is grossly contaminated.

Anaerobic gangrenous infections may result from injuries to the external genitalia, and in some instances there has been complete loss of genital skin as a result of secondary anaerobic infection. Therefore, systemic antimicrobial therapy should also be instituted. A surgical dressing should be loose, particularly if hemostasis has been achieved. Pressure dressings should be used only to minimize postoperative edema and hemorrhage. In any event, the wound should be inspected frequently for tenderness and inflammation. Drains should be removed when the drainage diminishes, or if infection has failed to develop.

Avulsions, Burns, and Radiation Injuries

Avulsions are those injuries in which there is partial or complete loss of epithelial covering from an acute tearing away of the genital skin, as in power take-off injury in which the skin is wrapped in the clothing of an individual who has become involved with the rotating or power take-off shaft of a tractor. As the clothing is ripped from the body, the enmeshed skin of the genitalia is also torn away.[4] Secondary losses of genital skin result from infection or other injuries such as burns, constricting bands, and radiation injury.

The immediate management of avulsions is to relieve the pain, which usually is not severe and can be controlled with analgesics. The skin, as it is ripped from the body, rarely produces a major bleeding problem. The nature of the vessel rupture and the twisting and contusion to the ends of vessels helps to control oozing and bleeding from them. The mobility of the skin covering the external genitalia protects the underlying surface, so they are not often involved in this type of injury. However, there are instances in which the glans penis along with the skin of the shaft has been avulsed. Immediately, warm saline packs should be applied to the denuded area. Broad-spectrum antimicrobials should be administered, and the patient should be sent to a hospital for immediate repair. Repair of avulsions should be carried out in 8 hr to 12 hr after the injury (Fig. 79-3). Delay is indicated only when the line of demarcation between viable and nonviable tissue cannot be determined, but this line is easily determined in the instances of traumatic avulsion of the skin from the shaft of the penis or the scrotum.

Split-thickness skin grafts are the best means for covering the avulsed area. Pedicle grafts from surrounding areas have been used but usually produce bulky, hairy, grotesque coverage. In many instances, pedicle grafts ultimately must be taken down and the area covered with split-thickness grafts. The remaining cuff of tissue attached to the corona should be trimmed so that only a sufficient epithelial cuff remains to anchor the graft. On occasion, the cuff of skin remaining may be sufficient in length to cover the entire shaft of the penis. When this is done, however, there is a great risk of secondary edema requiring removal of this edematous skin and recovering the area with a split-thickness graft.

It is not advisable to use the avulsed skin, which usually leads to secondary infection and necrosis and delays primary covering of the avulsed area. The donor site to be used is dependent upon the extent of injury to other areas of donor skin. Generally, the skin from the inner aspect of the thigh is preferable, but there are occasions when in the course of tearing away or avulsing the skin there is an abrasion of the skin of the thigh which prevents its use. In these instances it cannot be used. A graft of 10 cm by 20 cm is usually sufficient to cover any denuded penis. In an infected wound the thickness of the graft is 0.02 to 0.024 of an inch (0.51–0.610 mm), and in grossly contaminated wounds the thickness should not exceed 0.012 to 0.016 of an inch (0.305–0.406 mm).

Multiple anchoring sutures are inserted around the base and around the cuff at the corona, with the ends being left long in order to facilitate the application of a tie-over, or bolus, dressing. This dressing is constructed in such a way that the middle of the dressing is larger than the extremities. Thus, when the tie-over sutures are brought together from the corona and the base, the pressure exerted on the dressing is equal to all portions of the graft, keeping it in contact with its base. This is essential because if the graft is to survive, it must be in constant contact with the base from which it derives its blood supply (Fig. 79-3E). Once the tie-over dressing is in place, it is fixed to the abdomen to prevent motion of the graft. At all times, however, it is advisable to keep the glans visible at the end of the dressing. Any evidence of discoloration should be checked to be certain there is viability in the shaft of the penis. An indwelling urethral catheter prevents urinary soiling during the time in which the graft is healing. In 10 to 14 days the dressing is removed, and at this time most portions of the graft will have taken. Small portions of surface epithelium which have not survived should be treated with a nonirritating, water-soluble ointment. Within a week or two this too will be completely epithelialized.

The simultaneous loss of scrotal skin presents other problems. One should try to use scrotal skin to house the testes, even if it is tight, for this is a particular type of skin and provides a functional

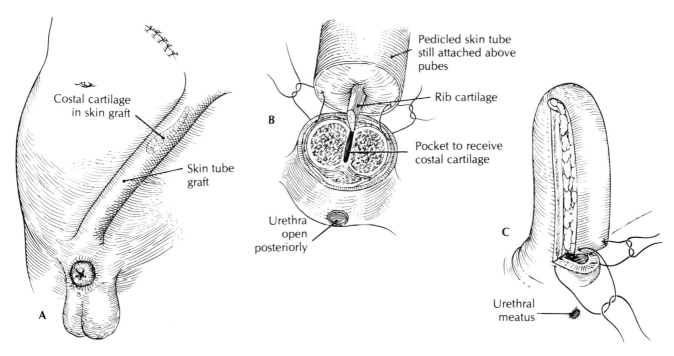

FIG. 79-4. Bergman's method of constructing an artificial penis.   **(A)** The skin tube is constructed.   **(B)** In joining the tube to the stump, the urethra may have to be brought out in the perineum.   **(C)** The artificial penis is contoured.

the extent of the injury (unsuccessful attempts at amputation are managed as lacerations), availability and condition of the distal segment, the patient's general condition, and the interval between injury and repair (must be less than 18 hr if reanastomosis is to be used).[14,16] Alternatives to primary anastomosis are plastic reconstruction or local reshaping measures.[9]

With the advent of microsurgical techniques, reanastomosis of the severed penis has been improved. The first successful reanastomosis was achieved by Best in 1962, after a prolonged healing period with mummification, débridement, granulation, and reepithelialization.[2] Fifteen years elapsed before the second successful repair was reported by Heymann in 1977, using microsurgical techniques.[10] The reader is referred to Chapter 80 for a discussion of surgical technique.

CONSTRUCTION OF ARTIFICIAL PENIS

In those patients in whom primary anastomosis is not feasible, a staged reconstruction using tubed pedicle grafts from the abdominal wall has been used to construct an artifical penis.[1] Bogoras first described this procedure in 1936 in the German literature.[3] It consisted of four stages requiring approximately 9 months to complete.

In the first stage, a phallic tube graft with an implanted segment of rib cartilage is constructed (Fig. 79-4A). An incision is made over the eighth or ninth rib from the sternum to the costochondral junction. A 6-cm piece of rib is removed and placed in normal saline until time for implantation. The tube graft is raised from two parallel incisions 6 cm to 7 cm apart, beginning at the lateral costal margins at the posterior axillary line continuing downward and anteriorly to a point anterior to the superior iliac spine. These incisions are deepened through the subcutaneous fat to the deep layer of the superficial fascia. The edges of the middle flap are sutured together with the epidermis outward. The cartilage is inserted into the cephalic portion of the flap graft with the concavity of the rib upward when the graft is turned to meet the penile stump. The first stage is completed by approximating the lateral skin margins of the original incisions.

After an interval of approximately 6 weeks, the second stage is undertaken. The urinary stream is diverted by a suprapubic cystostomy and the tube graft with the implanted cartilage is freed from its cephalic attachment, exposing the cartilage implant. Scar tissue is removed from the penile stump, and a pocket is developed in the septum between the corpora bodies into which the cartilage is anchored with a mattress suture. The remainder of the skin graft is approximated to the penile stump and the site of origin of the skin flap is closed, completing the second stage (Fig. 79-4*B*).

The third stage is undertaken after an interval of approximately 2 months. Before detaching the tube graft from its final abdominal attachment, the graft is conditioned by tying a rubber band about the tube graft close to its remaining abdominal attachment. Initially, this is done for 10 minutes every 3 hr. The time and the frequency of constriction are progressively increased until the day prior to release. The band should be able to remain in place for 15 hours without blanching the skin or lowering the temperature of the graft. Following release from the abdomen, the end of the tube graft and the site of its former attachment are closed (Fig. 79-4C).

The final stage is the advancement of the hypospadic urethral meatus. This is undertaken after it is certain that the tube flap graft has satisfactorily derived its blood supply from the penile stump.

More recently, a double tube flap procedure for penile construction has been described by Edgerton.* Originally the operation was developed for use in transsexual change, but it is conceivable that it could be used for repair of the traumatically amputated penis. Two tube grafts are constructed from the abdominal wall; one of 6 cm to 7 cm in width formed with the epidermis outward and a second one 3 cm to 3.5 cm in width formed with the epidermis inward for future use as a urethra to be inserted within the large tube graft. The details, complications, and success of this technique have not been published as yet.

Reanastomosis of a traumatically amputated testis is technically an extremely difficult undertaking and is rarely associated with success. Because of the vessel size, there is no chance of testicular survival unless microsurgical repair is used. The time interval between severance and repair is critical in a parenchymatous organ such as the testis. Ischemia time beyond 30 minutes usually leads to atrophy or secondary orchiectomy. In the vast majority of cases, it is much wiser to control the bleeding vessels and reconstruct the scrotum, foregoing any attempts at reanastomosis in favor of testicular prostheses and subsequent hormonal replacement therapy. When considering vascular

reanastomosis, the repair must be performed immediately. Obstructing clots in the distal vascular limbs must be irrigated from the testicular artery and vein, and the organ should be stored in iced Ringer's solution until the proximal limbs have been prepared in a similar manner. Following the reestablishment of blood flow, the scrotal compartment should be cleaned of extravasated blood and clots, the bleeding vessels should be secured, and the testis should be returned to its normal position. The scrotal wound is closed loosely with widely spaced sutures about a tissue drain.

REFERENCES

1. BERGMAN R, HOWARD AH, BARNES RW: Plastic reconstruction of the penis. J Urol 59:1174, 1948
2. BEST JW, ANGELO JJ, MILLIGAN B: Complete traumatic amputation of the penis. J Urol 87:134, 1962
3. BOGORAS NA: Uber die wolle plastische Wiederherstellung eines zym Koitus fahigen Penis (Penoplastica totalis). Zentralbl Chir 63:1271, 1936
4. CULLEN TH: Avulsion of the skin of the penis and scrotum. Br J Urol 38:99, 1966
5. CULP DA: Genital injuries: Etiology and Initial Management Symposia on Genito-urinary Trauma. In The Urology Clinics of North America, Vol. 4, No. 1, Philadelphia, W B Saunders, 1977
6. CULP DA, HUFFMAN WC: Temperature determination in the thigh with regard to burying the traumatically exposed testis. J Urol 76:436, 1956
7. ENGELMAN ER, POLITO G, PERLEY J et al: Traumatic amputation of the penis. J Urol 112:774, 1974
8. EVINS SC, WHITTE T, ROUS, S: Self-emasculation. Review of the literature, report of a case and outline of the objectives of management. J Urol 118:775, 1977
9. FLOCKS RH, CULP DA: Surgical Urology. Chicago, Year Book Publishers, 1954
10. HEYMANN AD, BELL–THOMSON J, RATHOD DM et al: Successful reimplantation of the penis using microvascular techniques. J Urol 118:879, 1977
11. HUFFMAN, WC, CULP DA, FLOCKS RH: Injuries of the external male genitalia. In Converse JM (ed): Reconstructive Plastic Surgery, Chap 70. Philadelphia, W B Saunders, 1964
12. HUFFMAN WC, CULP DA, GREENLEAF JS et al: Injuries to the male genitalia. Plast Reconstr Surg 18:344, 1956
13. JULIAN R, KLEIN MH, HUBBARD H: Management of a thermal burn with amputation and reconstruction of the penis. J Urol 101:580, 1969
14. MCROBERTS JW, CHAPMAN WH, ANSELL JS: Primary anastomosis of the traumatically amputated penis; Case report and summary of literature. J Urol 100:751, 1968
15. MENDEZ R, KIELY WF, MORROW JW: Self-emasculation. J Urol 107:981, 1972
16. SCHULMAN ML: Re-anastomosis of the amputated penis. J Urol 109:432, 1973

---

* Edgerton MT: Personal communication

Penile Replantation

80

David P. O'Brien III

Traumatic amputation of the penis is an uncommon but potentially devastating occurrence. Several case reports can be found in the literature, however, and recent enthusiasm for the use of microneurovascular anastomoses has prompted use of this technique for replantation of the penis.[1-8] It should be noted that an attempt to replant the penis should be made no matter what the time delay between amputation and repair.

Amputation of the penis occurs most commonly as an act of self-emasculation but has also been reported as resulting from assaults or accidental dismemberments. Self-emasculation has been reported in approximately 50 cases in the literature; traumatic amputation by assault or accidental means has been reported in fewer than 15 cases.[4] Many of these cases involve not only the penis but also to varying degrees the scrotum and scrotal contents.

Replantation of the penis has both anatomic (cosmetic) and functional objectives. The satisfactory appearance of the penis is of great importance to most patients, including those deranged few who attempt self-destruction. The psychologic aspects of penile appearance are obvious, and the functional aspects are of equal importance. Preservation of the penis as an erectile organ is desirable for the sexual and psychologic well-being of the patient. Maintenance of the urethra as a conduit for both urine and semen is also necessary.

Management of the Amputated Penis

Experience with organ transplantation has shown that cooling of an organ is essential if the organ is to sustain minimal damage during ischemia.[6] Suspension of the penis in a bag containing cool saline which is then placed in ice should decrease the metabolic requirements of the penis to a minimum and permit time for transportation of the patient to suitable operating facilities, transfusions, setting up the operation, and so forth. Care should be taken not to allow ice to touch the penis directly, because this may cause freezing of the tissue with

later necrosis. When microvascular procedures are to be used in the replantation, vessels should be handled as little as possible both in the penis and the amputated stump. If blood loss is not a problem the proximal vessels should be packed rather than clamped or tied.[2,3] Perfusion of the vessels should not be attempted to avoid damaging small vessels.

Technique of Replantation

Prior to the advent of microsurgery, the penis was attached as a free or composite graft.[1,3] When facilities are available, however, it appears conceptually sound to preserve and maintain neurovascular integrity by microsurgical means.[2,3,5,6] Use of microneurovascular reanastomosis is the only technique reported in the literature in which there have been no postoperative surgical complications in complete amputation of the penis. Free-graft anastomosis without neurovascular anastomoses should be used if microsurgical means are not available. The procedure, following inspection and cleaning of the respective surfaces of both the penis (Fig. 80-1) and amputated stump (Fig. 80-2), begins with débridement of any damaged or suspect tissue. The urethra and corpus spongiosum are anastomosed by conventional means using an interrupted absorbable suture of 4-0 chromic or Vicryl. Incorporation of the mucosa with this suture is our custom, but some authors recommend approximation without entering the mucosa. An indwelling Foley catheter at this juncture acts nicely as a splint to help stabilize the loosely attached penis. A few sutures are taken in the ventral portion of the fascia of the corpora cavernosa to continue to stabilize the penis. An absorbable suture of 3-0 chromic or Vicryl is suitable for this closure. It has not been necessary or technically possible in most cases to anastomose the central artery of the corpora cavernosum, although this was performed in the replantation done by Tamai.[8]

Microneurovascular anastomoses of dorsal arteries, veins, and nerves are performed next, using 9-0 or 10-0 vascular suture in the technique which

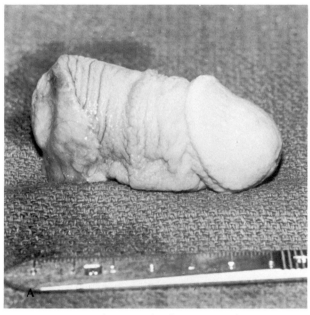
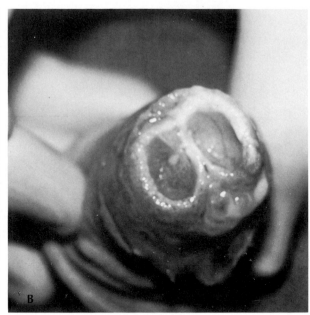

FIG. 80-1. **(A)** The completely transected penis.   **(B)** In this case there is an almost surgically clean edge.

FIG. 80-2. Base or stump of the amputation site. Care should be taken not to injure the small dorsal vessels if microneurovascular anastomoses are to be attempted.

FIG. 80-3. The completed replantation. Skin color is excellent and the glans demonstrates good capillary filling.

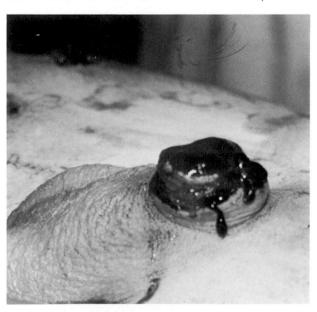

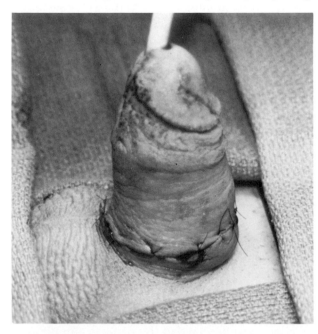

has recently become standard. It is recommended that as many vessels as can be found be reanastomosed, because these dorsal vessels are frequently multiple.[2,3] Nerves, when found, may be reapproximated with 10-0 suture material. The remainder of Buck's fascia is closed, and the skin is closed with interrupted sutures of 4-0 nylon (Fig. 80-3). Urinary diversion (suprapubic or perineal) should be performed so that the urethral catheter can be removed at the earliest moment possible. Initial use of the Foley for 3 to 4 days is helpful in splinting and keeping the penis elevated. Broad-

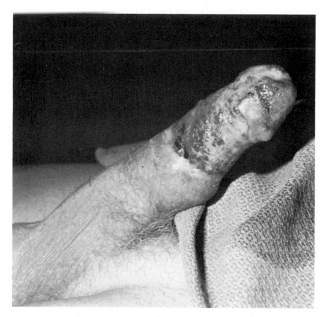

FIG. 80-5. Débridement of necrotic skin at 12 days post replantation. The underlying tissue is viable. Note the spontaneous erection during anesthesia.

FIG. 80-6. At 12 days, the penile shaft is grafted with split-thickness mesh skin. It is best not to graft the glans.

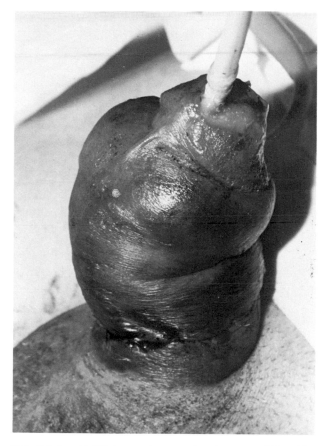

FIG. 80-4. At 72 hr, early necrotic changes of the skin are apparent. The glans retains good capillary filling.

spectrum antibiotic coverage is recommended, and heparin administration has been used by some authors.

Complications

Varying degrees of both skin and soft-tissue necrosis may occur as has been previously mentioned (Fig. 80-4). This usually occurs with free grafting, but necrosis has been reported in some cases in which successful microneurovascular anastomoses have been accomplished.[5,6] Early débridement promotes earlier grafting with split-thickness or meshed skin, and scrotal skin is not as satisfactory in appearance (Fig. 80-5, Fig. 80-6). The glans penis should not be grafted initially. The eschar which frequently forms on the glans will eventually peel off and leave appropriate glans tissue.[6] Grafting this area too soon may mar the cosmetic appearance.

Urethral strictures may occur at the anastomosis site. These are difficult to handle if skin loss has also occurred. Surrounding grafted skin is rarely

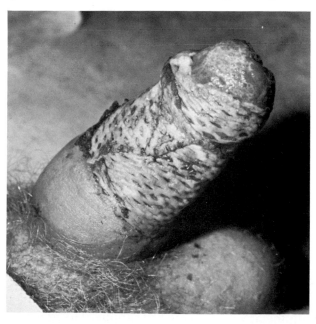

suitable for the types of procedures normally used in stricture repair. Use of scrotal skin as an island patch or inlay is of value, and burying the penis in a Cecil-type urethroplasty can be done. Minor strictures can initially be treated with dilation or visual urethrotomy. Fistulization at the anasto-

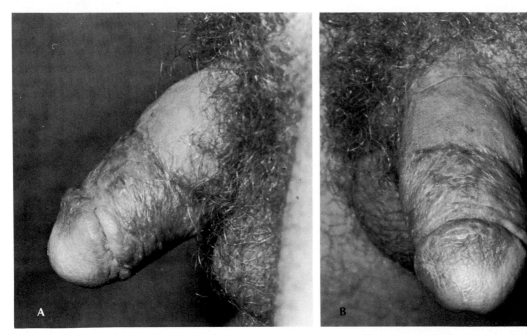

FIG. 80-7. The final result 6 months postreplantation is excellent cosmetically and functionally.

mosis site may occur but may be difficult to repair because of the lack of normal available skin surrounding the fistula.

Impotence as a complicating factor has not occurred in my two patients, nor is it commonly reported in the literature. It should be noted, however, that most of these injuries have resulted from severe psychologic disturbances in which subjective estimates of potency are difficult to evaluate. Pathologically, it would seem that the erectile tissues are at risk for necrotic change and fibrotic replacement with impotence resulting, as in some cases of priapism. It is a testament to the resilience of the cavernous bodies that erections occur at all, even after long periods of ischemia. Prosthetic insertion, either semirigid rods or inflatable prostheses, may be used to deal with impotence that might occur after penile replantation.

The psychiatric implications of self-mutilation are beyond the scope of this chapter. It is evident from the literature, however, that many patients who attempt self-emasculation are already receiving therapy which should continue. The group of patients who are of at least as much concern are those who traumatically, either by assault or accident, sustain amputation of the penis. Psychiatric consultation with these patients should be instituted so that anxieties and fears about the injury and treatment can be dealt with rather than repressed.

In summary, replantation of the penis is not only possible but also preferable to penile reconstruction procedures. Necrotic complications should be managed by early débridement. Reconstructive urethral procedures, although more difficult, are based on existing principles. Gratifying results (Fig. 80-7) are usually possible.

REFERENCES

1. BUX R, CARROLL P, YARBROUGH W: Primary penile reanastomosis. Urology 11:500, 1978
2. COHEN BE, MAY JW, DALY JSF et al: Successful clinical replantation of an amputated penis by microneurovascular repair. Plastic and Reconstructive Surgery 59:276, 1977
3. ENGELMAN ER, BLITO G, PERLEY J et al: Traumatic amputation of the penis. J Urol 112:774, 1974
4. EVINS SC, WHITTLE T, ROUS SN: Self-emasculation: A review of the literature, report of a case and outline of the objectives of management. J Urol 118:775, 1977
5. HEYMANN AD, BELL–THOMSON J, RATHOD DM et al: Successful reimplantation of the penis using microvascular techniques. J Urol 118:879, 1977
6. O'BRIEN DP, AMBROSE SS, NAHI F et al: Replantation of the penis following traumatic amputation: A report of two cases. in preparation
7. RANEY AM, MANEIS H, ZUMSKIND PD: Reanastomosis of completely transected penis in canine: Review of current concepts. Urology 6:735, 1975
8. TAMAI S, NAKAMURA Y, MOTOMIYA Y: Microsurgical replantation of a completely amputated penis and scrotum. Plast Reconstr Surg 60:287, 1977

Penectomy and Ilioinguinal Lymphadenectomy

81

Elwin E. Fraley

artial or total penectomy is most often done by urologic surgeons for the treatment of cancer and is usually followed by an ilioinguinal lymphadenectomy. This chapter describes these operations, focusing especially on the latter.

Penectomy

Small distal cancers can often be treated by partial penectomy, because recurrences in the stump are uncommon. The principal reason for selecting this operation is that afterward the patient can stand while urinating and can direct his stream; most patients do not have satisfactory sexual function, however.

The technique of partial penectomy is sufficiently well known not to require extensive description, but four points need emphasis. First, before any operation is performed on a primary penile carcinoma, the lesion should be cultured so that appropriate antibiotics can be given. Cancers of the penis are almost always infected, and the organisms usually travel to the regional lymph nodes. Second, for partial or total penectomy, the cancer should be covered before the operation so that it does not get implanted into the wound. Third, the margin proximal to the tumor must be examined by a pathologist, and the surgeon should try to obtain at least 2 cm of tumor-free margin. Finally, the urethra should be cut on a bias and spatulated to prevent postoperative stenosis.

The technique of total penectomy is illustrated in Figure 81-1. The specimen should include all the connective tissue at the base of the penis, because this tissue contains the lymphatics and nodes that provide the primary drainage of the organ. The scrotum should be left intact so that its lymphatics can help drain the legs after ilioinguinal lymphadenectomy.

Ilioinguinal Lymphadenectomy

The goal of a radical ilioinguinal node dissection is *en bloc* excision of all of the lymphatic tissue from the aortic bifurcation to the point where the femoral artery enters Hunter's canal. The urologic surgeon uses this operation in the treatment of cancers not only of the penis but also of the scrotum and the distal female urethra. In addition, it is sometimes necessary to do this procedure or some modification of it in men whose scrotum is contaminated with testicular tumors.[6]

ANATOMY OF THE ILIOINGUINAL AREA

In the past, there was a high incidence of serious complications with radical ilioinguinal lymphadenectomy. It may be that these occurred, at least in part, because the operation was conceived and carried out without proper consideration of the anatomy of the inguinal region.

The superficial abdominal groin fascia is composed of two layers. *Camper's fascia* is the superficial fatty layer and may be very thick in obese individuals. *Scarpa's fascia* is the deep fibroelastic layer, which begins in the lower abdomen, extends across the inguinal ligament, and becomes attached to the fascia lata. The two layers fuse medially and extend into the penis as the penile fascia. The same fused layer extends into the scrotum as the dartos fascia and then into the perineum as Colles' fascia.

The skin of the inguinal area is supplied by the superficial pudendal, superficial circumflex iliac, and superficial epigastric arteries. Branches of these vessels run within Camper's fascia parallel to the inguinal ligament. The skin overlying the inguinal lymphatics also receives a collateral blood supply from vessels that supply the lateral aspects of the thigh and abdominal wall. Thus, there is a transverse rather than a vertical orientation to the blood supply in this region. The three-incision skin bridge technique, described below, was evolved to preserve the blood supply to the skin of the inguinal region.[4]

The *femoral triangle* is a space below the inguinal ligament that is bounded by the adductor longus muscle, the inguinal ligament, and the sartorius muscle. Its floor is formed by the iliopsoas and

825

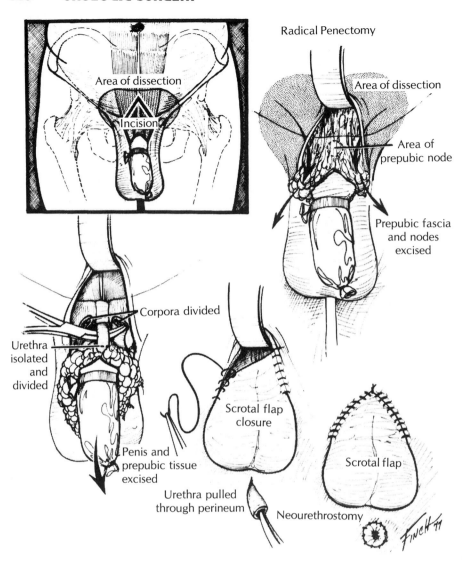

Radical Penectomy

FIG. 81-1. Technique of total penectomy, including removal of lymphatic tissue at the base of the penis. Note that tumor is covered to prevent it from seeding the wound. (Reprinted from Hoppmann HJ, Fraley EE: J Urol 120:393, 1978 with the permission of The Williams & Wilkins Co)

pectineus muscles and its roof by the fascia lata. It contains most of the lymph nodes in the groin region, which must be removed completely during a radical ilioinguinal lymphadenectomy.

The obturator artery arises as an anterior branch of the hypogastric artery and exits from the pelvis through the obturator foramen. It forms the medial boundary of the iliac node dissection. In approximately 25% of individuals, this artery arises from the inferior epigastric or external iliac artery and descends almost vertically into the obturator foramen, so that it lies on either the lateral or the medial side of the femoral canal. In such a position, the artery is prone to injury when the medial third of the inguinal ligament is divided or when a femoral hernia is repaired after the lymphadenectomy is complete.

The surface lymphatics below the umbilicus usually drain to the ipsilateral groin and iliac nodes. Midline structures, such as the genitalia and perineum, drain to both sides. Therefore, a bilateral ilioinguinal dissection is necessary for most tumors that are treated by the urologic surgeon.

The nodes in the inguinal area are divided by fascia lata into superficial and deep nodes; they are found either overlying the femoral triangle or attached to the femoral vessels. The superficial nodes, which number between 4 and 25, lie within Camper's fascia and drain into both deep inguinal and iliac lymph nodes. The deep inguinal nodes usually are fewer in number and form a continuous chain with the iliac nodes. The deep nodes are contained within the fibrofatty layer of the femoral sheath. Cloquet's node, the most cephalad and most constant deep inguinal node, is situated on the medial aspect of the femoral vein within or near the femoral canal.[9]

The prepubic node, which is present in only a few individuals, is located in the area of the pubis and drains the penis. It drains into the superficial inguinal nodes and should be removed when treating cancer of the penis by total penectomy.

INDICATIONS FOR RADICAL ILIOINGUINAL LYMPHADENECTOMY

Radical ilioinguinal lymphadenectomy is indicated for invasive epidermoid tumors of the penis, carcinoma of the distal urethra, melanoma of the urethra, carcinoma or melanoma of the scrotum, and contamination of the scrotum or inguinal region with testis cancer.[1,2,4-7] The procedure should be considered even if there is no clinical evidence of tumor, because the incidence of clinically normal, microscopically tumorous lymph nodes in patients with either epidermoid carcinomas or melanomas is as high as 50%.

The lymphadenectomy can be done either at the time the primary tumor is excised or later. There are those who argue that a delay between excision of the primary tumor and the groin dissection allows tumor cells in transit to complete their course and thus to be excised. However, despite the logical appeal of this idea, there are no data to indicate that survival rates improve when the lymphadenectomy is delayed. Delay is indicated, however, if the primary tumor is septic, as large fungating cancers of the penis often are. After the penectomy, antibiotics should be given for 2 weeks in an attempt to sterilize the lymphatics before the lymphadenectomy.

If it is necessary to do a bilateral operation, we prefer to do one side at a time and allow 4 to 6 weeks between procedures. We do bilateral operations in all cancers of the penis.

PREOPERATIVE EVALUATION AND CARE

We no longer do preoperative lymphangiography. The procedure adds very little to the preoperative evaluation; the result hardly, if ever, determines whether or not the operation is done; and the tissue reaction produced by the oily dye may cause a proliferative lymphangitis that could contribute to postoperative lymphedema of the legs.[3]

As with any other major operative procedure, the general preoperative condition of the patient must be satisfactory. There are, however, some special considerations related to this operation. For example, previous incisions in the groin area may affect the type of incision that can be used. Thus, if the patient has had a simple biopsy of a tumorous inguinal node, the biopsy incision must be excised widely as part of the definitive ilioinguinal lymphadenectomy. Furthermore, any open wounds, rashes, or infected areas over the groin should be treated preoperatively.

OPERATIVE TECHNIQUE

In order to expose the femoral triangle, the patient is placed on the operating table with the corresponding thigh slightly abducted and rotated externally and a small sandbag beneath the knee. The ipsilateral foot is anchored to the opposite leg for stability. The scrotum is sutured to the opposite thigh for better exposure. The major anatomic landmarks—such as the umbilicus, pubic tubercle, and anterosuperior iliac spine—should not be obscured by drapes.

Three types of skin incisions were used in the past. All of them crossed the groin crease and therefore were likely to become macerated and septic. The three-incision technique now recommended is designed to preserve the blood supply of the lower abdominal and inguinal skin (Fig. 81-2).

The operation is begun by assessing the lymphatics and lymph nodes in the pelvis. After the midline incision is made, the exposure of the iliac vessels is facilitated by division of the obliterated umbilical artery; this releases the peritoneum and facilitates its medial retraction. The patient must be completely relaxed and in the slightly head-down position. The ureter should be identified at the outset so that it can be retracted medially out of harm's way.

The proximal dissection is begun by incising the endopelvic fascia medial to the genitofemoral nerve from the inguinal ligament to the aortic bifurcation; this defines the lateral and superior limits of the dissection. All loose areolar and adventitial tissue surrounding the large vessels, which contains the lymph nodes and lymphatic vessels, is removed. The medial boundaries of the proximal dissection are the obturator vessels. If there is unilateral involvement of the nerve with tumor, the nerve may be resected; however, the patient would then have some difficulty walking postoperatively because of adductor muscle weakness.

When the medial dissection is completed near the inguinal ligament, the previously described anatomic variation in the obturator artery should be remembered; troublesome bleeding may occur

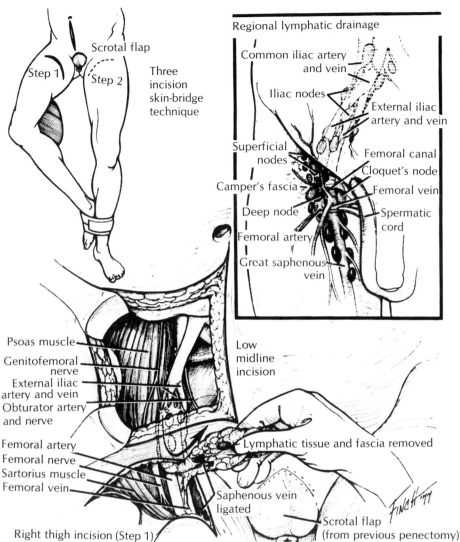

Step 1

Scrotal flap

Step 2

Three incision skin-bridge technique

Regional lymphatic drainage

Common iliac artery and vein

Iliac nodes

External iliac artery and vein

Superficial nodes

Femoral canal

Cloquet's node

Camper's fascia

Femoral vein

Deep node

Spermatic cord

Femoral artery

Great saphenous vein

Psoas muscle

Genitofemoral nerve

External iliac artery and vein

Obturator artery and nerve

Femoral artery

Femoral nerve

Sartorius muscle

Femoral vein

Low midline incision

Lymphatic tissue and fascia removed

Saphenous vein ligated

Right thigh incision (Step 1)

Scrotal flap (from previous penectomy)

FIG. 81-2. A three-incision approach to the inguinal and iliac lymph nodes provides excellent exposure. Skin bridge across the groin crease helps prevent some of the postoperative complications seen with other lymphadenectomy techniques. (Reprinted from Hoppmann HJ, Fraley EE: J Urol 120:393, 1978 with the permission of The Williams & Wilkins Co)

if this artery is divided accidentally. The proximal dissection is developed until all of the iliac and obturator lymph node groups and associated connective tissues connect to a pedicle of tissue that passes through the empty space in the femoral canal. As the dissection is completed, the various groups of nodes should be identified for the pathologist.

The second skin incision is made 10 cm below the inguinal ligament; the ends of the incision are curved away from the ligament to preserve the blood supply of the skin bridge. The incision is extended only a small distance into Camper's fascia so as not to disturb the *en bloc* dissection. A skin flap 2 mm to 4 mm thick is developed from the incision to a point just beyond the inguinal liga-

ment. This part of the dissection should include the prepubic node if the patient has cancer of the skin takes up the dye and fluoresces under an subcutaneous tissue from the skin bridge; in fact, every effort should be made not to devascularize the bridge. The edge of the skin bridge should be handled as gently as possible. The fatty subcutaneous tissue beneath the skin flap is then dissected off the underlying lower abdominal wall and the inguinal ligament.

To complete the dissection, the distal skin flap over the femoral triangle is developed. At the limits of the dissection, the subcutaneous tissue is incised through the fascia lata down to muscle. The saphenous vein and all of its major branches are identified and should be preserved. Interlocking mattress sutures are placed around the border to prevent the escape of lymph into the wound, and several mattress sutures are placed on the edges of the specimen to prevent retrograde escape of cancer cells.

The fatty lymphatic tissue is then dissected upward toward the inguinal ligament. Near the medial border of the sartorius, branches of the femoral nerve will be encountered; the muscular branches should be preserved, but the cutaneous branches may be transected. The femoral vessels are stripped of all surrounding tissues, including the vascular advential tissues. As the inguinal ligament is approached, the saphenous vein is ligated a second time. After the lymphatic-bearing tissues are dissected off the pectineus, the only remaining attachment is to the femoral canal.

The specimen is freed from the femoral vessels and the inguinal ligament so that it connects with the proximal specimen. The iliac and obturator lymphatic tissues are delivered through the empty space in the femoral canal, and the intact specimen is removed from below. Cloquet's node should be identified with a suture to assist the pathologist. The inguinal ligament does not have to be divided to complete the dissection. Before the wound is closed, the transversalis fascia is sutured to Cooper's ligament to prevent a postoperative femoral hernia.

There are two techniques for protecting the femoral vessels postoperatively. First, the sartorius is sectioned at its origin near the anterosuperior iliac spine and transposed to cover the femoral vessels. The transected end of the muscle is sutured to the medial edge of the inguinal ligament, and the borders of the muscle are sutured to nearby muscles to hold the ligament in place. As an alternative, the sartorius and adductor longus can be approximated so that most of the vessels are covered and the dead space is obliterated.

It is usually necessary to cut a small strip of skin from the edge of the distal skin flap to prevent postoperative skin necrosis. As an aid in determining the viability of various skin flaps, the patient can be injected with fluorescein. Viable skin takes up the dye and fluoresces under an ultraviolet lamp.[8]

Finally, two large suction catheters are placed in the area of the femoral dissection. The catheters are brought out through the skin in the midportion of the thigh, well away from the distal skin flap. The catheters should not be irrigated and are kept in place as long as they remain functional (usually 3 to 5 days).

The skin should be closed without tension. If the patient is kept in bed with the thigh slightly flexed, any existing tension on the distal suture line will be lessened. The wound is wrapped with loose dressings so as not to compress the skin flap; the dressings are removed on the second postoperative day. The legs are wrapped with compression bandages for at least 7 days. The patient is not mobilized until the sixth or seventh day after surgery and not until the wound suction has been removed.

POSTOPERATIVE COMPLICATIONS AND MANAGEMENT

Necrosis of skin is the most frequent early complication of radical ilioinguinal lymphadenectomy, with a reported incidence as high as 60%. Necrosis usually occurs in the midportion of the wound between the fourth and twelfth postoperative days. This problem is treated by debriding the dead skin and, after appropriate preparation of the underlying tissues, by covering the area with a split-thickness skin graft.

The most common late complication of this operation is lymphedema of the legs, with an incidence as high as 40%. Lymphedema is controlled during the early postoperative period with elastic bandages; later, fitted elastic stockings may be used. In anticipation of this problem, the patient can be fitted for an elastic stocking before the operation. The patient is also instructed to avoid injury to the legs and not to sit in one position with the legs dependent for long intervals.

Hemorrhage from the femoral vessels is perhaps the most frightening, and also the most lethal, complication of this procedure. It usually results from infection or skin slough. Fortunately, exsanguinating hemorrhage is infrequent if the femoral vessels are covered during the operation as described.

Moderate drainage of lymph may result from failure to ligate transected lymphatics. Continued use of suction catheters and immobilization and elevation of the legs usually resolves the problem. Occasionally, serum or lymph may collect under the flaps after wound suction has been discontinued. Seromas and lymphoceles usually can be managed by periodic aspirations and pressure dressings.

The incidence of postoperative hernia has been poorly documented in the literature. Hernia formation usually is associated with division of the inguinal ligament, especially at its midportion; therefore, the inguinal ligament should not be divided.

REFERENCES

1. BRYON RL, JR, LAMB EJ, YONEMTO RH et al: Radical inguinal node dissection in the treatment of cancer. Surg Gynecol Obstet 114:401, 1962

2. FORTNER JG, BOOHER RJ, PACK GT: Results of groin dissection for malignant melanoma in 220 patients. Surgery 55:485, 1964

3. FRALEY EE, CLOUSE ME, LITWIN SB: The uses of lymphangiography, lymphadenography and color lymphadenography in urology. J Urol 93:319, 1965

4. FRALEY EE, HUTCHENS HC: Radical ilio-inguinal node dissection: The skin bridge technique. A new procedure. J Urol 108:279, 1972

5. HOPPMANN HJ, FRALEY EE: Squamous cell carcinoma of the penis. J Urol 120:393, 1978

6. MARKLAND CM, KEDIA K, FRALEY EE: Inadequate orchiectomy for patients with testicular tumors. JAMA 224:1025, 1973

7. PACK G, REKERS P: Radical groin dissection. In Cooper P (ed): The Craft of Surgery, 2nd ed, p 1446. Boston, Little, Brown & Co, 1971

8. SMITH JA, JR, MIDDLETON RG: The use of fluorescein in radical inguinal lymphadenectomy. J Urol 122:754, 1979

9. WARWICK R, WILLIAMS PL (eds): Gray's Anatomy, 35th ed. Philadelphia, W B Saunders, 1973

Peyronie's Disease and Penile Curvature

Patrick C. Devine

82

Peyronie's Disease

Peyronie's disease begins as an inflammation in the areolar tissue between the tunica albuginea of the corpus cavernosum and its enclosed erectile tissue. The inflammation then involves the elastic tissue of the tunica albuginea but does not involve the overlying Buck's fascia or the underlying erectile tissue. The plaques usually occur on the dorsum of the penis and may be multiple. Peyronie's plaques may resolve spontaneously but they may also calcify or even ossify. The nodules can be acutely painful and sexually incapacitating, but more often the patient or his sexual partner notices painless penile induration.[4,14,18,24]

Curvature of the penis is not in itself an indication for surgical correction. The patient often perceives the deformity as a threat to his manhood and needs a frank and clear discussion of the cause of his problem and reassurance that it is neither a malignant disease nor a result of his sexual habits. Further, he needs reassurance that a surgical procedure for correction can be performed if necessary in the future.[18] Baseline evaluation of sexual function should include nocturnal penile tumescence (NPT) studies and examination by a competent sex therapy team.[10,16]

We treat the patients in the acute phase with vitamin E, 200 I.U. t.i.d., and recheck them at 6-month intervals for 18 to 24 months. Fifty percent to eighty percent of these patients note resolution or improvement during this period.[23,25,26] Treatment in the acute phase with potassium p-aminobenzoate (Potaba) or injection of anti-inflammatory medicines may be helpful when pain prevents intercourse.[*,5,17,22,27] We feel that radiation therapy should be avoided because it can cause further fibrosis.[6,8] The patient who fails to respond to nonoperative therapy within 18 months and has persistent and sexually incapacitating chordee is a candidate for surgical correction of Peyronie's disease.

---

* Marberger H: Orgotein, a new drug for the treatment of Peyronie's disease. Personal communication

SURGICAL TREATMENT

Lowsley excised the plaque and closed Buck's fascia over a free fat graft. He notes that his operation is unsuitable for the plaques that extend laterally to any considerable degree.[11–13] Poutasse divides the longitudinal dorsal fibrous cord and at times extends his operation to include the lateral plaques without interposition of any new tissue in the defect. This method may be adequate for a narrow bowstring band, but removal of a large plaque leaves a sizable defect in the tunica albuginea, which must either regenerate or contract. Healing by contracture could cause another chordee.[19,20]

I prefer the technique developed by Charles Devine and Charles Horton. In this approach the fibrosed or ossified plaque is removed along with the tunica albuginea and the tissue is replaced with a free graft of dermis that is rich in elastic tissue.[3,9,25] We also obtain baseline NPT studies and psychosexual evaluation of the patient and his wife. Most patients appreciate this interview, and many request subsequent discussions.[10]

We approach the Peyronie's plaque through a dorsal curvilinear or Z-incision and dissect the skin and dartos to expose completely the dorsal and lateral aspects of Buck's fascia (Fig. 82-1). After identification of the plaque, we produce an artificial erection to demonstrate the extent of the disease and remove the tourniquet from the base of the penis for the remainder of the operation (Fig. 82-2).[7] We incise Buck's fascia longitudinally on one lateral aspect of the penis and divide and fulgurate the encircling veins (Fig. 82-3). We carefully develop the plane between Buck's fascia and the tunica albuginea of the corpus cavernosum with its enclosed plaque. We elevate the dorsal vessels and nerves with Buck's fascia to avoid injury to those important structures (Fig. 82-4). After outlining the plaque on the diseased tunica albuginea with a marking pen, we incise and remove it. We incise the rim of diseased tunica albuginea to form a stellate defect (Fig. 82-5).

We then measure the defect, harvest an elliptical patch of skin from the lower abdomen, and excise

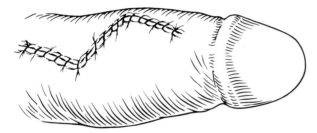

FIG. 82-1. Closure of dorsal Z incision

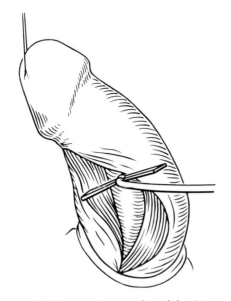

FIG. 82-2. Phallic erection produced by intracorporeal injection of sterile normal saline.

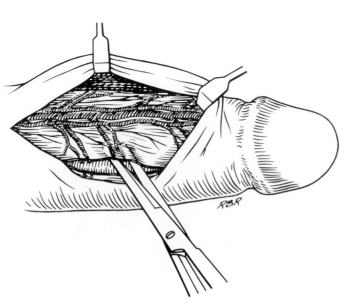

and discard epidermis and subcutaneous tissue. This leaves a piece of dermis of appropriate size to fill the defect. We close the donor site primarily and then attach the dermal graft over the defect in the tunica albuginea with interrupted sutures of 4-0 Dermalon at 2-cm intervals and continuous sutures of 4-0 Vicryl between the nonabsorbable sutures (Fig. 82-6). After the dermal graft has been secured, we confirm its adequacy with an artificial erection, reapproximate Buck's fascia laterally to support the graft, and close the wound. We use a moderate compression dressing for 2 hours followed by cold saline soaks. We drain the wound for 1 or 2 days with a "minivac" drain.†

We try to minimize erections with diazepam (Valium) during the first 2 postoperative weeks, and we discourage intercourse until 6 to 8 weeks after the operation. A dermal graft softens and becomes considerably more elastic by 12 to 18 weeks after operation.

The patient with Peyronie's disease who complains of impotence before operation needs a thorough evaluation of all possible causes. He should have NPT tracings to verify impotence, a glucose tolerance test, a review of all medications, and

---

† The "minivac" has been a valuable adjunct. We cut the Luer hub off a 16-gauge Butterfly needle and cut holes in the side of the tube so that blood and serum will drain, leaving the plastic tube long enough so that the needle end will reach the abdominal wall from the wound. The tip of this tube with the side holes is left in the wound. Plugging the other end of the needle into a sterilized Hemovac blood collection tube provides suction drainage.

FIG. 82-3. Elevation of Buck's fascia.

FIG. 82-4. Exposure of Peyronie's plaque by elevation and protection of dorsal nerves and vessels.

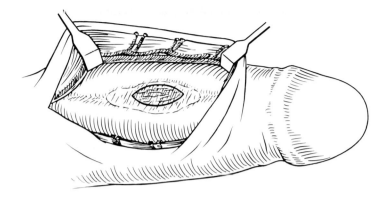

FIG. 82-5. Removal of Peyronie's plaque and stellate incisions in tunica albuginea.

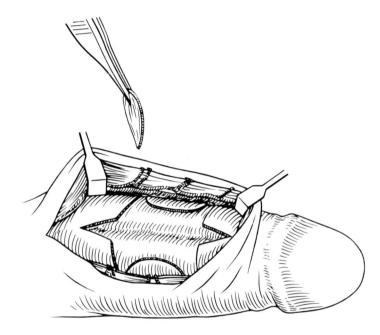

FIG. 82-6. We secure the graft in place with widely spaced sutures of 4-0 to 5-0 Prolene. We leave these long and, while applying traction, sew the interval edges with running sutures of 4-0 Vicryl.

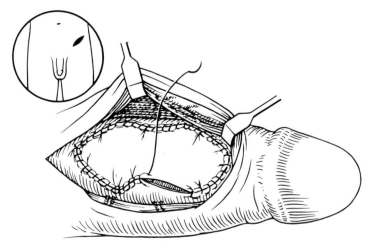

TABLE 82-1.   Causes of Abnormal Penile Curvature

Congenital
Ventral chordee
  Hypospadias
  Chordee without hypospadias
  Congenitally short urethra
Dorsal chordee
  Epispadias
  Exstrophy
Lateral chordee
  Torsion of penis
  Unilateral aplasia of the corpus cavernosum
  Unilateral hypoplasia of the corpus cavernosum
  Unilateral hyperplasia of the corpus cavernosum

Acquired
Trauma with scarring of:
  Skin
  Urethra
  Buck's fascia
  Tunica albuginea of the corpus cavernosum
Peyronie's disease

baseline endocrine tests. If these are normal, he should have noninvasive and, if necessary, invasive vascular studies. If these fail to show the cause of impotence, the patient may need psychological examination by a qualified sex therapist to determine the cause. We have not found the high percentage of impotence associated with Peyronie's disease that was reported by Raz and associates.[21,25] Patients with organic impotence and Peyronie's disease may require placement of an internal corporal prosthesis either at the time of surgical correction or as a second procedure at a later date. Because many of our initially impotent patients regain potency following correction of Peyronie's disease, we prefer to place the prosthesis at a second operation, if necessary.[25] Although 70% of our patients are potent and have a straight penis postoperatively, 30% are either impotent or have a degree of postoperative chordee. We make these facts clear to the patient and his wife before operation.[25]

Penile Curvature

Surgical correction of penile curvature should be reserved for those patients in whom congenital disease causes curvature when detumescent, or when congenital or acquired disease causes sufficient pain and curvature at tumescence to prevent intercourse.

Causes of abnormal penile curvature are listed in Table 82-1.

The ventral chordee associated with hypospadias is usually caused by fibrosis of the mesenchymal tissue that normally would have formed the corpus spongiosum and Buck's fascia if development had not been arrested (Fig. 82-7).[23]

The treatment of chordee must consist of the complete surgical removal of all constricting fibrosis, including that surrounding the urethral meatus, thereby allowing the corpora cavernosa to extend fully. The urethra must then be constructed and the penis recovered with pliable skin to prevent recurrence of chordee (see Chap. 76). The corpora cavernosa should be inflated with sterile normal saline before and after each of these operative procedures to ensure complete resolution of the chordee.[7]

Congenital chordee that occurs without hypospadias is one of four types.[1,2] **Type I** is caused by a band of dysgenetic mesenchymal tissue representing the undeveloped corpus spongiosum. The urethra consists of mucosa and is fused to the overlying penile skin. We make a longitudinal ventral, paramedian penile incision, carefully dissect the urethra from the corpora cavernosa, and make no attempt to separate the urethra from the skin. The flexible penile skin then allows the penis to straighten while the urethra remains intact.

Type II, which results from thickening and insufficiency of Buck's fascia, is approached through a circumcising coronal incision. We completely dissect the corpus spongiosum from the corpora cavernosa and remove the thickened Buck's fascia, including the fascia that lies in the groove between the corpus spongiosum and the corpora cavernosa. Removal of this inelastic tissue releases the corpora cavernosa and relieves the chordee. The corpus spongiosum with its enclosed urethra stretches easily to allow the increased ventral penile length.

Type III, caused by a thickened inelastic dartos fascia, is treated by removal of the offending tissue through a circumcising incision at the coronal sulcus.

Type IV is caused by scarring or congenital insufficiency of the tunica albuginea of the corpora cavernosa. We approach the area through a coronal circumcising incision or a ventral curved longitudinal incision. We incise the tunica albuginea on its short side at one or more sites, obtain dermis from the lower abdomen by excising an elliptical full-thickness segment of skin of appropriate size, and close the defect primarily. We remove the epithelium from the graft, discard it, and then

FIG. 82-7. Comparison of the normal and hypospadiac penis showing the dysgenetic tissue that causes chordee. (Converse JM (ed): Reconstructive Plastic Surgery, Vol 7, 2nd ed. Philadelphia, WB Saunders, 1977; *used with permission of WB Saunders)

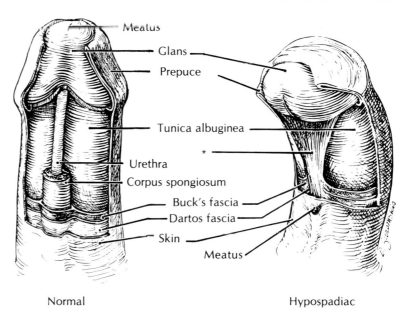

Normal   Hypospadiac

place the free dermal graft on the defects in the tunica albuginea of the corpora cavernosa. We use interrupted sutures of 5-0 Prolene at 2-cm intervals with continuous sutures of 5-0 Vicryl absorbable material in between. When lengthening of the short side of the tunica albuginea is not sufficient, plication of the tunica albuginea on the long side may be performed to obtain a straight but shorter penis.[15]

The congenitally short urethra is best treated by dissection of the urethra and corpus spongiosum from the corpora cavernosa, division of the urethra, and placement of a free full-thickness tube graft of preputial skin to lengthen the urethra sufficiently to allow straightening of the penis.

The dorsal chordee of epispadias and exstrophy may result from insufficient penile skin or urethra, from fibrosis of Buck's fascia or the dorsal aspect of the tunica albuginea of the corpora cavernosa, or from a combination of these factors. Release of this dorsal chordee consists of replacement of the insufficient tissue or removal of the fibrosis to allow free extension of the corpora cavernosa and urethra (see Chap. 65).

The treatment of lateral chordee should consist of complete exposure by a circumcising coronal incision with release of all fibrosis. This is followed by incision of the tunica albuginea and lengthening of the hypoplastic corpus cavernosum with a patch or patches of dermis; when this is insufficient to restore parity to the corpora, plication of the long side can be performed.

When there is congenital or traumatic absence of one corpus cavernosum, the best treatment is reassurance and patience until body growth is complete; if the patient has incapacitating chordee with erections or absence of erections, a single penile prosthesis can be installed.

Post-traumatic penile chordee can often be prevented by immediate surgical repair of the fracture of the penis. When post-traumatic fibrosis has occurred, surgical excision of the fibrotic tissue, with replacement of the urethra or tunica albuginea, allows straightening of the penis.

REFERENCES

1. DEVINE CJ, JR: Chordee without hypospadias. In Horton CE (ed): Plastic and Reconstructive Surgery of the Genital Area, p 383. Boston, Little, Brown and Co, 1973
2. DEVINE CJ, JR, HORTON CE: Chordee without hypospadias. J Urol 110:264, 1973
3. DEVINE CJ, JR, HORTON CE: Surgical treatment of Peyronie's disease with a dermal graft. J Urol 111:44, 1974
4. DEVINE CJ, JR, HORTON CE: Surgery of the male genitalia. In Devine CJ, Jr, Stecker JF, Jr (eds): Urology in Practice, p 943. Boston, Little, Brown & Co, 1978
5. FUREY CA JR: Peyronie's disease: Treatment by the local injection of meticortelone and hydrocortisone. J Urol 77:251, 1957
6. FURLOW WL, SWENSON HE, LEE RE: Peyronie's disease: A study of its natural history and treatment with orthovoltage radiotherapy. J Urol 114:69, 1975

7. GITTES RF, MCLAUGHLIN AP: Injection technique to induce penile erection. Urology 4:473, 1974

8. HELVIE WW, OCHSNER SF: Radiation therapy in Peyronie's disease. South Med J 65:1192, 1972

9. HORTON CE, DEVINE CJ, JR: Peyronie's disease. Plast Reconstr Surg 52:503, 1973

10. JONES WJ, JR, HORTON CE, DEVINE CJ, JR: Evaluation of surgical failures after operation for Peyronie's disease: Development of a prospective study. Presented at American Urologic Association, 1980

11. LOWSLEY OS: Surgical treatment of plastic induration of the penis (Peyronie's disease). NY State Med J 43:2273, 1943

12. LOWSLEY OS, BOYCE WH: Further experiences with an operation for the cure of Peyronie's disease. J Urol 63:888, 1950

13. LOWSLEY OS, GENTILE A: An operation for the cure of certain cases of plastic induration (Peyronie's disease) of the penis. J Urol 57:552, 1947

14. MCROBERTS JW: Peyronie's disease. Surg Gynecol Obstet 120:1291, 1969

15. NESBIT RM: Congenital curvature of the phallus: Report of three cases with description of corrective operation. J Urol 93:230, 1965

16. OSBORNE D: Psychologic evaluation of impotent men. Mayo Clinic Proc 51:363, 1976

17. PERSKY L, STEWART BH: The use of dimethyl sulfoxide in the treatment of genitourinary disorders. Ann NY Acad Sci 141:551, 1967

18. PEYRONIE F DE LA: Sur quelques obstacles qui s'opposent á l'éjaculation naturelle de la semence. Paris, Mem de l'Acad Roy de Chir, p 425, 1743

19. POUTASSE EF: Peyronie's disease. Trans Am Assoc Genitourin Surg 63:97, 1971

20. POUTASSE EF: Peyronie's disease. J Urol 107:419, 1972

21. RAZ S, DEKERNION JB, KAUFMAN JJ: Surgical treatment of Peyronie's disease: A new approach. J Urol 117:598, 1977

22. ROTHFELD SH, MURRAY W: The treatment of Peyronie's disease by iontophoresis of C_{21} esterified glucocorticoids. J Urol 97:874, 1967

23. SCARDINO PL, SCOTT WW: The use of tocopherols in the treatment of Peyronie's disease. Ann NY Acad Sci 52:390, 1949

24. SMITH BH: Peyronie's disease. Am J Clin Pathol 45:670, 1966

25. WILD RM, DEVINE CJ, JR, HORTON CE: Dermal graft repair of Peyronie's disease: Survey of 50 patients. J Urol 121:47, 1979

26. WILLIAMS JL, THOMAS GG: The natural history of Peyronie's disease. J Urol 103:75, 1970

27. ZARAFONETIS CJ, HORRAX TM: Treatment of Peyronie's disease with potassium para-amino-benzoate (potaba). J Urol 81:770, 1959

Surgery for Male Impotence

83

William L. Furlow

Male impotence is best defined as the inability to achieve or sustain an erection suitable for vaginal penetration and sexual intercourse. In the context of operative treatment currently available, this definition is better applied to the term *erectile dysfunction*.

A review of the urologic literature reveals the physician's long search for a reliable method of surgical treatment that would reestablish an acceptable penile erection by which the patient could achieve vaginal penetration and sexual intercourse.[6,8]

CLASSIFICATION OF ERECTILE DYSFUNCTION (IMPOTENCE)

In considering the appropriate treatment for the male with erectile dysfunction, it is essential that we differentiate between those forms of impotence that are psychogenic, and therefore potentially reversible by conservative means, and those that can be classified as organic, which are irreversible by conservative means. The clinical differentiation between organic and psychogenic impotence evolves in an orderly fashion by means of a complete patient history including a sexual history, physical examination, psychologic evaluation, laboratory investigation, and nocturnal penile tumescence monitoring. When applicable, the use of other phallodynamic studies such as the Doppler penile blood pressure determination, pulse volume recordings, and sacral reflex latency testing may be of value. For the interested reader, the literature has numerous articles detailing these studies and their interpretation in the differentiation of organic and psychogenic impotence.[1,3,5,10,12]

PENILE PROSTHESES IN THE SURGICAL TREATMENT OF MALE IMPOTENCE

Penile prostheses currently available for implantation can be divided into two major categories: rigid and semirigid prostheses and the Inflatable Penile Prosthesis.

The rigid and semirigid prostheses are either single, centrally placed devices or paired, semirigid, flexible or malleable rods; each is composed of medical-grade silicone elastomer. These devices have in common that, when implanted, they provide the patient with a permanent degree of penile rigidity suitable for vaginal penetration and sexual intercourse. The individual characteristics of each device are well described in the urologic literature.[2,4,7,9,11,13,15]

The hydraulically operated Inflatable Penile Prosthesis, by virtue of its mechanical function, is the only currently available device in the second major category of prosthetics.[14] This device is different from the semirigid prostheses because it permits a controllable erection, accomplished by voluntary inflation of the penile cylinders to the erect state and voluntary deflation of the cylinders to achieve the flaccid state. As with the semirigid and rigid prostheses, the inflatable penile device in the erect state provides an erection suitable for vaginal penetration and sexual intercourse.

Surgical Implantation of Penile Prostheses

PREOPERATIVE PREPARATION

The preoperative preparation of patients undergoing prosthetic implantation has been fairly well standardized for both semirigid prostheses and the inflatable penile prosthesis. Broad-spectrum antibacterial prophylaxis is begun the day before surgery. The night before surgery, the patient is instructed to take a povidone-iodine shower with special attention to the abdomen, genitalia, and perineum. A surgical shave is carried out in the surgical holding area or in the operating room on the day of surgery. Skin preparation of the patient consists of the standard 15-minute scrub. Similarly, the surgeon and all assistants carry out a 15-minute surgical hand scrub. Surgical hoods, although not mandatory, are considered advisable to minimize the shedding of hair. As a final precaution and in an effort to reduce unnecessary traffic within the operating room, signs may be posted at all entrances into the operating room, requesting the

reduction of unnecessary traffic in and out of the surgical theatre.

CHOICE OF SURGICAL APPROACH

The surgical approach may depend on the design of the prosthetic device to be implanted. The single, centrally placed rod prosthesis is best implanted through a dorsal penile shaft incision. Paired rigid and semirigid prostheses can be implanted through a pubic incision by means of the infrapubic approach, a dorsal penile shaft incision, or a perineal incision. The Inflatable Penile Prosthesis can be implanted through a pubic incision or a scrotal approach.

Surgical Procedures for the Various Devices

PAIRED SEMIRIGID ROD PROSTHESES

Perineal Approach

Paired semirigid rod prostheses of the Small–Carrion,* Finney,† or Jonas‡ design are easily implanted by the perineal approach (Fig. 83-1 and 83-2). The patient is placed in the lithotomy position. An inverted-U or a midline perineal skin incision is made. The bulbous urethra is identified and retracted laterally to either side, and the crus of each corpus cavernosum is exposed. A short 2-cm to 3-cm vertical incision is then made in the tunica albuginea of each crus, approximately 1 cm proximal to the bifurcation of the crura; the cavernosal tissue is thus entered. Traction sutures of 2-0 silk are used to separate the edges of the tunica while a tunnel is developed within the corpus cavernosum. Dilation and tunneling are gently carried out to the distal end of each corpus cavernosum with graded cervical dilators from 7 mm to 12 mm in diameter. Cavernosal dilations should extend distally to beneath the glans penis. Similarly, proximal dilation is carried out to the insertion of the crus. The degree of dilation can be determined by the diameter of the prosthesis selected for implantation. When semirigid and rigid prostheses are implanted, overdilation is unnecessary and, indeed, it may injure or perforate the tunica. Difficulty in achieving dilation may result

FIG. 83-1. Paired semirigid rod prostheses: **(A)** Small–Carrion, **(B)** Finney flexi-rod, and **(C)** Jonas silver-wire. (**A** from Fürlow WL: Diagnosis and treatment of male erectile failure. Diabetes Care 2:18, 1979. By permission of the American Diabetes Association)

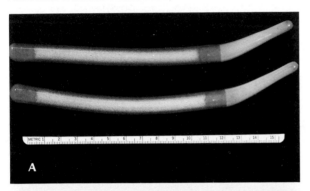

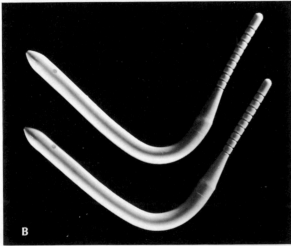

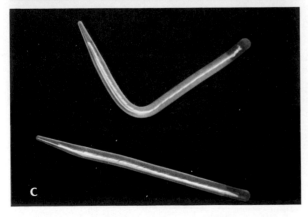

---

* Manufactured by Heyer–Schulte Corp, Goleta, California 93017
† Manufactured by Medical Engineering Corp, Racine, Wisconsin 53404
‡ Manufactured by Dacomed, Inc, Minneapolis, Minnesota 55346

FIG. 83-2. Inverted-U perineal incision, vertical crural incision, and implantation of paired semirigid rod prostheses.

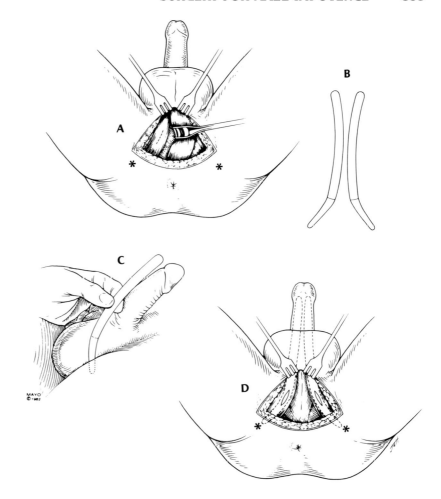

because of previous infection, partial fibrosis secondary to Peyronie's disease, vascular insufficiency, trauma, or priapism. Alternative methods of corporal tunneling include the initial use of the long Metzenbaum scissors followed by insertion of the graduated dilators or the prosthesis itself. In addition, several of the manufacturers of paired semirigid prostheses provide prosthetic sizers that are suitable for corporal tunneling and dilation.

After appropriate cavernosal dilation and before introduction of the prosthesis, each corpus is thoroughly irrigated with an antibacterial solution of polymyxin B and neomycin. The length of the prosthesis to be implanted is then determined in accordance with methods recommended by each manufacturer. Reusable measuring devices are provided for the Jonas and the Small–Carrion prostheses. These prostheses, as well as the Finney prosthesis, can be trimmed for precise sizing and fitting.

The size of the Finney prosthesis is best determined by measuring the distance from the pubic bone to a point near the middle of the glans penis (approximately 1 cm distal to the corona) and then selecting a size 2 cm shorter than this measurement. The resulting shaft length allows 2 cm of short hinge to extend beyond the pubis and gives the desired hinge effect characteristic of this specific design. When the Finney prosthesis is inserted by the perineal approach, a proper fit is determined by the fact that when the proximal tail is inserted into the crus, it does not buckle but holds the distal end of the prosthesis firmly beneath the glans. Accurate sizing is essential, because implantation of a prosthesis of sufficient size prevents proximal migration of the device and the subsequent flexing of the glans over the prosthesis.

With sizing and trimming completed, the distal end of the prosthesis is inserted into the corpus cavernosum and advanced to the distal limits of the corpus beneath the glans. The proximal end of the prosthesis is then flexed and inserted into the proper end of the crus. Once the device has been positioned accurately in each corpus, the

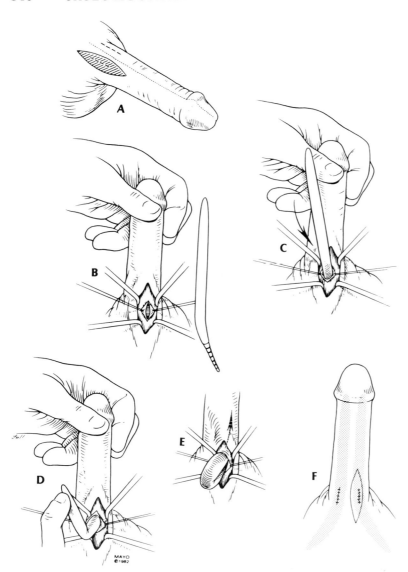

FIG. 83-3. Penile shaft approach for implantation of paired semirigid or flexible prostheses.

incision in the tunica albuginea is closed by means of a running absorbable suture of 4-0 Vicryl. After closure of the tunica, the distal ends of the prosthesis are again palpated through the soft tissues of the glans penis to ensure symmetry and proper positioning beneath the glans. The wound is then thoroughly irrigated with the antibiotic solution, and the subcutaneous tissues and skin are closed in layers. The perineal skin incision is closed with a continuous subcuticular 4-0 Vicryl suture.

Pubic Approach

Paired semirigid prostheses may also be implanted through a transverse or vertical pubic incision, as described below for implantation of the Inflatable Penile Prosthesis. The transverse incision is made slightly above the inferior border of the symphysis

pubis in order to expose the base of the penis and the dorsal surface of the corpora cavernosa. If a vertical incision is used for the paired prostheses, the inferior aspects of the incision should start at the base of the penis and need only be extended cephalad to the midportion of the symphysis or slightly higher.

Exposure of the base of the penis brings into view the corpora cavernosa and overlying Buck's fascia. Buck's fascia and the underlying loose areolar tissue are opened through parallel incisions to either side of the midline in order to avoid the midline neurovascular structures. Retraction of Buck's fascia and the neurovascular structures exposes the thick, glistening covering of the cavernosal tissue, the tunica albuginea. Parallel traction sutures of 2-0 Prolene placed full thickness

FIG. 83-4. Subcoronal approach for implantation of the Jonas silver-wire prosthesis.

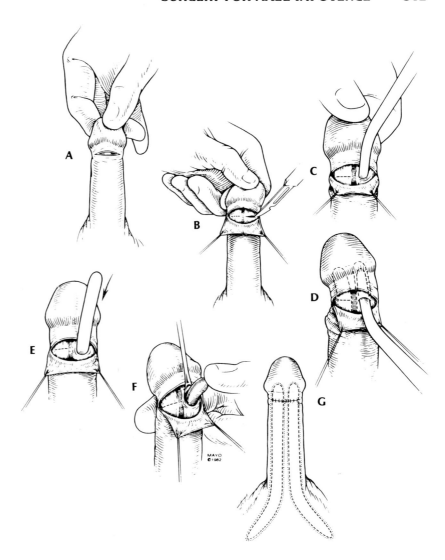

through the tunica albuginea aid in stabilizing the corpus cavernosum while the tunica is being incised.

The corpus cavernosum is opened by a 2-cm vertical incision through the tunica albuginea. Separate transverse incisions through the tunica of each corpus cavernosum may also be used; however, care must be taken to avoid transecting the neurovascular structures, which are not always precisely in the midline. With the cavernosal tissue exposed, proximal and distal cavernosal tunneling and dilation can be carried out in the same manner as previously described for perineal implantation. Determination of the size of the prosthesis, although similar in method to that described above, may require that the surgeon take into account the length of the incision made in the tunica. An incision of more than 2 cm in length may result in slightly shorter total measurements unless a por-

tion of the incisional length is taken into account in the overall measurements. Final trimming to the exact fitting length should be done gradually and may necessitate multiple reinsertions of the proximal end of the prosthesis to ensure a satisfactory fit. Closure of the tunica albuginea should be carried out with an absorbable suture such as 4-0 Vicryl.

Penile Shaft Approach

The penile shaft technique may be utilized for the implantation of any of the paired semirigid prostheses (Small–Carrion, Finney, and Jonas), although it is most suitable for the more flexible Finney prosthesis and the Jonas design. In this approach (Fig. 83-3), a single skin incision is made vertically to one side of the midline on the dorsum of the penis and is carried down to the tunica albuginea; care is taken to avoid the dorsal neu-

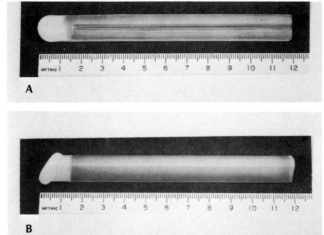

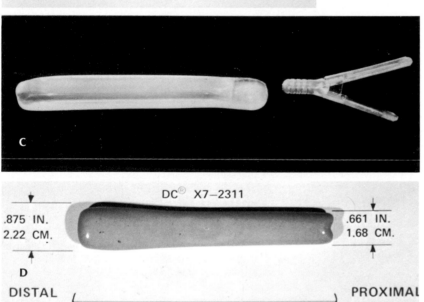

FIG. 83-5. Single centrally placed rod prosthesis: **(A)** Pearman, **(B)** Lash, **(C)** Loeffler, and **(D)** Gerow. (**B** and **C** from Furlow WL: Diagnosis and treatment of male erectile failure. Diabetes Care 2:18, 1979. By permission of the American Diabetes Association)

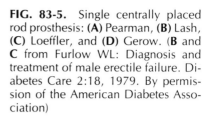

rovascular structures. The tunica albuginea of each corpus is incised vertically for a distance of 3 cm to expose the cavernosal tissue, and a tunnel is created distally to beneath the glans and proximally into each crus, as described previously in the section on perineal implantation. After appropriate sizing and trimming of the prosthesis, the proximal end of the prosthesis is placed into the crus and then flexed so that the distal end is positioned beneath the glans.

Subcoronal Technique

Although the Jonas silver-wire prosthesis can be implanted through any of the incisions previously described, the malleable design of the prosthesis permits it to be implanted through a modification

of the penile shaft approach, the subcoronal approach (Fig. 83-4). In the subcoronal approach, a radial skin incision is made approximately 1 cm proximal to the corona of the glans penis on the dorsum of the penile shaft; the tunica albuginea of both corpora cavernosa are exposed (see Fig. 83-7A). The tunica of each corpus is then incised transversely for a distance of 1 cm in order to enter the cavernosal tissue. Cavernosal dilation may be carried out by means of the prosthesis sizer that is available with this device from the manufacturer, by sharp scissor dissection, or by the use of graduated cervical dilators. The dilator, which is also a sizer, permits accurate selection of device length. Use of this incision requires that the proximal end of the prosthesis be inserted initially down to its

FIG. 83-6. Penile shaft approach for Implantation of single, centrally placed rigid and semirigid prostheses.

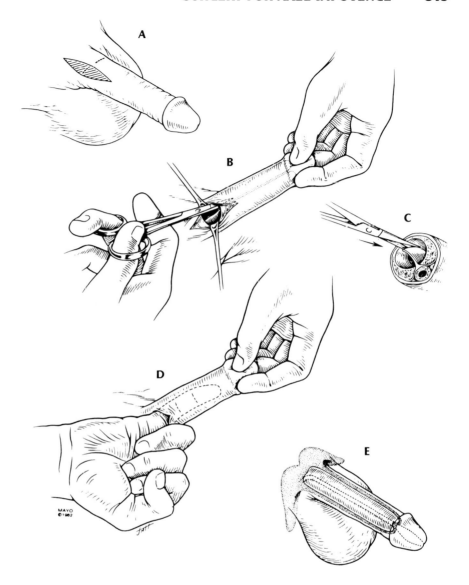

most proximal limit within the crus. The distal end is then flexed and positioned within the corpus cavernosum beneath the glans penis. The tunica is closed with a running absorbable suture. The overlying subcutaneous tissue and skin are closed in layers with absorbable suture.

SINGLE, CENTRALLY PLACED, RIGID PROSTHESES

The single, centrally placed, rigid prostheses have limited usefulness in the surgical management of impotence since the introduction of the paired, semirigid prostheses and the Inflatable Penile Prosthesis (Fig. 83-5). Several are limited in their availability; however, in the context of this chapter, it

is appropriate that the surgical technique for their implantation be described (Fig. 83-6).

These devices are designed to be positioned beneath the tunica albuginea on the dorsum of the penile shaft. A dorsal, vertical skin incision can be utilized to expose the underlying Buck's fascia and the tunica albuginea. Because these devices require central implantation beneath the tunica, it is necessary to make a transverse incision through the tunica albuginea of each corpus cavernosum and across the septal partition. The septal attachment is then freed from the dorsal tunica distally to the corona of the glans penis and proximally to the base of the penis; either blunt or sharp scissors may be used for the dissection. The distance from the base of the penis to the distal limit of the corpora is then measured, and a prosthesis of appropriate size is selected and trimmed to the final measured length. After insertion of these single prostheses beneath the tunica, the sheath is closed transversely by means of fine absorbable sutures; this is followed by layered closure of Buck's fascia and the penile skin.

This basic surgical approach is suitable for any of the single, centrally placed rigid rods, including the Pearman, Lash–Maser, Loeffler, and Gerow designs.

INFLATABLE PENILE PROSTHESIS

The Inflatable Penile Prosthesis§ (Fig. 83-7) can be implanted by the pubic approach or the scrotal approach.

Pubic Approach

The pubic approach requires either a 3-inch transverse skin incision over the midpoint of the symphysis pubis or a short vertical midline suprapubic incision extended inferiorly over the symphysis to its midpoint. The incision is carried through the subcutaneous tissue to the anterior rectus fascia. The rectus sheath is incised the length of the

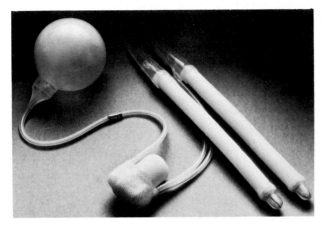

FIG. 83-7. Inflatable Penile Prosthesis consists of paired inflatable cylinders, an inflate–deflate pump, and a spherical reservoir.

§ Manufactured by American Medical Systems, Inc, Minneapolis, Minnesota 55343

FIG. 83-8. Implantation of the inflatable penile prosthesis: pubic incision and reservoir placement.

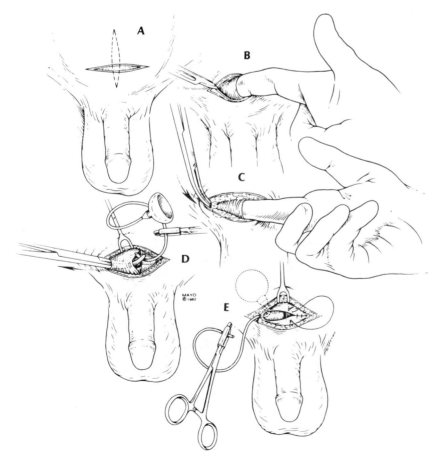

incision, and the midline between the rectus muscles is developed to expose the underlying prevesical space (Fig. 83-8*A*). Then, with the index finger, a small space is developed beneath the belly of the rectus muscle for placement of the spherical reservoir (Fig. 83-8*B*). Reservoir placement is accomplished first by locating the right pubic tubercle on the side corresponding to the side in which the inflate–deflate pump is to be positioned within the hemiscrotum. The external inguinal ring is identified. Subcutaneously a long, curved forceps is placed against the floor of the external inguinal ring in the region of Hesselbach's triangle, and the thin transversalis fascia is perforated with the blunt end of the forceps. The clamp is then passed into the paravesical space; the index finger of the opposite hand is used to guide the clamp through Hesselbach's triangle and medially beneath the belly of the rectus muscle into the exposed midline (Fig. 83-8*C*). The tubing from the reservoir is grasped in the jaws of the forceps and the forceps is withdrawn; the end of the tubing is thus brought out through the floor of Hesselbach's triangle into

the region of the external inguinal ring while the deflated reservoir is drawn into the right paravesical space (Fig. 83-8*D*). The collar of the reservoir is positioned snugly against the floor of Hesselbach's triangle. In this position the reservoir is filled with 65 ml of sterile 11.7% Iothalamate meglumine (Cysto-Conray II) solution. The reservoir tubing is clamped with a silicone-shod mosquito clamp and laid aside for later tailoring and connection to the appropriate tubing from the inflate–deflate pump. The anterior rectus sheath is then closed with a running suture of 1-0 Prolene (Fig. 83-8*E*).

The inferior border of the skin incision is retracted to expose the base of the penis and the corpora cavernosa (Fig. 83-9*A*). A 2-cm vertical incision is made through the tunica albuginea of each corpus cavernosum. This incision should be made in proximity to the inferior border of the symphysis and slightly lateral to the midline to avoid the neurovascular midline structures. Parallel traction sutures of 2-0 Prolene through the full thickness of the tunica albuginea are used to

FIG. 83-9. Implantation of Inflatable Penile Prosthesis: cavernosal body exposure, entry, and dilation.

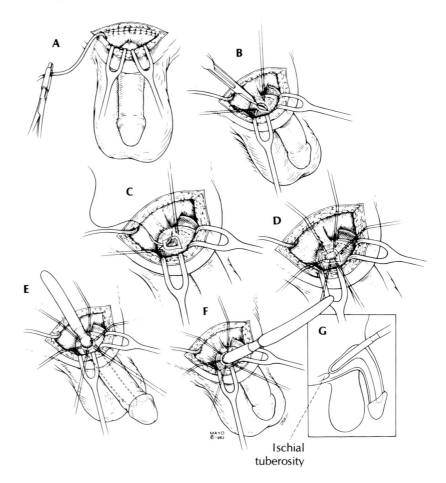

Ischial tuberosity

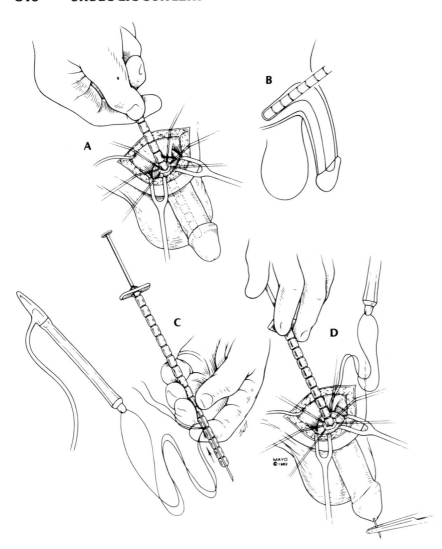

FIG. 83-10. Implantation of Inflatable Penile Prosthesis: measurement of distal and proximal cavernosal length and use of the Furlow cylinder insertion device.

stabilize the corpus for accurate positioning of these incisions (Fig. 83-9*B*). With the corpus cavernosum opened, a series of 2-0 Prolene sutures are placed through the full thickness of the tunica on each side to hold the incision open and to facilitate preparation of the corpus cavernosum for insertion of the inflatable cylinders (Fig. 83-9*C* and *D*). Proximal and distal dilation of the corpus cavernosum is carried out by initial gentle scissors dissection followed by gentle passage of graduated cervical dilators of 8 mm to 11 mm in diameter (Fig. 83-9*E* to *G*).

The corpus cavernosum is measured by means of the Furlow cylinder insertion tool (Fig. 83-10). It is important that this measurement be made before the length of the incision in the tunica is extended. The distal measurement is determined from the distal end of the tunica incision to the

distal end of the corpus cavernosum, whereas the proximal length is measured from the proximal end of the tunica incision to the proximal end of the crus (Fig. 83-10*A* and *B*). These values are then added together to obtain the total cylinder length needed for implantation.

Cylinder Size and the Use of Rear Tip Extenders. The proximal measurement of the corpus cavernosum must be done carefully so that proper use can be made of rear tip extenders. Rear tip extenders are needed in nearly all cases of penile implantation with the inflatable penile prosthesis to ensure proper direct exiting of the cylinder input tube from beneath the tunica albuginea. This prevents contact between the input tube and the inflatable portion of the cylinder. Direct contact of the two silicone surfaces can result in input-tube wear, a cylinder leak, and subsequent total loss of

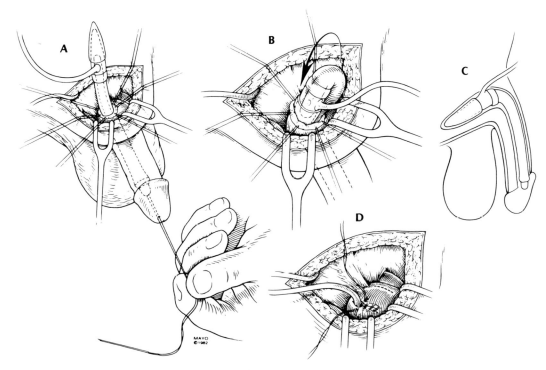

FIG. 83-11. Implantation of the Inflatable Penile Prosthesis: distal and proximal positioning of the inflatable cylinder.

fluid. Rear tip extenders of the proper length, added to the proximal end of the inflatable cylinder, prevent this from occurring by extending the distance from the proximal end of the cylinder to the input tube, corresponding to the measured length of the proximal portion of the corpus cavernosum. In other words, the size of the inflatable cylinder plus the length of the rear tip extender should equal the desired length of the device to be implanted within the corpus cavernosum. For example, if the overall length of the corpus cavernosum is 18 cm as determined by the insertion tool, and a 3-cm rear tip extender is required for direct exit of the input tube, a 15-cm inflatable cylinder should be used with a 3-cm rear tip extender to give an overall length of 18 cm.

The cylinder is implanted with the proper-sized rear tip extender attached by means of the Furlow cylinder insertion tool (Fig. 83-10C and D). The distal end of the cylinder is positioned at the distal end of the corpus and held with moderate traction on the suture attached to the cylinder (Fig. 83-11A). The proximal end with its rear trip extender is then passed into the proximal end of the crus (Fig. 83-11B and C). The tunica albuginea is closed by means of the previously placed interrupted 2-0 Prolene sutures (Fig. 83-11D). Implan-

tation of the opposite corpus cavernosum is carried out in a similar fashion.

The inflate–deflate pump is positioned subcutaneously in the hemiscrotum, usually on the same side as the implanted reservoir (Fig. 83-12). A subcutaneous pouch is developed in the hemiscrotum with the use of blunt finger dissection or a large (18-mm) cervical dilator (Fig. 83-12A). The tunnel leading to this pouch is best developed lateral to the spermatic cord and the testis. The pump is inserted with the deflate button located laterally and slightly anteriorly for easy patient access (Fig. 83-12B). The pump is held in place by Babcock clamps applied to the pump tubing, and individual tubing components are joined together with stainless steel connectors (Fig. 83-12C). All tubing is routed subcutaneously. The cylinder tubes from the cylinder are tailored to the desired length and joined to the cylinder tubes from the pump by means of right-angle connectors.

The reservoir tubing from the reservoir is tailored to the proper length and connected to the reservoir tubing from the pump by a straight stainless steel connector. Each tube is secured to its segment of the connector by means of a double tie of 3-0 Prolene (Fig. 83-12D); this completes the implantation. Before closure of the wound the

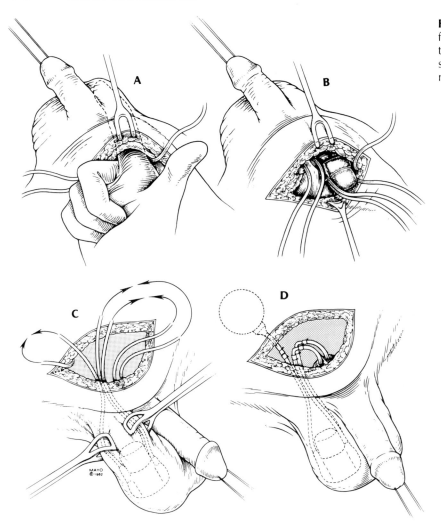

FIG. 83-12. Implantation of the In-flatable Penile Prosthesis: placement of the inflate–deflate pump in right hemiscrotum and completion of tubing connections.

prosthesis is tested for symmetric inflation of the cylinders, parallel position of the cylinder tips beneath the glans, and satisfactory deflation. The cylinder traction sutures are then removed by cutting one limb of the double suture close to the glans and withdrawing the suture. The wound is closed, usually in two layers over the tubing, and then the skin is closed with a running subcuticular suture of 4-0 Vicryl. A 12Fr Foley catheter is passed through the urethra into the bladder and left indwelling overnight. The cylinders are left deflated and the shaft of the penis is wrapped firmly in conforming gauze, which is removed on the day after surgery.

Scrotal Approach

The patient is positioned in a modified lithotomy position similar to that used for the perineal approach. The corpora are approached ventrally through a vertical midline incision 2 cm to 2.5 cm in length at the penoscrotal angle (Fig. 83-13A). The incision is made through the subcutaneous tissue and dartos fascia laterally to the urethra and down to the belly of the corpus cavernosum. The tunica is incised vertically for a distance of 2 cm to expose the cavernosal tissue of the corpus (Fig. 83-13B). Tunneling and dilation of the corpus are achieved in the same manner as previously described for the pubic approach.

Proximal and distal measurements are determined by means of the Furlow insertion tool. The appropriate length of the rear tip extenders to be added to the proximal end of the cylinder is then calculated. The sum of the rear tip extender and the inflatable cylinder should equal the overall measured length of the corpus cavernosum.

The inflatable cylinder is then inserted into the distal end of the corpus cavernosum with the

FIG. 83-13.   Implantation of Inflatable Penile Prosthesis: Scrotal approach and cylinder implantation.

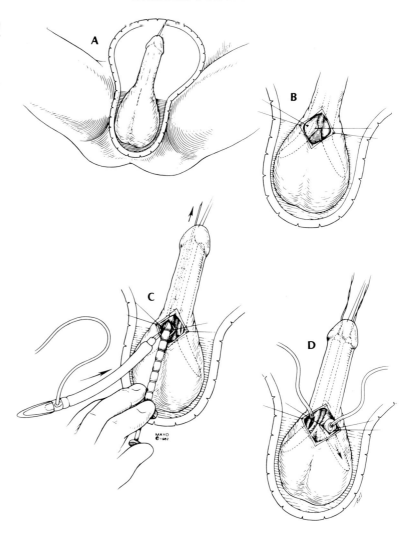

Furlow insertion tool (Fig. 83-13C). The rear tip extender is added to the proximal end of the cylinder, and this end is inserted proximally into the crus (Fig. 83-13D). When the scrotal approach is used, the edges of the tunica should be closed with an absorbable suture such as 2-0 Vicryl to avoid palpation of the suture knots on the ventral surface of the penis.

The reservoir can be implanted in one of two ways. A separate pubic incision can be used to enter the prevesical space, as described under the section on the pubic approach; or the reservoir can be inserted into the prevesical space through the scrotal incision. If the latter method is chosen, the pubic tubercle on one side or the other is palpated through the scrotal incision and the external inguinal ring is identified. The thin wall of the transversalis fascia is punctured with the blunt point of a long curved clamp or curved scissors to

gain entry into the prevesical space (Fig. 83-14A). By blunt dissection, the defect in the transversalis fascia is enlarged to admit the surgeon's index finger. With the index finger a pouch is gently developed in the prevesical space to accommodate the spherical reservoir. For reservoir positioning, a special reservoir insertion tool can be used (Fig. 83-14B). The reservoir is filled with 65 ml of 11.7% lothalamate meglumin (Cysto-Conray II) solution or sterile saline, and the collar of the reservoir is gently pulled out against the floor of Hesselbach's triangle. If the defect is too large and causes the collar to protrude into the inguinal region subcutaneously, it should be partially closed.

The pump mechanism is positioned in the ipsilateral hemiscrotum with the deflating button

---

‖ Manufactured by the Lone Star Instruments Company, Houston, Texas 77001

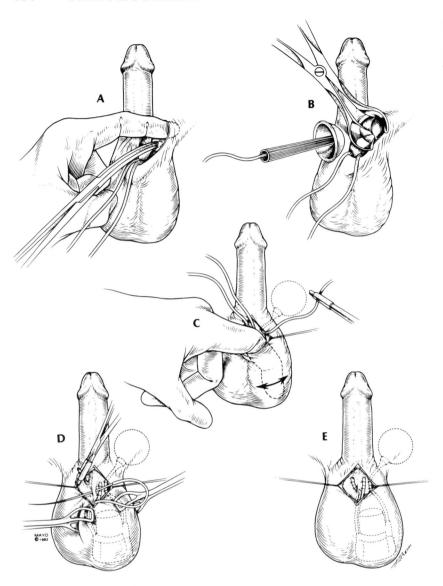

facing laterally (Fig. 83-14C). The cylinder tubing is shortened to allow for direct connection of the cylinder tubing from the pump by means of the straight stainless steel connectors. The reservoir tubing from the reservoir and the reservoir tubing from the pump are also shortened and connected with a straight stainless steel connector. The midline scrotal septum is perforated in order for the tubing connection from the cylinder on the side opposite the pump to pass across the midline (Fig. 83-14D and E). The subcutaneous tissue is closed in layers with 3-0 chromic suture, the skin with nonabsorbable 4-0 catgut, and the penoscrotal skin with a running subcuticular stitch of 4-0 Vicryl.

Postoperative Care

SEMIRIGID PROSTHESES

Although the period of wound healing varies, depending on the incision used for implantation, it is preferable to instruct the patient to avoid active sexual intercourse for at least 2 to 3 weeks after surgery. Patients are continued on antibiotic prophylaxis for 1 week after operation.

Early postoperative discomfort is usually confined to the area of the incision and generally subsides in a matter of days. Patients are usually advised to avoid tight, constrictive underclothes during the first 2 to 3 weeks postoperatively.

INFLATABLE PENILE PROSTHESES

The patient is kept in the Trendelenburg position for the first 24 hours. The scrotum is packed with ice. The urethral catheter is removed on the day after surgery.

The patient is maintained on broad-spectrum antibacterial prophylaxis for 7 to 10 days. The prosthesis is left in the deflated position (penis flaccid), and no attempt is made to begin pump instructions until at least the fifth to the seventh day postoperatively or until scrotal discomfort is minimal. Each day the pump is pulled down gently into the most dependent position of the scrotum in order to maintain a satisfactory pump position for later operation of the device by the patient. Tight underclothing, including jockey shorts and athletic supports, is to be avoided for the first few weeks after surgery. Once the patient is able to inflate and deflate the device, he is instructed to carry this out as a daily routine—leaving the device inflated for 10 to 15 minutes and then deflating it to the flaccid state. This procedure is best continued for a minimum of 4 to 6 weeks. Sexual intercourse should be deferred for at least 4 to 6 weeks after surgery.

REFERENCES

1. ABELSON D: Diagnostic value of the penile pulse and blood pressure: A Doppler study of impotence in diabetics. J Urol 113:636, 1975
2. APFELBERG DB, MASER RR, LASH H: Surgical management of impotence: Progress report. Am J Surg 132:336, 1976
3. BOHLEN JG: Sleep erection monitoring in the evaluation of male erectile failure. Urol Clin North Am 8:119, Feb 1981
4. FINNEY RP: New hinged silicone penile implant. J Urol 118:585, 1977
5. FURLOW WL: Diagnosis and treatment of male erectile failure. Diabetes Care 2:18, 1979
6. GEE WF: A history of surgical treatment of impotence. Urology 5:401, 1975
7. GEROW F: Dow Corning New Product Information Bulletin No. 51-453, May 1978
8. GERSTENBERGER DL, OSBORNE D, FURLOW WL: Inflatable penile prosthesis: Follow-up study of patient-partner satisfaction. Urology 14:583, 1979
9. KRANE RJ, FREEDBERG PS, SIROKY MB: Jonas silicone-silver penile prosthesis: Initial experience in America. J Urol 126:475, 1981
10. KRANE RJ, SIROKY MB: Neurophysiology of erection. Urol Clin North Am 8:91, Feb 1981
11. LOEFFLER RA, IVERSON RE: Surgical treatment of impotence in the male: An 18-year experience with 250 penile implants. Plast Reconstr Surg 58:292, 1976
12. OSBORNE D: Psychologic evaluation of impotent men. Mayo Clin Proc 51:363, 1976
13. PEARMAN RO: Insertion of a Silastic penile prosthesis for the treatment of organic sexual impotence. J Urol 107:802, 1972
14. SCOTT FB, BRADLEY WE, TIMM GW: Management of erectile impotence: Use of implantable inflatable prosthesis. Urology 2:80, 1973
15. SMALL MP: Small–Carrion penile prosthesis: A report on 160 cases and review of the literature. J Urol 119:365, 1978

Suprapubic Prostatectomy

84

Vincent J. O'Conor, Jr.

Suprapubic prostatectomy refers to the enucleation of adenomatous hyperplastic tissue from the prostate, performed through the cavity of the bladder after extraperitoneal incision of the anterior bladder wall. It may also be termed *transvesical prostatectomy* to distinguish it from the *transcapsular* or retropubic prostatectomy. These procedures are not true prostatectomies. They are more correctly considered adenomectomies because the true prostate (capsule) is left intact when they are properly performed.

Suprapubic prostatectomy is the procedure of choice in approximately 10% of patients with significant bladder neck obstruction. The operation described results in morbidity and mortality comparable to transurethral resection and provides a long-lasting, functionally satisfactory result.

History

Suprapubic cystostomy for the removal of bladder calculi was successfully performed in 1561 by Pierre Franco in France, who, despite his success, emphasized that he would not advise others to perform this procedure.[10] Franco's advice was accepted for the next 300 years. In 1868, Sir Henry Thompson, in his book *Diseases of the Prostate,* stated that cystotomy should only be considered a last-ditch measure to control intractable prostatic bleeding. The operation was considered so hazardous that Thompson favored "permitting nature to do her own work without any undue haste on our part to be officious in offering her assistance."[11]

In spite of this, in 1827, Amussat did remove a part of the prostate, a tumor the size of a hazel nut protruding from the bladder neck in a patient with a large bladder calculus; the patient survived. However, it was 58 years before an attempt was made to remove the obstructing prostatic tissue completely. This was performed by vonDittel in 1885, on a physician with bladder neck obstruction; unfortunately, the patient died on the sixth postoperative day. Probably the first planned and successful suprapubic prostatectomy was performed by William T. Belfield of Chicago in 1886.[1] Like Amussat and vonDittel, Belfield reported only one case, but he continued to perform suprapubic prostatectomy and, a few years later, reported on 80 cases.

In May 1894, Eugene Fuller of New York performed the first complete removal of a prostatic adenoma suprapubically; in 1895, he reported six successive and successful cases of prostatectomy. In 1900 Ramon Guiteras (Fuller's associate and founder of the American Urologic Association) described this technique in Paris and discussed the technique with Peter Freyer of London. Surprisingly, a year later, Freyer reported his experience with four patients and claimed originality for the procedure, failing to give credit to either Fuller or Guiteras. The subsequent controversy and debate led to a classic article, published by Fuller in 1905, which outlined the events as they occurred.[2] This important article is included in the volume *Classical Articles in Urology.*[5] Nonetheless, Peter Freyer should be given credit for popularizing the operation and subsequently publishing his results in 1600 cases with a relatively low mortality rate.

Subsequent developments to refine suprapubic prostatectomies have been directed toward achievement of hemostasis. In the early part of this century, suprapubic prostatectomy became the most widely used procedure and also the most lethal, with mortality rates of 25% to 30%. The operation was usually done blindly through a high bladder incision, and bleeding was controlled either by packing or by placement of large tubes for drainage. A classic statement by Edward L. Keyes summed it up, "No operation on the urinary tract is, in my opinion, *less* technically elegant than a thoroughly performed suprapubic prostatectomy . . . No matter how vigorous the operator or how brilliant his execution, a large amount of vital fluid (blood) must of necessity be lost during the operative maneuver alone."[6] Compressive balloon bags, such as those described by Pilcher and Hagner, were often used to control bleeding; however, visual ligation of arteries ultimately led to more accurate hemostasis. This was aided by retractors, as described by Judd, and detail to the bladder neck, as advocated by Lower of Cleveland and Harris of Australia in 1972.[9]

The most significant contribution to exposure and hemostasis was the description by Harvard in 1954 of the low transverse opening of the bladder, which allows direct visualization and control of bleeding in the prostatic fossa.[3] The use of this approach, with minor modifications, lowered the mortality of this procedure in our hospital from 8.4% in 1952 to 1.4% in 1972.[8] A recent review of the last 300 such operations revealed no deaths, and this compares favorably with a mortality rate of 0.3% for transurethral resection in our hospital.[*4]

Indications

The primary indicator for an open enucleation procedure, either suprapubic or retropubic prostatectomy, is the size of the gland. The surgeons in our department at Northwestern are comfortable doing a transurethral resection for glands weighing up to 60 g and reserve open prostatectomy for the larger gland. The result is that 90% of obstructing adenomas are handled transurethrally and only 10% are removed by the suprapubic or retropubic approach.

If a patient is returning to a remote part of this country, a foreign country, or an area where good urologic care is not available, we may advise open prostatectomy, because late bleeding rarely occurs after enucleation but is not uncommon weeks or months after transurethral resection.[4]

Other indications for open enucleation are large associated bladder diverticula, calculi such as jack stones that defy litholapaxy, severe stricture of the posterior urethra that cannot be bypassed by perineal urethrotomy, and ankylosis of the hips, which prevents positioning for proper endoscopic resection.

The selection of the proper procedure is made only after complete urologic evaluation: excretory urography with cystography and cystoscopic examination. Cystography is notorious for deceiving one about the size of the prostate; cystoscopy is the ultimate evaluation, with measurement of length and size and (most helpful) the palpation of the prostate with the instrument in place. We have used ultrasound evaluation for several years, but it is not as accurate in estimating size as direct observation.

---

* Hwong L, O'Conor VJ Jr: Unpublished data, 1981

Transvesical Prostatectomy

PREOPERATIVE TREATMENT

Proper preoperative care has significantly improved the results of prostatectomies in the past 50 years. Catheter drainage, to improve renal function in patients with azotemia resulting from chronic bladder neck obstruction, has played a large role in reducing postoperative complications. Approximately 30% of our patients have been admitted in acute urinary retention. Associated fluid and electrolyte replacement is essential, but most important is the recognition of associated systemic disease, which can be treated prior to surgery and supported postoperatively. The average age of patients undergoing open prostatectomy on our service is 72. Significant cardiovascular disease is present in 50%, pulmonary disease in 10%, and diabetes in 10% of our patients. The documentation of acute myocardial infarction interdicts any surgical procedure for a 6-month period.

ANESTHESIA

Spinal anesthesia is our choice for all operations on the prostate; only in rare instances is general inhalation anesthesia used. The relaxation during the operation and, more importantly, the lack of leg motion in the early postoperative period prevent undue pulling on the catheter, disruption of clots, and increased bleeding.

OPERATIVE PROCEDURE

The patient is placed in a supine position with shoulder braces to allow further Trendelenburg position. The abdomen, scrotum, and penis are scrubbed with antiseptic detergent and painted with similar antiseptic (povidone-iodine, Betadine). If a catheter is not in place, a soft 18 red rubber catheter is used to distend the bladder with 200 ml to 300 ml of sterile saline. The catheter is removed; rarely is there urethral leakage if the operation is indicated. A single folded towel is placed beneath the penis and three others are laid lateral and superior to the proposed incision. A final, doubly folded towel covers the penis so that it may be exposed later without contamination. Drapes are then applied and the transverse incision is made 2 finger-widths (4 cm) above the symphysis and is carried down to the anterior rectus sheath. At this point two Gelpi vaginal retractors are placed in the subcutaneous tissue to provide exposure.

The rectus sheath is incised in the midline and extended laterally with the Richter scissors, avoiding incision into the muscle itself. The edges of the rectus sheath are then grasped with Kocher clamps and, with elevation and scissor dissection, the sheath is separated from the underlying muscle (Fig. 84-1). The tendinous part of the rectus muscles is exposed but not divided. Careful incision of linea alba is made close to the pubis and the undersurfaces of the recti are freed bluntly, exposing the prevesical space. This is done cautiously to avoid injury to the deep inferior epigastric vessels that enter this area. Moist sponges are placed on the muscles and the muscle bellies are retracted laterally with a Balfour retractor. Minimal dissection is done on the anterior bladder; an area large enough for an incision is cleared off approximately 2 cm above the bladder neck and grasped with two Allis clamps. These clamps are elevated, a scalpel stab is made transversely in the midline, and the bladder contents are evacuated. At this point two mattress sutures of 1-0 chronic are placed above and below, left long, and secured by clamps (Fig. 84-2). These sutures aid us in the reintroduction of the exploratory finger later in the procedure.

The bladder opening is extended bluntly by stretching with fingers to the desired size, rather than incising the wall, which injures more vessels. The bladder is then inspected and, if diverticulectomy or removal of calculi are planned, this is done prior to prostatic enucleation. If limited assistance is available, a self-retaining Judd retractor is placed. We find the best exposure to be obtained by placing three loose sponges posteriorly, with a large Deaver retractor over them. Two narrower Deavers are then placed on either side of the bladder neck area, exposing the prostate.

At this point the ureteral orifices are identified and, with traction on the posterior retractor, removed from the area to be incised or coagulated. The mucosa over the prostate is circumcised either with a long-handle knife or with the Bovie cutting electrode (Fig. 84-3). This incision allows a clean break when the adenoma is enucleated and avoids tearing mucosa toward the ureteral orifices. This incision should be quite wide; otherwise difficulty will be encountered in removing the adenoma after enucleation. If there is a large amount of intravesical tissue, sponge sticks are used to expose the areas to be incised.

All retractors and sponges are removed prior to enucleation. At this point we check to be sure a 3-inch neuro head roll is available in case rapid packing is necessary after enucleation. In the very obese patient it is helpful to place two fingers in the rectum to elevate the prostate, but this is not done routinely. The index finger is placed into the urethra and, with forward pressure toward the symphysis, the urethral mucosa is broken and the plane between adenoma and capsule is defined.

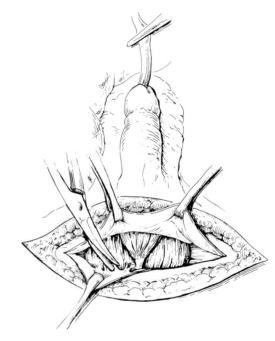

FIG. 84-1. Suprapubic prostatectomy; transverse incision in rectus sheath separating underlying muscle fibers

FIG. 84-2. Aspirating bladder contents; stay sutures in place

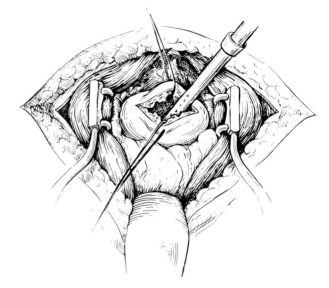

The mucosal attachments at the apex are freed early in the procedure, because later elevation of the adenoma or scissor dissection in this area can injure the external sphincter. Freeing mucosal attachments is generally done by pinching the tissue between the thumbnail and index finger, then sweeping the finger posteriorly, freeing first one and then the other lateral lobe (Fig. 84-4). With large adenomas, it is often easier to remove the lobes separately. When the right hand is being used, one may encounter difficulty in getting the left hand to perform complete enucleation properly. If the adenoma is markedly adherent, it is grasped with a lobe forceps or tenaculum and freed by scissors dissection under vision.

After removal of the adenoma, the retractors are replaced and the fossa packed tightly with the 3-inch, 5-yard head roll (Figs. 84-5 and 84-6). Pressure is applied over this packing and maintained for 5 minutes. If rectal pressure has been used, the surgeon then changes gown and gloves; this allows stabilization of the patient after a brisk blood loss. The 3-inch gauze is inched out slowly, exposing the posterior bladder neck, wich is grasped with long Kocher clamps at the 5 o'clock and 7 o'clock positions. Deep mattress sutures of 1-0 chromic are placed in these areas, grasped with clamps, and pulled upward to expose the bladder neck further (Fig. 84-7). Continued pressure is placed on the gauze packing with a long narrow Deaver. Meanwhile the bladder neck area is exposed on either side to the 11 o'clock and 1 o'clock areas; here again Kocher clamps elevate the tissue for placement of 1-0 chromic mattress sutures, which are held for elevation. The four sutures are now elevated, exposing the fossa.

Further exposure is systematic, visualizing first one side, then the other. This may be aided by inserting an empty ring holder and opening the blades or by using a sponge stick to pull laterally, first one side, then the other, obtaining hemostasis by spot coagulation or suture ligation. We rarely use a boomerang needle, because the small 5/8-inch curved needle with atraumatic suture can be placed deep in the fossa under direct vision.

When the arterial bleeding is controlled, a single loose sponge is placed deep in the fossa to control venous ooze, and attention is turned to the bladder neck. Redundant tags or mucosal flaps are trimmed; if a posterior contracture seems present, a wedge incision of the contracture is performed and often

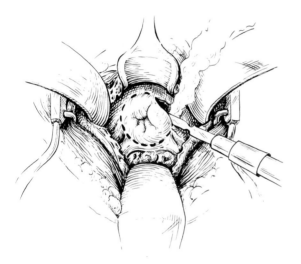

FIG. 84-3.   Incision of mucosa over the adenoma

FIG. 84-4.   Digital enucleation of adenoma

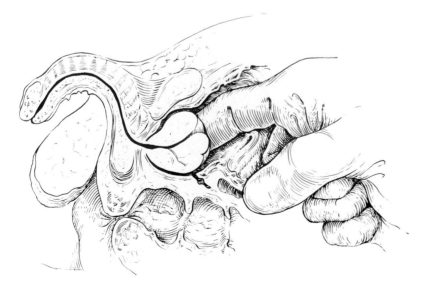

a running suture of 3-0 plain catgut is placed from 5 o'clock to 7 o'clock, approximating mucosa to the posterior capsule. On occasion the bladder neck is brought down to the posterior capsule in a method described by Harris in 1927 as "retrigon-

ilization." Generally at this point a mild venous ooze from the apex is present; if it is controlled by a single gauze sponge, one can expect it will be controlled by catheter pressure with or without a small piece of Surgical or another hemostatic substance. Occasionally, however, particularly with large adenomas, persistent and rather heavy bleeding appears from the posterior capsule with no obvious large arterial pumpers.

Historically, urologists have described a contraction of the prostatic capsule that in itself slows bleeding, much as the uterus contracts after delivery. When excessive bleeding persists, it appears that this contraction is not taking place, and we have utilized a suture technique that to our knowledge has not previously been described. Using the atraumatic 1-0 chromic on a ⅝-inch needle, we take a bite in the posterior capsule on the right wall, another on the left wall, and then tie it, crimping the capsule. If this is not immediately effective, a second similar suture is placed deep in the fossa (Fig. 84-8). The cessation of bleeding with these sutures is often dramatic.

A 24Fr Foley catheter is then placed, drawing back the towel on the penis, which had been draped to avoid rectal contamination. While the bag is being inflated, the gauze is left deep in the fossa. When the bag is inflated with volume milliliters of water greater than the weight in grams (a 30-ml bag will easily hold 100 ml), the gauze is removed. The bag is pulled snugly against the

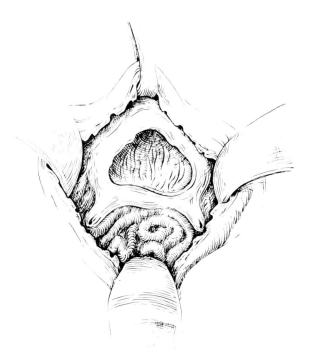

FIG. 84-5. View of empty prostatic fossa

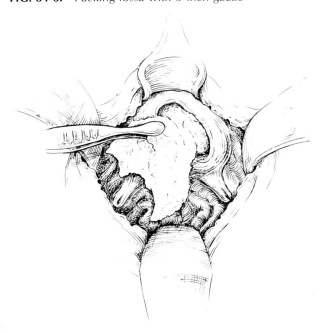

FIG. 84-6. Packing fossa with 3-inch gauze

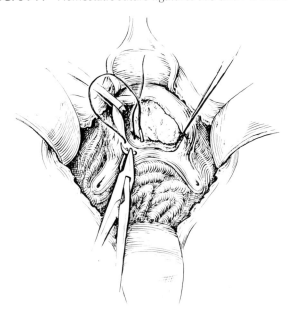

FIG. 84-7. Hemostatic suture ligatures at 5 and 7 o'clock

bladder neck. The bag must not be placed in the prostatic fossa because this prevents the normal contraction of the capsule, produces significant postoperative discomfort, and may contribute to postoperative incontinence. The double-bag Oddo

catheter designed to produce pressure in the fossa has only been used once in our hospital after a transurethral resection. We do not hesitate to slip a small piece of Surgical deep into the fossa to control venous oozing. The other hemostatic sub-

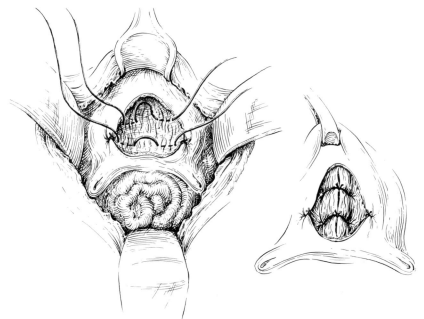

FIG. 84-8. Plicating sutures in posterior capsule

FIG. 84-9. Pursestring suture of bladder neck

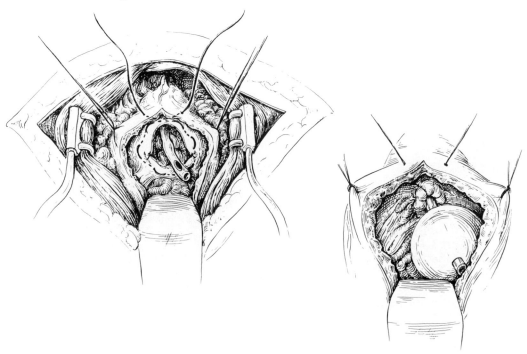

stances, Oxycel and Gelfoam, are relatively insol uble and may subsequently require endoscopic removal or irrigation with sodium bicarbonate to dissolve.

If all of the preceding fail to control bleeding, the pursestring suture around the bladder neck, as described by Malament in 1965, should be considered.[7] The pursestring is placed circumferentially around the bladder neck, closed tightly over the catheter, brought out to the skin, and fixed with buttons (Fig. 84-9). We have not resorted to packing for hemostasis for the past 20 years.

When hemostasis is ensured, a decision is made whether or not to use suprapubic tube drainage. Primary closure of the bladder with urethral Foley catheter drainage is often done, but the close supervision of the patient is mandatory to obviate clot retention, and our practice generally involves placement of a No. 32 right-angle Pezzer catheter, through which clots can pass easily and two-way irrigation can be instituted if necessary. The upper bladder flap is grasped with a Kocher clamp; a Kelly clamp is passed through the wall several centimeters from the margin after checking that the peritoneum has been pushed superiorly; and the Pezzer catheter is brought through. The bladder is closed in two layers with 1-0 or 2-0 chromic, usually with one continuous suture reinforced with interrupted sutures.

Irrigation is then performed and any small leak is repaired. A split rubber drain is led out from the prevesical space and the Pezzer catheter, brought out through a stab wound superior to the incision (Fig. 84-10). The angle of this catheter keeps the peritoneum up and also permits rapid closure of the sinus when removed. The rectus muscle bellies are loosely approximated, the rectus fascia closed with interrupted sutures, and the subcutaneous tissue and skin closed in the usual manner.

The dressing is applied using Montgomery or Senn straps to facilitate frequent changing for several days of the inevitably damp dressings.

POSTOPERATIVE CARE

Intravenous fluid therapy is fairly routine following prostatectomy. Most patients receive 1000 ml each 8-hour period for the first 24 hours. If not nauseated, most patients are allowed clear liquids when they are able to more their legs or when the anesthetic wears off. If fluids are tolerated, the intravenous fluids are discontinued the next morning and diet is advanced as tolerated. Deep breathing, coughing, and leg motion are encouraged and

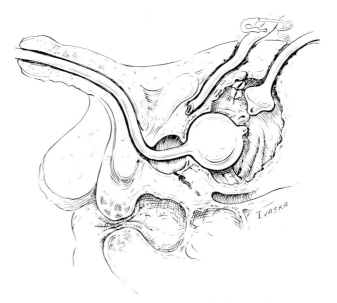

FIG. 84-10. Foley catheter snug at bladder neck; prevesical drain and Pezzer catheter

the former are actually forced upon our patients by respiratory-care personnel.

Ambulation is encouraged. The patients may sit up the night of surgery and progress to walking the next day. Antibiotics are not given routinely.

Care of the catheters has varied considerably over the years; however, in the past 15 years, our practice has been to remove the Foley catheter first. If bladder spasm is a problem, the fluid in the urethral Foley catheter is removed, leaving only 30 ml; this usually relieves the discomfort. The urethral catheter is removed on the second postoperative day, the suprapubic tube, on the fifth postoperative day. Generally the suprapubic drainage ceases within 24 hours. However, if it persists, a small Foley catheter is inserted for 24 hours, and most patients void without leakage after this. The drain is left in after removal of the suprapubic tube and usually is removed the following day. Most patients are discharged on the seventh or eighth postoperative day and are followed weekly as outpatients until the urine is clear, anywhere from 4 to 8 weeks.

COMPLICATIONS

As noted, postoperative late bleeding is rare with suprapubic prostatectomy compared to transurethral resection. The use of blood replacement for significant bleeding is less than 15% (compared to 3% for transurethral resection).

Epididymitis develops in about 3% of patients,

and we do not currently perform routine vasectomy.

Incontinence of a permanent nature is uncommon. Some patients have some stress incontinence early and often are placed on ephedrine or phenylpropanolamine to obtain relief.

Impotence should not result from this or any other patient prostatectomy, although *retrograde ejaculation* is common and accepted if explained to the patient preoperatively.

Urethral stricture is rare in our patients, probably the result of early removal of the urethral catheter.

REFERENCES

1. BELFIELD WT: Prostatic myoma—A so-called middle lobe of the hypertrophied prostate—Removed by suprapubic prostatectomy. JAMA 8:303, 1887
2. FULLER E: The question of priority in the adoption of the method of total enucleation suprapubically of the hypertrophied prostate. Am Surg 41:520, 1905
3. HARVARD BM: Low transvesical suprapubic prostatectomy with primary closure, In Campbell MF (ed): Urology, 1st ed, p 1965. Philadelphia, W B Saunders, 1954
4. IGNATOFF JM, O'CONOR VJ, JR: Transurethral resection: A review. Int Urol Nephrol 9:33, 1977
5. IMMERGUT M: In Classical Articles in Urology, p. 166. Springfield, Ill, Charles C Thomas, 1967
6. KEYES EL: An efficient method of controlling hemorrhage after suprapubic prostatectomy. Med Rec 42:331, 1892
7. MALAMENT M: Maximal hemostasis in suprapubic prostatectomy. Surg Gynecol Obstet 120:1307, 1965
8. NANNINGA J, O'CONOR VJ, JR: Suprapubic prostatectomy: A 28-year review, 1942–1970. Int Urol Nephrol 4:377, 1972
9. O'CONOR VJ, JR: The History of Suprapubic Prostatectomy. American Urological Association and Hoffman LaRoche, Inc, 1975
10. O'CONOR VJ, JR: Suprapubic and retropubic prostatectomy. In Harrison IH, Gittes RF, Perlmutter AD et al (eds): Campbell's Urology. Philadelphia, W B Saunders, 1979
11. THOMPSON H: Diseases of the Prostate. London, J & A Churchill, 1868

Retropubic Prostatectomy

85

Ralph A. Straffon

In the majority of urologic clinics, prostatectomy is most frequently performed by transurethral resection of the prostate gland. Certain patients, however, require an open prostatectomy. The retropubic prostatectomy is the most recently developed of the four present-day surgical approaches to the prostate.

Terrance Millin, who introduced and popularized the classic, simple retropubic prostatectomy, first reported his technique and results in 1945.[3] In 1947, he published a monograph entitled *Retropubic Urinary Surgery*.[4] However, the actual performance of some form of retropubic prostatectomy predated Millin's report. Weyrauch credits Van Stockum with performing the first retropubic prostatectomy in 1909.[6] Van Stockum entitled his operation "extravesicle suprapubic prostatectomy" and made a longitudinal capsular incision on one side of the midline. Subsequent surgeons, such as Hildebrand (1912), Maier and Mermingas (1923), and Jacobs and Casper (1933) all used capsular incisions to remove the prostate, but Millin deserves the credit for popularizing the technique.

In the ensuing years, Millin's technique of retropubic prostatectomy gained acceptance and was widely used. Surgeons realized the advantage of direct visualization of the prostatic fossa for improved hemostasis. In an attempt to improve hemostasis still further, various methods of suturing the visical neck were evolved, such as that recorded by Dittmer.[2] Riches advocated excision of the posterior prostatic capsule in routine retropubic prostatectomy to detect and remove an early focus of prostatic cancer.[5] Blue and Campbell stressed the importance of a wide resection of the vesical neck.[1]

INDICATIONS AND CONTRAINDICATIONS

Retropubic prostatectomy can be used whenever open prostatectomy is needed to treat prostatic obstruction. Our indications for an open prostatectomy are in those patients with any of the following: (1) a large prostate gland (more than 80–100 g), (2) a large prostate gland associated with one or more good-sized bladder diverticula, (3) a large prostate gland associated with a vesical calculus that is not amenable to litholapaxy, and (4) fixed hip joints that make placement in the lithotomy position impossible. Fewer than 5% of our prostatectomies are performed by an open surgical approach.

The retropubic prostatectomy is contraindicated in the small fibrous prostate or in the presence of carcinoma of the prostate. In either of these cases, enucleation of the obstructing prostatic tissue is very difficult.

Retropubic Prostatectomy Technique

PREOPERATIVE PREPARATION

As with all patients undergoing prostatectomy, the general health of the patient must be evaluated by a thorough history and physical examination. In addition to the usual laboratory studies, chest radiograph, and electrocardiogram, some specific urologic evaluation is required.

Renal function is evaluated with a simple serum creatinine or a creatinine clearance. A urinalysis should be done and if bacteria are present, urine culture and sensitivity studies are obtained to aid in selecting the appropriate antibiotic. This antibiotic is administered prior to and throughout the operative procedure and during the postoperative period.

An intravenous pyelogram, though not an essential part of the evaluation of a patient with prostatic obstruction, is usually obtained in our clinic, with a postvoiding film.

If the patient is not in acute retention, we avoid instrumentation of the urinary tract unless symptoms or findings suggest that the patient may have a neurogenic bladder or a bladder diverticulum. In these patients, a cystometric examination and a cystogram with both oblique views and a post-drainage film are important aspects of the preoperative investigation.

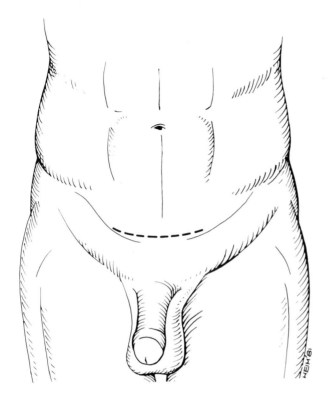

FIG. 85-1. The modified Pfannenstiel incision

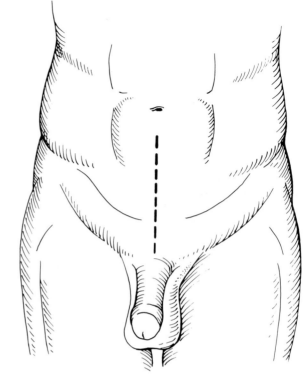

FIG. 85-2. The midline vertical incision

The patient who is admitted in renal failure associated with prostatic obstruction requires a period of catheter draining. In some patients, a postobstructive diuresis may ensure that demands careful monitoring of fluid and electrolyte therapy. Once the serum creatinine has stabilized, a cystometric examination and cystogram should be done to evaluate the status of the bladder, which has been chronically overdistended. These studies identify the patient with a large bladder diverticulum that should be removed at the time of prostatectomy. They also identify the patient with a large-capacity, decompensated bladder who may have difficulty emptying the bladder after the prostatic obstruction has been removed.

A cleansing enema is usually given the evening before the operation. Preoperative medications are administered on call to the operating room.

OPERATIVE PROCEDURE

The patient is placed in the supine position and the operating table is flexed somewhat to elevate the pelvis. The entire operative field, from midepigastrium to midthigh, is shaved and scrubbed with povidone-iodine (Betadine) solution. We pre-

fer a modified Pfannenstiel incision, placed about 2 cm above the symphysis pubis (Fig. 85-1). Equally good exposure can be obtained through a midline vertical incision as shown in Figure 85-2. After the skin incision is made, the subcutaneous tissue is divided in line with the incision down to the rectal fascia, and bleeding vessels are fulgurated. The rectal sheath is opened exposing the rectus and pyramidalis muscle on either side of the midline. The incision is then extended laterally and slightly upward on each side, incising the aponeurosis of the external and internal abdominal oblique muscles. The rectal sheath is freed upward from the underlying rectal muscle and downward to the symphysis pubis. The tendinous insertions of the rectus and pyramidalis muscles on either side of the midline are separated from their insertions into the symphysis pubis for a distance of several centimeters to provide better exposure to the space of Retzius. The rectal muscles are then separated in the midline to complete the exposure.

The extraperitoneal fat and peritoneum are swept off the anterior surface of the partially inflated bladder, exposing the anterior surface of the prostate and bladder. A self-retaining retractor can then be placed in the incision to obtain maximal exposure of the anterior surface of the prostate, vesical neck, and bladder. Frequently, there are several large veins present in the loose areolar tissue on the anterior surface of the prostate. These can be ligated and divided or even fulgurated to avoid troublesome bleeding (Fig. 85-3). The prostatic capsule can then be visualized by gently dissecting away this loose areolar tissue.

The vesical neck can easily be identified by palpation. To be certain of its location, the surgeon may exert gentle downward traction on the indwelling urethral catheter and palpate the position of the balloon in relation to the vesical neck. The site of the incision into the prostatic capsule is usually about 1 cm below the vesical neck. Two traction sutures are placed in the prostatic capsule above and below the selected site for the prostatic capsular incision. Once the traction sutures are in place, a transverse incision through the surgical capsule of the prostate is carried out (Fig. 85-4). The length of the incision varies with the size of the prostate gland and should extend far enough laterally on either side to afford maximum exposure of the prostatic fossa.

The transverse incision into the prostatic capsule extends into the prostatic adenoma. This affords direct visualization of the junction between the prostatic adenoma and the surgical capsule of the prostate. This cleavage plane can then be developed using the curved Metzenbaum scissors, shown in Figure 85-5.

The dissection of the adenoma from the prostatic

capsule can be continued with the curved scissors downward toward the membranous urethra. This technique is particularly useful in small prostatic adenomas, which tend to be more adherent to the prostatic capsule. The dissection may also be car-

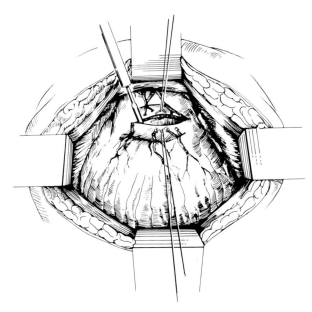

FIG. 85-4. Transfixion sutures placed on the capsule anteriorly with an incision being made transversely in the prostatic capsule

FIG. 85-5. Identification of the cleavage plane between the prostatic adenoma and the surgical capsule of the prostate

FIG. 85-3. The ligation and division of periprostatic veins over the prostatic capsule anteriorly

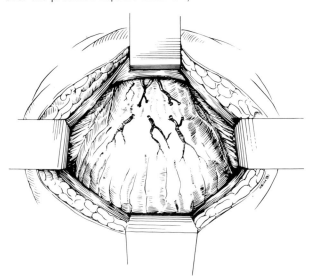

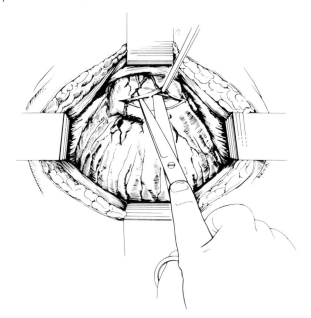

ried upward toward the vesical neck, freeing the prostate tissue in this area. In large adenomas, digital enucleation of the adenoma can easily be done once this plane of dissection is established. In digital enucleation, the dissection is best started at the apex of the prostate, freeing both lateral lobes and dissecting upward. Care must be taken at the apex of the prostate not to tear the urethra.

If the finger cannot break through the urethral mucosa in this area, sharp dissection with the scissors may be necessary to avoid tearing it. Once the lateral lobes are dissected upward, it is very simple to remove the median lobe as well. It is extremely important to avoid any trauma at the apex of the prostate because this may result in postprostatectomy urinary incontinence (Fig. 85-6).

After removing the entire prostatic adenoma, the vesical neck is identified, posteriorly. A figure-of-eight suture ligature of 2-0 chromic is placed at

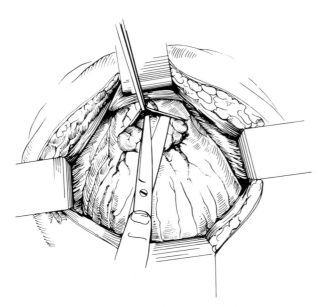

FIG. 85-6. Continuing the dissection of the prostate of the adenoma from the prostatic capsule using Metzenbaum scissors

FIG. 85-7. The figure-of-eight sutures applied at the vesicle neck at 5 and 7 o'clock to secure hemostasis

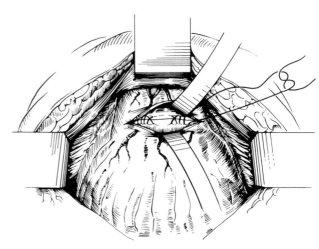

FIG. 85-8. Approximation of the mucosa to the prostatic capsule at the vesical neck

FIG. 85-9. Fulguration of bleeding points in the prostatic fossa under direct vision

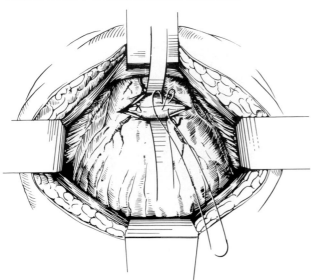

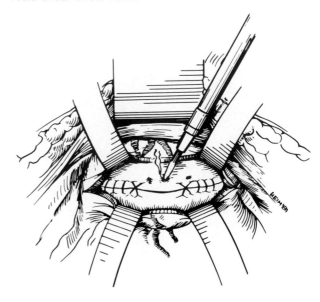

both 5 and 7 o'clock in the vesical neck to secure hemostasis (Fig. 85-7). A running suture of 2-0 chromic is then used at the vesical neck to approximate bladder mucosa to the prostatic capsule. This suture also aids in hemostasis in this area and is placed on both sides of the vesical neck under direct vision (Fig. 85-8).

Next, bleeding vessels in the prostatic fossa are coagulated under direct vision. Visualization of the prostatic fossa can be facilitated if the surgeon wears a head light for illumination and uses small ribbon retractors on either side of the fossa (Fig. 85-9). In some patients, the posterior lip of the vesical neck is very prominent and protrudes into the lumen. This can be removed by wedge resection of this area as diagramed in Figure 85-10. The area outlined can be grasped with an Allis forceps and then, using either scissors or knife, the wedge can be removed posteriorly. The ureteric orifices should be identified to be sure that the wedge is well away from this area. This wedged-out area is sutured as depicted in Figure 85-11.

A 24Fr Silastic-coated Foley catheter with a 30-ml retention balloon is inserted through the urethra into the bladder. The transverse incision of the prostatic capsule is then closed with interrupted sutures of 2-0 chromic, which are placed quite close together to ensure secure closure of the capsule (Fig. 85-12). Once this closure has been completed, the Foley catheter is pulled against the

vesical neck to tamponade the prostatic fossa and prevent venous oozing from the fossa into the bladder. The catheter is usually left on traction for several hours after the surgical procedure is completed. This traction can easily be achieved simply by taping the catheter to the thigh of the patient. A suprapubic catheter is used only if there is excessive bleeding. In the majority of patients, a urethral catheter provides sufficient drainage.

A Penrose drain is placed in the space of Retzius,

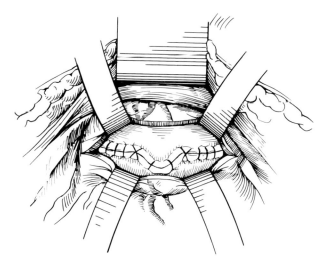

FIG. 85-11.   Closure of the wedge resection of the vesical neck with interrupted chromic sutures

FIG. 85-10.   The wedge resection of the vesical neck posteriorly

FIG. 85-12.   Closure of the incision of the prostate capsule anteriorly with interrupted chromic sutures

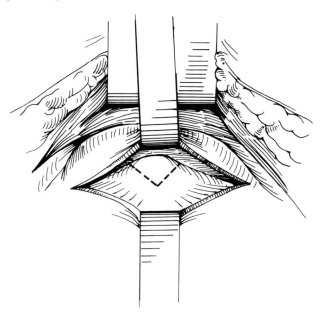

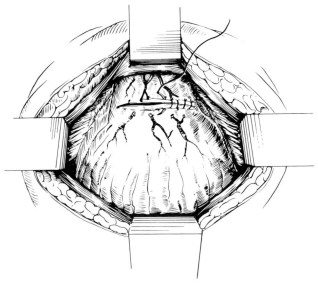

brought out through a stab wound below the incision, and sutured placed.

The tendinous insertion of the rectus and pyramidalis muscles are reapproximated to the symphysis pubis with interrupted chromic sutures. The rectal muscles are then approximated to the midline, and the incision is closed in layers using 1-0 chromic sutures. Subcutaneous tissue is approximated with interrupted 3-0 plain. We usually use staples for the skin closure.

POSTOPERATIVE CARE

At the end of the operative procedure, an intravenous injection of 20 mg of furosemide is given to ensure a good postoperative diuresis. This dose may be repeated in 60 minutes if an additional diuresis is required.

The catheter is usually removed on the sixth postoperative day. The Penrose drain is moved partially outward on this day and is finally withdrawn on the seventh postoperative day when the skin clips are removed.

Complications

The usual minor wound complications can occur in retropubic prostatectomy, as in any procedure in which a skin incision is used. Since we have been using skin staples in the closure, which tend to cause less of a reaction, the incidence of wound infections has been reduced.

Postoperative hemorrhage is relatively uncommon with this technique of prostatectomy because the exposure of the prostatic fossa allows good hemostasis with the fulgurating electrode. In addition, catheter traction in the immediate postoperative period helps cut down on venous oozing from the prostatic fossa into the bladder. Delayed bleeding may occur from time to time, as in any other form of prostatic surgery.

Postoperative urinary leakage through the prostatic capsule is rare if a good closure is secured. When it does occur, it usually responds to a period of indwelling urethral-catheter drainage.

The incidence of postoperative urinary incontinence is low, particularly if great care is taken in dealing with the apex of the prostate. Urge incontinence may occur in the postoperative period, as it can in all forms of prostatectomy; it usually responds to anticholinergic medications.

We have found that urethral strictures are uncommon when a Silastic Foley catheter is used. Bladder neck contractions are also rare following retropubic prostatectomy.

Osteitis pubis, which used to be quite common, is now rarely seen, particularly with the routine use of antibiotics especially in those patients who have urinary tract infections.

The retropubic prostatectomy is an excellent way of performing prostatic surgery in those patients requiring an open approach to the prostate gland.

REFERENCES

1. BLUE GD, CAMPBELL JN: A clinical review of one thousand consecutive cases of retropubic prostatectomy. J Urol 80:257, 1958
2. DITTMER H: Modification of technique for retropubic prostatectomy: Report of 100 cases. J Urol 81:558, 1959
3. MILLIN T: Retropubic prostatectomy: New extravesicle technique: Report on 20 cases. Lancet 2:693, 1945
4. MILLIN T: Retropubic Urinary Surgery. London, E & S Livingstone, 1947
5. RICHES E: Posterior capsulectomy in routine retropubic prostatectomy. J Urol 85:965, 1961
6. WEYRAUCH HM: Surgery of the Prostate. Philadelphia, W B Saunders, 1959

Perineal Prostatectomy

86

Herbert Brendler

The first operations for relief of urinary retention due to prostatic enlargement were probably done through the perineum, and early medical writings contain references to division of the bladder neck through the perineum for this purpose.[10]

Covillard, in 1639, however, was apparently the first to remove a hypertrophied middle lobe by tearing it away with forceps after perineal lithotomy. In 1848, Sir William Fergusson exhibited specimens of hypertrophied prostates he had enucleated through the perineum after removal of bladder calculi. Küchler, in 1866, formulated the first systematic technique for radical perineal prostatectomy, but his operations were done only in the cadaver. In 1867, Billroth used Küchler's method to carry out the first two intentional prostatectomies in living subjects. Apparently, however, the lobes were not entirely removed in these two patients.

In 1873, Gouley advocated systematic enucleation of the lateral lobes and excision of the median lobe through the perineum. However, Goodfellow is credited with being the first to perform perineal prostatectomy successfully on a routine basis.[4] His method involved the use of a midline vertical incision from the base of the scrotum to the anal margin, followed by incision of the membranous urethra, extension of the opening into the bladder, and complete enucleation of the prostatic lobes. His technique, although differing in certain respects from that used today, nevertheless forms the basis of current methods.[5]

During the next decade, a number of technical modifications were suggested by Nicoll, Alexander, Albarran, Proust, dePezzer, Legueu, and others. For the most part, those changes were concerned, with improving delivery of the prostatic lobes into the perineal incision for enucleation. In 1903, Young described the operative technique first developed by him at the Johns Hopkins Hospital, which probably is still the one most widely used.[9] In 1939, Belt introduced an important modification in the perineal approach to the prostate, which did much to reduce the risk of rectal injury inherent in the operations of Young and earlier surgeons. Belt's method of closure also was a great improvement over earlier methods and shortened convalescence considerably.[1]

Surgical Anatomy

STRUCTURE

The normal adult prostate is a firm, elastic organ located immediately below the bladder and resting on the superior layer of the urogenital diaphragm, to which it is firmly attached. Its shape is roughly pyramidal or conical, and it measures 3 cm to 4 cm from apex to base. Its greatest transverse diameter is 4 cm to 5 cm; anteroposteriorly, it measures approximately 2 cm. It is transversed throughout its length by the first portion of the urethra, and behind this, by the ejaculatory ducts (Figs. 86-1 and 86-2).

The anterior surface of the gland is convex. The posterior aspect, which lies immediately in front of the rectum and is easily palpated through its wall, possesses a distinct median furrow ending in a notch superiorly. It is customary to divide the gland into two lateral lobes, a median (or posterior commissural) lobe connecting these two, a posterior lobe (lying behind the plane defined by the ejaculatory ducts), and an anterior lobe. In actuality, the individual lobes are not clearly demarcated, as they are in lower animals.

On cross section, no true lobar pattern exists but rather two concentric layers, as described by Franks.[3] The outer one is quite thick and composed of long, branched glands—the prostatic glands proper—which drain into ducts curving posteriorly. These external glands are thought to be the site of origin or prostatic carcinoma. Separated from the outer gland layer by an indefinite capsule are the inner glands. These consist of a larger set of submucosal glanduloductal units and a smaller set of short glands lying immediately beneath the mucosa. It is from the inner gland layer that benign hyperplasia arises (Fig. 86-3).

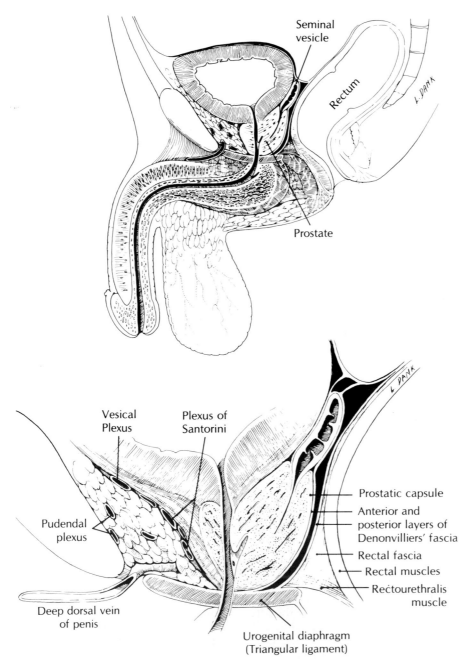

FIG. 86-1. Relation of prostate gland to surrounding structures

The epithelium of the acini consists of tall columnar cells. Beneath these is an indefinite layer of flattened basal cells. No histologic differences can be discerned between cells of the inner and outer glands. The ductal epithelium is also of the tall columnar type. The acini are surrounded by dense fibromuscular stroma containing some elastic fibers.

A tough capsule composed of fibrous tissue and muscular elements envelops the prostate com-

pletely and is densely adherent to it. Fibromuscular septa originating from the capsule penetrate the gland in a branching manner, forming trabeculae.

FASCIAL INVESTMENTS

The prostate is firmly fixed in position by reflections of the endopelvic fascia but remains somewhat movable at its base. Anteriorly, a fascial layer springing from the white line of the pelvis forms the two puboprostatic ligaments, beneath and between which lies the prostatic venous plexus (Santorini). These ligaments must be served in order to expose the apex of the prostate during total retropubic prostatectomy.

Two other fascial coverings invest the prostate and seminal vesicles posteriorly. These two layers are loosely attached to each other by areolar tissue and constitute what are generally termed the *anterior and posterior layers of Denonvilliers' fascia* (Fig. 86-1). Denonvilliers' original papers on the subject in 1836 and 1837 do not describe a posterior fascial layer, and Tobin and Benjamin have found that this actually arises from primitive mesenchyme around the rectum.[8] Nevertheless, because of its importance in the perineal approach to the prostate, the term *posterior layer* has achieved general acceptance among urologic surgeons.

The anterior layer of Denonvilliers' fascia is a dense tough covering that is continuous over the posterior aspect of the prostate and seminal vesicles and is closely attached to the underlying prostatic capsule. It can easily be differentiated from the posterior layer of Denonvilliers' fascia by its glistening appearance, aptly designated the *pearly gates*. The two layers are reasily separated; this is essential for proper surgical exposure of the posterior surface of the prostate and seminal vesicles and avoidance of injury to the rectum. The anterior layer of Denonvilliers' fascia constitutes an effective barrier to the backward extension of prostatic inflammatory and malignant disease. It is an important surgical landmark in total perineal prostatectomy and seminal vesiculectomy for cancer.

RELATION TO RECTUM

In perineal exposure of the prostate, the rectum is found to be attached near the apex of the gland by a small band of muscle fibers known as the *rectourethralis*. This structure extends from the urogenital diaphragm and membranous urethra anteriorly to the rectum posteriorly. It is short and often indefinite. The anterior portion of the levator ani fibers, which encircles the sides of the prostate, is more or less fused with it; indeed, the rectourethralis may merely represent the midline raphe of the levatores. In any event, it must be divided to permit retraction of the rectum and access to the space between the two layers of Denonvilliers' fascia.

ARTERIAL SUPPLY

The main artery to the prostate arises from the inferior division of the hypogastric (internal iliac) artery. It enters the prostate just below the bladder neck (Fig. 86-4). Flocks has described the intrinsic arterial distribution to the prostate as consisting of two groups of vessels: an external (capsular) and

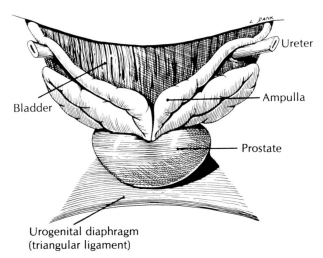

FIG. 86-2. Posterior view of prostate gland and seminal vesicles

FIG. 86-3. Cross section of normal prostate gland

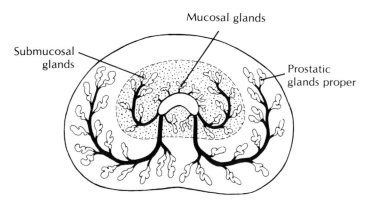

an internal (urethral).[2] The latter group enlarges with age, especially with prostatic hyperplasia. During enucleation, major branches of this group are apt to be injured in the posterolateral region of the bladder neck and can cause serious bleeding.

VENOUS DRAINAGE

The veins of the prostate constitute a well-defined plexus (Santorini), which occupies the anterior and lateral surfaces of the gland (Fig. 86-5). This plexus receives the dorsal vein of the penis in the pubo-prostatic space. Eventually it empties into the hypogastric (internal iliac) veins. The plexus of Santorini must be handled with great care in the retropubic approach to the prostate. Occasionally, venous tributaries may be encountered on the posterior aspect of the prostate during perineal exposure, but these usually are not a problem.

FIG. 86-4. Arterial supply of prostate gland

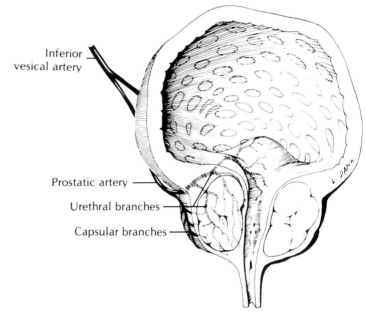

FIG. 86-5. Major venous drainage of prostate gland

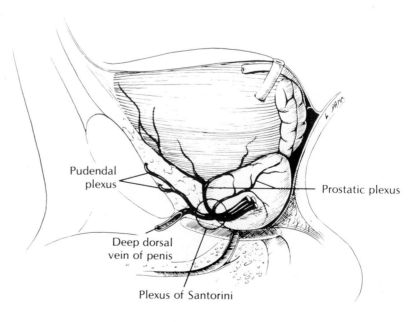

Pathology

Benign prostatic hypertrophy consists of multicentric nodules of hyperplastic epithelial and fibromuscular elements that originate in the periurethral area. This growth is unique to man; it has, moreover, never been experimentally reproduced in animals. Although endocrine factors are implicated in its development, its etiology remains obscure. Attempts to control benign prostatic hypertrophy clinically by hormonal means have not been conspicuously successful.

HISTOGENESIS

Early in adult life, the prostate undergoes certain involutional changes that are focal at first but later spread to involve the entire gland. Both epithelial and stromal elements in the inner and outer prostatic zones are affected, and to varying degrees. Hyperplasia of the inner layer leads to benign prostatic hypertrophy; associated atrophic changes are seen in the outer layer, or prostate proper, but secondary hyperplastic changes may also occur here. Although Morgagni was the first to note that benign enlargement of the prostate arose from the inner part of the gland, the question of whether the initial changes take place in the epithelium or in the stroma has never been satisfactorily answered.[6]

STRUCTURAL FEATURES

Progressive growth of the hyperplastic nodules leads to their coalescence into lobes that compress the outer prostate into a false, or "surgical," capsule. At operation, the hypertrophied lobes can be shelled out of this capsule with ease. The enlarged prostate varies considerably in size and consistency, depending on the relative amounts of glandular and fibromuscular components. Franks has described five types of hyperplastic nodules: stromal (fibrous or fibrovascular); fibromuscular; muscular (leiomyoma), an uncommon type; fibroadenomatous; and fibromyoepithelial, the most common type.[3] To these, Mostofi and Thomson have added a sixth type, the purely adenomatous.[7]

From the surgical standpoint, it is important to recognize which of the following anatomic types of prostatic obstruction is present:

1. Contracture of the bladder outlet
2. Median bar
3. Median lobe hypertrophy (when large, this elevates and may compress the lower ends of the ureters)
4. Lateral lobe hypertrophy, intraurethral in location (bilobar type)
5. Combined median and lateral lobe hypertrophy (trilobar type)
6. Subcervical (pedunculated, arises from the prostatic urethra and projects through the bladder neck, acting like a ball valve)
7. Subtrigonal
8. Anterior commissural hypertrophy (seldom seen)

Operative Procedure

The perineum, external genitalia, abdomen, and upper halves of both thighs are shaved the night before surgery. Cleansing enemas are given until the returns are clear. When varicose veins are present, the lower extremities are wrapped snugly with elastic bandages to midthigh.

Either spinal or general anesthesia can be used. Caudal block is also acceptable. With general anesthesia, tracheal intubation ensures adequate respiratory exchange.

The genitalia are cleansed thoroughly, after which cystoscopy is performed. The entire operative area from costal margins to midthigh is then painted with skin antiseptic. Bilateral vas ligation is carried out.

Perfect positioning is essential for the perineal operation. The patient is placed in the exaggerated lithotomy position on any ordinary operating table (Fig. 86-6). (We do not use the Young perineal table any longer because it has proved too uncomfortable for the patient.) Sandbags are placed beneath the sacrum to position the perineum as close to horizontal as possible. The table is then elevated to bring the operative area up to the level of the operator's chest. This makes the operation a good deal easier and improves visualization considerably. The perineum can usually be positioned adequately without resort to the Trendelenburg position, but occasionally a slight Trendelenburg position may be necessary. Under *no* circumstances should shoulder braces be used, for fear of postoperative brachial palsy. All other points where pressure is likely (*e.g.*, popliteal areas) are carefully padded.

The curved Lowsley tractor is passed through the urethra and held upright without opening the blades (Fig. 86-7). A curved skin incision is made approximately 1 cm from the anal margin. The anus is excluded from the operative field by covering it with a towel secured by three Allis clamps to the posterior edge of the incision. Using the index fingers, the ischiorectal fossae are developed

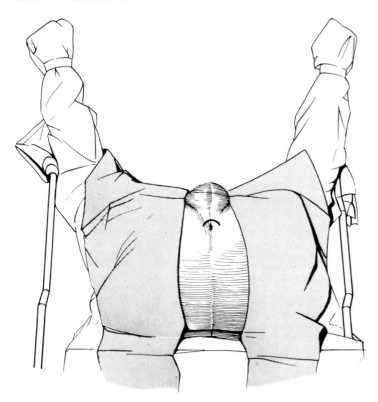

FIG. 86-6. Perineal prostatectomy. Standard operating table is used for exaggerated lithotomy position. Classic inverted-U incision is shown.

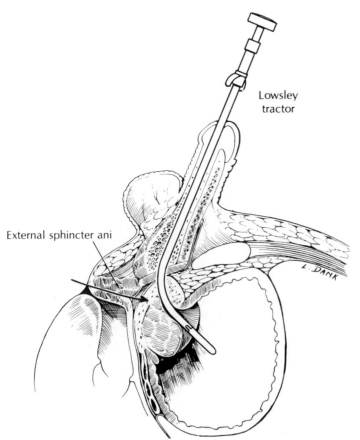

FIG. 86-7. Perineal prostatectomy. Curved Lowsley tractor is in place at the outset of the operation.

Lowsley tractor

External sphincter ani

perpendicular to the plane of the perineum. The central tendon is gently separated from the underlying rectum and cut across distal to the external anal sphincter, taking care not to disturb that structure (Fig. 86-8). A bifid posterior retractor is placed in the ischiorectal fossae, and gentle traction is exerted. The lateral fossae are developed next and held with two small lateral retractors. The rectourethralis muscle is identified and cut (Fig. 86-9).

By carefully incising the pararectal fascia (posterior layer of Denonvilliers), the rectum can be gently peeled posteriorly off the apex of the prostate. The Lowsley tractor is then passed fully into the bladder and the blades are opened. The bifid posterior retractor is replaced by a plain posterior one (the lipped Richardson is useful here), using a moistened pad to protect the rectum. The posterior layer of Denonvilliers' fascia is progressively incised and retracted posteriorly until a window appears through which the anterior layer of Denonvilliers' fascia—the ''pearly gates''—can be seen clearly.

At this point, the operator simultaneously depresses the handle of the Lowsley tractor toward the abdominal wall and exerts firm downward traction on the posterior Richardson retractor (Fig. 86-10). The remaining posterior fascial layer is thereby stripped away from the prostate, which comes clearly into view, now covered only by the glistening anterior layer of Denonvilliers. This is a most effective maneuver but it should not be done before dissection of the posterior fascial layer has been completed at the apex.

An inverted-V or curved prostatotomy is now made, and a plane of cleavage is established with the dissecting scissors (Figs. 86-11 and 86-12). Care is taken to peel back and preserve the posterior flap for subsequent closure of the prostatotomy. The urethra is incised, the curved Lowsley tractor removed, and the regular Young prostatic tractor inserted gently into the bladder through the prostatotomy, using a rotary motion. The blades of the tractor are then opened, the prostate is drawn down, and enucleation is begun.

As soon as possible, the urethra at the apex of the adenoma is cut across with the scissors, thereby facilitating enucleation distally and minimizing the danger of damage to the external urethral sphincter (Fig. 86-12). Enucleation is carried out essentially under direct vision, using the scissors and the finger. Enucleation can sometimes be facilitated by removing the Young tractor and grasping the lobes with forceps that are specially designed for this purpose. The lobes can then be drawn progressively into the operative field. The hypertrophied

lobes are cut away sharply from the bladder neck under direct vision (Fig. 86-13). With care, the bladder neck can be preserved intact, even after removal of a very large adenoma.

After enucleation has been completed, the bladder neck is grasped with Millin T-clamps, which were originally designed for the retropubic oper-

FIG. 86-8. Perineal prostatectomy. After the perineal incision, ischiorectal fossae are developed by blunt dissection. The central tendon of the perineum is isolated. The line of incision is shown.

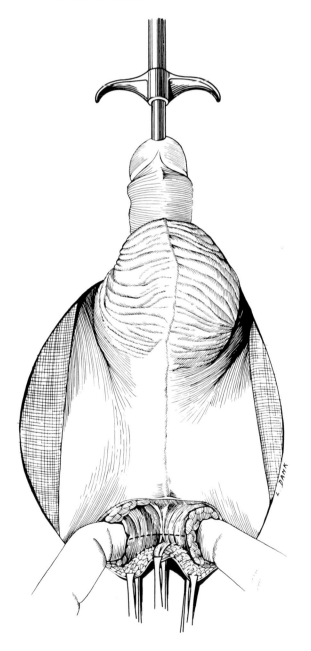

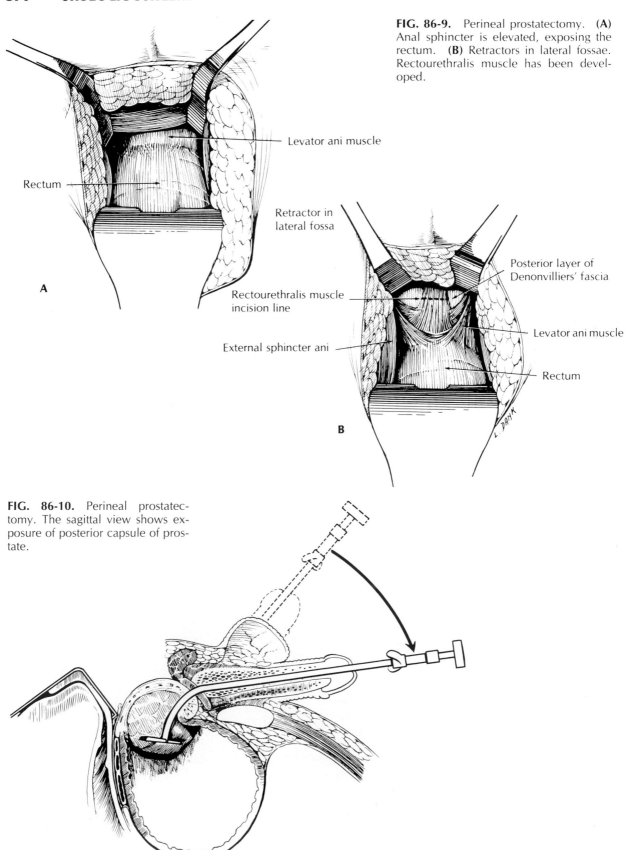

FIG. 86-9. Perineal prostatectomy. **(A)** Anal sphincter is elevated, exposing the rectum. **(B)** Retractors in lateral fossae. Rectourethralis muscle has been developed.

Levator ani muscle

Rectum

A

Retractor in lateral fossa

Rectourethralis muscle incision line

External sphincter ani

Posterior layer of Denonvilliers' fascia

Levator ani muscle

Rectum

B

FIG. 86-10. Perineal prostatectomy. The sagittal view shows exposure of posterior capsule of prostate.

ation. These have the advantage of being offset so that one can obtain an unimpeded view of the bladder neck (Fig. 86-14). A careful search is made for bleeding vessels (especially at 5 and 7 o'clock). Smaller ones are controlled effectively by electrocoagulation. Larger arteries require mattress sutures of 2-0 plain catgut. The interior of the bladder is explored with the finger, and any blood clots are removed. The entire prostatic fossa is inspected carefully for residual adenomatous tissue. Remaining tags of tissue are trimmed away from the bladder neck.

A 22Fr Foley catheter is passed through the urethra and into the bladder, where the bag is inflated with 30 ml to 45 ml of water. The bladder neck, which feels like a soft cervical os dilated to about 1 finger-width, will retain the bag nicely. Wedge resection of the posterior lip is generally unnecessary. If desired, a three-way Foley catheter

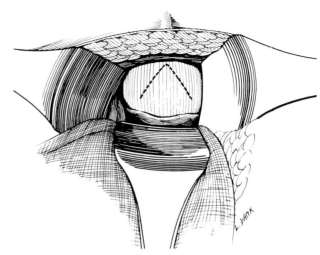

FIG. 86-11. Perineal prostatectomy. The usual inverted-V capsulotomy is used in perineal enucleation.

FIG. 86-12. Perineal prostatectomy. **(A)** Enucleation of an adenoma is initiated by developing a cleavage plane between capsule and adenoma. **(B)** An incision is made into the prostatic urethra. Young's tractor is placed into the bladder, enabling mobilization of the adenoma and amputation of the urethra at the apex.

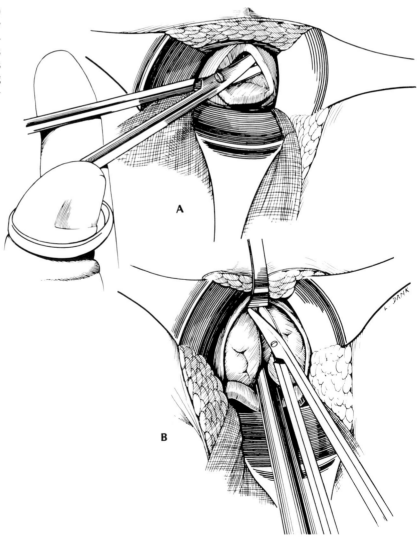

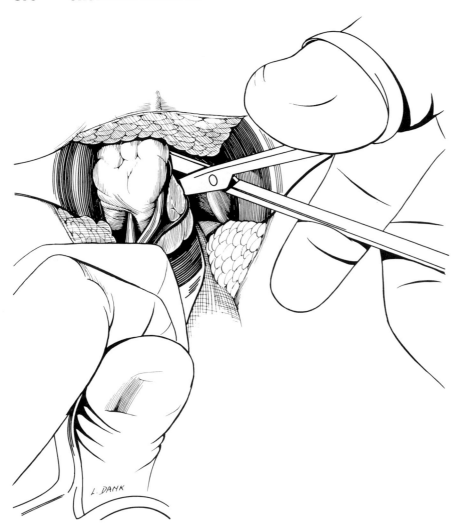

FIG. 86-13. Perineal prostatectomy. Adenoma is freed from the bladder neck by blunt and sharp dissection.

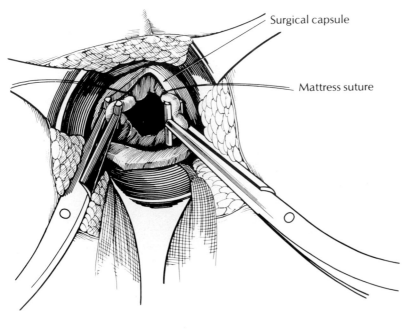

FIG. 86-14. Perineal prostatectomy. The vesical neck is grasped and drawn down with Millin T-clamps, enabling hemostatic mattress sutures to be placed.

Surgical capsule

Mattress suture

may be used to permit through-and-through irrigations postoperatively.

Closure is simple. The edges of the prostatotomy are approximated with interrupted 2-0 chromic catgut sutures (Fig. 86-15). The rectum is inspected for possible injury. No effort is made to bring the levator ani fibers together. A Penrose drain is left in the retroprostatic space. Skin edges are approximated with interrupted fine cotton or silk sutures (Fig. 86-16). A simple dressing is applied to the wound, using a split T-binder. The lower extremities are brought down simultaneously and gradually. Too-rapid depositioning may result in hypotension because of the sudden rush of blood into the legs, particularly if they have not been wrapped preoperatively.

Excessive bleeding is seldom encountered during perineal prostatectomy. If care is taken to obtain adequate exposure, bleeding vessels can usually be identified and secured without difficulty. The only other complication that may occur during the operation is laceration of the rectum, readily recognized from the characteristic appearance of the rectal mucosa. The injury should be completely mobilized and repaired with interrupted 4-0 chromic catgut sutures placed so that the mucosal edges are inverted. The muscularis should be closed in two additional layers, again using interrupted sutures of 4-0 chromic catgut.

If the injury is recognized *before* the urinary tract is opened, it is best to close the perineal incision and enucleate the gland through a suprapubic incision. If the rectal injury is not appreciated until *after* the urinary tract has been entered, the laceration should be repaired meticulously, as just outlined. Postoperatively, the patient should be maintained on a low-residue diet, and bowel activity should be completely suppressed with paregoric for 7 days.

POSTOPERATIVE CHANGES

After removal of the hypertrophied lobes, the raw surfaces of the prostatic fossa soon reepithelialize.

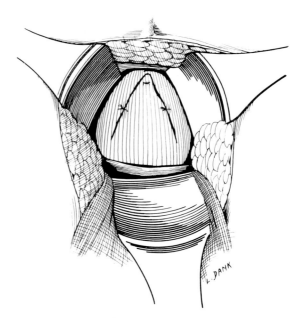

FIG. 86-15. Perineal prostatectomy. The surgical capsule is closed with interrupted sutures.

FIG. 86-16. Perineal prostatectomy; closure of muscles and subcutaneous fat of perineum. Penrose drain is left indwelling, and skin edges are approximated with interrupted sutures.

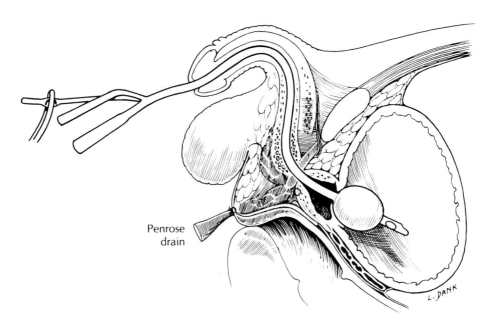

Penrose
drain

The compressed outer prostate (prostate proper, or surgical capsule) eventually reexpands to normal size. Scattered areas of induration usually persist indefinitely and can be detected by rectal palpation.

POSTOPERATIVE CARE

If a regular Foley catheter has been used, it is simply attached to straight bedside drainage. From time to time, gentle manual irrigation may be carried out to keep the system free of clots. The catheter is secured to the thigh, but no traction is necessary. If a three-way catheter has been used, it is attached to a through-and-through irrigating system containing sterile saline solution, which is run in just rapidly enough to keep the efflux reasonably clear. The patient is given appropriate antibiotics. Fluids may be given by mouth during the first day, and they are customarily supplemented by intravenous infusions to maintain a satisfactory intake.

The perineal Penrose drain is usually removed on the first postoperative day. At this time, the patient may be placed on a soft or regular diet and allowed out of bed. Early ambulation is encouraged.

The skin sutures are removed on the sixth or seventh day. Usually, the perineal wound heals benignly, but sometimes partial separation of the skin edges may occur. Healing may be promoted by removal of the dressing and exposure to a heat lamp. Warm sitz baths are also effective.

The urethral catheter is removed between the seventh and tenth postoperative days. Not infrequently, urinary leakage may occur from the wound for a day or two after the catheter has been taken out. If it continues longer than this, an 18Fr 5-ml Foley catheter may be reinserted for a day or two. Care must be taken in passing the catheter to be certain it does not curl up in the prostatic fossa. Sometimes a stylet is helpful, with the aid of a finger in the rectum.

It is extremely important during the immediate postoperative period that no rectal instrumentation be performed. No thermometers or rectal tubes should be inserted; this must be made clear to the nursing staff.

About 10% of patients experience some urinary incontinence for a few days after removal of the catheter. This disappears rapidly in the vast majority, but up to 6 months may be required for complete cessation of leakage in the occasional patient. Permanent incontinence is highly uncommon after uneventful perineal prostatectomy.

Persistent perineal urinary fistula has been feared by those unfamiliar with perineal surgery. Actually, this complication is rarely seen. Its occurrence should lead one to suspect some form of urethral obstruction, for example, a postoperative stricture. Occasionally, a stricture of the urethra may develop postoperatively. A single, gentle dilation with a urethral sound usually suffices to take care of this. Postoperative stenosis of the bladder neck is highly unusual.

If unexplained fever or signs of sepsis develop, the urethral catheter should be removed promptly. If this occurs early in the postoperative period, it is likely that profuse urinary leakage will continue from the perineal wound, necessitating intensive nursing care to keep the patient as comfortable as possible. Surprisingly enough, patients from whom the catheter has had to be removed prematurely, or from whom the catheter has inadvertently slipped out, may begin voiding satisfactorily as early as the second or third day.

Other complications such as vasitis, epididymitis, thrombophlebitis involving the lower extremities, pulmonary embolism, myocardial infarction, and cerebrovascular accidents occur about as frequently after perineal as after other types of prostatectomy.

REFERENCES

1. BELT E, EBERT CE, SURBER AC, JR: A new anatomic approach in perineal prostatectomy. J Urol 41:482, 1939
2. FLOCKS RH: The arterial distribution within the prostate gland: Its role in transurethral prostatic resection. J Urol 37:524, 1937
3. FRANKS LM: Benign nodular hyperplasia of the prostate: A review. Ann R Coll Surg Engl 14:92, 1954
4. GIBSON TE: George E. Goodfellow (1855–1910). Invest Urol 7:107, 1969
5. GOODFELLOW GE: Median perineal prostatectomy. JAMA 43:194, 1904
6. MORGAGNI GB: The Seats and Causes of Disease Investigated by Anatomy, Book 3. London, Johnson & Payne, 1760
7. MOSTOFI FK, THOMSON RV: Benign hyperplasia of the prostate gland. In Campbell MF (ed): Urology, p 1101. Philadelphia, W B Saunders, 1963
8. TOBIN CE, BENJAMIN JA: Anatomical and surgical restudy of Denonvilliers' fascia. Surg Gynecol Obstet 80:373, 1945
9. YOUNG HH: Benign hypertrophy of the prostate. In Young's Practice of Urology, Vol I, p 417. Philadelphia, W B Saunders, 1926
10. YOUNG HH: Surgery of the prostate. In Keen's Surgery, Vol IV, p 372. Philadelphia, W B Saunders, 1912

Principles of Electrosurgery

87

David W. Goddard

*E*lectrosurgery is the technique that uses appropriately developed and modified radio-frequency electric currents to cut tissues and control bleeding.[19] Electrosurgical generators and the accessories used with them continue to be improved and to become more sophisticated. Yet the manifold electrical apparatuses, especially various monitoring devices used by anesthesiologists, still provide potential hazards to the patient undergoing electrosurgery.[21,23,25] A simple understanding of the electrophysics, potential hazards, and necessary safety factors involved certainly is required, in order for the surgeon to be able to use electrosurgical techniques effectively and with maximum safety.

Basic Electrical Principles

As indicated in Table 87-1, one electrical stimulation of nerve or muscle per second causes an individual contraction of the muscle; at 15 stimulations/second, the response is clonic; at 40 stimulations, the muscle is in painful tetany; at more than 2500/second, tetany remains maximal to about 5000 stimulations/second but pain begins to disappear; by 15,000 stimulations/second, all responses have vanished other than the production of heat in the tissues.

Theoretically, one could use frequencies in the millions per second for electrosurgery, and there was a period when many investigators claimed outstanding characteristics for several specific high frequencies. However, current frequencies above 10 million cycles per second (10 MHz) tend not to remain confined to the cords designed to transport them and jump to the operator applying the current or to other conductors. This makes it virtually impossible to obtain proper control with ultrahigh frequencies. Present electrosurgical devices use frequencies somewhere in the range of 300,000 to 2,000,000 Hertz (300 KHz to 2 MHz). These large amounts of electrical energy may be passed safely through the body without producing any effect other than heat and without losing control of the current.

Electrical production of heat depends on the quantity of current flowing and the resistance offered to its flow. The heat produced in tissue is the direct result of the resistance offered by the tissue to the passage of the current. This principle is involved in both medical diathermy and electrosurgery. Figure 87-1 is a graphic comparison of the principles of medical diathermy and electrosurgery.

When large electrodes of approximately equal size are used to bracket a certain part of the body, the current density is quite evenly dispersed within the intervening tissue, and an increase in tissue temperature is produced that provides the beneficial effects of heat without sufficient concentration of heat anywhere to cause cell injury; this is *medical diathermy*. On the other hand, when one electrode is large and the other one is small enough, the current no longer is evenly dispersed but becomes sufficiently dense to cause cell destruction where the small electrode is applied; this is the application of *surgical diathermy* or, more properly, *electrosurgery*. The small electrode is called the *active electrode* and the large one is called the *indifferent electrode*, *return electrode*, or *patient plate*.

It is important to recognize that, except for current leakage, current division to monitors or other ground locations, or capacitive coupling, the same amount of current passes through both electrodes, but heat is generated at the patient plate. The difference at the two electrodes is simply a difference in current density and not a difference in total current.

Bipolar electrosurgery is a specialized technique in which two essentially identical small electrodes are used in close proximity to each other. As the radio-frequency current alternates, the two electrodes alternate between being active and indifferent electrodes. The current path and surgical activity is limited to the volume of tissue between and immediately surrounding each electrode. Typ-

TABLE 87-1. Electrical Stimulations Per Second

Stimulations/Second	Muscle Response
1	One contraction
15	Clonic contraction
40	Painful tetany
2500–5000	Tetany, progressively less pain
15,000 and up	Only heat in tissues

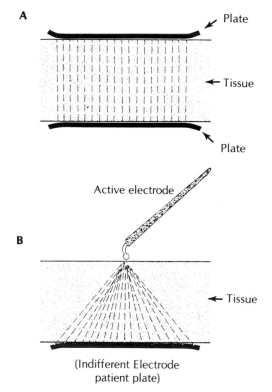

FIG. 87-1. Principles of diathermy: **(A)** medical diathermy, dispersing electrical energy through tissue, **(B)** surgical diathermy, with maximal electrical activity at the active electrode

ically, the two electrodes are tines of a bipolar forcep, which are used to affect relatively small amounts of tissue. The surgical effect is generally limited to dessication or simply denaturization of the tissue through heating, although sparking and carbonization can occur in some instances. This technique lends itself to the delicate control by coagulation of bleeding from small vessels; there is no danger of tissue injury elsewhere because no separate or remote return electrode is used and the current path is limited to the short distance between the two bipolar electrodes. To date, no successful cutting bipolar electrode has been made.

Neurosurgeons and plastic surgeons most commonly use bipolar techniques, but there is no reason why the advantages and inherent safety of bipolar electrosurgery cannot be used by all surgeons for delicate, small-vessel electrocoagulation. Many modern electrosurgical generators offer the connection of both monopolar and bipolar accessories simultaneously and so expand the applicability of the bipolar technique.

Radio frequencies are capable of being modulated; thus, it is possible to produce many different wave forms, all of which may have different effects upon tissues. The *wave form* refers to the graphic representation of the relationship between an electrical current and time. The *oscilloscope* is the instrument used to display the visual appearance of the wave form. Alternating electrosurgical currents reverse their direction of flow thousands of times a second, tracing a sinusoidal line on the oscilloscope that is the wave form. When the current is modulated, the oscilloscope also displays the modulation wave form (Fig. 87-2). Generally speaking, alternating electrical currents that trace a symmetric, continuous wave form at radio frequency on the oscilloscope are good cutting currents. Conversely, similar currents that are interrupted in some manner are good coagulating currents.

DEVELOPMENT OF ELECTROSURGICAL GENERATORS

The earliest and simplest radio-frequency, alternating-current generators employed the principle of capacitor discharge across a spark gap to an inductive coil. This type of oscillator produces what is known as a *damped wave form,* that is, with each capacitor discharge a series of oscillations is set up between the coil and the capacitor. The voltage peak of the first oscillation is the highest and each subsequent oscillation is diminished through energy loss down to the point where the spark gap opens, breaking the circuit; after this one process is repeated. This damping or fading of the wave form produces *interruption* of the current, a characteristic commonly required for coagulation or hemostasis (Fig. 87-3).

The main objection to spark gap-generated currents is that they have relatively high peak voltage ranging from 6,000 to 12,000 volts for cutting and coagulating; this destroys more tissue than is appropriate or necessary in accomplishing hemostasis.

Clark, in 1911, used a high-voltage electrostatic generator in a spark gap-tuned circuit unit; he apparently was the first individual to use radio-

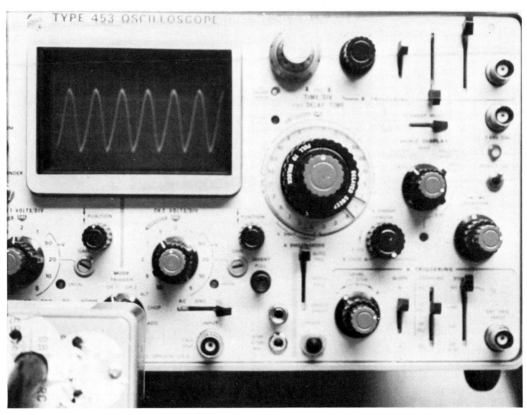

FIG. 87-2.   The oscilloscope provides visual demonstration of a pure sine wave form.

frequency current to cut and coagulate living tissue.[6] He not only initiated these techniques on readily available superficial lesions such as warts, granulations, pigmentations, tattoos, and so on, but also described treatment of a bladder papilloma aided by the catheterizing cystoscope.

De Forest's invention of the vacuum tube led not only to the development of radio, but also to a new kind of electrosurgical generator because he demonstrated that undamped, radio-frequency alternating currents produced by the vacuum tube have the ability to cut tissue. Although Bovie, Liebel, Flarsheim, Cushing, and McLean played important roles in the early development of electrosurgery; Wappler, Stern, McCarthy, Baumrucker, Nesbit, and Iglesias had much to do with the development and improvement of resectoscopic equipment.[3,5,8,17,18,24,26] Men such as Alyea, Alcock, Barnes, and Valk helped immensely to popularize transurethral prostatic and bladder tumor resection. However, it was Theodore M. Davis, a urologist from Greenville, South Carolina, who, with unbelievable skill and perseverance, perfected the techniques and equipment of both resectoscopes and electrosurgical generators that made modern-day transurethral surgery possible.[10,11]

Davis, above all, truly deserves the title Father of Transurethral Surgury.[12]

For the most part tube-generated, radio-frequency, alternating currents have been used exclusively for their excellent cutting qualities. However, it is important to point out that, unless something specific is done in the electronic circuitry to change the situation, all these currents take place within a 60-cycle envelope of the wall of line current with which they started. This fact is very significant and explains why the tube-generated current of the Bovie and other older units, as well as the cutting currents of many of the newer solid-state generators, have a definite coagulating effect: the 60-Hz current *interrupts* the radio-frequency current 120 times a second.[16]

Until recent years virtually all available electrosurgical generators provided an unrectified and unfiltered cutting current. That is to say, they provided (1) a tube-generated current wrapped in a 60-cycle envelope, a cutting current of a closely packed damped wave train from a spark gap generator, or both; and (2) a coagulating current of interrputed, damped waves from a spark gap generator. Gradually during the past decade improvements have been made in electrosurgical

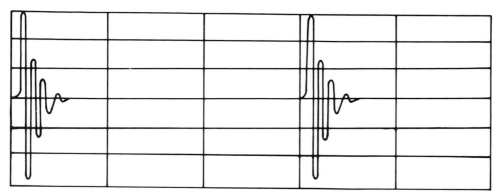

Spark gap coagulation waveform

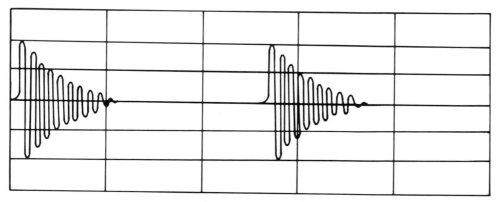

Spark gap cutting waveform

FIG. 87-3. Vertical, approximately 2kv/div; horizontal, approximately 10 μsec/div

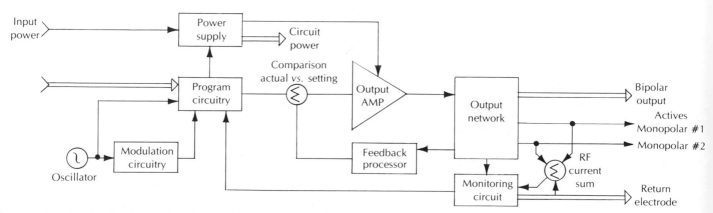

FIG. 87-4. Stock diagram of a modern electrosurgical generator.

generator design that reduce the size, increase the reliability and safety, and change the surgical behavior of the radio-frequency currents. Most designs use various solid-state technologies to generate the output current and use integrated circuits to control it internally. A great variety of specific techniques continue to be used in circuitry; the specific mechanization probably is of little consequence so long as the equipment capabilities match the intended application (Fig. 87-4).

The newer units provide the proper quality of currents at adequate but significantly lower voltages, all under good control. They cut and coagulate at about 500 to 2000 peak voltage, compared to the extremely high voltage of the spark gap generator; it follows that these units should produce less tissue damage per unit of use time. Given that the most important factor in producing coagulation or hemostasis is interruption of the current, it is fairly simple to interrupt the radio-frequency current in many ways. Various methods of wave form modulation are used, which react in a similar manner to the varying degree of wave form damping of spark gap equipment to produce cutting, coagulation, and blended currents. Virtually any wave form, along with precisely controlled voltage, can now be produced electronically, and there are

excellent solid-state generators now that cut and coagulate superbly well.

The "sharpest" cutting currrent one can use is that of a pure *uninterrupted* symmetrical wave form; these wave forms are very good for open surgery but are not the ones of choice for transurethral surgery because they produce no hemostasis (Fig. 87-5). Vacuum tube or solid-state generated pure sine waves are identical and fortunately, unless modified, are "wrapped in the envelope" of the 60-cycle line current. As noted, this envelope provides a certain element of hemostasis in the "pure" cutting currents as we know them, making the amount of bleeding tolerable until it can be controlled completely by a coagulating current. *Blended currents* are cutting currents that are specifically modulated to produce greater degrees of hemostasis than would be provided by the 60-Hz envelope alone.

Safety Considerations

Although modern surgery as we know it, in almost all disciplines, would not be possible without electrosurgery, there are inherent dangers in the use of electric currents of which the surgeon must be aware.[7,9] In the ever-increasing sophistication of the electrical environment in the operating room,

FIG. 87-5. Presently available wave forms. Electrosurgical units can provide various wave forms for cutting and coagulation. Manufacturer's representatives are able to demonstrate and explain the particular wave forms offered by respective electrosurgical units.

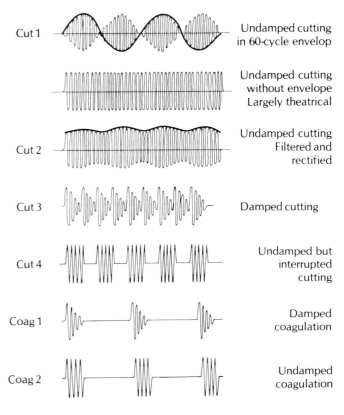

Cut 1 — Undamped cutting in 60-cycle envelop

Undamped cutting without envelope Largely theatrical

Cut 2 — Undamped cutting Filtered and rectified

Cut 3 — Damped cutting

Cut 4 — Undamped but interrupted cutting

Coag 1 — Damped coagulation

Coag 2 — Undamped coagulation

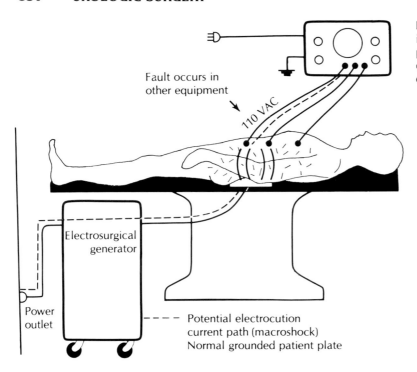

FIG. 87-6. Macroshock. An electrical fault in monitoring equipment may provide the potential for injury owing to dispersion of current through ground sites other than the electrosurgical unit.

Fault occurs in other equipment

110 VAC

Electrosurgical generator

Power outlet

--- Potential electrocution current path (macroshock)
Normal grounded patient plate

surgeons must be concerned with two different currents, the low-frequency line current from the power company and the radio-frequency current produced by the electrosurgical generator. Low-frequency current can produce shock, cause cardiac arrest, and kill. Radio-frequency current can produce burns.[20]

Most ground-referenced electrosurgical units made today and in the recent past have capacitive coupling between the return electrode connection and ground. Capacitive coupling prevents the significant conduction of low-frequency currents from whatever source to ground by way of the patient plate. When many electronic devices are connected to a patient, any one of the devices can develop a fault and become a source of low-frequency current.

Unfortunately, no matter how well an electrosurgical unit is designed and produced, it cannot always protect the patient from injury by low-frequency current introduced from another source, such as a monitoring apparatus (Fig. 87-6). Indeed, when one is using an electrosurgical unit that is designed to flow its radio-frequency current to power ground, the patient lying on a well-grounded patient plate and connected to another electrical apparatus is, according to one comparison, like a person using a two-wire electric shaver while sitting in a bathtub full of saline. The primary responsibility for the protection of the patient from

macroshock under this condition must lie with the designers and producers of the various electrical appliances other than the electrosurgical generator. Electrical isolation of these other electrical devices seems to be a good way to discharge this responsibility. To a considerable extent, this is being done not only with conventional methods, including the use of battery powered monitors, but also with more sophisticated telemetry monitors.

Unlike low-frequency currents, radio-frequency currents are not necessarily easy to control. When radio-frequency current flows through a wire, that wire has both electrostatic (capacitive coupling) and electromagnetic (inductive coupling) fields of electrical energy surrounding it. There is a constant need for meticulous attention to detail when the patient is the center of a highly complex field of electrical energy. Cardiac pacemakers constitute a special concern.[14] Radio-frequency safety consists of the prevention of burns either at the patient plate site or at sites remote from either the intended active electrode site or the patient plate.

Return electrode, radio-frequency safety basically is dependent upon proper selection and application of the patient plate. There is no question that *the most common cause of patient burns at sites other than the active electrode is either misapplication or faulty construction of the patient plate.*[2] There has been extensive work done recently on return electrodes. Urologic electrosurgical procedures, espe-

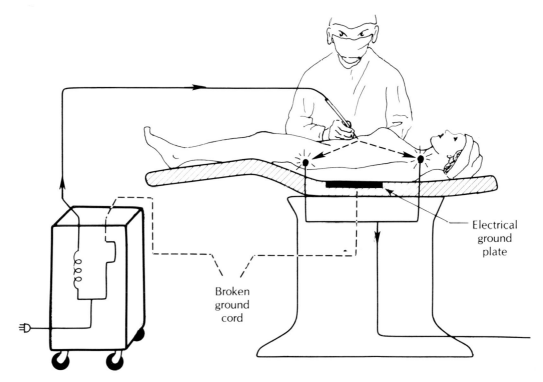

FIG. 87-7. Broken ground cord. If cord-to-patient plate is broken, high-frequency current would seek and flow to other ground locations such as monitoring devices, resulting in burn or other injury.

cially the transurethral resection (TUR), draw large radio-frequency currents; the selection and application of return electrodes that will definitely provide low temperature rise are especially critical in these procedures.

All older electrosurgical units and some of the new ones flow radio-frequency currents to power ground, and the patient plate is the designated connection of the patient to ground. If a broken cord or some other mishap disrupts the connection of the patient to ground in a grounded system, the electrosurgical current will seek the path of least resistance to ground, wherever it may be (Fig. 87-7). The current may flow through a point where the patient is in contact with the operating table; it may flow through monitoring electrodes; it may even flow through the surgeon or the anesthesiologist.

Several approaches presently are being taken by different manufacturers to try to solve or manage the problem of ectopic (alternate path) flow of radio-frequency currents to ground locations other than that provided by the patient plate. An early approach used the principle of a two-wire monitor between the patient plate and the electrosurgical

generator to ensure the integrity of the patient plate connection to ground, on the assumption that the current would not flow through other ground connections if the one provided by the patient plate was functioning correctly. The validity of this assumption may be questionable if monitoring electrodes or other contacts with ground from the patient are in a position closer to the active electrode than is the patient plate. Further, for this approach to solve the problem of ectopic current flow, the monitoring system must be failproof, a condition not necessarily true of the early monitors, but one that is correctable by updating.

"Total circuit monitors" have been used to some extent. Here a presumably innocuous monitoring signal is passed into the patient from the active electrode and also through the return electrode. This type of monitor verifies that there is some circuit present, but it does not give data on the adequacy of the circuit to carry the radio-frequency current load and it is not sensitive to the quality of the return electrode's connection.

In at least one widely marketed modern electrosurgical generator, ectopic current is directly measured and controlled. In this design, current emanating from the active electrode is compared with current flowing through the patient return electrode. If the difference is more than a nominal amount, an alert is generated, indicating that a burn hazard may be present at an alternating-path contact site such as a stirrup, resectoscope body, or a monitoring electrode.

The use of such a system provides obvious safety advantages for the operator and patient; however, certain precautions must be taken to ensure trouble-free performance. A large-area, low-impedance return electrode placed close to the site of surgery will ensure that the return electrode is the dominant current path and will discourage current division. The patient should be well insulated from grounded objects such as the table and stirrups. Some sort of isolation system for the ECG monitor should be used. When steps are taken so that "normal" requirements are satisfied, this system has been shown to provide superior protection against divided-current path burns.

A very recent series of developments has culminated in monitoring systems that use a patient plate divided into two or more parts. These systems make the patient a part of the monitoring circuitry which, in turn, ensures the integrity of the connection between the patient and the patient plate. Different systems allow such monitoring using resistance or capacitance; however, the concept in either case is to ensure the adequate connection of a return electrode to the patient's body.

It goes without saying that alternative-site, radio-frequency safety begins with the user.[1] The active electrode produces lesions at intended points within an incision and may produce lesions at unintended points remote from the incision if "hot" active electrodes are permitted to stray from the surgical site. This is particularly important to recognize when multiple active electrodes are connected to a single electrosurgical generator. Some designs allow only single or individually keyed electrodes to be "hot" at any given instant; these are recommended. If use of multiple active electrodes is contemplated, the surgeon should consult the manufacturer's manuals to determine specific equipment behavior under these conditions. The use of insulating holsters for unused electrosurgical accessories is a good idea in any case.

Radio-frequency current return division is a possibility in any electrosurgical procedure; this phenomenon is dependent in part upon equipment design and is probably best discouraged by electrical isolation techniques. Certain contact sites with the patient, other than the patient plate, may invite division of return to the generator of the high-frequency current; this is particularly true of

generators that are referenced to power ground. The "extra" contact site with the patient may not be well suited to conducting the current and, in some cases, extreme heating may occur. Components sensitive to division or return current flow are as follows:

1. *ECG electrodes*—Large surface-area electrodes, never needle electrodes, should be used. Commercially available ECG choke cables or electrically isolated or telemetrized ECG equipment should eliminate any problems in this regard.

2. *Grounded patient supports,* such as knee stirrups, may conduct significant currents; however, their relatively large area of contact usually keeps the current density low enough to avoid injury. Other patient contacts with ground may not be so forgiving.

3. *Insulation on active accessories*—Resectoscopes may be particularly sensitive. Insulation blocks should be of modern design and should be checked regularly. Loop insulation can be a problem, leading to conduction of radio-frequency current to the body of the scope with resulting urethral injury. It might be worth noting again that the surgeon can be affected by these extra or divided-current return paths, and burns to the surgeon's eye area have been reported.

Various other designs have been invoked to reduce the chance of significant division of current return flow; perhaps the most significant of these is *electrical isolation* of the electrosurgical generator. A battery probably is the best example of electrical isolation. It is common knowledge that an electric current flows from the positive pole of a battery only when it can flow to the negative pole of the same battery. Theoretically, in an electrically isolated electrosurgical generator, the radio-frequency current flows through the patient only to its own patient plate. It does not flow to ground and, if it cannot flow to its own patient plate, it simply does not work and no current flows. Furthermore, the patient plate of an electrically isolated electrosurgical system does not act as a "saline-filled bathtub" connection to power ground and does not serve as a pathway for the flow to ground of current entering the patient from other electrical devices.

Unfortunately, electrical isolation is not an absolute term. That is, it is possible for an electrosurgical system to be well-isolated or to be poorly isolated, but not to be completely isolated. Only a well-isolated system provides the degree of safety for the patient that we want.

The big problem in electrical isolation of radio-frequency current generators is capacitive coupling, which is caused by the electrostatic field produced by the flow of radio-frequency current. Capacitive coupling results in a leakage path to ground of a certain fraction of the radio-frequency current. This fraction, if sufficiently large, can cause burns.

The answer to this problem is to be found in superior design and quality production aimed at keeping the flow to the patient plate as large as possible and the leakage to ground as small as possible. Theoretically, there always will be some leakage to ground from capacitive coupling. However, electrically isolated electrosurgical systems with very small amounts of leakage are presently available. The current in these systems does not produce burns unless it is concentrated into a very small ground contact area such as would be provided by needle electrodes for patient monitoring; of course, it is common knowledge now that needle electrodes should not be used.

Essentially the same amount of radio-frequency current that flows into the patient at the active electrode flows out of the patient at the return electrode or patient plate. The difference is that the current density is highly concentrated at the active electrode but widely dispersed at the patient plate. It is important to remember that heat is generated at the patient plate. Blood, flowing through the tissues that are in contact with the patient plate, serves as a "heat sink," taking this heat away and cooling the tissue. Anything that tends to compromise blood flow to these tissues interferes with the cooling effect and could lead to tissue damage. This type of injury can occur if the nurse or orderly tries to shove or force a patient plate under the buttocks of a patient who has not been lifted clear of the table, particularly an older patient with loose, redundant skin over the buttocks. Such a maneuver can cause an overfolding of the skin, leading to both ischemic injury and a burn. The patient always should be lifted clear of the table and placed down directly and evenly on the patient plate when this type of return electrode is being used.

Thermal injuries at the patient plate also can occur whenever the patient plate is applied to the patient in such a way that does not ensure a broad contact between the patient and the plate.[4] If a bent or wrinkled plate is used or an adhesive plate is not applied properly, the uneven contact with the patient may produce areas of current density high enough to cause injury.

For years I have felt that a large patient plate beneath the buttocks offered the highest margin of return electrode safety; however, a very well-presented, thought-provoking paper by Gedron, a clinical engineer, has made me pause to consider.[15]

Gedron points out that many postoperative lesions thought to be burns are not burns at all but rather decubitus, pressure necroses. As previously pointed out, overfolding of skin and perhaps just prolonged direct pressure beneath a patient plate (called "shearing forces" by Gedron and previously discussed by Dinsdale[13] and Reichel[22] certainly can compromise circulation; they can not only lead to ischemic changes themselves but can also make the involved tissues more susceptible to thermal injury. It may very well be, especially in instances in which the surgery is prolonged (more than 2 hours), that a well-designed, well-produced, and properly applied adhesive patient plate may be better than a large patient plate (Fig. 87-8).

Smooth, undamaged, unwrinkled patient plates and monitoring electrodes of large surface area (to provide low current density) always should be used. Adhesive patient plates should be applied in strict compliance with the manufacturer's printed instructions. The patient plate (*i.e.*, primary and selected return electrode) should be placed closer than any monitoring electrodes to the area where the active electrode is to be used. Patient plates that have a large surface area and are disposable after one use seem to be best. All cords for the conduction of radio-frequency current should be in good condition; here again disposable, one-time use cords probably are best.

Dos and Don'ts

Certain simple precautions should be observed by the urologic surgeon to ensure maximal patient safety, minimal surgical complications, and the desired efficacy of both endoscopic and open electrosurgical procedures.

DOS

1. Learn to use and be competent with one integrated electrosurgical system; this should include familiarity with the manufacturer's printed operating instructions.
2. Make certain that all cords connecting the electrosurgical unit to the wall current, to the working element (active electrode), and to the patient plate are in good repair. Reusable cords should be checked before each use with an ohmmeter to ensure their integrity; disposable cords may obviate problems. Resectoscope blocks and loops should be tested similarly.
3. Use a patient plate of large surface area. Be sure the plate is not bent or wrinkled. Follow carefully the manufacturer's instructions when using adhesive patient plates. Disposable one-time use plates help to avoid problems.

FIG. 87-8.   Damaged ground or patient plate.   **(A)** The ideal patient plate is of large size, providing maximal contact area for dispersion of current density and heating effect.   **(B)** Wrinkled, bent, or otherwise deformed ground plates may minimize contact area, leading to localization of high-current density and potential tissue injury.   **(C)** ''Tenting'' of an adhesive return electrode results in inadequate surface contact with the patient. Improper application of the adhesive return electrode may permit this condition to occur.

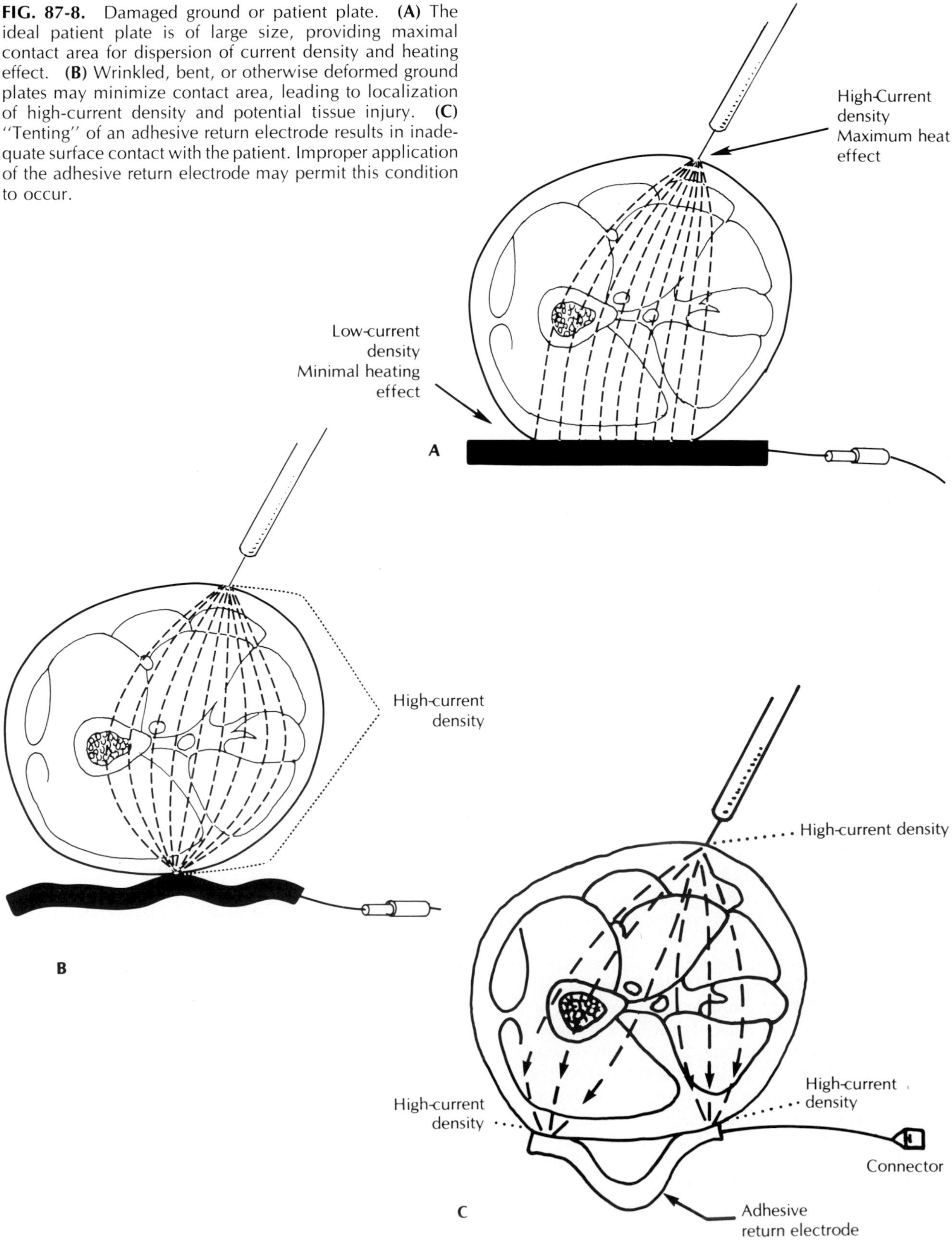

High-Current density
Maximum heat effect

Low-current density
Minimal heating effect

A

High-current density

B

High-current density

High-current density

High-current density

Connector

Adhesive return electrode

C

4. Use a modern, highly conductive gel between the patient and the patient plate. Most modern adhesive disposable patient plates have their own highly conductive gel incorporated into their structure.

5. Consider and discuss with your hospital safety engineer the possibility of using low-frequency electrical isolation techniques with all electrical equipment in your operating room.

6. If you are using an older electrosurgical system that has a patient plate continuity monitor, consult with the manufacturer to be sure that any recommended improvements in the monitoring system have been incorporated into your equipment.

7. Determine that there is compatibility between the electrosurgical generator and the patient plate you are using.

8. Use nonconductive lubricants in the urethra for transurethral electrosurgical procedures. Mineral oil and petroleum jelly are very satisfactory.

9. Use insulated holsters for all active electrodes at open surgery; this is particularly important when multiple active electrodes are in use.

DON'TS

1. Don't use old and untested cords, worn-out or outdated resectoscopic working units, or patient plates that are bent, distorted, or too small.

2. Don't use surgical lubricating jelly as a conductive gel between the patient and the patient plate.

3. Don't allow the skin to be wrinkled or folded under the patient plate.

4. Don't use surgical lubricating jellies to lubricate the urethra for transurethral electrosurgical procedures. These jellies are conductors, if not the best ones, and could encourage division of current to the urethra with resulting injury. However, if the urethra already is scared and strictured and an internal urethrotomy has been done, the objection to surgical lubricating jelly is not so strong, and lubricating jelly might have some theoretical preference.

5. Don't use higher power settings for cutting and coagulation than you need and don't struggle with lower power settings than are required. Start low when learning to use new equipment and increase power gradually until the electrosurgical unit is performing well for you, then go no higher. (All modern solid-state units with which the author has had experience have more than enough power and well-designed wave forms to cut and coagulate well).

6. Don't do a transurethral electrosurgical procedure with a new or unfamiliar electrosurgical system until you have read the manufacturer's instructive manual about it, examined it carefully, and found the answers to any questions you may have about it. An understanding of what to expect from the various available cutting modes (wave forms) probably is most important. Coagulation is not likely to cause any problems once you have learned to be precise in applying the loop for coagulation and have determined the proper power setting for you.

GLOSSARY

(These terms are defined here strictly as they apply to electrosurgery)

Active Electrode–The electrode that is applied to the patient for the purpose of generating a current of high density with significant heating and, therefore, cutting or coagulating ability.

Capacitance–The property of a system of conductors and dielectrics that permits the storage of electrically separated charges when potential differences exist between the conductors.

Capacitive Coupling–The association of two or more circuits with one another by means of mutual capacitance between them.

Capacitor–An electronic element consisting of two electrodes separated by a dielectric, used for introducing capacitance into an electrical circuit.

Coagulate–To denature the protein in tissue by a flow of interrupted radio-frequency current, usually to stop bleeding.

Conductive Gel–A material used to improve electrical conductivity of the return electrode through skin contact.

Current Density–The ratio of current to surface area, *e.g.*, amperes per square centimeter.

Current Division–A characteristic or tendency of electrosurgical current to flow back to the generator or to ground through paths other than the return electrode.

Damped Current–Current that has attenuated and interrupted flow particularly radio-frequency current modulated by a decaying exponential wave form.

Dessicate–To drive water from tissue by heating it with electric current.

Electrical Isolation–An output format in which there is no intentional coupling between the return electrode and the power ground.

Filtered Wave Form–Wave form made to have little modulation and to be uniform. Antithesis–unfiltered, not uniform, especially modulated by a multiple of the line frequency.

Fulgurate–To apply current to tissue through an electric spark or arc.

Hard Grounded–Connected directly to power ground with little or no impedance.

Hz:–Abbreviation of Hertz, a unit of measurement for frequency of alternating current; 1 Hertz is 1 cycle (2 reversals) per second.

Impedance–The total opposition a circuit offers to the flow of alternating current.

Inductance–Property of an electrical circuit that tends to oppose any charge of current because of a magnetic field associated with the current itself.

Inductor–A device used for introducing inductance into an electrical circuit.

Integrated Circuits–Devices in which many circuit elements are combined on a single silicon wafer.

KHz–Abbreviation for Kilo-Hertz, *i.e.*, 1000 alternating cycles per second.

Line Frequency–The frequency of the power line, usually 50 or 60 Hz.

Output Current–Current developed by the electrosurgical generator for the purpose of cutting or coagulating tissue.

Modulation–The process of modifying some characteristic of a radio-frequency wave so that it varies in step with the instantaneous value of another wave, *e.g.*, the power line frequency.

Power Ground–The common conductor in a power distribution system, usually connected to a building structure.

Radiofrequency Current–RF current. Alternating current with a frequency usually between 300 KHz and 10,000 KHz.

Rectified–A quality of voltage or current that has been converted from alternating current to unidirectional or direct current.

Return Electrode–Contact device used to complete the electrosurgical circuit, providing a low current density and minimal heating; also patient plate or indifferent electrode.

Sinusoidal–Varying in proportion to the sine of an angle as a function of time.

To "Sink" Current–To conduct current, usually to ground.

REFERENCES

1. ATKIN DH, ORKIN LR: Electrocution in the operating room. Anesthesiology 38:181, 1973
2. BATTIG CG: Electrosurgical burn injuries and their prevention. JAMA 204:1025, 1968
3. BAUMRUCKER GO: Transurethral Prostatectomy. Baltimore, Williams & Wilkins, 1968
4. BECKER CM, MAEHOTRA IV, HEDLEY-WHYTE J: The distribution of radiofrequency current and burns. Anesthesiology 38:106, 1973
5. BOWIE WT: The comparative efficiency of sources of radiation used in therapy. Boston Med Surg J 197:1509, 1928
6. BOVIE WT: New electrosurgical unit. Surg Gynecol Obstet 47:751, 1928
7. BRUNER JMR: Hazards of electrical apparatus. Anesthesiology 28:396, 1967
8. CUSHING H: Electro-surgery as an aid to the removal of intracranial tumors. Surg Gynecol Obstet 47:751, 1928
9. DANILEVICIUS Z: Editorial: Electrical safety in the operating room. JAMA 224:1287, 1973
10. DAVIS TM: A new cystoscope for retrograde fulguration. J Urol 26:491, 1931
11. DAVIS TM: Prostate operation. Prospects of the patient with prostatic disease in prostatectomy vs resection. JAMA 97:1674, 1931
12. DAVIS TM: Experience in transurethral resection. The Fifth Ferdinand C. Valentine Memorial Lecture. Bull NY Acad Med 43:152, 1967
13. DINSDALE SM: Decubitus ulcers in swine: Light and electron microscopy study of pathogenesis. Arch Phys Med Rehabil 54:51, 1973
14. FEIN RL: Transurethral electrocautery procedures in patients with cardiac pacemakers. JAMA 202:7, 1967
15. GEDRON F: "Burns" occurring during lengthy surgical procedures. Journal of Clinical Engineering 5:19, 1980
16. HEMINGWAY A, STENSTROM WK: Physical characteristics of high frequency current. JAMA 98:1446, 1932
17. MCLEAN AJ: The Bovie electrosurgical current generator: Some underlying principles and results. Arch Surg 18:1863, 1929
18. MCLEAN AJ: Characteristics of adequate electrosurgical current. Am J Surg 18:417, 1932
19. OTTO JF, JR: Principles of minor electrosurgery. Cincinnati, Liebel-Flarsheim, 1957
20. OVERMYER KM, PEARCE JA, DEWITT DP: Measurements of temperature distributions at electrosurgical dispersive electrode sites. Journal of Biomechanical Engineering 101:60, 1979
21. PRENTISS RJ, HARVEY GS, BETHARD WF et al: Massive adductor muscle contraction in transurethral surgery: Cause and prevention; Development of new electrical circuitry. J Urol 93:263, 1965
22. REICHEL SM: Shearing force as a factor in decubitus ulcers in paraplegics. JAMA 166:762, 1958
23. SEMANS JH: Electrosurgical complications of transurethral resection. J Urol 65:1056, 1951
24. STERN M: Resection of obstructions at the vesical orifice: New instruments and a new method. JAMA 87:1726, 1926
25. WALD AS, MAZZIA VDB, SPENCER FC: Accidental burns associated with electrosurgery. JAMA 217:916, 1971
26. WEYRAUCH HM: Surgery of the Prostate. Philadelphia, W B Saunders, 1959

Transurethral Prostatic Electroresection

William R. Fair

88

HISTORY OF TRANSURETHRAL RESECTION

Words from the Old Testament are one of the earliest references to urinary incontinence and retention. Although it was not until 1649 that Riolanus first suggested that bladder neck obstruction and the inability to pass urine could be due to the prostate, urethral catheters were known long before Christ.[11] *In 150 A.D. Galen reported attempting to destroy urethral "callosities" by* passing a catheter through the urethra.[20]

Early efforts at relieving prostatic obstruction were primarily focused on attempts to break through the urethral obstruction by passing catheters and sounds. In 1575 Ambrose Pare passed a sharp thin sound to "ream" an opening through the obstructing prostate. In the 19th century, a number of French surgeons who were skilled with the lithotrite modified their instrument in an attempt to relieve prostatic obstruction. In 1834, James Guthrie reported cutting the vesical neck with a knife concealed within a catheter. Mercier devised a urethrotome blade for incising the vesical neck and performed on more than 300 cases using this instrument in a blind fashion. In 1874, Bottini developed a technique of blind coagulation of the vesical neck using a galvanocautery. This instrument was also a modification of a lithotrite but consisted of a dull platinum blade instead of the sharp steel blade of the previous instruments. The platinum blade was connected to a source of electrical energy by insulated wires. The instrument was used blindly and designed to produce tissue destruction, with eventual sloughing and elimination of the prostatic obstruction. In 1877, Nitze developed the first cystoscope and in 1879, Edison revolutionized not only medical instrumentation but the world, when he developed the incandescent lamp that proved to be so valuable in later cystoscopes.[20]

In 1882 d'Arsonval fulgurated tissue with low-frequency current and observed that high-frequency current—that with more than 10,000 oscillations per second—could be passed through the body without causing harm, other than a feeling of heat. Later experiments, made possible by DeForest's invention of the vacuum tube in 1908, demonstrated that high-frequency current would destroy tissue when applied using a point electrode. These observations established the basic functions of the modern electrosurgical unit: the ability to fulgurate or coagulate tissue by use of low-frequency currents and the incision of tissue with high-frequency currents.[20]

Another landmark in the development of transurethral prostatectomy occurred in 1909 when Hugh H. Young introduced a fenestrated tube to popularize the cold punch operation for prostatectomy.[8] Although the instrument designed by Young was a major advance, it did not allow the surgeon to visualize the operating field while cutting and again was designed for a "blind" procedure. Braasch adapted these principles in developing a direct vision cystoscope for use with the Young punch; this permitted the operator to excise the tissue under direct vision but did not provide any means of controlling hemorrhage.[4]

In 1910 Edwin Beer was the first to apply high-frequency current in urology when he coagulated bladder tumors through a catheterizing Nitze cystoscope.[20]

The development of spark gap generators capable of producing highly damped coagulating current and relatively undamp cutting current was announced in 1924 by G.H. Liebel of Cincinnati and W.T. Bovie of Harvard. This invention was followed shortly after by a resectoscope developed by Maximilian Stern and instruments developed by Collings who, in 1925, reported incising a median bar under water. With the resectoscope it was possible to cut tissue with undamped current under vision; however, no provision was made for control of bleeding. It was Theodore M. Davis of Greenville, South Carolina, who first employed the Bovie generator, with both cutting and coagulating current, in the excision of large amounts of prostatic tissue. To Davis also goes the credit for developing the foot switch that made it possible to change easily from coagulating to cutting current.[16]

In 1932, Joseph McCarthy devised the McCarthy resectoscope, the forerunner of most of the modern instruments. Since that time a number of additional improvements have been added. Any history of transurethral resection would be incomplete without the mention of the names of such outstanding urologists as Gershom Thompson, the first to add continuous irrigation as an element of his cold punch instrument. Reed Nesbit, Iglesias, Baumrucker, Bumpus,[5] Wappler, and a number of other talented and creative individuals, all contributed to the development of our instrumentation from the early days of breaking through the prostatic obstruction to the modern continuous-flow instrument that allows excision and coagulation of tissue without the necessity of emptying the water periodically from the bladder.[17]

This, then, is the heritage of the urologist. When one considers the difficulties that still confront the modern-day resectionist with the wealth of equipment now available it makes one humble, indeed, to contemplate the feats of our predecessors, who faced the difficulty of relieving prostatic obstruction before the days of adequate anesthesia, the Foley catheter, antibiotics, and modern instruments.

The ability to do transurethral surgery well is the one characteristic that distinguishes urologists from other surgical specialists. Indeed, endoscopic diagnosis and transurethral surgery set the specialty of urology apart from other surgical specialties. Mastery of the diagnostic and surgical techniques involved in endoscopic diagnosis and treatment should be the primary concern of those entering training in urology, as well as those responsible for the teaching of urology residents.

No other area of surgery is more difficult to teach or to master. An improperly performed transurethral resection may not simply fail to improve the patient, but injudicious cutting may make him much worse. Severe hemorrhage, infection, and total urinary incontinence can result from transurethral surgery; at times, even the master resectionist is taxed to the utmost.

Transurethral resection is truly a procedure for an individual surgeon; hence the opportunity to learn by watching other surgeons perform, as at open surgery, is lost. For the resident in urology who is anxious to learn endoscopic surgery, there is no way better, nor more tedious, than sitting by an experienced resectionist in viewing the progress of the procedure from start to finish.

Despite the difficulties in learning the procedure and performing it well, all urologists share a special pleasure in having become adept at transurethral resection of the prostate. The ability to resect the prostatic adenoma completely with a minimum of blood loss and with no risk of making the patient incontinent is very much a personal triumph. To quote from Longfellow:

> In the elder days of art,
> builders wrought with utmost care,
> every small and unseen part,
> for the Gods see everywhere.

In doing a proper transurethral resection of the prostate, the modern urologist shares with these ancient craftsmen the satisfaction of performing excellent surgery without a visible incision, where no one else has the opportunity to view the results of his expertise. Like the craftsman in the poem, the urologist who has mastered transurethral surgery can take special pride in treating efficiently one of mankind's oldest afflictions.

Indications

Under indications we must consider both the general indications for prostatectomy and the specific indications for transurethral prostatectomy *versus* an open prostatectomy.

GENERAL INDICATIONS

Much has been written about the indications for surgical removal of the prostate. The chief indication for transurethral resection of the prostate (TURP) is an obstruction of the bladder neck causing impairment of the urinary stream. The etiology of the obstruction is most commonly benign prostatic hyperplasia (BPH) but other conditions, such as bladder neck contracture, the presence of a median bar (Marion's disease), prostatic cysts, removal of prostatic tags and remnants, chronic bacterial prostatitis, and carcinoma of the prostate are all occasional indications for transurethral resection. By far the most common condition requiring transurethral prostatectomy is BPH; the remainder of this section deals with the indications for TURP in this condition.

Although there is little disagreement over the need to relieve bladder neck obstruction, there is much controversy about what constitutes an obstruction. How is significant bladder neck obstruction best diagnosed? Symptoms, rectal examination, intravenous pyelography (IVP), residual urine determinations, ultrasound, and CT scanning have all been advocated. The routine measurement of residual urine to determine the need for prostatectomy appears to be an illogical approach. Given that most men over the age of 50 have some prostatic enlargement with some residual urine, how much residual urine is significant enough to indicate a need for surgery? To many urologists 100 ml of residual urine appears to be the "magic number." Yet it seems inconsistent to recommend surgery in an individual with mild to moderate symptoms and 100 ml of residual urine and to withhold surgery in another patient with identical symptoms but only 95 ml of residual urine. Even though the determination of residual urine may be of value as one factor to consider in determining the necessity for TURP, it should never be used as the sole determinant for surgical intervention. The indications for prostatectomy in benign disease can be considered as medical and social.

Medical Indications

The medical conditions indicating that relief of benign prostatic obstruction is required are relatively few: complete obstruction or urinary retention, azotemia or uremia secondary to obstruction uropathy, and hydronephrosis or ureteral dilation secondary to the outlet blockage.

Recurrent episodes of bacteriuria are not necessarily an indication for prostatectomy. Recurrent urinary tract infections are usually the result of a bacterial prostatitis. Although some men with this condition have benefited from surgery, TURP should not be done unless attempts at medical therapy have failed. In my experience, TURP is successful in eradicating bacterial prostatitis in only about one third of patients in whom it is performed. There is little or no evidence to support the commonly espoused statement that "a significant residual urine leads to recurrent infections." Again, what is significant? Once bacteria gain entrance to the bladder, there is no reason to believe that they will grow more readily in 200 ml of urine than they do in 20 ml. Since most men over age 50 carry some residual urine and, unless they have had urethral instrumentation, very few men have urinary tract infections, the evidence linking the mere presence of residual urine to an increased incidence of urinary tract infection is weak at best.

Social Indications

In essence, a patient without the above-mentioned medical indications requires TURP only when the symptoms are severe enough that the patient requests that something be done to relieve them. There is a great deal of individual variation in tolerance to urinary frequency and nocturia, the two most common symptoms of BPH, so no ab-

solute guidelines can be given about when TUR is required. Every busy urologist who has been in practice for at least 5 to 10 years has dozens, or perhaps hundreds, of patients being followed with varying degrees of symptoms as a result of BPH. The wise urologist delays surgery in these people until the patient himself feels that his symptoms are such that surgery is indicated. "Never be in a hurry to operate only on symptoms" is a proven adage that when adhered to, will save the young urologist much grief.

SPECIFIC INDICATIONS FOR TURP *VERSUS* OPEN PROSTATECTOMY

There are two kinds of prostatic outflow obstruction that demand TURP as opposed to open prostatectomy: the small, fibrous prostate and the obstructing malignant prostate. The rationale for the transurethral approach in these conditions can best be explained by means of histophotographic views of obstructing lesions in the prostatic urethra (Figs. 88-1 to 88-3). The tissue found in benign prostatic hyperplasia actually arises from the periurethral glands that lie between the normal prostate and the mucosa of the prostatic urethra. The elegant studies of McNeal have clearly established the histologic origin of the obstructing tissue and should be familiar to all with an interest in the histology of the prostate.[13]

As the hyperplasia progresses, the adenomatous tissue forms spheroids or nodules that compress the normal prostate and the musculature of this portion of the urethra. The normal glandular and muscular posterior urethral components form the surgical capsule, which can be separated from the adenomatous growth by enucleation or resection. In contrast, with the small fibrous gland, no clearcut delineation between adenoma and capsule is found. An open operation to enucleate the gland is fraught with difficulty and often involves sharp dissection in a field lacking landmarks of what should and should not be removed.

Prostatic cancer and chronic infection also obliterate the prostatic tissue planes; in these conditions enucleation by open surgery is inadvisable or impossible.

Contraindications

Transurethral resection is the method of choice for all but very large prostatic glands. In my practice, I prefer an open enucleation, usually by the retropubic route, for glands heavier than 50 g. Although many experienced resectionists will do TURs on

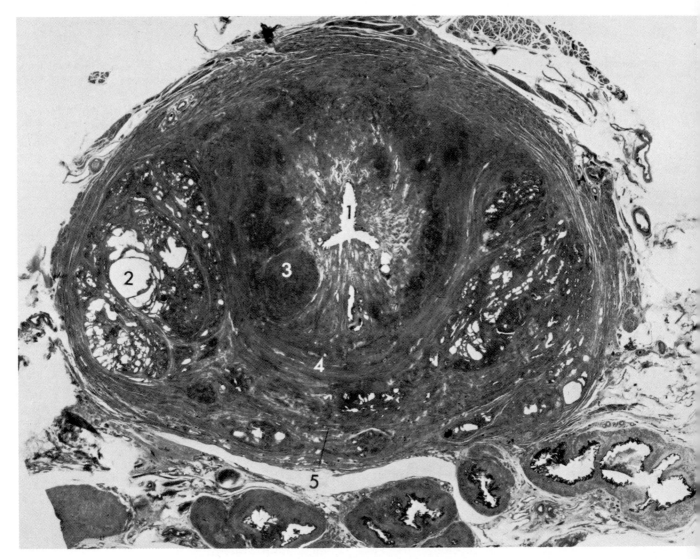

FIG. 88-1. Horizontal macrosection of base of prostate in region of bladder neck: **(1)** Urethral lumen at bladder neck; **(2)** adenomatous hyperplasia of lateral portions of cranial gland of prostate; **(3)** periurethral fibromyomatous spheroid within smooth-muscle sphincter; **(4)** sphincteric smooth muscle at vesical neck; **(5)** medial portion of cranial prostate without hyperplasia. (Courtesy Prof. S. Gil-Vernet, University of Barcelona)

larger glands, for most urologists it is quicker and easier to do an open enucleation than a TURP if the gland is more than 40 g to 50 g. Even in the hands of an experienced resectionist, a TURP on a massive gland is a time-consuming procedure that may be attended by considerable loss of blood.

The presence of a urinary tract infection should be considered an absolute contraindication to TURP or open prostatectomy. Some urologists proceed with surgery in a patient with an infection, if bacterial-sensitivity tests indicate that the infecting organism is sensitive to an antibacterial agent given preoperatively. I believe this is a dangerous practice. The correlation of clinical response to bacterial-sensitivity test results reveals that such testing is only about 60% accurate.[7] There is no compelling reason to operate in the presence of infected urine, and urine cultures should be sterile preoperatively.

Although it is possible to crush and remove large bladder stones with a lithotrite, an open operation avoids the possibility of urethral or bladder injury and is preferred by many surgeons.

Relative contraindications to TURP include a small-caliber urethra or the presence of urethral

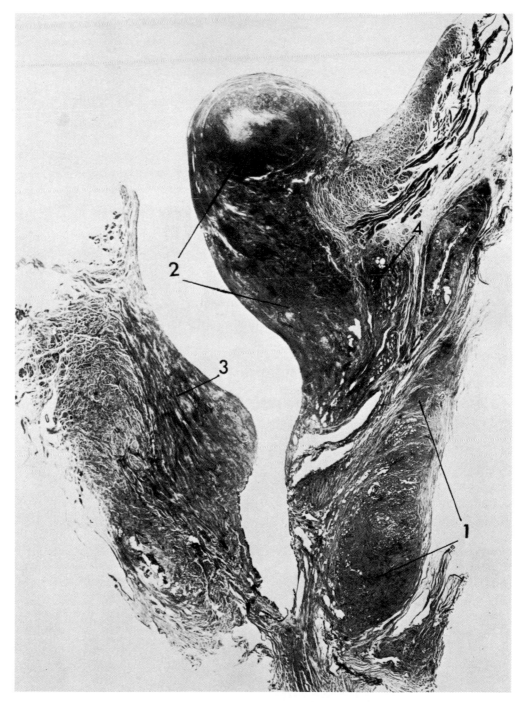

FIG. 88-2. Sagittal section of trigone, prostate, and seminal vesicles: **(1)** posterior (caudal) prostate with small areas of carcinoma; **(2)** adenomatous hyperplasia at vesical neck forming a pedunculated middle lobe; **(3)** hypertrophy of vesicocervical smooth muscle (opening fibers); **(4)** normal portion of cranial prostate. (Courtesy Prof. S. Gil-Vernet, University of Barcelona)

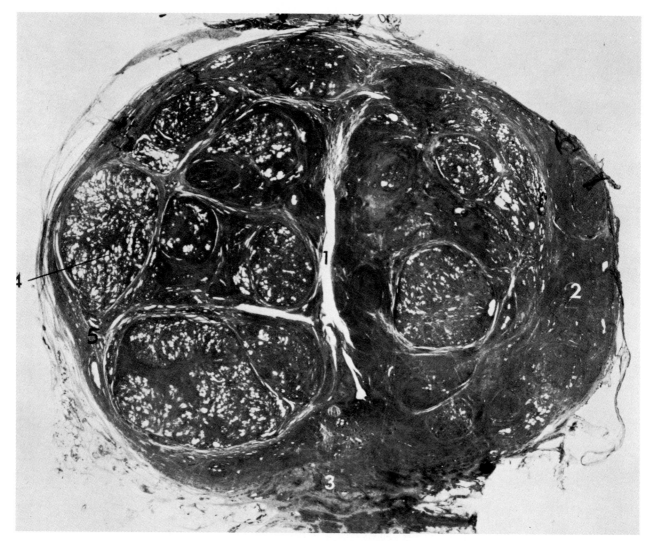

FIG. 88-3. Horizontal section at prostatic base and vesical outlet: **(1)** urethral lumen at bladder neck; **(2 and 3)** carcinomatous infiltration from posterior lobe; **(4)** benign adenomatous hyperplasia; **(5)** hypertrophied lateral lobe infiltrated by carcinoma. (Courtesy Prof. S. Gil-Vernet, University of Barcelona)

strictures. However, a TURP is easily accomplished through a perineal urethrotomy, and the performance of an internal urethrotomy prior to TURP adds little in time or morbidity to the procedure.[9]

Obviously, conditions that restrict the introduction or use of a resectoscope may make transurethral resection undesirable. Orthopedic problems that prevent proper positioning, such as ankylosis of the hip, and large, irreducible scrotal hernias are but two examples of such problems.

Preoperative Evaluation

Although transurethral surgical techniques for dealing with outlet obstructions have been at least

partially responsible for the diminution in the morbidity and mortality associated with prostatic surgery, the effect of proper selection and preparation of the patient for operation has been equally important. The cardiovascular, pulmonary, and general physiologic status of the patient is of obvious importance when prostatic surgery is contemplated, but the prime determinant of the safety or advisability of prostatectomy is the status of the patient's renal reserve.

I still consider the IVP essential in evaluating patients prior to prostatectomy. In recent years, several published studies have contended that the routine use of intravenous pyelography added little information to the preoperative evaluation. The difficulty with such studies is that they were retrospective analyses done on patients in whom the necessity for prostatectomy had already been determined. Thus, it is not surprising that the IVP did nothing to alter this decision. Probably a retrospective analysis of the chest radiograph, hemoglobin, or blood chemistries would yield similar results. A more appropriate test of the usefulness of the IVP would be to assess its value in determining the need for surgery in patients presenting with symptoms of bladder neck obstruction. The field of urology is unique in that through the combination of radiology and endoscopy we are able to visualize the entire urinary tract. My feeling is that, prior to performing surgery in patients with symptoms of urinary obstruction, good medicine dictates that we evaluate the entire genitourinary tract as much as is conveniently possible, just as an internist might examine the heart and lungs of a patient presenting with a headache.

A serum creatinine or blood-urea-nitrogen (BUN) is necessary for a total estimation of renal function. In the presence of azotemia resulting from obstructive uropathy, surgery should be postponed until catheter drainage has been used for a long enough period of time to maximize renal function. If there is a permanent loss of renal function after drainage, a different kind of operation, such as staged resection or internal cystotomy, may be considered or surgery may be contraindicated entirely.

The general medical and physical condition of the patient must be thoroughly evaluated. Cardiovascular disorders, except recent myocardial infarction and blatant defects in cardiovascular reserve, are not serious deterrents to surgery. The hazard is greater in the patient with a history of peptic ulcer or evidence of chronic emphysematous and infectious pulmonary disease, because the stress of surgery is likely to induce episodes of gastrointestinal bleeding or acute exacerbations of chronic pulmonary infection. The patient with a history or symptoms of ulcers is prepared for surgery with antispasmodics, absorbent demulcents, and cimetidine; the patient with pulmonary emphysema and infection is given an antibacterial agent, tracheobronchial cleansing, and intermittent positive-pressure therapy.

It is not my practice to do routine urodynamic studies in patients with symptoms of prostatism unless the symptoms are incompatable with the size of the prostate or careful neurologic examination reveals a possible neurologic deficit. Some urologists feel that preoperative flow rates are of value, particularly in documenting the changes before and after surgery.

In the vast majority of transurethral resections, cystoscopy should be done at the time of TURP and not as a separate procedure on a different day. Exceptions to this rule include cystoscopic examination to confirm prostatic enlargement that is not detectable on rectal examination. Also, whenever I am undecided about the need for an open operation, I feel it is better for the patient to have a cystoscopic examination under local anesthesia, with intravenous sedation if necessary, than for the surgeon to have the patient anesthetized for the combined cysto–TURP, only to find that the size of the gland makes a TURP inadvisable. In our and many other hospitals, it then becomes necessary to transport an anesthetized patient from the endoscopy room to an operating room suitable for an open procedure.

The practice of my general surgical colleagues of referring patients for evaluation of prostatism before hernia repair or hemorrhoidectomy has enabled me to distinguish those who probably will and will not have postoperative voiding difficulties. If the patient's urinary stream is feeble, the bladder architecture seriously altered, or renal function diminished, prostatectomy should be considered before elective herniorrhaphy or hemorrhoidectomy. In a mild urinary disorder, the decision about surgery is best settled according to the patient's own assessment of his urinary difficulties after he has been appraised of the possible retentive consequences of the proposed surgery. Postoperative retention is not common in patients with mild prostatism. Hemorrhoidectomy should be avoided in significant prostatism because the hemorrhoids may be markedly relieved by prostatectomy.

Occasionally, the urologist is confronted with the necessity of relieving prostatic obstruction in a patient with a terminal illness or in a patient confined permanently to bed. Although each patient must be evaluated as an individual, in general, I would not proceed with surgery in patients with a concurrent illness that is likely to be fatal in less than 6 months. Similarly, I see little benefit in doing a TURP in older men who are permanently bedridden and who may be more comfortable and more easily managed with long-term catheter drainage.

Routine preoperative blood work ordered on our service includes a complete blood count and differential, chemistry battery, prothrombin time, and partial thromboplastin test (PTT). Blood is drawn for a type and screen; because of the rarity of blood transfusion following TURP, we no longer routinely crossmatch blood prior to surgery.

PREOPERATIVE ANTIBIOTICS

Despite the widespread use of antibiotics prior to TURP, there are no prospective studies that confirm the need for prophylactic antibiotics in patients with sterile urine. However, the use of midstream urine specimens alone may not reflect accurately the bacterial flora of the urethra, the most likely source of any bacteria introduced during transurethral procedures. It is well documented that some men can void an absolutely sterile midstream urine despite the presence of high bacterial colony counts in the urethral specimen.

I routinely culture both the first voided 5 ml to 10 ml of urine (VB_1), which appears to be an accurate reflection of urethral bacteriology, as well as the midstream (VB_2) specimens. If potential urinary tract pathogens are not found in any quantity, in these cultures, I give the patient no antibacterial therapy, before, during, or after TURP. If only one preoperative culture is obtained, a collection technique that incorporates the first portion of urination (*i.e.*, a total specimen rather than a midstream collection) should be cultured. Using this technique, gram-negative or other potentially pathogenic bacteria that are present in small numbers may be assumed to originate from below the vesical neck, and preoperative antibiotics may be indicated. If antibacterials are used prophylactically, an aminoglycoside, carbenicillin, or an injectable cephalosporin given at least 1 hour prior to the start of surgery and continued for no more than 48 hours would be advisable. A sterile urine, as evidenced by a negative culture on the day prior to catheter removal, is essential before catheterization is discontinued.

Prerequisites to Surgery

Although the major prerequisite for the performance of transurethral surgery is a thoroughly trained, skilled endoscopist, it is probably more nearly true of transurethral than of open surgical procedures that the surgeon is no better than his equipment. A relatively uncomplicated operation can be turned into a nightmare for all concerned if serious or protracted difficulty is encountered in the functioning of the instruments or the electrosurgical unit.

The surgeon should never tolerate working elements that do not fit and function with absolute smoothness. Sheaths should be rejected if they impinge in any manner on the working element or cutting loop; lens and light systems cannot be faulty. A variety of factors concerned with trans-urethral surgery, such as type of table and chair, size of room, and a number of other conveniences, are of obvious importance, but the essentials are the resectoscope and the electrosurgical unit; these must always be in perfect repair.

INSTRUMENTS

In view of the number of abnormalities that may be encountered in the lower urinary tract in the course of diagnostic endoscopy preparatory to a surgical procedure such as TURP, a certain minimum number of instruments should routinely be available. Unsuspected conditions can force considerable delay if additional instruments must be sought and sterilized. Instruments appropriate for the more common conditions should be set out on the table, and instruments to deal with less common variations should be in sterile packs near at hand and ready for use.

Unless a right-angled lens with the lock for the resectoscope sheath is available, a cystoscope of appropriate size should be on the table, and another should be in a sterile box on the shelf in case of malfunction. Replacement bulbs for nonfibrotic cystoscopes and Foroblique lenses can be marshaled in a perforated metal case in a pan of cold sterilizing solution. At least two Foroblique or Vest lenses, a retrograde lens, and two working elements should be available for the resectoscope. Additional endoscopes, lenses, and working elements can be kept in wrapped boxes that have been gas sterilized.

Selection of the type of working element is primarily a matter of individual preference. Many surgeons trained in the use of the Stern–McCarthy instrument, the old "side-winder," have a stout affection for it and contend that the surgeon has a better 'feel' for the tissue he is cutting when using this instrument. Others, including myself, prefer a one-handed instrument such as the Iglesias, Nesbit, Baumrucker, Storz, or Olympus models. The use of such instruments frees the contralateral hand for use in the rectum or on the abdomen. I believe that the use of digital rectal pressure affords the surgeon valuable guidance to the amount of tissue still present and aids greatly in the ability to do a complete resection.

Refinement of fiberoptic endoscopes has progressed rapidly and these endoscopes are replacing instruments with a bulb lighting system. The major advantage of fiberoptic instruments is that they provide more intense and reliable illumination than ordinary light bulbs; in the new miniature instruments this is a truly significant advantage. The fiberoptic system also obviates replacement costs for burnt-out light bulbs. The newer glass-rod lens systems have greatly improved clarity of vision and have enlarged the field of view remarkably.

The continuous-flow resectoscope units have the great advantage of being able to do an entire resection without stopping and draining the bladder during the procedure. The use of the continuous flow resectoscope requires some training on the part of those who are unfamiliar with this instrument. Also, the 27Fr sheath required is viewed as unnecessarily large by some surgeons for the performance of a TURP.

The 24Fr, 26Fr, and 28Fr resectoscope sheaths should all be available on the instrument table, because an initially capacious urethra may not remain so as surgery progresses and the surgeon may wish to use a smaller sheath. The choice between Bakelite, steel-covered Bakelite, Teflon, or Fiberglas sheath covering appears to be a matter of individual preference; no one material seems to be superior to the others.

Whatever its composition, the sheath should be true, have a lock that works, and have a smooth beak. Tissues can readily be damaged if the beak is serrated or irregular. I believe that only the short-beaked sheath should be used. The long-beaked sheath is dangerous, even though perforations during transurethral resection are related more to the surgeon's training than to the length of the sheath beak. Sheaths should be replaced periodically because much-used ones tend to lose insulation, leak current, and dissipate cutting potency.

Two Timberlake obturators should be available, one plain-tipped and one with a screw-tip coupling to fit the thread of a filiform, so that a tortuous urethral lumen may be passed safely without damage to tissues.

Filiforms, LeForte sounds, or woven silk or nylon followers should be at hand, as should a set of bougies à boule (Otis bulbs). Ordinary sounds cannot properly calibrate a urethra; diminution in luminal size other than that produced by dense stricture can only be detected, on withdrawal of the bougie, by the hang of the boule at the point of narrowing.

The Conger perineal urethrotomy clamp can profitably be added to the instrument set for vas ligation and meatotomy, in the event that perineal urethrotomy is necessary.

A lithotrite should always be readily available because unsuspected calculi can be encountered. Because flexible grasping forceps are so useful in unhandy situations when something must be removed from the bladder that cannot quite be retrieved with the resectoscope loop, they should be instantly available. Two light cords, two water lines, and power cords should be on the table, and a device such as a metal ring attached to a spring clip by elastic bands should be suspended from the x-ray head carriage or some part of the table to keep cords and water lines disentangled and nonencumbering.

An Ellik evacuator or a Toomey piston syringe should be filled and in position in a deep pan of sterile irrigating solution. The Ellik evacuator should have hand-tailored hose connections of heavy rubber with a big bore; there should be no more than 2 finger-widths of tubing between metal tip and glass shank to provide stability and ease of handling.

The density of the current generated varies inversely with the surface area of the electrode. Hence, a fine-caliber loop, such as a size 10 or 12 (0.010 or 0.012 inch in diameter), results in more concentrated current and better cutting. Large-caliber loops, such as size 18 or 20, produce better hemostatis but inferior cutting action. The loop must be kept free of encrusted material during the performance of the TURP. Coagulated material effectively increases the diameter of the loop, and, as a result, less current is transmitted and cutting efficiency is impaired.

ELECTROSURGICAL CURRENTS AND UNITS

The choice of electrosurgical unit can be left to personal preference and availability of parts and service. The newer units with built-in warning lights to detect improper grounding, short circuits, or inadequate line current are generally most satisfactory. They must be inspected, cleaned, and adjusted if necessary; inspection should be routine and of a frequency dictated by amount of use. Individual settings for cutting and coagulating are governed by the machine, the surgical maneuver, and the type of lesion to be dealt with.

Different types of current produce different effects on tissue. Tissue destruction is caused by heat generated in the vicinity of the active electrode. The radius of the zone of destruction is directly related to the intensity of the current and the length of time it is applied. Three types of electrical currents are utilized in prostate resections: cutting, coagulating, and blended. *Cutting current* is the undamped current generated by a tube oscillation. *Coagulating current,* in contrast, is a highly damped current generated from a spark gap oscillator. *Blended current* is a combination of the two.

Each type of current has a different effect on tissue. Cutting current, applied briefly, causes little tissue destruction. Therefore, a higher setting for the cutting current increases greatly the efficiency of the cut while adding little to the danger of the procedure; no tissue destruction is found beyond 3 mm from the loop.[20] Tissue destruction is also minimized by the use of a rapid cutting stroke, which is possible by the use of a sufficiently high cutting current. A smooth, rapid, stroke also is effective in preventing charred tissue from adhering to the loop. Too much cutting current produces an arc, noticed as a blue flame between the electrode and the tissue, and should be avoided.

Because coagulating current leads to more tissue destruction, the intensity of the current should be as low as will adequately coagulate the tissue, and the time of application should be as small as possible.

Glands with a high moisture content cut more readily; moist vascular tissue is best handled by the resection using a blended current to maximize cutting and coagulating properties. In contrast, small fibrous glands or bladder neck contractures are best treated by using a small-caliber loop with a tube cutting current of high intensity.

In many hospitals newer electronic, solid-state electrosurgical units are replacing the older vacuum tube and spark gap machines. I prefer the solid-state units because they appear to produce a cleaner-cutting, more rapid operation with less specimen charring and tissue destruction.

Further detailed information regarding electrosurgery is found in Chapter 87.

LIGHTING SYSTEMS

A variety of lighting systems are available for endoscopic surgery. The dry cell battery box has the advantage of mobility but cannot compare with bulb or fiberoptic systems with respect to light intensity, and they have been totally eliminated in many hospitals. Battery box systems are still used for cystosopic examination in a surprising number of urology offices.

When using a bulb system, rheostat transformers are preferable to extend the useful life of the bulb.

Whenever available, a fiberoptic light source should be used. There is absolutely no comparison between the amount and adequacy of illumination obtained with fiberoptic sources and that obtained with incandescent bulbs. The actual type and power of fiberoptic instrumentation required depends on individual requirements. The advent of fiberoptic lighting has vastly improved endoscopic photography and has made possible the effective use of teaching attachments for the resectoscope. Special units are available to accommodate the need for these ancillary items.

IRRIGATING FLUIDS

Despite experimental and clinical evidence that has clearly established the superior safety of nonhemolyzing solutions over water during the performance of a TURP, some urologists still persist in its use.[6,10] Although water may enable better visibility, a point I am not ready to concede, absorption of a nonisotonic solution may cause hemolysis and hemoglobulinemia with subsequent renal failure. I thus recommend the use of nonhemolyzing solutions such as 1.1% glycine, 1.8% urea, 3% sorbitol, or a similar product.

The convenience of these sterile factory-bottled solutions and disposable tubing units has caused me to use them exclusively. Solutions should be cool to dissipate the heat that the electrical current causes in the tissues, but they need not be at the hypothermic levels some workers have used in an attempt to reduce bleeding.

ENDOSCOPY TABLE

The simple Young endoscopy table is quite satisfactory. It has a commodious drainage tray and can be fitted with posts for foot-sling support, as well as standard leg holders. If it is not used for roentgenography, it can be moved about in rooms used for both open and endoscopic surgery. Certain of the power-driven tables that raise and lower the patient and provide for Trendelenburg and Fowler positions can be equipped for image-intensifying radiographic studies and ordinary urographic procedures, but their drainage trays are unhandy in position and operation and are neither sufficiently long nor capacious. Endoscopy chairs such as that of Barnes, which can be raised and lowered semiautomatically, are less expensive, and they are quite satisfactory in providing the up-and-down mobility needed to expedite transurethral surgery of the bladder and prostate.[2]

Whatever table is used, the patient should be positioned so that the buttocks are slightly over the edge of the table when the legs are raised in the lithotomy position. If the patient is too far up on the table the resectionist will have to hunch forward throughout the procedure; this position rapidly leads to operator fatigue.

I am a firm believer in the value of the O'Conor

sheath, which allows the surgeon to evaluate the rectum periodically. Resection of the apical tissue is made much simpler when the surgeon can elevate the distal prostatic area by the rectal finger.

ENDOSCOPY ROOM

In many institutions the endoscopy rooms for performing transurethral surgery are small, cramped, dimly lit, and located off a major traffic corridor; such as near the outpatient clinic or x-ray areas. This fact, coupled with the absence of a visible surgical incision, has helped to create the idea in the minds of other surgeons and the lay public alike that transurethral surgery is almost an outpatient procedure requiring little skill and causing little risk to the patient.

I strongly believe that the endoscopic surgery unit should be in the operating room area for the following reasons: to ensure that the same rules required to maintain sterility in the operating rooms are required in the resection rooms, to have the facilities for open surgery readily available should a catastrophy occur during transurethral surgery, and to impress upon other hospital personnel and urology residents in training that a transurethral resection is a major surgical procedure requiring adequate preoperative evaluation, the administration of general or regional anesthesia, a high degree of surgical skill, and constant vigilance during and following surgery to ensure a successful outcome, as is required of any other surgical procedure of comparable magnitude. The room must be large enough to permit uncrowded positioning of the equipment and tools of the surgeon and anesthesiologist. Adequate lighting for both the surgeon and the anesthetist, as well as facilities for oxygen, suction, and hanging intravenous or irrigating solutions, must be available. X-ray film view boxes should be located within the room so that it is not necessary for the surgeon to leave the room to view the films if a radiograph should become necessary.

ANESTHESIA

Although the anesthesiologists summation of the physiologic status of the patient must be considered, the ultimate decision about the type of anesthesia administered must be a joint one. Some urologists strongly favor regional block or spinal anesthesia as the most satisfactory for transurethral surgery, because such anesthesia both leaves the patient alert enough to answer questions and cooperate as necessary and provides an extra modality by which physiologic response may be judged.

The degree of relaxation of the operative area is usually better, and the absence of postoperative nausea is desirable. Litigation-inspired hesitancy to use spinal anesthesia is understandable, but prohibition of spinal anesthesia has no more documented validity in a patient with carcinoma of the prostate than in any patient with a cancer that might metastasize to the spine.

Anesthesiologists who administer only enough regional anesthetic to dull sensation in the sacral nerves often do not realize that the patient and the urologist will be discomfited and the entire procedure prolonged and made more disagreeable if the patient can appreciate bladder distention. When not specifically contraindicated, I prefer to bring anesthesia to the ninth thoracic segment to obviate discomfort associated with distention of the bladder and afford a more reposed patient. I have not found that any of the acute abdominal consequences of lower tract perforation are masked with this level of anesthesia.

Because of the rigid limits of operating time propounded by many endoscopic surgeons, which really has had particular reference to the resident in training, anesthesiologists tend to curtail the length of anesthesia by avoiding adjuvants and diminishing the amount of agent administered. I prefer a more lengthy duration of anesthesia to avoid having to contend with an uncomfortable, restless, anxious patient during the sometimes painstaking terminal sequences of transurethral surgery. If the period of the regional anesthesia is too short, general anesthesia may be needed to allow completion of the task.

In our institution most prostatic resections are performed under general anesthesia. Having done TURPs using both general and spinal anesthesia, I believe that there is little to choose between the two. The condition of the patient and the skill and experience of the anesthesiologist involved should be considered in choosing the type of anesthesia. Although I recognize a potential advantage of spinal anesthesia in this setting, an incomplete or too brief spinal can add considerably to the difficulty encountered in performing the TUR.

Both the surgeon and the anesthesiologist must be aware of the amount of blood loss during the surgery. Because of the nature of the procedure, an appreciable blood loss can occur and be masked in the large quantities of irrigating fluid that are used. The surgeon's experience is generally an excellent guide to the degree of blood loss. In some situations, the method of Litin and Emmett, in which aliquots of irrigation fluid are used to estimate blood loss, can be of significant value.[12]

It is the responsibility of the urologic surgeon to familiarize the anesthesiologist both with the pulse and pressure changes characteristic of extravasation or excessive fluid absorption and with the consequences of vesical distention in the patient with neurologic abnormalities associated with autonomic hyperreflexia, so that appropriate prophylactic or therapeutic measures can be taken.

The most important prerequisites for transurethral surgery are the training and skill of the surgeon. Any reasonably adept person with interest in and temperament for surgery can be taught to perform transurethral procedures correctly and expeditiously, but the period of training in all phases of diagnostic and surgical endoscopy is long. Although there is obvious merit in the use of such training devices as electroresection of beef hearts and cow udders, the only practical method of learning transurethral surgery is to set up the transurethral surgical case, perform the diagnostic endoscopic examination, and gradually progress from observation to tentative use of the surgical unit to more extensive supervised experience.

Techniques

The initial step involves the introduction of the instrument, examination of the bladder, and familiarization with the landmarks that will guide the surgeon throughout the rest of the operation.

If a preoperative cystoscopic examination has not been done, it is my practice to pass the 17Fr Wappler cystoscope sheath, with the Foroblique lens in place, under direct vision. The practice of passing the cystoscope directly into the bladder with the obturator already inserted is to be condemned; urethral strictures and other abnormalities may be missed completely and the risk of creating a false passage is unacceptably high, especially for the beginning cystoscopist. Failure to examine the urethra while passing the instrument omits an essential part of the examination. The excuse that one can examine the urethra "on the way out" is simply not logical and ignores the well-established observation that even a single pass of the cystoscope can cause a significant inflammatory reaction in the urethra. Furthermore, if a urologist never has the occasion to visualize an intact, untraumatized urethra prior to instrumentation, how will he ever learn the appearance of a normal urethra? I believe that many cases diagnosed as "posterior urethritis" by cystoscopy alone in the absence of confirming cultures are the result of assessing the urethra after the cystoscopic examination, as the instrument is being withdrawn.

At the time of cystoscopic examination, the examiner must be sure to do a thorough visualization of the entire bladder. It is not uncommon to find calculi or even bladder tumors co-existing with benign prostatic hyperplasia.

If no urethral abnormalities exist a well-lubricated curved Van Buren sound should be passed gently into the bladder (Fig. 88-4) prior to passing the resectoscope. A good rule of thumb is that the urethra should comfortably accept a sound at least two sizes larger than the resectoscope sheath. I find no reason to use a sheath larger than 24Fr or 26Fr. Therefore, a 26Fr or 28Fr sound should be passed prior to the resectoscope.

Any one of a number of conditions may exist to impede the passage of instruments into the urethra; some of the more frequent problems are considered below.

Meatal Abnormality

One of the most common conditions that may impede the passage of instuments into the urethra or otherwise interfere with the performance of transurethral surgery is a small urethral meatus. This is encountered as a normal variant, a congenital anomaly, or a result of a variety of balanomeatal inflammatory or traumatic insults. It is, additionally, a common and distressing sequel of transurethral resection of the prostate. When the urethral meatus is snug to the No. 26 or No. 28 bougie, meatotomy should be done to prevent postoperative meatal stenosis, which may be more bothersome than the prostatic obstruction.

Meatotomy Technique

Meatotomy is often poorly and hurriedly performed. The extent of the incision of the meatus is frequently inadequate and fails to prevent the tissue damage that ensues when the rigid sheath of the instrument saws back and forth in too confined a lumen for an hour or more. Even when the incision is adequate, the surgical reconstruction may be so poorly carried out that dense scarring results and produces further meatal narrowing or the meatal incision is improperly realigned and causes a hypospadiac condition.

To obviate these problems, the extent and caliber of the urethral restriction must be delineated by means of the bougie à boule. When the bougie is withdrawn through the meatus, the point where the hang of the boule is first noted represents the proximal extent of the meatal narrowing and indicates the point to which the meatus must be opened (Fig. 88-5).

Several satisfactory techniques have been proposed for meatotomy, but inadequate incision and
(*Text continues on p. 905.*)

FIG. 88-4. Urethral dilation: **(A)** penile urethra being drawn over well-lubricated sound; **(B)** tip of sound in position for downward swing of sound; **(C)** completion of downward arc maneuver

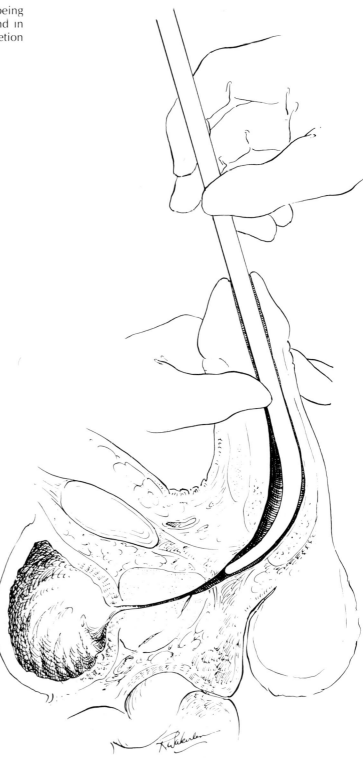

A

(Continued)

FIG. 88-4. (Continued)

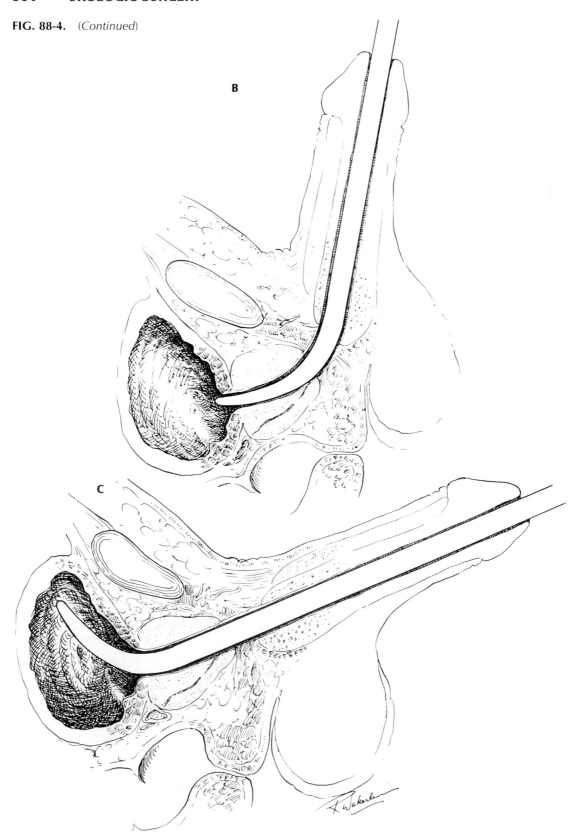

FIG. 88-5. **(A)** Hang of bougie in fossa navicularis indicates extent of meatal restriction. Meatotomy incision is made down to boule (bulb) of bougie, through restriction; **(B)** sutures appose cut margins and control bleeding; **(C)** transverse incision in loose frenular skin; **(D)** mobilization of frenular skin; **(E)** frenular skin flap approximated to cut margins of glans to obviate hypospadias

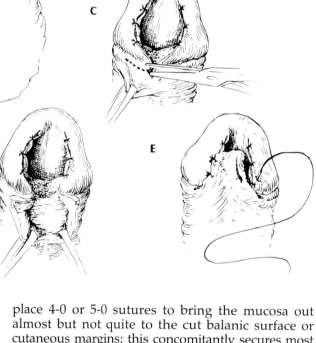

inappropriate repair, not the selection of a specific technique, pose the problem.

Meatotomy is adequate when a bougie of the desired size does not hang as it is withdrawn. Compression sutures may be taken at this point on either side of the incision to curtail bleeding, and the repair of the meatus may be left until the termination of the surgical procedure. Simple cautery fulguration of the cut surfaces is likely to produce eschar, which may slough repeatedly and cause narrowing.

I prefer to isolate the cut mucosal edges and place 4-0 or 5-0 sutures to bring the mucosa out almost but not quite to the cut balanic surface or cutaneous margins; this concomitantly secures most bleeding points (Fig. 88-5B). Check the meatal caliber again, and using fine Dexon suture, sew the more proximal balanic surface and cutaneous margins together so that only the deeper tissues remain separated. If this restricts the meatus, a transverse incision of the skin at the frenular area affords development of a skin flap that can be sewn to the cut balanic margins. In this fashion, a large meatus that is not hypospadiac is created

(Fig. 88-5*E*). If the meatotomy is carefully reconstructed, it heals without a scar. Dorsal meatotomy is usually unsatisfactory, because bleeding is difficult to control and an appropriate length of incision is difficult to judge.

Phimosis

A redundant or severely phimotic foreskin should be excised at the time of transurethral surgery because it can interfere with the procedure, trap secretions postoperatively, or pose the hazard of paraphimosis if inadvertently left retracted.

Urethral Abnormality

Stricture, a congenitally small urethra, priapism, a short suspensory ligament, severe Peyronie's disease, corporal fibrosis, thrombosis producing deviation, a very long penis, or prostatic urethra can produce an impediment to the passage of instruments (Fig. 88-6) or to their mobility during transurethral surgery. Short strictures can be handled easily by cutting the stricture at the 12 o'clock position using the visual urethrotome. For longer or multiple areas of stricture, the Otis urethrotome should be inserted beyond the strictured area, opened until it is held tightly, and withdrawn with the knife in the 12 o'clock position. This procedure may be repeated until the 24Fr or 26Fr sheath passes without difficulty.

In impassable strictures or patients with a short suspensory ligament, severe Peyronie's disease, corporal fibrosis, or an abnormally small urethra, surgery should generally be performed through a perineal urethrotomy. Although it is used less frequently than formerly, perineal urethrotomy should be considered whenever the instrument does not feel completely loose or move freely in the urethra. The teaching of Valk that perineal urethrotomy should be practiced when the operative procedure will take longer than average represents sound and experienced judgment.

Priapism is usually only transitory, but if it poses more than minor difficulty, perineal urethrotomy should be carried out. The very long penis and very long prostate can also be managed by urethrotomy. For simple endoscopy, the long panendoscope sheath and the short bridge are helpful.

Perineal Urethrotomy Technique

The use of the grooved sound and the Conger clamp simplifies and expedites the performance of perineal urethrotomy (Fig. 88-7). The sound is passed; its heel is depressed so that the urethra is made to bulge into the perineum; and the Conger clamp is then applied, grasping skin, sound, and urethra to prevent any sliding of tissues over each other. The groove of the sound is cut down on for 1 inch to 2 inches. The clamp is released slightly, repressed into the perineal skin a bit more firmly, and reapplied to make the margins of the incision bulge, enabling tag sutures to be placed on either side of the urethral incision. Bleeding points are spot coagulated.

At the termination of transurethral surgery, the catheter may be brought out through the perineal urethrotomy wound or through the urethra, depending on individual circumstances such as the need to avoid urethral irritation or the need for the inlying catheter to provide dilation of a urethral stricture. In most instances, unless there is substantial intolerance to the urethral catheter, it is not necessary to bring it out through the perineal urethrotomy wound. We use fine catgut to approximate the bulbar tissues and bring the skin together loosely with one or two fine Dexon sutures.

Surgery of Benign Prostatic Hyperplasia

A transurethral resection of the prostate can be thought of as consisting of several distinct phases. The first is endoscopic examination and identification of the all important landmarks. The second is resection of the adenoma, a step that is further subdivided into three phases: median lobe; left and right lateral lobes and anterior lobe; and the final trimming of apical tissue and obtaining of maximal hemostasis.[3,15,20]

ENDOSCOPIC EXAMINATION

In many ways the edoscopic examination is the most critical part of the procedure. Having a clear picture of the location of the verumontanum, the external sphincter, bladder neck, ureteral orifices, and the relative distances between these landmarks minimizes the possibility of subsequent damage to these structures. However, exclusive dependence on these landmarks is not enough to ensure complete removal of the adenoma nor to avoid damage to the urinary sphincter mechanism.

In residency training, special emphasis should be placed on the visual identification of adenomatous tissue and its differentiation from muscle and capsular fibers. If only adenoma is removed, the critically important smooth and striated muscular structures in the posterior urethra will not be molested. Before resection, careful visual and palpable delineation of landmarks or guide points

FIG. 88-6. Bouginage of urethral strictures: **(A)** boule of bougie hanging at sites of stricture along urethra; **(B)** bougie being withdrawn from urethra; **(C)** Bougie à boule with French caliber marking on flange

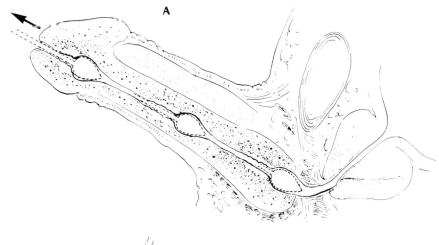

A

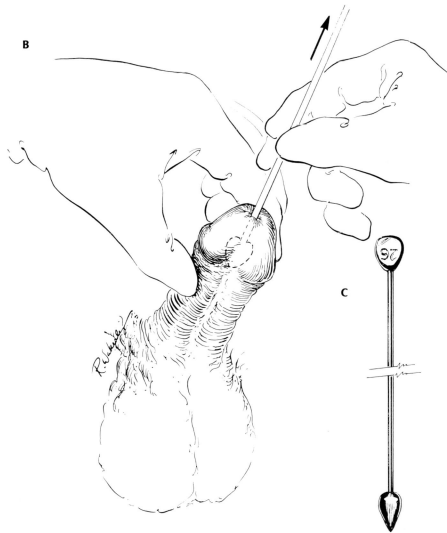

B

C

should be made to assess the disposition, depth, and breadth of the adenoma at each level of the vesicourethral outlet.

A pattern of examination must be developed. The examination should begin with inspection of the bladder, because manipulation of an instrument in the posterior urethra may induce consid-erable bleeding and cause the vesical examination to be less meaningful. Bladder evaluation can be carried out with the cystoscope or the resectoscope sheath fitted with the right-angled and retrograde lenses. The circular bladder walls can be inspected by quadrants for mucosal lesions or other abnor-malities and subjacent muscular derangements.

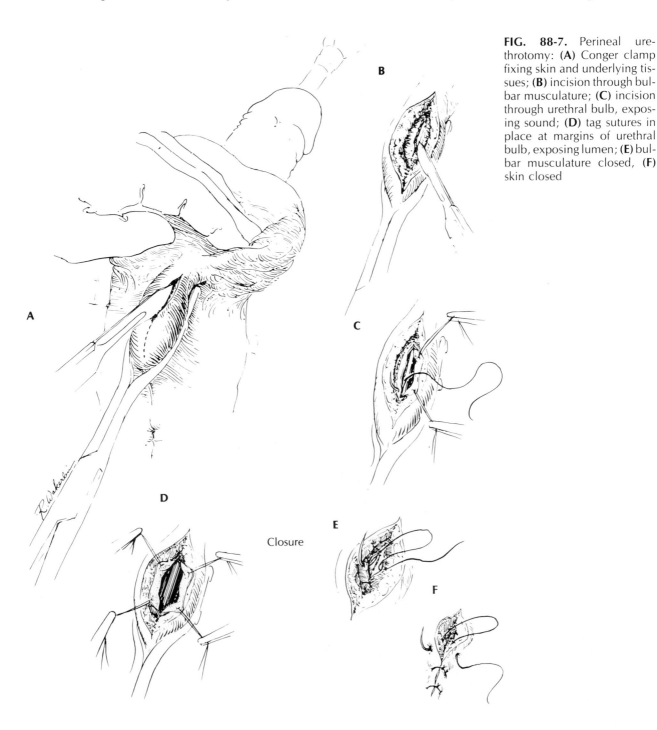

FIG. 88-7. Perineal ure-throtomy: **(A)** Conger clamp fixing skin and underlying tis-sues; **(B)** incision through bul-bar musculature; **(C)** incision through urethral bulb, expos-ing sound; **(D)** tag sutures in place at margins of urethral bulb, exposing lumen; **(E)** bul-bar musculature closed, **(F)** skin closed

Closure

In the bladder base (or posterior quadrants), the interureteric ridge or trigonal area should be traversed with particular reference to the distance between it and the bladder neck. When the trigone is significantly hypertrophied and the prostatic fossa is elongated, this distance is diminished and the cutting electrode may inadvertently encroach on the ureteral orifices. The recesses of cellules and diverticula should be inspected carefully for calculi or other lesions. A finger in the rectum helps this examination by pushing these areas into view.

After the walls have been evaluated, the bladder base can be traversed with the right-angled lens by depressing the eyepiece and moving the instrument with up-and-down strokes from one side to the other, as if one were painting longitudinal stripes with it. The instrument should then be turned over so that the process can be repeated on the anterior half of the bladder. The anterosuperior reaches of the bladder can often be better inspected by manual suprapubic pressure to bring the anterior wall closer to the lens and by a slower flow of irrigating fluid to slacken vesical distention. Before study of the posterior urethra, the retrograde lens may be used to view the vesical neck area and evaluate the extent of any intravesical intrusion of the prostate.

In the examination of the prostatic urethra, the first step is to inspect the extent and configuration of whatever middle lobe tissue is present. The examiner should measure its length and the length of loop excursion needed to go from its tip to the vesical neck. He should then observe how closely the middle lobe approximates the trigonal surface to estimate how carefully to lift middle lobe tissue off and away from the trigone before cutting it. The length of the adenoma should be measured in all quadrants; at the same time its thickness should be estimated by pressing the sheath gently against the finger in the rectum.

The verumontanum is carefully inspected to determine its configuration and prominence and to measure the distance between its most distal point and the circumference of the membranous urethra. The junction of the verumontanum and the membranous urethra can be palpated rectally as the finger comes down from the spongy prostatic adenoma and the soft spot below the verumontanum in the midline to encounter the firmer texture at the beginning of the membranous portion of the urethra. The junction can best be viewed endoscopically as the sheath is slipped and slowly rotated back and forth distal to the verumontanum. The mucosa is fixed over the adenoma in the prostatic urethra and is more mobile in the membranous portion. In some men, the mucosa at this junction resembles accordion pleating as the sheath is moved back and forth (Fig. 88-8).

FIG. 88-8. Orientation for endoscopic examination: **(A)** endoscopic view of mucosal fold at prostatic and membranous urethral junctions; **(B)** lateral view of sheath approaching prostatic membranous junction; **(C)** intrusion of sheath causing mucosa to form accordion pleats at junction

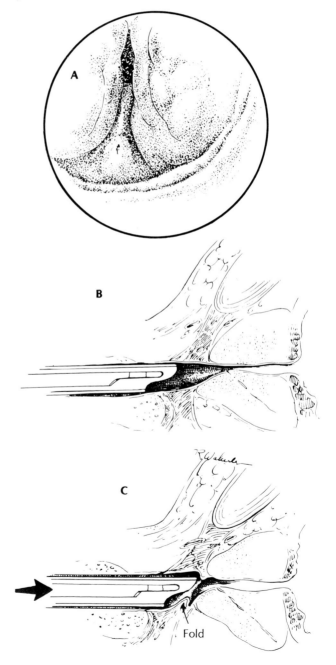

Fold

Visual differentiation between cut adenoma and muscular tissue is even more important. Not only may the adenoma be compressed and bunched lateral or distal to the verumontanum, but also, as it is cut, more spheroids can expand so that the spatial relations of the adenoma to the verumontanum and the membranous urethra change continually. The only safeguard is the surgeon's ability to differentiate between adenoma and other tissues on the basis of appearance. In essence, muscle is arranged in orderly fiber groupings, whereas adenoma is in whorls or more disorderly granular form.

RESECTION OF THE ADENOMA

The beginning point of a transurethral resection is often determined by personal preference, right-or left-handedness, and the type of adenoma encountered. Within the limits imposed by variations in adenomatous configuration, it is advisable for the surgeon to adhere to a routine pattern. Because right-handed surgeons often believe that the body positions and maneuvers required for resection on the right side of the prostate are more comfortable for them than those on the left, the resection may be begun on the left side of the prostatic urethra so that the less comfortable positions will be undertaken when the surgeon is fresher to his task. This, of course, is a personal preference.

As mentioned above, there are actually three steps in the resection of the adenoma.

Resection of the Middle Lobe

Unless there is very minor or no intravesical protrusion of the middle lobe, it is preferable to resect this part of the gland first. Removal of the middle lobe as a first step facilitates vision and aids fluid and tissue evacuation. The middle lobe adenoma is resected at the 6 o'clock position until the bladder neck fibers, which mark the lower end of the trigone, are visible. At this time no further resection of the bladder neck fibers is done. In some cases, these bladder neck fibers can form a rather heavy obstructing ring; then more resection in this area is required but is best left until near the completion of the operation to minimize the risk of undermining the area beneath the trigone. If intravesical

FIG. 88-9. Transurethral resection of middle lobe of prostate: **(A)** resection begins at free tip of middle lobe; **(B)** Anterior and lateral cuts made in middle lobe; **(C)** Cross-step resection on anterior surface of middle lobe

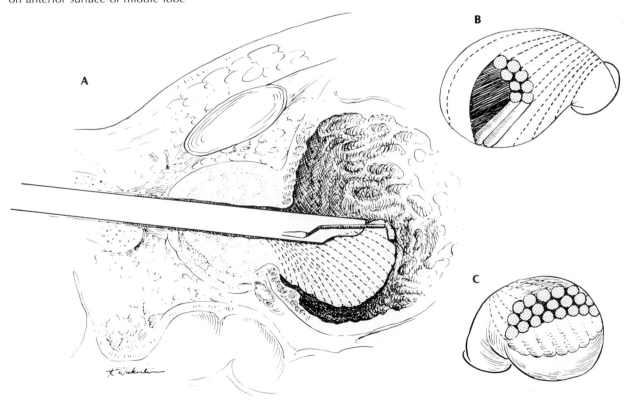

protrusion of the middle lobe is moderate to severe, it is often preferable to resect the entire thickness of one lateral aspect of the lobe at a time rather than to cross the lobe from side to side in successively deeper layers.

The most intravesical tip of the middle lobe is resected on its anterior and lateral surfaces successively (Fig. 88-9). The loop is caught on the most intravesical extremity of the lobe and is brought back along the anterior aspect with as deep a bite as is justified by the thickness of the lobe. If the lobe is long, the sheath may be moved with the loop as it is withdrawn so that longer pieces of tissue can be removed (Fig. 88-10). Movement of the sheath is stopped at the bladder neck and the loop is snapped home to disengage the cut tissue. The next loopful is then taken with the sheath canted to the side so that the loop picks up part of the anterior cut surface and part of the underlying lateral border tissue, reducing the breadth of the lobe from the lateral aspect (Fig. 88-9). This method avoids thinning the lobe in its anteroposterior diameter and prevents the development of a thin broad layer of adenoma, which can be difficult to remove because each loopful must be lifted carefully off the trigone so that the trigone and ureteral orifices will not inadvertently be cut (Figs. 88-11 and 88-12).

Because an intravesical middle lobe tends to be more bulbous at its free margin, each successive cut should be slanted to incorporate more of the free end tissue as resection progresses around the anterolateral margin. This prevents the intraprostatic fossa neck portion of the lobe from becoming so thin that the lobe is unmanageably mobile on its stalk; it also prevents the shearing off of a piece too large to evacuate. A large piece of middle lobe, inadvertently detached and lying free in the bladder, is often difficult to cut into pieces that can be readily evacuated. Under these circumstances, it is better to leave that portion of the lobe until the resectoscope sheath can be conveniently removed. The Lowsley biopsy forceps and Foroblique lens can then be inserted and the free middle lobe tissue can be grasped and extracted, because adenomatous tissue is usually sufficiently compressible to pass through the normal urethra without damaging it. If the lobe is too big for such simple extraction, the tissue can be fragmented with the Lowsley forceps.

When resection of one lateral aspect of the middle lobe has been completed, the same maneuver is repeated on the other lateral border so that the loop does not cut down directly on the thinned anterior surface of the lobe alone. The free tip of the lobe is again approached with canted strokes, taking a greater thickness of tissue at the tip than at the base. Approaching the lobe from both lateral aspects permits long strips of adenoma to be removed with less danger of inadvertent cutting of trigonal structures. Using the resectoscope on its side allows the operator to see the trigone and the clearance between it and the middle lobe with each stroke.

When the bulk of intravesical middle lobe has been resected, its base or pedicle can be quickly trimmed down flush with the bladder neck. As with the small median lobe, it is safer not to resect the pedicle down into the posterior urethra until later in the operation. To do so creates a recess, on which the beak of the sheath can easily catch with subsequent bladder neck damage resulting.

Resection of the Lateral Lobes

Before beginning the resection of the lateral lobe it is again necessary to ascertain the position of

FIG. 88-10. Sliding-sheath technique for resecting long strips of tissue: **(A)** cut is begun at tip of middle lobe; only the loop moves; **(B)** loop remains extended while sheath and working element are slid backward to cut a long tissue strip.

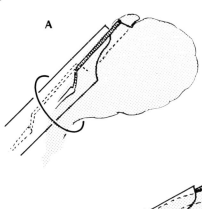

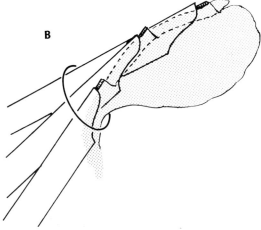

the verumontanum and the bladder neck. By rotating the sheath to the 12 o'clock position, the anterior commissure will be visible. There is usually very little adenomatous tissue directly in the region of the anterior commissure. The first cut is made not directly in the midline at the commissure but slightly to the left of center at the 1 o'clock position. Greater speed, greater accuracy in delineating the junction of adenoma and surgical capsule, and better control of bleeding can be achieved by beginning at the top and working down. Particularly when the adenomatous lateral lobes are large,

the process of *encirclement* (detaching the adenomatous lateral lobe tissue from the surgical capsule everywhere but at its base) is of such value in ensuring clean resection, rapid removal of devascularized tissue, and diminished bleeding that it outweighs any advantage of an initially more comfortable position for resection that might be gained by starting at the bottom.

Unless adenomatous tissue intrudes into the bladder, the initial cut of the loop should never extend past the bladder neck. The loop should be placed precisely at the junction of adenoma and

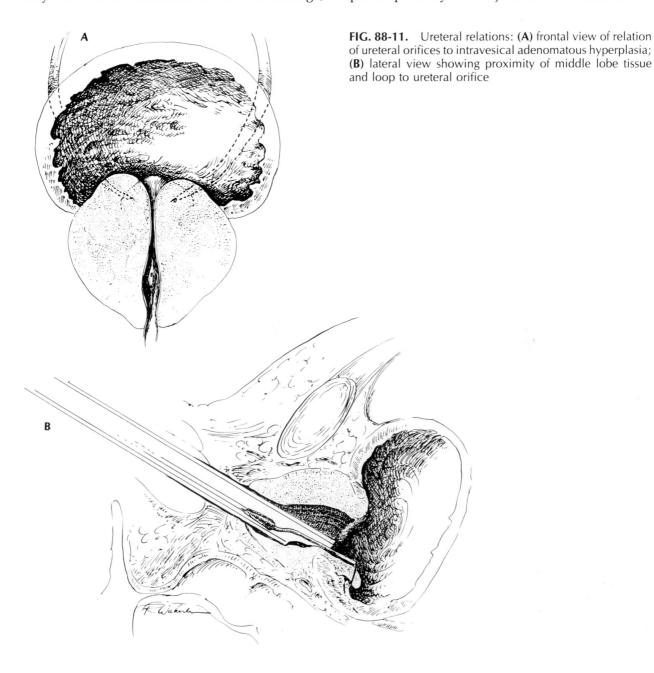

FIG. 88-11. Ureteral relations: **(A)** frontal view of relation of ureteral orifices to intravesical adenomatous hyperplasia; **(B)** lateral view showing proximity of middle lobe tissue and loop to ureteral orifice

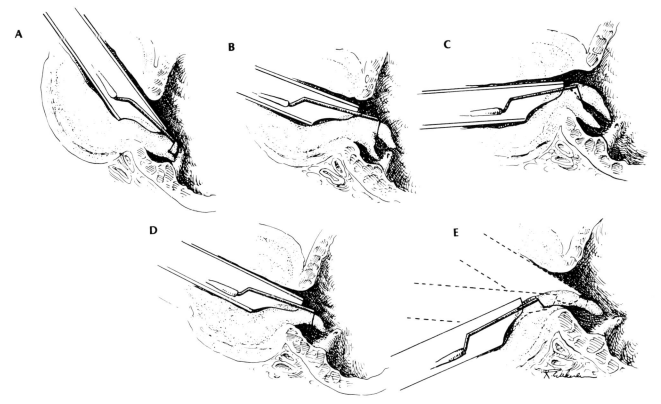

FIG. 88-12. Steps in resection of pedunculated middle lobe to avoid ureteral, trigonal, and vesical neck injury: (**A**) cut is begun; (**B**) tissue is lifted after initial bite of loop; (**C**) cut is completed; (**D**) deep layer of tissue is engaged; (**E**) sheath is withdrawn and tissue is lifted as loop excises remaining intravesical middle lobe tissue down into prostatic urethra.

bladder neck fibers and the cut made only into adenoma.

Irrespective of the size of the adenoma, the technique of resection on the roof of the fossa is the same. Beginning at the vesical neck successive relatively shallow bites are taken at 1 o'clock and then gradually back toward the membranous urethra in a fashion that keeps the surface smooth (Fig. 88-13).

At the bladder neck and a little to the left of the midline, deeper bites are taken until muscle fibers are bare from the neck to the distal extent of prostatic adenoma. Once muscle has been exposed in the midline, the thickness of adjacent lateral adenoma can be determined and deeper bites may be taken with each cut as the instrument is moved laterally. It is most important to leave the bared muscle as smooth as possible from bladder neck to external sphincter; this is accomplished by taking long, even strokes. Short, chopping loop movements inevitably leave a wavy, corrugated surface that becomes more difficult to trim as the adenoma gets thinner.

Tissue waves or corrugations hide bleeding points by canting the vessels so that they are at oblique angles to the wall; also, blood may glance off ridges and fan out, making location of the bleeding vessels more difficult. Removal of longitudinal strips, from the bladder neck to the prostatic apex down to the muscle, continues until the roof is cleared (Fig. 88-14A). At this point management of small and large adenomas differs somewhat.

Cross-Step Technique for Small Adenomas. If the adenomatous tissue on the lateral lobe does not appear to be thicker than 2 to 3 loop-widths, it can be removed in side-to-side, stepdown fashion (Fig. 88-14B) rather than by encirclement. In this method, the loop traverses the breadth of lateral lobe from midline to capsule and back again in cross-step fashion. Each stroke starts at the junction of adenoma and bladder neck and finishes just inside or proximal to the apex of the adenoma at its abutment on the membranous urethra. If the adenoma between these two points is longer than the excursion of the loop, the sheath can be moved simultaneously until the apex is reached, at which

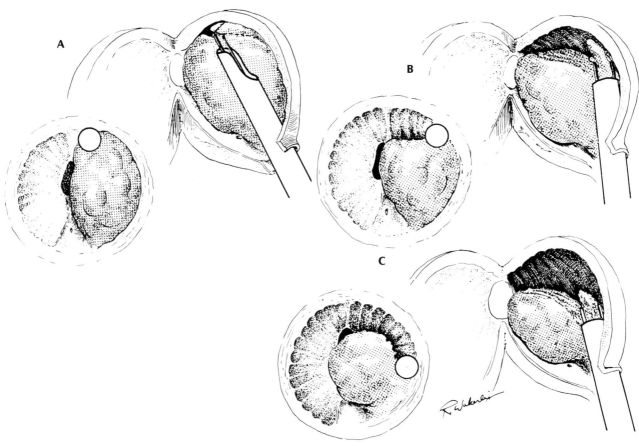

FIG. 88-13. Transurethral resection of lateral lobes of prostate: **(A)** resection begins at anterior commissure to clear tissue from roof of prostatic fossa; **(B)** left lateral lobe tissue is removed down to surgical capsule from anterior commissure to 2 o'clock position to allow encirclement of lobe; **(C)** encirclement of lateral lobe tissue

FIG. 88-14. Transurethral resection of lateral lobes of prostate: **(A)** resection of anterior portion of lateral lobe; **(B)** cross-step resection of lateral lobe tissue in small adenoma

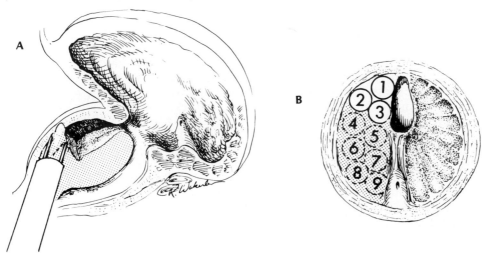

point the sheath is held stationary and the loop is allowed to finish its excursion and to cut off and detach the piece of tissue.

Sliding the sheath and working element as a unit after the extended loop has begun to cut to the desired depth has two advantages: First, it permits the excision of long pieces of tissue more quickly and with less movement than if the sheath remained stationary during each excursion of the loop; it thus diminishes blood loss and fluid absorption and decreases instrumentational trauma. Second, it allows a smoothness of stroke that is invaluable for correct sculpturing of the fossa. In using this method, the surgeon should take as long a stroke as possible in every instance; develop a slight forward and upward pressure of the sheath as the loop finishes its cut, so that a shearing motion is added to help the loop disentangle the tissue strip; and begin moving the sheath forward into position for the next stroke while the loop sends the cut strip of tissue into the bladder.

As the resection of the small adenoma is continued in horizontal cross steps from the surgical capsule toward the midline and back, the sheath must first be rotated so that the loop cuts on the concavity of the lateral wall with its full face rather than its side. The bared muscle on the roof is the best guide to the adenoma–capsule junction as resection proceeds down the lateral wall, until the thickness of tissue between sheath and the rectal finger can be palpatated more posteriorly.

After the cut into the adenoma at the vesical neck has been begun, the sheath is held lightly while the loop is kept as close as possible to the

depth indicated by the relation of the bared capsule of the lateral roof area and the uncut lateral-wall adenoma below it. As the loop bares the underlying tissue on the lateral wall, the surgeon can determine quickly whether the tissue represents muscle fibers or a further rim of adenoma. If it appears to be adenoma, more pressure is applied on the sheath to deepen the loop bite in an attempt to remain at muscle fiber level throughout the cut.

Any island of adenoma left proximally when the previous cut was adjusted to stay at capsule level can be trimmed off before the next stepdown cut is taken. It is often simpler to use the side of the loop (Fig. 88-15) to trim thin islands of tissue down to capsule, because the sheath can be leaned against the bladder neck or lateral walls to permit delicate shaving strokes.

The next layer of transverse steps crosses from the midline to the lateral wall and is accomplished in similar fashion. The terminal portion of the cutting stroke is made with a sweeping motion of the resectoscope as the apical region of adenoma is reached (Fig. 88-16). This brings the operator's

FIG. 88-16. Resection of apical tissue: **(A)** apical adenoma; **(B)** sweeping lateral to medial movement of loop and instrument as apical adenoma is removed.

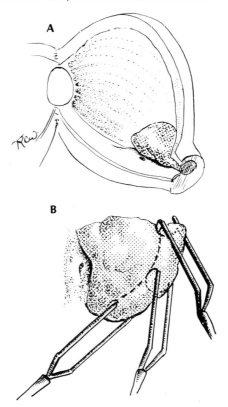

FIG. 88-15. Use of side of loop to shave thin layers of residual adenoma

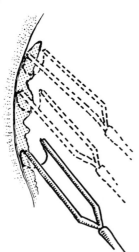

head closer to the patient's contralateral thigh because the hollow of the lateral lobe tapers toward the midline at the apex.

A rim of tissue is left at the apex until the bulk of adenoma between it and the bladder neck is removed. This tissue acts as a buffer against damage to the membranous urethra by the movements of the sheath and loop (Fig. 88-16). This method additionally enables expansion of the adenoma at the apex, making it more accessible for subsequent rapid removal.

Back-and-forth, steplike reduction of the lateral lobe mass is continued. The floor at the bladder neck must *not* be thinned down to bare muscle fibers at this time, to prevent the formation of a lip at the junction of bladder neck and posterior fossa. Such a lip can be a hazard during the early parts of resection, since the beak of the sheath can catch on it or the pressure of irrigating fluid can spread the muscle fibers. The floor tissue at the bladder neck, as well as the rim of adenoma at the apex, are left relatively undisturbed until the other half of the prostatic urethra has been dealt with. In small adenomas, the second half is resected in the same way as the first.

Encirclement Technique for Large Adenomas. Large adenomas may be managed in the cross-step fashion used for small ones, but an adenoma larger than 35 g to 40 g may be managed best by the encirclement technique.

The prostatic fossa is again divided into hemispheres and the left side is attacked first. After the first anterior longitudinal strip of tissue has been removed from bladder neck to apex, the resectoscope sheath is moved forward and canted to the left so that the juxtacapsular part of the lateral lobe junction with the roof can be engaged and a cut the length of the fossa can be made. Because the upper portion of the lateral lobe may be quite bulky, a few cross-step, side-by-side excursions of the loop may be needed to obtain sufficient room for the sheath to begin the encirclement of lateral wall tissue (Fig. 88-13).

After the anterior capsular wall has been exposed down to approximately 2 o'clock, the junction of the anterolateral capsule wall and the adenoma is attacked so that a groove can be cut between the bulk of the lateral lobe tissue and the capsule. The loop is placed so that its capsular edge just grazes the bare capsule above the tissue to be cut as it starts to make the cleavage between adenoma and capsule. If the fossa is long, the sheath should be moved with the loop after the bite has been started until the narrowing of the apical portion of the fossa is reached and the loop excursion can be concluded. The next cut is made

FIG. 88-17. Encirclement technique of lateral lobe resection: **(A)** outline of tissue resection for encirclement of lateral lobe; **(B)** cross-step resection of encircled, avascular lateral lobe tissue

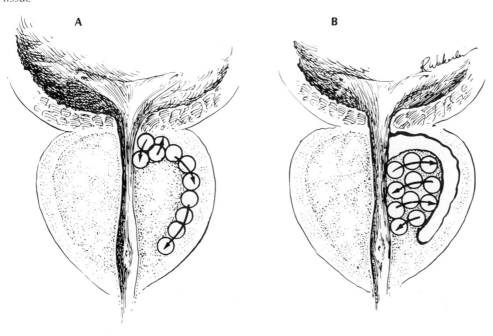

in the same juxtacapsular groove, which is delineated by brushing the sheath down the lateral capsule wall so that it slides between capsule and adenoma. The loop should be extended and ready to cut when the bottom of the groove is reached.

If the adenoma is long, the sheath is moved in a curve parallel to the concavity of the lateral capsular wall as it encircles the adenoma and tapers toward the apex. Successively deeper strips of adenoma are cut from this groove between capsule and lateral lobe, thus encircling the bulk of the lateral lobe and separating it from the fossa wall to avascularize it and prepare it for rapid removal (Fig. 88-17).

In a very long adenoma, if sliding the sheath as the cutting loop is withdrawn would disengage too cumbersome a strip of tissue, the cut can be terminated at the midpoint of the fossa. An upward maneuver will release the tissue, and the same level of adenoma can be returned to and cut out to the apical area without moving the sheath from the groove. When a large gland is being encircled, the sheath should be kept in the groove between capsule and lateral lobe as constantly as possible, because much time can be consumed by reorienting and repositioning the sheath if it is brought to the midline between the two lateral lobes. The sheath should be removed from the groove only when the bladder is being evacuated.

Islands of adenoma can be left until the cleaning up process after removal of the encircled lateral lobe. However, the amount of tissue left should not be so great as to obscure vision. Significant ridges or uneven spots should be resected before the groove is deepened into the next layer of adenoma, either by using the full face of the loop or by skiving thinner spots with the side of the loop. Care must be taken not to make the trench between the capsule and the mass of adenoma so deep as to cause the narrow strip of lateral lobe tissue to flop over in the midline and obscure vision. To prevent this from occurring, it is occasionally necessary to go back and resect the mass of encircled tissue from medial to lateral such as is described above for small adenomas. When the groove has been deepened to a point nearing the floor of the prostate, slanting cuts should be made toward the midline, just to the side of the verumontanum. Even the largest gland tapers near the apex, and care should be taken not to cut too deeply near the verumontanum at this time. After the lateral mass of tissue is removed, a cushion of apical adenoma remains that can be removed during the final trimming.

When the encirclement technique is used, bleed-ing points usually are prominent because the main feeding branches of the deep prostatic or adenomatous vascular system are encountered directly (Fig. 88-18). Fulguration of major bleeders minimizes blood loss and subsequently enables an almost bloodless removal of the encircled lateral lobe tissue.

The tissue separated from the lateral wall is now connected with the fossa only on the floor and can be attacked rapidly from the top down. By sliding the instrument as the loop is brought through the tissue, strips as long as can be conveniently handled are cut and evacuated through the sheath. If the isolated mass of adenoma is not particularly long but is fairly thick, to-and-fro cutting may be more advantageous (Fig. 88-19), because fewer sheath movements increase the speed of resection and diminish trauma to normal tissues. Under these circumstances the attack can be made in side-step fashion, back and forth across the adenomatous mass, cutting tissue on both forward and backward excursions of the loop and taking the whole mass down in layers until the capsule at the floor is approached. Here long unidirectional strokes are resumed, beginning with the adenoma just distal to the bladder neck, which was not previously disturbed.

The entire floor of the fossa is now hollowed out by deepening the bite as the bladder neck is left and as the rectal finger presses up on the posterior wall of the prostate. A rhythm of rectal pressure and sheath manipulation can keep each cut perfectly smooth so that as soon as capsule is bared at the beginning of the cut, the loop can remain at the adenoma–capsule junction through-

FIG. 88-18. Arterial supply to surgical capsule and adenoma. Encirclement deprives isolated tissue of its blood supply.

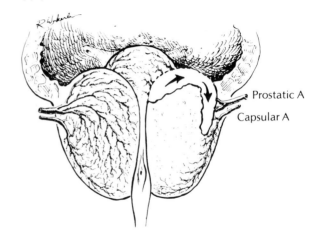

Prostatic A

Capsular A

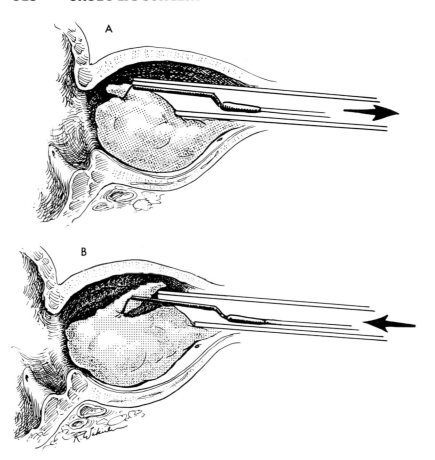

FIG. 88-19. Technique of electroresection: **(A)** standard excursion of cutting loop; **(B)** tissue being cut as loop is extended.

out its excursion (Fig. 88-20). Particular care must be taken at the bladder neck at the beginning of each cut to avoid thinning the vesicoprostatic muscle fibers. If there is subtrigonal adenomatous protrusion, a bit of tissue should be left here until the terminal stages of the resection to give the capsule a chance to contract and make the posterior vesical neck lip less prominent.

The contralateral half of the prostate is then dealt with according to its size, length, and configuration. Because adenomatous enlargement is usually symmetrical, the surgical approach is generally identical.

Final Trimming

After the middle and lateral lobes have been resected, the tissue remaining is found in the apical region on either side of the verumontanum and just adjacent to and below the posterior vesical neck. Because the apical adenoma has been allowed to expand, it can now be reached more easily because the rectal finger causes it to protrude from its lateral recesses. Only the final thin rim of apical tissue may have to be searched for. Very small

bites should be taken in this area and it is generally wise not to go distal to the verumontanum. Resecting too little tissue in this area is certainly the lesser of two evils when excessive resection beyond the verumontanum carries with it the risk of causing urinary incontinence. The entire apical circumference should be inspected from the more distal urethra as the resectoscope sheath is rotated, to determine completeness of removal of adenoma.

The remainder of the prostatic fossa is inspected and any irregular tags or islands of adenoma are removed; the end result should be smoothly concave fossa. Any remaining tissue on the floor at the vesical neck is trimmed down to muscle fibers. At this point, a general survey of the prostatic cavity is made. Any immediately apparent arterial bleeders are coagulated; any overlooked spheroid masses are trimmed away. The bladder is then thoroughly evacuated of chips and detritus. Sufficient time should be allowed for any residual adenoma to expand.

The final assessment of the fossa should now be done. Inspection of the prostatic cavity with the resectoscope sheath well out in the membranous

FIG. 88-20. Technique of electrosection. Finger in rectum presses tissue up for smooth removal as excursion of loop is terminated at prostatic apex.

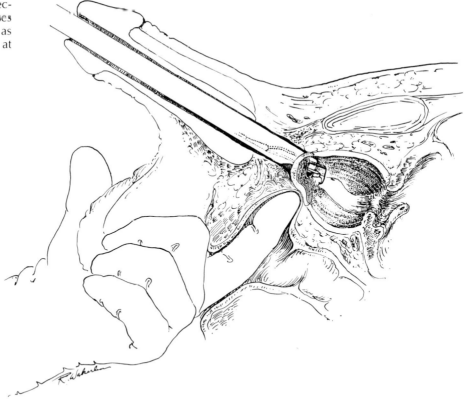

urethra is important. Elevation of the apical prostate with the rectal finger while the beak of the sheath is moved back and forth in the membranous urethra will demonstrate the membranoprostatic junction (Fig. 88-21) and enable the sheath to be fixed at that point so that the excursion of the loop into residual apical adenoma will be concluded without intrusion into the normal tissue around it. The anterior areas should be inspected carefully. Rarely is there any significant residual tissue in the area of the anterior commissure. If some is present in this area, tilting the table into the Trendelenburg position will make resection of this tissue easier. The anterior apical area should also be examined, keeping in mind that foreshortening often occurs in viewing this area, so that the excursions of the loop must be even more carefully restricted. During the final inspection phase, it is helpful intermittently to restrict or stop the flow of irrigating fluid so that small arterial bleeders and venous oozing can be identified and coagulated. Major arterial bleeding is characteristically encountered at any of four sites: 2 o'clock, 5 o'clock, 7 o'clock, and 10 o'clock. It is essential to cauterize all arterial bleeders; however, venous bleeding is usually controlled by gentle catheter traction.

It is important to be sure that all the chips are removed from the bladder, because large pieces of prostatic tissue can cause postoperative obstruction and their passage is a cause of concern to the patient. The chips are best removed by use of the Ellik evacuator or a Toomey piston syringe. After irrigation with these devices another visual inspection should be made to ensure that all tissue is removed.

At the termination of the procedure, a 22 Fr silicone Foley catheter with a 30-ml bag is inserted and filled with 30 ml to 45 ml of fluid, depending on the size of the gland. I am opposed to the routine use of three-way catheters in the postoperative period for the following reasons.

1. A three-way catheter drains less well than a two-way Foley of comparable size because of the need to accommodate the extra lumen.

2. I prefer not to have a large volume of fluid introduced into the bladder of a fresh postprostatectomy patient. Many patients undergoing TURP are old and debilitated; they may tolerate poorly any irrigating fluid absorbed through venous sinuses in the prostatic bed. Should the catheter drainage get blocked for any reason,

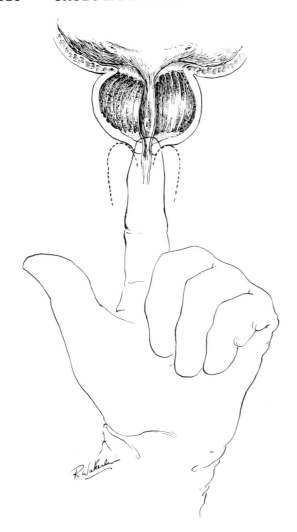

FIG. 88-21. Technique of electroresection. Finger in rectum distinguishes apical adenoma on both sides of midline soft spot below verumontanum.

the net effect is virtually a direct intravenous infusion of the irrigating solution through the open prostatic sinuses at a pressure equal to the height of the bottle above the level of the bladder; in most situations this is at least 100 cm water pressure.

3. Each time the irrigating solution is changed, the system of closed catheter drainage becomes open catheter drainage with an increased risk of inducing infection.

4. If the postoperative bleeding is so brisk as to block the catheter, I prefer to know it early rather than later.

5. Blood loss is more difficult to quantify in the presence of a continuous irrigation.

6. The routine use of postoperative irrigation is an unnecessary expense to the patient.

Before leaving the resection room the surgeon should irrigate the catheter while pulling the catheter down to apply moderate traction. If the irrigating fluid is not *completely clear* within 5 minutes of applying traction, the resectoscope should be reinserted and any bleeders, coagulated. Aside from assessing the control of bleeding in the immediate postoperative period, this little trick also ensures the surgeon that should bleeding recur over the next few hours it is likely that the reinstitution of traction will be sufficient to stop the bleeding.

In general, I prefer to use traction as sparingly as possible, although it appears that a moderate degree of traction can be tolerated by most patients for 6 hours to 8 hours without subsequent difficulty. After removal of traction the catheter should be taped to the lower abdominal wall to avoid the risk of pressure necrosis at the penile meatus.

The catheter is generally removed within 48 hours to 72 hours, but in patients with large bladders as a result of chronic retention it may be necessary to leave the catheter in for a longer time. The use of povadone-iodine (Betadine) ointment, applied to the urethral meatus twice daily for as long as the catheter is in place, helps to lubricate the meatus and may reduce the likelihood of urinary infection.

Complications

In addition to the meatal problems already discussed, the following problems deserve mention.

OBTURATOR NERVE STIMULATION

Obturator nerve stimulation during transurethral resection fortunately occurs infrequently. It is most commonly encountered when resecting lateral wall bladder tumors. It produces a sudden thigh movement that can cause the cutting loop to bite more deeply than desired and possibly to produce perforation. Although the curare-type drugs readily depress the reaction in the intubated patient under general anesthesia, this remedy is not suitable for the patient under regional block anesthesia. Local infiltration of anesthesics and the suggestions of Prentiss and associates may be required to prevent stimulation, but diminution of the cutting current, very careful paring of tissue, and cutting in the sensitive areas only at the very beginning of bladder filling will suffice in most instances.[19] Repeated light stimulation of the nerve can also fatigue it and abolish its response. The experienced surgeon has adjusted his reflexes so that the foot pedal is immediately released and the resectoscope is more loosely held the instant obturator stimulation occurs. This usually minimizes inadvertent cutting of tissue.

INSTRUMENT MALFUNCTION

Scrupulous attention to preoperative testing and the discarding of worn equipment usually keep instrument malfunction to a minimum. If the lighting system fails, the light cords and bulbs should be checked or changed. If the electrotome fails to cut or cuts improperly, the power cord should be changed and the irrigating fluid checked by taste to be sure that a current-conducting solution, such as saline solution, has not inadvertently been used. The substitute electrosurgical unit should be checked to make certain that the original unit is not at fault.

PERFORATION

Small perforations of the prostatic capsule are inevitable during the performance of a complete resection and are of no significance. A large perforation is often first detected by a change in the patient's blood pressure or respiration, failure of the return of irrigating fluid, or a palpable suprapubic mass. The resection should be terminated and a cystogram should be done if signs suggest a perforation. In most cases, the extravasation is extraperitoneal and can be managed by making a small suprapubic incision and inserting two drains in the space of Retzius. This is a simple procedure and does not require moving the patient to a major operating room. Intraperitoneal perforation requires closure of the wound.

EXCESSIVE HEMORRHAGE

Venous ooze can usually be controlled by traction as previously described. At times, the combination of filling the balloon to 50 ml to 60 ml and traction will be necessary to control bleeding. If, despite irrigation and traction, the blood loss continues to be excessive, it is necessary to take the patient back to the operating room. The resectoscope is reinserted and careful inspection is performed.

The prostatic fossa must be scraped clean of clot, quadrant by quadrant, until the entire resected surface is bare and can be seen clearly. The lens should then be withdrawn into the membranous urethra and the water inlet compressed to see if there are any obvious spurting vessels. This maneuver may also reveal intruding adenomatous tissue that may have expanded during this interval and that may be the source of bleeding.

Inspection of the entire vesical neck should then be undertaken with particular attention to the bladder side of the outlet. Vessels at the neck may be canted toward the bladder or actually be on the vesical side of the outlet if there is a drop-off at this point into the bladder. The fossa should then be carefully inspected quadrant by quadrant, side to side, back and forth, with particular attention to any excrescence or nubbin of residual adenoma that might be harboring a bleeding vessel under one of its margins. Very careful cleansing of the fossa usually suffices to clear the irrigation fluid return. If only venous bleeding is discovered, reinsertion of the catheter, with an appropriate amount of water in the balloon and variations of traction tension, usually facilitates clearing of the irrigant after a time.

Meticulous inspection and cleansing of the fossa should always be done before a coagulation defect is contemplated. A bleeding or coagulation disorder should, of course, be considered if the routine measures are unavailing, and the administration of epsilon aminocaproic acid (EACA), conjugated estrogen (Premarin), vitamin C, and other substances is usually harmless even if not often helpful. The best guarantee of hemostasis in transurethral prostatic surgery is clean removal of all adenoma, sparing of normal tissues, and careful terminal search for bleeding points.

POST-TUR SYNDROME

The post-TUR syndrome is a term applied to either of two conditions thought to be due to excessive absorption of irrigation fluid through the venous sinuses and into the general circulation. Avoidance of the use of sterile water as an irrigating agent will prevent the problem of hemolysis, hemoglobinuria, and possible renal shutdown.

A syndrome of increased blood pressure, tachycardia, muscle paralysis, and various degrees of mental disorientation may occur in some patients. This "low salt syndrome" is thought to be due to excessive absorption of fluid with a resulting dilution of the extracellular fluid. During the performance of a TURP the average patient absorbs about 900 ml of fluid.[14] In elderly and debilitated men this may lower the serum sodium to values of 120 mEq/liter or below and precipitate the rather bizarre mental and muscular symptoms which, unless promptly recognized and treated, can lead

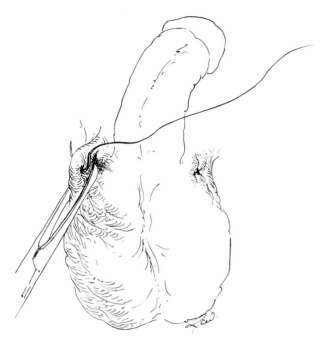

FIG. 88-22. Percutaneous method of vas ligation of Alyea and Valk

to death. The use of diuretics such as furosemide, or in life-threatening situations the infusion of hypertonic saline, should be instituted upon recognition.[18]

EPIDIDYMITIS

I do not routinely do a bilateral vasectomy in patients prior to TURP. Although the literature indicates that prophylactic vasectomy may indeed decrease the risk of postoperative epididymitis, in truth, the incidence of epididymitis is so low that little benefit appears to be gained by the routine performance of vasectomy. A better appreciation of the importance of sterile urine preoperatively, the judicious use of appropriate antibiotic prophylaxis in patients at high risk for infection, the use of smaller silicone or Teflon-coated catheters, and a decrease in the length of catheterization postoperatively, all have contributed to a decline in the overall incidence of epididymitis following TURP.

In those patients with long-term preoperative catheter drainage, urethritis or recurrent epididymitis vasectomy might be indicated, although the decision must be individualized.

Two methods of preoperative vasectomy have gained acceptance. In the percutaneous method of Alyea (Fig. 88-22), the vas is isolated by palpation through the scrotum and is encircled by passing a needle with swedged on 1-0 or 2-0 chromic catgut through the intact skin.[1] The suture is tied tightly and is left until the suture dissolves and the knot drops away. This procedure, although perhaps esthetically objectionable, appears to be effective as the standard ligation and resection technique.

In the standard technique the vas is isolated in the upper scrotum by running the fingers of both hands over the cord until the vas can be separated from the other scrotal structures. It is then held so that the fingers of one hand can keep it apart while an Allis clamp is placed around only the vas in its taut tunnel of scrotal skin (Fig. 88-23). An incision is made through the skin and scrotal layers that are being held between the limbs of the Allis clamp, down through the vasal sheath. The Allis clamp is then tilted to cause the incision to gape sufficiently to enable the tips of a mosquito clamp to pick the vas from its sheath bed and pull it gently out of the wound. The incision must be made through the vasal sheath so that a straight clamp can be slipped under only the vas itself. Two clamps are placed about 1 cm apart, and the vas is cut so that the portion between the clamps can be excised. After ligation, the clamps are released to permit the severed ends to retract up into the sheath so that there will be no adherence to surrounding tissues or the skin.

Simultaneous Conditions of the Prostate

CARCINOMA OF THE PROSTATE

When benign hypertrophy and carcinoma coincide, the technical aspects of transurethral resection are identical to those used for benign hypertrophy, because the areas of adenoma and normal capsule act as guidelines for the extent of resection in the carcinomatous areas. Capsular or peripheral extension of carcinoma negates an encirclement maneuver, but by using the depth of adjacent adenomatous tissue as a guide, a cross-step resection similar to that used for small adenomas can be done. Carcinoma usually has a fuzzy cottonwood appearance that differentiates it from the coarse nodules of the benign gland. Most carcinomas are relatively bloodless. Resecting them is technically an easier procedure than resecting a very vascular adenoma. The important difference is that in carcinoma, particularly an extensive one, the normal tissue plane that separates the adenoma from the prostatic capsule is lost. Because the carcinoma infiltrates the capsule and pericapsular tissues, the

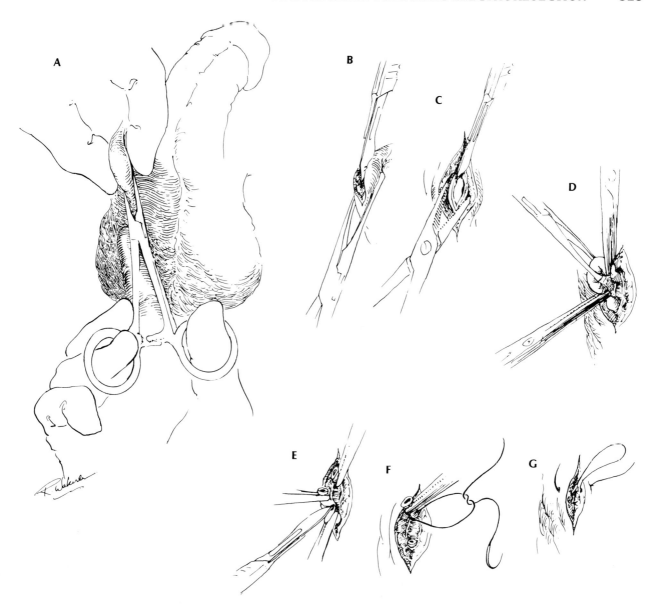

FIG. 88-23. Vasectomy: **(A)** vas is isolated and held with Allis clamp; **(B)** incision through scrotal skin; **(C)** incision deepened through vasal sheath; **(D)** vas delivered from its sheath and doubly clamped; **(E)** portion of vas excised; **(F)** proximal and distal ends of severed vas ligated; **(G)** skin closed

resection cannot continue out beyond the level of the adjacent adenoma-capsule junction lest perforation occur. Therefore areas of carcinoma are simply cut off flush in the same plane as the limit of removal of surrounding benign tissue (Fig. 88-24).

When the carcinoma is bulky and extensive, the technique of resection must differ from that used for benign hypertrophy. Here, aside from the bladder neck and the membranous urethra, there are often no precise landmarks to determine the ultimate depth of tissue resection. Endoscopic tactics depend on a sculpturing of the fossa to correspond to visual and palpable estimates of the thickness of tissue between rectal finger and resectoscope sheath. The movement of the sheath is restricted, and an experienced resectionist can often suspect the presence of malignancy from the "feel" of the sheath in the urethra. Under these circumstances the surgeon should remove readily

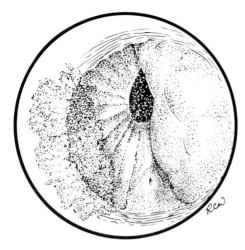

FIG. 88-24. Removal of carcinomatous tissue. As capsule is cleared of adjacent benign adenoma, carcinoma of prostate extending through capsule is cut off flush in same plane.

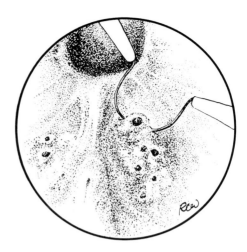

FIG. 88-25. Removal of seed calculi embedded in thin layer of adenoma

accessible tissue anywhere from the bladder neck to the verumontanum, which is often the only identifiable landmark. Because carcinoma tends to regrow locally I believe that a mere "channeling" procedure is not sufficient. An attempt should be made to remove as much tissue as possible to ensure a moderate concavity of the fossa from just beyond the bladder neck to the verumontanum. This is usually best accomplished by cross-step resection from medial to lateral. Many of these malignancies invade the area of the external sphincter and make it rigid, resulting in difficulties in urinary control. It is wise to avoid cutting too close to the external sphincter and, most importantly, to minimize the use of coagulating current in this area. When resecting prostatic malignancies the surgeon must be aware that in some patients the malignancy produces large amounts of circulating fibrinolysin that can lead to massive hemorrhage. The condition can be diagnosed by clotting studies and is treated by the administration EACA, an inhibitor of prostatic urokinase.

PROSTATIC CALCULI

There is no specific reason to remove prostatic calculi, although in some patients with chronic bacterial prostatitis, the infecting organism has been shown to reside within the stone protected from antibiotic, as happens with infected renal calculi. Prostatic stones are found most commonly in the plane between the adenoma and the capsule and serve as a good guide to the depth of the resection. The calculi can be unroofed by the

resectoscope loop (Fig. 88-25). A finger in the patient's rectum is very useful in providing pressure to push the calculi into the prostatic fossa where they can easily be removed. In doing a TURP for documented chronic bacterial prostatitis that is refractory to treatment, it is important both to try to remove all calculi and to remove all adenoma so that capsular fibers are visible in all areas of the prostate. This "radical TUR" has been reported to be effective in eliminating infection in only about one third of cases and only when virtually all prostatic tissue has been resected.

PROSTATIC ABSCESS

The classic prostatic abscess in which an entire lobe is virtually filled with pus is encountered infrequently. Most prostatic abscesses seen in surgical practice today are found as small pockets of purulent material (remnants of prior infections) encountered during the course of TURP for benign prostatic hypertrophy. No special adjustments in technique are required. In a true, bulging abscess, transurethral resection provides excellent drainage and is less morbid than transrectal evacuation. The bulging, fluctuant prostatic lobe is readily apparent at surgery. A single passage of the loop results in a gush of pus, and little else is required. A small urethral catheter is helpful in maintaining drainage for a few days after surgery.

REFERENCES

1. ALYEA EP: Vaso-ligation: A preventive of epididymitis before and after prostatectomy. J Urol 19:65, 1928

2. BARNES RW: Endoscopic Prostatic Surgery. St Louis, CV Mosby, 1943

3. BLANDY JP: Operative Urology, p 142. Oxford, Blackwell Scientific Publications, 1978

4. BRAASCH WF: Median bar excision. JAMA 70:758, 1918

5. BUMPUS HC, JR: Transurethral prostatic resection. Br J Urol 4:105, 1932

6. CREEVY CD: The importance of hemolysis during transurethral prostatic resection: A clinical investigation. J Urol 59:1217, 1948

7. EUDY W: Correlations between in vitro sensitivity testing and therapeutic response in urinary tract infections. Urology 2:519, 1973

8. EMMETT JL: Transurethral resection with the cold punch: Operative technique. J Urol 49:815, 1943

9. EMMETT JL, ROUS SN, GREENE LF et al: Preliminary internal urethrotomy in 1036 cases to prevent urethral stricture following transurethral resection: Caliber of the normal adult male urethra. J Urol 89:829, 1963

10. GLENN JF, JONES WR, HENSON PE, JR: Effects of intravenous administration of various irrigant solutions upon urine and blood of dogs. Invest Urol 2:530, 1965

11. LEWIS B: History of Urology. Baltimore, Williams & Wilkins, 1933

12. LITIN KB, EMMETT JL: Method for measuring blood loss during transurethral resection when nonhemolytic irrigating solutions are employed. Proc Mayo Clin 34:158, 1959

13. MCNEAL JE: Regional morphology and pathology of the prostate. Am J Clin Pathol 49:347, 1968

14. MADSEN PO, MADSEN RE: Clinical and experimental evaluation of different irrigating fluids for transurethral surgery. Invest Urol 3:122, 1965

15. MEBUST WU, FORET JD, VALK WL: Transurethral Surgery. In Harrison JH, Gittes RF, Perlmutter AD et al (eds): Campbell's Urology, Vol 3, p. 2361. Philadelphia, WB Saunders, 1979

16. NESBIT RM: Transurethral Prostatectomy. Springfield, Illinois, Charles C Thomas, 1943

17. NESBIT RM: A history of transurethral prostatic resection in Silber SJ (ed): Transurethral Resection, p 1. New York, Appleton-Century-Crofts, 1977

18. PARRY WL, SCHAEFER AF, MUELLER CB: Experimental studies of acute renal failure. I. The protective effect of mannitol. J Urol 89:1, 1963

19. PRENTISS RJ, HARVEY GW, BETHARD WF Massive adductor muscle contraction in transurethral surgery: Cause and prevention; Development of new electrical circuitry. J Urol 93:263, 1965

20. WEYRAUCH HM: Surgery of the Prostate. Philadelphia, WB Saunders, 1959

Transurethral Punch Prostatectomy

89

David C. Utz

Instruments based on the cold-punch principle and designed to remove a portion of the prostate were in use long before the development of the operating cystoscope. Guthrie, in 1834, described a catheter with an enclosed blade projecting from the end of it that incised tissue as it was introduced and withdrawn. Realizing the limitations of incision of tissue only. Mercier in 1847 designed a series of instruments incorporating a conical excisor which removed small pieces of prostatic tissue at the posterior commissure. This was the beginning of the evolution of transurethral prostatic resection.

In 1909, Young developed a similar knife instrument by modifying his posterior urethroscope so that the fenestra was on the convex rather than the concave surface, in the direction of the beak, of the Mercier excisor. Interest in transurethral surgery was aroused, and the word *punch* was added to urologic nomenclature.

Because of lack of visualization of the field and of any means of hemostasis, practical application of this technique was limited to median bar and cicatricial obstruction at the vesical neck. These disadvantages were partially overcome by Braasch, who incorporated an inner cutting tubular sheath into his direct-vision cystoscope, thus affording adequate observation of the tissue before and during excision.[1] To solve the problem of bleeding, Bumpus modified the Braasch instrument to include a guide carrying an electrode so that it was no longer necessary to replace the resectoscope with a cystoscope to electrocoagulate bleeders.[2]

Equipment

INSTRUMENTS

In 1935, Thompson described a direct-vision resectoscope that was a modification of the Braasch–Bumpus punch instrument.[10] The chief objections to the latter had been surmounted. With the Thompson direct-vision resectoscope, the tissue to be removed could be inspected more precisely and excised under observation. No longer was it necessary to change the sheath to close the fenestra and convert the instrument into a cystoscope or to introduce an electrode for fulguration of vessels. With the Thompson instrument* (Fig. 89-1), the tissue is excised when the tubular knife, attached to a sheath which slides inside the outer housing, closes the fenestra. The hollow central sheath transports irrigating fluid and is activated by a lever into which the fluid inlet valve is incorporated. Electrofulguration of blood vessels is accomplished with a plastic-covered electrode that passes within the wall of the outer housing. Irrigating fluid circulates through the eyepiece by entering a small aperture adjacent to the glass and flowing down a rubber tube which is weighted by a perforated metal ball or a Tuohy–Borst adaptor so that the tube remains in the pan of the operating table even when the instrument is rotated 180 degrees. This circulatory system prevents bubbles from forming in the eyepiece and can be interrupted when desired by closing a small cock on the eyepiece.

Frohmüller modified the Thompson resectoscope by substituting fiberoptic light illumination, adding the Lumina† telescopic system, and altering the beak and the washer mechanism (Fig. 89-2).[7]

SUCTION APPARATUS

One of the exceptional advantages of the cold punch is the facility with which excised pieces of tissue can be evacuated from the bladder. Bladder contents are emptied by way of the lumen of the inside sheath without removing the sheath. A fluid outlet valve as large as the central caliber of the

---

* Boehm Surgical Instrument Corp, 966 Chili Ave, Rochester, NY 14607 (distributed by V Mueller, 6600 W Touhy Ave, Chicago, Illinois 60648).

† Richard Wolf GMBH, 7134 Knittlingen, West Germany (in USA: Richard Wolf Medical Instruments Corp., 7046 Lyndon Ave, Rosemont, Illinois 60018).

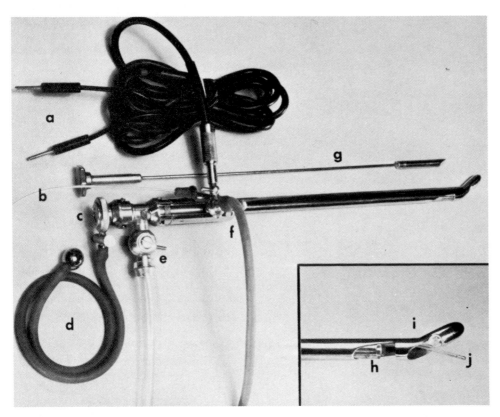

FIG. 89-1. Components of Thompson resectoscope: **(a)** light cord; **(b)** plastic-coated fulgurating electrode; **(c)** eyepiece with bubble eliminator; **(d)** fluid tube with weight; **(e)** fluid outlet valve with attached plastic suction tube; **(f)** fluid inlet valve mounted on inner sheath; **(g)** obturator; **(h)** knife blade partially withdrawn; **(i)** lamp; **(j)** fulgurating electrode

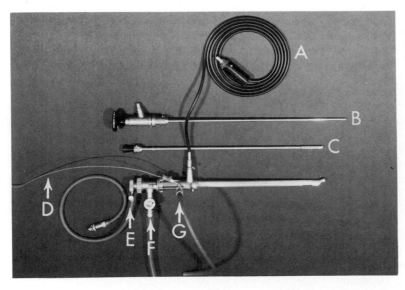

FIG. 89-2. Components of Frohmüller resectoscope: **(a)** fiberoptic light cord; **(b)** lumina telescope; **(c)** obturator; **(d)** fulguration electrode; **(e)** eyepiece with bubble eliminator; **(f)** fluid outlet valve with attached plastic suction tube; **(g)** fluid inlet valve mounted on inner sheath

FIG. 89-3. Suction apparatus used to evacuate tissue and irrigating fluid with Thompson resectoscope: **(a)** five-gallon collecting bottle (*dotted line*); **(b)** outlet tube that carries bloody irrigating fluid and cut pieces of tissue from bladder to collecting bottle; **(c)** suction tube connected to vacuum line; **(d)** trap that filters prostatic tissue from fluid. At conclusion of operation, trap is removed, lid **(e)** is unscrewed, and cut pieces of tissue are removed. (Litin RB, Emmett JL: Proc Staff Mtg Mayo Clin 34:158, 1959)

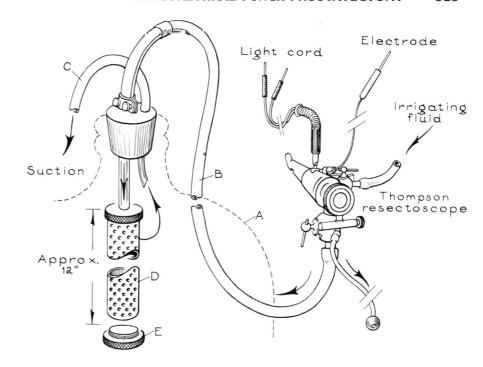

instrument accommodates the largest piece of tissue that can be resected. The bladder can be emptied by gravity supplemented by the expulsive force of the bladder and suprapubic pressure, or it can be evacuated by suction with the system described in 1948 by Doss (Fig. 89-3).[3] In this arrangement, a firm plastic or rubber tube is connected to the fluid outlet valve of the resectoscope and attached to a cylinder trap, which is stabilized inside a 190-liter (5-gal) glass bottle by a two-holed rubber stopper. A negative pressure is created in the bottle by means of a tube connected to a source of vacuum at 12.5 cm (5 in.) of mercury. Prostatic tissue collected in the trap is obtained for pathologic examination, at the conclusion of the operation, by removing a lid. The irrigating fluid accumulating in the bottle is measured and the blood loss is determined by the method of Litin and Emmett.[9]

IRRIGATING FLUID SUPPLY

The irrigating fluid systems used with direct-vision operative cystoscopy vary, but an essential requirement in all of them is a relatively high, constant pressure to ensure adequate flow, and thus, clear vision. The fluid transport system within the Thompson resectoscope accommodates a considerably larger volume than is possible in the lens instruments. This offers an outstanding advantage—namely, in the presence of sharp bleeding, vision is much clearer with the cold punch.

At the Mayo Clinic, two sources of irrigating fluid are available.[8] Tanks centrally located in the cystoscopic suite supply sterile warm (90° F) water by overhead conduits to each room at a pressure of 180 cm (6 ft) of water calculated from the level of the table. The capacity of each tank is 380 liters (100 gal), and the entire system is sterilized periodically by steaming.

The other source, the Emmett irrigating-fluid supply, is more versatile in that nonhemolytic (glycine, glucose sorbitol—Cytal) or isotonic solutions, as well as sterile water, can be provided.[5,11] Differential flow rates and pressures can be attained, by a simple adjustment, to accommodate varying operative conditions such as type of resectoscope used, height of operating table, severity of bleeding, and degree of bladder tonicity. The entire tank, which has a capacity of 33 liters, can be easily autoclaved and can be moved on casters from room to room (Fig. 89-4).

Although the Valentine flask system can be used as an irrigating-fluid source, the unit must be kept at least 120 cm (4 ft) above the bladder for the Thompson resectoscope and requires several fillings for the average prostatic resection.

PREPARATORY PROCEDURE

The conventional instrument organization for the operating table is shown in Figure 89-5.

The Otis bougies, sizes 24Fr to 30Fr, are passed

first to detect urethral narrowing. If the 24Fr Otis bougie does not pass, smaller ones are used to characterize the stricture. A retrograde urethrogram can be made while the patient is on the operating table if any doubt exists about the location and caliber of the stricture. Then, either the urethra is dilated with van Buren or LeFort sounds to 26Fr, or an internal urethrotomy is carried out to the same caliber with the Otis urethrotome.

Cystoscopy is performed and if the clinical

FIG. 89-4. Emmett irrigating-fluid supply for transurethral surgery: **(a)** air valve; **(b)** test alarm; **(c)** test safety; **(d)** pressure regulator knob; **(e)** pressure gauge; **(f)** foreign-material trap; **(g)** quick connect–disconnect air coupler with bacterial filter for compressed air; **(h)** funnel opening for filling tank; **(i)** outlet to resectoscope for fluid; **(j)** tank of cast aluminum, lined with Teflon; **(k)** sight gauge for fluid volume; **(l)** cart. (Farrall Instrument Co, Grand Island, NE 68801)

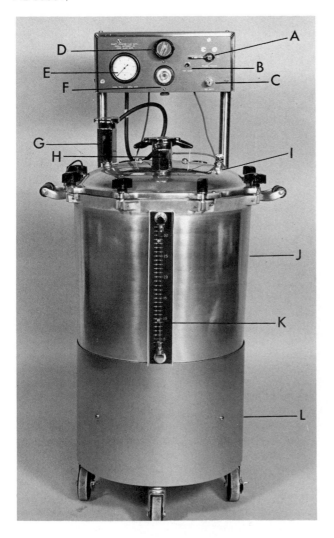

impression of significant prostatic obstruction is confirmed, the urethra is prepared for passage of the resectoscope. An internal urethrotomy is performed if a 30Fr Otis bougie encounters resistance in the urethra distal to the membranous segment.[6] If the urethral caliber is adequate, 20 ml of lubricant is injected by plastic syringe into the urethra and a 28Fr and then a 30Fr van Buren sound are passed.

There are three calibers of the Thompson resectoscope: 24Fr, 27Fr, and 30Fr. The 27Fr instrument is the most useful size, but, for adenomas larger than 100 g, the largest caliber is advantageous. The use of the 24Fr resectoscope is restricted primarily to younger patients with vesical neck contracture.

At the completion of the operation, either a 22Fr or a 24Fr irrigating retention catheter is introduced. The versatility of this catheter for continuous or intermittent irrigation or straight drainage is apparent.

Technique of Resection

The basic principles of transurethral resection are much the same, irrespective of the type of instrument used. However, a few unique features of the cold-punch operation require explanation.

Deserving special emphasis is the fundamental fact that prostatic tissue must be forced into the fenestra of the resectoscope. To accomplish this, pressure is exerted by the entire left arm on the instrument; using the urogenital diaphragm as a fulcrum, a lever action is obtained (Fig. 89-6). Mere application of pressure with the fingers on top of the resectoscope only results in bits of tissue being engaged and the operator becoming exhausted. In the final stages of the operation, resection of median lobe tissue in a pocketed urethra is expedited by digital rectal pressure against the posterior surface of the prostate.

There are four essential maneuvers of the cold-punch technique. In the first (Fig. 89-7A), the portion of tissue to be cut is observed. The inlet irrigating-fluid valve is opened fully, and the knife is in the home or closed position so that the fenestra is occluded. The next step (Fig. 89-7B) involves engagement of tissue. The instrument is advanced 2 cm or 3 cm and the blade is withdrawn, opening the fenestra. The tissue is engaged by pressure on the resectoscope, securing the prostate in the fenestra. In the third maneuver (Fig. 89-7C), the inner sheath containing the tubular blade is thrust forward with a rapid, determined movement, excising the prostatic tissue. The bite or piece of tissue is propelled by the stream of irrigating fluid through the opening adjacent to the beak of the

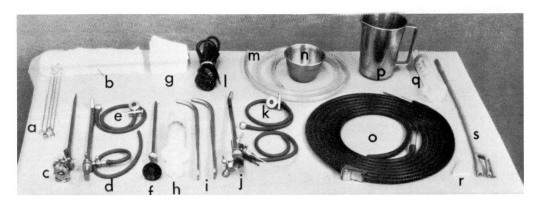

FIG. 89-5. Surgical table setup for transurethral prostatic resection: **(a)** Otis bougies (24, 26, 28, and 30Fr); **(b)** lubricant; **(c)** Otis urethrotome; **(d)** 24Fr Braasch direct-vision cystoscope with irrigating-fluid line attached; **(e)** eyepiece with bubble eliminator for cystoscope; **(f)** lens for Braasch cystoscope; **(g)** gauze sponges for wiping eyepiece and lens; **(h)** 50-ml plastic syringe containing lubricant; **(i)** 28 and 30Fr van Buren sounds; **(j)** 27Fr Thompson resectoscope assembled with electrode, obturator, and fluid supply line; **(k)** eyepiece with bubble eliminator and weight for resectoscope; **(l)** light cord for cystoscope and resectoscope; **(m)** line for suction system; **(n)** small receptacle for urine sample and special tissue collection; **(o)** irrigating-fluid line from overhead water supply or solution tank to short line on cystoscope and resectoscope; **(p)** graduated 500-ml container used for hand irrigation of catheter; **(q)** empty 50-ml plastic syringe for catheter; **(r)** metal (K-gar) catheter clamp; **(s)** 24Fr retention latex catheter for irrigation

FIG. 89-6. Resection technique with Thompson resectoscope. Engagement of prostatic tissue is accomplished by creating lever action with resectoscope, using urogenital diaphragm as fulcrum. (From Emmett JL: J Urol 49:815. Baltimore, The Williams & Wilkins Co, © 1943)

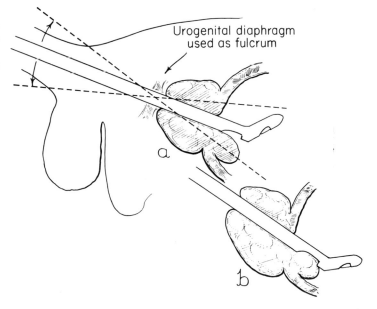

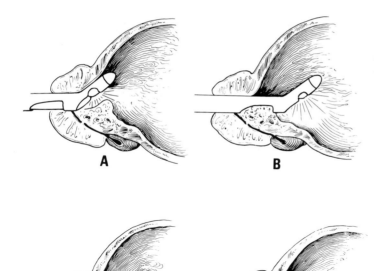

FIG. 89-7. Resection technique with Thompson resectoscope: **(A)** examination of prostatic tissue to be excised; **(B)** engagement of tissue in opened fenestra; **(C)** excision of tissue as knife is thrust forward to close fenestra; **(D)** electrofulguration of spurting vessels

instrument into the bladder. When the bladder is sufficiently distended, the tissue with the irrigating fluid is evacuated by closing the inlet valve and opening the outlet valve. Finally, the most active bleeding vessels are electrofulgurated (Fig. 89-7D). Aggressive desiccation of the prostatic urethra in an attempt to obtain perfect hemostasis is unnecessary and only results in a comprehensive slough accompanied by postoperative hemorrhage.

The Thompson resectoscope must be rotated 360 degrees to visualize the entire circumference of the prostatic urethra. Each operator develops his own style of handling the instrument, but generally the knife is activated by the right hand regardless of what sector is being resected. The electrode is held by the right hand when resecting the right lateral and median lobes and by the left hand when working on the left lateral lobe. Figure 89-8 illustrates a satisfactory manner of handling the instrument.[4]

Critique
Controversy over which type of resectoscope—the hot loop or the cold punch—is superior is only pedantic and trivial. Both instruments have their advantages and disadvantages, and excellent prostatic resections can be done by experienced urologists with either instrument. It is probably true, however, that few urologists are competent in the use of both instruments for prostatic resection. To those trained in direct-vision cystoscopy, use of the Thompson resectoscope is natural. The unmagnified, clear view of structures even in the presence of sharp bleeding, the tactile appreciation of tissue consistency, and the facility of removing resected tissue and irrigating fluid in the bladder seem to be distinct advantages.

REFERENCES

1. BRAASCH WF: Median bar excisor. JAMA 70:758, 1918
2. BUMPUS HC, JR: Transurethral prostatic resection. Br J Urol 4:105, 1932
3. DOSS AK: Transurethral prostatectomy assisted by suction apparatus. J Urol 59:211, 1948
4. EMMETT JL: Transurethral resection with the cold punch: Operative technique. J Urol 49:815, 1943
5. EMMETT JL, PAPANTONIOU A: Apparatus to supply isotonic irrigating fluid during transurethral prostatic resection. Proc Staff Meet Mayo Clin 33:446, 1958
6. EMMETT JL, ROUS SN, GREENE LF et al: Preliminary internal urethrotomy in 1036 cases to prevent urethral stricture following transurethral resection: Caliber of normal adult male urethra. J Urol 89:829, 1963
7. FROHMÜLLER H: Direktsichtinstrumente in der Urologie. Verh Dtsch Ges Urol 24:331, 1973

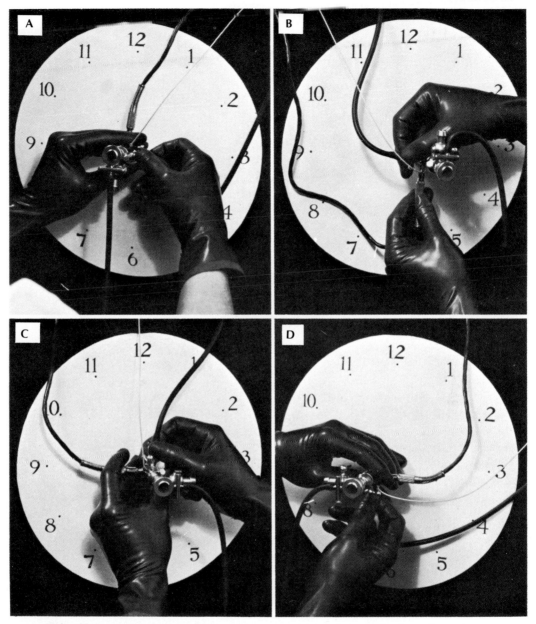

FIG. 89-8. Method of handling resectoscope to resect prostatic tissue in various sectors: **(A)** at 6-o'clock position for median lobe; **(B)** at 12-o'clock position for anterior lobe; **(C)** at 3-o'clock position for left lateral lobe; **(D)** at 9-o'clock position for right lateral lobe. (Emmett JL: J Urol 49:815. Baltimore, The Williams & Wilkins Co, © 1943)

8. GREENE LF, SEGURA JW: Transurethral Surgery. Philadelphia, WB Saunders, 1979

9. LITIN RB, EMMETT JL: Method for measuring blood loss during transurethral resection when nonhemolytic irrigating solutions are employed. Proc Staff Meet Mayo Clin 34:158, 1959

10. THOMPSON GJ: A new direct vision resectoscope. Urol Cutan Rev 39:545, 1935

11. WILSON JD, UTZ DC, TASWELL HF: Autotransfusion during transurethral resection of the prostate: Technique and preliminary clinical evaluation. Mayo Clin Proc 44:374, 1969

Prostatic Biopsy Techniques

90

Joseph W. Segura

There is general agreement that the urologist should consider biopsy of any prostate that does not feel normal on digital rectal examination. This sentiment recognizes both the ubiquitous nature of prostatic cancer and the inaccuracy of the examining finger in distinguishing tumor from other conditions of the prostate. Although confidence about the presence of cancer on rectal examination varies from "near certainty" to "mild suspicion," in one large series the examining finger resulted in an accurate prediction only half the time.[3]

Techniques

Biopsy of the prostate may be accomplished in five ways: transrectal needle biopsy, transperineal needle biopsy, suction biopsy, open prostatic biopsy, and transurethral biopsy. Because clinical situations requiring biopsy are so common, the ideal biopsy technique should be simple, safe, accurate, and easily repeatable. Transrectal and transperineal biopsy techniques fulfill these criteria, and most urologists in the United States use one of these as a standard method of obtaining biopsy material.[6]

TRANSRECTAL NEEDLE BIOPSY

At the Mayo Clinic, transrectal needle biopsy is the preferred technique for prostatic biopsy. It may be performed as an office procedure without an anesthetic or in the hospital with the patient under general or regional anesthesia. Transrectal needle biopsy probably is the most accurate of available procedures and has the advantages of simplicity and easy repeatability. Its particular advantage is that the finger can readily guide the needle to the suspicious area. Its chief disadvantage is the definite risk of bacteremia and sepsis despite preliminary rectal cleansing, although the risk is minimized by the preliminary use of antibiotics. Also, some patients cannot tolerate the discomfort, and an accurate specimen may be impossible to take. In others, discomfort precludes multiple speci-

mens. Both of these problems are obviated by doing the procedure with the patient under general anesthesia.

Oral antibiotics are given at least 2 hours before the biopsy specimen is taken. Trimethoprim-sulfamethoxazole (double strength), one tablet twice a day, is preferred, and this dosage is continued until 4 days after the biopsy. An alternative selection is nitrofurantoin, 100 mg four times a day, for the same time period. An enema is self-administered 1 hour before the biopsy. Whether the patient is placed in the knee–chest or lithotomy position is a matter of the physician's personal preference; inspection of the rectum through the anoscope and aspiration of any retained enema is much easier with the patient in the knee–chest position. The anoscope is inserted, and retained enema or watery stool is aspirated. If a large amount of stool is present, the procedure is best deferred pending a more thorough cleansing of the rectum. An iodophor-soaked swab is used to prepare the rectal mucosa.

With the index finger as a guide, the physician obtains a core of tissue using the Franklin modification of the Vim–Silverman needle or the Travenol Trucut needle (Fig. 90-1). My preference is the Vim–Silverman because a larger core of tissue can be obtained, but the Trucut needle is simpler and quicker to operate and is less traumatic. Multiple cores are obtained as necessary, a process that is easier with the patient under anesthesia. If more than one core of tissue is taken, the technique provides an accuracy of about 90%.[7] After the specimen has been taken, the rectal mucosa need not be inspected for bleeding.

Most patients tolerate transrectal needle biopsy well with few complications. About 6% of patients become infected despite adequate prophylaxis, and bacteremia is common but usually not clinically significant.[5] Urethral and rectal bleeding is very common, but usually it disappears spontaneously. Occasionally, urethral bleeding persists for a week or longer, and a rare patient may require a transfusion.[1] Acute urinary retention sometimes ensues,

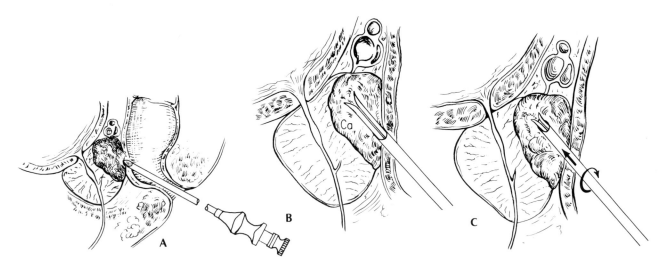

FIG. 90-1. Transrectal prostatic needle biopsy technique using the Franklin modification of the Vim–Silverman biopsy needle. Multiple cores may be obtained as necessary.

FIG. 90-2. Perineal prostatic needle biopsy. The Travenol needle is illustrated. Note that the course of the needle is entirely extrarectal.

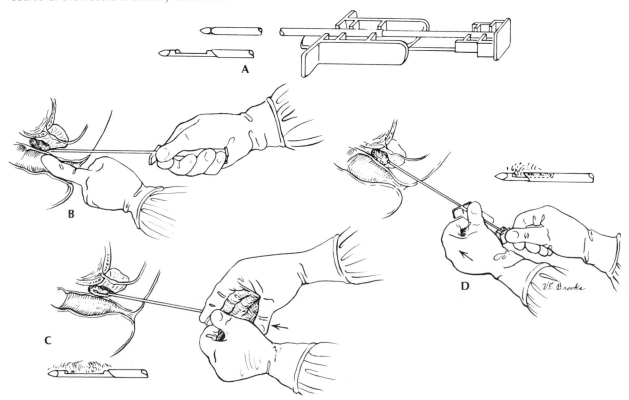

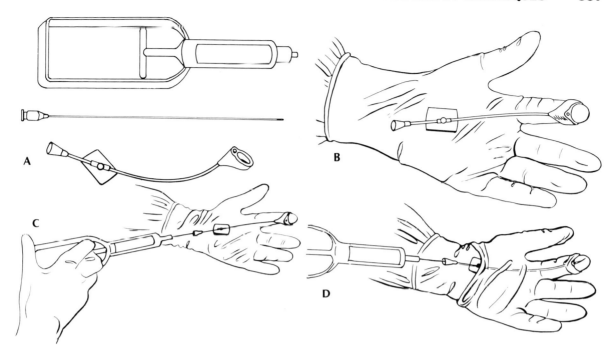

FIG. 90-3.   Transrectal suction prostatic fine-needle biopsy using the Franzén needle. (After photograph from Professor Kelâmi, showing his technique)

but this usually responds to conservative measures. Perirectal hematomas have occurred. Although very rare, death may ensue, usually from sepsis.

TRANSPERINEAL NEEDLE BIOPSY

This technique is usually done as an in-hospital procedure with the patient under anesthesia, but it can be performed as an office procedure using local anesthesia and sedation. Its major advantage is that the risk of sepsis is minimal because the needle does not pass through the rectal mucosa. However, the technique is somewhat less accurate than the transrectal method.

With the patient under general anesthesia or after the skin of the perineum has been infiltrated with 1% lidocaine, a Vim–Silverman or Trucut needle is inserted into the perineum above the anal sphincter (Fig. 90-2). A finger in the rectum guides the needle to the appropriate point in the prostate, and cores are taken as necessary. With this method, the false-negative rate is somewhat higher on the first biopsy than it is with the transrectal method, but because multiple cores are usually taken, this is not a disadvantage. Complications are similar to those with the transrectal technique, although the risk of bacteremia is considerably reduced. Despite this, antibiotics should be used prophylactically.

The seeding of tumor in the needle tract has been reported, but this complication is rare.[2]

SUCTION BIOPSY OF THE PROSTATE

In this method, the diagnosis of cancer is based on the pathologic examination of material aspirated from the prostatic nodule. After a preliminary enema and preparation of the rectal mucosa with iodophor, the Franzén biopsy needle is introduced directly into the nodule through the rectal wall, and material is aspirated from the nodule, utilizing the syringe (Fig. 90-3). The needle may be inserted many times into the suspicious area. The method is less traumatic than either of the needle biopsy methods, and its simplicity lends itself to common use. Interpretation of the material, however, requires an expert cytologist, and if such is not available, the technique is best not employed.[4] Although this technique has gained popularity in Europe, it has never been widely employed in the United States.

OPEN PROSTATIC BIOPSY

Open prostatic biopsy has been used to elucidate suspicious nodules in patients who are potential candidates for surgical cure of prostate cancer. As such, the method often has been followed by immediate radical prostatectomy. Because of the success in taking multiple specimens by the transrectal or the transperineal method, particularly when the accuracy of these specimens is monitored by frozen-section analysis of the pathology specimens, open prostatic biopsy is usually not necessary.

The patient is placed in the lithotomy position, and the posterior portion of the prostate gland is exposed in the same manner as for a perineal prostatectomy. The patient should be warned that impotence may accompany this attempted biopsy. A wedge-shaped piece of tissue is removed with a knife, and the defect is closed with catgut sutures. The tissue should be examined on frozen section, and if it is positive for cancer, a radical perineal or radical retropubic prostatectomy may be performed or the incision simply closed.

The biopsy specimen also may be taken through the retropubic approach. In this technique, the prostate is exposed in the same manner as for a retropubic prostatectomy; the prostate is then rotated laterally, and a wedge of tissue encompassing the suspicious area is removed. The technique is somewhat more difficult than the transperineal biopsy method.

TRANSURETHRAL BIOPSY

Because most carcinomas of the prostate occur in the posterior lobe, transurethral resection of the prostate may not remove the tumor-containing portion of the prostate. Therefore, one should not depend upon a transurethral resection for diagnosis of carcinoma when the posterior lobe feels suspicious. Extensive local disease with widespread prostatic or intravesical extension of tumor may be diagnosed easily by transurethral biopsy of the suspicious area.

REFERENCES

1. BISSADA NK, ROUNTREE GA, SULIEMAN JS: Factors affecting accuracy and morbidity in transrectal biopsy of the prostate. Surg Gynecol Obstet 145:869, 1977

2. DESAI SG, WOODRUFF LM: Carcinoma of prostate: Local extension following perineal needle biopsy. Urology 3:87, 1974

3. EMMETT JL, BARBER KW, JR, JACKMAN RJ: Transrectal biopsy to detect prostatic carcinoma: A review and report of 203 cases. Trans Am Assoc Genitourin Surg 53:85, 1961

4. LIN BPC, DAVIES WEL, HARMATA PA: Prostatic aspiration cytology. Pathology 11:607, 1979

5. RUEBUSH TK, II, MCCONVILLE JH, CALIA FM: A double-blind study of trimethoprim-sulfamethoxazole prophylaxis in patients having transrectal needle biopsy of the prostate. J Urol 122:492, 1979

6. TURNER BI, WARNER JJ, RHAMY RK: Prostatic needle examination: Current clinical concepts. South Med J 73:183, 1980

7. ZINCKE H, CAMPBELL JT, UTZ DC et al: Confidence in the negative transrectal needle biopsy. Surg Gynecol Obstet 136:78, 1973

Pelvic Lymphadenectomy

91

Gary Lieskovsky

Based on a collective series, the incidence of pelvic lymph node metastases from prostatic cancer at the time of staging lymphadenectomy is as follows: 22% for patients with clinical Stage A_2 disease, 16% for patients with clinical Stage B_1 disease, 35% with clinical Stage B_2 disease, and 50% for patients with clinical Stage C disease.[6,10,15,17,24,25,31] It is evident that tumor dissemination by lymphatics occurs in an orderly fashion with the primary drainage to the obturator–hypogastric lymph nodes. McLaughlin and co-workers reported that 87% of all patients with lymph node metastases had disease in the obturator–hypogastric nodes, whereas involvement only of the external iliac or common iliac lymph nodes occurred in 9% and 4% respectively.[15] More recently Morales and Golimbu have advocated extended pelvic lymphadenectomy to identify those patients with involvement of presacral and presciatic nodes since they discovered that these nodes contained metastases in approximately 50% of patients who had other positive pelvic nodes.[16] However, in only two of the 24 patients (8.3%) was there involvement only of the presacral or presciatic lymph nodes in the absence of other pelvic node metastases. Involvement of para-aortic lymph nodes in the absence of positive pelvic nodes (leap-frogging) rarely, if ever, occurs. McLaughlin and co-workers reported that in only three patients (5%) were the deep pelvic nodes skipped by tumor metastases.[15] Others have failed to witness any instance of periaortic involvement without concomitant pelvic node metastases.[18] Based on the incidence, location, and pattern of lymph node metastases we agree with Paulson and others that pelvic lymphadenectomy should be performed in selected patients, especially those with a Gleason histopathologic grading score of 6, 7, or 8, as a means of staging the disease accurately and providing information upon which treatment decisions can be based.[18]

The incidence of pelvic node metastases from transitional cell carcinoma of the bladder relates directly to the grade and depth of tumor infiltration.

Skinner and associates* in 1981 reported their experience with 131 consecutive patients undergoing radical cystectomy with pelvic lymph node dissection and urinary diversion following planned preoperative high-dose, short-course radiation therapy. Based on the preoperative clinical stage established by transurethral biopsy, 17% of patients with Stage T_1 disease had unsuspected nodal metastases and 42% of patients with muscle invasion (T_{2-3}) had lymph node involvement. When the relation of tumor infiltration into the bladder wall of the cystectomy specimen was compared to the incidence of positive nodes, 5% of patients with carcinoma in situ (P1S) or with invasion only of the lamina propria (P1) were found to harbor nodal metastases. Positive nodes were identified further in 30% of patients with superficial muscle invasion (P2), 30% with deep muscle invasion (P3A), and 64% with perivesical fat involvement (P3B). Based on the reported rate of metastases to the pelvic nodes in patients with bladder cancer, a thorough bilateral pelvic lymphadenectomy seems indicated. Current evidence suggests that pelvic node dissection in patients with minimal nodal disease provides a therapeutic advantage and further identifies those patients at risk for subsequent failure in whom the early use of systemic adjuvants based on chemosensitivity testing may improve their survival.

Dissemination of squamous cell carcinoma of the penis through lymphatics, with involvement of the regional lymph nodes of the groin and deep pelvis, represents one of the earliest routes of spread unless there is penetration of Buck's fascia and the tunica albuginea with early access to the vascular corpora cavernosa, predisposing to hematogenous metastases. Considerable controversy exists about the role of groin dissection and pelvic lymphadenectomy for those patients. The incidence of clinically false-negative nodes is approx-

---

* Skinner DG: Personal communication, 1981. Data presented at Annual Meeting, American Urological Association, Boston, MA, 1981

imately 50% at the time of initial presentation, and 20% of patients with clinically negative nodes at the time of presentation harbor occult inguinal metastases. Advocates of prophylactic groin dissection feel that identifying the 20% of patients at risk both reduces their potential for local recurrence leading to subsequent skin necrosis, infection, and hemorrhage from erosion of the iliac and femoral vessels, and decreases the potential for distant metastases.[3] In contrast, support for a more conservative approach is based on the reported 75% cure rate in patients in whom groin dissection is delayed until the nodes become clinically manifest.[11] Although survival in some patients with microscopic involvement of the pelvic nodes has been achieved by pelvic node dissection, the experience of Spaulding and Grabstald suggests that the presence of positive pelvic nodes is associated with a very limited survival despite aggressive surgical management.[27] Because the value of pelvic lymphadenectomy in patients with penile cancer remains to be established, its performance may be indicated from a staging or prognostic standpoint and may indicate the need for subsequent adjuvant chemotherapy.

Metastases to the pelvic lymph nodes from primary carcinoma of the urethra occurs often when the tumor involves the proximal two thirds of the urethra but is rare in distal lesions unless extensive invasive tumor is present.[28] The rationale for aggressive surgical excision including pelvic lymphadenectomy for proximal lesions is based on the observation that urethral cancer has the tendency to remain an aggressive regional or localized disease with a low incidence of distant metastases.

Predictability and Prognostic Significance of Positive Nodes

PREDICTORS OF NODAL PATHOLOGY

Preoperative assessment of pelvic and para-aortic lymphadenopathy in patients with tumors of the bladder, urethra, prostate, and penis has been attempted in the past by lymphangiography and more recently by the use of computed tomographic (CT) scanning. In prostatic cancer the high incidence of false-positive (32%–59%) and false-negative (22%–36%) results precludes the use of lymphangiography in the evaluation of nodal pathology.[13,19,21] Similarily, preliminary results employing CT scanning for identifying pelvic lymph node involvement indicate a significant degree of inaccuracy, approaching 40%.[9] Therefore, it seems reasonable to try to establish an accurate, reproducible predictor of nodal pathology and to obviate the need for a staging pelvic lymph node dissection in all patients. Recently, reports suggest that for cancer of the prostate such a system exists, based on the Gleason histopathologic grading score of the primary tumor.[8] According to the data, only an occasional patient with a Gleason score of less than 5 will be found to have evidence of lymph node metastases, compared to an incidence of more than 90% in patients with a Gleason score of 9 to 10.[18,21] Based on these reports it appears that lymphadenectomy is unnecessary in patients in whom the lymph node status is highly predictable, but should be considered in patients with whom uncertainty exists (Gleason score 6, 7, or 8).

In cancer of the penis, sentinel node biopsy has been recommended as a means of more appropriate selection of patients for prophylactic ilioinguinal lymphadenectomy. Cabanas reported that 80% of patients with positive sentinel nodes had no other positive nodes and, more importantly, when the sentinel nodes were negative, no other positive nodes were identified.[2] However, others have noted instances in which the sentinel nodes were negative in patients who were subsequently found to have metastases in the inguinal nodes.[20] At the present time it does not appear that sentinel node biopsy can be used as a reliable, reproducible predictor of the status of lymph node involvement in patients with cancer of the penis.

As with cancer of the prostate, accurate evaluation of pelvic nodal metastases prior to surgery in patients with bladder or urethral cancer is lacking. It, therefore, remains that pelvic lymphadenectomy is the best means of identifying positive nodes in patients with these tumors.

PROGNOSTIC SIGNIFICANCE OF POSITIVE NODES

Pelvic lymphadenectomy has been advocated to assist in accurate pathologic staging and in planning a more rational therapeutic approach based on the presence or absence of unsuspected nodal metastases. However, dispute continues about whether or not pelvic node dissection in patients with minimal lymph node metastases has any therapeutic benefit. For cancer of the prostate, McLaughlin and associates have reported that in patients with positive nodes, approximately one third demonstrated metastases limited to one or two nodes and half of these were micrometastases.[15] Therefore, it seems reasonable to proceed with definitive treatment of the primary tumor and adjunctive lymphadenectomy in hopes of achieving a therapeutic advantage. Flocks and associates were among the first to report an improved survival for patients with positive nodes treated aggressively by the combination of node dissection, radical prostatectomy, and radioactive gold implantation compared to similar patients treated conservatively.[7] Barzell and colleagues have reported that the extent or volume of nodal metastases is more important than their mere presence. In their series, patients with positive lymph nodes but less than 3 cm³ of tumor volume, when treated by lymphadenectomy and implantation of ^{125}I radioactive seeds, did equally as well at 5 years in terms of survival as did those patients with negative nodes who were treated in a similar fashion.[1] However, Whitmore and co-workers recently reported that the presence of positive nodes in these patients, regardless of extent, portends at 75% or greater probability of metastases within 5 years of surgery.[29] Recently Cline and associates reported that the median time to failure in patients with positive pelvic nodes following radical prostatectomy and pelvic node dissection was less than 2 years. Furthermore, there was no significant difference in the interval of time to failure, irrespective of treatment, between patients with only one positive node and those with involvement of more than one node. This seems to suggest that lymphadenectomy may not be therapeutically beneficial in patients with minimal lymph node involvement, but it emphasizes the need for further adjuvant therapy for these high-risk patients.

Similarly, in patients with bladder cancer who are undergoing radical cystectomy and pelvic node dissection for cure, approximately 25% will have evidence of lymph node involvement. This points up the need to treat the pelvic lymph nodes as well as the primary tumor. Based on the early results of 230 consecutive patients undergoing radical cystectomy and pelvic node dissection, Whitmore and Marshall failed to demonstrate any significant survival advantage in patients with positive nodes treated in this manner.[30] They reported that two of 13 patients with tumor involving one or two lymph nodes had survived 5 years, but none in the series survived with more than two involved nodes.

More recently, however, significant improvements in the 5-year overall survival rates have been reported in patients with positive nodes undergoing low-dose preoperative radiation therapy followed by radical cystectomy and pelvic node dissection. Skinner has recently reported a 5-year overall survival of 37% for 37 patients with proven pelvic nodal metastases following radical cystectomy and bilateral pelvic lymphadenectomy.* More

---

* Skinner DG: Personal communication, 1981. Data presented at Annual Meeting, American Urological Association, Boston, MA, 1981

than two thirds of those surviving 5 years demonstrated deep penetration by the primary tumor P3 (B₂–C) or direct extension into the prostate (P4). This compares favorably with the 5-year survival rate of 17% reported by Dretler, Ragsdale, and Leadbetter for 35 patients with positive nodes (33% for those with fewer than three positive nodes), and 21% reported by Reid and associates for 24 patients with pelvic lymph node involvement.[5,23] Based on these results, coupled with advances in surgical technique that have lowered its operative mortality and morbidity, pelvic lymphadenectomy is suggested whenever radical cystectomy is indicated for management of bladder cancer.

Surgical Principles and Techniques

PRINCIPLES

Previously a conventional pelvic node dissection included total removal of all lymphatic and fibroareolar tissue from the lateral pelvic side walls and complete skeletonization of the major pelvic vessels (Fig. 91-1). However, recently Paulson and associates reported their experience with conventional *versus* limited node dissection for patients with cancer of the prostate.[18] Their data indicate that although there is a greater amount of nodal tissue removed in conventional node dissection than in a limited lymphadenectomy, there was no significant difference in the number of positive nodes identified employing either technique. Because one of the major complications associated with external-beam radiation therapy following pelvic node dissection is chronic penoscrotal or leg lymphedema, it is our present policy to limit the extent of the node dissection in the management of prostate cancer (Fig. 91-2).[12]

For cancer of the prostate the lymph node of Cloquet or Rosenmüller at the femoral canal is the most distal node removed. The circumflex iliac artery and vein signify the distal limits of dissection. Laterally the surgical dissection is limited to the inferior margin of the external iliac artery, preserving the lymphatic channels that course along its upper border. Within the pelvis the lateral pelvic wall within the obturator canal continues to represent the lateral limits of the dissection in this area. Superior dissection begins at a point at which the ureter crosses the common iliac artery; the hypogastric artery represents the superior margin of the dissection. Medially a well-defined, thin fascial plane separates the bladder from the loose, fatty areolar tissue that is to be removed from the obturator hypogastric fossa. The proximal hypogastric artery and vein are dissected cleanly, as is

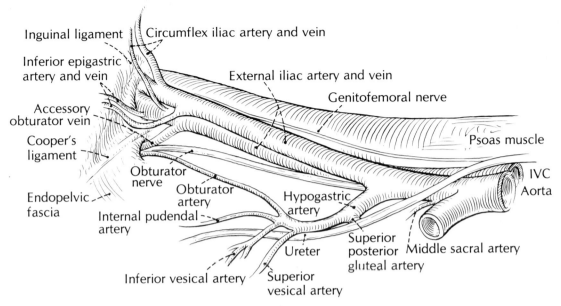

FIG. 91-1.   Right lateral pelvic wall. Anatomy of pelvic blood vessels and nerves encountered in a pelvic lymph node dissection is depicted.

FIG. 91-2.   Completed dissection; iliac and obturator nodes have been removed.

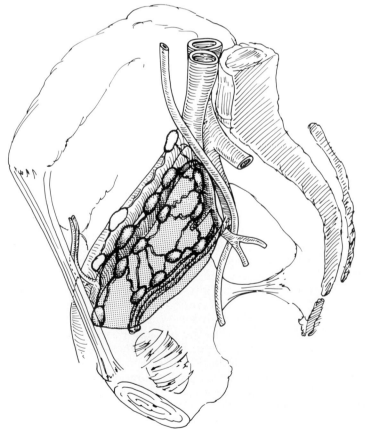

the obturator nerve. The posterior extent of the dissection is the ventral aspect of the hypogastric vein deep within the pelvis. Once these limits of dissection have been completed and the obturator nerve has been cleanly exposed and dissected, the *en bloc* fibroareolar lymphatic tissue containing the pelvic nodes is easily removed.

TECHNIQUE

In patients undergoing radical cystectomy with pelvic lymphadenectomy for bladder cancer, a lower midline and upper left paramedian incision is made extending from the pubis to a level 4 cm to 6 cm above the umbilicus. After careful intra-abdominal exploration has ruled out unresectable tumor, the ascending colon, peritoneal attachments to the small bowel mesentery, and descending colon are all mobilized. This allows packing of the intra-abdominal contents away from the operative site, except for the descending colon which can be retracted laterally in the deep pelvis. Both ureters are then isolated, clamped with large hemoclips, mobilized superiorly, and tucked up and out of the way.

Pelvic lymphadenectomy is then initiated at the level of the aortic bifurcation, clipping and dividing the proximal lymphatics with large or medium hemoclips. The fibroareolar and lymphatic tissue is stripped off the distal aorta and vena cava, with care not to avulse small vessels arising from the common iliac vessels as they course medially over the sacral promontory. Lateral extension from this point identifies the common iliac vein and extends to the genitofemoral nerve that represents the lateral limits of dissection. Once the proximal dissection is completed and the lateral peritoneum

including the vas deferens has been divided, the distal dissection is begun at the femoral canal. Here all tissue, including the lymph node of Cloquet or Rosenmüller, is swept from the canal proximally. It is essential to clip or ligate all small lymphatics draining into this node, as well as those running parallel and adjacent to the external iliac artery and vein, to prevent lymph accumulation and protein loss. This can be accomplished by using small hemoclips which, in addition, conserve time.

After identifying the circumflex iliac artery and vein, the most distal margin of dissection (Fig. 91-1), the external iliac artery and vein are circumferentially dissected. Commonly an accessory obturator vein inserts into the back wall of the external iliac vein just proximal and medial to the circumflex iliac vein; it should be clipped and divided to prevent the bothersome bleeding that can result should the vein be avulsed.

Once the distal limits of the dissection have been defined, the fibroareolar tissue is sharply and bluntly dissected off the undersurface of Poupart's and Cooper's ligaments and swept medially toward the obturator fossa. A constant small vessel that usually is found crossing over Cooper's ligament into the deep pelvis should be coagulated and care should be taken not to injure the inferior epigastric vessels in this region by vigorous retraction of the rectus muscles.

Having completed the proximal and distal lymphatic dissection, the fibroareolar tissue that is loosely adherent to the adventitia of the external iliac artery and vein is incised on the anterior aspect of both vessels (Fig. 91-3). This allows the artery and vein to be freed completely and divides the specimen in such a way that half of the specimen can be swept medial and the other half lateral to

FIG. 91-3. Incision of fibroareolar tissue loosely adherent to adventitia of iliac artery and vein. This allows a portion of areolar tissue to pass lateral to iliac vessels into the obturator fossa.

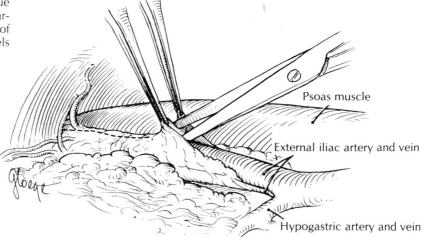

Psoas muscle

External iliac artery and vein

Hypogastric artery and vein

the iliacs into the obturator fossa. On the medial side between the hypogastric and circumflex iliac branches, there are no significant vessels that leave or enter the external iliac artery or vein, so rapid dissection of this portion is possible. However, laterally there is usually a small muscular arterial and venous branch, found along the proximal portion of the external iliac vessels, which should be clipped and divided to avoid accidental division and troublesome bleeding. Next the fascia overlying the psoas muscle can be incised medial to the genitofemoral nerve.

Because the tissue has been divided previously over the common and external iliac vessels, the medial portion of the specimen can be swept off the sacral promontory into the deep pelvis, and the lateral portion can be swept off the psoas muscle lateral to the vessels into the obturator

fossa. By retracting the external iliac vessels medially, a gauze x-ray sponge can be used effectively to sweep the entire lateral specimen into the obturator fossa. The vessels are then retracted laterally and the gauze sponge with the lateral specimen can be retrieved beneath the vessels, thus cleaning the lateral pelvic wall (Fig. 91-4A and B). Medial traction applied with the left hand assists in exposing the obturator nerve, which is then carefully dissected free and protected (Fig. 91-5). Once the nerve has been freed and retracted laterally, the obturator vessels located medial to the obturator nerve can be clipped and divided; this allows the obturator nodes to be swept medially with the entire specimen. At this point the hypogastric artery and vein are dissected until the superior vesical arteries are identified. It is unnecessary and perhaps unwise to dissect below or

FIG. 91-4. Gauze sponge. This is used to assist in sweeping the lateral fibroareolar tissue off the psoas muscle into the obturator fossa. **(A)** This maneuver is initiated by medial retraction of vessels. **(B)** Once gauze has been tucked into obturator fossa with the aid of tissue forceps, it is retrieved beneath the iliac vessels, thus dissecting all fibroareolar tissue from the lateral pelvic wall. Upward and lateral retraction of vessels by a vein retractor completes this maneuver.

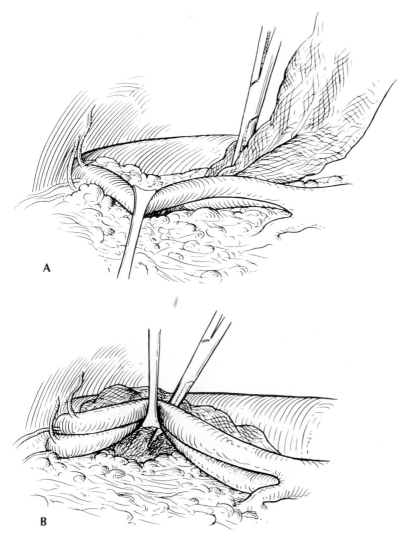

A

B

posterior to the superior and inferior vesical arteries, because hazardous bleeding from the venous complex forming the hypogastric vein may result.

At this stage, the entire *en bloc* specimen can be removed easily because there are only loose attachments to the smooth, thin fascia covering the bladder and prostate (Fig. 91-6).

Pelvic Lymphadenectomy with Radical Prostatectomy

In patients with prostatic cancer who are undergoing pelvic lymphadenectomy alone or in combination with radical prostatectomy a similar surgical technique is employed, albeit with some modifications.

The patient is placed in the extended supine position with 10 degrees Trendelenburg. Through a lower midline extraperitoneal incision extending from the pubis to the umbilicus, the peritoneum is dissected off the undersurface of the rectus and transversalis fascia; additional exposure is provided by dividing the posterior fascia above the semicircular line.

The peritoneum is then mobilized from the area of the femoral canal and freed from the spermatic cord, which is retracted laterally after the vas deferens is clipped and divided. The peritoneum should be mobilized above the point at which the ureter crosses the common iliac artery before proceeding with lymphadenectomy. In patients with

FIG. 91-5. Effect of medial traction on sponge. This technique is used in dissection of the lateral pelvic wall. Note the exposed obturator nerve.

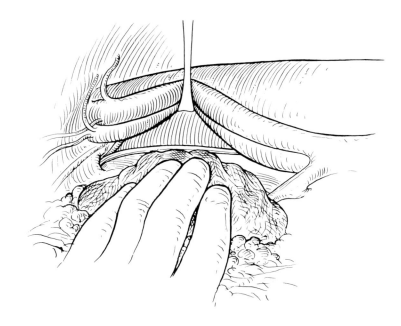

FIG. 91-6. Limits of dissection in patients with prostatic cancer who are undergoing pelvic lymphadenectomy. Note the lateral margin is the inferior aspect of the external iliac artery.

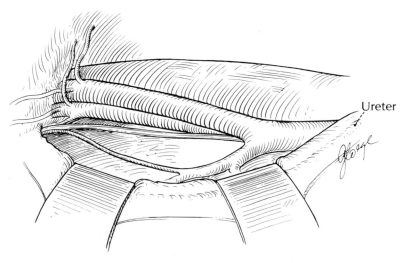

Ureter

prostatic cancer the entire dissection should be performed extraperitoneally to prevent the morbidity that follows when radiation therapy is added to transperitoneal lymph node dissection. Because it is our aim to be more selective and to remove only those nodes that are primarily involved in patients with cancer of the prostate, a more limited lymphadenectomy is performed than that previously described for patients with bladder cancer.

Dissection is initiated at the femoral canal with the lymph node of Cloquet again representing the distal limits of the dissection. Care should be exercised during dissection of this area not to interfere with the drainage of the lymphatic channels that course along the external iliac artery, which represents the lateral limits of the dissection. After completion of the distal dissection, attention is redirected to the proximal limits of the dissection, the point at which the ureter crosses the common iliac artery. Here the proximal lympathic channels are similarly clipped and divided, and the external iliac vein and proximal hypogastric artery are stripped. After the external iliac vein has been dissected completely, the obturator and hypogastric nodes are dissected in a fashion similar to that described previously.

Bilateral extraperitoneal lymphadenectomy alone or in combination with radical retropubic prostatectomy, using the technique described, can be accomplished with an average operating time of 75 minutes. Others prefer to perform staging pelvic node dissection with subsequent radical perineal prostatectomy based on the status of the lymph nodes.

Complications

The incidence of early complications following pelvic lymphadenectomy alone as a staging procedure for carcinoma of the prostate ranges from 12% in our series to 24% reported by Ray and coworkers, who performed the procedure transperitoneally.[12,15,17,22] When radical prostatectomy is combined with pelvic lymphadenectomy, the early complication rate ranges from 17% to 33%.[14,15,17] It seems unlikely that pelvic lymph node dissection increases the inherent morbidity of radical prostatectomy, except possibly by increasing the risk of thromboembolic complications especially among patients not prophylactically anticoagulated.[12]

Chronic penoscrotal or leg lymphedema represents the most significant late complication occurring in patients in whom pelvic radiation is added to lymphadenectomy. Of 17 patients undergoing pelvic lymphadenectomy and definitive external-beam radiation therapy, 7 (41%) had chronic lymphedema, compared to only 5 of 48 patients (10%) in whom pelvic lymphadenectomy was combined with radical prostatectomy.[12]

For patients with bladder cancer, Skinner has reviewed his experience in 131 consecutive patients undergoing high-dose, short-course preoperative radiation followed by immediate radical cystectomy and pelvic node dissection.[26] He reported an operative mortality of 0.7% ($\frac{1}{131}$), with an early complication rate of 28%. In his analysis of the data, he contended that the addition of a pelvic node dissection in these patients did not increase the operative mortality or morbidity as compared to procedures not incorporating a pelvic lymphadenectomy.

It, therefore, appears that, aside from the increased risk of thrombophlebitis and the occasional development of a lymphocele, pelvic node dissection does not significantly contribute to the complication rate but provides valuable information for future management, especially in patients with positive nodes.

REFERENCES

1. BARZELL W, BEAN MA, HILARIS BS et al: Prostatic adenocarcinoma: Relationship of grade and local extent to the pattern of metastases. J Urol 118:278, 1977
2. CABANAS RM: An approach for the treatment of penile cancer. Cancer 39:456, 1977
3. CATALONA WJ: Role of lymphadenectomy in carcinoma of the penis. Urol Clin North Am 7:785, 1980
4. CLINE WA, KRAMER SA, FARNHAM R et al: Impact of pelvic lymphadenectomy in patients with prostatic adenocarcinoma. Urology 17:129, 1981
5. DRETLER SP, RAGSDALE BA, LEADBETTER WF: The value of pelvic lymphadenectomy in the surgical treatment of bladder cancer. J Urol 109:414, 1973
6. DONOHUE RE, PFISTER RR, WEIGEL JW et al: Pelvic lymphadenectomy in stage A prostatic cancer. Urology 9:273, 1977
7. FLOCKS, RH, O'DONOGHUE EP, MILLERMAN LA et al: Management of stage C prostatic carcinoma. Urol Clin North Am 2:163, 1975
8. GLEASON DF, The Veterans Administration Cooperative Urological Research Group: Histologic grading and clinical staging of prostatic carcinoma. In Tannenbaum M (ed): Urologic Pathology: The Prostate, p 171. Philadelphia, Lea & Febiger, 1977
9. GOLIMBU M, MORALES P, SHULMAN Y et al: Computerized tomography for staging prostatic cancer (abstr 235). Paper presented at the American Urology Association Meeting, New York, May 1980

10. GOLIMBU M, SCHINELLA R, MORALES P et al: Differences in pathological characteristics and prognosis of clinical A2 prostatic cancer from A1 and B disease. J Urol 119:618, 1978

11. GRABSTALD H: Controversies concerning lymph node dissection for cancer of the penis. Urol Clin North Am 7:793, 1980

12. LIESKOVSKY G, SKINNER DG, WEISENBURGER T: Pelvic lymphadenectomy in the management of carcinoma of the prostate. J Urol 124:635, 1980

13 LOENING SA, SCHMIDT JD, BROWN RC et al: A comparison between lymphangiography and pelvic node dissection in the staging of prostatic cancer. J Urol 117:752, 1977

14. MCCULLOUGH DL, MCLAUGHLIN AP, GITTES RF: Morbidity of pelvic lymphadenectomy and radical prostatectomy for prostatic cancer. J Urol 117:206, 1977

15. MCLAUGHLIN AP, SALTZSTEIN SL, MCCULLOUGH DL et al: Prostatic carcinoma: Incidence and location of unsuspected lymphatic metastases. J Urol 115:89, 1976

16. MORALES P, GOLIMBU M: The therapeutic role of pelvic lymphadenectomy in prostatic cancer. Urol Clin North Am 7:623, 1980

17. NICHOLSON TC, RICHIE JP: Pelvic lymphadenectomy for stage B1 adenocarcinoma of the prostate: Justified or not? J Urol 117:199, 1977

18. PAULSON DF: The prognostic role of lymphadenectomy in adenocarcinoma of the prostate. Urol Clin North Am 7:645, 1980

19. PAULSON DF, Uro-Oncology Research Group: The impact of current staging procedures in assessing disease extent of prostatic adenocarcinoma. J Urol 121:300, 1979

20. PERINETTI EP, CRANE DB, CATALONA WJ: Unreliability of sentinel lymph node biopsy for staging penile carcinoma. J Urol 124:734, 1980

21. PISTENMA DA, BAGSHAW MA, FREIHA FS: Extended-field radiation therapy for prostatic adenocarcinoma. In Johnson DE, Samuels ML (eds): Cancer of the Genitourinary Tract, p. 229. New York, Raven Press, 1979

22. RAY GR, PISTENMA DA, CASTELLINO RA et al: Operative staging of apparently localized adenocarcinoma of the prostate: Results in fifty unselected patients. I. Experimental design and preliminary results. Cancer 38:73, 1976

23. REID EC, OLIVER JA, FISHMAN IJ: Pre-operative irradiation and cystectomy in 135 Cases of bladder cancer. Urology 13:247, 1976

24. SADLOWSKI RW: Early stage prostatic cancer investigated by pelvic lymph node biopsy and bone marrow acid phosphatase. J Urol 119:89, 1978

25. SALTZSTEIN SL, MCLAUGHLIN AP, III: Clinicopathologic features of unsuspected regional lymph node metastases in prostatic adenocarcinoma. Cancer 40:1212, 1977

26. SKINNER DG, CRAWFORD ED, KAUFMAN JJ: Complications of radical cystectomy for carcinoma of the bladder. J Urol 123:640, 1980

27. SPAULDING JT, GRABSTALD H: Surgery of penile cancer. In Harrison JH, Gittes RF, Perlmutter AD et al (eds): Campbell's Urology, p 2438. Vol 3, Philadelphia, WB Saunders, 1979

28. SULLIVAN J, GRABSTALD H: Management of carcinoma of the urethra. In Skinner DG, deKernion JB (eds): Genitourinary Cancer, p 419. Philadelphia, WB Saunders, 1978

29. WHITMORE WF, JR, BATATA M, HILARIS B: Prostatic irradiation: Iodine-125 implantation. In Johnson DE, Samuels ML (eds): Cancer of the Genitourinary Tract, p 195. New York, Raven Press, 1979

30. WHITMORE WF, JR, MARSHALL VF: Radical total cystectomy for cancer of the bladder: 230 consecutive cases five years later. J Urol 87:853, 1962

31. WILSON CS, DAHL DS, MIDDLETON RG: Pelvic lymphadenectomy for the staging of apparently localized prostatic cancer. J Urol 117:197, 1977

served if possible, but their dissection allows increased mobility of the bladder neck at the time of its anastomosis to the membranous urethra superior to the urogenital diaphragm. Small hemoclips are preferred as a means of lymphostasis and hemostasis for this dissection. Medium-sized arterial branches are ligated with 3-0 Prolene suture ligature if needed. Closure of the widely mobilized posterior parietal peritoneal flaps is accomplished by a running 3-0 chromic gut suture. The anterior peritoneum is left open until completion of the anastomosis of the bladder to the urethra after prostatectomy.

EXPOSURE AND RESECTION OF THE PROSTATE, SEMINAL VESICLES, AND AMPULLARY PORTION OF THE VAS DEFERENS

The extraperitoneal space is easily opened bluntly. Areolar tissue is cleaned from the anterior and lateral surface of the prostate, exposing the endopelvic fascia that sweeps laterally from the prostate superior to the urogenital diaphragm. The endopelvic fascia is incised vertically 2 mm lateral to the prostate (Fig. 92-2). This incision must be made very carefully, because the endopelvic fascia is only 1 mm to 2 mm in thickness and large veins of the retropubic (Santorini) plexus are immediately beneath it. Those veins that are in the path of dissection may be clipped and divided between hemoclips. One may then gently insert the index finger and separate the prostatic urethra from the rectum, using a long-handled curved clamp (tonsil or right angle) to establish the plane of dissection until the index finger can be passed between the prostate and rectum (Fig. 92-2).

The puboprostatic ligaments can then be easily divided. I prefer to divide these "ligaments" that contain smooth muscle, veins, and connective tissue between sutures of 2-0 chromic gut.[1] On each side of the prostate, one suture is placed against the periosteum of the posterior aspect of the symphysis and the other is placed in the capsule of the prostate (to secure the puboprostatic ligaments). There is usually room to cut the puboprostatic ligaments between the sutures on each side with a sharp blade. Usually the dorsal vein of the penis, which runs beneath the symphysis between the puboprostatic ligaments, is secured in this manner. If not, it must be secured and divided to minimize blood loss. Walsh has advocated securing the dorsal vein separately inferiorly and posterior to the symphysis pubis through a

small skin incision, prior to division of the prostate.[7]

The urethra is divided above the urogenital diaphragm by cutting across it flush with the apex of the prostate (Fig. 92-3). It is best to cut with the catheter in place and to put distal sutures of 1-0 chromic gut at the 2 o'clock and 10 o'clock positions in the urethra before the balloon is deflated and the catheter withdrawn. One may then complete the resection by placing two additional sutures distally in the posterior half of the urethra at the 5 o'clock and 7 o'clock positions. Once the circumference of the urethra has been cut completely, a small gauze pack for compression of venous oozing is placed distally excluding the urethra and distal sutures, and the prostate is mobilized bluntly (superiorly) to the prostatovesical junction. Occasionally, in patients who have had transrectal needle biopsy prior to radical prostatectomy, the prostate is quite adherent to the rectum. In these instances, further mobilization is deferred until division of the prostate at the bladder neck. Others prefer to divide the prostate from the bladder initially, performing the separation at the apex as the final step in removal of the prostate, seminal vesicles, and ampullary portions of the vas deferens.

The bladder neck is defined and the prostate is divided from it sharply, preserving the muscular

FIG. 92-3. The division of the prostatic urethra at the urogenital diaphragm may be facilitated by the use of a small elastic traction band, *i.e.,* Vesiloop. This band allows direct visualization of the urethra at the apex of the prostate prior to severing it immediately distal to the apex of the prostate.

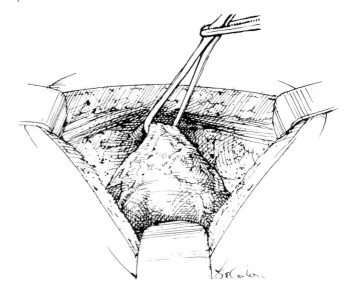

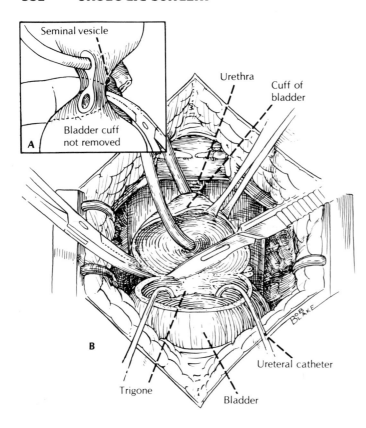

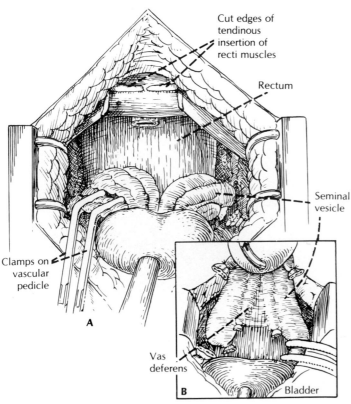

FIG. 92-4. Retropubic prostatovesiculectomy. **(A)** In order to preserve continence, the vesical neck is often retained. **(B)** If tumor invasion of the vesical neck is suspected, a cuff of bladder is removed. Considerable bleeding may be encountered when the trigone is divided, and indwelling ureteral catheters may be valuable in protecting orifices.

FIG. 92-5. Retropubic prostatovesiculectomy. **(A)** After division of the bladder from the prostate, the latter is elevated in the wound and the vascular pedicle is isolated. At this point the rectum is tented by traction; a guiding finger in the rectum is advisable to prevent injury when clamps are applied to the pedicle. **(B)** Traction on the prostate is shifted in the opposite direction and final attachments of vasa deferentia and seminal vesicles enclosed in their fascial envelope are divided at a high level above gross tumor extension if present.

collar of the vesical neck. Indigo carmine may be given intravenously at this point to aid in identifying the ureteral orifices so that No. 5 ureteral catheters may be passed to each kidney (Fig. 92-4). These are left in place until time for the anastomosis of the bladder to the urethra. As the incision is carried from anterior to posterior at the bladder neck, bleeding vessels are seen at the 2 o'clock and 10 o'clock and 5 o'clock and 7 o'clock positions, they are treated by suture ligature with 3-0 chromic gut.

The incision is carried posteriorly completely through the bladder until a distinct fascial plane posterior to the prostatovesical junction is seen. This fascia is substantial and covers the seminal vesicles and vas deferens. It may be incised or separated with a tonsil clamp, mobilizing medially the ampullary portion of the vas deferens on either side. The vas is dissected proximally until a preampullary portion is identified. The proximal portion is ligated with a suture ligature of 2-0 chromic gut and the ampullary tip is clamped with a large hemoclip. After the vas has been divided on each side, the pedicle of the seminal vesicle is dissected out. It is located just posterolateral and superior to the tip of the seminal vesicle on either side and is lateral to the vas deferens (Fig. 92-5). Once the artery to the seminal vesicle is secured on each side, two arterial branches on each side remain (Fig. 92-6). These come in laterally, one near the

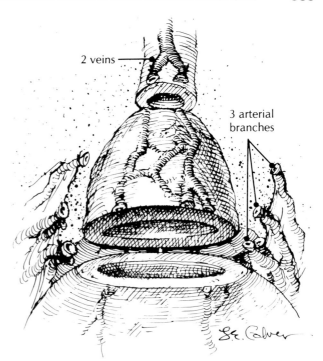

FIG. 92-6.   The vascular supply of the prostate is isolated prior to dissecting it free from the underlying rectum. Note, there are usually three arterial branches on either side, the first to the tip of the seminal vesicle, the second supplying the midportion of the prostate, and the third branching to the prostate and urogenital diaphragm just proximal to the endopelvic fascia.

FIG. 92-7.   Circumferential narrowing of the bladder neck is accomplished until the bladder neck is snug on the index finger of the operator. Ureteral catheters may be passed to protect the intramural ureter during placement of the vesicourethral sutures (usually four to six in number).

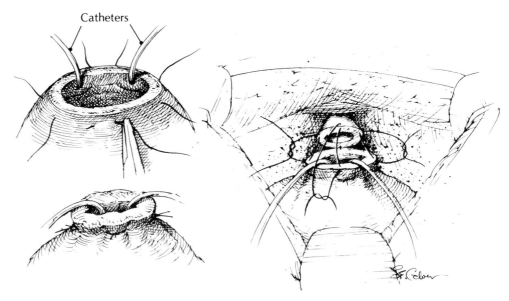

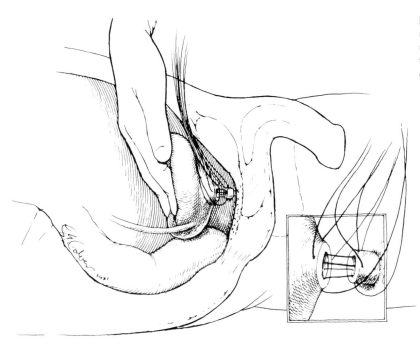

FIG. 92-8. The operator's hand may be used to compress the bladder against the urogenital diaphragm; this permits one to tie the sutures and complete the vesicourethral anastomosis without tension.

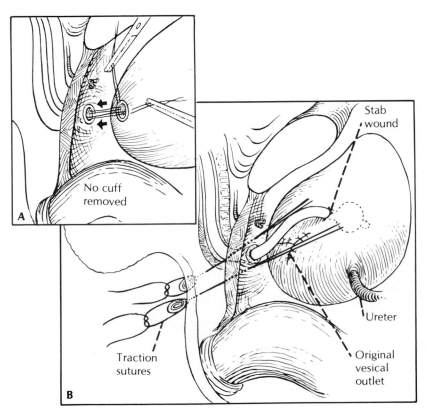

Stab wound

No cuff removed

A

Traction sutures

B

Ureter

Original vesical outlet

FIG. 92-9. Retropubic prostatovesiculectomy. **(A)** Direct vesicourethral anastomosis may be made when the vesical neck is retained. **(B)** When a cuff of bladder has been removed, it is sometimes difficult to make a vesicourethral anastomosis without tension. In such a case the original vesical outlet may be closed as indicated and replaced by a stab wound higher on the bladder wall. Under these circumstances traction sutures from the bladder through the perineum may aid in fixation during the healing process.

center and the other near the apex on each side. They are divided between clips or 3-0 chromic gut ligatures. The large veins in Figure 92-6, usually ligated with the puboprostatic ligaments, or separately as suggested by Walsh,[7] represent venous return from the dorsal vein of the penis. The remainder of the fascial and areolar attachments of the prostate to the rectum are sharply divided, and the prostate is removed.

RECONSTRUCTION OF THE BLADDER NECK, VESICOURETHRAL ANASTOMOSIS, AND CLOSURE

Circumferential narrowing of the bladder neck is accomplished by a series of seromuscular sutures passing from a subepithelial position around the circumference of the vesical neck (Fig. 92-7). The circumference of the vesical neck is decreased until it is about 1.5 cm in diameter (snug on the index finger). A 22Fr, 30-ml retention catheter is then passed into the bladder. The four chromic gut sutures which were passed "outside in" on the urethral end are now brought "inside out" at the vesical neck, taking good muscular bites with a minimum of bladder mucosa. An assistant places a hand intraperitoneally and pushes the bladder inferiorly. Such compression tends to "accordion" the bladder, pressing it against the urogenital diaphragm. This allows one to tie the sutures, uniting the bladder and urethra without tension on the anastomosis (Fig. 92-8). The catheter balloon is inflated to approximately 30 ml and is irrigated; returns should be clear. A 1.25-cm (½-in.) Penrose drain is placed near the anastomosis on the left side and brought out extraperitoneally through a separate stab wound in the groin. The author then takes a suture through the seromuscular layer of the bladder on each side, attaching it to the periosteum of the posterior aspect of the pubis. This serves further to reduce tension on the anastomosis. In cases in which the bladder cannot be mobilized because of scarring, in spite of intraperi-toneal compression and hypogastric artery branch dissection, one can consider the use of sutures through the adventitial muscle layer of the bladder neck, brought out through the perineum and tied over a button on the perineum, to hold the bladder against the urethra. Higher continence rates may be anticipated if direct anastomosis can be accomplished. The author has had to resort to the perineal button (Vest) technique on only one occasion in fifty cases since adopting the peritoneal surface compression of the urinary bladder and hypogastric pedicle dissection at the time of lymphadenectomy (Fig. 92-9).

REFERENCES

1. ALBERS DD, FALUKNER KK, CHEATHAM WN et al: Surgical anatomy of the pubovesical (puboprostatic) ligaments. J Urol 109:388, 1973
2. CHUNG RS, GURLL NJ, BERGLUND EM: A controlled clinical trial of whole gut lavage as a method of bowel preparation for colonic operations. Am J Surg 137:75, 1979
3. CLAYTON RS: A clean colon in one hour. App Radiol 9:69, 1980
4. DAVIS GR, SANTA ANA CA, MORAWSKI SA et al: Development of a lavage solution associated with minimal water and electrolyte absorption. Gastroenterol 78:991, 1980
5. MILLIN T: Retropubic prostatectomy. A new extravesical technic: Report of twenty cases. Lancet 2:693, 1945
6. PAULSON DF, PISERCHIA PV, GARDNER W: Predictors of lymphatic spread in prostatic adenocarcinoma, Uro-oncology research group study. J Urol 123:697, 1980
7. REINER WG, WALSH P: Anatomical approach to the surgical management of the dorsal vein and Santorini's plexus during radical retropubic surgery. J Urol 121:198, 1979
8. WAJSMAN ZEW: Lymph node evaluation in prostatic cancer. Is pelvic lymph node dissection necessary? Urology-[Suppl] 17:80, 1981
9. WALSH, PC: Radical prostatectomy for the treatment of localized prostatic carcinoma. Urol Clin North Am 7:583, 1980

Radical Perineal Prostatovesiculectomy

93

William L. Parry

The perineal approach for prostatovesiculectomy is no more difficult than other routes from a technical standpoint, and the surgeon who masters this operation is likely to use it for many of his patients. The procedure is regaining favor, along with the resurgence of interest in surgical *palliation* for a great number of patients with prostatic carcinoma. After prostatovesiculectomy the contiguous structures of the perineal cavity are highly resistive to local recurrence. A striking advantage of the perineal approach is the small degree of physiologic reaction it produces in older patients. Other advantages over the retropubic approach are the less vascular field of dissection, better exposure for the vesicourethral anastomosis, and optimal dependent drainage, especially for cases with known prostatic infection. It is the most direct route for open biopsy and is preferred for poor-risk, very obese, or emphysematous patients. Although I prefer a retroperitoneal exploration to evaluate more accurately the extent of the disease, a number of urologists deal with lesions judged relatively avirulent on clinical and histologic grounds by perineal prostatovesiculectomy alone.

The frequently quoted disadvantage of the perineal approach is that it requires two incisions to inspect or dissect pelvic lymph nodes. Often, for the advantages described above, the combined abdominal–perineal approach may be preferable; this approach is not associated with increased anesthesia risk, significant time difference, or extra morbidity. In fact, the perineal prostatovesiculectomy is viewed by many as the ideal second-stage operation after the assessment of the extent of the malignancy by permanent histologic sections of pelvic lymph nodes. Many surgeons who are experienced with this approach use it comfortably for the more difficult dissections encountered after an earlier subtotal operation for benign disease or after partial or total irradiation.

The principal contraindications to this operation are ankylosis of the hip and the rarer cases of younger men with invasion of the bladder base, for which more radical surgery with cystectomy and urinary diversion through an abdominal incision may be indicated.

Indications

GENERAL

Surgery is the only established means of curing prostatic carcinoma, and the hope for cure depends on early detection. Until it is possible to diagnose more of these cancers before extension has occurred, the emphasis must be on palliation for a larger number of patients, by surgical eradication of the local disease. Perineal prostatovesiculectomy offers the opportunity to remove the local source of continuing contamination of tumor in the manner that many other cancers are approached, usually with little physiologic disturbance of these older patients. Grossly removed prostatic carcinoma is much to be preferred over hormone therapy to control the disease and repeated transurethral resection to remove obstructing tissue.[35,44] Palliation, if not cure, has the potential of new dimensions of enhancement with adjuvant irradiation and chemotherapy and with increased host resistance by immunologic means. The sequela of impotence already is being alleviated with penile prosthetic devices, and the complication of permanent incontinence is being relieved with the improvement of surgically placed mechanical sphincters.

SELECTION BY STAGE AND GRADE

The treatment of prostatic carcinoma is guided by the *stage* of the neoplasm, which is judged clinically, and by the *grade* of biologic activity, which is determined microscopically. Increasing data indicate that a combination of these classifications affords a more reliable assessment of the lesion's virulence and the patient's prognosis.[30]

Four similar stages are generally recognized by

letter (Whitmore), by Roman numerals (American Joint Commission for Cancer Staging and End Result Reporting) or by the tumor, nodes, metastases (TNM) classification (International Union Against Cancer).[41] For simplicity the ABCD staging is used in this chapter.

Grading, which currently seems to give more accurate measurement of patient survival of prostatic neoplasms, regardless of the form of treatment, has different criteria of biologic activity. Gleason's System (VA Cooperative Urological Research Group) currently is the favored pathologic reference, taking precedence over the Mostofi (Armed Forces Institute of Pathology), Gaeta (National Prostatic Cancer Project), and Mayo Clinic Systems.[31] It takes into account the primary and secondary tumor patterns together with the glandular differentiation and tumor growth in relation to the stroma. Until a grading system can be accepted universally, each surgeon should understand his own pathologist's interpretation of whether the tumor is well differentiated, moderately well differentiated, or poorly differentiated (anaplastic).

Another advantage of prostatovesiculectomy is that the pathologic findings of removed tissue lead to correction of both understaging and overstaging of the classifications for end result reporting. The indications for radical prostatectomy by the evaluation of retroperitoneal exploration and pelvic node assessment to further stage and grade the extent of the disease certainly poses many new questions (see Chap. 91).[2,29,32,46]

Stage A Disease

Stage A_1 prostatic carcinomas generally should not be disturbed if it is reasonably certain that they are focal, well differentiated, and have only one cellular pattern. Most Stage A_1 disease apparently remains latent for an extended period, and the entire focus of cancer may have been removed by the original surgery at which the cancer was discovered.[9] Also, small series have not shown positive pelvic nodes or seminal vesical invasion.[46] Further, the increased incidence of complications may militate against prostatovesiculectomy after subtotal procedures in some instances. Patients who do not have radical surgery can be reassured by close follow-up and repeated needle biopsies. The prostatovesiculectomy is occasionally justified in those who are so concerned about the diagnosis itself that they desire the surgery with the full realization of possible sequelae.

Stage A_2 tumors tend to be more diffuse and have a higher grade of biologic activity. In fact,

several reports indicate a greater virulence here than in B_1 lesions.[14] Perineal prostatovesiculectomy for cure is considered strongly in these cases because pelvic node involvement is low.[46] Even though the dissection may be difficult, palliation seems better than following radiation therapy. Long-term treatment results of effective control are not holding up to earlier reports, and increased stricture complications in these cases are hard to manage.[40]

Stage B Disease

All Stage B_1 lesions should be considered biologically active and the ideal indication for perineal prostatovesiculectomy. The cure rate by radical surgery is better than any treatment modality for carcinoma of the prostate.[25] These tumors usually are confined within one lobe although they are multifocal histologically. The long-term cure rate is lower for high-grade lesions but substantial palliation may be expected for many, because the seminal vesicles and pelvic nodes seem to be involved in no more than 15% of the cases.[29,32,46] The fact that the prostate gland contains so few lymphatics until the capsule or perivesicular spaces are reached may account for the disparity between the clinically active and latent cancer.

Stage B_2 lesions remain good candidates for radical prostatectomy. By definition these tumors involve more than one lobe and often invade the capsule. Yet many have a well-differentiated or moderately well-differentiated grade, only about 20% extend into the seminal vesicles, and local recurrence after prostatovesiculectomy is less than 5%.[2,8,26,46] Retroperitoneal exploration is particularly valuable in planning additional therapy because approximately one third have positive pelvic nodes.[2,29]

Stage C Disease

Surgical removal of the primary lesion should be recommended more often than it now is for patients with extension of the cancer beyond the prostatic capsule but with no evidence of distant metastases. Prostatovesiculectomy is a far less extensive operation than is done for patients with invasive bladder cancer who are generally in the same age-risk group. The cure rate is low, of course, but the long-term improvement of the patient's comfort and function, as well as the decrease in complications from recurrent local disease associated with transurethral resections, has been striking in several reports.[35,37,43] Prostatovesiculectomy is recommended, especially when the biopsy shows a low grade of biologic activity and the local extension is judged to be removable. Such tumors often have a better prognosis than high-grade lesions confined to the gland. Study of the specimens removed at surgery for early Stage C disease indicates that extraprostatic extension has been mistakenly diagnosed in 10% or more of these cases. Local recurrence is less than 10%. Prostatovesiculectomy is generally contraindicated in patients with high-grade histopathology who usually prove to have extensive pelvic node involvement.[29]

At the University of Oklahoma Medical Center, we have been impressed with the results of performing an exploratory perineal operation whenever there seems any prospect of removing the local disease. Only rarely has it been necessary to abandon the operation because of fixation to adjacent structures, distortion of anatomy, or increased vascularity. Even when not all the tumor can be removed above the seminal vesicles, the results of prostatovesiculectomy—in terms of shorter hospital stay, fewer outpatient visits, and better palliative effect—are more satisfactory than those of transurethral resection.[35] In the future, additional palliation may be obtained by using adjuvant therapy.

Stage IV or D Disease

Radical surgery is rarely indicated in Stage IV or D disease, even for palliation. The exeption is the patient with a low-grade, locally operable lesion whose only criterion for the Stage D classification is a slightly elevated prostatic serum acid phosphatase determination.

INCONTINENCE

The decision about radical surgery of the prostate may hinge on the possibility of incontinence, because this is the principal undesirable sequela of prostatovesiculectomy. At one extreme, if it is necessary to remove a sizable cuff of bladder and all the prostatic tissue, the surgeon must expect a significant incidence of temporary and sometimes permanent incontinence. At the other extreme, if he preserves the bladder neck and leaves a button of prostatic *capsule* at the apex, the patient is usually continent soon after the catheter is removed.

The patient's domestic circumstances, as well as his mental and emotional outlook, should influence the decision about the extent of surgery. Most advocates of radical surgery prefer the classic prostatovesiculectomy when there is a good prospect for cure. Patients usually adjust to incontinence if it occurs because they have the satisfaction of

knowing that an effort has been made to remove the cancer. However, urologic surgeons particularly those just beginning practice in a community, may find it difficult to recommend radical surgery when more conservative measures are less likely to produce incontinence. For a great many patients in this age group prostatovesiculectomy may be primarily palliative but still preferable to transurethral resection, because recurrence of local disease is less likely. In such patients, altering the classic operation to minimize incontinence is often justified, because no significant difference in survival has been reported in controlled series as a result of such modifications.

Surgical disturbance of perineal innervation, as well as damage to the sphincter regions, is believed to contribute to incontinence after prostatovesiculectomy, although the mechanism is not well understood. Experience has shown that it is important to avoid dissection laterally in the ischiorectal fossa and in the region of the bulbous urethra, where branches of the perineal nerve supplying the sphincter region may be injured. Also, traction and transfixion sutures through the urogenital diaphragm generally should be avoided.

IMPOTENCE

Impotence is less and less a consideration in the decision for prostatovesiculectomy. The dread of cancer is real; men at this age are usually declining in sexual performance; and their wives are more concerned about survival. Moreover, if treated with estrogens or orchiectomy, these men would become impotent anyway. Men tend to exaggerate their sexual capabilities, and many are relieved to have an excuse for their decreased activity. Impotence usually follows perineal prostatovesiculectomy, but not invariably. Surgeons tend to emphasize the former preoperatively but often do not think about helping couples postoperatively. With time, 5% to 15% of men can achieve some degree of erectile satisfaction.

If there is serious concern about this aspect of a patient's life, it should be respected. Some prostatic lesions remain operable for several years, although procrastination is hazardous. If impotence is the chief factor in deciding against surgery, these men and their wives need to know that radiation therapy also leads to this sequela although the same amount of dysfunction usually occurs more gradually. Today the possibility of having a penile prosthesis inserted later by relatively minor surgery gives a number of patients enough encouragement that they are still a male and helps their spouses agree to proceed with prostatovesiculectomy.

SELECTION IN THE AGED GROUP

Urologic surgeons should be aggressive in recommending prostatovesiculectomy for Stages A_2, B, and C disease. Contrary to general opinion, old men succumb more rapidly to biologically active prostatic carcinoma than young men with the same grade of tumor. Physiologic differences in patients make it difficult to limit the age beyond which prostatovesiculectomy should not be advised, but the age 75 is now recommended as the reasonable upper limit when the surgeon is experienced and capable. The likelihood of death from unrelated causes obviously restricts the benefits that may be expected from surgery, but if a patient's physical condition and mental state indicate an expectancy of at least 3 years of worthwhile life, he should be considered for the operation. These older patients may live 5 years or longer with the cancer, of course, but their lives and their effect on the family are of an entirely different quality when the local manifestations of cancer have been removed.

SELECTION AFTER SURGERY FOR BENIGN DISEASE

A previous subtotal prostatectomy is a deterrent to prostatovesiculectomy.[20] If radical surgery is done within 4 or 5 days after a subtotal procedure, before the fibrous stage of wound healing begins, dissection is not difficult, even through the same wound, and complications are not increased. If the second procedure must be delayed for more than 7 days, however, it should be postponed at least 6 weeks, and usually longer, until the acute tissue reaction has subsided; otherwise, dissection is hazardous and sometimes impossible. Complications are more likely after a delayed secondary prostatovesiculectomy than after a primary procedure. A disturbed blood supply may impair healing at the vesicourethral anastomosis, and problems are often encountered in bringing the bladder down to the urethra. Prostatovesiculectomy may be as difficult after a transurethral resection as after an open subtotal operation, depending on the depth of the resection, the amount of fulguration, and the removal of muscular tissue at the vesical neck. Secondary prostatovesiculectomy is not a very satisfying cancer operation because tissue barriers have been opened already, and often the remaining prostate must be removed piecemeal. Local tumor recurrence, however, does not seem to be increased. Before deciding about such an operation, it is advisable for the patient to understand also the advantages and disadvantages of radiotherapy. The need for secondary surgery becomes less common as biopsy is more routinely performed before subtotal prostatectomy.

OTHER OPERATIVE CONSIDERATIONS

Preoperative endocrine treatment causes many prostatic cancers to become smaller, although microscopically the actual extent of the tumor seems to remain unchanged.[38,39] Today, if the tumor is operable, there seems little justification for delaying surgery by estrogen therapy. Currently the value of preoperative partial or total irradiation is being debated. In the future more specific chemotherapeutic agents or the immunologic increase of host resistance may justify delay of the surgery after diagnosis.

Diagnostic Studies

This chapter describes the technique of perineal prostatovesiculectomy based on the assumption that minimal diagnostic criteria have been met, as listed below:

A *clinical evaluation* should occur, including a rectal examination to determine the stage or extent of the local lesion and whether it is surgically removable grossly.

A positive *biopsy* for carcinoma is required, which can be graded histologically.

Cystoscopy is recommended, even in the absence of urinary symptoms, to determine whether there is intravesical extension of the tumor. Neoplastic invasion of the bladder neck proven by biopsy and the relation of the ureteral orifices to such extension are important in planning radical surgery.

A *prostatic serum acid phosphatase* determination currently is the preferred chemical marker of tumor aggressiveness and extraprostatic extension.

Intravenous urography is valuable for excluding ureteral obstruction, which is a grave sign when it is caused by cancer.

Scintillation photographic scans using radioactive pharmaceuticals detect bone metastases far earlier and more cheaply than standard roentgenographic surveys, although a special x-ray or bone biopsy may be indicated to check a "hot spot" of other reactive bone conditions.

Computed tomography (CT) and *ultrasound*, if available, are used to rule out large, unsuspected pelvic node involvement before retroperitoneal exploration. These will become more valuable noninvasive techniques for detection of smaller nodes with advancements of the resolution power of the equipment.

For surgical decisions, other diagnostic techniques, such as prostate fluid analysis; bone marrow aspiration; chemical, immune, or isotope-labeled assays; vasoseminal vesiculography, lymphangiography, pelvic angiography; and so on are not sufficiently reliable for routine clinical use.[7]

Preoperative Preparation

Frank, considerate discussion of the disease and the method proposed for its treatment are important preliminary considerations. Not only do patients and their families gain insight into the problem, but their confidence and cooperation are also improved. An explanation of the alternative methods of treatment, the immediate postoperative course, and the later convalescence may avoid misunderstanding and minimize anxiety. Patients can be encouraged by a reminder that radical surgery is proposed only for relatively early disease. There is some evidence that cancer patients, either because of their personality or as a result of fear brought on by the diagnosis, express their emotions poorly and are inclined to mask their feelings with a facade of pleasantness.[28] My own approach usually is to obtain the patient's permission to talk to him and his spouse or another family member together. This speeds up my understanding of his total position and avoids miscommunication. Definite treatment recommendations are proposed, and the patient is made aware that he shares the responsibility for making the decisions.

Preliminary studies for prostatovesiculectomy follow the general work-up for other surgery in the aged.[21] For more specific details see my chapter in *Surgery in the Aged.*[33] Careful systemic evaluation is important because patients in this group are likely to have other diseases. Study of the cardiovascular and respiratory systems is especially important because of the patient's positioning for perineal surgery. Unsuspected liver disease, hemorrhagic disorders, or recent treatment with drugs that are poorly tolerated during anesthesia should be investigated. Because elderly people do not tolerate blood loss well, anemia or a blood volume deficiency should be corrected at least 6 hr and preferabley 18 hr before surgery if whole blood instead of packed cells is given. Two units of blood should be available during surgery, but postoperatively it is not ordinarily necessary to keep blood

on call because bleeding is far less than after subtotal prostatic surgery.

Preliminary bowel preparation reduces the possibility of gross wound contamination at surgery and minimizes fecal impaction afterward when the rectal wall is susceptible to injury. Mechanical cleansing ordinarily consists of a liquid diet for 1 or 2 days and a cathartic plus a cleansing enema the day before operation. This is followed by a low enema to empty the rectum the next morning. Before the operation, 50 ml to 100 ml of a 5000 units/ml solution of polymyxin B sulfate, which is surface-active and bactericidal within 15 min to most organisms, is instilled into the rectum. In the operating room, this is drained, but it may be replaced with a smaller amount of the same solution. Some surgeons prefer a low-residue diet for several days before surgery combined with phthalylsulfathiazole (Sulfathalidine)/neomycin or erythromycin/kanamycin. These latter agents inhibit bacteria through metabolic pathways and so are slower in their effect. In the event of rectal injury, however, there is little evidence that preoperative bowel sterilization gives more protection than simple mechanical cleansing and it does increase the risk of postoperative enteritis.

Before the anesthetic is administered, intravenous fluids should be started to initiate and maintain a good urinary output during surgery and to overcome the release of antidiuretic hormone. These fluids must have an osmotic concentration exceeding 0.3% sodium chloride in 5% dextrose and distilled water. Ringer's lactate and 2.5% mannitol solution are readily available examples of such fluids. The resulting diuresis causes rapid excretion of indigo carmine, which is used during surgery to facilitate the location of the ureteral orifices, thus reducing the possibility of ureteral obstruction from edema caused by landmark catheters. In addition, fluid administration protects against acute tubular necrosis when blood transfusions are given; elderly people with impaired renal function tend to become excessively dehydrated and somewhat acidotic when fluids are withheld before surgery.

Most patients do not have an indwelling catheter or a urinary infection at the time of surgery. If a catheter is present, there may be some advantage to irrigating the bladder copiously with saline solution and instilling a rapid-acting antibacterial agent (polymyxin B sulfate) just before surgery. Systemic antibacterial medication, if given, should be prescribed to reach therapeutic blood levels at the time of operation, because gram-negative bacterial infection is a serious problem in the elderly.

Proper positioning of the patient should prevent hemostasis in the extremities and pressure on the

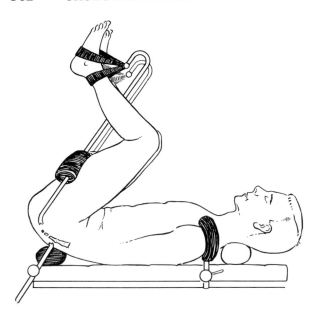

FIG. 93-1. Position of patient for perineal prostatovesiculectomy. Special Young table may be used, but a standard operating table is satisfactory with appropriate elevation of buttocks. Support must be placed under the sacrum as shown. To maintain optimal position, it is important that padded shoulder braces be placed laterally against acromial process so that there is no risk of brachial plexus injury.

popliteal spaces or calves of the legs. If the surgeon chooses to wrap the legs with elastic bandages, he should be aware that these bandages may actually cause venous stasis if they are not properly applied. The lithotomy position possibly has higher risk for peripheral venous thrombosis and subsequent pulmonary emboli, especially in patients with varicosities or a history of phlebitis. Minidose heparinization is done pre- and postoperatively on most perineal prostatovesiculectomies as part of a large study at the University of Oklahoma Medical Center.

ANESTHESIA

Either general or regional anesthesia is adequate for perineal prostatovesiculectomy; the choice depends on the characteristics of the patient and the judgment of the anestheiologist. General anesthesia with intubation and controlled respiration provides a greater margin of safety during the operation, but regional anesthesia requires less postoperative care to prevent respiratory complications and is probably used more often. The general condition of these usually older patients is of more concern to the anesthesiologist than the technical hazards of the surgery itself. The neces-

sary exaggerated lithotomy position further affects the ability of homeostatic mechanisms to adjust; hypoxia and changes in the blood volume and *p*H must be recognized rapidly so corrective measures can be instituted promptly. Even though the anesthesiologist today has many means of monitoring and supporting the patient to provide optimum surgical exposure, the urologic surgeon also has an obligation not to request extremes of position that offer little mechanical advantage when compared to the added burden on the patient's vital capacity.

HISTORY AND TECHNICAL PRINCIPLES

Surgical techniques and anatomic approaches for the treatment of malignant prostatic disease have evolved in a fashion roughly parallel to that of surgery for benign enlargement.[45] Total removal of a cancerous prostate was first undertaken by Billroth in 1867 through a midline perineal incision. The radical perineal prostatectomy, as described by Young in 1905, was intended to be curative.[47] His principles have become standards for the various prostatovesiculectomy procedures. These principles consist of removing the prostate and its capsule together with the seminal vesicles, the ampullae of the vasa deferentia, as much as possible of the adjacent fascia, and a cuff of bladder, all in a single block. Campbell and Hudson and Stout have advocated ligating the vascular pedicles of the prostate before manipulating a malignant gland (and in some respects this may be better cancer surgery).[10,23] This sequence in the perineal operation, however, risks more injury to contiguous anatomy and makes removal of structures above the prostate in their enveloping fascia more difficult. Experience has demonstrated no appreciable dissemination of prostatic carcinoma when dissections proceed from the apex. Today the perineal prostatovesiculectomy is advocated even more for palliation than cure. The operation is modified in certain situations to encourage its use by minimizing the chance of incontinence.

Surgical Technique

POSITION OF THE PATIENT

The exaggerated lithotomy position for perineal prostatovesiculectomy is the same as that for perineal prostatectomy for benign disease, and it can be achieved with the equipment on any standard operating table. Figure 93-1 demonstrates the essential aspects of good position. Before the foot of the table is lowered, the sacrum (not the coccyx) is brought to the edge of table; the buttocks are extend a few inches beyond.

Padded shoulder braces are then adjusted to stabilize the patient by counterpressure when the legs are flexed and to prevent shifting in the Trendelenburg position. It is important that these braces be placed carefully laterally against the acromial processes to prevent injury to the brachial plexus. Elevation of the sacrum on a sandbag or folded towels facilitates exposure of the deep perineal structures later in the operation.

As the last step in positioning the patient, the legs are elevated and the thighs are flexed to tighten the perineum. To maintain this position, padded poles are pressed against the inner aspects of the thighs, or the feet are suspended or held in a strap harness with the knees fixed to the poles by elastic bandages. Extreme flexion of the thighs to a point that the perineum is parallel to the floor improves exposure very little and may seriously compromise the vital capacity of the lungs. Surgical assistants are spared considerable discomfort if the table is raised and the surgeon stands to operate.

EXPOSURE OF THE PROSTATE

A modification of Young's perineal approach is described here. To displace the prostate toward the perineum, a Lowsley prostatic tractor is passed through the urethra into the bladder, and its blades are opened. If a tractor is not available, a sound may be used (Fig. 93-2). Traction on an inflated

FIG. 93-2. Perineal prostato-vesiculectomy. **(A)** Incision is made 1.5 cm anterior to the anal margin and extended to its lower border. **(B)** A curved Lowsley tractor or Van Buren sound may be used to displace the prostate to a more superficial position to facilitate exposure. **(C)** The central tendon of the perineum is exposed and isolated for division after the ischiorectal fascia has been incised in the angles of the wound.

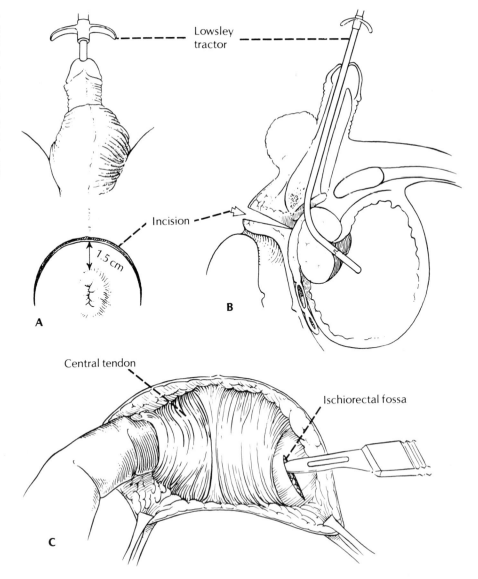

Foley catheter also is adequate if a guiding finger in the rectum is used to dissect its attachments off the prostate.

The skin incision is made 1.5 cm anterior to the anal opening and is curved downward on either side close to the medial borders of the ischial tuberosities. It is extended to the level of the inferior anal margin to facilitate mobilization of the rectum, which is needed for complete removal of the prostate and seminal vesicles. The superficial perineal fascia is incised laterally near the angles of the wound, and the underlying fat, which bulges upward, identifies the point for introducing each index finger slightly forward and upward along each side of the rectum. These ischiorectal fossae are developed only to aid in the division of the central tendon of the perineum. They should not be opened up to the bulb or sphincter region. If they cannot be entered easily, the surgeon should suspect that he is dissecting too high—within the transverse perineal muscle or above—where excessive bleeding from the bulb is encountered and there is danger of damage to the sphincter.

The central tendon extends from the transverse perineal muscle to the anal sphincter and may be divided easily after it is isolated by finger dissection. The location of the rectum is sensed with an index finger in each ischiorectal fossa; in penetrating from one fossa to the other behind the central tendon, the secret is to make certain that the separation is directly on the rectal fascia. If the surgeon is overly fearful of perforating the rectum, he tends to divide the central tendon only partially; without the rectal fascia as a landmark, his dissection often proceeds blindly too high in the perineum. The rectal wall is relatively tough and resilient, and the proper cleavage plane can be developed readily by finger dissection with reasonable safety. Some surgeons prefer to divide the central tendon by sharp dissection down to the characteristic sheen of the rectal fascia, aided by tension on the upper and lower wound margins. If there is any question concerning the identity of the rectal fascia, it should be checked with a finger in the rectum. The importance of this fascia cannot be overemphasized, because the next steps in the operation depend on this landmark.

In dissecting the rectum off the posterior surface of the prostate, it is essential to understand that the rectum makes a right-angle turn at the level of the apex of the prostate (Fig. 93-3). The key to the operation is in dividing the rectourethralis muscle, which tents the rectum at this strategic point. When this structure is divided, the rectum drops to a horizontal position, providing exposure of the prostate and seminal vesicles. If there is any mistake in identification, the rectum is most likely to be incised or torn at this point. To expose the rectourethralis, the rectal fascia is put under tension between a small bulb retractor under the transverse

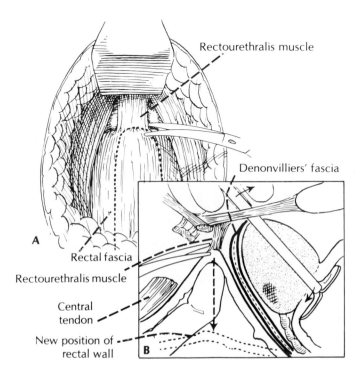

FIG. 93-3. Perineal prostatovesiculectomy. After the levator ani muscles have been displaced laterally, the rectourethralis muscle is identified and cut, with a guiding finger in the rectum, as close to the rectal fascia as is practical. The rectal wall is normally tented at this point until division of the rectourethralis muscle allows it to drop to a more horizontal position. Note the position of the central tendon as it joins the transverse perineal muscle; also note the relation of the latter to the genitourinary diaphragm. Denonvilliers' fascia is solidly fused at the apex of the prostate, then is separable for a cleavage plane 1–1.5 cm proximal.

Rectourethralis muscle

Denonvilliers' fascia

A

Rectal fascia

Rectourethralis muscle

Central tendon

New position of rectal wall

B

perineal muscle anteriorly and a bifid retractor or depressing traction over the rectum posteriorly. By blunt dissection, the levator ani muscles are teased aside upward, further exposing the shiny rectal fascia until fibers of the rectourethralis become visible in the midline.

The rectourethralis may be a well-developed muscle bundle or merely a few fibrous bands extending from the rectum to the urogenital diaphragm near the external urethral sphincter. Its location may be anticipated by pressing the Lowsley tractor outward to palpate the apex of the prostate deep in the wound. Its isolation for division is facilitated by grasping and tenting up the rectourethralis in the midline, bluntly dissecting downward and over the rectal fascia laterally on each side, and exposing the landmark white surface of the prostate at its apex.

Isolation and division of the rectourethralis muscle during perineal surgery were considered a special skill in the days before antibacterial agents, when rectal injury constituted a serious problem.

Today, unless the rectourethralis is quite distinct, it is recommended that the operator insert a finger in the rectum as a guide for severing the attachment very close to the rectal fascia. This maneuver reduces operating time and minimizes the chance of disturbing the adjacent sphincter region. The anus has been isolated from the wound by a drape, and contamination from a previously cleansed rectum is negligible. Evidence now suggests that the rectourethralis is really a part of the external urethral sphincter instead of a central portion of the levator ani, so its preservation should reduce the possibility of postoperative incontinence.

At this point the surgeon must decide whether to proceed by dissecting the rectum off the posterior surface of the prostate and seminal vesicles *between* or *beneath* the two layers of Denonvilliers' fascia (Fig. 93-4).[42] The first technique is the easier. A thin layer of the posterior fascia is incised transversely about 1 cm below the apex of the prostate (above this point, the layers are usually fused). This exposes the glistening inner surfaces of the

FIG. 93-4. Perineal prostatovesiculectomy. Dissection usually proceeds with incision of Denonvilliers' fascia 1 cm below the apex of the prostate, where the two layers are no longer fused. Within these ''pearly gates,'' blunt dissection is continued beyond the tips of the seminal vesicles. This space represents an obliterated portion of the peritoneal cavity. An alternate route of dissection lies between the rectal wall and the posterior layer of Denonvilliers' fascia. Note also the potential cleavage plane between the layers of Denonvilliers' fascia between the bladder and the seminal vesicles, to be established later in the operation.

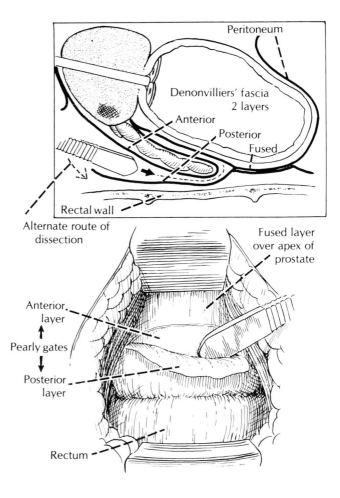

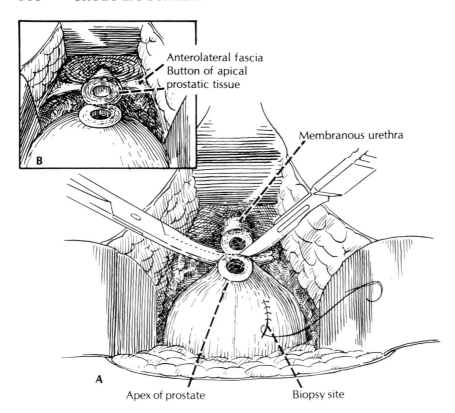

Anterolateral fascia
Button of apical
prostatic tissue

B

Membranous urethra

A

Apex of prostate   Biopsy site

FIG. 93-5. Perineal prostatovesiculectomy. Biopsy of the suspected area in the prostate is done by wedge excision; the site is cauterized or closed with a running suture. The prostate is divided from the membranous urethra either at the apex (**A**) or by transecting the prostate itself, leaving a small button of apical capsule (**B**). The latter is a safe procedure if the lesion is not located near the apex. Glandular prostatic tissue should be teased out from within the button and kept attached to the specimen.

fascial layers, the "pearly white gates" described by Young. The blunt dissection within Denonvilliers' fascia should be completed, separating the rectum to the tip of the seminal vesicles, before losing the advantage of tension from the intact anterior structures. Rarely is the peritoneum reached or entered with this deep dissection.

The alternate route of dissection is between the rectal fascia and the posterior layer of Denonvilliers' fascia. The posterior layer usually peels off the rectum without unusual difficulty. This method is not associated with increased bleeding, but it causes the rectum to become more vulnerable.

Many surgeons routinely use this route because the extra fascial investment around the neoplasm theoretically constitutes a better operation for cancer. It is indicated whenever the layers are adherent or the tumor is extensive. As the dissection is completed, the rectum may be protected with gauze and depressed further with a long-bladed posterior retractor if necessary, to provide optimum exposure of the prostate and seminal visical region. Occasionally, when a large gland is being removed, the levator ani muscles must be partly divided transversely on one or both sides at a point where the cut edges will be visible in case bleeding occurs.

BLOCK DISSECTION

The apex of the prostate is visualized with the aid of an anterior bulb retractor, and a curved, pointed clamp is maneuvered under the anterolateral prostatic (endopelvic) fascia precisely at the junction of the prostate with the membranous urethra (Fig. 93-5A). The prostate should be excised at this point if the lesion is near the apex. This point is identified by palpation of the indwelling prostatic tractor or catheter.

At the next step in the operation, when the remainder of the urethra is being divided, the clamp is used as a landmark and a safeguard to prevent the dissection from extending into an extremely vascular area. Halfway behind the urethra and the nearby palpable inferior margin of the pubis, the dorsal vein of the penis courses through the urogenital diaphragm. This vein immediately divides in three plexuses that course anteriorly and laterally over the prostate, the veins of Santorini. Great care in dissection around the urethra prevents injury to this vulnerable venous complex. Small arterial branches also often enter the apex of the prostate from the perineal artery through the urogenital diaphragm. If bleeding occurs, it may be aggravated by direct attempts to control it at this point of dissection. The division of the prostatourethral junction should be completed and hemostasis, secured. The use of a small clamp instead of a finger behind the urethra minimizes the chance for injury to the sphincter.

Opening the urethra at the prostatourethral junction is emphasized because if the urethra is incised more distally by pulling it from within the sphincter, the subsequent anastomosis is more difficult and the chance of stricture formation is greater. Involvement of the membranous urethra is rare in early cases, and roughly only 10% of malignant lesions are close to the distal apex.

Before the urethra is completely divided, the urethral instrument is removed and a Foley catheter with a 30-ml balloon is passed through the prostatic urethra into the bladder and used for traction. If one anticipates removing a cuff of bladder neck later in the operation, it is better to use a Young prostatic tractor. If only a margin of capsule sufficient to hold placement of sutures can be left with safety, this appears important. The membranous urethra, like the esophagus, is composed mainly of longitudinal muscle with few circular elements and thus it does not hold sutures well for a secure anastomosis.

If the malignant lesion is some distance away from the apex of the prostate, a portion of the distal prostatic capsule (less than 0.5 cm) may be left in place.*[4] Prostatic glandular contents are freed from within this capsular button and remain attached with the specimen to be removed. This capsular button provides better tissue for a secure anastomosis with less chance of stricture formation than does the friable membranous urethra. It also contains muscular and elastic fibers that contribute to urethral resistance and continence. This practice of retaining a small capsular button and teasing away any glandular tissue has not been associated with a reported higher incidence of local recurrence,[36] although microscopic foci are reported as high as 75% in the general apical area.[8]

After the urethra has been divided, downward traction is exerted on the catheter to facilitate dissection beneath the anterolateral prostatic fascia toward the vesical neck (Fig. 93-6A). The prostate can be mobilized safely beneath this layer because tumor rarely extends anteriorly. By keeping within this plane of cleavage, one avoids the dorsal vein of the penis, coursing between the puboprostatic ligaments and the veins of Santorini that divide

---

* Parry WL, Blankenship JB: Unpublished data

around them. If the veins above the anterolateral fascia are damaged, bleeding is troublesome and time consuming to control (Fig. 93-6B).

Unless this plane of cleavage is established, the operator also cannot easily dissect beneath the puboprostatic ligaments and he usually must divide them. The puboprostatic ligaments are avascular themselves, but ordinarily they are tied because of the veins coursing through and around them. These ligaments, which are condensations of the endopelvic fascia, do not insert into the prostate primarily, but instead contain muscle fibers in their proximal portion that arise from the vesical neck.[1] The concept that this part of the bladder support may be a factor in the mechanism of continence is another reason for preserving not only them but also the vesical neck whenever possible during perineal prostatovesiculectomy.

FIG. 93-6. Perineal prostatovesiculectomy. **(A)** Dissection usually continues beneath the anterolateral fascia; it is not necessary to divide the puboprostatic ligament. **(B)** Alternate route of dissection above the anterolateral fascia requires division of the puboprostatic ligament and increases the possibility of venous bleeding.

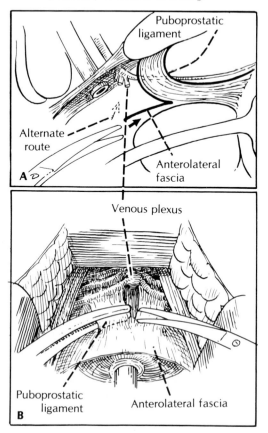

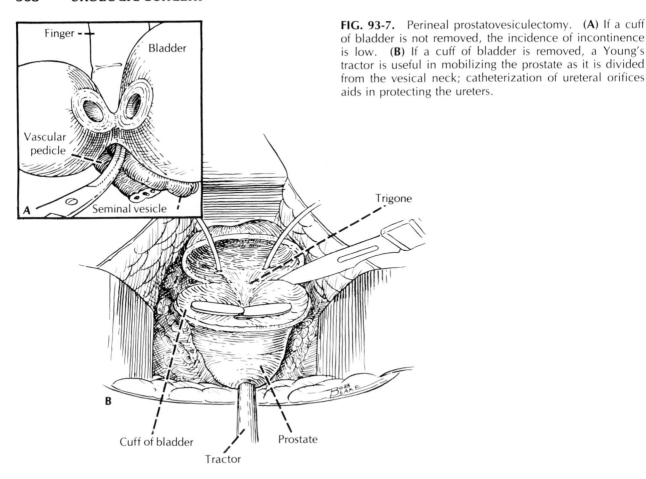

From this point, blunt dissection under traction to the vesical neck is a surprisingly short distance of only 1 cm to 2 cm, and the surgeon should feel for the catheter balloon or tractor instrument within the bladder to identify the prostatovesical junction. Invasion of the vesical neck is uncommon in early lesions.[44] Unless there is concern that the cancer extends into the bladder, the vesical neck should be preserved to minimize the chance of incontinence.[24] The proximity of the ureteral orifices actually limits the amount of trigone that can be removed posteriorly, and there is little justification for removing a cuff of bladder anteriorly because tumor extension rarely occurs in this area.

The attachments between the prostate and bladder anteriorly can be divided with little bleeding. Sharp dissection with scissors, by following the curvature of the prostate or by sensing the curvature of the Foley balloon on the bladder side, is continued down to the urethra, which is identified by its indwelling catheter. The urethra is incised partially transversely at the bladder neck. The deflated balloon end of the catheter is extracted,

clamped to its drainage end, and used for downward traction of the prostate. Another Foley catheter is inserted through the normal vesical neck opening, inflated to a much larger diameter, and used for upward traction (see Fig. 93-8). The remainder of the urethra circumference is divided and bleeding points are secured.

The final posterior attachments of the prostate are severed down to a distinct plane of cleavage between the fascial layers separating the bladder and seminal vesicles (Fig. 93-4). Finding the correct plane is most important in preventing dissection into layers of the trigone, where the ureters may be injured, and in preserving an important layer of fascia over the seminal vesicles. This plane of cleavage can be established medial to the vascular pedicle by maintaining downward traction on the prostate and upward traction on the bladder and then by hugging the bladder wall on one side with a finger and penetrating from the other side with a pointed clamp (Fig. 93-7A). Some experienced surgeons prefer to divide the final attachments at the vesical neck by perpendicular sharp dissection

FIG. 93-8. Perineal prostatovesiculectomy. **(A)** Both layers of fascia that envelop structures above the prostate are penetrated by blunt dissection against a finger underneath. **(B)** First vascular pedicles and then vasa deferentia are divided and ligated. This permits retraction of the specimen out of the wound and allows optimal exposure for ligation of the vascular pedicle well above each seminal vesicle. Ideally each of these structures should be removed in its enclosing fascia.

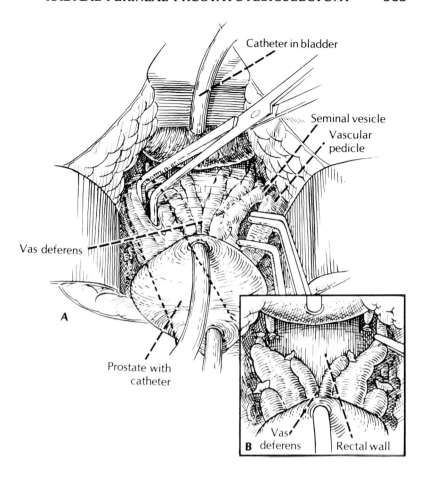

or cautery, estimating the proper depth by palpation with a finger from below and identifying the fascia covering the seminal vesicles as it comes into view (Fig. 93-7B).

When a cuff of bladder is to be removed, it is convenient to cut against the blade of a prostatic tractor to measure the width to be excised. Ordinarily a 1-cm cuff is removed anteriorly. Posteriorly, even though tumor extension is more likely, removal of a greater amount is usually impractical because of the nearby ureteral orifices. These are surprisingly close to the vesical neck, as compared to their magnified distance when seen cystoscopically. If the ureteral orifices are constantly visible (with or without the aid of indigo carmine dye given intravenously), ureteral catheters need not be inserted. Dissection across the trigone is associated with more bleeding and greater difficulty in defining the plane of cleavage between the bladder and seminal vesical fascia than is the case when a cuff of bladder is not removed.

In the pattern of local extension, most lesions first invade the prostatic capsule and then take the path of least resistance, often the ejaculatory ducts into the space between the seminal vesicals and the bladder. The growth outside the prostate is usually along the perivesical fascia rather than directly into the seminal vesicles. Therefore, it is important to remove at least the investing anterior layer of Denonvilliers' fascia (sometimes called the *genital fascia*), which lies between the bladder and the seminal vesicles, because adenocarcinoma is likely to extend beneath this plane. It is difficult to remove both layers of this fascia, because the layers are not clearly defined and dissection close to the bladder may injure the intramural ureters. In Figure 93-4, the fascial layers have been exaggerated for clarity.

If the proper plane has been established, the base of the bladder can easily be separated from this anterior layer of Denonvilliers' fascia, which encloses the seminal vesicles. This is accomplished by a combination of traction on the bladder neck, countertraction on the prostate, and blunt dissection against an underlying finger. Such dissection usually is not difficult even when the tumor extends beyond the prostate. Thus, if bleeding occurs or the separation proceeds poorly, the surgeon should make certain he is not entering layers of the trigone, where there is danger of ureteral-orifice or tunnel injury. An extra means of checking is to insert a finger in the bladder and, together with an outside digit, to sense the expected thickness of the trigone and bladder wall.

In order to obtain maximum exposure above the seminal vesicles, it is best first to divide the vascular pedicles with their fascia off the posterolateral margins of the prostate (Fig. 93-8). These contain the major arteries to the gland and are branches of the inferior vesical arteries. Release of these pedicles allows the specimen to be delivered significantly further out of the wound. The pedicles may be isolated on each side by penetrating both layers of fascia with a pointed clamp against the upward pressure of a finger from below. Occasionally, especially near the prostate where the vessels branch, the pedicle is so thick that it is more safely ligated in two parts. The proximal ends of the pedicle should be transfixed or doubly ligated before the clamp is released, because the vessels tend to retract not only within the fascia but also deep in the wound. Some surgeons prefer to ligate these major prostatic vessels early in the operation, before dividing the distal urethral attachments.

After the vascular pedicles have been divided, it is possible to expose the vasa deferentia well above the prostate. They are easily palpated bimanually near the midline, and although it is tempting to expose them by opening the fascia, they are friable if tied alone. Moreover, dissemination of malignant cells is less likely if the vasa are divided along with their surrounding fascia after isolation by penetrating both layers of fascia along each side of the vas with a guiding finger from below. The prostate can be then brought further out of the wound, and the upper extent of the seminal vesicles (which is surprisingly high) can be reached.

Uncertainty about the location of the ureters often obliges the surgeon to open the fascia longitudinally to visualize the tips of the seminal vesicles (Fig. 93-8) before dividing the attachments above. The tips lie loosely in the fascia, but their vascular supply to be ligated is located about 1 cm from the tips of the vesicles on the medial side. If a band or cord of induration suspected of tumor extends beyond the seminal vesicles, as much of it as possible should be removed. It is uncommon to expose a ureter during perineal prostatectomy; if the proper plane of cleavage has been established

between the bladder and seminal vesicles above the level of induration to be removed, there is practically no danger of ureteral injury. The position of the rectum is checked before the final clamps are applied. By this method of dissection and exposure, one usually can remove all gross evidence of extension in those cases selected for surgery, as outlined above.

After the prostate has been removed, the integrity of the ureters is confirmed either by injecting indigo carmine intravenously and inspecting both the inside and the outside of the bladder or by inserting ureteral catheters. With extensive dissection, it is not uncommon to open the peritoneal cavity; no particular hazard is involved as long as the occurrence is recognized. The openings may be closed without drainage.

The surgeon should tag the specimens with sutures to identify the vesical neck and apex regions and specifically request the pathologist to search for apical or vesical neck invasion. He should also perform the routine examination for extension into the seminal vesical region. In these ways, the surgeon will increase his own knowledge of the prognosis of radical surgery relative both to cure or palliation and to modifying the classic prostatovesiculectomy.

VESICOURETHRAL ANASTOMOSIS AND WOUND CLOSURE

Ordinarily, when a cuff of bladder has not been removed, direct anastomosis can be made between the small bladder opening and the membranous urethra or a button of capsule at the apex of the prostate (Fig. 93-9A). About six interrupted absorbable sutures, placed through all layers of both structures, usually provide a secure and watertight anastomosis over an indwelling 22Fr catheter with a 30-ml balloon. Because the membranous urethra is friable, mattress sutures are sometimes preferable. The anastomosis must be made without tension or ischemia; in patients who have had previous prostatic surgery, any fixation at the bladder neck must be released.

A similar type of vesicourethral anastomosis can be fashioned after a cuff of bladder has been removed (Fig. 93-9B). When approximating the posterior portion of the bladder outlet, the surgeon must be especially careful to avoid compressing the ureteral orifices; often ureteral catheters are kept in place until this approximation has been completed. Some surgeons believe that closure of the vesical neck with the urethral aperture posterior rather than anterior gives better results. Hutch

FIG. 93-9. Perineal prostatovesiculectomy. **(A)** Anastomosis of the bladder neck to the membranous urethra is accomplished by interrupted, absorbable sutures. This is readily done when the prostate has been transected just at the vesical neck. **(B)** If a cuff of the bladder has been removed, reduction of the vesical outlet is effected. **(C)** A penrose drain is placed between the bladder and the rectum and brought out through a stab wound. **(D)** The skin is closed by interrupted, nonabsorbable sutures after the levator ani muscles have been approximated.

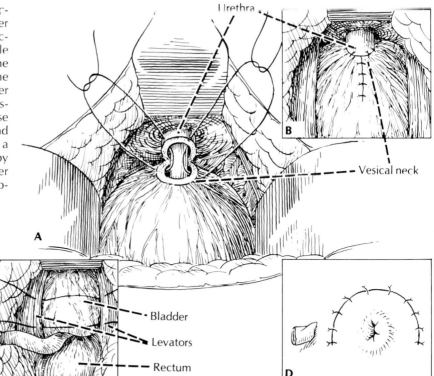

preferred to reduce the outlet circumferentially in an effort to preserve some of the internal sphincter. In all instances, the lumen of the new vesical outlet should measure approximately 1.5 cm in diameter. It is still uncertain whether there are advantages to mobilizing the anterior portion of the bladder to fashion a tube to increase the probability of continence. We have abandoned the use of traction sutures extending from the lateral aspect of the vesical neck to the perineal skin, which Vest described for reducing tension on the anastomosis.

Hemostasis is checked at the arterial sites described in this chapter. At times, small branches of the internal pudendal artery adjacent to the prostate are difficult to locate when severed, because they retract into the fat around the rectum in the vicinity of Alcock's canal. Other continued arterial bleeding may be found if dissection proceeded into the bulb area of the penis, the bladder wall or trigone, or the levator ani. A finger is inserted in the rectum, and the wall is inspected centimeter by centimeter to exclude injury.

The wound during closure is irrigated and a rapid-acting antibacterial (polymyxin B sulfate) is instilled as a precautionary measure against soiling from the rectum. A Penrose drain is placed beneath the bladder and may be brought out through a stab wound in the perineum. The levator ani muscles are approximated in the midline with interrupted absorbable sutures (Fig. 93-9C). It is advisable to approximate the central tendon to aid in anal control and to use interrupted, nonabsorbable sutures for skin closure in older individuals. For safety, the urethral catheter is sutured and taped to the penis and maintained at least until the patient is over any period of mental confusion and healing has proceeded to a point at which the reinsertion of a catheter would not likely injure the urethrovesical anastomotic site.

Transsacral Prostatovesiculectomy

Transsacral prostatovesiculectomy is a modification of the perineal approach in which part of the incision extends over the coccyx onto the sacrum, thus facilitating dissection above the seminal vesicles. This procedure was introduced in the late 1800s, revived in Europe in the 1940s, and first reported in the United States by Vallett in 1957.[27]

The chief advantages of this technique are that it provides the most direct approach to the seminal vesical region for removal of locally extended prostatic carcinoma, especially in obese individuals. Also it affords the best exposure free of bony

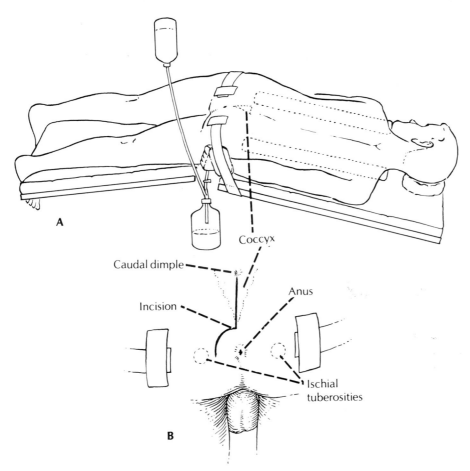

FIG. 93-10. Position of the patient for transsacral prostatovesiculectomy. **(A)** Patient lies prone on a slightly flexed operating table; legs are horizontal and separated. The trunk is elevated from the table with pads to minimize interference with respiration. An indwelling urethral catheter is connected to a fluid system for bladder distension later in the procedure. **(B)** Incision extends from the caudal dimple downward over the coccyx and laterally around the anus.

protuberances for reconstruction of the urethra by vesicourethral anastomosis or by replacing the length of the prostatic urethra. As with the perineal procedure, the postoperative course is relatively benign.

This posterior operation does not allow inspection or dissection of the pelvic lymph nodes. It may, however, be substituted for the perineal prostatovesiculectomy as a staged operation if there is ankylosis of the hip joints. The value of this approach is difficult to appreciate until one sees the technique of removing bone and displacing the rectum and senses the exposure clear of pelvic bone hindrance.

POSITION OF THE PATIENT

The patient is placed prone on the oprating table with legs separated; the penis and the urethral catheter emerge through an opening in the table (Fig. 93-10A). The table is flexed a few degrees, principally as an aid in maintaining position if the anesthesiologist must raise the patient's head or feet during the procedure. The legs are usually kept horizontal to prevent impaired venous drainage. A Trendelenburg or Fowler position does not alter the surgeon's working conditions. Laminectomy pads or rolled blankets are placed along both sides of the body, raising the trunk off the table so there will be minimal interference with respiration. Because the urethral catheter usually is not changed during the operation, a 22Fr catheter should be inserted before surgery. The balloon, inflated to 30 ml, should be drawn snugly against the vesical neck as an aid for later identification of the prostatovesical junction. The catheter is connected to a fluid system for distention of the bladder as needed to elevate structures in the wound. A small rubber balloon bag may be placed under the suprapubic region to elevate the bladder, but this should be used cautiously; if there is evidence of impaired venous drainage from the legs, contributing to hypotension, the bag should be deflated immediately. The perineal area is exposed by spreading the buttocks with wide strips of adhesive tape.

EXPOSURE OF THE PROSTATE

The skin incision is begun at the dimple of the caudal canal, extended downward over the coccyx, and curved around the anus medial to the ischial tuberosity (Fig. 93-10B). It is deepened to the periosteum in the superior portion and continued interiorly at this depth through the perineal fascia to expose the fat of the ischiorectal fossa lateral to the anus. Small self-retaining retractors placed in the superior and middle portions of the wound to expose the bone segment usually control all superficial bleeding.

The margin of the coccyx is quickly severed from the fibrous attachments of the gluteal musculature with heavy curved scissors (Fig. 93-11). No significant bleeding occurs because the dissection is kept close to the periosteum. To mobilize the curved coccyx, it is best to penetrate under this bone in its midportion and insert a finger to displace the rectum downward as the remaining lateral attachments are divided on either side. In the transsacral position, the rectum tends to fall away from the coccyx; by dissecting close to the periosteum, the surgeon need not take extra care for fear of rectal injury. The tip of the coccyx is elevated by a finger, and the final attachments of the coccygeal anal ligament are divided. It is not absolutely necessary to suture this ligament during closure to maintain competence of the rectal sphincter.

The removal of a 1-cm segment of sacrum provides easy access to the tips of the seminal vesicles unless the prostate is greatly enlarged, and it provides wider exposure than is afforded by removal of the coccyx alone. The sacrum is divided approximately 1 cm below the sacral canal, which is well below the exit of any important nerves. The rectum is protected with a finger or flat retractor while the sacrum is divided with light taps of a hammer on a medium osteotome. Only two or three cutting positions of the osteotome are necessary for the transverse division; then the lateral bony attachments are divided similarly, and the fibrous attachments are severed with scissors.

Bleeding from the bone edge is usually minimal; if it persists, bone wax is applied. Because terminal branches of the middle sacral vessels sometimes course downward over the inner surface of the sacrum to this level, it is safer to ligate the central posterior attachments of the sacrum, although these vessels rarely cause significant bleeding.

The inferior surface of one side of the levator ani muscle is exposed by developing the ischiorectal fossa until the prostate can be palpated (Fig. 93-12A). In a similar fashion, the superior surface of this levator ani is exposed by displacing the rectum toward the midline until the prostate can be palpated again. The levator ani sling on each side resembles the diaphragm that separates the pleural cavity from the peritoneal cavity. Sometimes it is attenuated or has a variable origin extending upward along the lateral margin of the wound from the obturator fascia. The muscle is divided, keeping it under tension with two fingers on either side, all the way down to the fascia covering the prostate (Fig. 93-12A). Occasional small arterioles must be transfixed; these serve as landmarks for approximating the muscle during closure. Cutting the levator ani on one side enables the opposite corner of the wound to be retracted widely (Fig. 93-12C).

FIG. 93-11. Transsacral prostatovesiculectomy. By blunt and sharp dissection, the sacrum and coccyx are exposed. With a protecting finger between the coccyx and rectum, the distal sacrum is divided by the osteotome. Middle sacral vessel branches should be anticipated in this area.

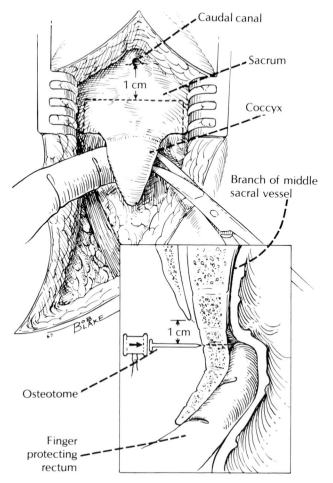

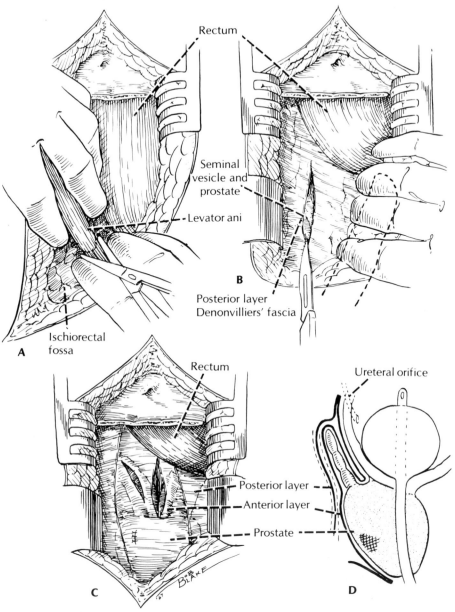

Rectum

Seminal
vesicle and
prostate

Levator ani

Ischiorectal
fossa

A

B

Posterior layer
Denonvilliers' fascia

Rectum

Posterior layer
Anterior layer
Prostate

Ureteral orifice

C

D

FIG. 93-12. Transsacral prostatovesiculectomy. **(A)** The levator ani muscle is divided down to the prostate after development of the ischiorectal fossa below and separation of the rectum above. This allows the opposite corner of the wound to be retracted widely. **(B)** The rectum is retracted off the fascia overlying the prostate and the seminal vesicles. This is facilitated by a guiding finger in the rectum. **(C and D)** The usual route of dissection is to open the posterior layer of Denonvilliers' fascia to expose the prostate; then additional incisions must be made in the anterior layer of Denonvilliers' fascia to isolate successively the vasa deferentia, the seminal vesicles, and the vascular pedicle above the prostate.

The rectum bulges into the wound, and a plane of cleavage can be developed quickly around its lateral border to the point at which it is to be separated from the prostate. It has already been explained that fused layers of peritoneum extend between the rectum and prostate. The surgeon may dissect between these posterior and anterior layers of Denonvilliers' fascia, where separation is easier and bloodless or dissect the rectum off both layers of this fascia. The second method is not risky in the transsacral operation, because even if the rectum is entered, the damage is usually on

the posterolateral side, where it can be repaired at a safe distance from the proposed vesicourethral anastomosis. The rectum has a greater circumference than is generally expected, so we use a guiding finger in the lumen to facilitate its separation from the prostate and seminal vesicles (Fig. 93-12B).

The rectum can be displaced by developing a cleavage plane on both sides before freeing the central portion, but the most expeditious technique is to palpate the margin of the prostate and then to make a separate longitudinal incision through the posterior layer of Denonvilliers' fascia (Fig. 93-

FIG. 93-13. Transsacral prostatovesiculectomy. After attachments of the vasa deferentia and the seminal vesicles are divided, these structures are separated from the base of the bladder and vascular pedicles are ligated. The prostate is then detached at its junction with the membranous urethra, or a small button of prostatic capsule may be left in place. The vesico-prostatic junction may be identified accurately by palpating the catheter balloon with the bladder.

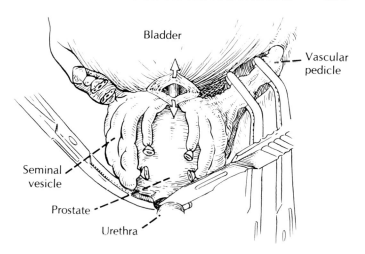

12B). Displacement of the rectum laterally is continued upward over the tips of the seminal vesicles, whose position can be judged by palpation of the Foley balloon within the bladder. When the rectum has been mobilized throughout the length of the wound, it can be retracted easily, almost out of sight, by a large Deaver retractor, and it is not necessary to disturb the sphincter area or to divide the rectourethralis attachment. The structures cephalad to the prostate are not visible at this time, even if the dissection has been done within Denonvilliers' fascia, because the seminal vesicles and the vasa deferentia are enveloped in an additional layer of anterior Denonvilliers' fascia (Fig. 93-12C and D).

A particular advantage of the transsacral approach is that the surgeon is better able to determine the amount of extension of the cancer beyond the prostate, especially in the seminal vesical region, before he commits himself to proceed with prostatovesiculectomy. Fixation of local tissues or abnormal venous patterns often give a clue to the extent of involvement.

BLOCK DISSECTION, VESICOURETHRAL ANASTOMOSIS, AND CLOSURE

These techniques basically are the same as for the perineal prostatovesiculectomy (Fig. 93-13) and were detailed in the second edition of this text.[34] The differences to remember are that the posterior structures are now anterior in the wound. The original urethral catheter is deflated; later it is reinflated but not removed from the wound. The most troublesome bleeding usually comes from the anterior veins now, in this position, coursing posteriorly over the prostate and bladder. This bleeding ceases with packing and the tamponade of

closure. Finally, if desired, the length of prostatic urethra can be replaced with a tube fashioned from a flap of the bladder wall (Fig. 93-14).[16]

Postoperative Management

The course after perineal prostatovesiculectomy is remarkably benign compared with that after retroperitoneal surgery or an enucleation operation for benign prostatic enlargement. The most important aspect is observation of cardiorespiratory status. Coronary insufficiency is rare, but it is still the most common cause of death after surgery. The critical period is after the patient is moved out of the exaggerated lithotomy position. This should be done slowly to avoid a sudden increase in the vascular space. Such an increase might be produced mechanically by resuming the normal position or chemically by release of acidotic agents from large masses of relatively ischemic tissue.

The patient is usually able to walk within 24 hr and requires few analgesics or sedatives. It is surprising how quickly the patient can sit comfortably on a ring after perineal or transsacral surgery. A stool softener is given the second night after surgery and a few nights thereafter to prevent fecal impaction and unnecessary straining. The use of rectal tubes, rectal thermometers, or enemas is forbidden during the immediate postoperative period, when the rectum is most susceptible to injury. When the wound is clean and dry, the patient may be released from the hospital without specific restrictions, and he should be able to resume his usual activities within 3 weeks.

As a precautionary measure, antibacterial agents are given by most surgeons during the first few days after surgery. Perineal and sacral incisions tolerate contamination remarkably well.

Removal of the Penrose drain is not begun until

at least 4 and usually 7 days after surgery, so that a potential sinus tract can be established. It is left longer if drainage continues or if the urethrovesical anastomosis is questioned.

Cleansing the perineal wound after each bowel movement with an antiseptic solution (benzalkonium chloride—aqueous Zephiran 1:10,000—povidone-iodine—Betadyne ½%), local heat, and warm sitz baths, even while the drain is in place, are ordered customarily. These measures may aid wound healing and are welcomed by the patient.

Skin sutures are usually not removed from perineal and transsacral incisions until at least 8 to 9 days after surgery because of the age of the patient and the increased possibility of wound separation. If perineal traction sutures have been used, they are left in place 10 days or longer.

Catheter irrigation is needed only occasionally because bleeding is not often a problem. In the immediate postoperative period, the patient in effect irrigates his own catheter if adequate diuresis is maintained. The catheter is removed in 7 to 10 days if the vesicourethral anastomosis has been made securely; it may be left 2 to 3 weeks, if the

FIG. 93-14. Transsacral prostatovesiculectomy. **(A)** Ordinarily the prostate is separated from the bladder at the vesical neck. (See Fig. 93-6 inverted for removal of the prostate with or without dividing the puboprostatic ligaments.) When a cuff of bladder is removed, it should be remembered that the ureters lie on the upper side of the bladder in the wound and that there are many large veins in the vicinity. **(B, C,** and **D)** The technique is illustrated for replacing a length of prostatic urethra.

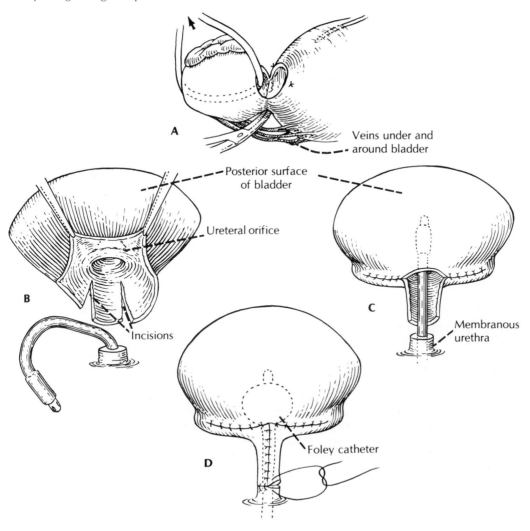

structures have not been well approximated, if practical. Antibacterial agents are given for at least 1 week after removal of the catheter because of edema that persists at the anastomotic site.

If the vesicourethral anastomosis has been made precisely, the patient continues to void with a good stream and the urine returns to normal promptly. In such cases, the urethra is calibrated in approximately 3 months and later only if indicated. If the flow rate is decreased, the usual practice is to calibrate the urethra beginning 2 weeks after the catheter is removed and doubling the time interval until it is certain that the junction remains adequate. After prostatovesiculectomy, the course of the urethra is displaced and the location of the vesicourethral anastomosis is very close to the rectum. This crucial junction may be identified by rectal palpation after first passing a small catheter. Its calibration is far safer with soft rubber catheters than standard curved sounds. If rigid instruments are necessary, filiforms and followers are preferable.

Complications

IMMEDIATE COMPLICATIONS

Hemorrhage after prostatovesiculectomy is rare unless the patient has been hypotensive at the time of wound closure. Gentle traction on the catheter balloon controls intravesical venous bleeding, but traction sufficient to control arterial bleeding at the vesical neck leads to incontinence if left continuous for longer than 4 hr. If intravesical bleeding cannot be controlled, transurethral fulguration should be attempted before the wound is opened. Extravesical bleeding generally is controlled by the tamponade effect of Fowler position.

Rectal injury is not a problem if it is recognized and treated promptly. These defects are usually small and should be closed with interrupted sutures of fine permanent interrupted sutures on an atraumatic needle, preferably including all layers of the bowel wall. The primary closure should be reinforced by one or two additional layers of fine interrupted sutures imbricating the muscularis and serosa without tension.

Whether to proceed with prostatovesiculectomy after rectal injury is a question that arises only when the injury occurs before the urethra is divided. Rather than risk rectourinary fistula, some surgeons prefer to close the wound and proceed again about 2 weeks later, sometimes by a different route. Most surgeons, however, continue the operation after the defect has been repaired. Before closure, the wound may be irrigated with a rapid-acting antibacterial solution (5000 units/ml polymyxin). Antibacterial solutions may be instilled in the rectum and continued on a daily basis as an added precaution. Some surgeons dilate the anal sphincter excessively or leave rectal drains in place to keep the intraluminal pressure low. Although keeping the bowel at complete rest is no longer advocated, the patient should be kept on a liquid, low-residue diet for several days. Later, a stool softener is given to prevent straining. If the bowel has been mechanically cleansed before surgery, there is questionable advantage in beginning oral bowel sterilization; sterilization may cause diarrhea and proteolytic enzymes from the small intestine are detrimental to wound healing, especially if absorbable sutures have been used to close a defect. There appears to be more risk with rapid sterilization (neomycin) than with a longer program (phthalylsulfathiazole—Sulfathalidine).

Replacing the urethral catheter during the immediate postoperative period may be difficult if the urethrovesical anastomosis has not been made precisely. A guiding finger in the rectum and lubricant injected in the urethra may be helpful. Before resorting to wound opening, one should anesthetize the patient and make an attempt to introduce the catheter under endoscopic vision.

Ureteral obstruction is a rare complication of prostatovesiculectomy. The ureters are above the usual level of dissection, and the surgeon is alert to their position because of their great importance and small size. In the past, edema from the use of landmark catheters (usually larger than 6Fr) was the cause of most ureteral obstruction, but today the use of diuretics has virtually eliminated this problem. When diuresis is maintained during surgery, intravenous indigo carmine dye appears quickly, ordinarily eliminating the need for such catheters. If the ureteral orifices are compromised during closure by sutures within the bladder, the sutures may be released cystoscopically a few days later, when it is practical to pass a rigid instrument. Even in the presence of complete bilateral obstruction, the patient may be managed conservatively during this period without demonstrable renal damage if infection is not present. In the very rare instance when a ureter has been divided, it should be reimplanted from an abdominal approach.

DELAYED COMPLICATIONS

Urinary leakage through the drain tract is not uncommon after the catheter is removed. If it does

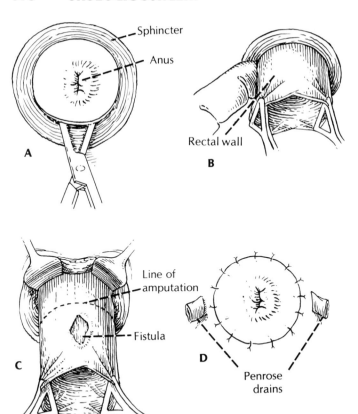

Sphincter

Anus

Rectal wall

A

B

Line of
amputation

Fistula

C

D

Penrose
drains

FIG. 93-15. Young–Stone operation for urethrorectal fistula. This procedure is accomplished by **(A)** circumferential incision around the anus, **(B)** mobilization of the terminal portion of the rectum beneath the external sphincter, and **(C)** amputation of the distal rectum including the site of fistula. The fistula is generally found with 2 cm of the anal margin, necessitating relatively minimal amputation of rectum. Closure of the incision **(D)** is done with multiple interrupted sutures with drains placed through lateral stab wounds.

not subside within 1 or 2 days, the catheter should be replaced for a few days longer. A cutaneous urinary fistula that requires curettage or excision is very rare.

Superficial inflammation is rather frequent in perineal or transsacral wounds because of continuing local contamination. It is best to leave the permanent type of skin sutures an extra few days until inflammation has subsided, rather than to chance wound separation, which heals slowly. Incisional hernias do not occur after perineal or transsacral operations. Infrequent deep-space infections are more likely to occur when the drain comes out too early and there is continued extravasation of urine. This problem should be anticipated and treated promptly.

Most urethrorectal fistulas occur after unrecognized rectal injury. The first treatment should consist of replacing the urethral catheter, minimizing the rectal flora by the local instillation of antibacterial solutions, and reducing bowel activity. If such measures are not successful within a few days, we fulgurate the opening transurethrally and transrectally. If the fistula persists, it is the usual practice to do a diverting colostomy and

suprapubic cystostomy. Repair is undertaken after 3 weeks or longer, when the inflammatory reaction is at a minimum. The first attempt is extremely important because secondary procedures are less likely to be successful.

We have been so impressed with the modification of the Young–Stone operation that today we would not hesitate to repair a urethrorectal fistula without a preliminary colostomy.[48] In this procedure ureteral catheters are inserted preoperatively to protect the ureters, which are often near the point of closure. In the classic operation, an incision is made around the mucocutaneous junction of the anus (Fig. 93-15A), and a plane of cleavage is established between the rectal wall and sphincter at 6 o'clock, where there is a natural defect in the decussation of muscle fibers. Pennington clamps are attached to the rectal wall for traction, and by blunt dissection the rectum is freed posteriorly and laterally (Fig. 93-15).

Sharp dissection anteriorly is necessary to free the rectum up to and beyond the fistulous tract. This dissection is facilitated by a guiding finger in the rectum. The fistulous opening is usually less than 2 cm from the anal margin, but dissection must be continued an equal distance beyond it. Ordinarily there is very little tract to excise.

The urethral edges are freshened, and although actual closure of the defect is not undertaken, an attempt is made to cover it with interrupted sutures of fine absorbable material, keeping in mind the location of the ureteral catheters (Fig. 93-16). If possible, a second layer of closure is made, including fragments of the levator ani.

A Penrose drain is placed on each side of the area of closure and brought out through stab wounds lateral to the anus. The distal portion of the rectum containing the defect is excised in portions, as the mobilized proximal portion is advanced and sutured to the adjacent skin margins without tension (Fig. 93-15). The drains are removed in approximately 1 week. The suprapubic catheter, which was present either preoperatively or was inserted by punch technique, can be clamped for a trial voiding after 3 weeks, although many surgeons wait considerably longer.

LATE COMPLICATIONS

Stenosis of the vesical neck, earlier reported as approximately 6%, has become uncommon with increased greater efforts to effect and maintain a good vesicourethral anastomosis. It is least likely when a button of apical prostatic capsule is left in place. If stenosis does develop, however, it can usually be remedied by dilations at increasing intervals. If this is unsuccessful, an internal urethrotomy of the vesical neck can be considered. Unfortunately, with the fixation of tissues, incontinence may result or the enlarged outlet may again be susceptible to contracture. Plastic revision of the vesical neck, which is located deep in the pelvis after prostatovesiculectomy, is nearly impossible from a suprapubic approach, although it might be feasible if the symphysis pubis were removed. A perineal or transsacral approach is our choice for a revision attempt.

Continence is regained almost immediately after removal of the urethral catheter if a cuff of bladder has not been removed and a button of apical prostatic capsule has been used for anastomosis. Urinary leakage great enough for the patient to wear an appliance occurred in fewer than 5% of patients in the author's series. Continence ordinarily returns within a few days if the vesical neck has been left intact but the entire prostate has been removed (persistent incontinent rate of less than 10%). In the classic prostatovesiculectomy, when all the prostate and a cuff of bladder are removed, complete continence is variable. More than 50% of

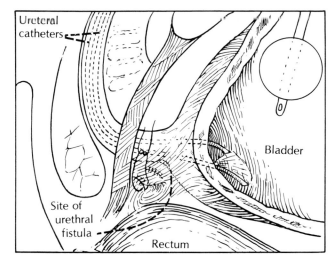

FIG. 93-16. Young–Stone operation. Closure of the urethral defect in the Young–Stone procedure is usually accomplished in two layers of interrupted absorbable suture material. As indicated in this sagittal view, ureteral catheters are inserted for landmarks during operation; postoperatively urine is diverted with a suprapubic catheter.

patients regain control within 3 weeks; 80% within 3 months; and 90% within 6 months.* Today this pattern of improvement is accelerated with trials of various pharmacologic agents. After 6 months, patients rarely regain satisfactory control, and corrective surgical measures should be considered. Sphincter exercises are of doubtful value in speeding the return of continence. but by learning how to "set" the muscles, those with stress incontinence may be spared some accidents. All patients with persistent incontinence should have cystourethrographic–endoscopic examinations and urodynamic studies to exclude remediable disorders and to select the most efficacious drug therapy.

Local tumor recurrence develops in no more than 5% of patients in whom local extension is only microscopic, and in fewer than 10% of those with obvious local extension who have not had postoperative radiotherapy. The recurrence occurs more often with high-grade lesions. Even then patients often succumb to other causes than their prostatic carcinoma before urethral or ureteral obstruction occurs. If unilateral or bilateral upper tract obstruction develops, placement of indwelling ureteral stents is considered first. Operative urinary diversion is reserved for selected cases in which the patient seems to have at least 6 months of quality living and enjoys an important family role.

---

* Parry WL, Blankenship JB: Unpublished data

END RESULT REPORTING

I have purposely omitted treatment results in this text because a number of management programs with many variables are being explored. Current perineal prostatovesiculectomy data may be gleaned from selected references in the bibliography.[3,5,6,11–13,15,17,19,22,26,37,39] In this age of computer analysis, the urologic surgeon who believes radical surgery has treatment importance for carcinoma of the prostate is invited to record and make available his individual case data in some accepted manner for future teaching and practice.[41]

REFERENCES

1. ALBERS DD, FAULKNER KK, CHEATHAM WN et al: Personal communication and surgical anatomy of pubovesical (pubo-prostatic) ligaments. J Urol 109:388, 1973

2. ALYEA EP, DEES JE, GLENN JF: An aggressive approach to prostatic cancer. J Urol 118:211, 1977

3. ARDUINO LJ, GLUCKSMAN MA: Lymph node metastases in early carcinoma of the prostate. J Urol 88:91, 1961

4. BELT E: Radical perineal prostatectomy in early carcinoma of the prostate. J Urol 48:287, 1942

5. BLACKARD CE: The Veterans Administration Cooperative Urological Research Group studies of carcinoma of the prostate: A review. Cancer Chemotherapy Reports 59:225, 1975

6. BOXER RJ, KAUFMAN JJ, GOODWIN WE: Radical prostatectomy for carcinoma of the prostate: 1951–1976. A review of 329 patients. J Urol 117:208, 1977

7. BRUCE AW, O'CLEIREACHAIN F, MORALES A et al: Carcinoma of the prostate: A critical look at staging. J Urol 117:319, 1977

8. BYAR DP, MOSTOFI FK, Veterans Administration Cooperative Urological Research Group: Carcinoma of the prostate: Prognostic evaluation of certain pathologic features in 208 radical prostatectomies. Cancer 30:5, 1972

9. BYAR DP, Veterans Administration Cooperative Urological Research Group: Survival of patients with incidentally found microscopic cancer of the prostate: Results of a clinical trial of conservative treatment. J Urol 108:908, 1972

10. CAMPBELL EW: Total prostatectomy with preliminary ligation of the vascular pedicles. J Urol 81:464, 1959

11. CANTALONA WJ, SCOTT WW: Carcinoma of the prostate: A review. J Urol 119:1, 1978

12. CANTALONA WJ, SMOLEN JK, HARTY JI: Prognostic value of the host immunocompetence in urologic cancer patients. J Urol 114:922, 1975

13. CARSON CC, III, ZINCKE H, UTZ DC et al: Radical prostatectomy after radiotherapy for prostatic carcinoma. J Urol 124:237, 1980

14. DE VERE WHITE R, PAULSON DF, GLENN JF: The clinical spectrum of prostate cancer. J Urol 117:323, 1977

15. FLOCKS RH: The treatment of stage C prostatic cancer with special reference to combined surgical and radiation therapy. J Urol 109:461, 1973

16. FLOCKS RH, CULP DA: A modification of technique for anastomosing membranous urethra and bladder neck following total prostatectomy. J Urol 69:411, 1953

17. FLOCKS RH, O'DONOGHUE EPN, MILLEMAN LA et al: Surgery of prostatic carcinoma. Cancer 36:1975

18. GLEASON DF, MELLINGER FT, Veterans Administration Cooperative Urological Research Group: Prediction of prognosis for prostatic adenocarcinoma by combined histological grading and clinical staging. J Urol 111:58, 1974

19. GLENN JF: Surgical therapy of cancer of the prostate. In Skinner DG, deKernion JB (eds): Genitourinary Cancer, Chap. 18. Philadelphia, W B Saunders, 1978

20. GOODWIN WE: Radical prostatectomy after previous prostatic surgery: Technical problems encountered in treatment of occult prostatic carcinoma. JAMA 148:799, 1952

21. GREENFIELD LJ. In Greenfield LF (ed): Surgery in the Aged. Philadelphia, W B Saunders, 1975

22. HANASH KA, UTZ DC, COOK EN et al: Carcinoma of the prostate: A 15 year followup. J Urol 107:450, 1972

23. HUDSON PB, STOUT AP: Indications for radical perineal prostatectomy. In An Atlas of Prostatic Surgery, p 65, Philadelphia, W B Saunders, 1962

24. HUTCH JA: A new theory of the anatomy of the internal urinary sphincter and the physiology of micturition. IV. The urinary sphincteric mechanism. J Urol 97:705, 1967

25. JEWETT HJ: Radical prostatectomy for palpable clinically localized, nonobstructive cancer: Experience at the John Hopkins Hospital, 1909–1963. J Urol 124:492, 1980

26. JEWETT HJ: The present status of radical prostatectomy for stages A and B. Prostatic cancer, Symposium on the prostate. Urol Clin North Am 2(1):105, 1975

27. MARESCA GM, VALLETT BS: Parasacral prostatectomy. Del State Med J 29:31, 1957

28. MATHIS JL: Psychological treatment of the patient with cancer. Clinical Medicine 78:521, 1971

29. MCLAUGHLIN AP, SALTZSTEIN SL, MCCULLOUGH BL et al: Prostatic cancer: Incidence of and location of unsuspected lymphatic metastases. J Urol 115:89, 1976

30. MELLINGER GT, GLEASON DF, BAILAR J, III: The history and prognosis of prostatic cancer. J Urol 97:331, 1967

31. MURPHY GP, WHITMORE WF, JR: Report of the workshops on the current status of the histologic grading of prostate cancer. Cancer 44:1490, 1979

32. NICHOLSON TC, RICHIE JP: Pelvic lymphadenectomy for stage B_1 adenocarcinoma of the prostate: Justified or not? J Urol 117:199, 1977

33. PARRY WL: Management of renal, urinary and genital problems. In Greenfield LF (ed): Surgery in the Aged, p 74. Philadelphia, W B Saunders, 1975

34. PARRY WL: Prostate Malignancies. In Gleen JF, Boyce WH (eds): Urologic Surgery, 2nd ed, Chap. 40. Hagerstown, Harper & Row, 1975

35. PARRY WL: Prostatovesiculectomy relative to palliation for carcinoma of the prostate. Presented at the South Central Section of American Urological Association, October 1978

36. PUTENNEY REH, LAMSON BG: Cancer of the prostate gland: A clinical and pathological evaluation of patients treated by radical prostatectomy. J Urol 85:649, 1961

37. SCHROEDER FH, BELT E: Carcinoma of the prostate: A study of 213 patients with stage C tumors treated by total perineal prostatectomy. J Urol 114:257, 1975

38. SCOTT WW: An evaluation of endocrine therapy plus radical perineal prostatectomy in the treatment of advanced carcinoma of the prostate. J Urol 91:97, 1964

39. SCOTT WW, BOYD HL: Combined hormone control therapy and radical prostatectomy in the treatment of selected cases of advanced carcinoma of the prostate: A retrospective study based upon 25 years of experience. J Urol 101:86, 1969

40. SEWELL RA, BRAREN V, WILSON SK et al: Extended biopsy followup after full course radiation for resectable prostatic carcinoma. J Urol 113:371, 1975

41. Task Force on Urologic Sites (Parry WL): Prostate. In Beahrs OH, Carr DT, Rubin P (eds): American Joint Committee for Cancer Staging and End-results Reporting, p 119. Chicago, 1977

42. TOBIN CE, BENJAMIN JA: Anatomical and surgical restudy of Denonvilliers' fascia. Surg Gynecol Obstet 80:373, 1945

43. TOMLINSON RL, CURRE DP, BOYCE WH: Radical prostatectomy: Palliation for stage C carcinoma of the prostate. J Urol 117:85, 1977

44. VICKERY AL, JR, KERR WS, JR: Carcinoma of the prostate treated by radical prostatectomy. A clinicopathological survey of 187 cases followed for 5 years and 148 cases followed for 10 years. Cancer 16:1598, 1963

45. WEYRAUCH HM: Surgery of the Prostate. Philadelphia, W B Saunders, 1959

46. WILSON CS, DAHL DS, MIDDLETON RG: Pelvic lymphadenectomy for the staging of apparently localized prostatic cancer. J Urol 117:197, 1977

47. YOUNG HH: The cure of carcinoma of the prostate by radical perineal prostatectomy (prostato-seminal vesiculectomy): History, literature and statistics of Young's operation. J Urol 53:188, 1945

48. YOUNG HH, STONE HB: An operation for urethro-rectal fistula: Report of three cases. Trans Am Assoc Genitourin Surg 8:270, 1913

Interstitial Radiotherapy of the Prostate

94

Bernard Lytton

The treatment of early stage prostatic cancer remains controversial. Assessment of treatment failure indicates that at 10 years about 16% of patients, treated either by radical prostatectomy or radiation therapy, have died of cancer and that another 6% to 8% are alive with evidence of persistent or recurrent disease.[6,8] It is estimated that of patients who were treated conservatively or with some form of hormonal manipulation, 24% died of cancer within 10 years.

The figures for cancer deaths are probably underestimates, because many recorded noncancer deaths are likely to be related to the underlying disease. Moreover, the various groups are not strictly comparable since the mode of selection, staging, and tumor grading is different. Staging by pathologic examination of the specimen following radical prostatectomy is obviously more accurate than clinical staging, which is usually associated with a significant degree of understaging but is the only method available in patients treated by radiation therapy. The conservatively treated group includes a large number of stage A lesions that would tend to decrease the number of treatment failures. Thus the evidence suggests that either radical prostatectomy or curative radiation therapy is indicated for early-stage prostatic cancer. It is still unclear, however, which of these modalities provides more favorable results. The present evidence, based on 10-year survival rates, suggests that they are comparable.

Each form of treatment is associated with significant morbidity.[4] Radical prostatectomy results in some degree of urinary incontinence in about 5% of patients and impotence in all of them. External-beam radiation, with a dose of 6000 rads to 7000 rads,* causes significant and persistent proctitis or cystitis in 3% to 5% of patients and impotence in 30% to 50%. Because the treatment must be delivered daily over 6 to 7 weeks, it is socially disruptive and requires prolonged absence from work.

---

* Rads/millicuries is 1.1 to 1.2.

Interstitial radiation, by implantation of radium needles, was used extensively in the treatment of prostatic cancer prior to the advent of hormonal therapy. This high-energy radiation caused problems similar to those with external beam, and special precautions for the attendants and patients were necessary. Radioactive gold, either in the colloidal form for injection or in platinum-coated seeds, is used for interstitial radiation, usually as a supplement to radical prostatectomy (in more advanced cases) or in conjunction with external-beam therapy.[2,3] The use of this isotope also requires special precautions both by the surgeons and patients.

^{125}I is an isotope with a low-voltage γ emission, a half-life of 60 days, and half-value layer for tissue of only 2 cm, where gold has a half-life of 2.7 days and a half-value layer for tissue of 6 cm. The half-value layer for tissue of radium is 10 cm. The interstitial implantation of ^{125}I seeds into the prostate for early-stage cancer by a retropubic approach was first introduced by Whitmore and his associates in 1970.[9] There is now a fairly extensive experience with this method and the preliminary results suggest that its continued use is well justified.[7] Ambrose has advocated a transcoccygeal implantation technique.[1]

Advantages and Disadvantages

ADVANTAGES

1. Complications of treatment are uncommon. They tend to be less severe than with other forms of radiation because of the low energy and low half-value layer for tissue of the ^{125}I.
2. Proctitis and cystitis do occur but are usually temporary and subside spontaneously.
3. Loss of potency occurs less frequently and is seen in about 10% to 15% of patients who are sexually active prior to the procedure.[5]
4. The treatment can be completed in a realtively short period of time. No special precautions are

required for the surgeons, nursing personnel, or family. The long half-life of the isotope allows a relatively long period of storage of the seeds.

5. A staging lymphadenectomy can be performed at the time of the implantation.

DISADVANTAGES

1. The treatment requires an operative procedure.
2. The low half-value for tissue requires an even distribution of seeds to obtain a relatively homogeneous dose of radiation to the gland. Some centers have undertaken to correct this by supplemental treatment with external-beam radiation. This should be confined to the prostate because inclusion of the pelvic area after lymphadenectomy may produce severe lymphedema. Supplemental treatment has resulted, however, in a number of serious complications, such as rectal ulceration or stenosis that required fecal diversion by colostomy in some instances. Very careful dosimetry is required by an experienced radiotherapist if interstitial radiation with ^{125}I is to be supplemented by external-beam therapy.

Patient Selection

Interstitial radiation for early-stage prostatic cancer is generally advocated for patients under 70 years of age with no evidence of metastatic disease, with a life expectancy of a least 5 to 10 years, and with a general condition that does not preclude a major surgical procedure. Early-stage prostatic cancer includes patients with A_2 and B stage disease, A_2 being defined as three or more foci of tumor in a prostatectomy specimen. Also included are early C lesions, in which the tumor extends to the limits of the prostate with no tumor palpable beyond it, although microscopic capsular invasion is probably present. Patients with seminal vesical involvement are best treated by external-beam therapy, which covers a wider field, because a satisfactory seed implant cannot be performed.

Patients are evaluated by chest radiograph, bone scanning, and estimation of serum prostatic acid phosphatase by an enzymatic method. Lymphangiography is not performed because of the unacceptably high percentage of false-positive and false-negative results. It is extremely difficult to detect microscopic nodal metastases by lymphangiography. When there is concern about seminal vesical involvement, computed tomographic (CT) scanning of the pelvis may help to determine whether this has in fact occurred.

Following transurethral resection of the prostate, evaluation for seed implantation should be deferred for 3 to 4 months to allow the prostatic fossa to heal and tissue reaction to resolve. The amount of residual tissue can be determined by

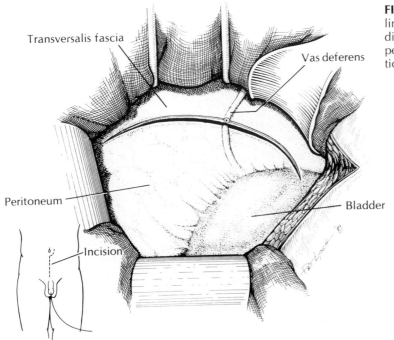

FIG. 94-1. Exposure on the left, showing the line of incision in the transversalis fascia with division of the vas deferens for reflection of the peritoneum. The inset depicts the preferred vertical abdominal incision for the procedure.

Transversalis fascia

Vas deferens

Peritoneum

Bladder

Incision

endoscopic examination and palpation of the prostate over the cystoscope. Should it be decided that insufficient tissue remains to allow an effective implant for interstitial radiation, the patient should be treated by external-beam irradiation or radical prostatectomy.

Surgical Procedure

Surgery involves a pelvic lymphadenectomy together with direct implantation of ^{125}I seeds into the prostate under direct vision.

The patient is placed supine on the operating table with legs slightly apart to allow a finger to be inserted into the rectum during the seed implantation. Some surgeons prefer to place the legs in low stirrups and to use an O'Conor drape to provide easy access to the rectum. A No. 18Fr Foley catheter is placed in the bladder to define the position of the prostatic urethra. A Bucky diaphragm is placed under the patient so that a radiograph can be taken intraoperatively to check the distribution of the seeds at the completion of the implant. The table is placed in 10 degrees to 15 degrees of Trendelenburg to allow the abdominal contents to fall away from the pelvis.

A lower midline incision is made from the symphysis pubis to the umbilicus (Fig. 94-1). It is preferred to a transverse incision because it can more easily be extended if wider access to the retroperitoneum is required. The rectus fascia is divided in the midline (marked by the decussation of the aponeurotic fibers) and the muscles are separated right down to the pubic bone to provide maximal access to the retropubic space. The extraperitoneal space is entered at the lower end of the incision to avoid injury to the peritoneum, and the transversalis fascia is then divided just above the pubis. The division of the fascia is extended laterally behind the rectus muscles to allow the peritoneum and its contents to be displaced upward and medially on each side to expose the iliac vessels and lymph nodes (Fig. 94-1). The vas deferens is identified on each side and divided proximal to the inguinal ligament; the gonadal vessels are preserved, if possible, because their division may cause testicular ischemia with pain and swelling in the immediate postoperative period.

A self-retaining retractor is used to maintain exposure and the peritoneum is retracted cephalad to expose the origin of the common iliac artery (Fig. 94-2). The ureter should be identified and is usually found loosely adherent to the overlying peritoneum with which it is retracted. The lymph node dissection is begun by dividing the perivascular fascia and lymph channels over the origin of the common iliac artery. Major lymph channels are occluded with silver clips. The dissection is continued down over the iliac vessels, removing the lymph nodes and lymphatics along with the perivascular fascia, which provides an easy plain of separation from the vessels. The external iliac

FIG. 94-2. Exposure of the left lateral pelvic wall at completion of the lymphadenectomy

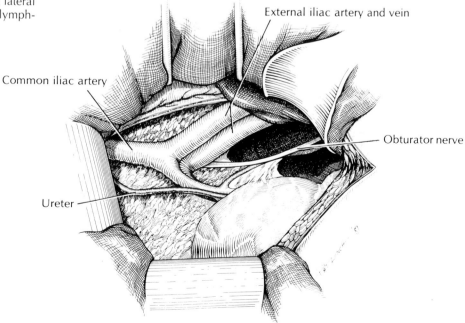

Common iliac artery

External iliac artery and vein

Obturator nerve

Ureter

artery and vein are dissected free; the genitofemoral nerve on the lateral side marks the lateral boundary of the dissection. The lymphadenectomy is carried down to the inguinal ligament. All obvious lymphatic channels are occluded with silver clips, which helps to prevent the formation of a lymphocele.

The dissection is continued down the internal iliac artery as far as its first division. The obturator fat pad and node are now located over the antero-medial aspect of the obturator foramen. The fatty tissue is gently separated from the lateral pelvic wall to expose the obturator nerve, which should be identified clearly before the obturator lymph node is removed. Injury to this nerve produces a fairly severe disability due to paralysis of the adductor muscles. The obturator nerve is freed by blunt dissection with the end of the scissors. There are some large friable veins laterally that must be controlled by silver clips and divided to enable the obturator nodes and fat pad to be dissected free from the obturator fossa. The dissection is completed by removing the nodal and fatty tissue as far back as the division of the internal iliac vessels (Fig. 94-2). The same dissection is carried out on the opposite side.

Removal of the sacral lymphatics on the lateral side of the common iliac vessels has been advocated but is not the general practice and probably adds to the morbidity of the procedure. It has been argued that pelvic lymphadenectomy should not be performed as a routine procedure in patients with early-stage prostatic cancer because it is probably only of prognostic, but not of therapeutic, value and is associated with significant morbidity. It appears to bring about a relatively high incidence of pulmonary embolus, as well as hematoma, lymphocele formation, and genital edema. It has been our practice to use low-dose heparin, 5000 units, SC, twice daily as prophylaxis against venous thrombosis (although a recent study indicates that this is ineffective) and to avoid removal of all the deep inguinal nodes to obviate genital edema. To date, there has been little morbidity and no mortality in more than 100 patients who have undergone pelvic lymphadenectomy. There were two cases of pulmonary embolus that responded well to anticoagulants and two patients developed a significant hematoma. Evidence of lymphatic metastasis has been detected in 20% to 30% of patients with early-stage prostatic cancer. Frozen section is not done because they frequently miss metastases, and the seed implant is performed in any event, to provide local control of tumor growth.

Following the lymphadenectomy the prostate is exposed retropubically by sweeping away the periprostatic fat with two small gauze packs that are placed laterally on each side of the gland (Fig. 94-3). The preprostatic veins are ligated and divided. A finger is inserted into the rectum so that the

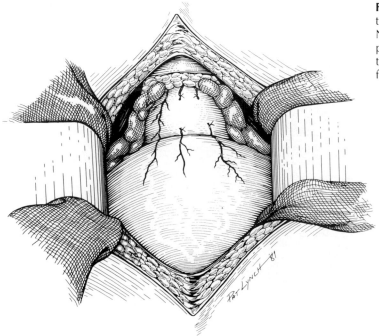

FIG. 94-3. Exposure of the anterior surface of the prostate in preparation for insertion of needles. Note sponges on each side of the prostate, improving exposure, and the divided prostatic veins that allow distal displacement of the preprostatic fat.

placement of needles, through which the seeds are implanted, can be carried out more accurately (Fig. 94-4). The length and width of the prostate are determined by use of a small right-angled measure (Fig. 94-5) and the depth is measured by inserting a 15-cm needle into the thickest portion of the gland as far as the posterior capsule.

The implant is calculated to provide a minimum tumor dose of 18,000 rads to 20,000 rads, delivered to decay, although some areas within the tumor may receive a total dose of 35,000 rads. The half-life of the isotope is 60 days. The total tumor dose is calculated by obtaining the mean dimension of the gland (*i.e.*, the sum of the length, width, and depth divided by three). A standard nomogram is then used to calculate the number of millicuries required to treat the tumor adequately. The number of millicuries needed to deliver the required dose is approximately six times the mean gland dimension. This provides the correct number and appropriate spacing of the seeds to be implanted based on their radioactivity.

Eighteen to twenty-four hollow bore 17-gauge needles, 15 cm in length, are inserted through the anterior surface of the gland at intervals of 8 mm to 10 mm, depending on the calculated dosimetry for the seeds. The finger in the rectum allows the needles to be placed as far as the posterior capsule of the prostate. Needles are inserted at the apex and along the lateral borders of the gland, then along the medial side of each lobe at the side of the urethra, and finally into the remaining portion of each lobe at the appropriate intervals.

The ^{125}I seeds are made of titanium, 0.5 mm in diameter and 5 mm long. They contain the isotope, absorbed onto an ion-exchange rosin located between two radiopaque gold markers loaded into small magazines. These are implanted through the needles using a modification of the introducer originally designed by Henschke (Fig. 94-6). It is important to withdraw the needle 0.5 cm with the graduated introducer before inserting the first seed, in order to prevent radiation injury to the rectum. The seeds are implanted at 1-cm intervals through the depth of the gland so that, depending on the measured thickness of the prostate at that site, one to three seeds are implanted through each needle.

A radiograph is taken at the conclusion of implant to demonstrate the distribution of the seeds; if necessary, extra seeds are implanted wherever there do not appear to be an adequate number.

The packs are then removed and all bleeding is carefully controlled by coagulation or clips. The rectus sheath is approximated with a continuous 1-0 Prolene suture and the skin is closed with staples or interrupted 3-0 nylon sutures. The Foley catheter is left indwelling for 24 hours postoperatively. Drains are not used. Should a lymphocele form, it is nearly always absorbed spontaneously

FIG. 94-4. The 17-gauge needles (15 cm) are in position under digital control in preparation for ^{125}I seed implant.

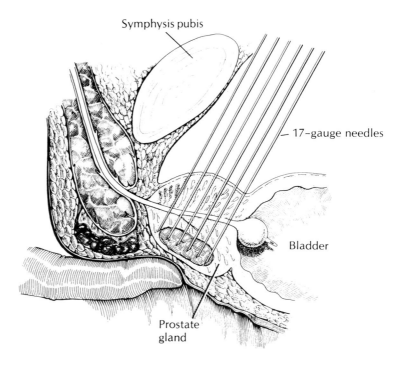

Symphysis pubis

17–gauge needles

Bladder

Prostate gland

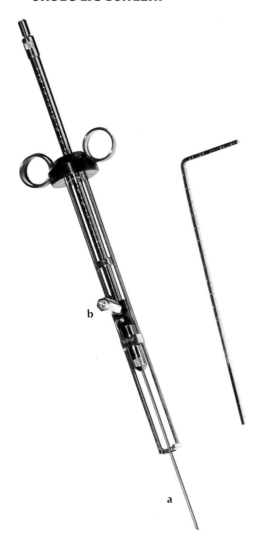

FIG. 94-5. Graduated seed introducer with 17-gauge needle mounted **(a)**, magazine for 12 seeds **(b)** and graduated right-angled measure

after several months; whereas, in the presence of a drain, there is prolonged discharge that usually becomes infected secondarily. Moreover, significant bleeding is not usually drained adequately, and the presence of a drain may lead to infection of the hematoma.

The preliminary results after 5 years indicate that more than 90% of the patients with Stage B disease are alive and 63% remain free of disease. Patients with lymph node metastases have received an additional 4500 rads of external-beam irradiation to the iliac and para-aortic lymph nodes with shielding of the prostate. The efficacy of this procedure is doubtful because preliminary results

indicate that it does not prevent progression of the disease.

A perineal approach with exposure of the posterior surface of the prostate has been advocated for seed implantation. The advantage of this approach is that the needles can be placed more precisely at right angles to the gland; the disadvantage is that digital control of the distal end of the needle is not possible. Moreover, pelvic lymphadenectomy must be performed through a separate incision if this is thought to be indicated. This approach has not been widely accepted. Implants have been performed through percutaneous perineal insertion of needles under digital control, but this approach is generally used for supplemental irradiation. Perhaps more direct is the transcoccygeal posterior approach to the prostate (Fig. 94-6), as recommended by Ambrose.[1]

Radioactive gold grains can be implanted in a similar manner through a hollow needle. The seeds are 0.5 mm in diameter and 2 mm long and deliver a dose of 30 to 35 millicuries. Implantation is performed to achieve a tumor dose of between 2500 rads and 3500 rads. This is usually supplemented by external-beam radiation 8 to 10 days later using a dose of between 4000 rads to 5000 rads delivered to the prostate and periprostatic area through a rotational or opposing field technique. This gives a combined tumor dose of 6500 to 8000 rads.

Patients with obstructive symptoms frequently improve after interstitial radiation. Should these symptoms persist or become worse it is best to manage the patient by intermittent self-catheterization for 4 to 6 months, to allow the maximum radiation effect to take place before performing a transurethral resection. This procedure is not contraindicated following irradiation of the prostate and does not appear to be associated with any increase in complications or morbidity.

REFERENCES

1. AMBROSE SS: Transcoccygeal [125]iodine prostatic implantation for adenocarcinoma. J Urol 125:365, 1981
2. CARLTON CE, JR, HUDGINS PT, GUERRIERO WG et al: Radiotherapy in the management of stage C carcinoma of the prostate. J Urol 116:206, 1976
3. FLOCKS RH: The treatment of stage C prostatic cancer with special reference to combined surgical and radiation therapy. J Urol 109:461, 1972
4. HERR HW: Complications of pelvic lymphadenectomy and retropubic prostatic ^{125}I implantation. Urology 14:226, 1979

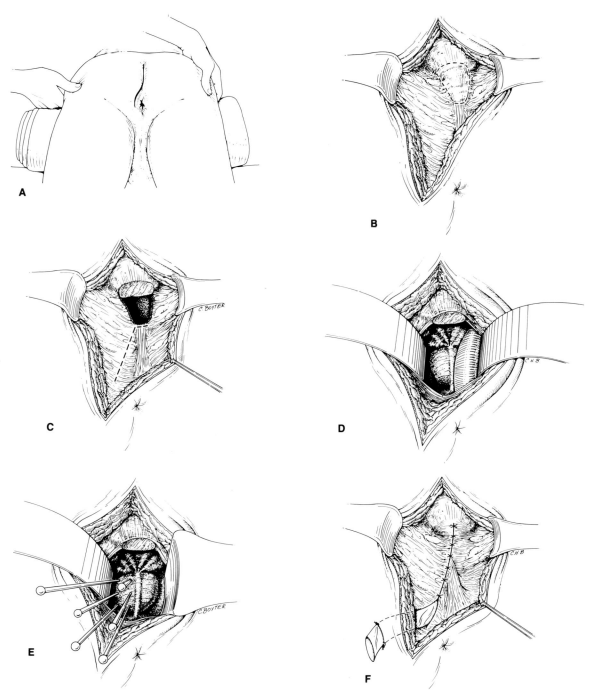

FIG. 94-6. Transcoccygeal implantation technique of Ambrose. **(A)** With the patient in a modified jackknife position, the buttocks are spread and taped and the incision is made as shown. **(B)** The posterior surface of the coccyx and the levator ani are exposed. **(C)** The coccyx is removed, giving access to the pelvis above the levators. **(D)** The endopelvic fascia is incised at the lateral margin of the prostate. **(E)** The posterior surface of the prostate is completely exposed with carrier needles placed. **(F)** The deep layers are closed and a Penrose drain is brought out lateral to the incision. (J Urol 125:365, 1981; © 1981, The Williams & Wilkins Co, Baltimore)

5. HERR HW: Preservation of sexual potency in prostatic cancer patients after pelvic lymphadenectomy and retropubic ^{125}I implantation. J Urol 121:621, 1979

6. JEWETT HJ, BRIDGE RW, GRAY GF, JR et al: The palpable nodule of prostatic cancer: Results 15 years after radical excision. JAMA 203:403, 1968

7. LYTTON B, COLLINS JT, WEISS RM et al: Results of biopsy after early stage prostatic cancer treatment by implantation of ^{125}I seeds. J Urol 121:306, 1979

8. RAY GR, CASSADY JR, BAGSHAW MA: Definitive radiation therapy of carcinoma of the prostate: A report on 15 years of experience. Radiology 106:407, 1973

9. WHITMORE WF, JR, HILARIS B, GRABSTALD H: Retropubic implantation of iodine 125 in the treatment of prostatic cancer. J Urol 108:918, 1972

Prostatic Abscess

95

Alvin D. Couch

Current medical literature is devoid of extensive reported series of acute prostatic abscess, and chronic abscess formation is hardly mentioned.

However, not infrequently during the course of a transurethral resection of a large hyperplastic lateral prostatic lobe in a patient with mild prostatism, one encounters a small quantity of dark brown watery fluid followed by a sudden reduction in the size of an otherwise large lobe. These so called chronic abscesses are usually sterile but the wall of the abscess does reveal inflammatory cells. Whether this represents a true abscess or liquefaction of an area of prostatic infarction is not clear. The resection is completed without difficulty and the recovery is uninhibited.

Similarly, one may encounter inspissated debris accumulated around the prostatic calculi or in prostatic ducts. The debris produces a "chronic prostatic duct abscess" which, on urethroscopic visualization when incised during a prostatic resection, reveals a purulent discharge or a ribbon of thick puttylike material. Again this is not thought to be a true abscess but instead one of inspissation of scattered ductal debris with occlusion.

The treatment of both of these so-called chronic abscesses is drainage and obliteration of the ducts (and cavity, if present) by the transurethral route.

Symptomatology in this group is usually nothing more than a mild prostatism without systemic manifestations and occasional mild perineal pain.[8]

Since the advent and wide utilization of modern antimicrobial drugs, acute prostatic abscess has become a rarity in urologic practice.[7] Not only has the early use of antibiotic therapy lessened the incidence of this entity, but the etiology has changed as well from primarily Neisseria gonorrhaeae to Enterobacteriaceae infection, which is the most frequent organism encountered.[5,15,22] In the majority of cases, the abscesses arise from an acute prostatitis resulting from an infection of the posterior urethra.[1,4,6] However, metastatic abscesses do arise from a wide number of infectious processes that are staphylococcal in origin. Many disease processes have been incriminated involving pyemias, bacteremias, febrile illnesses such as typhoid, paratyphoid, and erysipelas, and recently cases of anaerobic infections of the prostate associated with transrectal needle biopsies have been reported.[5,11] Bladder neck outlet obstruction is often a contributing factor to the development of an acute prostatic abscess because residual urine, when infected, continually bathes the posterior urethra with a pool of infected urine.

Abscesses tend to occur in the periphery of the prostate gland near the apex. There is conjecture that during micturition there is turbulence in the area caused by the rigidity and slight narrowing of the membranous urethra, which in turn, is caused by the external urethral sphincter. Introduction of infected urine directly into the perpendicular ducts of the peripheral zone of the gland occurs, resulting in acute prostatitis and abscess formation.[3]

Other predisposing factors are diabetes mellitus—in which there is a higher incidence of abscess formation, instrumentation, and indwelling urethral catheters. Increased morbidity and mortality resulting from the prostatic abscess are definitely accentuated by the diabetic state. Likewise, urethral instrumentation and indwelling catheters have served as a contributing factor to at least half of the reported cases of acute prostatic abscess.[2,15]

Acute prostatic abscess may occur at any age, the youngest reported case being in a 46-day old infant.[9] The highest incidence occurs in the fifth and sixth decades of life, when prostatic disease is most common.[22]

Presentation and Diagnosis

SYMPTOMATOLOGY

Symptomatology is widely variable, ranging from mild fever and general malaise to a full-blown picture of lower urinary tract disease characterized by frequency of urination, dysuria, suprapubic or

991

perineal pain, and varying degrees of prostatism and urinary retention associated with fever, chills, sweating, and leukocytosis. The earlier symptoms, however, may be entirely constitutional and have little relation to the urinary tract. Usually the symptoms are present for less than a week, but the process may be prolonged for 2 weeks before localization is possible.[17]

PHYSICAL EXAMINATION

On physical examination the gland may be asymmetrically enlarged, tender, hot, and edematous and fluctuation may be elicited. Periprostatic induration extending to the pelvic side wall may fix the gland, suggesting malignancy. Fluctuation may be difficult to elicit, particularly if there is a fulminating prostatitis. Therefore, it is difficult to distinguish acute prostatitis, with sepsis and bladder neck obstruction, from prostatic abscess with sepsis and bladder neck obstruction; the symptoms are similar and the local findings are ambiguous or nonspecific.[2,15]

The diagnosis may depend either upon a sudden change in the clinical course of a presumed acute prostatitis or upon sequential changes in the consistency or size of the gland, severe perineal or suprapubic pain, and associated rectal or urinary tenesmus. A sudden onset of low-grade fever often suggests the presence of a prostatic abscess, and fluctuation within the gland is pathognomonic. Diagnosis and a definitive therapeutic approach should not wait for the development of a localized fluctuation. In the presence of an actual abscess, continued antibiotics without drainage is of little value and may in fact mask the systemic manifestation of the disease process.

Rupture usually is into the urethra because the gland is encapsulated and supported posteriorly by Denonvilliers' fascia and inferiorly in the midline by the triangular ligament, the rectourethralis muscles, and the central perineal tendon. Owing to these anatomic barriers, rupture into the rectum, ischioanal space, perivesical area, or peritoneum is rare.[13,14,24]

Radiographically one would expect to find on urethrogram an elongated, straight prostatic urethra, which may also be characteristic of prostatic carcinoma. A deviation of the urethra may be demonstrated, but after the acute process has subsided, the urethra returns to a normal appearance.

Occasionally an acute prostatic abscess encroaches upon the bladder and causes displacement, particularly if there is seminal vesical or perivesical space extension. Dilation of multiple prostatic ducts communicating with multiple old abscess cavities that have drained spontaneously may be demonstrated radiographically.

DIAGNOSIS

An awareness of the possibility of a prostatic abscess formation in the differential diagnosis of lower urinary tract pathology is paramount. Percutaneous perineal needle biopsy and aspiration of a suspected abscess for pus and culture material may afford an early diagnosis, may be accomplished in an atraumatic fashion, and may even result in a resolution of the abscess.[2,4,16,25] A biopsy specimen of the gland should be obtained at the time of aspiration, in order to exclude an associated carcinoma that may present symptoms and physical findings compatible with abscess.[10]

Treatment

Once the diagnosis of prostatic abscess is made, incision and drainage should be performed. Various therapeutic modalities have been used, including conservative treatment consisting of rest, antibiotic therapy with expectation of resolution, and natural rupture of the abscess into the urethra.[19]

TRANSURETHRAL TECHNIQUE

Surgical intervention with appropriate antibiotic therapy is the treatment of choice. It is generally agreed that the transurethral route with resection or saucerization of the abscess is preferable.[12] Perineal drainage and prostatotomy is still applicable, particularly when the abscess is located deep within or extends within the gland or into the periprostatic area.

In the past a transvesical or retropubic incision for drainage has been used, with the predictable complications of massive bleeding, delayed hemorrhage, and poor drainage. Some have preferred to rupture the abscess over a sound into the urethra (Steven's technique).[18]

If the transurethral route is utilized, endoscopically the involved area or lobe may be bulging and its surface may reveal inflammatory changes, bullous edema, hyperemia or papillary excrescences, and, in some cases, purulent draining ducts. In this instance a resection of the overlying tissue is made.[21] Usually with the first cut there is an escape of purulent material. In view of the frequent occurrence of multiple loculi, the resection should be carried far enough to allow saucerization of the abscess cavity and to remove any overhanging edges.[8] The resection should not transgress the base of the cavity.

There are some, however, who advocate a full prostatic resection because multiple loculi may occur. They advocate this particularly when there is a history of antecedent bladder neck outlet obstruction associated with significant prostatic hyperplasia.[20] Once prostatic resection has been accomplished, catheter drainage is established for 2 or 3 days and intensive antibacterial therapy is continued.

YOUNG TECHNIQUE

There is still a place in the urologic armamentarium for perineal drainage of a prostatic abscess, particularly if the abscess cannot be reached endoscopically or extends into the periprostatic tissues. This is accomplished by the Young technique. The patient is placed in an exaggerated lithotomy position and the perineum is elevated in the usual fashion. After sterile preparation of the genitoperineal area, an inverted-U incision is made 3 cm above the anal edge. The superficial fascia is incised and the central perineal tendon is divided. The rectourethralis muscle is then divided and the levator ani muscles are retracted laterally overlying the involved area of the prostate. Care is taken to avoid unnecessary dissection into the ischiorectal area and to prevent unnecessary violation of tissue planes. The area of fluctuation is identified, a longitudinal incision is made into the abscess, and the cavity is explored in order to destroy all loculi.

A small Penrose drain is sutured into the cavity with 2-0 plain catgut suture. The drain is brought out through the incision and anchored with a stitch. The incision is closed using chromic catgut technique. Catheter drainage with a 22Fr, 5-cc Foley catheter is established. Intensive antibacterial therapy is indicated during the pre- and postoperative course. The catheter is removed in 1 week; the drains usually fall out spontaneously after 7 or 8 days.[23]

OTHER TECHNIQUES

On occasion, when the diagnosis was not apparent, the retropubic and suprapubic approaches have been used to attempt a subtotal prostatectomy. In these cases enucleation was virtually impossible, bleeding was excessive, and, in general, the postoperative course was complicated by profuse bleeding and delayed hemorrhage in most instances.[18]

Discussion

It is apparent that the transurethral route for drainage of prostatic abscess is preferred and is most frequently used today. However, there are advocates of perineal needle aspiration of the abscess cavity with intracavitary instillation of antimicrobial drugs at the time of aspiration. However, because of the lack of adequate drainage it would appear that this should not be relied upon as a treatment of choice and that this modality should be limited primarily to diagnostic use.

If there is spontaneous rupture of the abscess into the urethra, there is still the possibility of overhanging edges that prevent adequate drainage. Again it seems feasible that resection of this tissue, if not a complete resection of the gland, should be carried out.

Although there may be symptomatic relief with spontaneous rupture of the abscess into the rectum, it is felt that drainage is often incomplete. The abscess cavity should be examined for loculi, these should be broken down, and a drain should be inserted.[10] Transvesical or retropubic drainage does not appear to be dependent and is not recommended, particularly because of the profuse operative and postoperative hemorrhage.[10,22] Rupture of the abscess over a sound has been described early in the literature by Stevens.[18] However, this also could lead only to inadequate drainage.

When prostatic abscess is not associated with cancer the prognosis is good.

REFERENCES AND SUGGESTED READING

1. BARLETT JG, WEINSTEIN, WM, GORBACH SL: Prostatic abscesses involving anaerobic bacteria. Arch Intern Med 138:1369, 1978
2. BECKER LE, HARRIN WR: Prostatic abscess: A diagnostic and therapeutic approach. J Urol 91, No. 5:582, 1964
3. BLACKLOCK NJ: The significance of the prostate in urinary tract infection in the male. Proc R Soc Med 68:505, 1975
4. CHITTY K: Prostatic abscess. Br J Surg 44:599, 1957
5. CORRADO ML, SIERRA MF, ENG R et al: Anaerobic prostatic abscess. NY State J Med p 652, March 1980
6. DAJANI AM, O'FLYNN JD: Prostatic abscess. Br J Urol 40:736, 1968
7. DRACH GW, KOHNER PW: Prostatitis. In Tannenbaum M (ed): Urologic Pathology: The Prostate, p 57. Philadelphia, Lea & Febiger, 1977
8. GREENE LF, SEGURA JW: Transurethral Surgery, p 229. Philadelphia: W B Saunders 1979
9. HEYMAN A, LOMBARDO LJ, JR: Metastatic prostatic abscess with report of a case in a newborn infant. J Urol 87:174, 1962

10. JAMESON RM: Prostatic abscess and carcinoma of the prostate. Br J Urol 40:288, 1968

11. MEARES EM, JR: Campbell's Urology, 4th ed, Vol 1, p 532. Harrison JH, Gittes RF, Perlmutter AD et al (eds): Philadelphia, W B Saunders, 1978

12. MITCHELL JP: The Principles of Transurethral Resection and Hemostasis, p 216. Baltimore, Williams & Wikins, 1972

13. MITCHELL RJ, BLAKE JRS: Spontaneous perforation of prostatic abscess with peritonitis. J Urol 107:622, 1972

14. MOSTOFI FK, LEESTMA JE. In Anderson WAD (ed): Pathology, 6th ed, Vol 1, p 844. St Louis, C V Mosby, 1971

15. PAI MB, BHAT HS: Prostatic abscess. J Urol 108:599, 1971

16. PERSKY L, AUSTEN G, JR, SCHATTEN WE: Recent experiences with prostatic abscess. Surg Gynecol Obstet 101:629, 1955

17. ROBBINS SL: Pathologic Basis of Disease, p 1190. Philadelphia, W B Saunders, 1974

18. SARGENT JC, IRWIN R: Prostatic abscess. Am J Surg 11:334, 1931

19. SMITH RB: Prostatic Abscess. In Kaufman JJ (ed): Current Urologic Therapy, p 284. Philadelphia, W B Saunders, 1980

20. SMITH RB, SKINNER DG: Complications of Urologic Surgery, Prevention and Management, p 293, Philadelphia, W B Saunders, 1976

21. THOMPSON IM: Transurethral Surgery, In Glenn JF (ed): Urologic Surgery, 2nd ed, p 515. Hagerstown, Harper & Row, 1975

22. TRAPNELL J, ROBERTS M: Prostatic abscess. Br J Surg 57:78, 1970

23. WEYRAUCH HM: Surgery of the Prostate, p 64. Philadelphia, W B Saunders, 1959

24. YOUNG HH, DAVIS DM, JOHNSON FP: Young's Practice of Urology, Vol. 1, p 160; Vol. 2, p 476. Philadelphia, W B Saunders, 1926

25. YOUNGER R, MAHONEY SA, PERSKY L: Prostatic abscess. Surg Gynecol Obstet 124:1043, 1967

Seminal Vesiculectomy

96

David M. Drylie

The seminal vesicles are among man's more ignored organs because of their obscurity; they are inaccessible to examination, and little is known about their meaningful function. Recent activity in the general study of reproductive biology has allowed those working in the laboratory to gain a better understanding of these organs than is generally possible for the clinician, because the seminal vesicles are more accessible in some species, such as the rat, than in humans.

In the clinical situation, these vesicles are among the few organs to remain firmly ensconced within the urologist's purview. Consequently, every urologist should be completely familiar with their anatomy and anatomic relationships, as well as with the disease states that may affect them. It would also seem to be prudent to be alert to any findings from the research laboratories that may alter the clinical relevance of the seminal vesicles. The only complication that is almost invariable (93%) after seminal vesiculectomy is infertility.[7] Perhaps the burgeoning male infertility clinics will become a source of heretofore unrecognized seminal vesical pathology.[11]

Surgical Indications

Surgical removal of the seminal vesicles is not difficult if the principles of more commonly performed urologic procedures, such as cystectomy, cystotomy, and perineal prostatectomy, are applied. The challenge rests with determining preoperatively that there is sufficient disease to justify the operation.

In the modern practice of urology, few indications exist for seminal vesiculectomy. The vesicles are most often removed during either a radical cystectomy or a radical prostatectomy; their removal is considered part of the primary procedure. Disease states for which seminal vesiculectomy might be indicated fall into several categories: inflammation, neoplasia, cystic disease, and congenital anomalies.

INFLAMMATION

Inflammation constitutes the most commonly encountered problem and is usually a manifestation of primary inflammation elsewhere (e.g., tuberculosis and prostatitis). Treatment is aimed at the primary focus and is primarily medical. Fibrotic obstruction of the tubular vesicle can occur anywhere along its length and cause impaired drainage, decreased response to medical therapy, varying degrees of infected or sterile cyst formation, and symptoms that are now related to a complication of the primary disease.

Instead of seminal vesiculectomy, drainage of an obstructed organ may be performed using a transrectal or percutaneous needle with digital, radiologic, or ultrasonographic guidance.[1] Drainage thus accomplished often supplements further medical therapy. Drainage by way of transvesical seminal vesiculostomy has been described but creates a functional bladder diverticulum and does not appear to be a totally acceptable form of therapy.[13] Seminal vesiculectomy is indicated in occasional cases of seminal vesiculitis if the foregoing therapy is ineffective.

NEOPLASIA

The most common neoplastic process involving the seminal vesicles is direct extension from prostatic adenocarcinoma, and treatment again revolves about one's choice of treatment for the primary lesion. Primary malignant neoplasms of the seminal vesicles are very rare; only 34 cases were reported as recently as 1973.[4] Benign neoplasms are even more rare. Seminal vesiculectomy alone would be considered only if preoperative or intraoperative evaluation revealed a benign mass confined to the seminal vesicle. With primary malignant disease, radical cystoprostatectomy to include the seminal vesicles and accompanying lymph node dissection would usually be indicated.

CYSTIC DISEASE

Cysts of the seminal vesicles are rare. These cysts must be distinguished from cysts arising from the müllerian duct remnant (*e.g.,* prostatic utricle), ejaculatory duct, or prostate. Needle aspiration of fluid for microscopy, culture, and cytologic analysis may be followed by injection of water-soluble radiopaque contrast media for cystography to assist in diagnosis. Seminal vesiculectomy may be indicated, if warranted by symptoms caused by cystic disease.

CONGENITAL ANOMALIES

Ectopic ureters in the male usually drain a complete renal unit.[2] They drain into the seminal vesicle in 28% of cases and are usually part of a dysgenetic total renal unit.[8,10] Seminal vesiculectomy may become necessary for symptoms related to the mass lesion produced, but removal of the abnormal renal unit with low ureteral ligation is usually easier and may suffice.

Diagnosis of Seminal-Vesicle Disease

Symptoms relating to seminal vesicular disease are nonspecific. Inflammation may cause symptoms of irritative voiding because adjacent structures, such as the bladder trigone and prostate, are also likely to be involved. Localized inflammation may irritate the overlying peritoneum and mimic an acute abdominal emergency. In some instances, vague lower abdominal or perineal pain may be the only symptom. Hematospermia, pyospermia, or both may occur, just as they may occur with prostatitis.

Rectal examination can detect seminal-vesicle disease if the vesicles are palpable. One must be able to palpate beyond the prostatic base. Normally, the soft character of the vesicles makes them indistinguishable from the equally soft ampullary vas and base of the bladder. Cystic dilation, thickened fibrotic walls, calcification, or tumor growths may be palpated and may heighten the examiner's index of suspicion. Inflammatory disease of the seminal vesicles may be detected as tenderness to palpation and is usually accompanied by a tender prostate. This finding again should cause one to suspect seminal vesiculitis. Cystic lesions must be distinguished from other causes of pelvic-floor cystic masses. Typically, a cyst of the seminal vesicles is not in the midline and does not reach the huge size that occurs with the midline müllerian duct cysts.

Visualization of the seminal vesicles until very recently has been accomplished primarily with seminal vesiculography, either by transurethral cannulation and injection of the ejaculatory ducts or by surgical exposure and injection of the intrascrotal vas deferens.[6] The former procedure proves less than satisfactory in the hands of most urologists. Operative injection, although easily accomplished, is believed to have a definite risk of subsequent vas obstruction from scarring or granuloma formation.

Catheterization perhaps should not be done by any method other than microscopic vasotomy. With the operating microscope, one can incise the exposed vas deferens either transversely or longitudinally, identify the mucosa, and atraumatically insert a 22- to 24-gauge blunt needle or small polyethylene cannula. Intravenous contrast material diluted 1:4 with sterile normal saline is then slowly injected during fluoroscopic monitoring. The procedure can be recorded on videotape or x-ray film exposed at appropriate times. Vesiculography has been described as an adjunct for staging carcinoma of the prostate.[1] In the population at risk for prostate cancer, however, one would presumably not be concerned with subsequent obstruction of the vas deferens.

Transrectal seminal vesiculography with aspiration of lesion contents for study is highly feasible.[5] This procedure can be accomplished with or without radiographic or ultrasonographic control.

Ultrasonography may become the most precise diagnostic tool for studying the seminal vesicles.[12] A rectal probe was first used.[2] Recent studies use an abdominal skin probe.[9] Further experience with this technique holds much promise, because it is noninvasive and precise.

Computerized tomographic (CT) scanning appears to offer another precise tool for diagnosing seminal vesicular lesions, but experience is not yet sufficient to allow critical comment. CT scanning has proved disappointing in evaluating other pelvic disease of interest to urologists.

Indirect information about the seminal vesicles can be gained from intravenous pyelography or cystography, which may disclose ureteral deviation, bladder base distortion, or calcification. Cystoscopy may also reveal abnormalities of the verumontanum or prostatic urethra. Marked distortion of the bladder base may accompany cystic lesions of the seminal vesicles. Localized or generalized inflammatory changes in the prostatic urethra or bladder may be seen.

FIG. 96-1. Surgical anatomy of seminal vesicles, posterior view

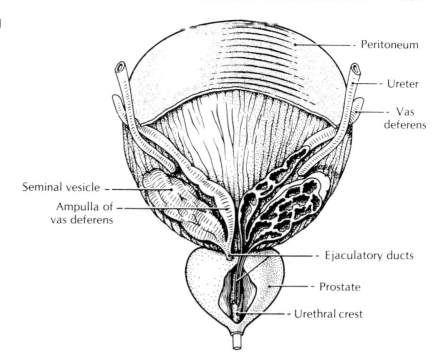

Peritoneum

Ureter

Vas deferens

Seminal vesicle

Ampulla of vas deferens

Ejaculatory ducts

Prostate

Urethral crest

FIG. 96-2. Retrovesical approach, peritoneal incision

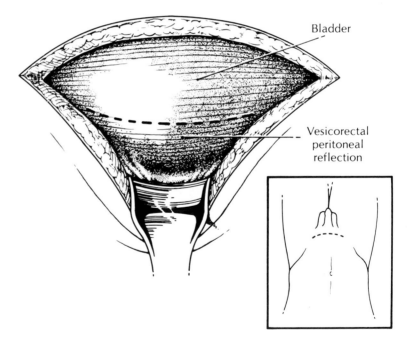

Bladder

Vesicorectal peritoneal reflection

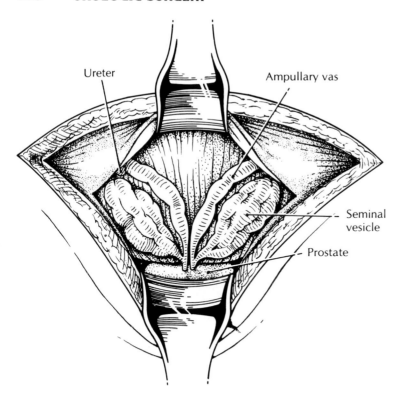

Ureter

Ampullary vas

Seminal
vesicle

Prostate

FIG. 96-3. Retrovesical approach, anatomic relationships of seminal vesicles

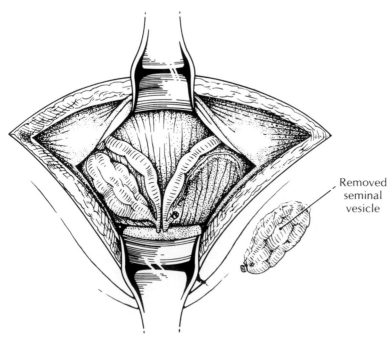

Removed
seminal
vesicle

FIG. 96-4. Retrovesical approach, ligation of vesicle base

Anatomy and General Surgical Considerations

The fact that there are various surgical approaches to the seminal vesicles demands that the surgeon be thoroughly familiar with the surgical anatomy of these organs. Their most intimate relationship is to the vas deferens, particularly its dilated terminal ampullary portion (Fig. 96-1). Both the seminal vesicles and the vas derive from the mesonephric duct and the considered by most to be mesodermal in origin. Surrounding them are the endodermally derived rectum and bladder. Distal fusion of the seminal vesicles and the ampullary vas deferens forms the ejaculatory duct, which courses through the largely endodermal prostate.

When normal in size (5–6 cm long and 1–2 cm thick), the rounded proximal tips of the seminal vesicles may be in close proximity to the lower ureter. Whereas the vas deferens passes anterior to the ureter at its lateral-to-medial crossing, the seminal vesicles do not maintain this constant relationship. Therefore, great care must be given to freeing these tips surgically, preferably while keeping the ureter under constant observation.

The individual seminal vesicle consists of a thin-walled tube, 15 cm long, which has coiled upon itself to achieve its normal organ size. The tube has a muscular wall identical to that of the vas deferens but much thinner, similar to the wall of the ampullary vas. A variable number of diverticula arise from the main lumen of the seminal vesicle, creating the grossly convoluted appearance of the vesicle. This often branched, tortuous, and relatively thin-walled tube is contained within a filmy adventitial envelope composed of blood vessels, collagen, and elastic fibers. A constant relationship to this adventitia is difficult to maintain when dissecting the vesicles.

Blood supply to the seminal vesicles derives primarily from small arterial branches of the prostatic artery and, to a lesser extent, from small branches of the inferior vesical, superior rectal, and middle rectal arteries. Venous drainage is to the inferior vesical plexus and the prostatic plexus, both of which lie lateral to the seminal vesicles. The blood vessels investing the seminal vesicles are small enough that hemostasis can be achieved rapidly and easily by electrocautery during dissection.

Dissection of the seminal vesicles from surrounding structures is most easily accomplished posteriorly, where the fused (or unfused) peritoneal reflection separates them from the rectum. Peritoneal fusion occurs at a variable level in relation to the superior aspect of the tips of the seminal vesicles.

No such definite structure separates the vesicles anteriorly from the bladder, but a definite surgical cleavage plane between bladder and seminal vesicles is easily developed in the absence of fibrosis or neoplastic cellular infiltration. Perhaps the ease

FIG. 96-5. Perineal surgery of the seminal vesicles. The approach is similar to that used for radical perineal prostatectomy.

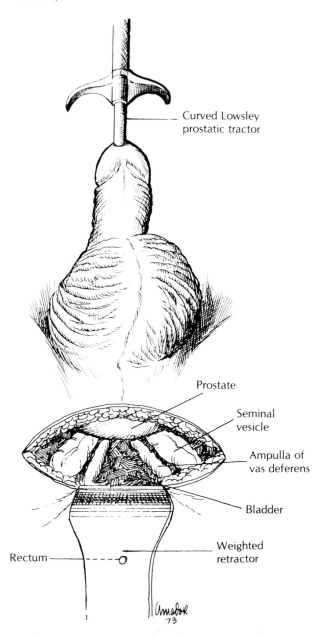

Curved Lowsley prostatic tractor

Prostate

Seminal vesicle

Ampulla of vas deferens

Bladder

Weighted retractor

Rectum

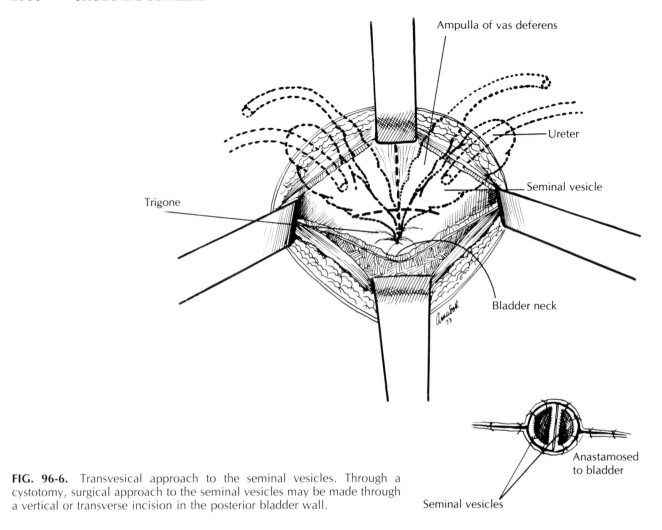

FIG. 96-6. Transvesical approach to the seminal vesicles. Through a cystotomy, surgical approach to the seminal vesicles may be made through a vertical or transverse incision in the posterior bladder wall.

of developing this dissection plane results from the different embryologic derivation of the bladder and seminal vesicles.

The most difficult dissection is the separation of the vesicles from the ampullary vas lying adjacent to their medial aspect. Fortunately, the thick-walled vas deferens can usually be traced from a lateral position cephalad to the vesicle tips. The orientation thus achieved allows the surgeon to separate the thin-walled ampullary vas gently from the laterally placed seminal vesicles. This dissection can be carried caudad to the point where the seminal vesicle joins the vas to form the ejaculatory duct.

The total length of the ejaculatory duct varies, as does the length contained within the prostate. The entrance of the seminal vesicles into the ampullary vas to form the ejaculatory duct often occurs within the prostate substance, so that caudal dissection of the isolated vesicles may, for practical considerations, terminate at or just within the prostate. Removal of the seminal vesicles, sparing the vas deferens, results in two paired surgical specimens.

Surgical Approach and Techniques

Urologists have been ingenious in devising approaches to the seminal vesicles. Removal of the vesicles has been periodically in and out of fashion. Some of the surgical approaches described were only possible because the glands were often relatively normal. Modern antibiotic therapy for inflammatory diseases involving the vesicles has obviated most of the nonneoplastic indications for seminal vesiculectomy. The remaining indications call for removal of large glands, most often densely adherent to surrounding structures. In the case of primary neoplasia, radical surgery with lymph node dissection as for bladder carcinoma is indicated and is described elsewhere. The only approach that meets virtually all needs is described in detail below in the section concerning the retrovesical (retropubic[14]) approach. The transvesical approach can be combined with the retrovesical approach and can be an option.[13] Previous surgery or trauma may have rendered the anterior procedures impossible, so every urologist should also consider the perineal approach. It has been reported that perineal seminal vesiculectomy does not result in impotence.[3]

RETROVESICAL SEMINAL VESICULECTOMY

The patient should have both mechanical and chemical preoperative preparation of the bowel. A Foley catheter is placed to keep the bladder empty. With the patient in the supine position on the operating table, a low transverse or vertical midline incision is made to approach the bladder as for a simple cystectomy. One may elect to reflect the bladder forward gradually with dissection of the peritoneum from the dome. However, an easier method is the transperitoneal approach with access to the posterior surface of the bladder and the seminal vesicles by way of a transverse peritoneal incision between the bladder and rectum (Fig. 96-2). The cleavage plane between the bladder and rectum is developed, and the posterior bladder is retracted anteriorly.

When the level of the prostate base is reached, the seminal vesicles can be identified adhering to the bladder. The vas deferens can then be located and traced to where it dilates and its wall thins, thus identifying the ampulla of the vas. During this identification, the corresponding ureter should be recognized passing beneath the vas as it approaches the midline. An enlarged seminal vesicle will lie over the ureter (Fig. 96-3). The superior and middle vascular pedicles to the bladder may be clamped and ligated on either one or both sides without compromising future bladder function. This additional dissection may be necessary to afford the exposure to accomplish removal of the vesicle as previously discussed (Fig. 96-4).

PERINEAL SEMINAL VESICULECTOMY

Perineal seminal vesiculectomy is useful for removal of smaller lesions and is performed as though one were doing a radical perineal prostatectomy (Fig. 96-5). Again, one must methodically identify the ampullary vas and its conversion to the muscular vas, the ureter, and the complete

posterior surface of the seminal vesicle before proceeding with the dissection of the vesicle.

TRANSVESICAL SEMINAL VESICULECTOMY

Smaller lesions may be removed successfully by transvesical seminal vesiculectomy (Fig. 96-6) according to principles previously discussed. Transvesical and retrovesical approaches may be combined in difficult situations, and the bladder may be opened completely in a bivalvular fashion if necessary.

REFERENCES

1. BECK PH, MCANINCH JW, LEWINSKY B et al: Vasoseminal vesiculography in staging adenocarcinoma of prostate. Urology 11:239, 1978
2. CREMIN BJ, FRIEDLAND GW, KOTTRA JJ: Ectopic ureterocele in single nonduplicated collecting system: Diagnosis by radiography. Urology 5:154, 1975
3. DILLON JR, BLAISDELL FE: Surgical pathology of the seminal vesicles. J Urol 10:353, 1923
4. GOLDSTEIN AF, WILSON ES: Carcinoma of the seminal vesicle—With particular reference to the angiographic appearance. Br J Urol 45:211, 1973
5. MEYER JJ, HARTIG PR, KOOS GW et al: Transrectal seminal vesiculography. J Urol 121:129, 1979
6. PALMER JM: Surgery of the seminal vesicles. In Harrison JH, Gittes RF, Perlmutter AD et al (eds): Campbell's Urology, p 2385. Philadelphia, W B Saunders, 1979
7. PANG SF, CHOW PH, WONG TM: The role of the seminal vesicle, coagulating glands, and prostate gland on the fertility and fecundity of mice. J Reprod Fertil 56:129, 1979
8. RIBA LW, SCHMIDLAPP CJ, BOSWORTH NL: Ectopic ureter draining into seminal vesicle. J Urol 56:332, 1946
9. RONNBERG L, YLOSLATO P, JOUPILA P: Estimation of the size of the seminal vesicles by means of ultrasonic B-scanning: A preliminary report. Fertil Steril 30:474, 1978
10. SCHNITZER BJ: Ectopic ureteral opening into seminal vesicle: A report of four cases. J Urol 93:576, 1965
11. SMALL MP: The seminal vesicles. In Glenn JF (ed): Urologic Surgery, p 416. New York, Harper & Row, 1975
12. TANASHI Y, WATANABE H, IGARI D et al: Volume estimation of the seminal vesicles by means of transrectal ultrasonotomography: A preliminary report. Br J Urol 47:695, 1975
13. WALKER WC, BOWLES WT: Transvesical seminal vesiculostomy in treatment of congenital obstruction of seminal vesicles: Case report. J Urol 99:324, 1968
14. WITHERINGTON R, RINKER JR: Retropubic seminal vesiculectomy for chronic seminal vesiculitis with preservation of potency. J Urol 104:463, 1970

Male Urinary Incontinence

97

Thomas P. Ball

There are few medical conditions more distressful to the male than the uncontrolled leakage of urine. Many pharmacologic and surgical approaches have been developed to cope with this problem, but it is only in recent years that the development of synthetic materials that are well tolerated by the human body has revolutionized surgery for the correction of urinary incontinence.

The availability of silicone rubber materials has made possible the development of the implantable artificial sphincter and urethral compression techniques that now have the capacity to effect the cure of many patients thought to be hopelessly incontinent and destined for urinary diversion. Although not without complications, these procedures have enabled many to return to a fully functional existence. In spite of this, or perhaps because of persistent mechanical problems associated with artificial devices, the search continues for methods of recreating physiologic voiding and control without the need for implantation of foreign materials.

Mechanism of Continence in the Male

Urinary continence in the male is the result of the combined function of two separate areas of sphincter activity. The proximal sphincter combines the action of the smooth muscle of the bladder neck and that of the prostatic urethra proximal to the verumontanum. The distal urethral sphincter is made up of the smooth muscle distal to the verunontanum and the striated muscle of the external sphincter in the membranous urethral area.

In the normal male, continence is maintained at the bladder neck or proximal urethral sphincter. The distal urethral sphincter acts voluntarily to stop the stream and as a backup system in cases of urgency and stress; it does not become the primary mechanism of continence unless the proximal sphincter is damaged by trauma or surgery, such as with prostatectomy or a Y–V plasty. This is graphically demonstrated in the patient who remains continent after elective sphincterotomy or surgery to bypass a severe membranous urethral stricture. In these cases, continence is maintained by the proximal sphincter unless a prostatectomy or similar proceddure damages the competency of the bladder neck area.

In the postprostatectomy patient, the bladder neck is no longer capable of maintaining continence, and it is only in the distal 2 cm of the prostatic fossa and membranous urethra that sphincter activity exists. Minor damage to the smooth muscle of the distal prostatic urethra may produce stress incontinence only, but the patient who has both smooth- and striated-muscle damage will be likely to suffer total incontinence.

Most of the patients we encounter with surgically correctable forms of urinary incontinence fall into one of four categories: postsurgical (postprostatectomy being the most common), traumatic (pelvic fracture or perineal trauma), congenital (epispadias or spinal dysraphism), or neurogenic (including hyperreflexia secondary to infection or tumor) and primary nervous system. With the exception of some cases of overflow incontinence secondary to overdistention of the hypotonic bladder, most forms of neurogenic incontinence are managed pharmacologically and with intermittment catherization. Postoperative hyperreflexia in the male usually represents only the hyperirritability secondary to chronic overdistention and detrusor hypertrophy seen with prostatic obstruction; symptoms generally abate in a matter of a few weeks. Should this condition persist, one must consider the possibility of carcinoma *in situ*, persistent infection, or a neurogenic cause.

When neurogenicity is felt to be the etiology, drugs that decrease bladder contractility may be of considerable benefit. One may approach these cases by decreasing bladder contractility or increasing the tone of the bladder neck and posterior urethra. Bladder contractility is a function of cholinergic activity and this activity may be decreased by the use of anticholinergics such as the belladonna alkaloids, quaternary ammonia drugs such as propantheline bromide (Pro-Banthine) and methantheline bromide (Banthine), and drugs that exert a direct effect on smooth muscles such as oxybutinin (Ditropan), flavoxate (Urispas), and imipramine (Tofranil). Imipramine has a dual action; it affects the bladder muscle directly and also blocks the re-uptake of noradrenalin, which increases the tonicity of the bladder neck.

Because alpha receptors are prevalent in the bladder neck and posterior urethra, the tone of these two areas can be improved by using alpha stimulators like ephedrine, pseudoephedrine, or imipramine (Tofranil). Though sometimes quite effective in mild cases, this form of therapy seldom produces satisfactory continence in the postprostatectomy patient. The poor results in this group of patients have necessitated the vigorous surgical attack that has produced the recent advances in management.

As mentioned previously, detrusor–sphincter imbalance may produce temporary incontinence in the early postoperative period. For this reason, no surgical approach should be undertaken prematurely, and it is generally felt to be advisable to wait a full year before surgery. The exception to this, of course, is endoscopy to rule out the presence of retained adenomas that could be preventing proper closure of the distal sphincter. Once it has been established that incontinence is not due to retained tissue, tumor, or infection, and that it is not secondary to neurologic dysfunction, surgical correction should be considered. The methods commonly employed for this purpose include primary reconstruction of the bladder neck, implantation or injection of materials to produce urethral compression, and implantation of an artificial urinary sphincter device. Each method is considered here in turn.

Surgical Management

Early attempts to control urinary leakage are documented in the literature of the middle 1700s.[10] The use of clamps and external compression devices to maintain continence has persisted through the years. Many continue to use devices such as the Cunningham or more recent Baumrucker clamps, which have been modified only slightly since the development of the prototypes more than 250 years ago.[2]

Young was probably the first to develop a surgical procedure for the correction of urinary incontinence.[28] His method, described in 1907, increased urethral resistence by narrowing the membranous urethra and covering it with the approximated transverse perineal and levator mus-

cles. Lowsley plicated both the bulbocavernosal and ischiocavernosal muscles with some success, then used a similar procedure combined with ligation of the deep dorsal veins of the penis in an attempt to cure erectile impotence.[15,16]

Hauri reported, in a preliminary study, that 10 of 11 patients operated on for the first time for postprostatectomy incontinence could be cured by imbedding the urethra between the corpora cavernosa.[9] This procedure resembles the Kaufman I, except that rather than plicating the crura across the bulb, Hauri frees the entire bulbous urethra from the corpora after cleavage of the bulbocavernosa, separates the corpora, and embeds the urethra between them. The corpora are united over the urethra with nonabsorbable sutures. A median rotation and adaptation of both ischiocavernosus muscles is then performed. This procedure bears further investigation.

Attempts to use the anal sphincter to produce continence have resulted in the development of several procedures, none of which has given consistent long-term results. The most popular of these procedures is the Mathisen procedure, which involves transection of the urethra in the distal bulb, tunneling of the proximal segment beneath the anal sphincter, and reanastomosis of the urethra after mobilization of the distal segment to gain length.[17] Indications for this procedure have diminished with the development of newer techniques.

Other nonimplantation attempts to achieve continence have included the use of muscle and fascial slings, vesicourethral suspension, urethral plication and twists, crural crossing procedures, and electrical stimulation. The most successful of these approaches to date have been the urethral lengthening and bladder flap procedures and these will be discussed in some detail.

Reconstruction of Internal Sphincter

Primary nonimplantation-type procedures attempt to correct incontinence by tubularizing the bladder neck to elongate the posterior urethra. The Young–Dees, Leadbetter, and Thompson procedures are similar in that they use trigonal muscle to form a tube after incising and mobilizing bladder muscle in the region of the anterior bladder neck.[6,14,18] Ureteral reimplantation is often required and is an integral part of the Leadbetter operation. These procedures were nicely described by Cook in a recent edition of the *Urologic Clinics of North America*.[5]

For the adult male, the procedure of Flocks and

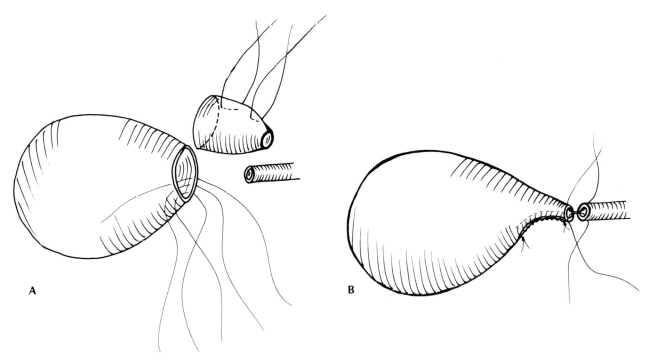

FIG. 97-1. **(A)** Radical prostatectomy. Bladder neck is closed in the midline with running or interrupted sutures. **(B)** Six sutures are usually used to approximate the urethra to the tubularized bladder neck.

Culp and Tanagho and Smith's adaptation of the same have become the most popular methods of bladder neck revision, providing successful control of incontinence in over 50% of properly selected cases.[7,26] This latter procedure is often effective for posttransurethral resection (post-TUR) incontinence, incontinence following radical prostatectomy, and epispadias. One must be careful to ensure that the patient has a nonscarred, healthy detrusor muscle and that there is no element of neurogenic bladder. The Tanagho procedure has provided continence when combined with a pull-through procedure to bridge an area of severe membranous urethral stricture. We have used it to create a bladder tube around which we subsequently placed an inflatable urinary sphincter, with restoration of continence until erosion occurred 1 year later due to excessive pressure in the device.

Schoenberg and Gregory reported the use of the Tanagho–Smith anterior bladder flap as a primary procedure for anastomosis of the bladder neck and urethra at the time of radical retropubic prostatectomy.[21] They felt that if the procedure was successful as a secondary method to cure incontinence, results should be even better when it was used primarily as a preventive measure. Although initial results were encouraging, the uncomplicated success rate was no improvement over that found in most large series of retropubic prostatectomies. Simple tubularization of the bladder neck by closing the defect in the midline beginning at the 6 o'clock position on the bladder neck has produced continence rates in excess of 90% (Fig. 97-1).

TANAGHO–SMITH PROCEDURE

The patient is placed in the supine position and the bladder is partially distended through a No. 18Fr, 5-ml Foley catheter. Suprapubic exposure is obtained through a midline or Pfannenstiel incision. The peritoneum is reflected upward from the anterior bladder surface and the retropubic space is dissected carefully to expose the vesicoprostatic junction. In male subjects, two thirds of the prostate is exposed. The puboprostatic ligaments are incised, and the anterior and lateral aspects of the vesicoprostatic junction are dissected.

After accurate delineation of the internal meatus, a 1-in. wide and 1-in. long flap is outlined by four stay sutures (Fig. 97-2). The parallel incisions on the anterior wall of the bladder extend from the vesical neck cephalad. The length of the rectangular flap is the same as the width. These dimensions should be determined with the bladder half full of saline. The inside of the bladder is inspected, especially to identify the apex of the trigone and ureteral orifices.

The initial transverse incision at the level of the internal meatus of the bladder is extended from within, around the vesical neck. In male patients, the incision is continued as deep as Denonvilliers'

fascia or until the seminal vesicles and the ampullae of the vasa are exposed. It is easy to slide the base of the bladder upward as soon as the proper plane is reached.

The vesical neck is separated from the prostate. A suprapubic Malecot catheter is placed as high as possible in the anterior bladder wall, close to the bladder apex and to one side of the midline away

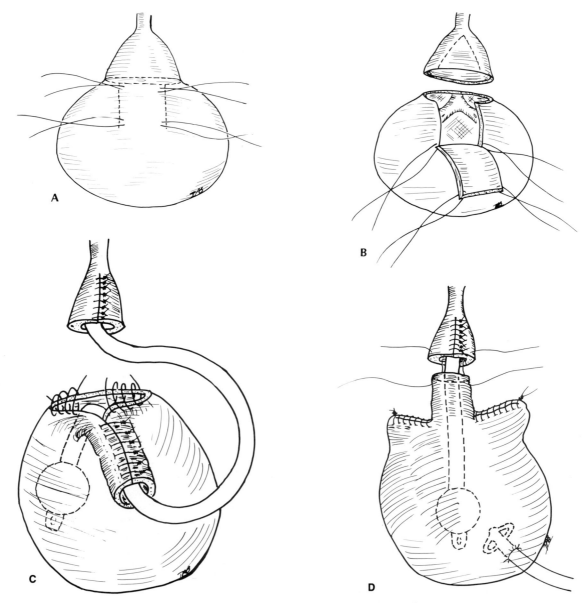

FIG. 97-2. **(A)** One-inch anterior bladder flap and circumferential bladder neck incision are outlined. **(B)** The flap is elevated and the bladder neck severed. The wedge to be removed from the anterior prostate is outlined. **(C)** Prostatic wedge is resected and closed. Tube is formed and bladder neck closure is begun. **(D)** Bladder is closed and tubes are inserted. Anastomosis is begun.

from the base of the bladder flap. The flap is ready for formation of a tube. The flap usually looks narrower and longer than it was originally, because of the contraction of its transverse fibers. In suturing the flap, one should be careful to include the retracted middle circular fibers. A one-layer closure of interrupted 2-0 chromic catgut is used. The apex of the trigone is sutured to the base of the tube with a mattress suture, restoring the normal anatomic relationship between the trigone and bladder outlet. The closure of the bladder is completed on either side with interrupted, full-thickness, 2-0 chromic catgut. The final suture line is Y-shaped; the straight limb corresponds to the tube and the lateral branches correspond to the closed vesical neck. The shape usually results in a dog-ear formation on either side.

The apex of the tube is anastomosed to the cut end of the proximal urethra. As soon as the posterior part of the anastomosis is completed, the surgeon reinserts a No. 16Fr to 18Fr Foley catheter and, thereafter, completes the anterior part of the anastomosis.

In postprostatectomy cases, a wedge from the prostatic capsule is first resected anteriorly to reduce the wide prostatic cavity. The cone-shaped prostatic urethra is thus converted into a tubular-shaped urethra. It is important to support the new vesicoprostatic junction. The tube is attached by two sutures between the anterior bladder wall close to the base of the tube and the upper margin of the pubic bone. Penrose drains are placed deep to the posterior suture line.

Postoperative Care

The suprapubic tube and urethral catheter are left in place for 2 or 3 weeks to ensure complete healing of the suture line. The Malecot tube is removed first, and after healing of the cystotomy wound, the Foley catheter is withdrawn from the urethra. Regaining urinary continence usually requires several weeks, so one should avoid making premature forecasts about the postoperative results. In his 1980 report to the American Urologic Association (AUA) of 10 year's experience with bladder neck reconstruction for total urinary incontinence, Tanagho reported 56 cases with a success rate of 70% for all causes.

Urethral Compression Procedures

In 1961, Berry reported success with implantation of an acrylic prosthesis for compression of the bulbous urethra.[3] Although implantation was temporarily successful in some cases, the incidence of urethral erosion, migration, and poor results dampened initial enthusiasm, and the procedure was abandoned. Based on the fact that initial success was achieved, Kaufman developed a series of urethral compression procedures, first using crural crossing and approximation, then implantation of polypropylene (Marlex) mesh, and achieving a success rate of about 60%.[11] In 1976, the Kaufman III procedure was reported, in which he and his associates replaced the Marlex mesh wad with an injectable silicone-gel prosthesis.[12] This prosthesis continues to produce success rates of about 60% with a relatively low complication rate. The newer prosthesis has a smooth silicone-gel dome that is placed against the urethra. It is reinforced on the sides and at the base by velour mesh and has Dacron straps by which it is fixed with staples to the bones of the pubic arch. The following is the operative procedure as described by Kaufman.[13]

KAUFMAN III SURGICAL PROCEDURE

The patient is given a broad-spectrum antibiotic, usually of the aminoglycoside group, on the morning before surgery. This is repeated on the morning of the operation and continued every 8 hr during hospitalization. An enema is given the night before operation and the perineum is washed carefully with hexachlorophene the night before and the morning of operation.

At surgery the patient is placed in a standard lithotomy position, the scrotum is elevated onto the pubis, and a midline perineal incision is made. The incision is carried precisely through the midline to the bulbocavernosus muscles. The bulbocavernosus muscle is exposed, and on either side the crura are exposed but not dissected. The superficial neurovascular bundles on either side of the midline are retracted to either side; care is taken during the operation and wound closure to avoid incorporating nerves, which may produce annoying hypesthesia and paresthesia of the scrotum and penis. The central perineal tendon is divided and the dissection continues behind the bulb to mobilize it from the central perineal tendon and to allow its compression upward against the urogenital diaphragm by the prosthesis (Fig. 97-3). We believe that this step provides the best compression of the urethra by approximating it to the urogenital diaphragm.

Serrated bone staples are driven into the pubis above the origin of the ischiocavernosus muscles. The staple is inserted on the medial side of the pubic bone near the ischium and hammered into the bone on each side in a lateral direction. Lacing

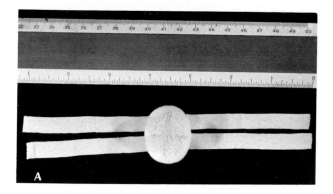

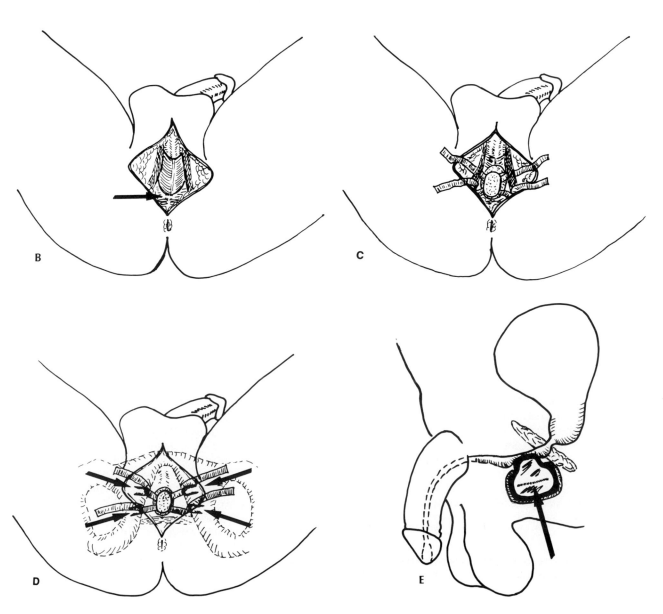

FIG. 97-3. **(A)** The Kaufman prosthesis is available from Heyer–Schulte Corporation, 5377 Overpass Road, Santa Barbara, California, 93111. **(B)** Midline incision is made. The central perineal tendon is divided (*arrow*) and the bulbocavernosus is exposed. **(C)** Kaufman prosthesis is in position. Straps are tied after the staples are firmly seated. **(D)** Cutaway view shows position of staples in the pubic bone (*arrows*). **(E)** Proper position of prosthesis against urethra, *arrow* shows the route of injection and the position of the needle stop.

the straps of the prosthesis under the staples results in a pulling upward of the prosthesis and a compression of the bulb against the urogenital diaphragm. The distal two straps of the prosthesis are placed about or through the crura with the modified ligature carrier or a sharp-pointed, right-angle clamp. If this appears to give inadequate fixation, two additional bone staples can be used; these are driven into the pubic arch on either side of the ischiocavernosus muscles.

The extra-large, silicone-gel prosthesis is used most commonly. The medium-sized prosthesis is used on the small bulbous urethra. The prosthesis is washed and autoclaved for use before emersion in an antibiotic solution of 1% neomycin or kanamycin for at least 5 minutes before use. The wound is irrigated frequently with this solution during the operation.

After the straps have been laced through the crura or through the staples, the position of the dome of the prosthesis against the bulbous urethra is ascertained, the straps are pulled up, and the staples are impacted. The staples are left slightly disimpacted to allow some adjustability of the tension on the straps. The straps are tied over the base of the prosthesis and, usually, the anterior and posterior straps are attached loosely to each other to prevent them from slipping over the end of the prosthesis.

The wound is irrigated again and closed with absorbable interrupted sutures. The subcutaneous tissue is approximated with 3-0 absorbable sutures, after which the skin edges are closed with the subcuticular suture. The wound is sprayed and a urethral pressure profile is repeated. Almost invariably, moderate tension with the straps results in a closing pressure of 70 cm to 90 cm of water. If a closing pressure of less than 60 cm of water is found, the prosthesis is injected immediately with radiographic contrast medium to bring the closing pressure to between 70 cm and 90 cm of water. Only rarely does pressure exceed 120 cm of water. The surgeon should consider opening the wound and relaxing tension in the straps if this should occur.

A 12Fr or 14Fr Foley catheter is left in the bladder for 48 hours. Occasionally, a suprapubic cystostomy with a cystocatheterization is done if a urethral catheter cannot be passed easily. The patient usually voids well on removal of the catheter, but 30% or so require a replacement of the catheter because of transient retention. In such cases, the catheter is left in place for another 48 hours. Sitz baths 3 times daily are begun 1 day postoperatively and continued for 10 days or so. Antibiotics are used postoperatively—aminoglycosides until the patient is discharged from the hospital and then cephalosporins. Perineal pain generally is not severe, and by the time of discharge from the hospital, 4 or 5 days postoperatively, the patient is quite comfortable.

Results

Of 184 cases done between 1972 and 1977, there were 169 cases that had excellent or very good results up to 6 weeks postoperatively. Fifteen patients failed to be improved. At 6 months, however, there was a significant loss of continence in the early improved group, with only 72 patients (about 40%) improved. One hundred thirteen patients had regressed to the point of requiring more than four changes of pads or an appliance. However, with one or more injections of the prosthesis and at 1 year or longer, 33% were considered excellent, 28% good, and 39% of the cases were considered failures. Postoperative injections, usually monitored by urethral pressure profile, are done with a 23- or 24-gauge needle using radiographic contrast medium, customarily injecting 5 ml to 10 ml each time. It is easy to palpate the prothesis and the perineum and to gauge when the needle has punctured the thick base of the prosthesis. The needle should not be advanced deeply into the prosthesis to prevent puncture of the unveloured dome. A disc of firm plastic has been incorporated within the capsule to act as a needle stop and to prevent the needle from puncturing the dome of the prosthesis (Fig. 97-3E).

Complications

In this series, there were 20 major complications, including 12 urethral or perineal skin erosions, two of which were associated with osteomyelitis requiring prolonged hospitalization for parenteral aminoglycoside therapy. In two cases, erosions of the Small–Carrion prosthesis and the silicone-gel prosthesis occurred. Of the two patients with urethral erosion, three required supravesical diversion. One had a ureterosigmoidostomy, and two had ureteroileal cutaneous diversion. Eight patients had infection in which draining sinuses ultimately required removal of the prosthesis. Minor complications occurred in 45 patients and were primarily in the form of urinary retention requiring replacement of the catheter for several days.

PERIURETHRAL TEFLON INJECTIONS

Teflon paste has been used for a number of years by the otolaryngologist for intracordal injection in

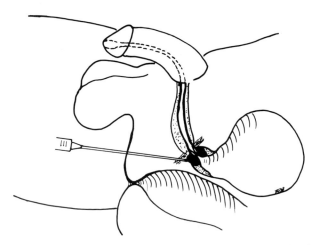

FIG. 97-4. Needle injects Teflon paste into paraurethral tissue and the sphincter area.

the treatment of paralytic vocal dysphonia. Politano has used this material for periurethral injection in incontinent patients since 1965 and has reported his experience with 125 patients, in which he achieved good to excellent results in more than 70% of the cases.[19]

A 4-in., 17-gauge needle is used with a Lewy pressure syringe to inject the Teflon paste. The external genitalia and the perineum are carefully cleansed and draped. The urethra is calibrated to be certain that strictures are not present. Urethrograms are obtained when necessary. The bladder and urethra are inspected with careful attention to the prostatic and membranous urethra. The panendoscope is left in the urethra, while a 17-gauge needle is inserted into the perineum and advanced toward the apex of the prostate.

By gentle to-and-fro motion, one can observe the tip of the needle advancing toward the region of the external sphincter. Care is taken to avoid penetration of the urethral lumen, which would provide an escape for the Polytef paste. When the needle has been advanced into its proper position, the Lewy syringe is attached and the injections are started. The needle is advanced, withdrawn, or moved to a new position as may seem appropriate in order to produce a complete closure or narrowing of the prostatic urethra, as well as of the sphincter area (Fig. 97-4). The injection can be monitored through the panendoscope and the blebs produced by the Polytef injections are clearly visualized. Generally, some 10 cc to 15 cc of the paste is injected. Early failures were generally the result of injection of too little Teflon paste.

Complications have been minimal and have generally consisted of symptoms of urethritis with burning and discomfort on voiding. Occasionally some perineal discomfort exists that subsides in several days to a week with warm sitz baths and analgesics. Some patients have exhibited a febrile response to the Teflon material. All such patients were placed on broad-spectrum antibiotics for approximately 1 week following the Teflon injection.

Indwelling catheters have not been used routinely, but intermittent catheterization has been used for those patients unable to void. In no instance has the patient been unable to void after a few days, and no patient has required any type of diversion or manipulation of the injected Teflon paste. There have been no reactions to the Teflon paste and embolization has not occurred in patients. However, migration of Teflon remains a possibility. The procedure is relatively simple and patients are usually discharged from the hospital within 48 to 72 hours. Injections can be repeated several times, and one patient in Politano's series was injected as many as five times.

Normally, however, it is advisable to wait from 4 to 6 months before repeating an injection. It has not been unusual for the patient to begin leaking urine several days after the injection, to remain wet for several months, and then suddenly to become dry. Therefore, several months should elapse before a repeat injection. In no instance has stricture formation been attributable to the Teflon procedure. The use of Polytef paste does not exclude a later open surgical procedure or the use of a prosthesis should it become necessary.

Even though initial reports with this procedure were encouraging, the reported results have not always been reproducible and enthusiasm has decreased somewhat in many areas.

Artificial Urinary Prostheses

The first artificial sphincter implantation in a human was performed by Scott in 1972.[22] This device was produced by American Medical Systems and was designated the AS-721 (Fig. 97-5). It consisted of a silicone rubber cuff that encircled the bladder neck, a reservoir containing fluid to fill the device, and two pumps that were used to inflate and deflate the system. A pressure-regulating valve maintained the proper pressure in the cuff while allowing excess fluid to be returned to the reservoir.

The early success with this prosthesis spurred the search for other simpler devices, and there are three that are currently used: the Swenson spring compression loop, a mechanical device that is still considered experimental; the Rosen inflatable clamp, and the AMS AS-791/792 prosthesis, which is an

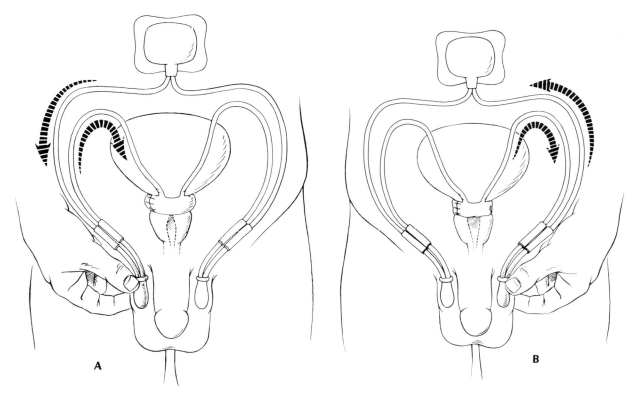

FIG. 97-5. Four parts of prosthetic urinary sphincter: reservoir, inflatable cuff, and two pumps. **(A)** Squeezing pump on right transports fluid from reservoir into cuff. **(B)** Squeezing pump on left deflates cuff into ''open'' position. Bulbs are implanted in labia of the female or in the scrotum of the male. (Scott FB et al: Urology 1·253, 1973)

outgrowth of the earlier AS-721 implanted by Scott.[20,25] Owing to its experimental nature, the Swenson device is not covered in detail in this text. A good review is available in the recent article by Cook.[5] We discuss the Rosen and newer Scott prostheses in some detail.

ROSEN INCONTINENCE DEVICE

In 1976, Rosen introduced a very simple implantable, artificial sphincter device.[20] It consisted of an occluder balloon which, when inflated, compressed the urethra against two contramember arms (Fig. 97-6). The fluid for compression was squeezed from a Silastic reservoir placed in the scrotum. When voiding was desired, the fluid was returned to the reservoir by squeezing a deflation valve in the upper part of the reservoir. Rosen reported a 77% success rate using this device, with no urethral erosion. Thirteen percent of the successful devices had to be replaced owing to rupture or mechanical difficulty, and there was an overall 23% failure rate. These statistics have been dupli-

cated by Small, who reported a 79% success rate in his series of 19 patients.*[24]

These success rates have not been confirmed by others, however. Giesy and co-workers recently reported that 42% of his patients developed urethral erosion and that there was a 6-month failure rate of 50% using this device.[8] Only 2 of 13 patients remained totally dry and 3 others experienced stress incontinence. Two other authors have reported similar experience. Carrion and associates reported only 3 successes out of 12 patients, with 7 mechanical failures in 16 insertions and 5 urethral erosions.[4] Augspurger reported an overall success rate of 60%; his longest success at that point was 22 months.[1] Our own experience was limited to the earliest models and was equally discouraging.

The original Rosen device has been improved by the development of a thicker, self-sealing scrotal reservoir that can be injected to add fluid to the system. The valve mechanism has been made more prominent to permit easier identification and ma-

---

* Small MP: Personal communication, February 1981

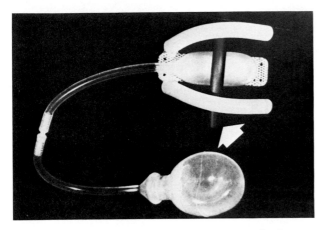

FIG. 97-6. Rosen inflatable incontinence prosthesis

nipulation by the patient, and the contramember arms have been reinforced and cushioned with additional silicone rubber to lessen the likelihood of urethral erosion. Most important, the device is now being produced in three sizes. This makes stable implantation far easier than with the original large-size device, which was very difficult to fit within the bulbocavernosus muscle and to implant in a patient with a narrow pelvis. All three sizes should be available at the time of surgery to ensure a proper fit.

Sterile procedure and antibiotic prophylaxis are absolutely essential when using prostheses, and the implantation procedure is preceded by administration of an aminoglycoside antibiotic on call to the operating room. Two thirds of the daily dose, as determined by body weight, is received at surgery. On the evening of surgery, the remaining one third is given as an intravenous infusion. Doxycycline; 200 mg, is given in the recovery room, and the aminoglycoside and doxycycline are continued parenterally through the second postoperative day. Oral doxycycline is then continued through day 10. The sphincter devices are soaked in an antibiotic solution of polymyxin B sulfate and neomycin sulfate prior to implantation, and the same solution is used copiously to flush the wound during the procedure. This regimen, combined with meticulous surgical technique, careful tissue handling, and hemostasis, has reduced the infection rate for both the Rosen and Scott devices to very acceptable levels.

ROSEN IMPLANTATION PROCEDURE

The surgical procedure as performed by Small is as follows. The patient is placed in the lithotomy position and after a 15-minute povidone-iodine scrub, the anus is draped out of the surgical field. A number 16Fr Foley catheter is placed in the bladder for identification of the urethra and a midline incision is made through the perineum down to the bulbocavernosus muscle. After this muscle has been freed of overlying fat, the corpus spongiosum and urethra are identified at the distal aspect, then the bulbocavernosus muscle is gently dissected off the corpus spongiosum with a right-angle clamp and opened in the midline to expose the deep bulbous urethra. The corpus spongiosum and urethra are gently mobilized to reveal the dense midline, fibrous attachments of the urethra to the underside of the symphysis pubis. This fibrous tissue is dissected sharply away from the pubis for a distance of about 1½ cm to open a plane for placement of the perineal member of the Rosen. Care is taken to avoid devascularization and skeletonization of the urethra during this process.

After the incontinence device has been placed around the deep bulbous urethra, the baseplate with its occluder balloon is sutured to the inside bulbocavernosus muscle through the predrilled holes in the baseplate and contramember arms (Fig. 97-7). A nonreactive, nonabsorbable suture material must be used. The flexible contramember arms are easily molded to fit the bulbous urethra. Four sutures are used to anchor the baseplate into the bulbocavernosus muscle. On one side, the sutures are placed through the baseplate and muscle only; on the other, the sutures are tied fixing the contramember arms to the baseplate, then passed through the muscle and retied for fixation. This fixation is essential to avoid twisting and displacement that could prevent proper compression and contribute to pinching of the urethra and erosion.

The inflate tube is then passed through a stab wound in the bulbocavernosus muscle (on the right side in right-handed individuals). Following copious irrigation with antibiotic solution, the muscle is closed with a continuous suture of 1-0 chromic catgut.

Blunt dissection of the scrotum is accomplished through the perineal wound in such a manner as to leave the scrotum with adequate subcutaneous tissue to maintain blood supply, yet thin enough to permit the patient to identify and manipulate the scrotal reservoir and deflation valve. Orchiectomy may be necessary in some patients but is no longer routinely performed because it is usually easy to place the scrotal reservoir above the testicle.

The reservoir is filled with either sterile saline

or the antibiotic solution in a concentration of 85% to 15% radiopaque contrast material. This permits adequate postoperative visualization of the device without sufficient concentration to allow crystallization, which could cause malfunction of the deflate valve. The reservoir is then placed in the scrotum, excess tubing is excised, and the connection is made to the perineal occluder after ensuring that all air has been removed from the system. A small stainless steel connector is used to connect the tubing and is fixed in place with nonabsorbable suture material. A pursestring suture may be used,

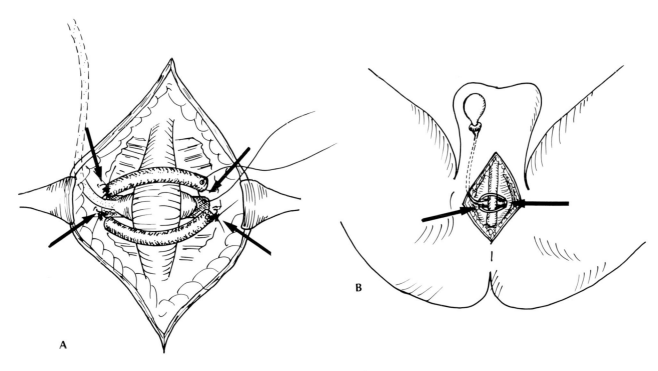

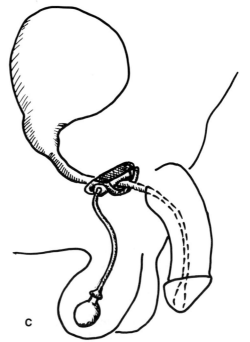

FIG. 97-7. **(A)** Rosen device in position: contramember arms are sutured into the bulbocavernosus muscle at four points using two sutures at each end (*arrows*). Tubing is routed subcutaneously to the scrotum. **(B)** Reservoir bulb is placed in the scrotum. The bulbocavernosus will be closed over the device. **(C)** Functional position of Rosen device is shown.

if desired, to fix the reservoir in the scrotum, but it is usually unnecessary.

The device is actuated to check proper function then the wound is closed with 3-0 plain catgut irrigating each layer with antibiotic solution. The 3-0 chromic catgut interrupted sutures are used to close the skin and a collodion dressing is applied. The 16Fr catheter is replaced by a No. 10 and 12 Fr silicone catheter, which is left in place for 7 to 10 days. *The device is not inflated* during this period.

Once the catheter is out, an external collecting device is used and the patient is allowed to transfer fluid in small amounts for 5 to 10 minutes at a time, three or four times a day. After 2 weeks, a pseudocapsule will have begun to develop to fix the device in place and the urethra will have become revascularized. At this time, sufficient fluid can be transferred to maintain continence. The patient is cautioned not to leave the device inflated while sleeping and is taught to use only the smallest amount of fluid necessary to maintain continence. When the occluder is inflated, the reservoir will have a persistent depression in its surface. Patients learn to judge the level of filling by the size of this depression. Using this method, urethral necrosis has reportedly been no problem.

Use of the Rosen and Scott devices may be contraindicated in patients who have had extensive pelvic or perineal radiation, perineal trauma, or urethral stricture disease requiring dilation. Its use is also not advised in individuals whose mental or physical status does not permit proper manipulation of the scrotal reservoir or pump.

AS-791/792 ARTIFICIAL SPHINCTER

The most popular and perhaps the most reliable method of managing urinary incontinence today is through the use of the AS-791/792 artificial sphincter produced by American Medical Systems. The success of this sphincter is the result of extensive clinical research and refinement of implantation techniques by Scott and by Furlow of the Mayo Clinic, who popularized the primary deactivation technique that is most commonly used today.[23]

Attempts to produce a sphincter that would maintain continence without urethral erosion, while compensating for variations in intra-abdominal pressure, resulted in many changes in the original models proposed by Bradley and Timm in the 1960s.[27] The AS-721 device, which required a pump in each side of the scrotum for inflation and deflation, was plagued by valve failure. This spurred the development of the AS-761, which was basically the same but inserted a pressure balloon into the system to maintain a constant level· of pressure and compensate for increases in intra-abdominal pressure with stress. From this pressure-balloon concept came the AS-742 model (Fig. 97-8), which replaced the old reservoir entirely with a new balloon reservoir of appropriate constant pressure. This model also eliminated the inflate pump in favor of a control assembly that would permit emptying of the cuff with the remaining pump and allow automatic refilling from the pressure balloon. This device has now been redesignated the AS-791/792. The AS-791 is used as a cuff around the bulbous urethra; the AS-792 has its cuff around the bladder neck. The only difference in the two devices is the position of the tubing ports on the control assembly (Fig. 97-9).

Implantation of the AS-791/792 can be performed either abdominally, with the cuff around the bladder neck, or perineally, with the cuff around the bulbar urethra. In females, the bladder neck is always used, whereas in males the bladder neck approach is reserved for children and adult males in whom the prostate and bladder neck have not been surgically altered. All patients must be free of infection prior to implantation, and positive urine cultures are treated with appropriate antibiotics until sterility is confirmed. All evidence of obstruction should be eliminated and any necessary corrective surgical procedures should be performed and allowed to heal prior to attempting implantation.

Bladder Neck Approach

A transverse lower abdominal incision is made, incising the rectus muscles to gain adequate exposure of the bladder neck area. With a catheter in the bladder, the balloon can be palpated to delineate the bladder neck. Incisions are made in the transversalis fascia on either side of the bladder neck. By use of combined sharp and blunt dissection, a plane is created between the posterior bladder neck and trigone, and the vas deferens, ampulla, and seminal vesicles. One should be able to palpate the trigone and the catheter at the bladder neck. If any question exists as to proper placement of the cuff, cystoscopy can be performed or the bladder can be opened for confirmation. I have experienced no difficulty in opening the bladder with this procedure, but must emphasize that a watertight closure must be achieved in each case.

Once the passage has been created around the bladder neck, a large right-angle clamp is used to dilate the passage sufficiently to permit the place-

FIG. 97-8. AMS AS-792, artificial sphincter. The artificial sphincter (AS-791 or 792) consists of four parts: **(1)** the cuff, which encircles and occludes the urethra; **(2)** the pressure balloon, which fills the cuff with sufficient pressure to occlude the urethra without strangulating the blood supply; **(3)** the pump, which is implanted in the scrotum and is used to empty the cuff by pumping its fluid back into the balloon; **(4)** the control assembly, which regulates the rate of filling of the cuff permits fluid to be transferred from the cuff to the balloon by squeezing at the pump and releases pressure from the cuff in response to abnormally high bladder pressure.

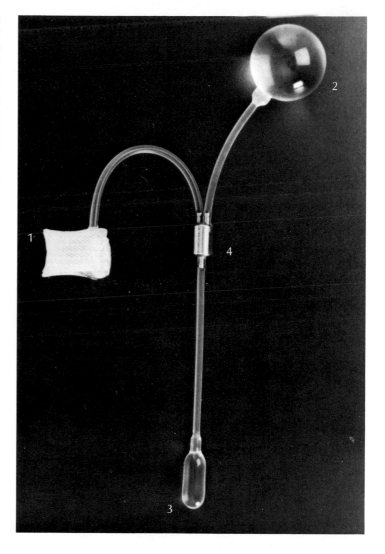

ment of a 2-cm cuff. Careful hemostasis is obtained; then an umbilical tape is passed around the bladder neck and clamped loosely to measure the circumference for selection of the proper length cuff. The tape is cut, measured, and a cuff of the same length is selected. This cuff is passed around the bladder neck and tied into place.

AS-791 pressure balloons come in five different pressure ranges varying from 50–60 cm H_2O to 90–100 cm H_2O. The object is to select the lowest pressure balloon available that will maintain continence. We do this by attaching a spinal manometer to an IV pole that can be raised or lowered to permit measurements between 50 cm and 100 cm H_2O above the bladder neck. The cuff is filled and connected to the manometer, which has been filled to the 100-cm level. The bladder is filled and the catheter is removed. Gentle pressure is placed on the bladder and the fluid is gradually drained from the manometer. The pressure at which leakage occurs is recorded and the proper pressure balloon is selected. In most cases, pressures of less than 90 cm H_2O are quite adequate.

The cuff is emptied and its tubing is clamped with a rubber-shod clamp. The pressure balloon is filled to 18 ml and connected to the cuff to permit the cuff to fill. The volume required to fill the cuff is determined by withdrawing all of the fluid from the balloon and subtracting that volume from 18 ml; this volume is recorded. The balloon is refilled to 16 ml (the volume at which it exerts its design pressure) and then implanted in the prevesical space adjacent to the bladder. Using a blunt tubing needle supplied by the manufacturer, the tubing from the cuff and balloon is passed through the inguinal canal to the external ring, where the

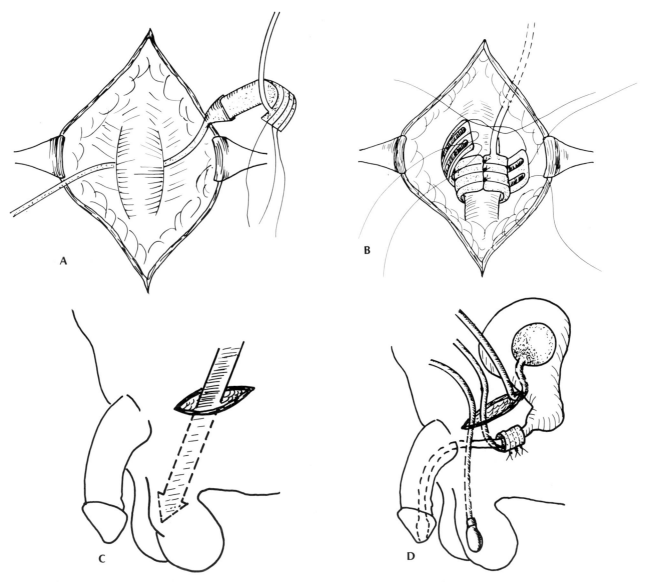

FIG. 97-9. **(A)** Midline perineal incision. Bulbous urethra is mobilized and the cuff inserter is being used to pass the cuff around the urethra. **(B)** The cuff is tied in place and a malleable cuff protector is positioned. Tubing is routed subcutaneously to the inguinal incision. **(C)** A finger or blunt clamp is used to develop a subcutaneous pocket in the scrotum for the pump. **(D)** A pressure balloon is placed in the prevesical space. The cuff and pump are in position and all the tubing is routed subcutaneously to the inguinal incision for connection to the control assembly in the region of the external ring.

connections to the control assembly can be made subcutaneously.

With a Kelly clamp, a pocket is dissected into the scrotum. This pocket should be deep enough to allow the pump to lie comfortably in the scrotum just behind the skin in a position that will permit easy manipulation by the patient. Tubing connections are made to the appropriate nipples on the control assembly with 3-0 Prolene suture. The system can be tested by applying uniform pressure over the abdomen. No leakage should occur. Squeezing of the scrotal pump should permit free voiding. Throughout this procedure, the wound is irrigated with a mixture of 50,000 units of bacitracin and 1 g of kanamycin sulfate (Kantrex) dissolved in 300 ml of normal saline. Careful

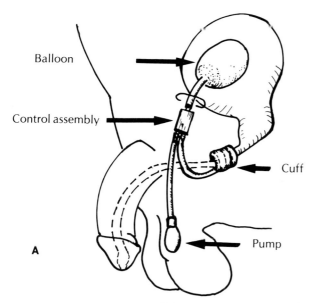

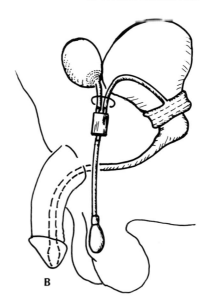

FIG. 97-10.   **(A)** AS 791 device; the cuff fits the bulbous urethra.   **(B)** AS 792 device; parts on the control assembly are rearranged to permit implantation at the bladder neck.

hemostasis is maintained, no drains are used, and the wound is closed with 1-0 Prolene suture. The stapling gun is used for the skin.

Bulbous Urethra Approach

The approach for perineal cuff insertion is identical to that described for the insertion of the Rosen device. A 5-cm cuff is usually appropriate for all adult male urethras (Fig. 97-9). A malleable metal protector has been designed to fit around the cuff to prevent fluid from being forced out when the patient sits. Tubing from the cuff is threaded subcutaneously from the perineum to a small incision placed over the external ring.

The incision over the external ring allows dissection through the ring for placement of the pressure balloon intra-abdominally adjacent to the bladder. The tubing should be brought out through a puncture wound in the fascia adjacent to the ring to prevent displacement of the balloon. The pump is implanted into the scrotum as previously described and the tubing is connected to the control assembly in the prescribed manner. A running nonabsorbable suture is used to close the perineal incision and the wound is sealed with a collodion dressing (Fig. 97-10).

RESULTS

Brantley Scott's overall long-term success rate for this newer prosthesis is in the range of 78%. Erosions have occurred but have been far less

frequent with the switch to lower pressure balloons. In Scott's most recent series of 203 patients, there were a total of 26 mechanical failures, most of which occurred in the first 6 months. There were very few pump or balloon failures. Most of the failures were in the early series cuffs. Recent model cuffs have been made more reliable, and statistics now indicate that patients who reach 6 months without experiencing a failure have a 96% chance of continuing to do well. Furlow recently reported to the AUA that 41 of 47 patients were doing well with the newer sphincter. Improvements in technique would doubtlessly improve the statistics of others as well. Our own experience with the new prosthesis has been most gratifying, and insertion of the AS-791/792 remains our procedure of choice in all cases of total incontinence.

Scott has formulated a number of basic principles of sphincter implantation that bear repeating:[23]

1. Avoid any instrumentation of the lower urinary tract within 48 hours of implantation.
2. All patients should have protective blood levels of antibiotics at the time of surgery, and this should continue until there is no postoperative threat of wound infection.
3. Allow recent surgery to heal completely before proceeding with implantation.
4. Relieve all obstruction before implantation.
5. Measure penile blood pressure in the elderly patient. If lower than brachial blood pressure,

use lowest pressure balloon and delay activation until after recovery (several months).

6. Use no balloon with a pressure greater than 90 cm H_2O.

7. Inspect the urethra carefully after dissection to rule out injury before proceeding with implantation.

8. Avoid use of surgical drains.

9. When combining implantation with reconstructive surgery, delayed activation should always be used.

The past decade has seen remarkable advances in the management of urinary incontinence. Further advances in technique and technology are inevitable. Urologists in training today can look forward to vast improvement in the outlook for management of this most unfortunate group of urologic patients.

REFERENCES

1. AUGSPURGER RR: Careful consideration required for Rosen prosthesis. Urology Times, January 1980

2. BAUMRUCKER GO: A new male incontinence clamp. J Urol 121:201, 1979

3. BERRY JL: A new procedure for correction of urinary incontinence. Preliminary report. J Urol 85:771, 1961

4. CARRION HM, LOBO J, POLITANO VA: Complications seen with incontinence device. Urology Times, September 1980

5. COOK WA: Incontinence in children. Symposium on male incontinence. Urol Clin North Am. 5:353, 1978

6. DEES JE: Congenital epispadias with incontinence. J Urol 62:513, 1949

7. FLOCKS RH, CULP DA: A modification of technique for anastomosing membranous urethra and bladder neck following total prostatectomy. J Urol 69:411, 1953

8. GIESY JB, FADIS EF, BARRY JM, FUCHS EF et al: Initial experience with the Rosen incontinence device. J Urol 125:794, 1981

9. HAURI D: An operation for cure of post-prostatectomy incontinence. Urol Int 32:284, 1977

10. HEISTER DL: Institutions chirurgicae. Amsielaedami: Janssonio Waesbergios, p 112, 1950

11. KAUFMAN JJ: Surgical treatment of post-prostatectomy incontinence. Use of the penile crura to compress the bulbous urethra. J Urol 107:293, 1972

12. KAUFMAN JJ, RAZ S: Passive urethral compression with a silicone gel prosthesis for the treatment of male urinary incontinence. Mayo Clin Proc 51:303, 1976

13. KAUFMAN JJ, RAZ S: Urethral compression procedures for the treatment of male urinary incontinence. J Urol 121:605, 1979

14. LEADBETTER GW, JR: Surgical correction of total urinary incontinence. J Urol 91:281, 1964

15. LOWSLEY OS: New operation for the relief of incontinence in both male and female. J Urol 36:400, 1936

16. LOWSLEY OS, BRAY JT: Surgical relief of impotence. JAMA 107:2029, 1936

17. MATHISEN W: A new operation for urinary incontinence. Surg Gynecol Obstet 130:606, 1970

18. MICHNER FR, THOMPSON IM, ROSS G: Urethrovesical tubularization for urinary incontinence. J Urol 92:203, 1964

19. POLITANO VA: Periurethral teflon injection for urinary incontinence. Urol Clin North Am. 5:415, 1978

20. ROSEN M: A simple artificial implantable sphincter. Br J Urol 48:676, 1976

21. SCHOENBERG HW, GREGORY JG: Anterior bladder tube in radical retropubic prostatectomy. Urology, 7:495, 1976

22. SCOTT FB, BRADLEY WE, TIMM GW: Treatment of urinary incontinence by an implantable prosthetic sphincter, Urology 1:252, 1973

23. SCOTT FB, LIGHT JK, FISHMAN I et al: Implantation of an artificial sphincter for urinary incontinence. Contemporary Surgery, 18:11, 1981

24. SMALL MP: The Rosen incontinence procedure: A new artificial urinary sphincter for the management of urinary incontinence. J Urol 123:507, 1980

25. SWENSON O: Internal device for control of urinary incontinence. J Pediatr Surg 7:542, 1972

26. TANAGHO EA, SMITH DR: Clinical evaluation of a surgical technique for the correction of complete urinary incontinence. J Urol 107:402, 1972

27. TIMM GW: An implantable incontinence device. J Biomed 4:213, 1971

28. YOUNG HH: Suture of the urethral and vesical sphincters for cure of incontinence of urine, with report of a case. Trans South Surg Assoc 20:210, 1907

Imperforate Anus

98

A. Barry Belman

The implementation of a preventive approach to the practice of medicine requires an awareness of potential relationships between various pathologic states. A classic example is myelodysplasia and its associated neurologic, orthopedic, and urinary abnormalities. Multidisciplinary clinics have been developed throughout the world to coordinate more effectively the care of children born with this abnormality, and the overall health of this unfortunate group has improved. Another entity in which the care of affected individuals can be improved by an awareness of the extent of the multisystem involvement is imperforate anus.

Duhamel first recognized the regional error in embryologic organization that resulted in fusion of the lower extremities (symmelia), sacral agenesis, imperforate anus, and absence of the entire genitourinary tract other than the gonads. He placed this constellation of abnormalities at the end of a spectrum and labeled the phenomenon "the syndrome of caudal regression."[5] If one assumes that a fetal injury occurred between the fourth and fifth weeks of gestation to produce this monster, one might better appreciate the frequent association of both sacral and urinary anomalies seen in the neonate who manifests its less severe form: imperforate anus. It is at this early stage in embryologic development that the ureteral buds and the lumbosacral spine are forming and the cloacal septum is dividing the urogenital sinus from the rectum. The risk of multisystem abnormalities is great in the child with imperforate anus.

Classification

Ladd and Gross introduced the first classification of anorectal anomalies in 1934.[9] They divided the abnormality into four types: stenosis or incomplete rupture of the anal membrane (Type I), persistent anal membrane (Type II), imperforate anus with a blind-ending pouch (Type III), and atresia of the rectum with an intact distal lumen and anus (Type IV) (Fig. 98-1). In 1970 Santulli, Kiesewetter, and Bill introduced a classification that divides anorectal

anomalies into four major types based primarily on the level of the imperforation relative to the pelvic floor or puborectalis muscle.[14] On this basis the grouping includes the low or translevator lesions; intermediate lesions; high or supralevator lesions; and a fourth, miscellaneous group, which is made up of the rare imperforate anal membrane, cloacal exstrophy, and the cloacal abnormality (rectocloacal fistula).

The two major classifications of imperforate anus, namely, high or supralevator lesions and the low or translevator type, represent the bulk of those seen clinically. They correspond respectively to Types III and I as defined by Ladd and Gross (Fig. 98-1). Armed with the knowledge of the level of the imperforate anus, the urologist can predict the incidence of associated urinary abnormalities and develop a more objective approach toward recommendations for evaluation and treatment.

In the miscellaneous groups two exceedingly rare forms are of urologic interest. Cloacal exstrophy (vesicointestinal fissure) presents as a lower abdominal wall defect consisting of two halves of an exstrophic bladder separated by a zone of intestinal mucosa (Fig. 98-2).[18] Each ureteral orifice is found in relationship to the two lateral areas of bladder mucosa. An orifice at the upper end of the intestinal zone usually leads to the terminal ileum, which is frequently prolapsed. The remainder of the large bowel other than this exstrophic colon and much of the small bowel may be absent. A blind loop of colon may extend into the pelvis but remains imperforate.

Additional commonly associated abnormalities include paired vermiform appendices, omphalocele, duplication of the internal genitalia in females, and a bifid phallus in both sexes. On this basis sex determination may be difficult and in the majority the sex of rearing should be female. Upper urinary anomalies are present in 60% and may be bizarre.[20]

Another rare abnormality, the rectocloacal fistula (cloacal abnormality), is the female variant of the high imperforate anus.[17] The child exhibits a single perineal opening into which the urethra,

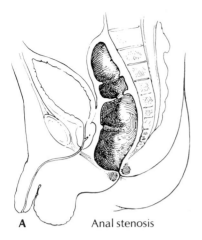

A   Anal stenosis

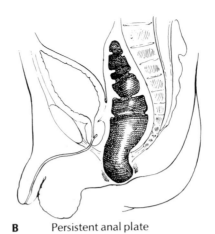

B   Persistent anal plate

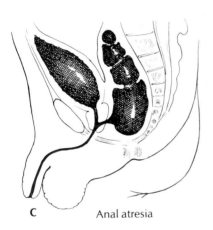

C   Anal atresia

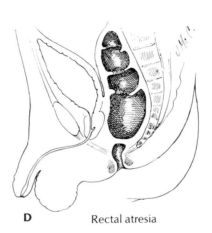

D   Rectal atresia

FIG. 98-1. Ladd and Gross's classification of imperforate anus: **(A)** type I, anal stenosis; **(B)** type II, persistent anal plate; **(C)** type III, anal atresia, type noted as supralevator lesion in this chapter; **(D)** type IV, rectal atresia.

distal vagina, and rectum enter proximally. An abdominal mass secondary to a muco- or hydrocolpos is frequently present. This is often the result of stenosis of the vaginal orifice. Embryologically the distal sinus is thought to represent a persistent urogenital sinus anterolaterally and residual cloaca posteriorly.[7]

Embryologic and Anatomic Considerations

The nephrogenic cord (renal blastema) appears caudally at the level of the future second and third sacral segments as a product of the metanephros in the fourth gestational week. In conjunction with the infolding of the urorectal septum, ureteral buds protrude from the anterior or urogenital segment at the level of the 28th somite (the future first sacral vertebra). These buds then meet the mesonephrogenic tissue and form the collecting system.[1] By the sixth or seventh week the urorectal septum

reaches the cloacal membrane where it meets the perineum and is classically thought to rupture, creating two separate excretory orifices.[3] Stephens suggests that lateral ingrowth completes the caudal separation of the urinary and intestinal tracts, and failure of development in this area results in the persistent rectourethral or rectovesical fistula.[17] Following cutaneous eruption it then moves posteriorly to its expected position. Failure of this migration is thought to be the underlying cause of imperforate anus.

Obviously an explanation that takes into account the entire multisystem spectrum is conjectural; however, if one postulates a regional injury in the area of the 28th somite at 4 to 5 weeks of fetal life, the frequent association of sacral, renal, and ureteral abnormalities found with the supralevator type of imperforate anus can be appreciated. Additionally, with limitation of completion of the urorectal septum and failure of rupture of the cloacal membrane, one would expect persistence

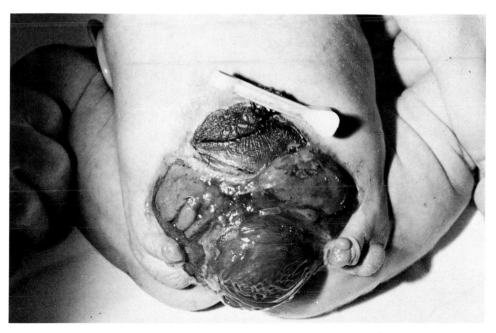

FIG. 98-2.   Cloacal exstrophy. Note bifid phallus and scrotum and bladder mucosa separated by colonic mucosa (inferior portion of exstrophy). Cutaneous termination of the small bowel, located inferiorly, is not visible.

of a communication between the posterior and anterior compartments of the cloaca at its most caudal aspect. This holds true in almost all cases with the supralevator type of abnormality and is reflected in the fistulous communication between the blind-ending rectal pouch and urethra or bladder in the male (Fig. 98-3A).

In the female the müllerian ducts fuse and interpose themselves in the inferior aspect of the urorectal septum (Müller's tubercle).[1] It is from this point that the female internal genital system develops. The vagina then migrates caudally and, in normal circumstances, becomes interposed between the urinary and intestinal tracts. However, when the persistent communication between distal rectum and bladder is encountered, it is likely that the vagina then incorporates the urinary portion of the fistulous tract. The result is a rectovaginal fistula (Fig. 98-3C).

Rectovesical fistulae occur rarely in females. In fact, supralevator lesions in females with a fistulous communication between the proximal vagina and rectal pouch with an otherwise normal urinary tract are rare. Apparently this anomaly manifests itself primarily as the more rare cloacal abnormality in which a single perineal opening is present from which the urinary, genital, and intestinal tracts meet (Fig. 98-4).

It is likely that in those patients with a low or infralevator imperforate anus, the injury occurs later in fetal development after rupture of the anal opening into the perineum but prior to completion of its posterior migration. Failure of complete separation of the cloaca by the urorectal septum is not likely because there is no communication between the intestinal and urinary tracts in this group.[1] It is not uncommon, however, for the rectal fistula to open into the distal dorsal vagina or posterior fourchette in girls or at the posterior scrotal raphe in boys (Fig. 98-3C).

CLINICAL ASPECTS

The therapeutic approach is dependent upon the level of the lesion. Careful examination of the perineum, posterior fourchette, inferior vagina, scrotal raphe, and ventral aspect of the penis for signs of a fistulous opening or meconium staining is essential to identify the presence of an infralevator lesion. Primary anoplasty is the treatment in children with infralevator lesions, whereas a diverting colostomy is generally preferred in those with a supralevator lesion. Rectal pull-through is delayed in the latter group until the child weighs at least 15 lb.[19]

To gain as much information as possible, complete urologic evaluation should ideally be carried out as the initial step. However, in most centers

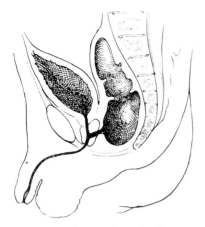

A   Supralevator imperforate
anus

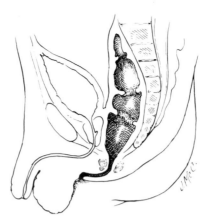

B   Infralevator with cutaneous
fistula at base of scrotum

FIG. 98-3.   Lesions in the male and the female.   **(A)** A supralevator lesion in the male with an entero-prostatic fistula.   **(B)** An infralevator lesion in the male. A cutaneous fistula is present at the base of the scrotum anterior to the anal dimple. **(C)** A suprelevator lesion in the female; this is a rare form with a rectal pouch entering high into the vagina.   **(D)** An infralevator lesion in the female; the cutaneous lesion is found at the posterior fourchette.

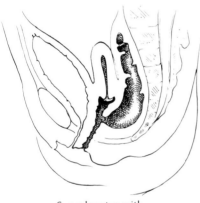

C   Supralevator with
upper vaginal fistula

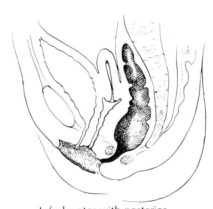

D   Infralevator with posterior
fourchette fistula

this evaluation is delayed until the child has recovered from the intestinal procedure. In the problem case, cystography may be helpful in demonstrating the urethrorectal fistula and blind rectal loop, thereby clarifying the level of the blind pouch. Unfortunately, inspissated meconium plugging the fistulous tract frequently interferes with complete visualization.

ASSOCIATED URINARY ANOMALIES

There have been many recent reviews of genitourinary abnormalities associated with imperforate anus.[2,6,8,10–13,15,16,23] The overall sex incidence is 58% males, 42% females. Exclusive of the rectourethral fistula, which should not be considered a separate abnormality, the frequency of genitourinary anomalies is high in all reports, with a sig-

nificantly high incidence of anomalies in patients with supralevator lesions. In our review of 174 previously untreated patients with imperforate anus presenting to Chicago Children's Memorial Hospital between 1965 and 1970, 143 of the total 174 had sufficient evaluation for urologic assessment.[2] Sixty-five (45%) had supralevator lesions, whereas 74 (52%) had infralevator lesions. Four patients exhibited cloacal exstrophy. Of the 65 patients with high-level lesions, 34 (52%) had associated genitourinary anomalies. Only 12 of the 74 (16%) with low-lying or intermediate lesions had associated genitourinary lesions (Table 98-1).

This compares favorably with the report of Santulli and associates, who noted urologic malformations in 40% of the males and 48% of the females with supralevator lesions, and 21% of the males and 14% of the female with infralevator or intermediate lesions.[15] Seventy-nine percent of the patients in their survey classified as miscellaneous (including cloacal exstrophy) had urinary abnormalities. Of the six additional patients subsequently surveyed by us who had a cloacal abnormality, three had upper tract abnormalities.* All were on the right side; two involved duplicated systems with ectopic upper pole ureters, and the third had an ectopic insertion of the ureter into the right horn of a duplicated uterus. Tank and Lindenauer found upper urinary anomalies in 60% of this group.[20]

Based on embryologic development and the theory of caudal regression advanced by Duhamel, one would expect a higher incidence of urinary anomalies with supralevator lesions (including cloacal abnormalities) than with the infralevator type.[5] One would also predict a higher incidence of upper than lower urinary tract anomalies. This corresponds to the theory of a regional error in organization and is underscored by the finding that the single most common urogenital abnormality associated with imperforate anus is unilateral renal agenesis.[2]

In our series 20 of the 34 patients with supralevator lesions having genitourinary anomalies had these abnormalities confined to the upper tract.[2] Eight had unilateral renal agenesis, whereas an additional six had either unilateral renal hypoplasia or dysplasia. Therefore 14 of 20 upper tract abnormalities were significant anomalies of renal formation. This was, in all likelihood, a response to abnormal budding of the ureter. On the other hand, there is not a single case of renal absence and only one case with a dysplastic kidney in the 12 patients with infralevator imperforation. Two patients with infralevator lesions had duplication, two demonstrated malrotation, and a pelvic kidney was noted in another.

As one might have anticipated, recent reviews have revealed vesicourteral reflux to be common. In those in whom cystography was routinely done, vesicoureteral reflux was found in 30% to 40% of those with high lesions. The incidence of reflux in those with low lesions is much more variable and the true incidence has not as yet been demonstrated.[10,12]

The rectourethral fistula, previously noted as a natural concomitant of high imperforate anus in the male, may also provoke urologic problems. Following bowel diversion urinary tract infection is generally not a problem and if present can be

---

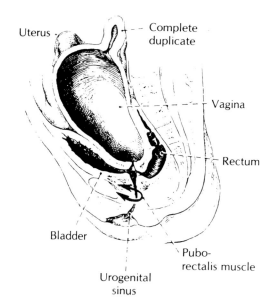

FIG. 98-4. Cloacal anomaly, a single perineal opening that communicates with the urethra, vagina, and rectum. *Double arrow* depicts level of puborectalis muscle. (Raffensberger JG: Chapter 18. In Kelalis, King, Belman [eds]: Clinical Pediatric Urology, Vol 2. Philadelphia, WB Saunders, 1976)

TABLE 98-1. Relationship of Level of Imperforation to Incidence of Urogenital Anomalies in 143 Patients

Level of Imperforation	No. of Patients	Patients with Associated GU Anomalies
Supralevator	65 (45)*	34 (52)
Infralevator	74 (52)	12 (16)
Cloacal exstrophy	4	4 (100)

* Number in parentheses indicates percentage

controlled with suppressive medication. However, rarely, because of this communication chronic urinary stasis may occur in the blind-ending rectal pouch leading to electrolyte imbalance.[4,21] Additionally urethral diverticulae with their associated risk of urinary stasis, infection, and calculus formation may result when an excessive length of fistula is allowed to remain attached to the urethra after a rectal pull-through (Fig. 98-5). Finally, the urethra may also be tented up at the time of ligation of the fistula, producing a urethral narrowing and secondary urinary outflow obstruction.[23]

Neurogenic bladder in these patients is mostly secondary to the associated sacral abnormalities.[24] Hall and co-workers reported 5 of 88 patients with

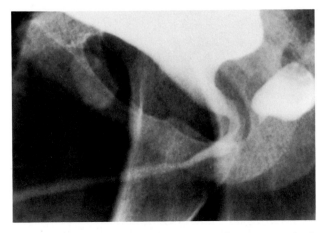

FIG. 98-5. Diverticulum at the site of a rectourethral fistula in a boy with supralevator imperforate anus. This was lined by nonmucus-producing mucosa and may represent a diverticulum secondary to a postoperative leak.

neurogenic bladders and imperforate anus.[6] In our own experience roughly 10% of these patients have neurogenic bladders, some of which can be attributed to surgical dissection and pelvic nerve damage.

Urologic Management

Most of the care given by urologists is consultative. Excretory urography and cystography done as routine procedures in all of these patients will reveal surprisingly high numbers and unusual types of abnormalities.

Occasionally immediate urologic care becomes necessary in this group of patients. Cutaneous vesicostomy as a temporary means of protecting the upper urinary tract may become necessary in those with electrolyte abnormalities or uncontrollable urinary tract infection associated with vesicoureteral reflux. Clean intermittent catheterization may ultimately be required in those with severely deranged neurogenic bladders.

Basically, the chief responsibility of the urologist is to impress upon our surgical colleagues the need for initial urologic evaluation and long term concern about the urinary tract. Radiographic evaluation, including cystography, is essential in all. During this procedure, awareness of the complications that result when dealing with the rectourethral fistula and the risk of bladder denervation associated with rectal pull-through must be foremost. Periodic urine cultures and notation of voiding patterns will identify those with associated lower urinary tract problems.

The management of cloacal exstrophy has ad-

vanced significantly in recent years with survival becoming the rule rather than the exception. Better management of the intestinal tract with incorporation of the small blind-ending colon may substantially improve absorptive capability and reduce diarrhea. Closure and turn-in of the previously united bladder halves (vis-à-vis bladder exstrophy), with a hope for urinary continence by means of clean intermittent catheterization, is the goal we are currently pursuing. However, the majority of the survivors will in all likelihood require urinary diversion.[22]

The role the urologist plays in these problems can be significant. Ultimately the surgical care may rest in our hands. The complex of problems that includes imperforate anus is complicated and requires a heavy investment by physicians, as well as use of the full range of paramedical support services.

REFERENCES

1. AREY LB: Developmental Anatomy. A Textbook and Laboratory Manual of Embryology, 7th ed. Philadelphia, WB Saunders, 1965
2. BELMAN AB, KING LR: Urinary tract abnormalities associated with imperforate anus. J Urol 108:823, 1972
3. BILL AH, JOHNSON RJ: Failure of migration of the rectal opening as the cause for most cases of imperforate anus. Surg Gynecol Obstet 106:643, 1958
4. CALDAMONE AA, EMMENS RW, RABINOWITZ R: Hyperchloremic acidosis and imperforate anus. J Urol 122:817, 1979
5. DUHAMEL B: From the mermaid to anal imperforation: The syndrome of caudal regression. Arch Dis Child 36:152, 1961
6. HALL JW, TANK ES, LAPIDES J: Urogenital anomalies and complications associated with imperforate anus. J Urol 103:810, 1970
7. JOHNSON RJ, PALKEN M, DERRICK W et al: The embryology of high anorectal and associated genitourinary anomalies in the female. Surg Gynecol Obstet 135:759, 1972
8. KIESEWETTER WB, TURNER CR, SIEBER WK: Imperforate anus. Review of a sixteen year experience with 146 patients. Am J Surg 107:412, 1964
9. LADD WE, GROSS RE: Congenital malformations of anus and rectum: Report of 162 cases. Am J Surg 23:167, 1934
10. PARROTT TS, WOODARD JR: Importance of cystourethrography in neonates with imperforate anus. Urology 13:607, 1979
11. PUCHNER PJ, SANTULLI TV, LATIMER JK: Urologic problems associated with imperforate anus. Urology 6:205, 1975
12. RICKWOOD AMK, SPITZ L: Primary vesicoureteral reflux

in neonates with imperforate anus. Arch Dis Child 55.149, 1980

13. SANTULLI TV: Malformation of the anus and rectum. In Mustard WT, Ravitch MM, Synder WH, Jr et al (eds): Pediatric Surgery, 2nd ed, p 983. Chicago, Year Book Medical Publishers, 1969

14. SANTULLI TV, KIESEWETTER WB, BILL AH, JR: Anorectal anomalies: A suggested international classification. J Peditr Surg 5:281, 1970

15. SANTULLI TV, SCHULLINGER JN, KIESEWETTER WB et al: Imperforate anus: A survey from the members of the surgical section of the American Academy of Pediatrics. J Pediatr Surg 6:484, 1971

16. SMITH ED: Urinary anomalies and complications in imperforate anus and rectum. J Pediatr Surg 3:337, 1968

17. STEPHENS FD: Congenital malformations of the Rectum, Anus and Genitourinary Tracts. Edinburgh; London, Livingstone, 1963

18. STEPHENS FD, SMITH ED: Anorectal Malformations in Children, p 334. Chicago, Year Book Medical Publishers, 1971

19. SWENSON O, DONNELLAN WL: Imperforate anus. In Swenson O (ed): Pediatric Surgery, vol. 2, 3rd ed, p 948. New York, Appleton-Century-Crofts, 1969

20. TANK ES, LINDENAUER SM: Principles of management of exstrophy of the cloaca. Am J Surg 119:95, 1970

21. TANK ES, WATTS H: Hyperchloremic acidosis from urethrorectal fistula and imperforate anus. Surgery 63:837, 1968

22. WELCH KJ: Cloacal exstrophy. In Ravitch MM, Welch KJ, Benson CD et al (eds): Pediatric Surgery, p 802. Chicago, Year Book Medical Publishers, 1979

23. WILLIAMS DL, GRANT J: Urological complications of imperforate anus. Br J Urol 41:660, 1969

24. WILLIAMS DL, NIXON HH: Agenesis of the sacrum. Surg Gynecol Obstet 105:84, 1957

Ambiguous Genitalia

99

R. Lawrence Kroovand

Is it a girl or a boy? This simple question is the first to be asked by parents, yet, when the genitalia are ambiguous, it is most difficult to answer. Ambiguity of the external genitalia presents an urgent problem that must be treated as a medical and social emergency requiring a thoughtful and systematic approach. Of the many complex management decisions that are essential in the evaluation and management of these infants and their families, the most important is the appropriate choice of gender as soon as possible after birth. Undue procrastination, a temporary choice, or inappropriate gender assignment at birth are unacceptable and may lead to disturbances in psychosexual development and lifetime repercussions for both family and child.

This chapter summarizes the important aspects of the embryology of sexual differentiation as they relate to an understanding of the classification and management of children with ambiguous genitalia. It includes the indications and techniques for surgical correction of these disorders, including the creation of a vulva for the male pseudohermaphrodite with phallic inadequacy. It does not discuss those conditions in which phenotypic sex is firmly established (*e.g.,* Klinefelter's syndrome or Turner's syndrome). Chapter 100, Adrenogenital Syndrome, emphasizes reconstructive techniques appropriate for feminizing the female pseudohermaphrodite, using girls with congenital virilizing adrenogenital syndrome as the prototype.

Normal Sexual Differentiation

Normal sexual differentiation results from an orderly sequence of changes occurring at three levels: differentiation of the gonad from the genital ridge, the development of the internal genital ducts from the mesonephric (wolffian) and paramesonephric ducts (müllerian), and the formation of the external genitalia. To appreciate the pathophysiology of disordered sexual differentiation, one must first have a clear understanding of the progression of normal sexual differentiation. Chromosomal factors direct the development of the primordial gonad either into a testis or into an ovary. Differentiation of the internal duct structures and external genitalia is completed under the stimulus of hormones from the fetal testis.

THE GONAD

At 3 weeks to 5 weeks after conception the gonads in both male and female fetuses are bipotential. Primordial germ cells migrate from the yolk sac to the urogenital ridge where male germ cells take up a medullary position and female germ cells, a cortical position. The chromosomal sex of the fetus directs development of the gonad into either a testis or an ovary.[13,14] Gonadal differentiation occurs independently in each of the paired genital ridges and is a function of the presence or absence of the information carried on the Y chromosome.

For development of a testis, factors located on the Y chromosome, on the X chromosome, and possibly on the autosomal chromosomes are necessary.[28] The most important of these factors is H–Y antigen, a cell-surface antigen presumably from the short arm of the Y chromosome near the centromere.[4,5,17] Testicular differentiation occurs when H–Y antigen interacts with somatic cell receptors on the genital ridge causing the medullary cords to differentiate into seminiferous tubules; the cortex regresses.[22] In the absence of a Y chromosome (and therefore H–Y antigen) and in the presence of two X chromosomes, ovarian differentiation occurs at 11 weeks to 12 weeks after conception, with proliferation of the cortex and regression of the medulla.

Chromosomal translocations involving the short arm of the Y chromosome can occur, resulting in XX males or XX true hermaphrodites without an evident Y chromosome, who are H–Y antigen positive.[27]

INTERNAL GENITAL DUCTS

At 7 weeks to 8 weeks after conception and prior to genital duct differentiation, two sets of paired primordial duct systems are present in both male and female fetuses: the mesonephric and the paramesonephric ducts. In the male, development of the internal ducts is induced by hormonal action. Sertoli cells of the seminiferous tubules of the fetal testis produce a nonsteroidal hormone called müllerian inhibiting substance (MIS) —a specific fetal regressor glycoprotein—which acts locally to cause regression of the paramesonephric ducts.[4,12] Slightly later, testosterone secreted by the Leydig cells of the fetal testis acts locally causing the mesonephric ducts to differentiate into the epididymis, vas deferens, and seminal vesicles.[26] If secretion of MIS is impaired or absent, paramesonephric regression is incomplete or does not occur, and to varying degrees a fallopian tube, a hemiuterus or uterus, and a vagina may develop on the side of the testis.

In the female the paramesonephric ducts persist, differentiating into the fallopian tubes, uterus, cervix, and upper vagina. The mesonephric ducts regress. These changes do not depend on gonadal stimulation and, therefore, in the absence of a gonad, paramesonephric differentiation similarly occurs.

EXTERNAL GENITALIA

Differentiation of the external genitalia occurs during the 7th through 16th weeks after conception. Prior to this time the genitalia of both sexes are bipotential, consisting of a genital tubercle, urethral folds, genital swellings, and the urogenital sinus (Fig. 99-1). In the male, virilization of the genital tubercle, fusion of the urethral folds, and scrotalization of the genital swellings are dependent upon circulation of fetal testosterone and its conversion to its active form 5-dihydrotestosterone by 5-alpha reductase, an enzyme that is present in the cells of the external genitalia and the urogenital sinus. The urethral folds fuse to encompass the anterior urethra, and the genital swellings migrate dorsally and fuse to form the scrotum. The prostate develops from the urogenital sinus. In the female and in the absence of androgen influence, the genital tubercle forms the clitoris, the urethral folds form the labia minora, and the genital swellings form the labia majora. The lower vagina arises from the urogenital sinus. With absent or deficient 5-alpha reductase or with abnormal androgen-receptor binding or action, the differentiating external genitalia either develop along female lines to form the clitoris, labia minora and majora, and the lower vagina or varying degrees of incomplete virilization may occur.[3]

In correlating normal sexual development with the clinical presentations that occur with genital ambiguity, certain concepts are important and are summarized as follows:

1. Initially the gonad is bipotential in all fetuses.
2. Initially both mesonephric and paramesonephric ducts are present in all fetuses.
3. Virilization of the internal ducts requires specific direction involving H–Y antigen and testosterone. This expression of a male direction is local in influence and may be unilateral in expression.
4. External genital development along a female line is autonomous, occurs in the absence of H–Y antigen or androgen, and does not require the presence of an ovary. The exact role of the ovary in development is unclear but appears to be negligible.
5. Masculinization of the external genitalia can occur in the presence of endogenous or exogenous androgen and requires conversion of testosterone to 5-dihydrotestosterone as the active form plus normal receptor activity.

Classification of Ambiguous Genitalia

Any alteration of the orderly process of sexual differentiation may result in genital ambiguity. The three most common causes of ambiguous genitalia are the following: chromosomal anomalies that result in abnormal gonadal differentiation (true hermaphroditism, mixed gonadal dysgenesis); excessive androgen production in a genetic female resulting in virilization of the external genitalia (female pseudohermaphroditism), and defective androgen production or action in a genetic male resulting in incomplete virilization or feminization of the external genitalia (male pseudohermaphroditism).[6]

This section considers the four categories into which ambiguous genitalia in the neonate are classified: true hermaphroditism, mixed gonadal dysgenesis, female pseudohermaphroditism, and male pseudohermaphroditism (Fig. 99-2).[2]

TRUE HERMAPHRODITISM

True hermaphroditism, in which both ovarian and testicular tissues are present, is a rare cause of ambiguous genitalia in newborn infants. These infants may have a testis on one side and an ovary on the other (lateral type), a unilateral ovotestis in

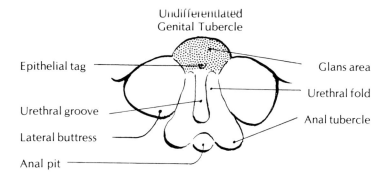

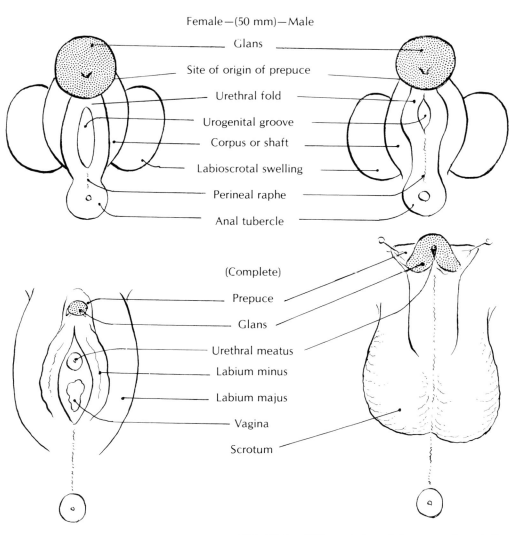

FIG. 99-1. Differentiation of the external genitalia.

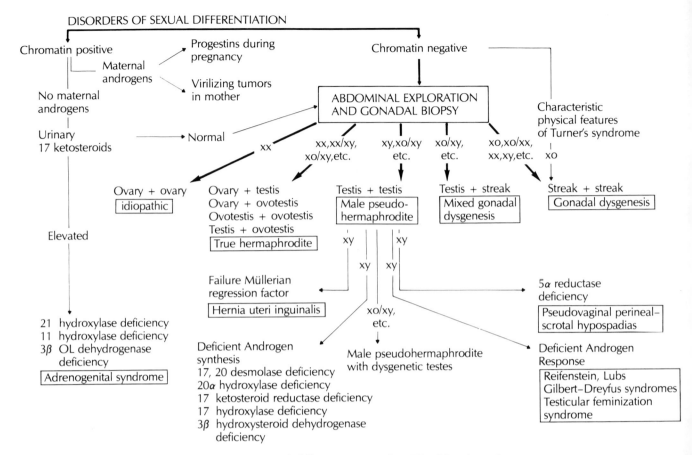

FIG. 99-2. Flow sheet depicts disorders of sexual differentiation. (Allen TD: Disorders of sexual differentiation. Urology (Suppl) 7:1, 1976)

combination with an ovary or testis (unilateral type), or bilateral ovotestes (bilateral type). In most true hermaphrodites a uterus is present. On each side the genital duct tends to conform to the sex of the ipsilateral gonad: a fallopian tube on the side of an ovotestis or ovary and a vas deferens on the side of a testicle. Virilization of the external genitalia in the true hermaphrodite is quite variable, although most have a large phallus with chordee and varying degrees of labioscrotal fusion; three fourths of these infants have been assigned a male gender because of phallic size. Gonadal tissue is often palpable in the labioscrotal fold or groin on one or both sides and most often represents testicular tissue, although ovotestes or ovaries may descend into the labioscrotal folds.

Even though the majority of true hermaphrodites have a 46XX karyotype, most are H–Y antigen positive, indicating the presence of Y chromosomal material.[8,28] Fertility is unusual, but pregnancy has been reported.[15]

MIXED GONADAL DYSGENESIS

Mixed gonadal dysgenesis (MGD) is second only to congenital adrenal hyperplasia as a cause of ambiguous genitalia in the neonate. Infants with MGD usually have a streak gonad on one side and a testis on the other.[5] All have an infantile uterus, cervix, and at least one fallopian tube; mesonephric duct structures may be present on the side of the testis. All patients with MGD are chromatin negative; most have a mosaic karyotype, 46XX/46XY. The appearance of the external genitalia is quite variable; however, most are poorly virilized and therefore raised as females.[15] Untreated, most tend to virilize at puberty. Although some have a phallus adequate for reconstruction, short adult stature is the rule in these children, with the height rarely above 148 cm; therefore, when a male gender assignment is considered, this outcome should be kept in mind. Because of a great tendency for malignant degeneration of the gonadal tissue, occasionally in early childhood (gonadoblastoma in the testis and seminoma–dysgerminoma in the streak gonad), early gonadectomy is usually recommended.[1]

FEMALE PSEUDOHERMAPHRODITISM

Female pseudohermaphroditism results when a chromatin positive 46XX female fetus is exposed to endogenous or exogenous androgen *in utero.* The most common etiology for female pseudohermaphroditism is congenital adrenal hyperplasia (CAH), which accounts for more than 60% of children with ambiguous genitalia.[23] This autosomal recessive condition, called the *adrenogenital syndrome,* is associated with a deficiency of one of several adrenal enzymes required for cortisol synthesis. As a result, excessive levels of precursors of cortisol with androgenic effects are produced, resulting in virilization of the external genitalia.

Adrenal differentiation occurs at 8 weeks to 10 weeks after conception, well after the paramesonephric ducts differentiate but during the time of urogenital sinus differentiation. It produces a varying degree of urogenital sinus fusion, hypoplasia of the lower vagina, and clitoromegaly. Also, because there is no testis there is neither MIS nor a local testosterone to affect the internal ducts, the mesonephric ducts regress. The extent of virilization of the external genitalia depends upon the stage of development at the time of androgen exposure. Because of the normal internal genital structures, girls with CAH should be raised as females with feminization of the external genitalia, as discussed in the following chapter.

MALE PSEUDOHERMAPHRODITISM

Male pseudohermaphrodites are genetic males with testis tissue and incomplete virilization of the external genitalia. This may be the result of deficient testosterone synthesis, a 5-alpha reductase deficiency, or an abnormal androgen receptor binding in the target tissues. Cryptorchism and defective paramesonephric duct regression may also be associated with some forms of male pseudohermaphroditism.

Deficient testosterone synthesis is an unusual cause for male pseudohermaphroditism. Defective testosterone action may result in the testicular feminization syndrome (TFS) or pseudovaginal perineoscrotal hypospadias (PPH).[29] TFS presents the appearance of a phenotypically normal female with short or absent vagina. TFS is caused by deficient androgen receptor binding and is diagnosed at puberty when amenorrhea is investigated or earlier at the time of inguinal hernia repair. PPH is associated with a 5-alpha reductase deficiency. The interested reader is referred to the literature for more information. Defective paramesonephric duct regression (hernia uteri inguinale) is a condition in which phenotypic males, usually with cryptorchism, are found to have a rudimentary uterus and fallopian tubes with variable development of the vasa differentia.

Owing to similar diagnostic and therapeutic considerations, several additional disorders of sexual differentiation in genetic males with normal gonads and diminutive or ambiguous genitalia are included here under male pseudohermaphroditism (*i.e.,* micropenis and penile agenesis). Those genetic males with severe exstrophy of the bladder and an extremely small epispadiac penis and those with cloacal exstrophy and a hypoplastic bifid penis generally should be considered for a female gender assignment and should be feminized appropriately.[6]

Differential Diagnosis and Gender Assignment

Because of the serious psychosocial consequences that can result if the sex of rearing is changed after age 18 months, it is very important to assign the proper sex of rearing as soon after birth as possible.[24] A multidisciplinary approach, typically including a pediatrician or neonatologist, a psychiatrist, an endocrinologist, and a reconstructive surgeon, is required not only in arriving at the diagnosis and the proper gender assignment but also in developing an appropriate plan of management.[30]

As part of the initial discussion with the family of a child born with ambiguous genitalia, the family should be told that the external genitalia are underdeveloped or incompletely formed and that further tests are necessary to establish the sex and the direction for future development. The assigning of a neuter name for the child should be avoided because this admits ambivalence and casts doubt on the final decision that is made. Gender choice should be based on the infant's anatomy and not on the chromosomal karyotype or the prospects for fertility, except for girls with CAH whose functional potential is unimpaired regardless of the severity of virilization. Because it is easier to construct a vagina than a satisfactory penis, only those infants with a phallus of adequate size should be considered for a male gender assignment.

TABLE 99-1. Evaluation of the Neonate with Ambiguous Genitalia

| Diagnosis | Buccal Smear | | Karyotype | H–Y antigen | Paramesonephric ducts |
	BARR BODY	FLUORESCENT Y STAINING			
Female pseudohermaphroditism	+	−	46XX	−	+
True hermaphroditism	±	±	46XX + mosaics	+	±
Male pseudohermaphroditism	−	+	46XY	+	−
Mixed gonadal dysgenesis	−	+	45XY/XO	+	+
			46XY	+	+

Evaluation of the newborn with ambiguous genitalia should include a careful history and physical examination. A history of an unexplained infant death in the neonatal period, of maternal ingestion of potentially androgenic substances during pregnancy, or of a family history of maternal aunts with sterility, amenorrhea, or an inguinal hernia containing a gonad may provide the diagnosis.

Physical examination of the infant should record the symmetry or asymmetry of the gonads, the presence of gonads and their position above or below the external inguinal ring, the presence of an epididymis on the gonad, a bifid scrotum, scrotal rugosity, hyperpigmentation of the labioscrotal folds, hypospadias, chordee, a midline uterus or rectal examination, or the presence of vaginal epithelial cells with estrogen effect on smear of the urethral discharge produced after massage of the neonatal uterus and vagina during rectal examination.

Diagnostically a buccal smear for Barr bodies and fluorescent Y staining, measurement of the H–Y antigen, a karyotype, biochemical evaluation for ketosteroid excretion, and contrast studies of the urogenital sinus to demonstrate a vagina attached to the urogenital sinus should be done.[6] Pelvic ultrasound may demonstrate a corpus uteri; endoscopy may show a small vagina or a narrow vaginal attachment to the urogenital sinus not filled by genitography. Laparoscopy and gonadal biopsy also may be indicated. A flow sheet to the differential diagnosis of disorders of sexual differentiation is shown in Figure 99-2.[2]

An important early laboratory test in the differential diagnosis of genital ambiguity is the buccal smear for Barr bodies. Based on the presence (chromatin positive) or absence (chromatin negative) of Barr bodies and the presence or absence of fluorescent Y staining, the four major conditions most commonly causing ambiguous genitalia at birth—female pseudohermaphroditism, true hermaphroditism, male pseudohermaphroditism, and mixed gonadal dysgenesis—can be identified (Table 99-1).

The chromatin positive infant with ambiguous genitalia is either a female pseudohermaphrodite or a true hermaphrodite. Female pseudohermaphrodites are chromatin positive (Barr body present), have a karyotype of 46XX, and are fluorescent Y negative and also H–Y antigen negative. Paramesonephric duct structures are always present and the urinary 17-ketosteroid and pregnanetriol excretions are elevated in those girls with CAH.

Most infants with true hermaphroditism (80%) are chromatin positive and generally have a karyotype of 46XX, although all are H–Y antigen positive; paramesonephric duct structures are usually present on at least one side. The 17-ketosteroid and pregnanetriol excretion are usually normal (not elevated).

With a chromatin negative buccal smear and ambiguous genitalia, the infant is either a male pseudohermaphrodite or has mixed gonadal dysgenesis. Male pseudohermaphroditism results from insufficient androgen synthesis or action; here the karyotype is 46XY and no paramesonephric duct structures are present. In mixed gonadal dysgenesis the karyotype is a mosaic 45XO/46XY, and paramesonephric duct structures are always present on the side of the streak gonad; mesonephric structures may be present on the side of the testis. Differentiation between male pseudohermaphroditism and mixed gonadal dysgenesis may require laparotomy and gonadal biopsy.

The current role of laparotomy in the management of the neonate with ambiguous genitalia is controversial. Laparotomy in the neonatal period should be done only if gonadal biopsy would influence the sex of rearing, as with true hermaphrodites or the infant with mixed gonadal dysgenesis in whom early gonadectomy is usually indicated. With recent advances in the diagnostic accuracy of ultrasonography, neonatal laparotomy may become unnecessary, and laparectomy and gonadectomy may be deferred until later in infancy when anesthetic and surgical considerations are less critical.[11] At the time of laparotomy all structures contrary to the assigned sex should be removed.

Management

FEMALE PSEUDOHERMAPHRODITISM

The management of the female pseudohermaphrodite and the feminization of her external genitalia are discussed in the following chapter, Adrenogenital Syndrome.

TRUE HERMAPHRODITISM

The true hermaphrodite with an inadequate phallus should be raised as a female. Although laparotomy is unnecessary during the newborn period, it is required sometime in early childhood to remove any testicular tissue that is present. For the true hermaphrodite with both a well-developed phallus and a vagina, gender assignment should be based upon the findings at laparotomy. Fertility may be possible in some of these children when they are raised as females.[15] However, it should be emphasized again that fertility and, for that matter, hormonal function should not be a consideration in gender assignment, except for the virilized female pseudohermaphrodite with adrenogenital syndrome.

The child with paramesonephric duct structures, a normal ovary on one side, and either a testis or ovotestis on the contralateral side should be raised as a female and the testis or ovotestis, removed. Further feminization may be done at a later time using the techniques described in Chapter 100. If there is an inadequate phallus and a testis that can be placed into the scrotum, the child might be raised as a male and the contradictory gonadal and paramesonephric structures, removed. Later, hypospadias repair and scrotoplasty using standard techniques should complete the masculinization.

MIXED GONADAL DYSGENESIS

In managing the infant with mixed gonadal dysgenesis, five factors favoring a female role must be considered when making a gender assignment:

1. The phallus is usually inadequately masculinized and a uterus and vagina are always present.
2. Short stature is the rule; approximately half of the patients will be shorter than 148 cm.
3. Even if the phallus appears adequate, the degree of development at puberty usually correlates well with phallic size at birth, Thus, the ultimate stature in terms of both genital and physical size is generally less than the mean and may pose serious psychological problems.
4. Although fertility is not a consideration, the testes are dysgenetic and lack germinal elements.
5. Malignant gonadal tumors—seminomas and gonadoblastomas—may develop in up to 20% of patients with mixed gonadal dysgenesis, often prior to puberty.[5]

Thus, most infants with mixed gonadal dysgenesis are best raised as females and should undergo early laparotomy and bilateral gonadectomy and feminization of their external genitalia. Later hormonal replacement and vaginal construction will complete feminization.

MALE PSEUDOHERMAPHRODITES

Male pseudohermaphrodites include those with testicular feminization syndrome, pseudovaginal perineoscrotal hypospadias, and isolated microphallus. Also listed here, because the decisional and surgical considerations are similar, are phenotypic males with penile agenesis, severe exstrophy of the urinary bladder, and cloacal exstrophy. Because of the uncertain potential for phallic growth at puberty, gender assignment in the male pseudohermaphrodite is often difficult. Generally the degree of phallic size at birth correlates well with the degree of growth achievable at puberty, thus gender assignment should be based on the phenotypic appearance of the external genitalia at birth. Prospects for fertility should not influence gender assignment since most male pseudohermaphrodites are infertile, even if raised as males.[8]

Testicular Feminization

These phenotypically normal females are diagnosed in adolescence or early adulthood, when primary amenorrhea or infertility are investigated, or occasionally at an earlier age, upon discovery of a testicle in an inguinal hernia or in the labia majora. Despite the presence of testes, these children undergo excellent feminization at puberty. Gonadectomy should be done once puberty is complete, because the potential for development

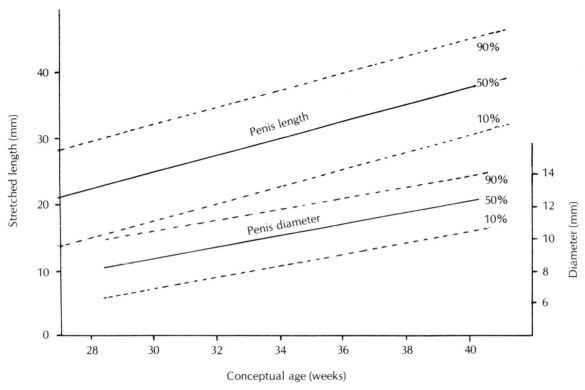

FIG. 99-3. Chart shows fetal phallic growth and penile standards for newborn male infants. (Feldman KW, Smith DW: Fetal phallic and penile standards for newborn male infants. J Pediatrics 80:395, 1975)

of malignant gonadal tumors, usually seminomas, after age 14 is great. Gonadectomy at the time of herniorraphy rather than at a later time may avoid the possible psychological consequences of this type of surgery in adolescence; it also avoids the risk that these patients might refuse gonadectomy or learn of their gonadal sex in a nontherapeutic setting. However, many experts feel that gonadectomy should be delayed until spontaneous puberty is complete. Estrogen replacement then induces normal pubertal changes and maintains feminization. If the vagina is too short after puberty, it may be augmented from either a skin graft or an isolated segment of sigmoid colon. Vaginal augmentation or construction is discussed in Chapter 101, Transsexual Surgery.

Pseudovaginal Perineoscrotal Hypospadias

In PPH there is typically a severe perineoscrotal hypospadias with a urethral opening at the base of the phallus and a blind vaginal pouch. The testes and mesonephric derivatives are normal. Because of the extreme severity of the genital ambiguity, most children with PPH should be raised as females and gonadectomy should be done prior to puberty to prevent virilization that otherwise would occur at puberty. Estrogen replacement is indicated to induce appropriate feminization. If virilization has occurred prior to gonadectomy, reduction clitoroplasty and vaginoplasty can correct the virilization, as discussed in the following chapter. In those raised as males, hypospadias repair should be done using standard techniques, as described in Chapter 76, combined with excision of the vaginal pouch.

Isolated Micropenis

Micropenis, a disorder of uncertain etiology, is probably related either to inadequate testosterone production or to utilization. It is defined as a penis in an otherwise normal newborn term male with a stretched length well below the 10th decile but otherwise normally developed (2.5 cm in length or less).[19] Figures 99-3 and 99-4 show the normal range of penile size for premature and term infants and young children.[7,25]

Because of an unknown growth potential, the newborn with micropenis presents a particular

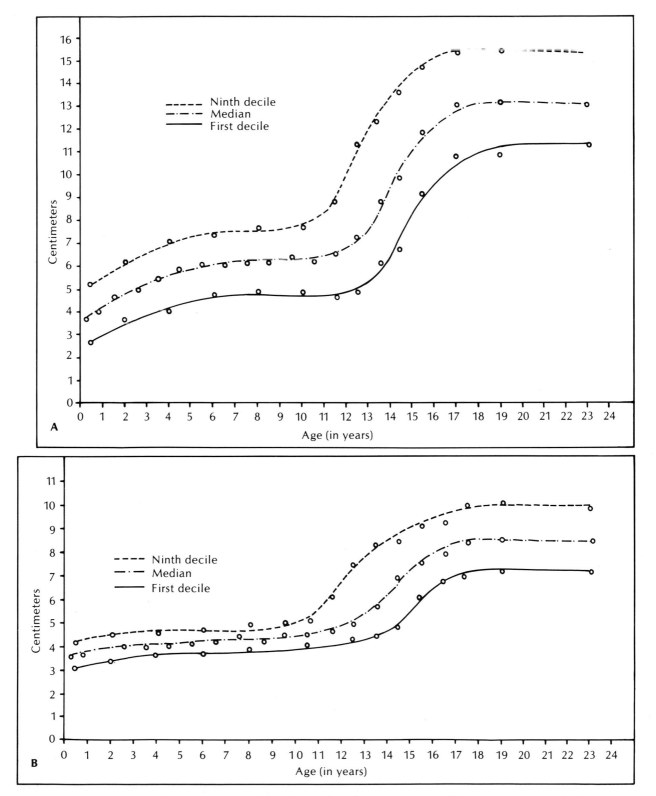

FIG. 99-4. Normal penile size from birth to maturity: **(A)** curve shows growth of the penis in length; **(B)** curve shows growth of the penis in circumference. (Schoenfeld SA, Beebe GW: Hormonal growth and variation in the male genitalia from birth to maturity. J. Urol 48:759, 1942)

problem in clinical decision making, especially when the testes appear to be normal. An extremely small phallus, such as one 1.5 cm in length with no palpable erectile tissue, poses no difficulty. However, a small penis of slightly larger size creates a management dilemma about whether a male gender assignment and repeated courses of testosterone therapy will result in a functionally adequate adult male or gender reversal will offer a more acceptable long-range solution.[16]

To determine if the penis is androgen sensitive, a diagnostic and therapeutic trial of androgen can be considered before making a gender assignment. Either systemic sustained action testosterone (Depo-Testosterone, 25–50 mg IM q 3 weeks for 3 months) or topical testosterone cream (5% testosterone propionate compounded in an aqueous base, applied locally bid for 3 weeks) may induce sufficient penile growth to simplify the decison. The use of injectable testosterone results in more dependable systemic levels and is generally more advisable, except in those with less severe conditions such as severe hypospadias within a small phallus, where the decisions of gender assignment are not in question but phallic enhancement may be beneficial. In those boys with adequate penile growth, a male gender assignment can be made following either topical or systemic testosterone. In the child with extreme microphallus, poor corporal tissue development, and rudimentary testes where there is poor prospect for penile growth, or in those in whom hormonal treatment has had an unsatisfactory response, a female gender reassignment should be made.

Penile Agenesis

In this unusual disorder the penis is absent and the urethra opens in the perineum just anterior to the anus. Associated anomalies of the genitourinary and gastrointestinal systems are frequent and at times are incompatible with life. In those infants who survive, construction of a functional penis is an unrealistic goal; thus, these children are best raised as females with early orchiectomy and later vulvoplasty (creation of a vulva). Hormonal supplementation and vaginal construction will complete feminization.[20]

MANAGEMENT OF THE MALE PSEUDOHERMAPHRODITE WITH AN INADEQUATE PHALLUS

The male pseudohermaphrodite with severe micropenis is the prototype for the description of the surgical approach to genital reconstruction to feminize the external genitalia. The same surgical techniques with minor modification can be applied to those patients with severe hypospadias and micropenis or to those who have suffered traumatic loss of the penis.

For family and social reasons, gender reassignment and the initial surgical procedures preferably should be done during the initial or referral hospitalization or at least by 18 months of age.[21]

The surgical objectives of gender reassignment are as follows:

1. Vulvoplasty including feminization of the perineum, repositioning of the urethral meatus to a feminine location, and clitoroplasty with preservation of sensation
2. Removal of the testes
3. Later construction of a vagina

Vulvoplasty (Fig. 99-5) involves an extended external urethrostomy to exteriorize the penile and bulbar urethra to simulate the mucosal appearance of the vulva (Fig. 99-5A). The extended midline urethrostomy is completed with a Y extension (Fig. 99-5A, *insert*) at the midperineum to permit defatting of the perineal portion of the labia majora, creating a flatter and more feminine contour of the external genitalia (Fig. 99-5B).

V flaps are created from inferolateral preputial or shaft skin and are advanced posteriorly and inferiorly on either side of opened urethra to form labia minora (Fig. 99-5B, *arrows*). This maneuver also pulls the phallus downward, enhancing the appearance of the clitoroplasty.

The inferior V flap of perineal skin can be turned into the deep bulbar urethra to avoid perineal contracture during healing, or, if a small vaginal pouch is present, the V flap can be turned into the vagina at the time of urethral exteriorization (Fig. 99-5C).

The clitoroplasty is usually done at the time of vulvoplasty. The techniques for clitoroplasty are described in Chapter 100.

The testes can be removed by small inguinal incisions. If they are located intra-abdominally, they can be removed by laparotomy.

Construction of a vagina can be accomplished either by use of a split-thickness skin graft or with an isolated segment of sigmoid colon, as described in Chapter 101, but it usually should not be attempted prior to puberty and only after full growth has been attained.[20] This procedure normally is not done by the urologist.

In the male with micropenis who has been inappropriately assigned a male gender role or

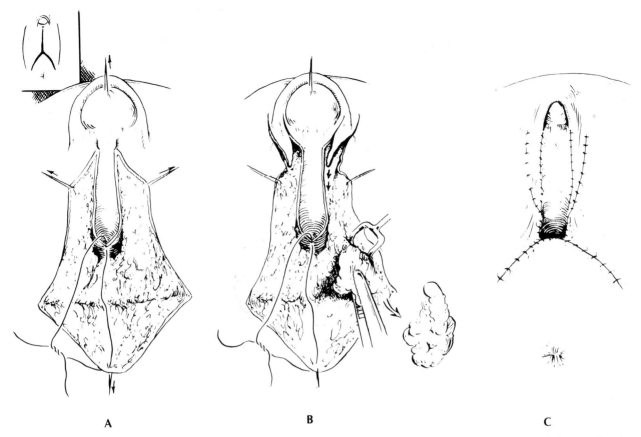

A   B   C

FIG. 99-5.   Technique for vulvoplasty (creation of a vulva) in the male pseudohermaphrodite with ambiguous genitalia or micropenis: **(A)** a midline extended urethrostomy with Y extension in the perineum (*insert*) to exteriorize the dorsal urethral mucosa that simulates the mucosa of the vestibule; **(B)** defatting of the lateral flaps to flatten and further feminize the contour of the labia majora; V-flaps created from the lateral prepuce (*arrows*) at the base of the phallus are advanced posteriorly on either side of the vestibule to create the labia minora. This also pulls the phallus downward, enhancing clitoroplasty. **(C)** Complete repair. The inferior V-flap from the Y extension of the extended urethroplasty may be turned into the deep bulbar urethra or into the vaginal pouch, when present.

who is diagnosed after infancy when gender reassignment is inappropriate, surgical improvement in the appearance of the small penis may be beneficial. Apparent penile length may be enhanced by defatting of the mons pubis as diagramed in Figure 99-6.

A small transverse incision is made above the penis, and the fatty subcutaneous tissue around the base of the penis and over the mons is excised (Fig. 99-6B). The remaining dermal layer is sutured carefully to the periosteum of the pubis to fix this skin in place and to reduce the chances of seroma formation (Fig. 99-6C). A bulky compression dressing and catheter drainage for several days postoperative is advisable.

Circumcision generally should be delayed be-

yond infancy because this skin may be required during later reconstructive surgery. Further, the redundant prepuce contributes to visual penile size.

Hinman has described a two-stage technique to increase the apparent size of the penis (Fig. 99-7).[10] In the first stage the shaft of the penis is lengthened and buried in the scrotum; in the second stage the penile shaft is freed from the scrotum.

A traction suture is placed through the glans penis and a circumferential incision is made around the base of the penis (Fig. 99-7A), leaving sufficient inner prepuce for later reapproximation with the scrotal skin. The penis, down to Buck's fascia, is mobilized from all surrounding tissues and back

(*Text continues on p. 1040.*)

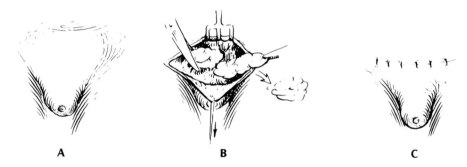

FIG. 99-6. Technique for defatting the mons in the male with micropenis: **(A)** micropenis; **(B)** a transverse incision above the penis permitting defatting of the mons and the base of the penis; **(C)** closure, with suture of the remaining dermal layer to the periosteum fo the pubis and careful skin closure.

FIG. 99-7. Hinman's plastic penile reconstruction in microphallus. **(A)** The first-stage incision is outlined. **(B)** The shaft of the penis is isolated from the surrounding tissue; a subcutaneous tunnel in the scrotum is dissected with scissors. **(C)** The shaft is placed through the scrotal tunnel. **(D)** A broad U-shaped incision is made for the second stage. **(E)** The wound is closed, using beaded sutures. (Hinman F Jr: J Urol 105:901–904. Baltimore, Williams & Wilkins Co., © 1971)

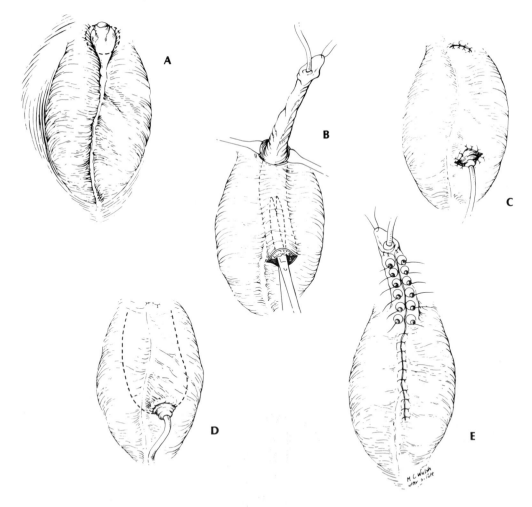

FIG. 99-8.   Glenn and Anderson's correction of penoscrotal transposition: **(A and B)** partial penoscrotal transposition in hypospadias;
(C) transverse incision; **(D)** incision around base of penis; catheter
in hypospadic orifice; **(E)** chordee excised; **(F)** lateral flaps approximated; **(G)** closure. (Glenn JF, Anderson EE: J Urol 110:603–605.
Baltimore, Williams & Wilkins Co, © 1973)

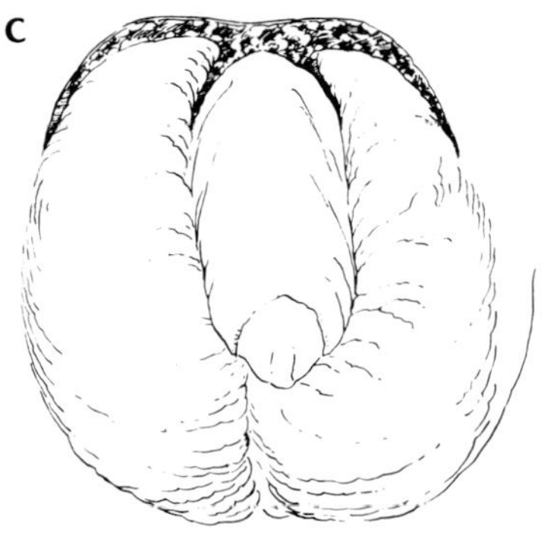

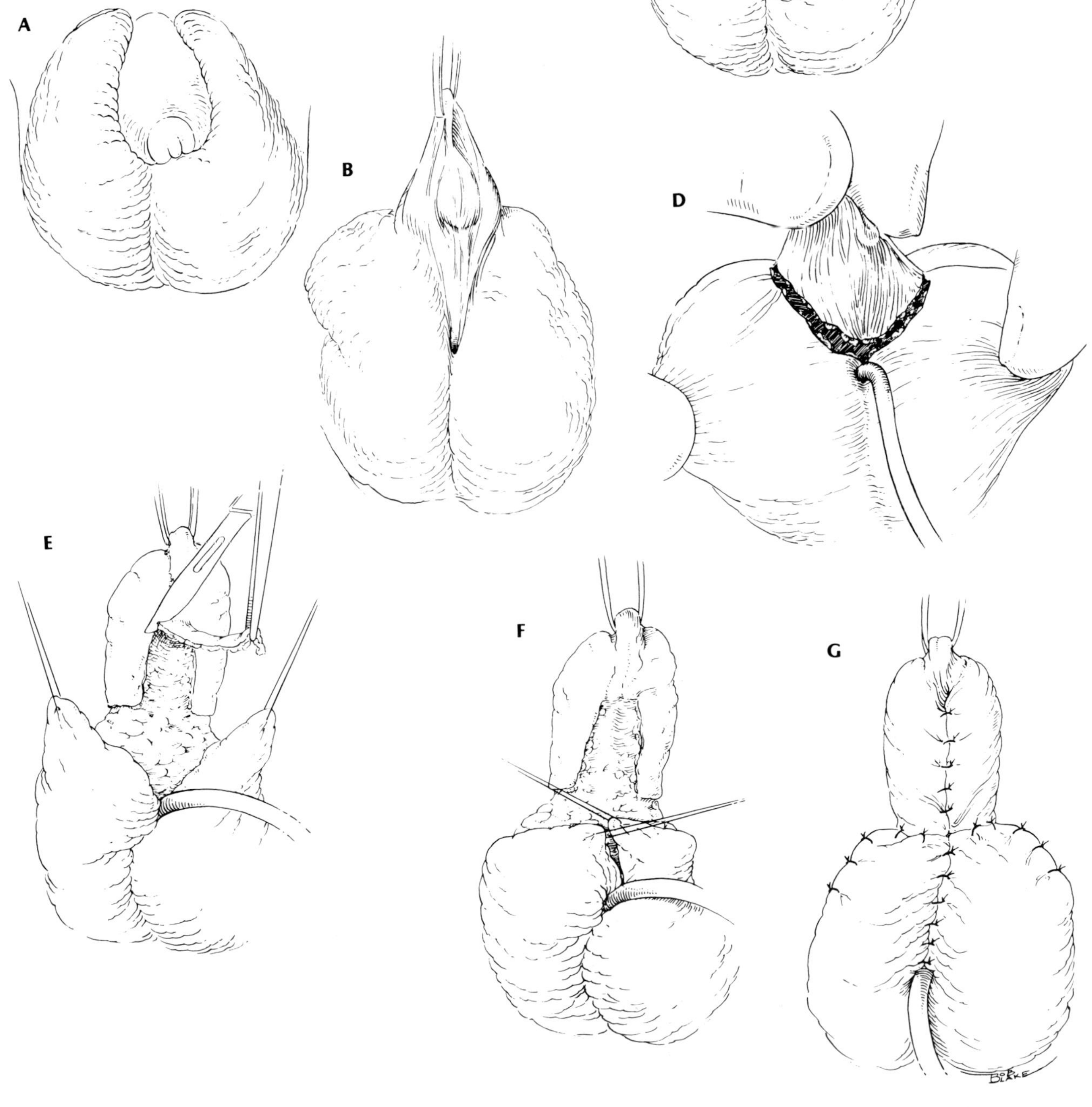

to the bifurcation of the corpora cavernosa. A subcutaneous tunnel of sufficient length to accommodate the penile shaft is made in the scrotum and the penis is drawn through it and sutured to the scrotal skin using fine absorbable suture material (Fig. 99-7C).

Three or four months later, after appropriate healing, the penis is freed from the scrotum. After measuring penile length and computing penile circumference, a generous U-shaped incision providing sufficient tissue for penile shaft coverage is made from the former penile base, and the penis is freed from the scrotum (Fig. 99-7D). The ventral penile skin may be closed with absorbable subcuticular suture material, a removable monofilament suture, or sutures held in place with lead shots. The scrotal skin is best closed with fine absorbable suture material (Fig. 99-7E). At each stage, a

FIG. 99-9. The author's preferred method for correction of penescrotal transposition. A child has penoscrotal transposition **(A)** and severe hypospadias **(B).** **(C)** After correction of the hypospadias, the penis is placed on traction with a suture through the glans. **(D)** The incisions are made on either side of the base of the penis; alternatively, when the penoscrotal transposition is very severe, the skin over the entire dorsum of the penis may be incised and mobilized (*insert*). **(E)** The initial V-incisions are carried ventrally around the entire base of the penis; the scrotal halves are excised for correction of a bifid scrotum, if present. **(F)** Closure is accomplished with midline approximation of the skin edges or, alternatively, with multiple Z-plasties (*insert*). **(G)** Completed repair is shown.

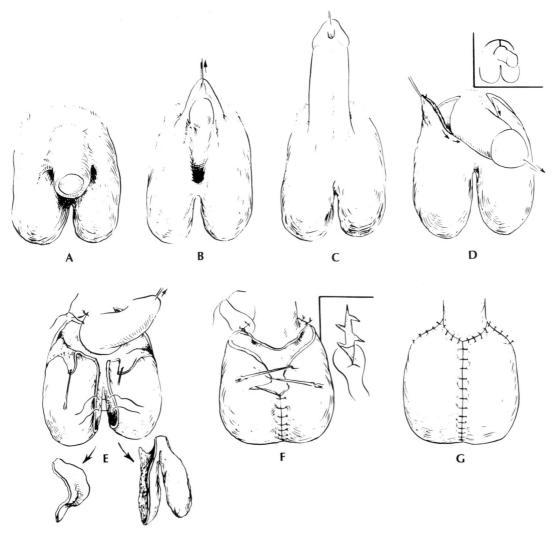

compression dressing and catheter drainage are advisable for several days postoperatively.

PENOSCROTAL TRANSPOSITION

In many boys with micropenis or in those with severe hypospadias and chordee, all or part of the scrotum is located anterior to the penis, partially or totally obscuring the penis from view (Figs. 99-8*A* and 99-9). In addition, the scrotum is frequently bifid (Fig. 99-9*A* and *B*). To correct penoscrotal transposition Glenn and Anderson have described a technique involving lateral mobilization of the malpositioned scrotum and repositioning of the scrotum below the penis (Fig. 99-8).[9] If associated with hypospadias and chordee, the chordee is corrected at the time of scrotoplasty and the hypospadias is corrected later as a planned second stage.[18]

Glenn and Anderson place the child in the lithotomy position, catheterize the bladder, and make a transverse incision across the top of the scrotum (Fig. 99-8*C*), continuing this incision ventrally around the base of the penis (Fig. 99-8*D*). The incision is completed by a midline extension vertically down the median raphe of the scrotum to permit development of lateral flaps (Fig. 99-8*E*). Any fibrous tissue is excised from the ventral surface of the penis, correcting the chordee, if present (Fig. 99-8*E* and *F*). The scrotal flaps are mobilized and brought together in the midline beneath the penis, using several layers of fine absorbable suture material (Fig. 99-8*F* and *G*). A compression dressing and catheter drainage are used for a few days postoperatively. If necessary, a urethroplasty is done as a separate second stage using one of the standard techniques of hypospadias repair, described in Chapter 76, Chordee and Hypospadias.

Glenn and Anderson recommend the initial surgery during the first few weeks or months of life; however, unless the anomaly is very severe and because correction of penoscrotal transposition is usually not an emergency, we prefer to delay surgery until a later time, allowing the infant to grow and lose much of the infantile prepubic fat pad. We also prefer to correct the chordee and hypospadias prior to correction of the penoscrotal transposition. This allows more optimal judgment about the need to correct the transposition and does not interfere with the use of scrotal or shaft skin during the hypospadias repair; after hypospadias repair a less extensive scrotoplasty may be necessary.[18]

Our technique is represented in Figure 99-9. In the child with penoscrotal transposition and severe hypospadias, the penile abnormality (chordee and hypospadias) is usually corrected in a planned two-staged procedure leaving the penoscrotal transposition and correction of the bifid scrotum, if present, as part of the second stage of the hypospadias repair.[18] If necessary, a planned third operative procedure can be performed.

For correction of the penoscrotal transposition the child is placed in the frog-leg position on the operating table with a folded towel under the buttocks. The penis is placed on traction with a suture through the glans (Fig. 99-9*C*). A V-shaped incision is made on either side of the base of the penis at the abdominal wall, leaving a bridge of midline dorsal skin intact (Fig. 99-9*D*). Alternately, for more severe anomalies the skin on the entire dorsum of the penis may be incised and mobilized for placement ventrad to the shaft of the penis (Fig. 99-9*D*, *insert*). The initial incision is carried ventrally around the penis (Fig. 99-9*E*), and closure is done in two layers using fine absorbable suture material (Fig. 99-9*G*).

If a bifid scrotum is part of the anomaly and requires correction, the midportions of the scrotal halves are excised when the scrota are redundant, and closure is done in layers as diagramed (Fig. 99-9*G*). Alternately, multiple small Z plasties may be done to assist in scrotal closure (Fig. 99-9*F*, *insert*).

REFERENCES

1. AARSKOG D: Clinical and cytogenetic studies of hypospadias. Acta Paediatr Scand (Suppl) 203:7, 1970
2. ALLEN TD: Disorders of sexual differentiation. Urology (Suppl 4) 7:24, 1976
3. BENGMARK S, FORSBERG JG: On the development of the rat vagina. Acta Anat (Basel) 37:106, 1959
4. BLANCHARD MD, JOSSO N: Source of the anti-mullerian hormone synthesized by the fetal testis: Mullerian-inhibiting activity of fetal bovine Sertoli cells in tissue culture. Pediatr Res 8:968, 1974
5. DAVIDOFF F, FEDERMAN DD: Mixed gonadal dysgenesis. Pediatrics 52:725, 1973
6. FEDERMAN DD: Abnormal Sexual Development: A Genetic and Endocrine Approach to Differential Diagnosis. Philadelphia, WB Saunders, 1968
7. FELDMAN KW, SMITH DW: Fatal phallic growth and penile standards for newborn male infants. J Pediatr 80:395, 1975
8. GLASSBERG KI: Gender assignment in newborn male pseudohermaphrodites. Urol Clin North Am 7:409, 1980
9. GLENN JF, ANDERSON EE: Surgical correction of penoscrotal transposition. J Urol 110:603, 1973

10. HINMAN F: Surgical management of microphallus. J Urol 105:901, 1971

11. HALLER JO, SCHNEIDER M, KASSNER EG et al: Ultrasonography in pediatric gynecology and obstetrics. American Journal of Roentgenography 128:423, 1977

12. JOSSO N: Interspecific character of mullerian inhibiting substance: Action of the human fetal testis, ovary, and adrenal on the fetal rat. J Clin Endocrinol Metab 32:404, 1971

13. JOST A: Problems of fetal endocrinology: The gonadal and hypophyseal hormones. Recent Prog Horm Res 8:379, 1953

14. JOST A, VIGIER B, PREPIN J et al: Studies sex differentiation in mammals. Recent Prog Horm Res 29:1, 1973

15. KIM MH, GUMPEL JA, GRUFF P: Pregnancy in a true hermaphrodite. Obstet Gynecol 53: (Suppl):415, 1979

16. KOGAN SJ: Micropenis: Etiologic and management considerations. In Kogan SJ, Hafez ES (eds): Clinics in Andrology—Pediatric Andrology. Boston, Martinus Nijhoff, 1981

17. KOO G, WACHTEL S, BREG W et al: Mapping the locus of the H–Y antigen. Birth Defects 12:175, 1976

18. KROOVAND RL, PERLMUTTER AD: Extended urethroplasty in hypospadias: A description and evaluation of a two-stage technique. Urol Clin North Am 7, No. 2:431, 1980

19. LEE PA, MAZUR T, DANISH R et al: Micropenis I: Criteria, etiologies and classification. Johns Hopkins Med J 146:156, 1980

20. MCINDOE A: Treatment of congenital absence and obliterative conditions of the vagina. Br J Plast Surg 2:254, 1950

21. MONEY J, HAMPSON JC, HAMPSON JL: Hermaphroditism; Recommendations concerning assignment of sex, change of sex and psychologic management. Bull Johns Hopkins Hosp 97:284, 1955

22. OHNO S, NAGAI Y, CICCARESE S et al: Testis—Organizing H-Y antigen and the primary sex determining mechanism of mammals. Recent Prog Horm Res 35:449, 1979

23. PERLMUTTER AD: Management of intersexuality. In Harrison, Gittes, Perlmutter (eds): Campbells Urology, 4th ed. Philadelphia, W B Saunders, 1979

24. ROSENFIELD RL, LUCKY AW, ALLEN TD: The diagnosis and management of intersex. In Gluck L (ed): Current Problems in Pediatrics. Chicago, Year Book Medical Publishers, 1980

25. SCHONFELD WA, BEEBE GW: Normal growth and variation in the male genitalia from birth to maturity. J Urol 48:759, 1942

26. SIITERI PK, WILSON JD: Testosterone formation and metabolism during male sexual differentiation in the human embryo. J Clin Endocrinol Metab 38:113, 1974

27. WACHTEL S, KOO GC, BREG W et al: Expression of H-Y antigen in humane males with two Y chromosomes. N Engl J Med 293:1070, 1975

28. WACHTEL S, KOO GC, BREG W et al: Serologic detection of a Y-linked gene in XX males and XX true hermaphrodites. N Engl J Med 295:750, 1976

29. WALSH PC, MADDEN JD, HARROS MS et al: Familial incomplete male pseudohermaphroditism, type 2: Decreased dihydrotestosterone formation in pseudovaginal perineoscrotal hypospadias. N Engl J Med 291:944, 1974

30. WALSH, PC: The differential diagnosis of ambiguous genitalia in the newborn. Symposium in congenital anomalies of the lower genitourinary tract. Urol Clin North Am 5:213, 1978

Adrenogenital Syndrome

100

Alan D. Perlmutter

The most common cause of genital ambiguity in the newborn is the adrenogenital syndrome (AGS), also described as virilizing congenital adrenal hyperplasia (CAH) because not all types of CAH cause virilization of the female fetus. Congenital adrenal hyperplasia is an autosomal recessive, inborn error of metabolism. Although both sexes are affected equally, in the most commonly encountered form, which involves virilization of the female fetus, the males have normal genital development.[5]

Virilizing congenital adrenal hyperplasia is clinically important for three reasons. It is not rare; it is the only other intersex condition besides nonadrenal female pseudohermaphroditism in which both an entirely normal sex role and fertility are usually possible; and it is the only intersex state, unrecognized and untreated, that threatens survival of the infant.[1] Because of the prominence of the adrenogenital syndrome among the causes of intersexuality, a separate chapter is devoted to this condition.[4] The surgical procedures for restoring normal female morphology and sexual function have evolved, in the main, from management of the adrenogenital syndrome, and these techniques can serve as prototypes for the correction of other intersex conditions whenever a female gender assignment has been made.[19]

Pathophysiology

Congenital adrenal hyperplasia is caused by a deficiency in one of the several enzymes necessary for adrenal steroidogenesis. This results in defective cortisol biosynthesis, common to all forms of CAH. As a result, ACTH secretion is elevated and increased levels of various cortisol precursors result. Several forms of CAH with different clinical manifestations have been described, depending upon the particular enzyme defect in the cortisol biosynthetic pathway. For some forms, accumulation of these precursors results in excessive testosterone production and fetal virilization (Fig. 100-1). A recent review of CAH provides excellent and detailed descriptions of its several clinical and biochemical manifestations, beyond the scope of this presentation.[12] This chapter considers only those forms associated with genital ambiguity and likely to be encountered by urologists.

The vast majority of patients (95%) with female virilization from CAH have a 21-hydroxylase deficiency that exists in two forms, mild and severe. In the mild form the enzyme activity is reduced, with a partial decrease in cortisol synthesis; despite virilization, signs of adrenal insufficiency appear only with severe stress. In the severe form the marked deficiency of 21-hydroxylase activity results in greater virilization and greater degrees of cortisol and aldosterone deficiency, with associated salt wasting. The severity of the cortisol deficiency, when untreated, can result in symptoms of marked clinical adrenal insufficiency within 1 week to 2 weeks after birth. These consist of anorexia, vomiting, dehydration, and ultimately circulatory collapse.

With 11-beta-hydroxylase deficiency, by contrast, salt and water retention occur and hypertension can result. Increased secretion of desoxycorticosterone, a sodium retaining steroid, is responsible.

An earlier block in the adrenal steroidal pathways, 3-beta-hydroxysteroid dehydrogenase (3-beta-OL) deficiency results in a deficiency of testosterone as well as of cortisol and aldosterone and is associated with severe salt wasting and a high mortality. Female infants show minimal virilization from increased levels of dehydroepiandrosterone, which is only weakly androgenic. The 3-beta-OL male infants have markedly incomplete virilization with severe hypospadias, cryptorchidism, and bifid scrotum—a form of male pseudohermaphroditism due to inadequate testosterone—because the 3-beta-OL deficiency also involves the Leydig cells of the testis.

Another early block, 17-hydroxylase deficiency, is a rare cause of male genital ambiguity. The other rare forms of CAH are unlikely to be encountered by urologists.

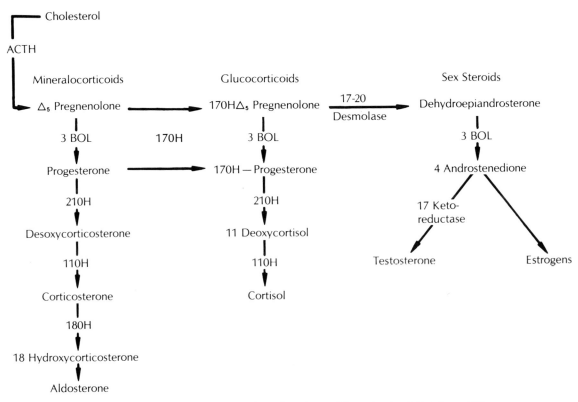

FIG. 100-1. Simplified diagram of pathways for adrenal steroid synthesis. (Mininberg DT, Levine LS, New MI: Current concepts in congential adrenal hyperplasia. Invest Urol 17:169, 1979. Reproduced by permission. Baltimore, Williams & Wilkins Co, © 1979)

EMBRYOLOGY

The embryogenesis of the reproductive tract is reviewed in Chapter 99. In summary, girls with virilizing CAH are genetically normal except for their hereditary adrenal enzyme deficiency; their ovarian and internal (müllerian) ductal development is normal. In the absence of fetal testicular tissue, there is no müllerian inhibiting factor to prevent the paramesonephric ducts from differentiating normally into the fallopian tubes, uterus, and upper vagina; the mesonephric duct appropriately regresses because this event occurs before adrenal function begins. The onset of embryonic adrenal function is during the somewhat later time of urogenital sinus differentiation. The abnormal steroidogenesis provokes a varying degree of urogenital sinus fusion, hypoplasia of the lower vagina, and clitoromegaly.

CLINICAL FEATURES

A family history of other siblings with ambiguous genitalia who died in early infancy or who were diagnosed with CAH is helpful in suspecting the condition. Virilized female neonates can present a spectrum of findings from minimal clitoromegaly and a normal or near-normal appearing vestibule to varying degrees of clitoral hypertrophy and chordee, labial and urogenital sinus fusion, and narrowing of the distal vagina.[1,18] The presence of hyperpigmentation of the genital skin is a clue that the virilization may be due to CAH. In its most extreme degree, virilization associated with salt-losing AGS can in rare cases result in a phallus with the size and configuration of a normal neonatal penis, a glandular urethral meatus, complete labioscrotal fusion with scrotal rugation (but empty of gonads), and a tiny suprasphincteric vaginal opening into the posterior urethra through identifiable prostatic tissue (Fig. 100-2).[19]

Physical examination should include rectal palpation, which will invariably identify a palpable cervix. Radiographic studies are generally unnecessary when CAH is diagnosed with certainty. In cases with severe virilization, ultrasonography can demonstrate the uterus and ovaries and genitography can be helpful in outlining the size and insertion of the lower vagina; the proximal vagina

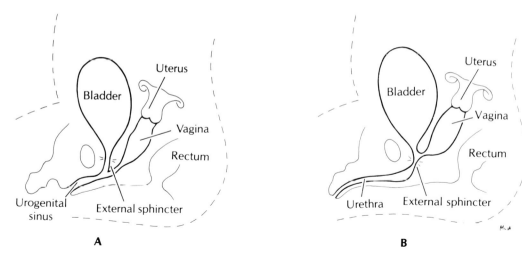

FIG. 100-2. Anatomic variations of the urogenital sinus in girls with adrenogenital syndrome. **(A)** In the most common form, the vagina enters the urogenital sinus distal to the external urethral sphincter. **(B)** The vagina enters the posterior urethra at the site of the verumontanum in a patient with complete phallic urethra. This is a rare type that is present in some patients with complete 21-hydroxylase deficiency (salt losers).

is invariably normal. Endoscopy is helpful mainly in evaluation of the completely virilized girl. Here the lower vagina tapers down to a narrow tract that joins the suprasphincteric urethra in a small punctum, similar to a seminal colliculus and normal utriculus. The vagina often does not fill retrograde by genitography, owing to the small opening. In this situation, intraoperative endoscopy is particularly useful for passage of a ureteral catheter or a Fogarty balloon catheter into the vagina as an aid in dissection.

Laparotomy, although useful for some other forms of intersex diagnosis and management (Chap. 99), has no place in the adrenogenital syndrome because the ovaries and internal reproductive structures are invariably normal, regardless of the severity of external genital virilization.

Laboratory studies for the diagnosis of CAH are described in review articles and in standard pediatric texts; these have included measurements or urinary 17-ketosteroid, 17-hydroxysteroid, and urinary pregnanetriol excretion. A 21-hydroxylase deficiency can now be diagnosed by an elevated serum 17-hydroxyprogesterone level, which can be taken from cord blood. For additional details of laboratory diagnosis and metabolic management, including steroid replacement, the reader should consult the literature.

Surgical Management

For the incompletely masculinized male with rare forms of CAH, management considerations are as outlined in Chapter 99, once the primary condition has been diagnosed and treated. Because the condition in these rare cases is due to androgen insufficiency rather than to insensitivity, one can expect appropriate penile growth with androgen therapy, assuming that the phallus is considered adequate for male gender assignment in the neonatal period.

For typically virilized females with CAH, the surgical considerations are both functional and cosmetic. Establishment of an adequate vaginal inlet will allow sexual intercourse and, because these girls are fertile, it will even allow pregnancy. A reduction clitoroplasty will provide a suitable feminine appearance. The steps involved to achieve these goals are described in the following text. The optimal timing of surgery remains controversial. Arguments exist for initiating reconstruction in infancy, even as early as the neonatal period, but certainly the surgery should be done before the age of 3 or 3½ years, when sexual awareness is appearing.[11]

In favor of surgery in early infancy, correction of conspicuous ambiguity may reduce the parents' anxiety about the infant's sex and ease their acceptance of a female sexual assignment. On the other hand, any corrective surgery in early infancy must be very meticulous, the maximum cosmetic improvement by clitoral reduction may not be realized, the chance of vaginal injury or stenosis is great, and, if done late in the first year at a time of physiologic obesity, the ability to establish the proper vestibular size and appropriate anatomic

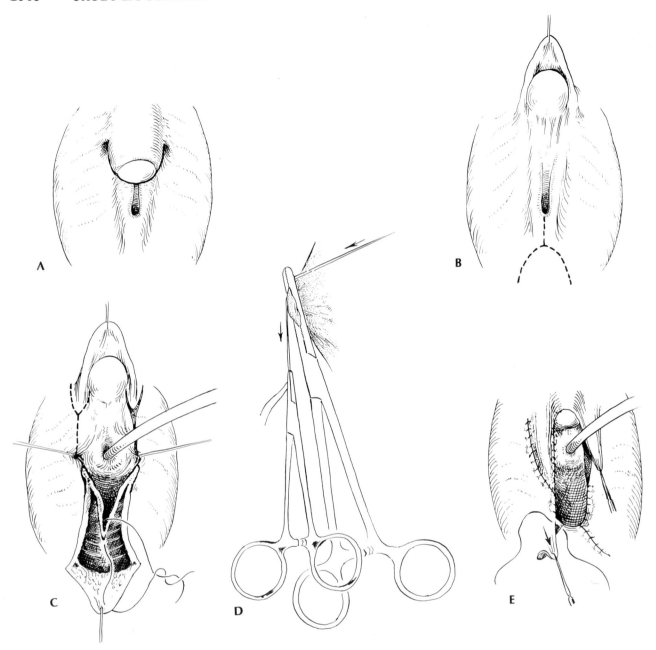

FIG. 100-3.   Technique of flap vaginoplasty: **(A)** preoperative appearance of genitalia; **(B)** outline of skin incisions to open midline planes and to develop short, broad-based U flap; **(C)** posterior wall of congenitally narrow, lower vagina has been exposed. At times it is surrounded by corpus spongiosum that, after division, requires hemostasis by cautery or by oversewing with fine catgut. A midline incision has been made in narrow vaginal segment which should be carried into the wider, thicker, müllerian-derived portion of the vagina, after blunt dissection and exposure of the posterior wall in the midline. This diagram also shows incisions around ventral preputial folds, which will be advanced inferiorly to create labia minora.   **(D)** *Insert* shows use of a heavy clamp on the perineal drape, lateral to the genitalia, as a hook over which traction sutures can be placed to provide lateral traction for symmetrical exposure during dissection and repair.   **(E)** Details of labial advancement and vaginal flap suturing. If labioscrotal skin is redundant, this tissue can be pulled downward as diagramed and trimmed if necessary to flatten the rugae and to give the labia majora a more appropriate appearance.

clitoral–vaginal relationships may be compromised. An alternative is early clitoroplasty with delay of the vaginoplasty until later childhood or even puberty. Although this corrects the gross ambiguity and avoids the risks of a vaginal stricture, it has the disadvantage of a not positioning the clitoris in a known relationship to the remainder of the vulva.

It is my personal preference to perform a vaginoplasty before the clitoroplasty, with plans to complete both steps during the same operation whenever feasible. This allows the clitoral reduction to be accomplished readily in appropriate relation to the vestibular anatomy, even if staged. The reconstruction is easily accomplished at 15 to 18 months of age, although I have been willing to operate in the first 6 months for more severe ambiguity or when parental anxiety requires it. Most parents, however, adjust surprisingly well after working with the intersex team, and are quite willing to delay the surgery until the time recommended as most suitable.

SURGICAL TECHNIQUES

Vaginoplasty

The principles of vaginoplasty include some form of incision of the urogenital sinus to expose the vulva plus an inlay flap of perineal skin to enlarge the outer vaginal barrel.[2,14] For a minimal degree

FIG. 100-4. Techniques of clitoral shaft plication. (**A** and **B**) The Stefan technique of through-and-through plication of the erectile bodies shortens the phallus and limits erectile expansion. A degloving incision behind the glans provides exposure. A 2-0 or 3-0 nonabsorbable suture is used, with the knots placed ventrally. Care is taken dorsally to avoid the neurovascular bundles. When the shaft skin and midline mucosa are reattached, these tissues can be trimmed down as appropriate to avoid redundancy and to establish the appropriate relationship of the glans to the other vestibular structures. Labia minora can also be fashioned as in Fig. 100-7 3 C and E. (**C** and **D**) Glassberg and Laungani use Nesbit's plication technique for shortening the phallus. They also recommend immobilizing the shaft by attaching the dorsal tunica albuginea to the inferior symphyseal periosteum, but if this is done, attempts should be made to identify and avoid the dorsal neurovascular bundles.

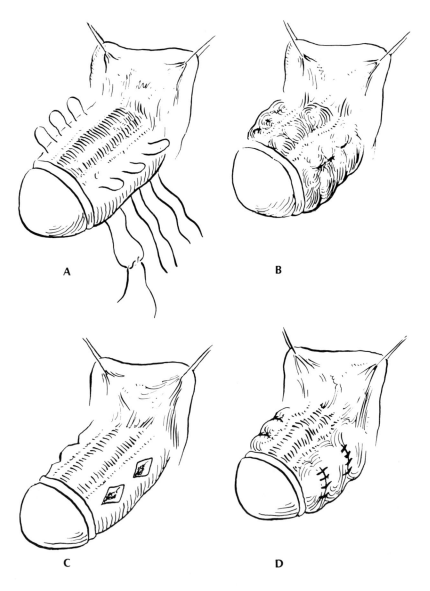

of urogenital sinus fusion, a simple midline cutback in the form of an episiotomy may be sufficient. However, with the more usual degrees of virilization, the lower, urogenital sinus-derived portion of the vagina is narrow and underdeveloped; here the insertion of a well-vascularized perineal skin flap creates an adequate vaginal lumen and minimizes the likelihood of secondary stenosis from contracture of overlapping suture lines.

Although the flap can be eccentric, based laterally or posterolaterally, I prefer a short, midline, posteriorly-based U flap with a fairly broad base just within the ischial tuberosities.[14] After mobilizing the flap and incising midline perineal and perivaginal tissues, the posterior vaginal midline is incised to the level of normal vaginal tissue with its normal lumen. Because the flap is elastic and hinged and drops into the posteriorly incised and separated perivaginal space, its length in the infant or very young child need not exceed 2½ cm or, at most, 3 cm. Figure 100-3 outlines the steps involved in flap vagionoplasty.

Because of the rarity of total female virilization, its reconstruction is not detailed here; the interested reader is referred to the original articles.[9,10]

Clitoroplasty

For a number of years, clitoral amputation was the preferred approach for restoring a feminine appearance because it was an easy and effective way to deal with a very large phallus. Initial experiences with clitorectomy had involved young women, once cortisone replacement became available; reported sexual gratification postoperatively was encouraging.[8] However, study of adolescent girls and young adult women who had been treated in early childhood by clitorectomy revealed the late onset of dating and romance and the inhibition of erotic arousal or expression, or both.[13] Although the authors suggested that these observations might be related either to the effects of antenatal androgen on the developing brain or to unknown effects of long-term steroid replacement, a possible role of early clitorectomy in this later behavior has not been assessed because a comparable group treated by clitoroplasty has not been reported.

Alternatives to clitoral amputation have in common the goal of preserving the innervation of the glans. Clitorectomy should now rarely, if ever, be necessary. Therefore, this chapter does not include a description of clitoral amputation.[7,14] These al-

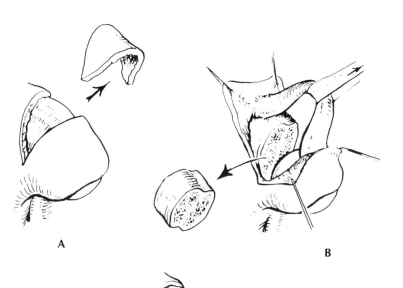

A

B

C

FIG. 100-5. Spence and Allen's segmental amputation of the clitoral shaft by a dorsal approach. **(A)** Excision of a transverse wedge of dorsal shaft skin. The midline mucosal strip is left intact, to ensure an adequate blood supply to the glans. **(B)** Isolation of the neurovascular bundle with a tape or Penrose drain and resection of a segment of phallic shaft. The proximal stump must be well ligated. **(C)** Closure. The glans can also be attached to the priosteum of the inferior symphysis, but this may entrap the dorsal nerves.

ternative procedures can be described as clitoral recession or reduction and can be selected depending upon the length and width of the phallus. The literature contains numerous such procedures and their modifications, from which I have selected those procedures that should be particularly useful and versatile.

When the phallus is very large, recession by relocation of the clitoral shaft under the mons pubis by attaching it to the pubic periosteum may result in a conspicious bulging of the shaft, especially during sexual arousal.[15] Therefore, the descriptions of recession here are limited to shaft plication and shaft resection. Methods for reduction of a large glans are also presented.

All techniques of clitoral surgery should have in common the preservation of at least some shaft skin and prepuce. These are used to fashion adequate labia minora, which tend to be very tiny in virilizing CAH, and to keep skin centrally as a clitoral hood. Figure 100-4 outlines procedures for shaft plication. Suture plication of the cavernosa (Fig. 100-4A and B) shortens the shaft and partially obliterates the erectile bodies.[17] This is particularly useful in preventing marked enlargement with erection. Alternatively, excision of ellipses of tunica albuginea (Fig. 100-4C and D) shortens the shaft without preventing engorgement and is therefore more suited to a lesser degree of clitoral hypertrophy.[3]

FIG. 100-6.   Goodwin's segmental amputation of the clitoral shaft by a ventral approach: **(A)** the completed vaginoplasty; **(B)** subglandular incision—a wedge of the midline mucosal strip can be excised to restore the proper vestibular relationships; **(C)** isolation of the shaft, with preservation of the dorsal neurovascular web; **(D)** shaft resection and beginning repair: **(E)** completed repair

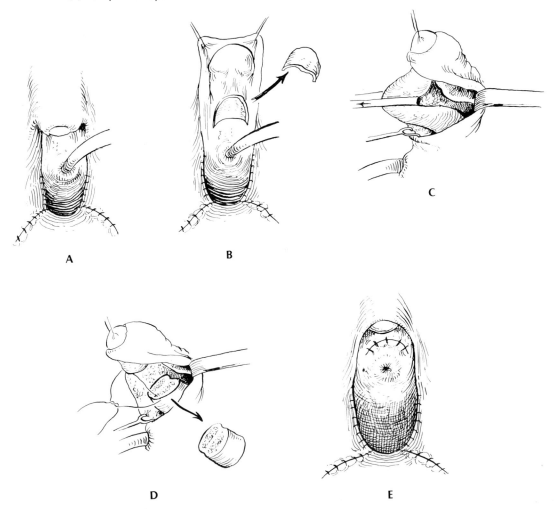

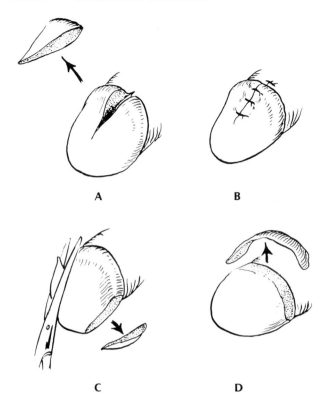

FIG. 100-7. Methods of glans reduction: (**A** and **B**) central wedge excision; (**C**) lateral glans trimming; (**D**) dorsal glans trimming. Any of these techniques can be combined with the other methods of clitoral plasty, as appropriate.

Figure 100-5 shows the Spence–Allen technique of shaft resection with preservation of the glans and its neurovascular supply.[16] Figure 100-6 is an alternate method by a perineal approach, described by Goodwin.[6] Shaft resection is particularly suited to concealing a long phallus. Figure 100-7 diagrams a variety of ways to reduce a large glans, which can be done at the time of clitoral recession or resection, when indicated.

Operative and Postoperative Management

An increased dosage of maintenance adrenal steroid replacement is required for the day of surgery and for 2 or 3 days postoperatively, as determined in consultation with the pediatric endocrinologist. A preoperative enema keeps the child more comfortable for the first few days after surgery. Infants can be positioned intraoperatively in a mildly exaggerated lithotomy position, by suspending the lower extremities with slight divergence. This exposes the perineum without creating excessive lateral tension on the genital tissues, which would tend to distract and distort the repair. Older children can be placed in pediatric gynecologic strap stirrups, similarly taking care to avoid excessive abduction of the thighs.

A loose petroleum jelly pack of 1-inch gauze in the vagina for 24 hours postoperatively helps to provide local hemostasis. A bulky perineal dressing is applied with gentle compression to minimize swelling. This can be changed when the vaginal pack is removed and can be discontinued in 48 hours. A small Foley catheter, which helps to keep the suture lines clean and dry, can be left for 2 to 4 days, depending on the degree of tissue edema. Sitz baths can be started 4, 5, or 6 days after surgery.

Several weeks postoperatively, if the vaginal flap is not clearly visualized, a sound or large catheter can be passed gently into the vagina to rule out the presence of synechiae or early stenosis at the apex of the flap. The use of a broad-based, short U flap minimizes the likelihood of a vaginal stricture; if the vagina has not been injured, a focal vaginal stenosis at the tip of the flap can be easily revised after puberty.

REFERERENCES

1. FEDERMAN DD: Abnormal Sexual Development: A Genetic and Endocrine Approach to Differential Diagnosis. Philadelphia, W B Saunders, 1967
2. FORTUNOFF S, LATTIMER JK, EDSON M: Vaginoplasty technique for female pseudohermaphrodites. Surg Gynecol Obstet 118:545, 1964
3. GLASSBERG KI, LAUNGANI G: Reduction clitoroplasty. Urology 17:604, 1981
4. GLENN JF: A practical approach to intersex problems. J Irish Coll Phys Surg 3:14, 1973
5. GLENN JF, BOYCE WH: Adrenogenitalism with testicular adrenal rests simulating interstitial cell tumor. J Urol 89:456, 1963
6. GOODWIN WE: Partial (segmental) amputation of the clitoris for female pseudohermaphroditism. Society for Pediatric Urology Newsletter, January 21, 1981
7. GROSS RE, RANDOLPH JG, CRIGLER FR, JR: Clitorectomy for sexual abnormalities: Indications and technique. Surgery 59:300, 1966
8. HAMPSON JG: Hermaphroditic genital appearance, rearing and eroticism in hyperadrenocorticism. Bull Johns Hopkins Hosp 90:265, 1955
9. HENDREN WH, CRAWFORD JD: Adrenogenital syndrome: The anatomy of the anomaly and its repair. Some new concepts. J Pediatr Surg 4:49, 1969
10. HENDREN WH, CRAWFORD JD: The child with ambiguous genitalia. Curr Probl Surg 1–64, November 1972

11. LEWIS VG, MONEY J: Adrenogenital syndrome: The need for early surgical feminization in girls. In Lee PA, Plotnick LP, Kowarski AV et al (eds): Congenital Adrenal Hyperplasia, p 463. Baltimore, University Park Press, 1977

12. MININBERG DT, LEVINE LS, NEW MI: Current concepts in congenital adrenal hyperplasia. Invest Urol 17:169, 1979

13. MONEY J, SCHWARTZ M: Dating, romantic and non-romantic friendships, and sexuality in 17 early-treated adrenogenital females, aged 16–25. In Lee PA, Plotnick LP, Kowarski AV et al (eds): Congenital Adrenal Hyperplasia, p 419. Baltimore, University Park Press, 1977

14. PERLMUTTER AD: Management of intersexuality. In Harrison JH, Gittes RF, Perlmutter AD et al (eds): Campbell's Urology, p 1535. Philadelphia, W B Saunders, 1979

15. RANDOLPH JG, HUNG W: Reduction clitoroplasty in females with hypertrophied clitoris. J Pediatr Surg 5:225, 1970

16. SPENCE HM, ALLEN TD: Genital reconstruction in the female with the adrenogenital syndrome. Br J Urol 45:126, 1973

17. STEFAN H: Surgical reconstruction of the external genitalia in female pseudohermaphrodites. Br J Urol 39:347, 1967

18. VERKAUF BS, JONES HW, JR: Masculinization of the female genitalia in congenital adrenal hyperplasia. Relationship to the salt losing variety of the disease. South Med J 63:634, 1970

19. WALSH PC: Intersex States. In Glenn JF (ed): Urologic Surgery, 2nd ed, p 35. Hagerstown, Harper & Row, 1975

Transsexual Surgery

101

J. William McRoberts

Transexualism is a psychiatric syndrome characterized by dissonant gender identity in which the individual attempts to deny his or her biologic sex.[7] These individuals seek, by surgical or hormonal means or both, to change their physical appearance permanently to conform to the image they have of themselves as a member of the opposite sex.

Although normal anatomically, the patients feel that their psychosexual identity differs from their anatomic sex because of a "trick of nature" that has them trapped inside the body of the opposite sex.[8] Unfortunately, psychiatric treatment and behavior therapy have not been successful in reorienting the adult transsexual's gender identity to one consistent with his or her anatomic sex.[3] Accordingly, surgical and hormonal therapy are presently the accepted means of treating transsexuals who meet the selection criteria.[3,6] Nevertheless, the role of the psychiatrist is central in evaluating the suitability of patients for possible sex reassignment surgery, in directing their overall rehabilitation program, and in providing continuity of care and emotional support prior to and following surgery.

A Gender Dysphoria Clinic was established in 1968 as an active clinical and research unit at the University of Washington School of Medicine. It only closed its doors when the author of this chapter moved to the University of Kentucky Medical Center in 1972. During the time of its activity, the multidisciplinary group constituting the Gender Dysphoria Committee screened more than 250 applicants seeking sex reassignment surgery. From this group of applicants 17 biologically male transsexuals were diagnosed and treated surgically. The selection criteria and long-term psychiatric and rehabilitative follow-up of these 17 patients have been reported previously.[3,4] Using similar selection criteria, since 1972 an additional 31 biologically male transsexual patients have undergone male-to-female sex conversion surgery at the University of Kentucky Medical Center. Twenty-seven of these 31 patients have been followed for at least 2 years.

These 27 patients, plus the 17 University of Washington patients, comprise the 44-patient study group reported here, from which has evolved the one-stage operation for biologically male transsexuals to which this chapter is devoted.

Surgical Procedure

EVOLUTION

The surgical procedure described here originated from the operation originally developed by Jones and his colleages, excepting that the copora cavernosa were not sacrificed.[5] Instead they were preserved as part of the reconstructed labia majora for the purpose of retaining erectile tissue to increase sensation during sexual arousal.

The complication rate was high initially. This was due to a combination of inexperience and the use of hard commercial vaginal molds. As these problems were resolved, it was apparent that there still remained the cosmetic and functional problems of scrotal hair within the neovagina and a tendency, with time, toward loss of vaginal depth. The latter problem was addressed by extending the depth of the perineal dissection even further beyond the prostate to a point beneath and beyond the bladder trigone. A split-thickness skin graft was then required to augment the most distal aspects of the perineal dissection, which could no longer be covered entirely by the scrotal and penile pedicle skin grafts.

Although these technical improvements had solved the functional problems, we were still not satisfied by the less-than-optimal cosmetic appearance of the introitus (caused by a round rather than vertical orientation of the vestibule) and by the presence of hair-bearing scrotal skin lining the posterior vagina. Both problems were solved by modifying Edgerton's two-stage procedure using penile skin as a pedicle graft flap into a one-stage operation and by retaining the corpora cavernosa as previously described.[1] After hearing of Granato's

1053

innovation, subsequently published in 1974, the operation was improved further by mobilizing the lower abdominal skin and subcutaneous tissues caudad and dorsally towards the rectum in order to reduce tension on the invaginated pedicle penile skin graft.[2] Excepting for minor refinements, our one-stage operation for biologically male transexuals has been standard since 1973.

PREOPERATIVE PERIOD

Our selection criteria for sex reassignment surgery have already been published.[3,4] Briefly they include a thorough psychiatric evaluation, a physical appearance convincing enough to allow the biologically male patient to fulfill the role of a female in society, sufficient intelligence to understand the limitations and possible complications of the surgery, an age of at least 21 years, having cross-dressed and been on hormonal treatment for at least 1 year and preferably 2 years prior to surgery, and having secured steady employment as a female. Among the selection criteria, the best predictor of successful rehabilitation following surgery is the extent to which the patient has already, prior to surgery, made adjustments to cope with a new gender identity. Especially important is the patient's ability to secure gainful employment as a female. For these patients, the surgery itself is but one of the many adjustments made along the way to complete social and sexual rehabilitation and does not loom disproportionately large as a factor in this ongoing process.

Once the patient is admitted to the hospital, she is instructed in hexachlorophene (pHisohex) scrubs of the lower abdomen, external genitalia, and perineum to be completed the night before and the morning of surgery. The patient is also started on an 18-hour mechanical bowel preparation, a clear liquid diet, and prophylactic broad-spectrum antibiotics and low-dose heparin. Following reexplanation of the details of the surgical procedure in front of two witnesses, the patient signs a special, unusually comprehensive operative permit detailing the operation itself, its goals, limitations, and all possible complications imaginable.

SURGICAL TECHNIQUE

After induction of general endotracheal anesthesia, the patient's perineum is positioned near the end of the operating table in a modified dorsal lithotomy position with the legs wrapped and supported on straight leg boards suspended by leg straps. The abdomen, thighs, external genitalia, and perineum are shaved, surgically scrubbed, and prepped for at least 10 minutes. The draping of the surgical field includes the addition of a rectal sheath cut from a disposable O'Conor drape. The rectal sheath is placed over the rectum and its edges are secured by skin sutures (Fig. 101-1A). Following these preparations, the table is tilted in the Trendelenburg position in order to place the patient's perineum in a more horizontal plane.

The surgery itself is initiated with a 4-cm to 5-cm vertical midline perineal skin incision. This extends a few centimeters above the scrotal perineal margin downward to 2 cm above the anal verge (Fig. 101-1A).

The skin incision is deepened and both testicles are in turn delivered through the wound (Fig. 101-1B). With traction on the testicles, the vasa deferentia and spermatic vessels are separately clamped, suture ligated, and amputated near the external inguinal ring, allowing the proximal ends of the spermatic cords to retract up into the inguinal canal.

Following bilateral orchiectomies, a curved Lowsley prostatic tractor is placed in the bladder for two purposes: to assist in urethral identification and to facilitate the deep perineal dissection by displacing the prostate superficially toward the perineum. The perineal surgery proceeds by blunt finger dissection on either side of the midline, developing the ischiorectal fossa laterally and cephalad along each side of the rectum. During the dissection, the central tendon and transverse perinei muscles are identified and transected (Fig. 101-1B). After displacing the levator ani muscles laterally, the dissection proceeds deeper into the perineum to expose the rectourethralis muscle, which is carefully divided (Fig. 101-C). Because the rectum is tented up by the rectourethralis muscle almost to a right angle at the level of the prostatic apex, once the rectourethralis muscle is divided the rectum is allowed to drop back more posteriorly, thus providing access to the prostate gland (Fig. 101-1D). At this point, additional width is obtained by incising the medial fibers of the levator ani muscles.

Continued deep dissection requires that the rectum also be separated off the posterior surface of the atrophic prostate, seminal vesicles, and bladder base. The safest route is between the two layers of Denonvillier's fascia. This is accomplished by transverse incision of the thin layer of the posterior fascia, which exposes the inner surface of the two fascial layers. By blunt and occasional sharp dissection, the neovaginal cavity is ultimately extended well past the posterior aspect of the

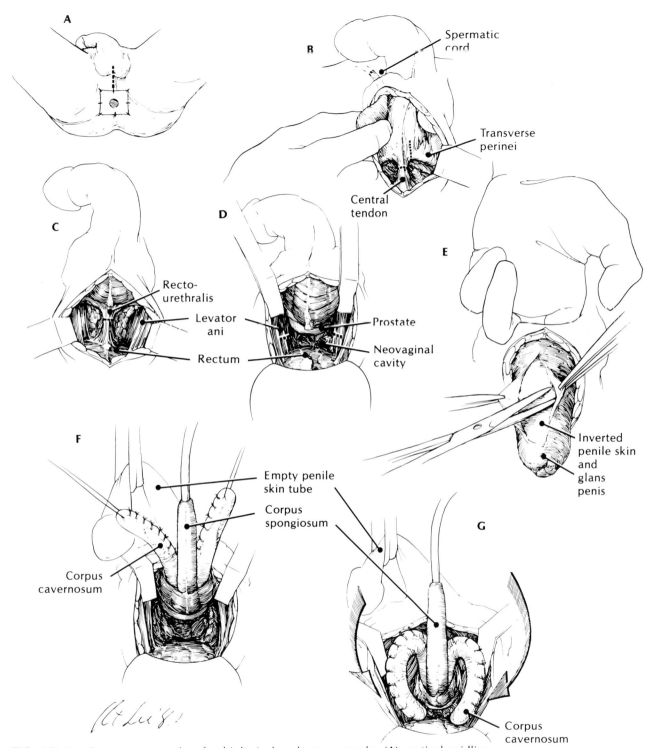

FIG. 101-1. One-stage operation for biological male transsexuals: **(A)** vertical midline perineal skin incision with an O'conor rectal sheath; **(B)** bilateral perineal orchiectomies in which the central tendon and transverse perinei muscles are transected; **(C)** retrourethralis muscle transected; **(D)** rectum drops back, medial fibers of levator ani muscle incised; **(E)** glans and penile skin inverted, subcutaneous fascia and fat incised and dissected off the inverted penile skin; **(F)** three corporal bodies separated, corpora cavernosum reduced in circumference and excess length removed; **(G)** corpora cavernosum swung laterally and posteriorly on either side of introitus. The buildup of tissue simulates the labia majora.

atrophic prostate to a point beyond the bladder trigone (see Fig. 101-2B).

At the completion of the perineal dissection, the newly formed vaginal cavity should be reasonably capacious, that is, it should be able to accept a soft vaginal mold measuring 5 cm in diameter and 15 cm in length. Because these dimensions vary with the local pelvic anatomy, a series of slightly smaller and larger molds should be available. After satisfactory hemostasis has been obtained, the Lowsley tractor is removed and replaced with an 18Fr Foley catheter. The neovaginal cavity is temporarily packed with moist gauzes.

Attention is now directed to the penile aspects of the surgery and to the dissection of the lower abdominal skin and subcutaneous tissues. Through the original midline perineal incision, blunt finger dissection is extended cephalad, first beneath the skin of the scrotum and then under the skin of the penile shaft. Once the skin has been mobilized from the underlying corpus spongiosum and the corpora cavernosa, the three corporal bodies are sharply severed just beneath the glans. The suspensory ligament of the penis is ligated and divided, and the corpora are brought out into the perineal wound. As a result, the glans and penile skin are preserved as an empty tube that is then turned inside out. The inverted tube is supported by two fingers and the subcutaneous fascia and fat are incised and dissected off the penile skin (Fig. 101-1E). The inverted penile skin nearest the glans is thinned further by rubbing with gauze, leaving only a very thin layer of skin in the distal third of the penile skin tube. Thinning of the penile skin serves to double its width and increase its length by approximately 50%. In addition, thinning of the periglandular skin facilitates capillary ingrowth into that segment of the graft; this allows it to function as a split-thickness skin graft, whereas the proximal two thirds remains as a pedicle skin graft. The glans penis usually does not survive intact but is retained for added skin coverage and as a buttress against pressure from the distal end of the vaginal mold.

With a tourniquet around the base of the three corporal bodies, the corpus spongiosum is freed by sharp dissection from the corpora cavernosa to the level of the proximal bulbous urethra. The corpora cavernosa are separated from each other by sharp midline dissection and are reduced to about two thirds of their normal circumferential diameter by filleting them medially and oversewing them with continuous 3-0 polyglycolic acid sutures (Fig. 101-1F). The narrowed corpora are then swung laterally and posteriorly on either side of the introitus and, after excess length is removed, they are secured to the lateral perineal fascia with several interrupted 3-0 polyglycolic acid sutures (Fig. 101-1G). By these surgical maneuvers, the corpora cavernosa are thus separated to the level of the midbulb, reduced in caliber by a third, and shortened in length by about 25%. When the skin is brought over the corpora, the buildup of the lateral introital margins by the underlying corporal bodies simulates labia majora (Fig. 101-2C).

Although the transection of the suspensory ligament of the penis aids in caudal mobilization of the base of the penile skin tube, further mobilization is required to reduce tension on the invaginated penile skin graft (Fig. 101-2B). The additional mobilization is accomplished by sharp and blunt dissection of the lower abdominal skin and subcutaneous tissue from the underlying fascia of the rectus and external oblique muscles (Fig. 101-2A). Dissection is carried to about the level of the umbilicus and, if need be, even more cephalad by severing the umbilical attachments. The base of the penile skin tube is thus mobilized caudad toward the rectum some 8 cm or 9 cm to overlie the newly formed introitus of the vagina. In order to prevent retraction of the abdominal flap, two 2-0 wire retention sutures are secured on either side of the symphysis pubis through its periosteum and tied over dental rolls on the abdominal skin (Fig. 101-2C).

While the penile skin flap is temporarily inverted into the perineal cavity (Fig. 101-2B), an appropriate exit site for the new urethra meatus is selected. The skin is incised and the urethra is brought out and amputated on the bias about 1 cm above the skin level to allow retraction. The urethral urothelium is sutured to the skin with interrupted 4-0 chromic catgut sutures (Fig. 101-2C). The urethral catheter is replaced by a suprapubic 12Fr cystocatheter to avoid the risk of pressure necrosis by the urethral catheter against the vaginal mold. Two large hemovac drains are inserted beneath the lower abdominal skin flap and placed to low suction. Through separate perineal stab wounds, two small Penrose drains are brought out to drain the wound. The skin margins are closed with running 4-0 polyglycolic acid sutures (Fig. 101-2C). A soft, individually selected Silastic mold is placed in the neovagina, and a sturdy compression dressing is applied over the perineum.

POSTOPERATIVE CARE

The patient is kept on antibiotics and low-dose heparin during the postoperative hospitalization, which, in the absence of complications, is 8 or 9 days in length. Intravenous fluids are maintained for the first 2 postoperative days, and a clear liquid dict is started on day 3 to reduce the need for bowel movements. In order to minimize abdominal pressure on the vaginal mold, the patient is in-structed to lie recumbent in bed or to sit in a chair, restricting ambulation to the bathroom only. When walking, the patient is encouraged to apply firm manual pressure upward on the perineum in order to support the perineal dressings and the vaginal mold.

FIG. 101-2. Completion of one-stage operation for biological male transsexuals: **(A)** mobilization of hypogastrium; **(B)** penile skin flap, including glans, inverted into perineal cavity; **(C)** operation completed (vaginal mold not in place)

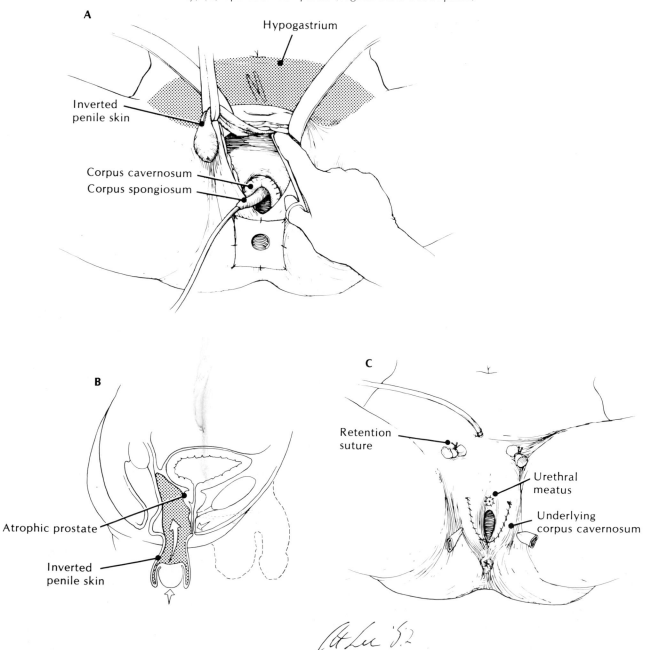

TABLE 101-1.   Surgical Complications in 44 Patients Undergoing Male-to-Female Sex Conversion

Early
Rectovaginal Fistula	2
Urethrovaginal fistula	1

Late
Urethral Stenosis	1
Urethral meatus placed too high, later revised	1
Vaginal stenosis, moderate, requiring revision	2
Vaginal stenosis, moderate, but surgery declined	1
Vaginal stenosis, minor	4
Total	12

12 complications in 9/44 (20%) patients

On the seventh postoperative day, the dressings are changed, the wire retention sutures are removed, the vaginal mold is changed, and the suprapubic catheter is removed. If there are no complications, the patient is discharged the next day.

As an outpatient, the vaginal mold is kept in the vagina at all times excepting when voiding, defecating, or taking a bath. The patient is seen again at 3 weeks; if the wounds are healing well, sexual intercourse is permitted in 6 weeks.

RESULTS

From 1968 through 1980, 48 biologically male transsexual patients have undergone male-to-female sex conversion surgery. Four of these patients, who were doing well when seen at 3- and 6-month postoperative office visits, were nevertheless lost to follow-up beyond 2 years and are accordingly not included in this series which requires a minimum 2-year follow-up.

There were twelve surgical complications, three occurring within 30 days and nine occurring later (Table 101-1). Three patients had two complications each, namely, two of the fistula patients also developed vaginal stenosis and one of the patients with minor vaginal stenosis also had the urethral meatus placed too close to the symphysis pubis, resulting in the patient's voiding over the edge of the toilet bowl. The meatus was subsequently repositioned down toward the introitus to a more functional site.

Eight of the complications were distributed among the first six patients. The high complication rate early in the series was due to a combination of inexperience and the use of hard commercial vaginal molds. Pressure necrosis of the hard mold

against an indwelling urethral catheter probably contributed to the development of the urethrovaginal fistula. Early patient abandonment of the uncomfortable molds contributed to three vaginal stenoses. The remaining four complications, consisting of three mild vaginal stenoses and one urethral stenosis, occurred in the next grouping of 17 patients. There were no surgical complications in the last 21 patients. This salutary trend appears to be a reflection of increased operative experience and the use of soft, individually tailored Silastic vaginal molds. The molds are constructed in our laboratory using biomedical grade Silastic, layered over a foam rubber center. The molds are soft and compressible, leading to improved patient tolerance and acceptance. A new generation of soft but expensive ($250) vaginal molds are also available commercially.*

CONCLUSIONS

A one-stage operation for biologically male transsexuals has been presented and the results and complications discussed. The surgical procedure as presently developed has a low complication rate and results in a vagina that is entirely functional for sexual intercourse and in an introitus with a cosmetic appearance that is nearly indistinguishable from that of the normal female perineum.

Although there still remains some controversy about the precise role of surgery in treating the transsexual patient, it is evident that surgery will continue to offer a select group of patients the best means of coping with the transsexual dilemma. Furthermore, it is important to retain the perspective that the therapeutic approach to transsexuals must be one of long-term physical, social, and psychological rehabilitation; sex reassignment surgery is only one, relatively modest aspect of the overall rehabilitative process.

It is absolutely essential for any surgeon contemplating treatment of transsexual patients to do so as part of a therapeutic team. It is as foolhardy to do transsexual surgery without the support of interested psychiatrists and committed social workers as it is ill-advised to transplant kidneys without the backup of hemodialysis and nephrologic consultation. With such an approach, properly screened and treated transsexual patients can now adapt to most aspects of life that were previously precluded by their psychoanatomic incongruity.

---

* Vaginal stents, Heyer–Shulte, 600 Pine Avenue, Galeta, California 93017

REFERENCES

1. EDGERTON MT, BULL J: Surgical construction of the vagina and labia in male transsexuals. Plast Reconstr Surg 46:529, 1970
2. GRANATO RC: Surgical approach to male transsexualism. Urology 3:792, 1974
3. HUNT DD, HAMPSON JL: Follow-up of 17 biological male transsexuals after sex-reassignment surgery. Am J Psychiatry 137:432, 1980
4. HUNT DD, HAMPSON JL: Transsexualism: A standardized psychosocial rating format for the evaluation of results of sex reassignment surgery. Arch Sex Behav 9:255, 1980
5. JONES HW JR, SCHIRMER HK, HOOPES JE: A sex conversion operation for males with transsexualism. Am J Obstet Gynecol 100:101, 1968
6. PAULY IB: The current status of the change of sex operation. J Nerv Ment Dis 147:460, 1968
7. PAULY IB: Adult manifestations of male transsexualism. In Green R, Money J (eds): Transsexualism and Sex Reassignment, p 37. Baltimore, The Johns Hopkins Press, 1969
8. WOLF SR, KNORR NJ, HOOPES JE et al: Psychiatric aspects of transsexual surgery management. J Nerv Ment Dis 147:525, 1968

Orchiopexy and Herniorrhaphy

Donald P. Finnerty

102

Cryptorchidism is the most common congenital anomaly of the male reproductive system, with many complications. Two percent to ten percent of newborn term infants are found to be cryptorchid. This incidence can be as high as 21% in premature infants.[39] At age 1 year the incidence approaches 1.0% and this figure remains constant through adolescence and adulthood.[6,39] The etiology of cryptorchidism is unknown. Anatomic theories have included gubernacular failures, shortened spermatic artery, tight inguinal ring, and abnormal attachments between the testes and the anterior abdominal wall. Approximately 6% of patients with cryptorchidism have endocrine disorders causing hypogonadism. Testicular dysgenesis may prevent the testes from responding normally to the stimulus for descent.[26,42] Genetic factors may play a role; there are reports of increased incidence of cryptorchidism in families.[40]

Based on its location the cryptorchid testis can be classified as *abdominal* (inside the internal ring), *canalicular* (in the inguinal canal), or ectopic (outside the normal path of testicular descent). The most common site of ectopia is the superficial inguinal pouch of Denis Browne.[8] A testis that can be manipulated into the scrotum is a retractile testis that is due to an active cremasteric reflex. From a therapeutic point of view this entity should be distinguished from a true cryptorchid testis.

Reasons for Therapy

Carcinogenesis

The relationship between cryptorchidism and testicular tumorigenesis is well established. Between 2% and 12% of testicular tumors arise in cryptorchid testes.[8,25] It is estimated that the cryptorchid testes is 20 to 50 times more likely to develop malignancy than the normally descended testis.[1,3] Position of the testis also plays a role, because an abdominal testis is 5 to 6 times more likely to develop malignancy than an inguinal testis.[8,30] Many authors suggest a link between testicular dysgenesis and subsequent tumor formation.[42,44] It is not surprising, then, to note that 20% of testicular tumors reported occur in the contralateral scrotal testis.[9,38]

The use of orchiopexy as prophylaxis against subsequent malignant degeneration of the testes has been questioned by many.[11,17,43] However, Martin and Menk, in a recent review of 166 cases of testicular tumors after orchiopexy, found only five cases of tumor in boys who had undergone orchiopexy before 10 years of age.[30] This could suggest that early repair may decrease the malignant potential of the cryptorchid testis.

Spermatogenesis

Histologic studies show that the germinal elements of the cryptorchid testis do not develop normally.[31] Differences between the cryptorchid and the normal testis become evident during the second year of life, characterized by decreased spermatogonium content and diminished tubular growth.[32] Hadzielimovic and associates have also recently identified a deficiency in DNA synthesis in the cryptorchid testis after 1 year of age.[21] These differences between the descended and cryptorchid testis increase in magnitude until puberty, after which time the cryptorchid testis generally loses all spermatogenic function.

Some discussion does exist about whether orchiopexy at any age improves fertility. Several authors have shown 70% to 80% fertility in patients who have undergone orchiopexy for bilateral cryptorchidism prior to the age of 10 years.[5,18] Kiesewetter had demonstrated histologic improvement in the appearance of the germinal cells on biopsies obtained some months after orchiopexy.[28] Hecker and Heinz, on the other hand, report fertility in only 35% of patients with uncorrected unilateral cryptorchidism.[23] Even more surprisingly, only 40% of patients with corrected unilateral cryptorchidism have contralateral descended testes that have matured normally. Lipschultz and colleagues have demonstrated abnormal spermatogenesis in 29 males who underwent orchiopexy between ages 4 and 12, suggesting an abnormality in the descended contralateral testes.[29]

Evaluation of fertility after orchiopexy is complicated both by a lack of long-term follow-up studies and by the varied timing of the orchiopexy itself. The literature at present seems to suggest that early orchiopexy probably offers at least a reasonable chance of improved fertility and should be undertaken.

Torsion

The undescended testis is particularly prone to torsion. The reader is referred to Chapter 103 for further discussion of this subject.

Inguinal Hernia

Many authors have suggested that there is from 65% to 90% association between a patent processus vaginalis and a cryptorchid testis.[19,27] In the majority of these patients the hernia is asymptomatic, and elective repair of the patent sac should be accomplished at the time of orchiopexy.

Trauma

The cryptorchid testis is particularly vulnerable to trauma. This is particularly true if the testis is located just above the pubic tubercle.

Psychologic Factors

The absence of a scrotal testis may cause anxiety and embarrassment in a young child, particularly once he comes under the scrutiny of his peers.[20] Psychologic factors constitute yet another indication for early orchiopexy.

Associated Anomalies

Cryptorchidism is commonly associated with abdominal wall defects such as exstrophy and the prune belly syndrome. Some authors have found a 20% association between cryptorchidism and the unsuspected upper tract anomalies.[10,14] This incidence increases to 25% when it is associated with hypospadias. Abnormal development of the epididymis and vas deferens are common in cryptorchidism.[40] Chromosomal abnormalities, particularly in patients with cryptorchidism and intersex anomalies, have been reported by Miniberg and Bingol.[33]

Diagnosis

The diagnosis of true cryptorchidism is occasionally difficult. The cryptorchid testis must be distinguished from the retractile testis. The true cryptorchid patient has an empty hemiscrotum that may be underdeveloped. The testis is usually palpable, most often within the inguinal canal. The nonpalpable testis is occasionally located by herniography, computed tomography, ultrasound, or spermatic venography.[2,12,46] Anorchia can be identified by a diagnostic course of human chorionic gonadotropin (HCG) followed by the measurement of serum testosterones. HCG is also useful in identifying the retractile testis.[36]

Therapy

Therapy is directed toward normal placement of the testes in the scrotum. Histologic studies have suggested that the ideal age for repair is during the second year of life.

Endocrine

Considerable interest has been focused on the hormonal treatment of cryptorchidism. Administration of HCG causes descent in 33% of bilateral cryptorchids and 16% of unilateral cryptorchids in some series.[13] In addition to satisfactory position of the testes, 46% of these successfully treated patients were fertile.[15]

Recently some authors have advocated the use of luteinizing hormone–releasing hormone (LH–RH) for the treatment of cryptorchidism. Happ and co-workers, in a recent study, treated a small series of patients with intranasal LH–RH and achieved complete descent in 64% of unilateral and bilateral cryptorchids.[22] Descent in unilateral cryptorchids is 3% according to Pirazzoli and associates.[36]

Surgical

Important points in the surgical repair of cryptorchidism include isolation and ligation of the hernia sac, adequate mobilization of the cord structures without injury to the vessels or vas, and placement of the testis in the scrotum without tension.

In 1899 Bevan established many of the basic surgical principles in the repair of cryptorchidism.[4] Many authors since that time have made modifications in the mobilization and the fixation of the testes.[7,34,35]

The basic principle of effective orchiopexy is the acquisition and maintenance of adequate cord length. Excessive tension on the mobilized testis and cord can cause ischemic atrophy and loss of the testis. The object of the repair is to abolish the triangle consisting of the renal pedicle, internal ring, and external ring and to replace it with a direct line from the pedicle to the scrotum.

An oblique incision in the inferior skin fold is made on the affected side. The subcutaneous tissue and Scarpa's fascia are incised, exposing the external inguinal ring. Care must be taken during this part of the procedure to avoid injury to the ectopic testis in Denis Browne's pouch. The external oblique aponeurosis is incised in the direction of its fibers, and the testis and cord are freed from the surrounding tissue to the level of the internal inguinal ring. The cord is then skeletonized by excising the fibers of the cremaster muscle (Fig. 102-1). The hernia sac is identified on the anteromedial surface of the cord and dissected free to the level of the internal inguinal ring. Here it is ligated with a nonabsorbable suture (Fig. 102-2).

The internal oblique muscle superior to the internal ring is retracted to allow better exposure of the retroperitoneal space. The dissection is continued by elevating the peritoneum from the spermatic vessels. The lateral spermatic fascia is divided laterally, thus allowing medial displacement of the vessels and, therefore, additional cord length (Fig. 102-3).

Other maneuvers to obtain additional length include incision of the internal ring superiorly, division of the inferior epigastric vessels, and division of the floor of the inguinal canal. The vas deferens may be mobilized for a short distance behind the bladder but this structure is rarely the limiting factor in obtaining adequate length. After adequate dissection is accomplished, a new internal ring is created medial and inferior to the original ring either by tunneling beneath the floor of the inguinal canal or by repairing the inguinal floor lateral to the new ring (Fig. 102-4).

The ipsilateral scrotal sac is stretched bluntly to

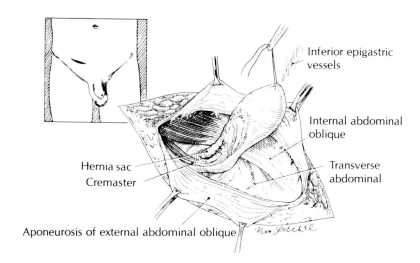

Inferior epigastric vessels

Internal abdominal oblique

Transverse abdominal

Hernia sac
Cremaster

Aponeurosis of external abdominal oblique

FIG. 102-1. Aponeurosis of the external abdominal oblique has been opened and the gubernaculum has been detached. The testicle is invested by the tunica vaginalis (*insert*).

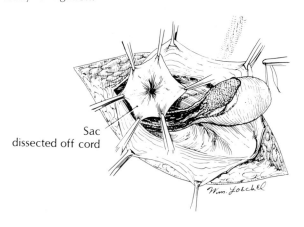

Sac dissected off cord

FIG. 102-2. Hernia sac has been dissected free and is ready for ligation.

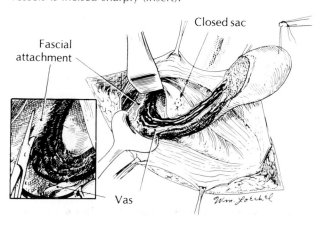

Closed sac

Fascial attachment

Vas

FIG. 102-3. Fibers of cremasteric muscle have been dissected from the cord. The vessels and vas are easily identified. The lateral fascial attachment of spermatic vessels is incised sharply (*insert*).

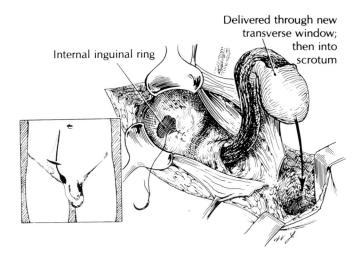

FIG. 102-4. The cord structures have been moved medial to the inferior epigastric vessels. The *insert* demonstrates how extra length can be obtained with this maneuver.

Internal inguinal ring

Delivered through new transverse window; then into scrotum

FIG. 102-5. Preferred methods of placing and fixing the testicle in the scrotum

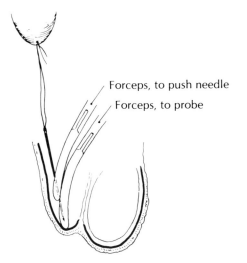

Forceps, to push needle

Forceps, to probe

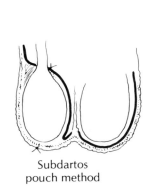

Subdartos pouch method

tear the dartos fibers. Final fixation of the testis in the bottom of the scrotum is done by means of suture fixation of the tunica albuginea to the dartos fibers or creation of a subdartos pouch (Fig. 102-5). The inguinal incision is closed using a standard inguinal ligament hernia repair.

Options for the management of the high undescended testis include staged orchiopexy, long-loop vas operation, microvascular surgery, or orchiectomy. Persky and Albert reported a 67% success rate using the standard orchiopexy procedure followed by a similar procedure 8 to 16 months later.[35] The long-loop vas procedure was popularized by Fowler and Stephens in 1959.[16] The procedure involves high ligation and division of the main vascular pedicle to the testes. This allows scrotal placement of the testes, with survival of the organ dependent on collateral circulation from

the vessels of the vas deferens, deep epigastric vessels, and gubernaculum testis. This procedure should be carefully thought out, because excessive dissection of the cord and its structures disrupts this collateral circulation. Silber and Kelly have reported success in autotransplantation of testes using microvascular techniques.[41] Hinman has recommended orchiectomy in the unilateral abdominal testis for defects of urogenital union, and in the symptomatic unilateral cryptorchid testes after puberty.[24]

COMPLICATIONS

The complications of orchiopexy result primarily from injury to the spermatic vessels or vas deferens. Ischemic injury to the testes can result from direct injury to the vessels or undue tension on the cord after the repair. Injury to the vas is uncommon. Long-term complications in the event of testicular tumor formation are altered lymphatic drainage pathways and possible involvement of uncommon regional nodes.

REFERENCES

1. ALTMAN BL, MALAMENT M: Carcinoma of the testes following orchiopexy. J Urol 97:498, 1967

2. AMIN M, WHEELER CS: Selective testicular venography in abdominal cryptorchidism. J Urol 115:760, 1976

3. BATATA MA, WHITMORE WF, JR, HILARIS BS et al: Cancer of the undescended or maldescended testes. Am J Roentgenol 126(2):302, 1976

4. BEVAN AD: Operation for undescended testicle and congenital inguinal hernia. JAMA 33:773, 1899

5. BRUNET J, DEMOWBRAY RR, BISHOP PMF: Management of the undescended testes. Br Med J 5084:1367, 1958

6. BUEMANN B, HENRIKSEN H, VILLUMSEN AL et al: Incidence of undescended testes in the newborn. Acta Chir Scand (Suppl) 283:289, 1961

7. CABOT H, NESBIT RM: Undescended testes. Arch Surg 22:850, 1931

8. CAMPBELL HE: The incidence of malignant growth of the undescended testicle. Arch Surg 44:353, 1942

9. CAMPBELL HE: The incidence of malignant growth of the undescended testicle: A reply and re-evaluation. J Urol 81:663, 1959

10. COOK GT, MARSHALL VF: The association of undescended testes and renal abnormalities. Presented at the annual meeting of the American Academy of Pediatrics, Washington, DC, November 1968

11. DOW JA, MOSTOFI FK: Testicular tumors following orchiopexy. South Med J 60:193, 1967

12. DWOSKIN JY, KUHN JR: Herniagrams in undescended testes and hydroceles. J Urol 109:520, 1973

13. ERLICH RM, DAUGHERTY LV, TOMASHEFSKY P et al: Effect of gonadotropin in cryptorchidism. J Urol 102:793, 1969

14. FELTON LM: Should intravenous pyelography be a routine procedure for children with cryptorchidism or hypospadias? J Urol 81:335, 1959

15. FONKALSRUD EW, MENGEL W: The Undescended Testis, p 162, 1981

16. FOWLER R, STEPHENS FD: The role of testicular vascular anatomy in the salvage of high undescended testes. In Webster R (ed): Congenital Malformations of the Rectum, Anus and Genito-Urinary Tracts. London, E & S Livingstone, 1963

17. GILBERT JB: Studies in malignant testes tumors; Tumors developing after orchiopexy. J Urol 46:740, 1941

18. GROSS RE: The Surgery of Infancy and Childhood, Its Principles and Techniques. (Philadelphia, W B Saunders, 1953

19. GROSS RE, JEWETT TC, JR: Surgical experiences from 1222 operations for undescended testes. JAMA 160:634, 1956

20. GROSS RE, REPLOGLE RL: Treatment of the undescended testes. Postgrad Med J 34:266, 1963

21. HADZISELIMOVIC F, HERZOG B, SEGUCHI H: Surgical correction of cryptorchidism at 2 years: Electron microscopic and morphologic investigation. J Pediatr Surg 10:19, 1975

22. HAPP J, KOLLMAN F, DRAWEH C et al: Treatment of cryptorchidism with pernasal gonadotropin-releasing hormone therapy. Fertil Steril 29:546, 1978

23. HECKER W, HEINZ HA: Cryptorchidism and fertility, J Pediatr Surg 2:513, 1967

24. HINMAN F, JR: Unilateral abdominal cryptorchidism. J Urol 122:71, 1979

25. JOHNSON DE, WOODHEAD DM, POHL DR et al: Cryptorchidism and testicular tumorigenesis. Surgery 63:919, 1968

26. JOHNSTON JH: Undescended testes. Arch Dis Child 40:113, 1965

27. KIESEWETTER WB: Undescended testes. W Va Med J 52:235, 1956

28. KIESEWETTER WB, SCHOLL WR, LETTERMAN GH: Histologic changes in the testes following anatomically successful orchiopexy. J Pediatr Surg 4:59, 1969

29. LIPSHULTZ LE, CAMENOS-TORRES K, GREENSPAN CS et al: Testicular function after orchiopexy for unilaterally undescended testes. N Eng J Med 295:15, 1976

30. MARTIN DC, MENK HR: The undescended testes: Management after puberty. J Urol 114:77, 1975

31. MCCALLUM DW: Clinical study of the spermatogenesis of undescended testes. Arch Surg 31:290, 1935

32. MENGEL W, HIENZ HA, SIPPE WG et al: Studies on cryptorchidism: A comparison of histological findings in the germinative epithelium before and after the second year of life. J Pediatr Surg 9:445, 1974

33. MININBERG DT, BINGOL N: Chromosomal abnormalities in undescended testes. Urology 1:98, 1973

34. OMBREDANNE L: Indication et technique de l'orchidopexie transscrotale chez l'enfant. Presse Med 18:745, 1910

35. PERSKY L, ALBERT DJ: Staged orchiopexy. Surg Gynecol Obstet 132:43, 1971

36. PIRAZZOLI P, ZAPULLA F, BERNARD F et al: Luteinizing hormone-releasing hormone nasal spray as therapy for undescended testicle. Arch Dis Child 53:235, 1978

37. REA, CE: Further report on the treatment of the undescended testes by hormonal therapy at the University of Minnesota Hospitals; A discussion of spontaneous descent of the testes and an evaluation of endocrine therapy in cryptorchidism. Surgery 7:828, 1940

38. SCHWARTZ JW, REED, JF, JR: The pathology of cryptorchidism. J Urol 76:429, 1956

39. SCORER CG: The descent of the testes. Arch Dis Child 39:605, 1964

40. SCORER CG, FARRINGTON GH: Congenital Deformities

of the Testes and Epididymis. New York, Appleton-Century-Crofts, 1971

41. SILBER SJ, KELLY J: Successful autotransplantation of
an intraabdominal testes to the scrotum by microvascular technique. J Urol 115:452, 1976

42. SOHVAL AR: Testicular dysgenesis as an etiologic
factor in cryptorchidism. J Urol 72:693, 1954

43. SOHVAL AR: Testicular dysgenesis in relation to neoplasm of the testes. J Urol 75:285, 1956

44. SUMNER WA: Malignant tumor of testes occurring 29
years after orchiopexy. J Urol 81:140, 1959

45. TOREK F: Orchiopexy for undescended testicle. Ann
Surg 94:97, 1931

46. WHITE JJ, SHAKER IJ, OH KS et al: Herniography: A
diagnostic refinement in the management of cryptorchidism. Am Surg 39:624, 1975

Testicular Torsion

103

Richard H. Harrison III

Dominating the surgical emergencies of the scrotum in infants, boys, and men is torsion of the spermatic cord, although no fatal cases have been reported either with or without operation. Early diagnosis and prompt treatment are essential if the testis is to be saved.

Although torsion has been reported numerous times at birth and in a few cases in older men, torsion is less common under the age of 10 and after the age of 40. The vast majority of cases arise within the second decade of life, just after puberty, when the testis is growing (Fig. 103-1). Over 450 articles on torsion have appeared in the world literature since the first reported case in 1840.[1] Jones's article on torsion during childhood is one of the more complete reviews in recent years.[19] O'Conor observed that torsion of the spermatic cord is not a rare clinical entity and that the many cases of atrophy of the testis following orchitis may in fact be the end result of torsion.[27]

Anatomy

Under normal conditions, the internal oblique muscle, its conjoined tendons, and the transversalis muscle act as a sphincter to prevent the return of the testis into the abdomen during the later months of intrauterine life. The cremaster muscle completely envelops the coverings of the testis and spermatic cord (Fig. 103-2A). When the cremaster contracts, it pulls the testis toward the external inguinal ring and, if there is no resistance, into the inguinal canal. If the cremaster is an unusually well-developed muscle with a large inguinal canal, cremaster retraction may bring the testis back into the abdomen. Toward puberty, such an ability of the testis to wander up and down lessens. In the normally descended and attached testis, the common mesentery is formed by the reflection of the parietal layer of the tunica vaginalis onto the epididymis and testis. The upper limit of this mesentery is usually about the center of the globus major, while the lower limit is the lower pole of the testis or the tip of the globus minor.

In Young's review of the earlier literature prior to 1926, the association of trauma with torsion is stressed, suggesting that extravaginal torsion occurs when there is sufficient trauma to cause tearing to the loose areolar connections between the exterior surface of the tunica vaginalis and the dartos muscle of the scrotum. This may occur at birth or in ectopic testes (Fig. 103-2B).

ETIOLOGY

Experimental Torsion

Probably the best controlled studies recording cellular changes from testicular ischemia were done by Smith.[37] Thirty-three dogs were subjected to periods of ischemia ranging from 2 to 14 hours. The results were as follows: the spermatogenic cells were slightly damaged by 2 hours, severely injured by 4 hours, and destroyed by 6 hours of ischemia; the Leydig cells were severely injured by 4 hours, nonviable after 8 hours of ischemia, and were destroyed by 10 hours; 10 hours or more of ischemia resulted in nearly complete fibrotic replacement of the testis.

Predisposing Factors

The presence of many abnormalities observed in various torsion cases has frequently overshadowed the most important factor in the pathology of torsion. This factor involves the high investment of the testis and adnexa by the visceral tunica vaginalis with a very capacious tunica vaginalis and the absence of the gubernaculum testis and posterior mesorchium, the scrotal ligaments (Fig. 103-2C).

Exciting Causes

Uffreduzzi, an Italian surgeon, suggested in 1912 that a normally attached testis would not undergo torsion and that torsion was caused by twisting of the spermatic cord as the result of contraction of the cremasteric muscle fibers caused by stimulants such as sudden cold. Differential diagnosis is more

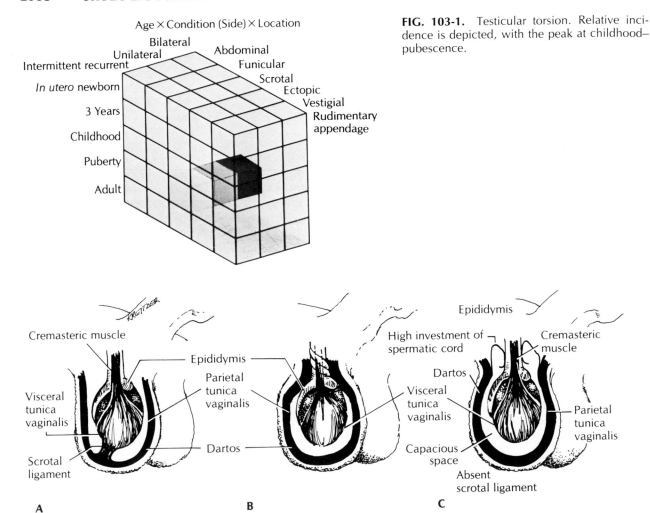

FIG. 103-1. Testicular torsion. Relative incidence is depicted, with the peak at childhood–pubescence.

FIG. 103-2. Mechanics of torsion: (**A**) scrotal ligament (gubernaculum); (**B**) extravaginal torsion; (**C**) bell clapper anomaly

fully elaborated in the monograph *Torsion in the Male*.[16]

PATHOLOGY

At surgery, the process may vary from congestion with edema to bluish-black hemorrhagic necrosis. In chronic, relapsing, or recurrent torsion, the inflammatory process is less acute and, on histologic section, there is usually an increase in fibrosis. Ormond best describes the pathogenesis: the first effect in early rotation is the flattening of the veins with partial obstruction of venous return. As the twisting continues, successive obliteration of the veins, partial obstruction of the artery, and finally obliteration of the artery occur.[29] If the venous return in entirely obstructed, the congestion is

greater and necrosis occurs in a short time. With obliteration of the artery, total infarction occurs.

Treatment of Torsion

MANUAL DETORSION

Two thirds of torsion of the spermatic cord occurs from without, as in crossing one's own legs: therefore, manual attempts should be made to rotate the testis on a vertical axis from within outward. No great force should be used, and the rotation should be continued until relief is experienced tactilely by the examiner in decrease of pain, as expressed by the patient. If the pain and resistance increase, obviously the wrong direction has been taken and rotation should be accomplished on a vertical axis in the opposite direction. Injecting the spermatic cord above the lesion with local anesthetic may afford sufficient relief for successful manual detorsion.

SURGICAL MANAGEMENT

The cardinal rule of testicular swelling should be, *unless you are positive that you are not dealing with torsion, explore.*[20] If the patient is young, you must be all the more positive because of the tragic consequences associated with misdiagnosis. There is a difference of opinion about whether the incision for torsion should be inguinal, inguinoscrotal, or scrotal, and, if scrotal, whether it should be in the median raphe or a separate scrotal incision.[9] My personal preference is an inguinal incision when-

ever I suspect associated hernia; however, when the pathology is clearly in the scrotum, I prefer an anterolateral crease incision on the affected side, avoiding obvious blood vessels (Fig. 103-3A). The opposite side is explored and fixed through a similar incision. Ottenheimer emphasized the necessity of testicular fixation, opening the parietal tunica vaginalis, everting it, and suturing the cut edges around (behind) the epididymis as in bottle hydrocelectomy (Fig. 103-3B to E).[30]

Definitive surgery depends upon the degree of viability of the affected structure and the location of the testis.[25] As a general rule, scrotal edema is marked when hemorrhagic infarction has already taken place and is absent or minimal when the hemorrhagic infarction is less complete and there is a better chance of salvage. When the fluid in the tunica vaginalis is sanguineous, one may anticipate

FIG. 103-3. Surgical correction of testicular torsion: **(A)** anterior, crease-following scrotal incision; **(B)** incision carried to tunica vaginalis; **(C)** tunica vaginalis entered, testis delivered from scrotum, and torsion reduced; **(D)** excess tunica vaginalis excised; **(E)** edges of parietal tunica vaginalis everted around epididymis with hemostatic suture; **(F)** dependent scrotum evaginated with index finger, inferior tunica albuginea sutured to dependent dartos pouch

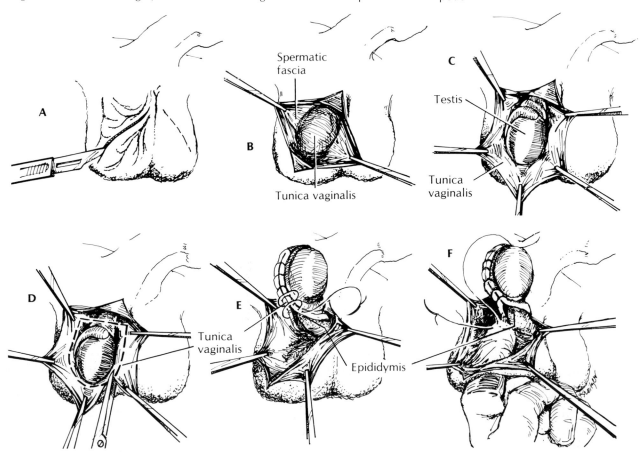

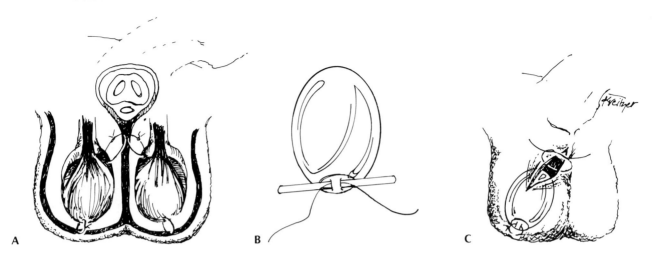

FIG. 103-4.   Bilateral testicular fixation and insertion of testicular prosthesis: **(A)** bilateral scrotal fixation; **(B)** Silastic gel-filled testicular implant II (Lattimer design); **(C)** Silastic prosthesis in place

that hemorrhagic infarction is present; when the fluid is clear, the torsion is usually less advanced. Incision through the tunica albuginea usually clarifies whether arterial infarction has occurred; if it has, there will be no bleeding. When the seminiferous tubules can still be differentiated from a globular blood clot equivalent, one should consider returning the probably infarcted hemorrhagic testis back into the scrotum. If the testis has returned to normal color, suggesting viability, it should be fixed to the scrotum by at least two widely spaced sutures (Fig. 103-3F). If the testis is not viable and the opposite testis is normal, orchiectomy should be carried out.

If the testis occupies an anomalous position and if the remaining opposite testis is in the normal descended position, orchiectomy should be done. If a maldescended or undescended testis is viable and the youngster is under 3 years of age, orchiopexy may be attempted. Simultaneous exploration of the opposite scrotum should be carried out, with excision of any redundant parietal tunica vaginalis and attachment to the scrotum with at least two nonabsorbable sutures.[16,27,30,38] Retorsion has occurred on the sides previously detorsed at open surgery, but also on the opposite side. Follow-up examination invariably reveals mobile, obviously pexed, testicles without hydrocele, because the serous fluid created by the remaining visceral tunica is absorbed by adjacent dartos muscle. When fixation of the opposite side is not done, metachronous torsion of the contralateral testicle occurs in 5% to 10% of the cases.[1]

The strongest argument for contralateral or-

chiopexy was made by Campbell, who reported two college boys rendered eunuchs through torsion of the contralateral testicle.[6] It is imperative that contralateral orchiopexy be carried out on any occasion when there is torsion on one side and that it not necessarily be limited to the bell-clapper deformity. The patient and parents should be informed that if torsion is found, a second incision will be made on the opposite scrotum for the purpose of excising any of the rudimentary appendages. A bottle hydrocelectomy will be performed with fixation in at least two separate sites, one dependent and one posteromedial, suturing the tunica albuginea to the dartos muscle and septum with nonabsorbable suture (Fig. 103-4A). Lyon, "reading between the lines in the surgical literature," gains the impression that a major reason for the reluctance to explore the second testicle is fear of damaging it; such fear is unfounded when orchiopexy is done correctly.[24]

If torsion occurs in an undescended testis after puberty, the organ should be removed; the internal ring should be closed; and if the patient desires, a Dow–Corning synthetic prosthesis should be sutured into the scrotum (Fig. 103-4B and C). Recent evidence suggests that attempting to salvage intra-abdominal testes is likely to be futile and that there is little hope for effective spermatogenesis; since there is also a higher incidence of malignant degeneration, orchiectomy should be the procedure of choice. Torsion of an undescended testicle after 3 years of age is best treated by orchiectomy immediately, if the opposite testis is normal.[8]

If the symptomatic testis grossly appears normal

and mobile at surgery, a diligent search for segmental areas of infarction should be made. If there are none, the parietal tunica should be everted around the epididymis, excising any rudimentary appendages and fixing it at two sites. Under these circumstances, and when the opposite testis is in normal anatomic position, contralateral exploration need not be done.

NONSURGICAL TREATMENT

In every case of sudden severe pain in the testis, the clinician should immediately strive to detorse manually for abatement of pain; however, manual detorsion alone is not sufficient treatment. Although one cannot insist upon surgery, the surgeon should attempt to overcome ignorance and the fear of anesthesia and surgery.

Miscellaneous Types and Treatments of Torsion

RECURRENT OR INTERMITTENT TORSION

Numerous reports of recurrent torsion of the spermatic cord have appeared in the world literature.[1,16,27] From the prognostic viewpoint, these are probably the more important cases, because they are the ones in which early surgical correction produces a higher percentage of preserved spermatogenesis. In 1931, Ormond addressed recurrent torsion of the spermatic cord, emphasizing that it occurs in all decades from infancy to old age, although most commonly about the age of puberty and early adult life.[29] Often the clinician does not see the patient until the intermittent pain from relapsing or recurrent torsion has abated. Upon examination, there is only slight edema, which may involve either the globus majus (if the spermatic artery had been involved in the partial torsion) or the globus intermedius or minus (if the artery and veins of the vas have been compromised, simulating epididymitis). When the cord untwists itself within a few minutes to an hour, there may often be no residual edema.

TORSION OF INTRA-ABDOMINAL TESTIS

If the mesorchium in the fold of peritoneum that covers the testis in its developmental position below the kidney is unduly lax, allowing the testicle to fall away from the internal ring and not become engaged in the inguinal canal, the testis could eventually become pedunculated. The first reported case of intra-abdominal torsion had an associated malignancy. Any male with an untreated undescended testis who presents with abdominal pain must be suspected of having not only torsion of the testis but also associated malignant degeneration, recalling Campbell's axiom that the higher the undescended testicle the greater the incidence of malignant degeneration.[4] Seminoma is the predominant tumor and embryonal carcinoma, the next most frequent. One teratoma has been reported and several of the earlier cases were reported to be sarcomas.

LOCALIZED (SEGMENTAL) INFARCTION OF THE TESTIS

Infarction of only a part of the testis is uncommon.[18] The area of the obvious infarction should be incised, evacuating the old blood and resuturing the tunica albuginea. Clinical symptoms may resemble torsion of one of the appendages more closely, because the symptoms might not be as severe as in torsion of the spermatic cord, and usually the former will be the clinical diagnosis. At the time of operation localized infarction may be mistaken for orchitis or even for testicular neoplasm, although incision of the tunica albuginea makes the correct diagnosis immediately clear. Because the infarct does not involve the entire testis, local incision and drainage may be undertaken and orchiectomy, avoided. Infarction produced by a thrombus originating from trauma is likely to be the most common cause. Undoubtedly segmental septic infarctions do occur but they are treated without surgery and managed as acute or subacute epididymo-orchitis.

TORSION OF THE SPERMATIC CORD IN THE NEWBORN INFANT

Torsion may occur as an intrauterine phenomenon. Torsion in the newborn infant presents quite a different clinical picture from torsion in older patients. Campbell was the first American to describe this as a separate entity, labelled *idiopathic hemorrhagic infarction*.[6] Subsequently several authors postulated that his case may originally have been torsion that had detorsed later, too late to prevent necrosis and gangrene.

Qvist's study of 158 cases of swelling of the scrotum in infants and children over a 5-year period, averaging 32 cases per year, included 12 cases of nonspecific epididymitis (two per year), usually associated with incarcerated hernia.[35] Of 61 cases of incarcerated hernia, 12 had nonspecific epididymitis. One third of the cases of swelling of the scrotum in infants and children were due to torsion of a rudimentary appendage or the testicle, with 20% idiopathic edema and only two cases of acute primary orchitis. The conclusion was that operation was the routine practice in cases of swelling of the scrotum in infants and children, except in clear-cut cases of idiopathic edema of the scrotum.

Nonspecific epididymitis occurs in boys of all ages and, may be hematogenous in nature, but most commonly is due to incarcerated hernia. Usually the infant presents an enlarged, hard, reddish-purple-black, nontender mass that does not transilluminate. Seldom do babies present with gastrointestinal disturbances; there is no vomiting, minimal or no fever, and no sign of toxicity or pain. The differential diagnosis in the newborn is different from those in older infants and children because of the lack of symptoms. Consideration of testicular tumor, although rare, is the first concern. The diagnosis of orchitis or epididymitis is unlikely. Torsion of a rudimentary appendage or strangulated inguinal hernia must be considered. The first case of synchronous neonatal bilateral torsion of the spermatic cord was reported in 1967 by Frederick and colleagues, the second by Papadatos and Moutsouris in Greece in 1976.[13,31] In the latter case, both testicles were of the extravaginal variety, both were unwound and replaced in the scrotum. Upon detorsion the color improved, and on examination 4 months later, they were firm in consistency and approximately normal in size.

Intra-Abdominal Intrauterine Testicular Torsion

Torsion of an intra-abdominal testis is a most uncommon event. It may easily be classified as intrauterine torsion of an intra-abdominal testis. None of the case reports had malignant degeneration, although one case was that of a 3-day-old youngster who had calcifications that were clearly visible on x-ray film.[7] Various authors emphasize the possibility of intrauterine intra-abdominal torsion in a neonate presenting with an undescended testicle and an abdominal mass.[2,5]

Surgery for Neonatal Torsion

Surgical exploration with reduction of the torsion should be performed immediately under nipple sucking "anesthesia" along with routine circumcision, meatotomy, and frenulectomy when indicated. Because the pathogenesis of extravaginal torsion need not be associated with testicular anomalies, it is logical to question the advisability of bilateral exploration. However, morbidity on examination is negligible; further, one should be certain the other testicle might not be lost at a later time, because there are several reported cases of the intravaginal variety with the typical bell-clapper deformity on the opposite side. Routine scrotal exploration with modified bottle hydrocelectomy should be carried out to guarantee adhesions with fixation into the proper anatomic position.[3] If there is synchronous bilateral torsion in a newborn, each testicle should be detorsed and placed back in the scrotum after freeing whatever was constricting.

FIG. 103-5.   **(A)** Separation of epididymis from testis, with elongated mesorchium; **(B)** site and action of torsion (*arrow*); **(C)** excision of excess parietal tunica vaginalis and suture of epididymis to tunica albuginea on either side

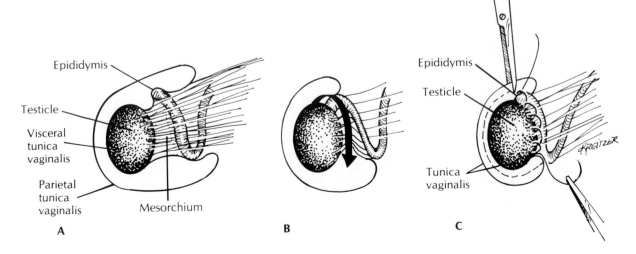

A prosthesis may be placed. Fixation of the opposite testis is a prophylactic measure against metachronous torsion. Those who declare surgery of the contralateral testis unessential have not had the clinical experience and responsibility of explaining metachronous torsion with resulting eunuchoidism.[6]

Although the spermatogenic or hormonal function after torsion of the spermatic cord is questionable, a better cosmetic result occurs if the lump of necrotic tissue is allowed to become atrophic; this may be of psychologic importance during adolescence.[23] Complete atrophy of both testes as a consequence of neonatal torsion may be the explanation of anorchism.[14]

TESTICULAR INFARCTION ASSOCIATED WITH INCARCERATED INGUINAL HERNIA

Testicular infarction as a complication of progressive symptomatic inguinal hernia with incarceration and strangulation is uncommon. At surgery, there is no torsion, yet the spermatic cord is compromised because of the edema secondary to the strangulated hernia. This becomes an academic point because, in both instances, the proper approach is immediate inguinal exploration.[15]

TORSION OF THE TESTICLE ON THE EPIDIDYMIS (TRUE TESTICULAR TORSION)

This uncommon category was emphasized by Parker and Robison in the review of their experience at Wilford Hall several years ago.[32] There is no

attachment or an elongated mesorchium distal to the branch of the spermatic artery that supplies the head of the epididymis (Fig. 103-5A and B). The epididymis should be sutured to the tunica albuginea with 4-0 chromic gut or equivalent material (Fig. 103-5C). The previously described surgical repair follows.

TORSION OF MALDESCENDED (ECTOPIC) TESTIS

The largest series in the American literature is reported in two papers coauthored by Holmes, the latter in 1972.[17,33] These cases occurred in patients with spastic neuromuscular disease, who usually were paraplegic. The mechanism suggested is abnormal contraction or spasm of the cremaster muscle. The important consideration is in the differential diagnosis of epididymitis, which is so common from chronic urinary tract infection. Orchiectomy is probably the surgical procedure of choice if the remaining testis is in the scrotum or the patient desires no children and is past puberty (Fig. 103-6).

TORSION OF A RUDIMENTARY VESTIGIAL APPENDAGE

Giovanni Battista Morgagni was professor of surgery at Padua for more than 50 years. He published his many observations on surgical pathology in *De Sedibus et Causis Morborum* in 1769.[26] Morgagni concluded that the flat, disclike corpuscles within the tunica vaginalis were ruptured versions of

FIG. 103-6. Sites of ectopic or maldescended testes

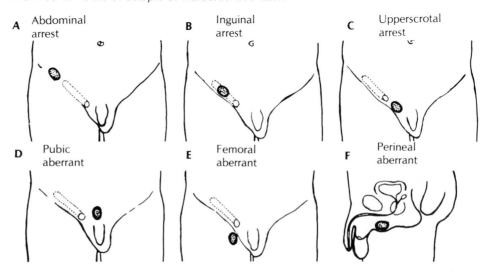

| A | Abdominal arrest | B | Inguinal arrest | C | Upperscrotal arrest |

| D | Pubic aberrant | E | Femoral aberrant | F | Perineal aberrant |

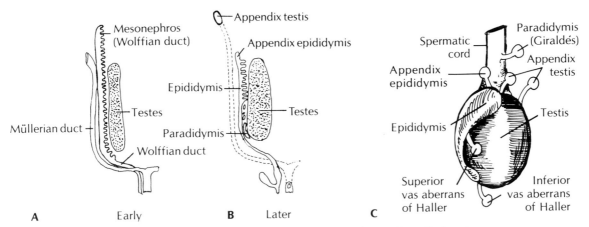

FIG. 103-7. Development of the male genital tract: **(A)** embryonal gonad, müllerian duct, and mesonephros; **(B)** involution of the müllerian duct and mesonephros illustrating site of origin of intrascrotal gonadal appendices; **(C)** types of rudimentary vestigial appendages

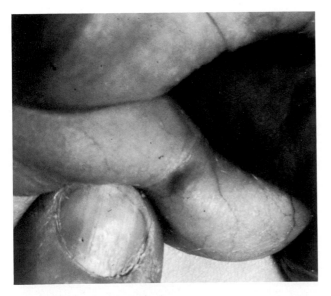

FIG. 103-8. The blue dot sign

cystic rudimentary appendages, which accounted for the fluid in the tunica vaginalis. In clinical parlance, many authors refer to the rudimentary appendages as sessile hydatids of Morgagni, pedunculated, predisposed to torsion, occurring most frequently around puberty, and thought to be due to hormonal influence with growth of both the testes and epididymides.

Embryology of Rudimentary Vestigial Appendages

The cranial end of the Müllerian duct persists as the appendix testis in approximately 90% of males;

the middle becomes the vas deferens; and the most caudal end persists as the prostatic utricle. The mesonephric (wolffian) duct in the cranial end may persist rarely as the organ of Giraldés (paradidymis), the appendices of epididymis in approximately 25% of adult males, and the superior or inferior organ of Haller in 1% to 2% (Fig. 103-7*A* to *C*). On occasion there may be two appendices testis and rarely one may be located lower down on the testicle, rather than in the customary position in the groove between the epididymis and testis or on the superior pole of the testis itself. Presman describes the various eponyms for rudimentary appendages; these are used interchangeably in the literature and are confusing to student and clinician alike.[34] Figure 103-8*A* lists the various embryonic structures in the middle section, their adult counterpart in the male on the left side, and their counterpart in the female on the right.

The predisposing factor is a sufficiently long stalk capable of twisting. The pathogenesis must be either subtle or violent trauma or contraction of the cremaster muscle. Symptoms are similar to torsion of the spermatic cord but much less severe, with pain the predominant symptom early in the process before the development of hydrocele. The purplish or "blue dot" sign mentioned by Fillis and Meyer in 1953, was more recently emphasized by Dresner (Fig. 103-8*B*).[10,11] Constitutional symptoms are usually less severe than with torsion of the spermatic cord, although there may be referred pain to the lower abdomen, some nausea and vomiting, and occasional shocklike symptoms. Hours later, the entity is indistinguishable from torsion of the spermatic cord.

Incidence

By far the most common torsion is that of the appendix testis, although cases have been reported on all the rudimentary appendages. The earliest report of a case of torsion of the appendix testis was by Ombredanne in 1913.[28] The largest series to date is that of Qvist, in a series of 121 operated over a 10-year period, with the largest number of cases between the ages of 10 and 11.[35] Torsion of the appendix testis may be an athletic injury, and because the condition is often misdiagnosed, it may result in prolonged discomfort with intermittent torsion recurring.

Surgical Treatment of Torsion of Rudimentary Appendages

Surgery is the accepted form of treatment because it provides prompt relief from pain, prevents recurrence, and may rule out torsion of the spermatic cord. Since appendiceal torsion is relatively uncommon, scrotal exploration is essential whenever there is doubt, particularly in the prepubertal youngster. If the diagnosis is torsion of a rudimentary appendage, then exploration of the opposite side becomes a matter of the urologist's own individual judgment. The same operation is carried out on all cases of suspected torsion. We endorse the bilateral surgical approach, in competent hands, using a standardized procedure for exploration of the contralateral side.

Conservative Management

The conservative management of intrascrotal appendiceal torsion has been suggested.[10,12,22] When the entity may be identified before scrotal swelling and edema mask the pathognomonic physical findings, immediate exploration offers no diagnostic advantage and only trades whatever operative risk there is for the diminished postoperative discomfort from the pain and natural resolution. Historically, urologists have recommended immediate exploration regardless of the certainty of the diagnosis or the degree of discomfort.[21,24]

We must conclude that this condition is more common than realized. We can agree with Fitzpatrick that early surgery reduces the subsequent period of morbidity, although nonsurgical management usually results in an uncomplicated recovery.[12] The arguments in favor of surgical excision of the rudimentary appendage are as follows: freedom from complications, painless and rapid convalescence, the guarantee of nonrecurrence, elimination of the possibility that the case is really one of torsion of the spermatic cord with an increased chance of survival and decreased amount of future atrophy, and prompt surgical excision that allows early resolution of any reactive changes in the epididymis and avoids tubular scarring and obstruction.

The Testis after Torsion

Torsion, though not fatal, is a matter of grave importance, for unless it is recognized early, the result is atrophy. When reviewing the literature and attempting to correlate testicular salvage with the number of hours of pain or swelling prior to surgery, one is impressed with the improving prognosis. Remarkable salvage rates are experienced in patients operated on within 6 hours after the onset of pain.

We can agree with the recommendation of Rajfer and Walsh, principally based upon the histologic work of Cooper in 1929, that the sooner a nondescended testis can be fixed into its normal anatomic dependent scrotal position, the better the statistical chance for a more normal semen count and for procreative manhood.[8,36]

The exceptions to atrophy in numerous cases explored more than 24 hours after the onset of pain probably fall into the category of partial or incomplete torsion of the spermatic cord. These are the ones in every series which should approach 100% viable testis capable of procreation. Krarup's remarkable long-term follow-up, of 48 of 74 patients (65%) in his series explored for torsion of the spermatic cord, was evaluated, graded, and grouped into four categories.[23] This study showed a clear correlation between the duration of torsion and the degree of subsequent atrophy.

Krarup noted a tendency for the manually reduced testes to remain full size more often than those he could not detorse manually before surgery. In his series, 30% of those contralateral testes that were not explored and fixed became symptomatic at a later time, and at least one required orchiectomy. Although all patients after puberty had normal libido and potency, semen analyses were quite variable. The lowest counts were among those who had had a testis removed, suggesting that patients who were operated on for unilateral torsion may have had congenital bilateral testicular spermatogenic abnormality.

REFERENCES

1. ABESHOUSE B: Torsion of the spermatic cord: Report of three cases and review of the literature. Urologic and Cutaneous Review 40:699, 1936

2. ARKIN R, SHAFER AB: Torsion of an intra-abdominal testicle in a neonate. J Pediatr Surg 8:551, 1973

3. BIORN CL, DAVIS JH: Torsion of spermatic cord in the newborn. JAMA 145:1236, 1951

4. CAMPBELL HE: Incidence of malignant growth in undescended testes: A critical and statistical study. Arch Surg 44:353, 1942

5. CAMPBELL JR, SCHNEIDER CP: Intrauterine torsion of an intra-abdominal testis. Pediatrics 57:2, 1976

6. CAMPBELL MF: Torsion of the spermatic cord in the newborn infant. J Pediatr 33:323, 1938

7. CHO SK: Infarction of an abdominal undescended testis presenting as a calcified abdominal mass in a newborn. Radiology 110:173, 1974

8. COOPER ER: The histology of the retained testis in the human subject at different ages and its comparison with the scrotal testis. J Anat 64:5, 1929

9. DEMING CL, CLARKE BG: Torsion of the spermatic cord. JAMA 152:6, 1954

10. DRESNER ML: Torsed appendage: Diagnosis and management: Blue dot sign. Urology 1:63, 1973

11. FILLIS BE, MEYER WC: Torsion of the hydatid of Morgagni. J Urol 69:6, 1953

12. FITZPATRICK RJ: Torsion of the appendix testis. J Urol 79:521, 1958

13. FREDERICK PL, NICKOLAS D, ERAKLIS AJ et al: Simultaneous bilateral torsion of the testis in a newborn infant. Arch Surg 94:299, 1967

14. GLENN JF, MCPHERSON HT: Anorchism: Definition of a clinical entity. J Urol 105:265, 1971

15. HAINES C: Torsion of the spermatic cord. Am J Surg 43:799, 1939

16. HARRISON RH, III: Torsion in the Male. A Monograph. Norwich NY, Norwich-Eaton Laboratories, 1981

17. JOHNSON MC, HOLMES TW, JR: Torsion and the ectopic testis. Surgery 55:854, 1964

18. JOHNSTON JH: Localized infarction of the testis. Br J Urol 32:97, 1960

19. JONES P: Torsion of the testis and its appendages during childhood. Arch Dis Child 37:214, 1962

20. KAPLAN GW: Acute scrotal swelling in children. J Urol 104:219, 1970

21. KING LM, SEKARAN SK, SAUER D et al: Untwisting in delayed treatment of torsion of the spermatic cord. J Urol 112:217, 1974

22. KOFF SA, DERIDDER P: Conservative management of intrascrotal appendiceal torsion. Urology 8:482, 1976

23. KRARUP T: The testes after torsion. Br J Urol 50:43, 1978

24. LYON RP: Torsion of the testicle in childhood. JAMA 178:702, 1961

25. MOORE TS, HOLLABAUGH RS: The "window" orchidopexy for prevention of testicular torsion. J Pediatr Surg 12:237, 1977

26. MORGAGNI GB: De sedibus et causis morborum. In Alexander B (trans): Seats and Causes of Diseases. London, Miller and Cadell, 1769

27. O'CONOR VJ: Torsion of the spermatic cord. Surg Gynecol Obstet 17:242, 1933

28. OMBREDANNE L: Torsion of the spermatic cord. Bulletin de Memorial Societe de Chirurgie 39:779, 1913

29. ORMOND JK: Recurrent torsion of the spermatic cord. Am J Surg 12:479, 1931

30. OTTENHEIMER EJ: Testicular fixation in torsion of the spermatic cord. JAMA 101:116, 1933

31. PAPADATOS C, MOUTSOURIS C: Bilateral testicular torsion in the newborn. J Pediatr 71:249, 1976

32. PARKER RM, ROBISON JR: Anatomy and diagnosis of torsion of the testicle. J Urol 106:243, 1971

33. PHILLIPS NB, HOLMES TW, JR: Torsion infarction in ectopic cryptorchidism: A rare entity occurring most commonly with spastic neuromuscular disease. Surgery 71:335, 1972

34. PRESMAN D: A morphologic study of the appendix testis. Invest Urol 1:312, 1964

35. QVIST O: Swelling of the scrotum in infants and children and nonspecific epididymitis. Acta Chir Scand 110:417, 1955

36. RAJFER J, WALSH PC: Testicular descent. Urol Clin North Am 5:1, 1978

37. SMITH GI: Cellular changes from graded testicular ischemia. J Urol 73:355, 1955

38. YOUNG HH, DAVIS DM: Torsion of the spermatic cord. In Young HH (ed): Practice of Urology, p 164. Philadelphia, W B Saunders, 1926

Infertility and Vas Reconstruction

104

Bruce H. Stewart

The idea of using surgery to prevent fertility in the male is not new. Procedures such as urethral subincision have been practiced by primitive tribes since antiquity. As the anatomy of the male reproductive system became better understood, bilateral partial vasectomy emerged as the procedure of choice for male sterilization.[7,19] Vasectomy has been used increasingly in recent decades and except for circumcision it is the most commonly performed male surgical procedure. It is estimated that between 800,000 and 1,000,000 vasectomies were done in the United States for male sterilization in 1972. However, since the work of Alexander, indicating a possible increase in generalized atherosclerosis following vasectomy, the number of elective vasectomies appears to have declined somewhat in this country.[2] Although this link may exist to a degree in experimental primate studies, there is thus far no good clinical evidence that vasectomy increases the risk of atherosclerotic or immunologic disease in man.[13,42]

Vasectomy should be reserved for well-motivated, emotionally stable individuals, preferably those having the full knowledge and consent of their marital partner. Psychologic and medicolegal complications can be minimized by using an information brochure and consent form such as that developed by Abel Leader of Houston, Texas, and that now used routinely at the Cleveland Clinic Foundation.[41] Consent of the wife is highly desirable, but because many of these patients are either in the process of a divorce or have no current spouse, it is generally believed that vasectomy should be a medical matter to be decided by the physician and his patient.

The operation should result in permanent sterilization with minimum risk and minimum postoperative complications. The procedure should also make possible future vasovasostomy without technical difficulties in the rare patient who changes his mind about permanent sterilization. A number of surgical techniques for vasectomy have been described (Chap. 105). The technique of Schmidt fulfills the ideal criteria, and it is therefore here described in some detail.[36]

The procedure should be done in a well-equipped pavilion and, in most cases, it is performed easily under local anesthesia. The midportion of the vas deferens is palpated between thumb and fingers, and it is elevated by digital compression to lie just beneath the anterior scrotal skin. To facilitate future vasovasostomy, vasectomy should be performed at the highest level in the spermatic cord that is technically possible. The skin, subcutaneous tissue, and fascia surrounding the vas deferens at the level selected are infiltrated with a local anesthetic agent sufficient to anesthetize a 3-cm or 4-cm segment of the vas deferens.

A 1-cm to 2-cm skin incision is made longitudinally over the exposed vas, and the subcutaneous tissues surrounding the vas are separated gently with a hemostat. The vas is then grasped firmly with an Allis forceps and delivered into the operating field, where a longitudinal incision is made through surrounding fascia to expose the vas (Fig. 104-1). Still holding the vas with the Allis forceps, the urologist carefully dissects the muscular wall of the vas free from surrounding structures with a hemostat, taking care to deliver only the vas deferens and not to include its adjacent blood vessels. After a 2-cm or 3-cm segment has been exposed by blunt dissection, the midportion of the exposed vas is grasped with a hemostat and elevated further into the operative field, and the Allis forceps is removed.

Firm downward traction on this hemostat places the distal vas on tension as it courses upward toward the inguinal ring. Palpation of the entire vas at this time confirms the side on which vasectomy is being performed. Repeating this maneuver on both sides helps avoid the error of ligating the vas deferens twice on the same side. The distal segment of the vas is then grasped with a smooth forceps, and the vas is transected with the scalpel about 1 cm from the forceps. A needle electrode or Vasector is inserted 3 mm or 4 mm into the lumen of the distal vas, and the lumen of the vas is then lightly fulgurated (Fig. 104-2). The recently developed battery-powered (Vasector) electrode has proven ideal for light fulguration of the vasal

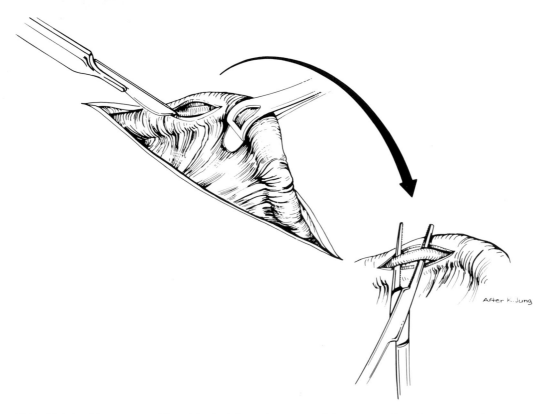

After K. Jung

FIG. 104-1. Vasectomy. After skin incision, the vas and its surrounding tissues may be grasped, isolated, and incised to isolate the vas deferens.

lumen during vasectomy and has proven safe, convenient, and effective in this regard.*

Small vessels coursing over the surface of the vas are also controlled by electrocautery. The distal vas is then dropped back within its fascial sheath, which is closed tightly with interrupted 4-0 chromic catgut sutures (Fig. 104-3). The proximal vas is then grasped 1 cm or 2 cm from the original hemostat and is transected next to the hemostat. This results in the removal of a 1-cm segment of vas, which is sent to the pathologist for microscopic confirmation of the accuracy of the procedure. The needle electrode is then inserted into the vas, and the lumen is again lightly fulgurated. Hemostasis is completed with light electrocautery, after which the vas is returned to the scrotum and the skin is sutured loosely with fine chromic catgut. A collodion dressing is applied and the procedure is repeated on the opposite side.

The Schmidt technique is preferred because of the relatively high incidence of sperm granulomas after conventional ligature techniques.[36] If the lig-

atures are applied too loosely, they may slip free; if applied too tightly, pressure necrosis of the proximal vas can occur. Extravasation of sperm cells, with formation of a sperm granuloma, can result in either case. Through these granulomas recanalization of the vas deferens can occur, with the subsequent appearance of sperm cells in the ejaculate and failure of the sterilization procedure. The fulguration of both cut ends of the vas deferens, combined with the interposition of fascia between the two severed ends, has virtually eliminated the problem of recanalization, and the incidence of spermatic granulomas has been reduced to less than 1%.

As Freund and Davis have demonstrated, 6 to 10 ejaculations are required to clear the ductal system of sperm cells following vasectomy.[12] For this reason, the patient is instructed to continue contraception and to return for checkup examination 4 to 6 weeks after vasectomy.[21] If physical examination at that time does not indicate a complication such as a sperm granuloma, and only if the ejaculate is free of sperm cells, then the patient is discharged.

Considerable research has been done recently

---

* Vasector electrode, Concept Incorporated, US 19 South, Clearwater, Florida 33516

FIG. 104-2. Vasectomy. After clamping and dividing the vas, the cut ends are fulgurated.

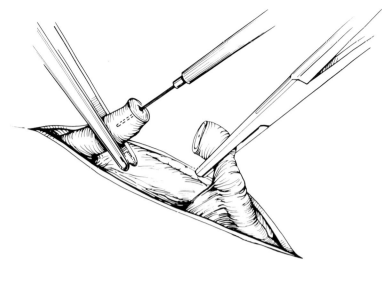

FIG. 104-3. Vasectomy. After fulguration and the resection of approximately 1 cm of vas length, the ends of the vas are returned to separate tissue planes.

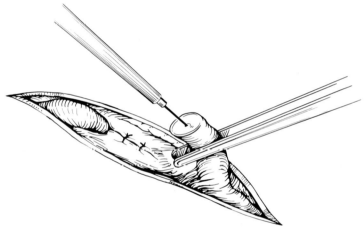

on techniques of reversible vasectomy.[8] To date, most of the procedures involving the insertion of an intravasal occlusive device have resulted in excessive inflammation and scarring at the site of the procedure, precluding successful recanalization after removal of the occluding device. Davis has developed an ingenious reversible intravasal valve of stainless steel and gold, but he has not yet demonstrated whether fertility can be restored after the valve has been in the closed position for prolonged periods. The incidence of complications after bilateral vasectomy has been low when the procedure was meticulously performed by experienced surgeons.[14,19] Long-term psychologic and immunologic sequelae of vasectomy have yet to be defined, although currently available studies indicate that these sequelae are probably not clinically significant in the human.[2,42,44]

Operations to Restore Fertility

Diagnostic Procedures

Testis biopsy should in general be performed only in the severely oligospermic or azoospermic person in whom other studies do not confirm a definitive diagnosis.[3,27,37] Endocrine assays and techniques of semen analysis are now sufficiently well developed to render testis biopsy unnecessary in most infertile patients. Biopsy may be performed using either local or general anesthesia, and it is best performed according to the technique described by Rowley and Heller.[34] The anterior surface of the testis is exposed through a small scrotal incision, using a hemostat or palpebral retractor.

Care should be taken to avoid accidental incision of the epididymis. Infiltration of the testicular substance by needle injection of local anesthetic solution should be avoided because it can cause unnecessary distention of the tunica albuginea, pain, and distortion of the testicular architecture. When necessary, the topical application of local anesthetic to the tunica albuginea is preferred.

The tunica albuginea is opened 2 mm or 3 mm, and the extruded testicular tissue is cut free with a fine scissors or a sharp razor blade. At no time should tissue forceps be used to handle the specimen, and under no circumstance should the tissue be placed on a sponge or cloth surface, which might tear its delicate architecture asunder. The specimen should be placed immediately into a freshly prepared fixative, using either Cleland's or Helly's solution. The commonly used 10% formalin fixative causes severe artifactual distortion of testicular anatomy and should never be used for fixing testis biopsy specimens.

The tunica albuginea is closed with interrupted 4-0 chromic catgut sutures, and the scrotal incision is closed in layers. Scrotal support is advised for several days after the procedure.

Scrotal Exploration. If the frozen section report from the testis biopsy should reveal normal seminiferous tubular architecture in the azoospermic patient, then surgically correctible ductal obstruction should be ruled out. To achieve maximum efficiency and minimal morbidity, the patient should be prepared for additional surgery; under the same anesthetic the scrotal incisions should be enlarged and the testes and spermatic cord structures delivered into the operative incision. At this point in time, the majority of patients with ductal obstruction are found to have the lesion located at the level of the mid- to caudal aspects of the epididymis, owing either to scarring from previous inflammatory disease or to congenital absence of the cauda epididymis. Obstructions in the mid-vas in the nonvasectomized patient or at the level of the ejaculatory ducts further down the system are most unusual. With early diagnosis and active antibacterial therapy for inflammatory diseases involving the lower urinary tract and male reproductive system, the relative incidence of congenital obstructive disease is now increasing.

Visual inspection of the epididymis, usually with the aid of opthalmologic loupes, is of critical importance in identifying obstructive epididymal disease. In the typical case, the epididymal ductule in the caput and midportion of the epididymis is greatly dilated, giving a yellowish-tan appearance to that portion of the epididymis, which is grossly enlarged when compared to the normal. In fact, a palpably enlarged caput epididymis in the azoospermic patient with otherwise normal testes is strong evidence that a surgically correctible epididymal obstruction exists; after examination in the office the patient can usually be told to expect not only a testis biopsy but definitive ductal reconstructive surgery as well.

The epididymis is followed downward until dilated ductules can no longer be identified. This usually occurs in the mid- to caudal aspects of the epididymis where the ductal system may either be partially or completely absent on a congenital basis or be involved in dense scar tissue if the underlying disease process was inflammatory in nature. The vas deferens should then be palpated carefully, since some cases of congenital ductal obstruction are associated with partial or complete agenesis of the vas deferens. Should the vas be palpably normal, the lowest portion of the dilated epididymal ductule is transected transversely, and fluid from this portion is examined immediately for the presence of spermatozoa. If they are present, the vas deferens is then dissected free from surrounding structures and brought into apposition with the lowermost portion of the transected epididymis. Epididymovasostomy is indicated unless the distal vas deferens is totally obstructed or absent. This can be determined by incising the vas deferens transversely at the epididymal level, leaving about one third of the muscular wall intact for better control during subsequent vasography. From a practical standpoint, if a No. 22 blunt-tipped needle can be inserted into the distal vas and 20 ml of sterile saline is injected without impediment, distal ductal patency can be assumed and the surgeon can proceed with epididymovasostomy without delay. Should any question of ductal patency remain, formal vasography or injection of methylene blue into the distal vas with identification of blue fluid emerging from a Foley urethral catheter can further clarify the situation. Once the presence of distal ductal patency has been confirmed, epididymovasostomy should be carried out forthwith, using microscopic techniques that will be described later.

Vasography is very rarely indicated nowadays, and is usually reserved for special cases of otherwise unexplained azoospermia. Should the testis biopsy be normal, the epididymis prove normal by visual inspection and palpation, and the vas deferens be palpably normal at the time of scrotal exploration, then vasography is indicated. This is done most easily by making a tranverse incision about 60% of the way through the vas deferens, enough to expose the lumen of the vas and yet preserve the integrity of the remaining muscular wall of the vas deferens. A 21- or 22-gauge, blunt-tipped needle is then inserted into the distal vas; 10 ml of dilute contrast medium is injected; and x-ray films are taken. Should the distal vas, seminal vesicles, and ejaculatory ducts appear normal and additional contrast medium be seen entering the bladder, then a proximal injection is made using at most 0.5 ml of contrast material. Actually, less than half this volume is all that is required to fill the convoluted portion of the vas deferens and the tail of the epididymis. Obstructions at the level of the convoluted vas that cannot be determined by prior visual inspection of the caput epididymis are extremely rare and this aspect of vasography is usually done only for the sake of completeness.

On rare occasions, such as in patients who have undergone prior herniorrhaphy with damage to the vas deferens in the inguinal canal, a block can be demonstrated by vasography and corrected surgically in some cases. Obstructions at the level of the ejaculatory duct are not surgically correctible in most cases in light of current knowledge, but at

least a diagnosis can be made and the patient and his family appropriately counseled following such studies. An example of a normal vasogram is shown in Figure 104-4. It should go without saying that testis biopsy, epididymal exploration, and vasography should always be done bilaterally unless structures on one side or the other are palpably absent.

VASOEPIDIDYMOSTOMY

Vasoepididymostomy is indicated in azoospermic patients with normal spermatogenesis and obstruction of the epididymis below the level of the entry of the vasa efferentia into the epididymal ductule in the caput epididymis. The vas deferens must be patent at least from the level of the midscrotum distally through the ejaculatory ductal system. The diagnosis may be suspected preoperatively with the finding of a firm testis of normal volume associated with enlarged, sometimes soft, but rarely

FIG. 104-4. Normal vasogram: **(A)** antigrade injection with free flow into prostatic urethra and bladder; **(B)** retrograde injection demonstrating normally patent system with inability to demonstrate epididymis beyond its most distal portion, the normal limitation of this procedure.

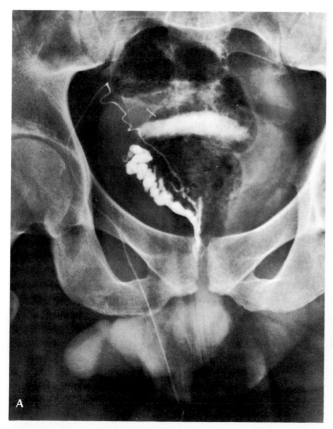

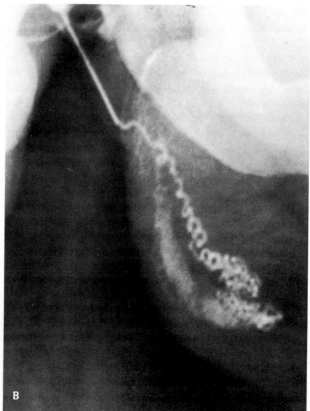

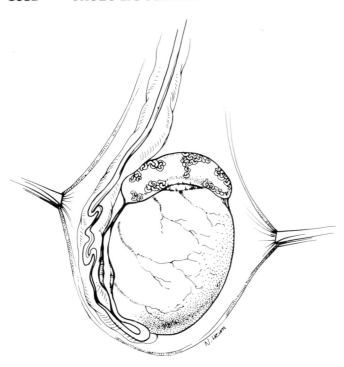

painful caput epididymis and palpation of a normal vas deferens. The diagnosis is confirmed by normal seminal fructose levels and serum follicle stimulating hormone (FSH), luteinizing hormone (LH), and testosterone. It is confirmed by testes biopsy, exploration of the epididymal and cord structures, and demonstration of distal vasal patency as described above. Whether the diagnosis is postinflammatory or congenital, surgical reconstruction is essentially the same. Examples of congenital and postinflammatory epididymal obstructive conditions are illustrated in Figures 104-5 and 104-6. Congenital partial agenesis of the tail of the epididymis and vas deferens is not uncommon. This may vary from segmental areas of partial or complete atresia, as shown in Figure 104-5, or it may be manifested by complete agenesis of the ductal system below the level of the caput epididymis. Postinflammatory epididymal obstruction (Fig. 104-6) usually involves the lower half of the epididymis and part of the convoluted vas.

In the past, the best results from vasoepididymostomy have been achieved with the laterolateral technique. This principle involved the creation of a fistula between transected epididymal ductules above the point of obstruction and a longitudinal incision made into the lumen of the vas deferens distal to the epididymal obstruction. For this reason, even under optimal surgical circumstances, only about one patient in five could be expected ultimately to achieve fatherhood. More recently, direct anastomotic techniques, joining the epididymal ductule proximal to the obstruction end-to-end to the transected distal vas deferens, using microsurgery, have been described by Silber and by Dubin.[11,38,39]

Because of its relative simplicity and satisfactory postoperative results, a modification of the Dubin technique is described here. Although the operating microscope may be used, six-power ophthalmologic loupes usually give adequate magnification for performance of the procedure, which in essence is a three-layer technique providing ductal patency in addition to a strongly supported anastomosis.

Technique of Vasoepididymostomy

The ductal system includes the tightly coiled epididymal ductule leading from the caput epididymis down into the convoluted portion of the vas. It is in this region that the majority of epididymal obstructions occur, shown here in shaded area (Fig. 104-7A). The testis, epididymis, and lower vas deferens are delivered into the operative incision, and by palpation and direct observation the potential site of obstruction is identified. The presence of tortuous and dilated, tan-to-yellowish colored ductules usually indicates the level at which sperm-containing fluid will be found; whitish, firm, fibrotic areas below this point usually indicate the

FIG. 104-6. Postinflammatory epididymal obstruction, also involving the convoluted portion of the vas

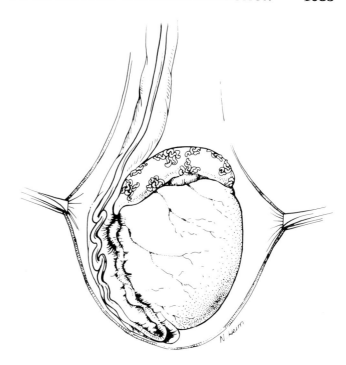

area of obstruction. The entire procedure should be performed after replacing the testis into the scrotal pouch, so that only the epididymis and vas deferens are exposed in the operative incision.

A transverse section is made in the epididymis at a point estimated to be just above the point of fibrotic epididymal obstruction (Fig. 104-7B). The severed proximal epididymal surface is inspected carefully for emission of creamy fluid, which is placed upon a sterile glass slide and inspected immediately for the presence of viable spermatozoa. Should this be the case, the particular ductule that is emitting the sperm-containing fluid can be identified by use of the six-power Designs for Vision opthalmalogic loupe.* There may be significant bleeding from surrounding vessels; if so, these are controlled with light, pinpoint cauterization using the bipolar electrode. Care should be taken not to fulgurate excessively or immediately adjacent to the ductule emitting the sperm-containing fluid.

The vas deferens is brought into apposition with the severed end of the epididymis, and transected sharply. Then either the proximal vas can be ligated or its lumen can be fulgurated with a needle electrode. The lumen of the vas deferens is dilated gently, and the distal ductal system is checked for patency by injecting 20 ml of sterile saline into the

---

* Designs For Vision, 120 East 23rd Street, New York, New York 10010

distal vas deferens with an ordinary syringe. If there is any resistance to injection of this volume of fluid, a conventional vasogram may be performed. After confirming patency of the distal ductal system, two to five sutures of 6-0 or 7-0 Prolene are placed meticulously through the lumen of the vas deferens and through the lumen of the sperm-containing epididymal ductule. Double-armed sutures are used, so that each bite is carefully placed from inside to outside the lumen. Each suture is carried for a millimeter or so into the surrounding epididymal tissue on the epididymal side and through the entire thickness of the wall of the vas deferens. These sutures are tied securely, once the surgeon is sure that there is no tension at the anastomotic site (Fig. 104-7C).

The wall of the vas deferens is then further secured to surrounding epididymal tissue with interrupted 6-0 Prolene sutures as illustrated here. The diameter of the severed epididymis is always greater than that of the vas deferens, so some exposed epididymal tissue will remain between the outer layer of the wall of the vas deferens and the adventitial layer of the transected epididymis. The outer muscular wall of the epididymis is then further secured to the millimeter or two of exposed epididymal tissue with interrupted 6-0 Prolene sutures (Fig. 104-7D). Care should be taken here not to enter the lumen of the vas or to cause kinking or angulation of the anastomosis. The adventitia of the transected epididymis is brought

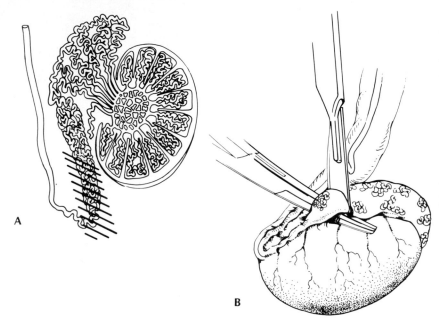

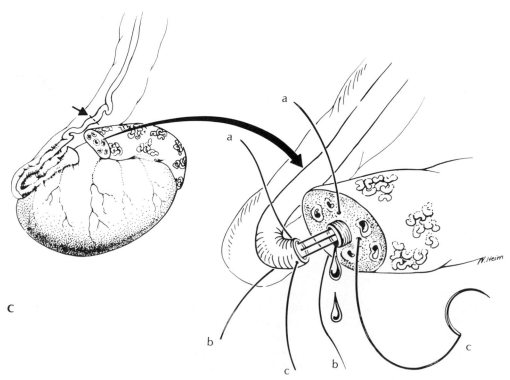

FIG. 104-7. Diagram of the ductal system. **(A)** The majority of epididymal obstructions occur in the shaded area. **(B)** Such an involved and fibrotic area of epididymis and proximal vas may be incised. **(C)** The cut epidiymal surface will exhibit a ductule emitting sperm-containing fluid; this is anastomosed to the severed end of the vas, utilizing magnification with operating loupe. **(D)** Further security is achieved by a second layer of 6-0 sutures. **(E)** Adventitia of both epididymis and vas are then secured with interrupted sutures.

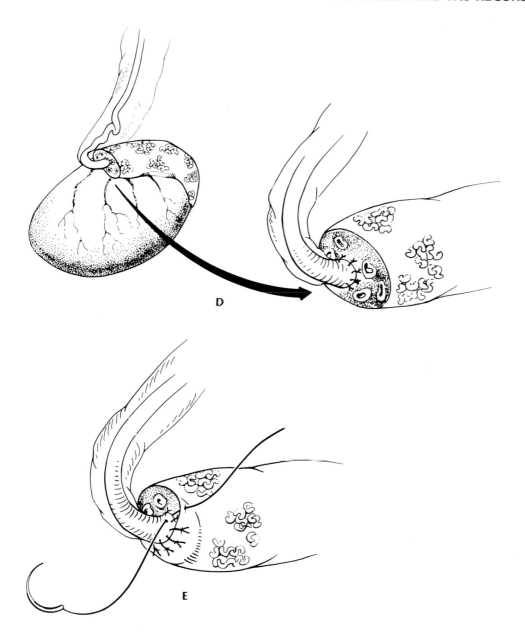

down over the outer portion of the vas deferens, perhaps 2 mm to 3 mm from the site of original vasoepididymostomy, with additional interrupted 6-0 or 7-0 Prolene sutures, thus completing a fluid-tight anastomosis and further reducing tension on the original anastomosis between the epididymal ductule and the lumen of the vas deferens (Fig. 104-7E). These structures are then dropped back into the depths of the scrotal pouch, and the scrotal incision is closed in layers in the usual fashion.

A light fluff dressing is applied and scrotal support is continued for several days following surgery. Routine antibacterial therapy can be em-

ployed if there is any suggestion of an underlying inflammatory cause for the original epididymal obstruction. Sexual abstinence is advised for 2 or 3 weeks following surgery, and a routine semen analysis is obtained between 1 and 3 months after operation. It is too soon to evaluate the efficacy of this technique *versus* that of Silber and of the laterolateral fistulization technique, but the principles of the technique are appealing and it is the procedure of choice of this author until further data become available. Hopefully, long-term experience with large numbers of cases will demonstrate superior results in terms of patency and pregnancies with the end-to-end technique described herein.

The surgical treatment of male sterility is often fruitless, but it nevertheless permits some hope for success. The procedure should be reserved for use by a limited number of specialists in order to give this group the opportunity to gain adequate experience. If one performs a single epididymal–deferential anastomosis every other year, good results will never be obtained and the already meager chances of success for the patient will be reduced still further.

To summarize this intricate and sometimes confusing field, the following points should be borne in mind:

1. Epididymal pathology is a potentially recognizable cause of subfertility in up to 20% of males, especially those with azoospermia or severe oligospermia.

2. Spermatogenesis in the testis remains unaltered regardless of the level of epididymal block.

3. Epididymal patency is a matter of degree. Epididymal pathology can cause both incomplete and complete blocks, leading to oligospermia as well as to azoospermia.

4. Not to inspect the epididymis while performing testicular biopsy may result in the loss of at least half of the value of scrotal exploration.

5. Microsurgical epididymovasostomy is best reserved for azoospermic men; it potentially results in fatherhood in roughly one of every five or six patients. With new microsurgical techniques the eventual rate of fatherhood hopefully will be much higher.

VASOVASOSTOMY

It is estimated that vasectomy for sterilization is currently being performed at a rate of 750,000 to 1,000,000 per year in the United States. The widespread use of this operation has resulted in a steadily increasing number of requests for restoration of fertility. Vasovasostomy was first performed clinically more than 60 years ago, and multiple techniques have since been employed in the hope of obtaining better patency and pregnancy rates.[10,16,22,24,25,29,31–33,35] The state of the art in 1972 was depicted by the results of a questionnaire sent to members of the American Urological Association. Of 1363 urologists who responded, 821 (60%) stated that they had never attempted vasovasostomy, and 542 (40%) had performed this operation.[9] Follow-up data were reported on 1630 patients undergoing vasovasos-

tomy, with postoperative patency rates. Advances in the surgical techniques for performing vasectomy reversal have recently led to improved results.[28,39] Nevertheless, a persistent discrepancy between postoperative patency and pregnancy rates suggests that nontechnical factors may also play an important role in determining whether fertility is ultimately restored.[2,3,4,37]

Following vasectomy, spermatozoa continue to be produced in most patients, but at a slower rate than normal. Testicular biopsy at the time of vasovasostomy thus generally reveals ongoing spermatogenesis with occasional mild focal tunica propria thickening, mild interstitial fibrosis, or intratesticular sperm granulomata.[38] In some patients in whom vasectomy was performed in the remote past, spermatogenesis may be severely impaired, whereas in others secondary epididymal obstruction may have developed. Both of these are sequelae of increased intraductal pressure from long-standing obstruction, and they limit the chances for successful restoration of fertility.

In approximately one third of men who undergo vasovasostomy, a sperm granuloma is found at the site of vasectomy. This is the result of a specific inflammatory response to extravasated sperm and it appears to be one mechanism by which autoimmunity to sperm develops following vasectomy. Silber has attached favorable prognostic importance to the presence of a postvasectomy sperm granuloma; he suggests that it indicates "venting" of the increased intraductal pressure, which can suppress spermatogenesis.[40] An equally common histologic finding in the vas deferens at the time of vasovasostomy is vasitis nodosa, which consists of proliferating small ductules within the wall of the vas associated with intramural fibrosis.[6]

The postulated pathogenetic sequence leading to these histologic findings in the vas deferens after vasectomy is as follows: continued muscular contraction of the vas deferens followed by breaks in the mucosa, sperm leakage, continued sperm penetration, and sperm granuloma formation. Proliferation of epithelium through the breaks in the mucosa, following natural tissue pathways in the wall of the vas deferens, results in vasitis nodosa. It is also important to note that the mechanism of spermatozoal removal after vasectomy is not explained by histopathologic findings in the vas deferens or testis, although phagocytosis undoubtedly plays an important role.

Current methods of performing vasovasostomy can be distilled into three basic techniques: single-layer reanastomosis with 6-0 sutures over an internal or exteriorized intravasal stent, single-layer reanastomosis with 6 0 sutures without a stenting device, and microsurgical single- or double-layer reanastomosis with 9-0 sutures.

In general, vasovasostomy can be performed comfortably by using a 2-inch upper scrotal incision over the palpated site of vasectomy on each side of the median raphe. After dividing the scrotal fascia, the vas is grasped with an Allis clamp and delivered through the incision. Small rubber tapes are used to isolate the vas both proximal and distal to the site of vasectomy. The vas is mobilized for a short distance proximal and distal to the area of vasectomy, taking care to preserve its neurovascular sheath. In some patients, identification of the transected ends of the vas is difficult because of scar tissue or granuloma formation. In this event, mobilization of the proximal and distal vas is performed following delivery of the testis and cord from the scrotum. After excising the scarred ends of the vas, patency of the distal vas is verified by injecting normal saline into it with a 23-gauge blunt needle. Patency of the proximal vas is confirmed by efflux of spermatic fluid that may or may not contain sperm. In a small percentage of cases, spermatic fluid cannot be expressed from the proximal vas, owing to epididymal obstruction. In this case, the head of the epididymis is exposed and, if dilated tubules containing sperm are found, vasoepididymostomy is carried out. It is

not uncommon to find that vasectomy has been performed in the convoluted portion of the vas. Reanastomosis is then performed between a carefully isolated proximal tubule and the straight distal vas.

In performing vasovasostomy, it is helpful to use an approximating clamp to stabilize apposed ends of the vas. The lumen of the obstructed proximal vas is usually dilated, although its outside diameter is unchanged. Whichever method of reanastomosis is employed, it is essential that the ends of the vas be brought together without tension and that accurate mucosa-to-mucosa approximation be achieved. In addition to obtaining a patent repair, a watertight anastomosis is also needed to prevent postoperative extravasation of sperm with inflammation and scarring.[15] Several approximating clamps are available and should be employed in performing vasectomy reversal. Regardless of the method employed, the operation should be done with microsurgical instruments, including the bipolar electrode, which is considerably less tissue-destructive than the standard electrocautery. Optical magnification is also recommended, using 3.5- to 6-power ophthalmologic loupes or the operating microscope. A modification of microsurgical techniques originally described by Silber and later simplified by Novick and others is described in Figures 104-8 through 104-11.

FIG. 104-8. Vasovasostomy. The vas is sharply transected proximal and distal to the sites of previous ligation or division.

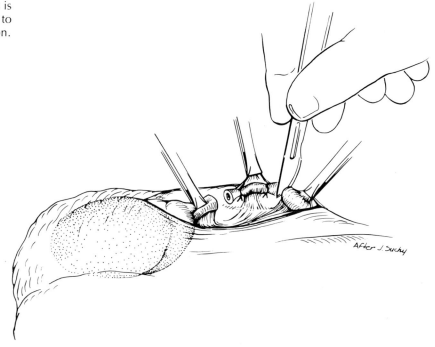

After J Suchy

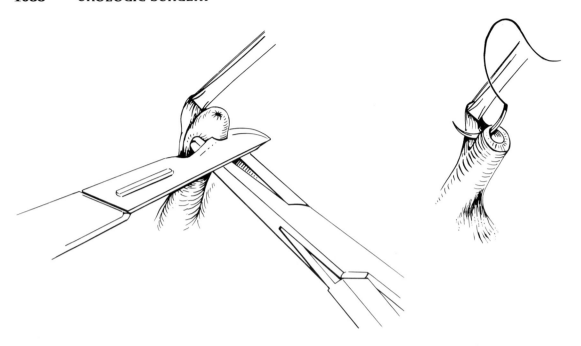

FIG. 104-9.   Vasovasostomy. After freshening the ends of the vasa, the double-armed sutures are passed from the lumen to the outside of the vas.

FIG. 104-10.   Vasovasostomy. As many as six or eight sutures are required for the approximation.

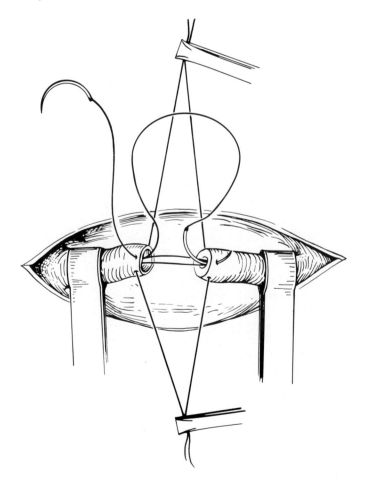

FIG. 104-11. Vasovasostomy. After placing the last approximating sutures, the fascia is reapproximated around the line of anastomosis.

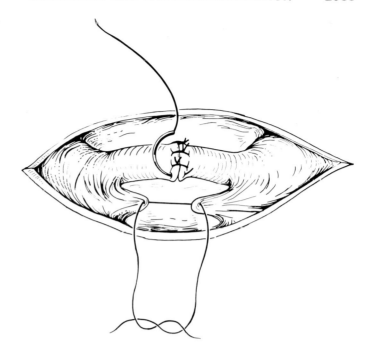

Technique of Vasovasostomy

The vas deferens at the point of its previous vasectomy is identified, dissected free from surrounding structures, and delivered into the operative incision. The surgeon, while preserving adventitia surrounding the vas and elevating the scar tissue and suture material as well as the remnants of the vas involved in the previous vasectomy procedure into the operative field, transects the vas sharply proximal and distal to the previous site of vasectomy (Fig. 104-8). By grasping the vasal adventitia, trauma to the segments of the vas to be anastomosed is minimized and blood supply to each remaining end of the vas deferens is preserved as completely as possible.

The surgeon freshens the ends of the vas, making sure the vas is sharply transected transversely and all occluding scar tissue has been removed. The first suture is passed through the lumen of the vas from the inside to the outside (Fig. 104-9).

Using the operating microscope under 16- to 25-power magnification and holding the severed ends of the vas deferens in approximation with specially designed atraumatic clamps, the surgeon brings the ends of the vas deferens together with interrupted 9-0 nylon sutures (Fig. 104-10). Each suture is double-armed and is passed from inside the lumen through the entire thickness of the vas deferens, with the needle close to the cut edge of the lumen of the vas. The suture is passed through the entire thickness of the vas deferens in a triangular fashion, thus achieving precise mucosal alignment and avoiding protrusion of muscle into the lumen of the vas. Several of these sutures are placed through the entire thickness of the vas; they are tied down without tension yet firmly enough to approximate accurately the ends of the vas deferens.

After releasing the clamps and ensuring proper alignment of the partially anastomosed vas, the surgeon inserts additional 9-0 nylon sutures through the partial thickness of the outer wall of the vas deferens to complete a watertight anastomosis and ensure maximum strength at the anastomotic site (Fig. 104-11). After the repair is complete, the fascia is reapproximated over the anastomosis and the scrotal incisions are closed without drainage. A pressure dressing or scrotal support is applied and maintained in place for several days following the operation.

Following vasovasostomy, patients are instructed to wear a scrotal support for 10 days and to abstain from sexual intercourse for 21 days. Postoperative semen analyses often demonstrate sperm at 1 month, although their appearance may be delayed for up to 6 months. In the initial specimens, sperm motility and morphology are commonly subnormal; however, these generally improve during the ensuing months. For this reason, pregnancy in the spouse may not occur for up to 1 year postoperatively.

TABLE 104-1.   Clinical Results with Vasovasostomy

Series	Number of Patients	Suture Method	Stent	Sperm in Ejaculate (%)	Pregnancy (%)
O'Conor, Sr. (1948)	48	Single-layer 6-0	External gut	60	—
Phadke (1967)	76	Single-layer 6-0	External nylon	83	55
Rowland and O'Conor, Jr. (1977)	21	Single-layer 6-0	External gut	67	29
Mehta (1970)	22	Single-layer 6-0	External nylon	91	—
Pai (1973)	21	Single-layer 6-0	External nylon	95	24
Dorsey (1973)	129	Single-layer 6-0	External Dermalon	88	19
Pardanani (1974)	13	Single-layer 6-0	External Silastic	92	—
Rowland and O'Conor, Jr. (1977)	20	Single-layer 6-0	External catgut	90	27
Banowsky (1978)	10	Single-layer 6-0	Internal catgut	90	50
Schmidt (1975)	117	Single-layer 6-0	None	80	30
Amelar and Dubin (1977)	93	Single-layer 6-0	None	84	33
Middleton (1978)	72	Single-layer 6-0	None	94	39
Silber (1977)	41	Two-layer 9-0	None	100	71

Table 104-1 lists the clinical results with vasovasostomy when employing the various techniques. Single-layer reanastomosis over an exteriorized intravasal stent has largely been abandoned because of the potential for sperm leakage and infection. Of the remaining available methods, a sufficient body of data is currently lacking to enable comparison of their relative long-term efficacy. Microsurgical reanastomosis under the operating microscope is a promising approach; however, this should not be attempted until sufficient practice has been obtained in an experimental laboratory. The skill and experience of the individual surgeon with a particular technique remain an important determinant of the outcome of the repair.

Regardless of the method employed, there continues to be a discrepancy between the presence of sperm after vasovasostomy and the pregnancy rate. Although the reasons for this are not entirely known, there are several nontechnical factors that appear to be of prognostic importance in determining whether fertility is ultimately restored:

The prevasectomy semen quality and fertility of the spouse are obvious considerations, which should be assessed preoperatively.

The interval between vasectomy and its reversal may also be significant because irreversible suppression of spermatogenesis occasionally results from longstanding ductal obstruction especially if longer than 10 years.

Conversely, the presence of sperm fluid at the time of vasovasostomy indicates ongoing spermatogenesis and is a favorable prognostic sign.

It is known that circulating sperm-agglutinating or sperm-immobilizing antibodies develop in 30% to 50% of vasectomized men. Although clinical data on the relation of sperm autoimmunity to the outcome of vasovasostomy are lacking, there are experimental data to suggest that persistence of these antibodies following reanastomosis may impair restoration of fertility.

Finally, vasectomy leads to division of the inferior spermatic nerve, which carries sympathetic fibers to the vas. The implications of this remain poorly understood, but diminished peristalsis of the vas after reanastomosis may also predispose to failure of the procedure.

Certainly recent advances in the methods of performing vasovasostomy have led to improved patency and pregnancy rates. Nevertheless, although technically satisfactory reanastomosis is a critical prerequisite to a successful repair, it is obvious that multiple factors determine whether pregnancy is ultimately achieved. Further improvement in the results of vasovasostomy procedures awaits a more complete understanding of the functional and anatomic changes that occur following vasectomy and their relation to fertility.

ORCHIOPEXY

The technique of orchiopexy is described in Chapter 105. Insofar as prevention of subsequent sterility is concerned, the operation is best performed between the ages of 1 and 3 years. From the psychologic standpoint, it is best to complete the operative correction of cryptorchidism before school age whenever possible. The classic Bevan procedure uses rubber band traction from testis to inner thigh, but it has the disadvantage of inadequate traction because of excessive thigh movement in most normally active children. Ultimate retraction of the testis into the upper scrotum occurs in most patients because of inadequate long-term downward fixation of the testis.

The Torek operation, in which the testis is fixed to the fascia of the inner thigh, results in testicular atrophy owing to impairment of the blood supply in many cases and always requires a second operation. The optimal technique of orchiopexy is that originally described by Ombrédanne.[30] This operation utilizes transseptal fixation of the undescended testis; it does not require a second operative procedure. Excellent results have been reported by those who perform large numbers of these procedures.[23]

Technique of Orchiopexy

The testis and spermatic cord are mobilized through an inguinal approach, and the associated hernia is repaired in the usual fashion; care is taken to preserve the testicular blood supply and to avoid undue angulation of the cord structures. An ipsilateral scrotal pouch is developed by blunt dissection, and a counterincision is made in the contralateral scrotal wall to expose the scrotal septum. A 2-cm to 3-cm incision is then made in the midpor-

tion of the septum, and the mobilized testis is brought through this opening to lie comfortably in the contralateral scrotal compartment. The testis is fixed in the contralateral compartment with several interrupted 3-0 silk sutures passed through the tunica albuginea of the testis and the septum itself. The incisions are closed in layers in the usual fashion without drainage.

On follow-up examination, the operated testis seems to lie in the ipsilateral scrotal compartment (Fig. 104-12), and it is prevented from further upward retraction by fixation to the scrotal septum. The ultimate cosmetic result is excellent (Fig. 104-13) and if proper operative technique is observed, testicular atrophy is rare.

Unfortunately, a great many children with unilateral cryptorchidism have abnormal contralateral testes. The subsequent fertility rate in this group of patients is considerably less than that in the normal population.[43] Nevertheless, for cosmetic reasons, for the modest improvement in fertility potential, and because of the slightly increased incidence of neoplasm in untreated cryptorchid testes, orchiopexy should be advised in all cases

FIG. 104-12. Orchidopexy. The transseptal technique is shown here.

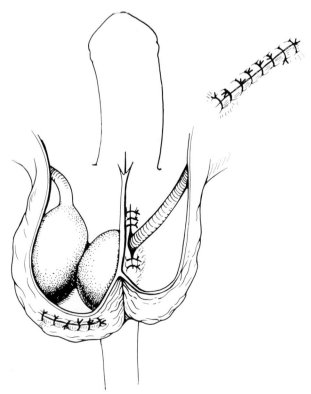

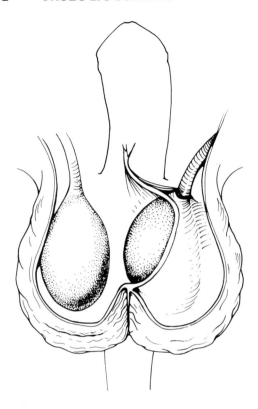

FIG. 104-13. Orchidopexy. Ultimately, the Ombrédanne technique results in slight retraction of the operated testis, bringing it back across the midline in good cosmetic and functional position.

initially seen before puberty. Management of intra-abdominal testes and other complicated situations requires special surgical procedures that are beyond the scope of this chapter.

HYDROCELECTOMY

Hydrocele results in infertility only in rare cases.[18] The operative technique, adequately described in another chapter, is indicated only in patients with significant oligospermia without other apparent cause and in patients in whom the usual attempts at medical management have failed.

SURGERY FOR VARICOCELE

Recent experience has shown that the varicocele is the most frequently encountered, surgically correctable condition causing male infertility.[3] Although operations to correct this condition have been done for nearly a century, Tulloch first drew attention to the salutory effects on patients with infertility in 1952. Since that time, many studies have confirmed the causal relationship between the varicocele and male fertility. Improvement in seminal quality after surgical correction of varicocele has been reported in most patients so treated. The rate of fatherhood after surgical correction of varicocele in patients with a "stress pattern" on semen analysis has averaged 40% to 50% in most large series.[11,37] In this author's personal experience, a control series of unoperated patients with varicocele has a rate of fatherhood of only 7%, as compared to 55% in patients treated surgically.

The majority of patients with oligospermia due to varicocele are afflicted only on the left side. However, Brown and others have shown the profuse cross-circulation between veins draining into the left internal spermatic vein and the veins draining the right testis.[5] Surgery, therefore, has usually been necessary only on the left side, except in those cases in which a right varicocele is palpably present.

In this regard, very recent additional innovations have been made in the diagnosis of subclinical bilateral varicocele by Narayan and associates utilizing a transjugular technique of catheterizing the spermatic veins on both the right and left side.[26] Incompetence of not only the left but also the right internal spermatic vein was demonstrated in a significant percentage of cases (60%). Interestingly enough, the majority of incompetent right internal spermatic veins drain either into the right renal vein or at an unusual level of the vena cava, at the L1–L2 level.

Dubin and Amelar, in a recent report of more than 900 patients treated by resection of the internal spermatic veins at the level of the internal inguinal ring, have reported an overall rate of fatherhood exceeding 60% in patients with left-sided varicocele in whom the preoperative sperm count exceeded 10 million cells/ml.[11] Results were less impressive when the preoperative count was below 10 million cells/ml, but the rate of fatherhood could be increased from 25% to over 40% by the routine postoperative use of chorionic gonadotropin, in the form of APL 4000 I.U. twice weekly by intramuscular injection for a total of 3 months. Amelar and his associates are now exploring the efficacy of performing bilateral spermatic vein ligation in those patients demonstrated to have bilateral varicoceles, in the presence of oligospermia with a typical stress pattern on semen analysis. Of 400 patients undergoing operation for varicocele in 1980, 232 underwent bilateral procedures. It is too early to assess the final results of this approach, but if successful it could represent another significant advance in the management of oligospermic patients.

The indications for bilateral varicocele repair are still unclear. Amelar simply employs physical examination, with great care to examine the right side with the patient in the upright position in a warm room, using Valsalva maneuvers and coughing to elicit small varicoceles. Whether or not long-term results of bilateral varicocele repair and the need for routine catheterization of the spermatic veins will significantly improve the prognosis for bilateral varicocele remains to be demonstrated. However, it would appear that the field is undergoing significant change with the passage of time, and that results of surgery in patients with oligospermia as the result of varicocele hopefully will continue to improve as further experience is gained.

The optimal age at which varicocelectomy should be done is also controversial.[31] Experience with adolescent patients with varicocele suggests that varicocele results in testicular growth arrest rather than atrophy, and that the onset occurs between the ages of 8 and 14 years in most cases.

Our preferred operative technique in slender patients has been essentially the one originally described by Ivanissevich in 1918 and subsequently popularized by Lewis.[17,20] This procedure has the advantage of approaching the internal spermatic vein at a level where danger of damage to the vas deferens and arterial blood supply to the testis is minimal. The inguinal approach, exposing the vessels near the inguinal ring, is preferred in obese or heavily muscled persons; it is used routinely by Amelar and associates.[3] Although occasional cases of testicular loss due to damage of the arterial blood supply during inguinal varicocelectomy have been reported, the recently modified technique described by Amelar and associates has been reliable, has resulted in superior postoperative results, and is technically simpler than the classical Ivanissevich approach. Because of these reasons and the significant decrease in postoperative morbidity, we now favor the Amelar–Dubin approach.

Amelar–Dubin Approach to Varicocele Repair

With the patient in the supine position, the surgeon first locates the external inguinal ring by inserting the index finger upward along the lateral scrotal wall just lateral to the pubic tubercle, where the vas deferens and cord structures can be palpated easily as they emerge from the external ring. The medial aspect of the skin incision is then started over this point and carried laterally for 2 or 3 inches, the length of the incision depending upon the obesity of the patient (Fig. 104-14).

Using rake retractors the skin edges are separated laterally and tented upward, thus separating

FIG. 104-14. Varicocele repair. The incision is over the midportion of the inguinal canal and tissue layers are divided to expose the cord.

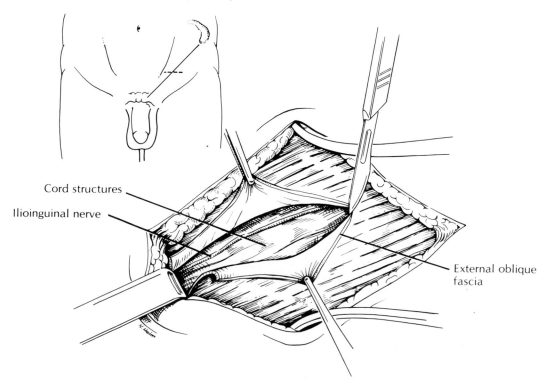

Cord structures

Ilioinguinal nerve

External oblique fascia

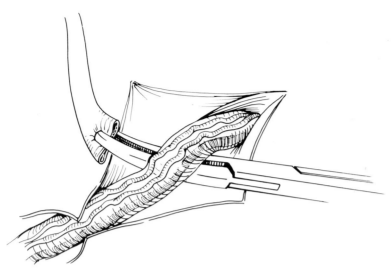

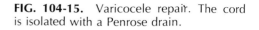

FIG. 104-15. Varicocele repair. The cord is isolated with a Penrose drain.

the subcutaneous tissues and allowing an easier identification of the two or three subcutaneous veins that course in a cephalad direction. These veins are rather constant; they are usually located in the midportion of the incision and must often be divided and ligated rather than simply fulgurated. Scarpa's fascia is then incised and the external oblique fascia is exposed, and by a sweeping motion downward with a sponge toward the base of the scrotum, the entire external fascia and the exernal inguinal ring are easily identified. The midportion of the external oblique fascia is incised in line with its fibers, and edges of the external oblique fascia are elevated into the incision by hemostats.

A self-retaining retractor is then inserted in the midportion of the incision down to the level of the fascia, and a right-angle retractor is inserted medially to allow the external oblique fascial incision to be continued medially to the level of the external ring. It is apparent that there are no contributing vessels to cord structures at this level, and by incising directly through the external ring maximum exposure of cord structures can be easily attained. The external oblique fascia is incised laterally to a point 1 cm or 2 cm medial to the internal ring, with care being taken to avoid injury to the underlying ilioinguinal nerve. Again by gentle upward traction on the hemostats attached to the external oblique fibers, the entire cord structures can easily be seen and separated from the inguinal canal by blunt dissection. Use of a right-angle retractor medially and laterally creates excellent exposure and minimizes incisional length.

Once the midcord structures have been mobilized, a curved hemostat is placed beneath the cord. A Penrose drain is drawn beneath (Fig. 104-15) and attached to the drapes above and below with Kelly hemostats to elevate the cord well into the incision.

The cremasteric fascia is then incised, and the anterior aspect of the cord is elevated toward the ceiling with a Babcock forceps. The varicosities that form the varicocele and drain upward into the internal spermatic vein lie anterior at this level, with the vas deferens and its associated vasculature situated posteriorly, near the floor of the inguinal canal. By blunt dissection the vas and its associated vessels are swept backward out of the operative field, and each individual tributary of the internal spermatic vein is dissected carefully from the surrounding structures (Fig. 104-16). There are usually two or three major branches at this level and once they are identified, the dissection can be continued both sharply and bluntly to expose the veins for a distance of 3 cm or 4 cm upward to within 1 cm or 2 cm of the internal ring and downward nearly to the level of the external ring.

The veins are cross-clamped individually or as a vascular bundle, a 3-cm or 4-cm section of the venous bundle is resected, and each bundle or vein is doubly ligated proximally and distally with 2-0 chromic catgut sutures (Fig. 104-17). Cremasteric and vasal vessels are left undisturbed by this technique and serve as normal collateral venous drainage following division of tributaries of the internal spermatic vein. The Penrose drain is then removed, the cord is allowed to resume its normal position, and the external oblique fascia is closed with interrupted 2-0 chromic catgut sutures.

By starting at the lateral aspect of the external oblique fascial incision and exerting upward trac-

FIG. 104-16 Varicocele repair. The cremasteric fibers are divided to expose the tributaries of the internal spermatic vein.

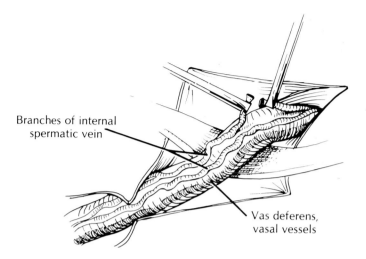

Branches of internal spermatic vein

Vas deferens, vasal vessels

tion on each suture, succeeding sutures can be placed more easily and the ilioinguinal nerve can more easily be avoided. The last suture should complete the closure of the external ring. At this point a Babcock or "peanut" forceps can be used to depress the cord structures downward and prevent inadvertent inclusion of cord structures in the last suture, which closes the external ring. The subcutaneous and Scarpa's fascial layer is then closed with a few interrupted plain catgut sutures, and the skin, with interrupted nonabsorbable or running subcuticular absorbable suture material. The subcuticular method is preferred when the patient lives at a distance and would be inconvenienced by a routine return visit for suture removal.

The inguinal approach to microsurgical ligation of the internal spermatic veins has proven to be easier to perform, with less postoperative morbidity than other approaches and continued satisfactory results in terms of subsequent fatherhood. These advantages are particularly important in patients with bilateral varicocele and when early return to full physical activity is desirable. With the passage of time, the retroperitoneal Ivanissevich approach will probably be reserved for those patients in whom extensive inguinal surgery has previously been performed or in whom inguinal surgery has failed to correct the varicocele.

There has been recent interest both in South America and in the United Staqtes in a new technique of treatment for varicocele. It involves the percutaneous insertion of a catheter through the femoral vein into the left internal spermatic vein and occlusion of the vein, either by injecting a sclerosing material or by inflating and then detaching a small inflatable balloon that thus occludes the left internal spermatic vein.[45] Robert

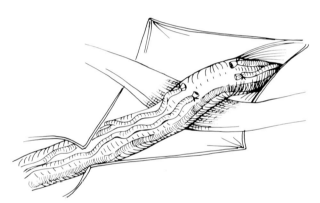

FIG. 104-17. Varicocele repair. All identified branches of the spermatic vein are doubly ligated and divided.

White, Professor of Cardiovascular Radiology at Johns Hopkins University, in consultation with Patrick Walsh, has now performed more than 50 of these procedures in patients with oligospermia thought to be secondary to varicocele. To date there have been no complications, but it is too early to assess the therapeutic effect of the procedure in terms of fatherhood. There is natural concern over potential malfunction of the "mini-balloon" device,* and early or late pulmonary embolism could also become a recognized complication of this procedure. The presence of collateral vessels below the level of the inguinal ring and preliminary clinical data would indicate that the recurrence rate will probably be much higher following this technique. The ultimate role of this ingenious technique will be determined with the passage of time, and at present we still consider

---

* Becton-Dickinson & Co, Rutherford, New Jersey 07070

surgery the standard form of therapy for this condition.

SURGICAL CORRECTION OF RETROGRADE EJACULATION

In rare cases, infertility can be due to retrograde ejaculation caused by previous Y–V plasty or transurethral resection of the vesical neck. In milder cases, conservative therapy using sympathomimetic medication such as ephedrine, 25 mg to 50 mg 1 hour before intercourse, or phenylpropanolamine hydrochloride (Ornade), 1 spansule b.i.d., can correct the situation. However, in most cases surgical revision of the vesical neck is the only way to correct the condition.

The procedure involves exposure of the end of the bladder neck through an anterior cystotomy incision and resection of a 1-cm strip of mucosa from the anterior vesical neck from 9 o'clock to 3 o'clock, creating an inverted horseshoe-shaped area of denuded raw tissue involving the anterior circumference of the vesical neck. This is then simply closed vertically with interrupted 2-0 chromic catgut sutures over a 20 F Foley catheter, leaving the posterior vesical neck intact and reducing the lumen of the bladder outlet to perhaps 22Fr or 24Fr. The anterior cystotomy is then closed in layers in the usual fashion, and Foley urethral catheter drainage is maintained for 21 days following surgery. The procedure has been extremely well illustrated by Abrahams and colleagues,[1] and illustrative material will therefore not be repeated here.

Although the condition is uncommon and experience has admittedly not been great in terms of patient numbers, the results of this technique have thus far been encouraging. The unfortunate sequelae in terms of fertility potential in patients undergoing surgery of the bladder neck at an early age emphasizes the point that a conservative approach should be considered unless significant obstruction is judged to be the cause of potentially serious urinary retention or deterioration of renal function.

Miscellaneous

Hypospadias, epispadias, and congenital chordee can prevent satisfactory intromission, thereby causing infertility. Operative correction of these defects is definitely indicated whenever satisfactory sexual or urinary function is impaired. The various techniques of repair have been described adequately in other chapters, as have those to correct organic impotence.

Many operative procedures, if performed when indicated and with proper techniques, can improve the fertility potential in patients who in the past have been thought to be essentially untreatable. The field of infertility and family planning, although distasteful to many urologists, is expanding rapidly. Application of the latest and best methods of diagnosis and treatment of these problems is necessary if our patients are to be properly served.

REFERENCES

1. ABRAHAMS JI, SOLISH GI, BOORJIAN P et al: The surgical correction of retrograde ejaculation. J Urol 114:888, 1975
2. ALEXANDER NJ: Vasectomy and vasovasostomy in rhesus monkeys: The effect of circulating anti-sperm antibodies on fertility. Fertil Steril 28:562, 1977
3. AMELAR RD, DUBIN L, WALSH PC: Male Infertility. Philadelphia, WB Saunders, 1977
4. ANSBACHER R: Sperm antibodies in vasectomized men. Fertil Steril 24:788, 1973
5. BROWN JS, DUBIN L, HOTCHKISS RS: The varicocele as related to fertility. Fertil Steril 18:46, 1967
6. CIVANTOS F, LUBIN J, RYWLIN AM: Vasitis nodosa. Arch Pathol 94:355, 1972
7. DAVIS JE, JULKA JF: Elective vasectomy by American urologists in 1967. Fertil Steril 21:615, 1970
8. DERRICK FC, JR, FRENSILLI FJ, KANZUPARAMBAN S et al: Results of vas deferens studies: Reversible vas plug—13 cases. J Urol 111:523, 1974
9. DERRICK FC, YARBROUGH W, D'AGOSTINO J: Vasovasostomy: Results of questionnaire of members of the American Urological Association. J Urol 110:556, 1973
10. DORSEY JW: Surgical correction of post-vasectomy sterility. J Urol 110:554, 1973
11. DUBIN L, AMELAR RD: 986 cases of varicocelectomy: A 12 year study. Urology 10:446, 1977
12. FREUND M, DAVIS JE: Disappearance rate of spermatozoa for the ejaculate following vasectomy. Fert Steril 20:163, 1969
13. GOLDACRE MJ, CLARKE JA, HEASMAN, MA et al: Follow-up of vasectomy using medical record linkage. Am J Epidemiol 108:176, 1978
14. HACKETT RE, WATERHOUSE K: Vasectomy reviewed. Am J Obstet Gynecol 116:438, 1973
15. HAGAN KF, COFFEY DS: The adverse effects of sperm during vasovasostomy. J Urol 118:269, 1977
16. HANLEY HG: Results of vasal anastomosis following voluntary vasectomy. Br J Urol 44:721, 1972
17. IVANISSEVICH O: Left varicocele due to reflux; Experience with 4,470 operative cases in 42 years. J Inter College Surgeons 34:742, 1970
18. KRAHN HP, TESSLER AN, HOTCHKISS RS: Studies of the effect of hydrocele upon scrotal temperature, pressure, and testicular morphology. Fertil Steril 14:226, 1963

19. LEADER AJ, AXELRAD SD, FRANKOWSKI R et al: Complications of 2,711 vasectomies. J Urol 111:365, 1974

20. LEWIS EL: The Ivanissevich operation. J Urol 63:165, 1950

21. MARSHALL S, LYON RP: Variability of sperm disappearance from the ejaculate after vasectomy. J Urol 107:815, 1972

22. MIDDLETON RG, HENDERSON D: Vas deferens reanastomosis without splints and without magnification. J Urol 119:763, 1978

23. MILLER HC: Transseptal orchiopexy for cryptorchism. J Urol 98:503, 1967

24. MOON KH, BUNGE RG: Splinted and nonsplinted vasovasostomy: Experimental study. Invest Urol 5:155, 1967

25. MONTIE JE, STEWART BH, LEVIN HS: Intravasal stents for vasovasostomy in canine subjects. Fertil Steril 24:877, 1973

26. NARAYAN P, AMPLATZ K, GONZALES R: Varicocele and male subfertility. Urology Prize Paper presented at the American Fertility Society Meeting, Houston, Texas, March 18–22, 1980. Fertil Steril 1982 (in press)

27. NILSSON S, OBRANT KO, PERSSON, PS: Changes in the testes parenchyma caused by acute nonspecific epididymitis. Fertil Steril 19:748, 1968

28. NOVICK AC: Vasovasostomy. In Stewart BH (ed): Operative Urology, Vol 2, Surgery of the Bladder, Pelvic Structures and Male Reproductive System. Baltimore, Williams & Wilkins, 1982

29. O'CONOR VJ: Anastomosis of the vas deferens after purposeful division for sterility. J. Urol 59:229, 1948

30. OMBREDANNE L: Indications et technique de l'orchidapexie transcrotale. Press Med 18:745, 1910

31. PARDANANI DS, KOTHARI ML, PRADHAN SA et al: Surgical restoration of vas continuity after vasectomy: Further clinical evaluation of a new operative technique. Fertil Steril 25:319, 1974

32. PHADKE GM, PHADKE AG: Experiences in the reanastomosis of the vas deferens. J Urol 97:888, 1967

33. ROWLAND RG, NANNINGA JB, O'CONOR VJ: Improved results in vasovasostomies using internal plain catgut stents. Urology 10:260, 1977

34. ROWLEY MJ, HELLER CG: The testicular biopsy; Surgical procedure, fixation and staining technics. Fertil Steril 17:177, 1966

35. SCHMIDT SS: Vas anastomosis: A return to simplicity. Br J Urol 47:309, 1975

36. SCHMIDT SS: Vasectomy; Indications, technique and reversibility. Fertil Steril 19:192, 1968

37. SCHMIDT SS, STEWART BH, SCHOYSMAN R: Surgical approaches to male infertility. In Hafez ESE (ed): The Human Semen and Fertility Regulation In the Male. St. Louis, CV Mosby, 1976

38. SILBER SJ, GALLE J, FRIEND D: Microscopic vasovasostomy and spermatogenesis, J Urol 117:299, 1977

39. SILBER SJ: Microscopic vasectomy reversal. Fertil Steril 28:1191, 1977

40. SILBER SJ: Epididymal extravasation following vasectomy as a cause for failure of vasectomy reversal. Fertil Steril 31:309, 1979

41. STEWART BH: Vasectomy. In Stewart (ed.): Operative Urology, Vol 2, Surgery of the Bladder, Pelvic Structures and Male Reproductive System. Baltimore, Williams & Wilkins, 1982

42. WALKER AM, HERSCHEL J, HUNTER JR et al: Hospitalization Rates in Vasectomized Men. JAMA 245:2315, 1981

43. WOODHEAD, DM, POHL DR, JOHNSON D: Fertility of patients with solitary testes. J Urol 109:66, 1973

44. ZIEGLER FJ, RODGERS DA, PRENTISS RJ: Psychosocial response to Vasectomy. Arch Gen Psychiatry 21:46, 1969

45. ZERHOUNI EA, SIEGELMAN SS, WALSH PC et al: Elevated pressure in the left renal vein in patients with varicocele: Preliminary observations. J Urol 123:512, 1980

Scrotal and Intrascrotal Surgery

105

Paul L. Bunce

Scrotum

Congenital Abnormalities

The most common congenital anomaly of the scrotum is the cleft or bifid scrotum, which is usually associated with hypospadias or exstrophy of the bladder. Surgical repair is effected quite simply at the time of repair of the primary process by freeing and uniting the two halves. The cosmetic results are satisfactory. Transposition of the external genitalia, a condition in which the scrotum lies anterior to the penis, occurs in several variations and the surgical repair depends entirely on the extent of the malformations.[15,38]

Inflammatory Lesions

In addition to the usual disease found in the skin and subcutaneous tissue elsewhere on the body, the scrotum is also subject to specific diseases peculiar to itself. Gangrene of the scrotum, most frequently caused by urinary extravasation, will be dealt with in the paragraph on trauma. A second type of gangrene peculiar to the scrotum has been termed *idiopathic* or *Fournier's gangrene*.[11] Although usually confined to the scrotum and penis, it may extend up over the abdominal wall and even to the thorax. The testes and spermatic cords are usually spared. Treatment consists of wide débridement of all necrotic tissue and massive antibiotic therapy. The wound may have to be debrided every few days in the operating room until healthy granulation tissue appears.[5,32] The postoperative period may be reduced by the judicious use of skin grafts after a clean bed has been obtained.[2]

Elephantiasis

In some of these patients the scrotum may attain heroic size. Plastic operations to restore a degree of normalcy involve radical excision of the skin and brawny subcutaneous tissues down to the testicular tunics with a reapproximation of the edges (Fig. 105-1).[6,8]

Benign Tumors

The most common benign tumor of the scrotum is the sebaceous cyst, which may be simply locally excised. Multiple sebaceous cysts may be more easily handled by amputating a portion of the scrotum. Other rare benign tumors include fibromas, lipomas, and myxomas, all of which are treated by local excision.

Malignant Neoplasms

Sir Percival Pott in 1775 recognized epidermoid cancer of the scrotum (chimney-sweeps' cancer) as the first occupational cancer. Also called mule spinner's disease among the cotton mill workers, this epithelial tumor generally develops slowly and spreads by way of the lymphatics. The surgical treatment consists of wide local excision with resection of the involved regional lymph nodes.[12,36]

Trauma

Most simple lacerations can be débrided and closed primarily. Where there is severe loss of scrotal skin, as in a traumatic avulsion, reconstruction necessarily depends on the imaginative use of all of the remaining viable skin tags. The magnificent regenerative powers of the scrotum are often ignored or underestimated.[31] Primary repair is often feasible, even though the defect may need to be closed with tension.[21] If the testes have been spared and yet have been completely denuded, they may be placed in temporary pockets developed in the thigh or in the groin. The wound is then covered with a split-thickness skin graft. At a second procedure a new scrotum can be constructed from this skin plus flaps raised from each inner thigh. It is important to remember that a small bit of scrotal skin can be made to go a long way, so that what seems inadequate at the initial operation may prove more than satisfactory when the testes are brought back from their temporary sites. When there is complete loss of the testes as well as the scrotum, the defect can usually be closed in an

1099

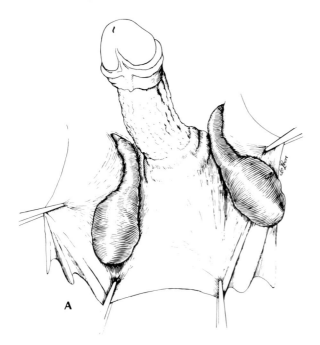

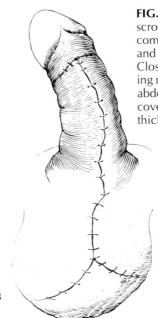

FIG. 105-1. Elephantiasis of the scrotum. **(A)** Genitalia after complete débridement of penile and scrotal lymphedema. **(B)** Closure has been effected by sliding normal tissue from thighs and abdomen. Often penis must be covered by free graft of split-thickness skin.

irregular fashion by using tissue that remains along the margin and by undermining flaps as necessary. These wounds require good dependent drainage and intelligent use of antibiotic therapy.

Traumatic inflammatory or instrumental perforation of the penile or bulbous urethra usually involves rupture of the deep fascia of the penis (Buck's fascia), so that the extravasating urine immediately enters the superficial perineal compartment of the scrotum. This compartment is bound by Colles' fascia, a continuation of the superficial fascia of the abdomen that extends over the penis and scrotum. Colles' fascia attaches firmly to the ischial and pubic rami, preventing spread to the thighs; it closely approximates the posterior border of the urogenital diaphragm, limiting spread posteriorly.[16] However, it is continuous with Scarpa's fascia of the abdomen, permitting extravasation to extend upward over the pubis with only minor resistance.

Urinary diversion by suprapubic cystotomy is the first step. Then dependent drainage of the areas of extravasation must be established with débridement of all necrotic tissue. When extravasation is extended over the abdomen and onto the thoracic wall, drainage may be a formidable task (Fig. 105-2). It is safer to place too many drains than too few; massive antibiotic therapy reduces mortality and morbidity.[13] After the inflammatory reaction has subsided there is usually adequate scrotal skin for satisfactory closure.

For the chronic urethral cutaneous fistulae, as in the classic watering-pot perineum secondary to urethral stricture disease, all tracts must be excised to healthy tissue. Again, there is usually adequate scrotal skin for satisfactory closure.

Testis

Congenital abnormalities of position of the testis are covered in Chapter 102 on orchiopexy and herniorrhaphy.

INFLAMMATORY CONDITIONS

The testis may be primarily involved in systemic diseases such as mumps and syphilis. Mumps orchitis has been treated in the past by multiple incisions in the tunica albuginea, but there is little evidence that this procedure has any merit. Most untreated suppurative processes of the epididymis eventually extend into and destroy the testis. The only treatment for this is orchiectomy.

Simple Orchiectomy—Surgical Technique

After suitable anesthesia (local, spinal, or general), preparation of the skin, and draping of the scrotum, a 4-cm to 5-cm incision is made between the visible surface blood vessels on the anterolateral scrotal wall while the assistant maintains pressure to immobilize the testis against the skin.[10] The incision is carried down through the dartos and cremasteric layers until the tunica vaginalis testis is reached. Blunt dissection with a sponge then allows the testis to be delivered from the wound. With slight traction on the testis, the cord is exposed proximal to the testis by blunt dissection, the vessels of the cord are secured with a suture ligature of 2-0 chromic, and the vas is tied separately to ensure hemostasis (Fig. 105-3). The wound at this point should be completely dry and may then be closed in layers without drainage. A pressure dressing reduces the postoperative edema. A subcapsular orchiectomy for the treatment of prostatic cancer would leave Leydig-like cells on the tunica albuginea and therefore has no rational place in therapy.[23]

TUMORS

Testicular tumors are the most common neoplasms occurring in males between the ages of 20 to 35 years. Therefore, any mass within the testis proper must be considered a malignant neoplasm. The treatment for any such mass is a radical orchiectomy.

Radical Orchiectomy—Surgical Technique

In radical orchiectomy for a testicular tumor, the incision is made in a skin line above the inguinal ligament exactly as for an inguinal herniorrhaphy and is carried down through the fascia of the external oblique until the inguinal canal is reached. The spermatic cord is dissected free and isolated. If there is some question whether a testicular tumor

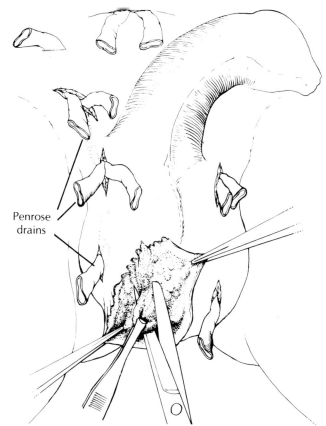

Penrose drains

FIG. 105-2. Treatment of urinary extravasation. Through-and-through drainage has been established and necrotic tissue is being removed.

FIG. 105-3. Simple orchiectomy. **(A)** Scrotal incision made between visible blood vessels on anterolateral aspect of scrotum. **(B)** Testis with intact tunics and cord has been delivered by sharp and blunt dissection. **(C)** Suture ligature is placed about the vascular pedicle and the vas has been ligated separately.

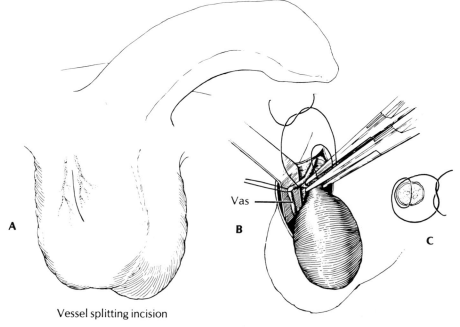

A

Vas

B

C

Vessel splitting incision

actually exists, a rubber-shod clamp should be placed across the vascular pedicle at this point and the testis should be brought up from the scrotal wound (Fig. 105-4). If an intratesticular mass is present, biopsy is usually not advisable because of

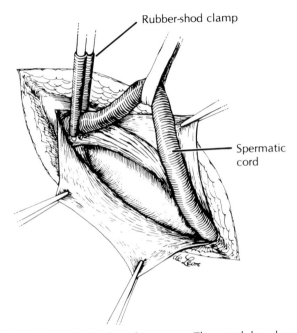

Rubber-shod clamp

Spermatic cord

FIG. 105-4. Radical orchiectomy. The cord has been isolated in the inguinal canal and a rubber-shod clamp has been placed on the spermatic cord prior to delivery of the testis from the scrotum. If a tumor of the testis is found, the cord and vas are secured at the internal ring without disturbing the clamp.

the danger of spreading tumor cells. The cord is suture ligated and divided at the internal ring. If a benign lesion is found, the rubber-shod clamp is removed, the testis is replaced in the scrotum, and the wound is closed in layers. When a simple orchiectomy has been done for testicular cancer, the old scrotal incision must be excised with a wide margin and the cord must be taken to the level of the internal ring as described above. The same wide excision is needed for the rare extratesticular sarcoma.[4]

TRAUMA

Trauma to the testis may be either a simple contusion or a complete rupture. Contusions may be treated expectantly with bed rest and scrotal support, but any repture requires surgical correction.

Rupture of the Testis—Surgical Technique

A standard scrotal incision is carried down through the tunica vaginalis, and blood clots are removed, and bleeding points are ligated. Every effort should be made to salvage remaining viable testicular tissue. Necrotic tubules can be resected back to fresh tissue without difficulty. After the bleeding points have been ligated and the edges freshened, the defect in the tunica albuginea is closed with a running suture of fine catgut and the wound is closed without drainage.[9]

There are now a few reports of successful reimplantation of the testes after autoemasculation and of autotransplantation by use of standard microvascular techniques.[1,34,37]

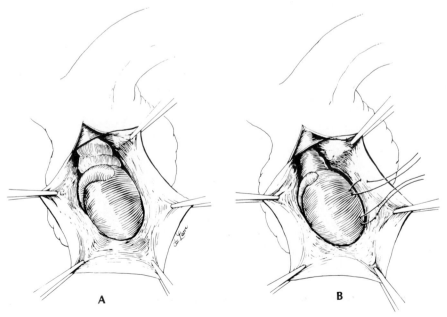

FIG. 105-5. Torsion of the spermatic cord. **(A)** Typical intravaginal torsion. **(B)** Cord has been straightened and sutures placed through the testis and scrotal wall.

A

B

TORSION OF THE SPERMATIC CORD

When torsion of the spermatic cord occurs there is only a short time available in which to save the testis. None of the physical signs or diagnostic tests, such as the Doppler or the radionucleotide examination, is infalliable. Occasionally, with mild sedation, the testis can be untwisted manually. As a rule, however, when the diagnosis of torsion is entertained, the patient should be prepared for the operating room as rapidly as possible.[7]

Under general anesthesia the scrotum is surgically prepared and draped. An incision is made (as for simple orchiectomy) and carried down through the tunica vaginalis. As the sac is being opened, the cyanotic testis usually starts to untwist and the color should return promptly. If the time interval from the onset of symptoms is more than 4 hours the testis may remain black, indicating that infarction has occurred and that the testis should be removed. If it becomes pink, the testis should be fixed firmly with three or four nonabsorbable sutures through the tunica albuginea to the scrotal wall (Fig. 105-5).[25] Some advise removing the tunica vaginalis or making a window in it to ensure stronger adhesions and thus prevent recurrence.[26,30]

At this point the surgical operation is just half finished, because a similar operation must be done on the opposite side to prevent torsion there at a later date.[20] The anatomic condition that permits torsion to occur is almost always bilateral. The wounds are closed in layers and a pressure dressing is applied for 24 hours.

Torsion of the appendix testis and appendix epididymis is similar to torsion of the spermatic cord in all respects, but it occurs on a smaller scale.[24] The operation consists simply of ligating the base of the appendage and excising it. The wound is closed in layers without drainage.

SPERMATIC CORD, VAS, AND EPIDIDYMIS

Congenital abnormalities of the vas and epididymis are discussed in Chapter 104, Infertility and Vas Reconstruction.

EPIDIDYMECTOMY—SURGICAL TECHNIQUES

The testis with its tunics is delivered through the scrotum as for simple orchiectomy and the tunica vaginalis is then opened for examination of the epididymis. The epididymis is separated from the testis beginning at the lower pole, using a combination of sharp and blunt dissection. As the dissection proceeds upwards, the vascular pedicle will be met at about the junction of the upper and middle third of the testis, where care must be taken to preserve the vessels of the testis (Fig. 105-6). The branches to the epididymis are ligated and divided, and the remainder of the epididymis can be freed without difficulty. A few small bleeders on the testis may need to be controlled with fine ligatures at this time. The tunica vaginalis can then be either resected or sutured loosely, and the remainder of the wound can be closed in layers with a small drain out the lower portion of the incision. A pressure dressing should be applied to the scrotum.

When an abscess has ruptured through the skin, wide débridement of the scrotum must be performed, along with total epididymo-orchiectomy.

Neoplasms and Trauma

Most tumors of the epididymis are benign adenomatoid tumors, but occasionally such a tumor has been reported as malignant. A simple orchiectomy is usually adequate treatment.

Trauma to the epididymis is most often merely a contusion that will respond to appropriate conservative therapy.

HYDROCELECTOMY

There are many satisfactory surgical methods for the care of a hydrocele.[17] After preparation of the skin and adequate local, spinal, or general anesthesia, an incision is made between the superficial scrotal vessels and dissection is carried down until the tunica vaginalis is reached. At this point the hydrocele appears as a blush cyst and pressure on the scrotum delivers the hydrocele from the wound with almost no bleeding. A sponge frees the hydrocele of any adherent tissue, and tiny bleeding points can be controlled with a cautery. The Andrews or "bottle operation" is performed by making a 2-cm to 3-cm incision at the upper end of the hydrocele sac, extruding the testis through this small opening, and then everting the remainder of the sac around the cord (Fig. 105-7A).[3] In the Jaboulay or Winkleman procedure, a small cuff of the hydrocele sac is left along the borders, everted about the cord, and closed with a single running suture of fine plain catgut (Fig. 105-7B). This has the advantage of rapid control of all of the small vessels along the edge of the sac. The testis is replaced in the scrotum, a small Penrose drain is led out of the lower portion of the incision, and the skin is closed in two layers with 3-0 plain

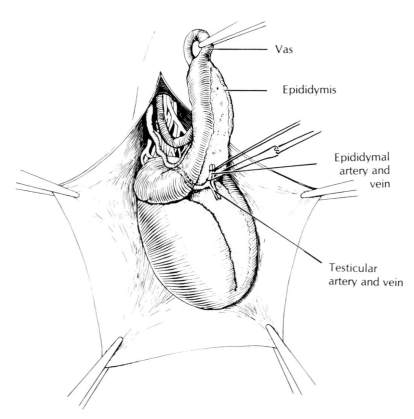

Vas

Epididymis

Epididymal
artery and
vein

Testicular
artery and vein

FIG. 105-6. Epididymectomy. Epididymis has been separated up to the vascular pedicle of the testis. Branches to the epididymis are ligated and divided carefully to preserve the testicular blood supply. The vas may be ligated and divided at any convenient site.

FIG. 105-7. Hydrocelectomy. **(A)** The Andrews operation; a small incision is made high in the sac prior to inversion of the sac about the cord. **(B)** Jaboulay or Winkleman technique; most of the sac is excised and a running suture closes the free edges loosely about the cord. This is a rapid method of controlling troublesome bleeding.

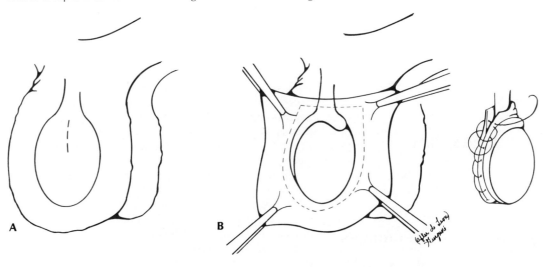

A   B

sutures for subcutaneous tissue and 2-0 chromic sutures on the skin. A pressure dressing is applied and the drain is removed in 24 hours. In another variation, the sac is opened and the parietal layer is dissected back flush with the epididymis and testis. Bleeders along the edge are either ligated or cauterized (Fig. 105-8*A*).

In the Lord procedure for hydrocelectomy, a small scrotal incision just large enough to permit delivery of the testis itself is made.[14,19] The incision is carried down until the tunica vaginalis is reached and incised, and the edges all around are grasped with Allis forceps. The testis is delivered from the wound, and the edges of the sac are plicated around the periphery with interrupted 2-0 or 3-0 chromic sutures about 1 cm apart (Fig. 105-8*B*).

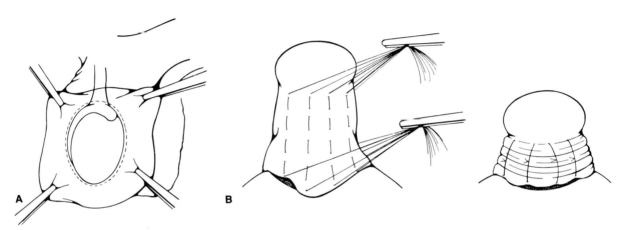

FIG. 105-8. **(A)** The sac is excised flush and bleeders are ligated or fulgurated individually. **(B)** The Lord operation. The testis is extruded through a small incision in the middle of the sac and then the sac is plicated with multiple sutures.

FIG. 105-9. Spermatocelectomy. The spermatocele is being separated from the head of the epididymis by sharp dissection.

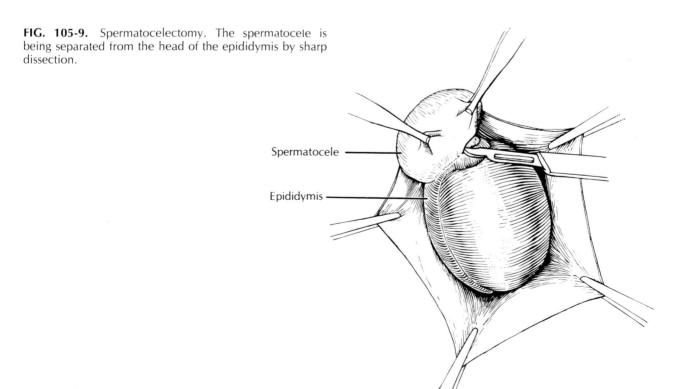

Spermatocele

Epididymis

The testis is replaced in the scrotum and a two-layer closure of the skin is performed as before.

A communicating hydrocele is an indirect inguinal hernia without the presence of any bowel in the hernia sac. The operation is basically an inguinal herniorrhaphy with division and high ligation of the hernial sac. The tunica vaginalis around the testis and lower portion of the cord does not have to be disturbed.

A hydrocele of the cord requires only local excision.

SPERMATOCELECTOMY

The testis is delivered through the scrotum as for simple orchiectomy and the hydrocele sac is opened to reveal the spermatocele. With sharp and blunt dissection, the cyst can be separated from the epididymis (Fig. 105-9). The few bleeders may be controlled with fine catgut ligatures or the cautery. Occasionally, with longstanding spermatoceles, it is necessary to resect the tunica vaginalis along with the spermatocele. The attachment to the epididymis is closed with a running 3-0 plain catgut

suture, and the wound is closed in layers. A small Penrose drain for 24 hours is usually helpful.

Sclerosant treatment of hydroceles or spermatoceles carries the risk of serious complications.[35]

HEMATOCELECTOMY

Hematoceles demand surgical exploration to determine whether there is also traumatic rupture of the testis.[22] The incision in the scrotum is carried down through the tunica vaginalis, the blood clots are removed, and any bleeding points are controlled. The operation then proceeds as for a simple hydrocelectomy.

Testicular Prosthesis

The key to the successful insertion of a testicular prosthesis is an inguinal incision. A scrotal incision, even a high one, is almost sure to lead to extrusion of the foreign body. The operation consists of an inguinal incision, the development of a scrotal pouch by blunt dissection, and an inversion of the lower portion of this pouch into the operative field so that the tab at the tip of the prosthesis can be

FIG. 105-10. Isolating the vas: (**A**) areas to be infiltrated with local anesthetic; (**B**) incising to the vas; (**C**) clearing the vas with iris scissors

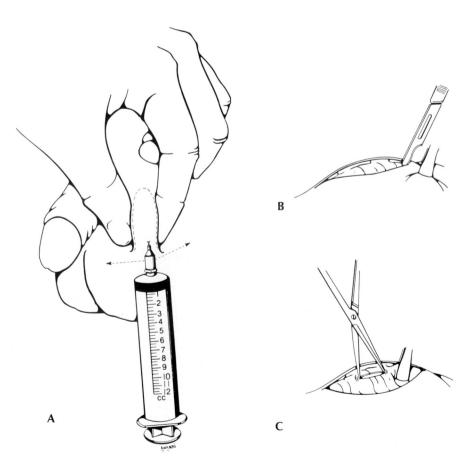

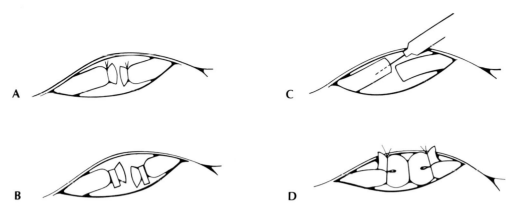

FIG. 105-11. Methods of sealing the vas: **(A)** simple ligature with a heavy catgut; **(B)** closing ends with hemoclips; **(C)** fulgurating 2 cm of lumen at each end; **(D)** ligature with the vas doubled back

firmly attached to the bottom of the scrotum with nonabsorbable suture.[18,19] The prosthesis is pushed back into the scrotum, a pursestring suture is placed around the neck of the pouch, and the inguinal incision is closed in layers.

VASECTOMY

Except under extenuating circumstances, vasectomy is most often performed in the outpatient clinic under local anesthesia. Another variation in surgical technique is presented in Chapter 104.

After suitable preparation of the skin and draping, the vas can be identified, isolated from the other elements of the cord, and brought up under the skin where it is held between the thumb and forefinger. Local anesthesia is infiltrated into the skin over the vas and into the surrounding tissue (Fig. 105-10A). After surface anesthesia is obtained, a tiny bit of the anesthetic should be injected around the vas itself. Then the vas is anchored to the skin with an Allis clamp.

An incision is made directly down to the vas, which can then be grasped with a second Allis clamp (Fig. 105-10B). When palpation has determined that this is indeed the vas, the first Allis can be removed, the adventitia over the vas can be stripped away with sharp iris scissors for a centimeter or so, and the vas can be elevated and doubly clamped (Fig. 105-10C). The vas is then divided and either ligated with 2-0 chromic (a heavy ligature which will not cut into the vas wall) (Fig. 105-11A) or closed with a medium-sized hemoclip (Fig. 105-11B).[27,33] An alternative method is to fulgurate the lumen of the cut ends of the vas with a needle electrode (Fig. 105-11C). After checking to be sure that there is no bleeding from small

vessels along the vas, the two ends can be dropped back into the wound or isolated from each other by interposition of a tissue layer. The wound is closed with a single absorbable suture. The patient is sent home wearing an athletic supporter to hold a small bandage in place. Flushing the vas with various solutions has been recommended to reduce the interval between surgery and sterility, but it is not always effective.[28] The patient must be warned that postoperatively he has to be considered fertile until an aspermic ejaculate is obtained.

REFERENCES

1. ABBON C, SERRANT M, BONNET F et al: Reimplantation du pénis et des deux testicules apres auto-émasculation complète: Revue de la litérature à propos d'un cas. Chirugie 105:354, 1979
2. ALTCHEK ED, HOFFMAN S: Scrotal reconstruction in Fournier syndrome. Ann Plast Surg 3:523, 1979
3. ANDREWS E, WYLLY S: The "bottle operation" for radical cure of hydrocele. Ann Surg 46:915, 1907
4. ASAADI M, NAJMI J, CARTER H et al: Spindle cell sarcoma of scrotum. Urology 16:525, 1980
5. BISWAS M, GODEC C, IRELAND G et al: Necrotizing infection of scrotum. Urology 14:576, 1979
6. BULKLEY GJ: Scrotal and penile lymphedema. J Urol 87:422, 1962
7. CASS AS, CASS BP, VEERARAGHAVAN K: Immediate exploration of the unilateral acute scrotum in young male subjects. J Urol 124:829, 1980
8. DICKSON RW, HOFSESS DW: Nontropical genital elephantiasis. J Urol 82:131, 1959
9. EDSON M, MEEK J: Bilateral testicular disruption with unilateral rupture. J Urol 122:419, 1979
10. ELÍAS J: The splitting scrotal incision. J Urol 86:117, 1961
11. FOURNIER JA: Étude clinique de la gangrene Fou-

droyante de la verge. Semaine Médicale (Paris) 4:69, 1884

12. GRAVES RC, FLO S: Carcinoma of the scrotum. J Urol 43:309, 1940

13. GRAY JA: Gangrene of the genitalia as seen in advanced periurethral extravasation with phlegmon. J Urol 84:740, 1960

14. HAAS J, CARRION H, SHARKEY J et al: Operative treatment of hydrocele. Another look at Lord's procedure. Urol 12:578, 1978

15. HINMAN F, JR, SPENCE HF, CULP OS et al: Panel discussion: Anomalies of external genitalia in infancy and childhood. J Urol 93:1, 1965

16. HOLLINSHEAD WH: Anatomy for Surgeons, Vol 2, 2nd ed, p 830. Hagerstown, MD, Harper & Row, 1971

17. LANDES RR, LEONHARDT KO: The history of hydrocele. Urol Surv 17:135, 1967

18. LATTIMER JK, VAKILI BF, SMITH AM et al: A natural-feeling testicular prosthesis. J Urol 110:81, 1979

19. LORD PH: A bloodless operation for the radical cure of idiopathic hydrocele. Br J Surg 51:914, 1964

20. LYON RP: Torsion of the testicle in childhood: A painless emergency requiring contralateral orchiopexy. JAMA 178:702, 1961

21. MANCHAUDA R, SINGH R, KESWANI R et al: Traumatic avulsion of scrotum and penile skin. Br J Plast Surg 20:97, 1967

22. MCCORMACK JL, KRETZ AW, TOCANTINS R: Traumatic rupture of the testicle. J Urol 96:80, 1966

23. MCDONALD JH, CALAMS JA: Extraparenchymal Leydig-like cells: Observations following subcapsular orchiectomy. J Urol 82:145, 1959

24. MCFARLAND JB: Testicular strangulation in children. Br J Surg 53:110, 1966

25. MCNELLIS DR, RABINOVITCH HH: Repeat torsion of "fixed" testis. Urology 16:476, 1980

26. MORSE TS, HOLLEBAUGH RS: The window orchiopexy for prevention of testicular torsion. J Pediatr Surg 12:237, 1977

27. MOSS WM: A sutureless technique for bilateral partial vasectomy. Fertil Steril 23:33, 1972

28. MUMFORD SD, DAVIS JE: Flushing of distal vas during vasectomy: Current status and review of literature. Urology 15:433, 1979

29. PRENTISS RJ, BOATWRIGHT DC, PENNINGTON RD et al: Testicular prosthesis: Material, methods and results. J Urol 90:208, 1963

30. REDMAN JF, STALLINGS JW: Torsion of testicle following orchiopexy. Urol 16:502, 1980

31. ROTH R, WARREN K: Traumatic avulsion of the skin of the penis and scrotum. J Urol 52:162, 1944

32. RUDOLPH R, SOLWAY M, DEPALMA RG et al: Fournier's syndrome: Synergistic gangrene of the scrotum. Am J Surg 129:591, 1975

33. SCHMIDT SS: Technics and complications of elective vasectomy. Fertil Steril 17:467, 1967

34. SILBER S, KELLY J: Successful autotransplantation in an intra-abdominal testis to the scrotum by microvascular technique. J Urol 115:452, 1976

35. THOMSON H, ODELL M: Sclerosant treatment for hydroceles and epididymal cysts. Br Med J 2:704, 1979

36. TUCCI P, HARALAMBIDIS G: Carcinoma of the scrotum: Review of literature and presentation of 2 cases. J Urol 89:585, 1963

37. WACKSMAN J, DINNER M, STRAFFON R: Technique of testicular autotransplantation using microvascular anastomosis. Surg Gynecol Obstet 150:399, 1980

38. WILSON MC, WILSON CL, THICKSTEN JN: Transposition of the external genitalia. J Urol 94:600, 1965

Index

Numbers followed by an *f* indicate a figure; *t* following a page number indicates tabular material.